Consultations in

FELINE
INTERNAL MEDICINE

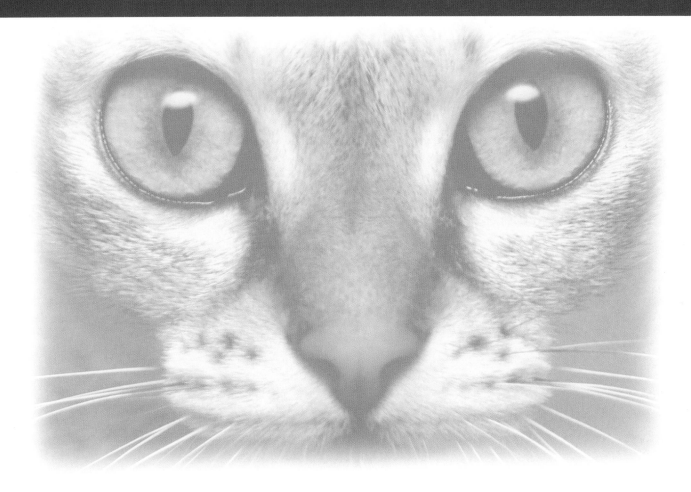

Consultations in
FELINE
INTERNAL MEDICINE

Volume 6

John R. August, BVetMed, MS, MRCVS, Diplomate ACVIM

Professor of Feline Internal Medicine

Department of Small Animal Clinical Sciences

College of Veterinary Medicine and Biomedical Sciences

Texas A&M University

College Station, Texas

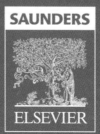

SAUNDERS

ELSEVIER

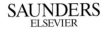

3251 Riverport Lane
St. Louis, MO 63043

Previous volumes copyrighted 2006, 2001, 1997, 1994, 1991

International Standard Book Number 978-1-4160-5641-6

Vice President and Publisher: Linda Duncan
Senior Acquisitions Editor: Anthony Winkel
Senior Developmental Editor: Shelly Stringer
Publishing Services Manager: Catherine Jackson
Senior Project Manager: David Stein
Design Direction: Charlie Seibel
Cover Art: Olek Kuperberg

Printed in China.

Last digit is the print number: 9 8 7 6 5 4 3 2 1

This book is dedicated to the memory of my mother,
Andrée August.

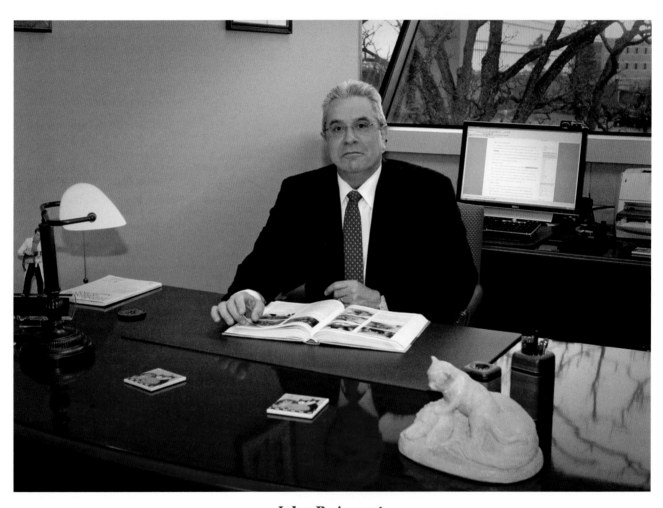

John R. August

Preface

There always seemed to be a cat in my home when I was growing up in southeast England in the 1950s and 1960s. At that time, cats were more popular as companion animals in Europe than in the United States. It was no surprise then that I should be tagged as the person who would be willing to see the feline patients when I arrived in the United States for my internship in the early 1970s. The label stuck, and I have enjoyed riding the wave of the surging popularity of cats as companion animals and family members ever since. By sheer luck, I was in the right place at the right time. Over the years, I have had the good fortune to travel to South America regularly, and I have watched with great interest how cats are now assuming new roles in the family and society in those countries. I owe a special thanks to my colleagues in South America who have invited me to their beautiful countries, and who have provided me with such gracious hospitality during my professional visits. It has been a special privilege for me to watch feline medicine evolve as a discipline internationally during my career.

Each volume of *Consultations in Feline Internal Medicine* takes 3 years to prepare, and carefully complements previous books in the series. Purposefully, this book is not a comprehensive treatise on feline medicine. Rather, it is an in-depth collection of timely topics that will be of unique interest to progressive feline practitioners when the book is published and beyond. I entrust the responsibility of choosing the subject matter and contributing authors of each volume to the eleven section editors, who are international leaders in their respective disciplines. Reflecting my own belief as an internist that scientific nutrition is a foundation of good health, we have included a new section in this volume devoted to the relationship between nutrition and health and disease.

Organizing sections and authoring chapters within strict time deadlines for a book like *Consultations in Feline Internal Medicine* takes an enormous amount of time and intellectual effort, and the section editors and authors all deserve my very sincere thanks for their contributions to this project. During the final year of preparation of this book, I have had the opportunity to edit all of the chapters three times, and I continue to be very impressed by the complexity and scope of the chapters. That these authors should go well beyond the call of duty when writing their chapters is a testament to the seriousness with which they took their invitation to contribute to this book, and also to the breadth of their expertise and experience in feline medicine. From a slightly selfish standpoint, I also like to think that it has a little to do with the evolving recognition of *Consultations in Feline Internal Medicine* as a respected resource for our profession.

Some other important recognitions are in order for my colleagues at Elsevier. Dr. Anthony Winkel, Senior Acquisitions Editor, Veterinary Medicine, deserves my special thanks for the guidance, mentorship, and motivation that he has provided me throughout the preparation of this volume. I also want to recognize Tony for his special commitment to the striking design and professional layout of this book. Ms. Shelly Stringer, Senior Developmental Editor, has been a tower of strength, making sure that the loop has been closed on thousands of details during the processing of all of the manuscripts, and maintaining communications among the more than one hundred contributors and section editors. Lastly, it has been a pleasure working again with David Stein, Senior Project Manager; I always know that the project will be completed with immaculate attention to detail and deadlines when it is placed in David's hands.

I must thank my wife Janet who once again tolerated my insistence that obligations to this book should supersede projects around our house and family vacations during the past year. My university has been generous this year in providing me with some extra time away from clinic duty to complete this project, and for that I am very grateful. Texas A&M University continues to give priority to the health and welfare of cats in its professional and postgraduate programs, offering a rotation in feline internal medicine for fourth-year students. In July 2008, we initiated a 3-year small animal internal medicine residency with a feline focus, with the intent of preparing the next generation of feline internists.

In closing, I hope that the sixth volume of this series exceeds your expectations and that it will become an important resource for your professional activities. A project of this size truly is a team effort, and it is a real privilege for me to contribute in this way to the rapidly evolving discipline of feline internal medicine.

John August
College Station, Texas

Section Editors

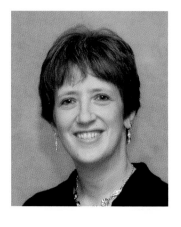

Ellen N. Behrend, VMD, PhD, Diplomate ACVIM Professor
Department of Clinical Sciences
College of Veterinary Medicine
Auburn University
Auburn, Alabama, USA
Endocrine and Metabolic Disease

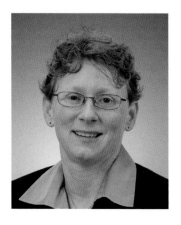

Joan R. Coates, DVM, MS, Diplomate ACVIM (Neurology)
Associate Professor
Department of Veterinary Medicine and Surgery
College of Veterinary Medicine
University of Missouri
Columbia, Missouri, USA
Neurology

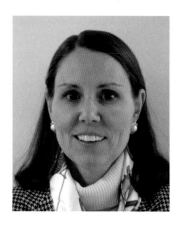

Ann E. Hohenhaus, DVM, Diplomate ACVIM (Oncology, Internal Medicine)
Chairman
Department of Medicine
The Animal Medical Center
New York, New York, USA
Hematopoietic and Lymphatic Systems

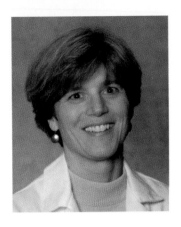

India F. Lane, DVM, MS, EdD, Diplomate ACVIM
Associate Professor, Director of Educational Enhancement
Department of Small Animal Clinical Sciences
College of Veterinary Medicine
The University of Tennessee
Knoxville, Tennessee, USA
Urinary System

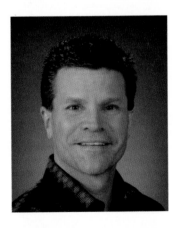

Julie Levy, DVM, PhD, Diplomate ACVIM
Maddie's Professor of Shelter Medicine
Department of Small Animal Clinical Sciences
College of Veterinary Medicine
University of Florida
Gainesville, Florida, USA
Infectious Diseases

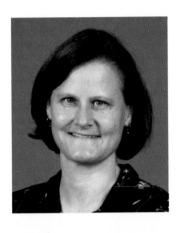

Matthew W. Miller, DVM, MS, Diplomate ACVIM (Cardiology)
Professor
Department of Small Animal Clinical Sciences
College of Veterinary Medicine and Biomedical Sciences
Texas A&M University
College Station, Texas, USA
Cardiology and Respiratory Disorders

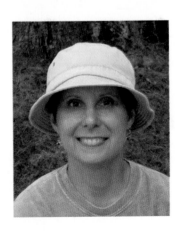

Karen A. Moriello, DVM, Diplomate ACVD
Clinical Professor of Dermatology
Department of Medical Sciences
School of Veterinary Medicine
University of Wisconsin
Madison, Wisconsin, USA
Dermatology

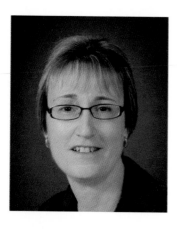

Kenita S. Rogers, DVM, MS, Diplomate ACVIM (Internal Medicine, Oncology)
Professor, Associate Dean for Professional Programs
Department of Small Animal Clinical Sciences
College of Veterinary Medicine and Biomedical Sciences
Texas A&M University
College Station, Texas, USA
Oncology

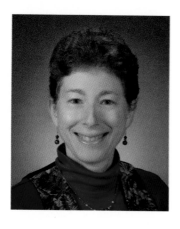

Margaret R. Slater, DVM, PhD
Senior Director of Epidemiology
Animal Health Services
ASPCA
Urbana, Illinois, USA
Population Medicine

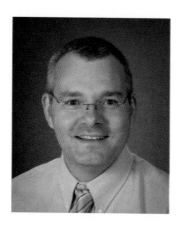

Jörg M. Steiner, medvet, Drmedvet, PhD, Diplomate ACVIM, ECVIM-CA
Associate Professor
Department of Small Animal Clinical Sciences
College of Veterinary Medicine and Biomedical Sciences
Texas A&M University
College Station, Texas, USA
Gastrointestinal System

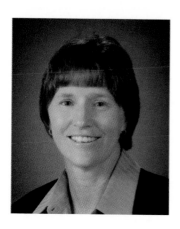

Debra L. Zoran, DVM, PhD, Diplomate ACVIM
Associate Professor
Department of Small Animal Clinical Sciences
College of Veterinary Medicine and Biomedical Sciences
Texas A&M University
College Station, Texas, USA
Nutrition in Health and Disease

Contributors

Hasan Albasan, DVM, MS, PhD
Research Associate
Department of Veterinary Clinical Sciences
College of Veterinary Medicine
University of Minnesota
St. Paul, Minnesota, USA
Purine Uroliths

Heidi S. Allen, DVM, Diplomate ACVIM
Staff Internist
The Internal Medicine Department
The Hope Center for Advanced Veterinary Medicine
Vienna, Virginia, USA
Therapeutic Approach to Cats with Chronic Diarrhea

Karin Allenspach, DrMedVet, PhD, FVH, Diplomate ECVIM-CA
Lecturer
Department of Veterinary Clinical Sciences
The Royal Veterinary College
University of London
Hatfield, Hertfordshire, United Kingdom
Antiemetic Therapy

Eva Axnér, DVM, PhD, Diplomate ECAR
Associate Professor
Department of Clinical Sciences
Division of Reproduction
Swedish University of Agricultural Sciences
Uppsala, Sweden
Catteries: Reproductive Performance and Problems

Kerry Smith Bailey, DVM, Diplomate ACVIM (Neurology)
Staff Neurologist
Oradell Animal Hospital, Inc.
Paramus, New Jersey, USA
Novel Anticonvulsant Therapies

Claudia J. Baldwin, DVM, MS, Diplomate ACVIM
Associate Professor
Department of Veterinary Clinical Sciences
College of Veterinary Medicine
Iowa State University
Ames, Iowa, USA
Shelter Population Health Management

Vanessa R.D. Barrs, BVSc (Hons), MVCS, FACVSc (Feline Medicine)
Senior Lecturer in Small Animal Medicine
Valentine Charlton Cat Centre
Faculty of Veterinary Science
The University of Sydney
Sydney, New South Wales, Australia
Pyothorax
Upper Respiratory Tract Aspergillosis
Diagnosis and Treatment of Low-Grade Alimentary Lymphoma

Joseph W. Bartges, DVM, PhD, Diplomate ACVIM, ACVN
Professor of Medicine and Nutrition
The Acree Endowed Chair of Small Animal Research
Department of Small Animal Clinical Sciences
College of Veterinary Medicine
University of Tennessee
Knoxville, Tennessee, USA
Dietary Therapy of Diseases of the Lower Urinary Tract

Julia A. Beatty, BSc (Hons), BVM, PhD, FACVSc (Feline Medicine), MRCVS
Senior Lecturer in Small Animal Medicine
Faculty of Veterinary Science
Hospital Director, Valentine Charlton Cat Centre
University of Sydney
Sydney, New South Wales, Australia
Pyothorax
Upper Respiratory Tract Aspergillosis
Diagnosis and Treatment of Low-Grade Alimentary Lymphoma

Allyson C. Berent, DVM, Diplomate ACVIM
Staff Veterinarian
Department of Clinical Studies—Philadelphia
School of Veterinary Medicine
University of Pennsylvania
Philadelphia, Pennsylvania, USA
Urological Interventional Techniques in the Feline Patient

Barbara Bighignoli, PhD
Department of Animal Science
University of Milan
Milan, Italy
Blood Types of the Domestic Cat

Paul B. Bloom, DVM, Diplomate ACVD, ABVP (Canine and Feline)
Assistant Adjunct Professor
Department of Small Animal Clinical Sciences
College of Veterinary Medicine
Michigan State University
East Lansing, Michigan, USA
Anatomy of the Ear in Health and Disease

Mark W. Bohling, DVM, PhD, Diplomate ACVS
Assistant Professor
Department of Small Animal Clinical Sciences
College of Veterinary Medicine
University of Tennessee
Knoxville, Tennessee, USA
A Review of Neutering Cats

Scott A. Brown, VMD, PhD, Diplomate ACVIM
Josiah Meigs Distinguished Professor and Head
Department of Small Animal Medicine and Surgery
College of Veterinary Medicine
University of Georgia
Athens, Georgia, USA
Linking Treatment to Staging in Chronic Kidney Disease

Christine M. Budke, DVM, PhD
Assistant Professor
Department of Veterinary Integrative Biosciences
College of Veterinary Medicine and Biomedical Sciences
Texas A&M University
College Station, Texas, USA
Understanding Population Dynamics Models: Implications for Veterinarians

Daniel L. Chan, DVM, MRCVS, Diplomate ACVECC, ACVN
Lecturer
Department of Veterinary Clinical Sciences
The Royal Veterinary College
University of London
Hatfield, Hertfordshire, United Kingdom
Critical Care Nutrition
Antiemetic Therapy

Ruthanne Chun, DVM, Diplomate ACVIM (Oncology)
Clinical Associate Professor
Department of Medical Sciences
School of Veterinary Medicine
University of Wisconsin
Madison, Wisconsin, USA
Urinary Tract Tumors

David B. Church, BVSc, PhD, MACVSc, MRCVS
Professor
Department of Veterinary Clinical Sciences
The Royal Veterinary College
University of London
Hatfield, Hertfordshire, United Kingdom
Acromegaly

Joan R. Coates, DVM, MS, Diplomate ACVIM (Neurology)
Associate Professor
Department of Veterinary Medicine and Surgery
College of Veterinary Medicine
University of Missouri
Columbia, Missouri, USA
Tremor Syndromes

Leah A. Cohn, DVM, PhD, Diplomate ACVIM
Associate Professor
Department of Veterinary Medicine and Surgery
College of Veterinary Medicine
University of Missouri
Columbia, Missouri, USA
Cytauxzoon Infections

Audrey K. Cook, BVMS, MRCVS, Diplomate ACVIM, ECVIM-CA
Clinical Associate Professor
Department of Small Animal Clinical Sciences
College of Veterinary Medicine and Biomedical Sciences
Texas A&M University
College Station, Texas, USA
Gastrointestinal Function Testing

Cynda Crawford, DVM, PhD
Maddie's Clinical Assistant Professor of Shelter Medicine
Department of Small Animal Clinical Sciences
College of Veterinary Medicine
University of Florida
Gainesville, Florida, USA
Progress on Diagnosis of Retroviral Infections

Curtis W. Dewey, DVM, MS, Diplomate ACVIM (Neurology), ACVS
Associate Professor
Department of Clinical Sciences
College of Veterinary Medicine
Cornell University
Ithaca, New York, USA
Novel Anticonvulsant Therapies

Alison Diesel, DVM
Resident in Dermatology
Department of Medical Sciences
School of Veterinary Medicine
University of Wisconsin
Madison, Wisconsin, USA
Medical Management of Otitis

Brian A. DiGangi, DVM
Resident in Shelter Medicine
Department of Population Medicine and Diagnostic
    Sciences
College of Veterinary Medicine
Cornell University
Ithaca, New York, USA
A Review of Neutering Cats

Joan Dziezyc, DVM, Diplomate ACVO
Associate Professor
Department of Small Animal Clinical Sciences
College of Veterinary Medicine and Biomedical Sciences
Texas A&M University
College Station, Texas, USA
Ocular Tumors

**Danielle M. Eifler, DVM, Diplomate ACVIM
    (Neurology)**
Staff Neurologist
Maine Veterinary Referral Center
Scarborough, Maine, USA
Tremor Syndromes

**Denise A. Elliott, BVSc (Hons), PhD,
    Diplomate ACVIM, ACVN**
Director of Scientific Affairs
Royal Canin USA Inc.
St. Charles, Missouri, USA
*Nutritional Management of Chronic Kidney
    Disease*

Michael A. Estrin, DVM, Diplomate ACVIM
Graduate Student
Boston University School of Public Health
Boston, Massachusetts, USA
Disseminated Intravascular Coagulation

**Lisa J. Forrest, VMD, Diplomate ACVR
    (Radiology, Radiation Oncology)**
Associate Professor,
Department of Surgical Sciences
School of Veterinary Medicine
University of Wisconsin
Madison, Wisconsin, USA
Diagnostic Imaging of the Ear

**Philip R. Fox, DVM, MS, Diplomate ACVIM
    (Cardiology), ECVIM, ACVECC**
Director
Caspary Research Institute
The Animal Medical Center
New York, New York, USA
Pathology of Primary Myocardial Disease

Lutz Froenicke, PhD
Department of Population Health and Reproduction
School of Veterinary Medicine
University of California
Davis, California, USA
Blood Types of the Domestic Cat

**Michele C. Gaspar, DVM, Diplomate ABVP
    (Feline)**
Consultant in Feline Internal Medicine
Veterinary Information Network
Davis, California, USA
Alternative Modalities in Feline Practice

Andrew Gendler, DVM
Resident in Radiology
Department of Surgical Sciences
School of Veterinary Medicine
University of Wisconsin
Madison, Wisconsin, USA
Diagnostic Imaging of the Ear

**Virginia L. Gill, DVM, Diplomate ACVIM
    (Oncology)**
Staff Oncologist
Katonah Bedford Veterinary Center
Bedford Hills, New York, USA
Plasma Cell Disorders

Josephine S. Gnanandarajah, BVSc, MS
Graduate Student
Department of Veterinary and Biomedical Sciences
College of Veterinary Medicine
University of Minnesota
St. Paul, Minnesota, USA
Purine Uroliths

**Richard E. Goldstein, DVM, Diplomate
    ACVIM, ECVIM-CA**
Associate Professor
Department of Clinical Sciences
College of Veterinary Medicine
Cornell University
Ithaca, New York, USA
Commercial Pet Food–Related Nephrotoxicity

**Thomas K. Graves, DVM, PhD, Diplomate
    ACVIM**
Associate Professor
Department of Veterinary Clinical Medicine
College of Veterinary Medicine
Associate Professor
Division of Nutritional Sciences
College of Agricultural, Consumer and Environmental
    Sciences
University of Illinois
Urbana, Illinois, USA
Hyperthyroidism and the Kidneys

Brenda Griffin, DVM, MS, Diplomate ACVIM
Assistant Professor
Department of Population Medicine and Diagnostic
    Sciences
College of Veterinary Medicine
Cornell University
Ithaca, New York, USA
A Review of Neutering Cats

**Meret E. Ricklin Gutzwiller, DVM,
    Diplomate ECVD**
Department of Clinical Veterinary Medicine
Dermatology Unit
Vetsuisse Faculty
University of Bern
Bern, Switzerland
Use of Interferon Omega for Skin Diseases

**Katrin Hartmann, DVM, DMVH, Diplomate
    ECVIM-CA**
Professor
Clinic of Small Animal Medicine
College of Veterinary Medicine
Ludwig Maximilian University
Munich, Germany
Influenza Infections
*Diagnosis and Treatment of Feline Infectious
    Peritonitis*

**Andrea M. Harvey, BVSc, DSAM (Feline),
    Diplomate ECVIM-CA, MRCVS**
Feline Advisory Bureau Clinical Fellow in Feline
    Medicine
Department of Clinical Veterinary Science
University of Bristol
Bristol, North Somerset, United Kingdom
Primary Hyperaldosteronism

Rebecka S. Hess, DVM, Diplomate ACVIM
Associate Professor
Department of Clinical Studies—Philadelphia
School of Veterinary Medicine
University of Pennsylvania
Philadelphia, Pennsylvania, USA
Diabetic Emergencies

Mark E. Hitt, DVM, MS, Diplomate ACVIM
Chief of Medicine
Atlantic Veterinary Internal Medicine
Annapolis, Maryland, USA
Inflammatory Liver Diseases

Margarethe Hoenig, DVM, PhD
Professor
Department of Veterinary Clinical Medicine
College of Veterinary Medicine
University of Illinois
Urbana, Illinois, USA
Metabolism, Diet, and Obesity

**Ann E. Hohenhaus, DVM, Diplomate ACVIM
    (Oncology, Internal Medicine)**
Chairman
Department of Medicine
The Animal Medical Center
New York, New York, USA
Selection of Treatment Protocols for Lymphoma

Edward Jazic, DVM, Diplomate ACVD
Dermatology for Animals
Campbell, California, USA;
Dermatology Clinic for Animals
Gilbert, Arizona, USA
Acne

**Lynelle R. Johnson, DVM, MS, PhD,
    Diplomate ACVIM**
Associate Professor
Department of Medicine and Epidemiology
School of Veterinary Medicine
University of California
Davis, California, USA
Bronchoscopy

**Mark C. Johnson, DVM, Diplomate ACVP
    (Clinical Pathology)**
Clinical Associate Professor
Department of Veterinary Pathobiology
College of Veterinary Medicine and Biomedical Sciences
Texas A&M University
College Station, Texas, USA
*The Dilemmas of Cytological Evaluation of the
    Feline Lymph Node*

Robert J. Kemppainen, DVM, PhD
Professor
Department of Anatomy, Physiology, and
    Pharmacology
College of Veterinary Medicine
Auburn University
Auburn, Alabama, USA
*Answers to Commonly Asked Endocrine
    Diagnostic Questions*

**Claudia A. Kirk, DVM, PhD, Diplomate
    ACVIM, ACVN**
Professor and Head
Department of Small Animal Clinical Sciences
College of Veterinary Medicine
University of Tennessee
Knoxville, Tennessee, USA
*Dietary Therapy of Diseases of the Lower Urinary
    Tract*

Barbara Kohn, DVM, Diplomate ECVIM-CA
Professor
Clinic for Small Animals
Faculty of Veterinary Medicine
Free University of Berlin
Berlin, Germany
Immune-Mediated Hemolytic Anemia

Laura Helen Kramer, DVM, PhD, Diplomate EVPC
Associate Professor
Animal Production
University of Parma Veterinary School
Parma, Italy
The Role of Wolbachia in Heartworm Infection

Dorothy P. Laflamme, DVM, PhD, Diplomate ACVN
Veterinary Nutritionist
Research and Development
Nestlé Purina Pet Care
St. Louis, Missouri, USA
Dietary Therapy of Chronic Diarrhea

Cathy E. Langston, DVM, Diplomate ACVIM
Head of Nephrology, Urology and Hemodialysis
The Animal Medical Center
New York, New York, USA
Survival and Outcome of Kidney Disease
Clinical Use of Erythropoietin in Feline Medicine

Michael R. Lappin, DVM, PhD, Diplomate ACVIM
The Kenneth W. Smith Professor
Department of Clinical Sciences
College of Veterinary Medicine and Biomedical Sciences
Colorado State University
Fort Collins, Colorado, USA
Gastrointestinal Protozoal Infections

Jennifer A. Larsen, DVM, PhD, Diplomate ACVN
Associate Professor
Department of Clinical Nutrition
School of Veterinary Medicine
University of California
Davis, California, USA
Unconventional Diets

Nicole F. Leibman, DVM, Diplomate ACVIM (Oncology)
Staff Oncologist
The Animal Medical Center
New York, New York, USA
Plasma Cell Disorders

Dawn Logas, DVM, Diplomate ACVD
Staff Dermatologist
Veterinary Dermatology Center
Maitland, Florida, USA
How to Treat Common Parasites Safely

Jody P. Lulich, DVM, PhD, Diplomate ACVIM
Professor
Department of Veterinary Clinical Sciences
College of Veterinary Medicine
University of Minnesota
St. Paul, Minnesota, USA
Purine Uroliths

Leslie A. Lyons, PhD
Associate Professor
Department of Population Health and Reproduction
School of Veterinary Medicine
University of California
Davis, California, USA
Blood Types of the Domestic Cat
Genetic Testing in Domestic Cats

Stanley L. Marks, BVSc, PhD, Diplomate ACVIM (Internal Medicine, Oncology), ACVN
Professor
Department of Medicine and Epidemiology
School of Veterinary Medicine
University of California
Davis, California, USA
Probiotics in Feline Medicine

Julia Marschall, DVM
Clinic of Small Animal Medicine
College of Veterinary Medicine
Ludwig Maximilian University
Munich, Germany
Influenza Infections

Kathryn M. Meurs, DVM, PhD, Diplomate ACVIM (Cardiology)
Professor, Richard L. Ott Chair of Small Animal Medicine and Research
Department of Veterinary Clinical Sciences
College of Veterinary Medicine
Washington State University
Pullman, Washington, USA
Genetic Screening of Familial Hypertrophic Cardiomyopathy

Matthew W. Miller, DVM, MS, Diplomate ACVIM (Cardiology)
Professor
Department of Small Animal Clinical Sciences
College of Veterinary Medicine and Biomedical Sciences
Texas A&M University
College Station, Texas, USA
Rhythm Disturbances: Recognition and Therapy

Nicholas J. Millichamp, BVetMed, PhD, DVO, MRCVS, Diplomate ACVO, ECVO
Associate Professor
Department of Small Animal Clinical Sciences
College of Veterinary Medicine and Biomedical Sciences
Texas A&M University
College Station, Texas, USA
Ocular Tumors

Karen A. Moriello, DVM, Diplomate ACVD
Clinical Professor of Dermatology
Department of Medical Sciences
School of Veterinary Medicine
University of Wisconsin
Madison, Wisconsin, USA
Medical Management of Otitis

Daniel O. Morris, DVM, Diplomate ACVD
Associate Professor
Department of Clinical Studies—Philadelphia
School of Veterinary Medicine
University of Pennsylvania
Philadelphia, Pennsylvania, USA
Methicillin-Resistant Staphylococci

Carolina Naranjo, LV, MS
Resident in Anatomical Pathology
Department of Pathobiological Sciences
School of Veterinary Medicine
University of Wisconsin
Madison, Wisconsin, USA
Ocular Tumors

Heide M. Newton, DVM, Diplomate ACVD
Staff Dermatologist
Animal Dermatology Clinic
San Diego, California, USA
Rush and Conventional Immunotherapy

Stijn J.M. Niessen, DVM, MRCVS, Diplomate ECVIM-CA
Department of Veterinary Clinical Sciences
The Royal Veterinary College
University of London
Hatfield, Hertfordshire, United Kingdom;
Diabetes Research Group
Newcastle Biomedicine
Newcastle University
Newcastle, United Kingdom
Acromegaly

Dennis P. O'Brien, DVM, PhD, Diplomate ACVIM (Neurology)
Professor
Department of Veterinary Medicine and Surgery
College of Veterinary Medicine
University of Missouri
Columbia, Missouri, USA
Metabolic Encephalopathy: Organic Acidurias

Carl A. Osborne, DVM, PhD, Diplomate ACVIM
Professor
Department of Veterinary Clinical Sciences
College of Veterinary Medicine
University of Minnesota
St. Paul, Minnesota, USA
Purine Uroliths

Sean D. Owens, DVM, Diplomate ACVP
Assistant Professor
Department of Pathology, Microbiology and Immunology
School of Veterinary Medicine
University of California
Davis, California, USA
Blood Types of the Domestic Cat

Mark A. Oyama, DVM, Diplomate ACVIM (Cardiology)
Associate Professor
Department of Clinical Studies—Philadelphia
School of Veterinary Medicine
University of Pennsylvania
Philadelphia, Pennsylvania, USA
Cardiac Blood Tests

Rebecca A. Packer, MS, DVM, Diplomate ACVIM (Neurology)
Assistant Professor
Departments of Basic Medical Sciences and Veterinary Clinical Sciences
School of Veterinary Medicine
Purdue University
West Lafayette, Indiana, USA
Metabolic Encephalopathy: Organic Acidurias

Philip Padrid, DVM
Family Pet Animal Hospital
Chicago, Illinois, USA
Asthma

Sally C. Perea, DVM, MS, Diplomate ACVN
Senior Nutritionist
Natura Pet Products, Inc.
Davis, California, USA
Unconventional Diets

Jean-Paul Petrie, DVM, Diplomate ACVIM (Cardiology)
Staff Cardiologist
Hudson Valley Veterinary Cardiology
Sloatsburg, New York, USA
Diastolic Dysfunction in Feline Cardiomyopathies

Jacqueline S. Rand, BVSc, PhD, Diplomate ACVIM
Professor and Director, Centre for Companion Animal Health
School of Veterinary Sciences
The University of Queensland
Brisbane, Queensland, Australia
Use of Long-Acting Insulin in the Treatment of Diabetes Mellitus

Kent R. Refsal, DVM, PhD
Professor, Endocrine Section
Diagnostic Center for Population and Animal Health
Michigan State University
Lansing, Michigan, USA
Primary Hyperaldosteronism

Claudia E. Reusch, DVM, PhD, Diplomate ECVIM-CA
Professor
Clinic for Small Animal Internal Medicine
Vetsuisse Faculty
University of Zurich
Zurich, Switzerland
Home Monitoring of Blood Glucose in Cats with Diabetes Mellitus

Kenita S. Rogers, DVM, MS, Diplomate ACVIM (Internal Medicine, Oncology)
Professor, Associate Dean for Professional Programs
Department of Small Animal Clinical Sciences
College of Veterinary Medicine and Biomedical Sciences
Texas A&M University
College Station, Texas, USA
Facilitating Client Grief

Risa M. Roland, DVM, Diplomate ACVIM (Cardiology)
Staff Cardiologist
Metropolitan Veterinary Associates
Valley Forge, Pennsylvania, USA
Congenital Heart Disease

John H. Rossmeisl, Jr., DVM, MS, Diplomate ACVIM (Neurology, Internal Medicine)
Assistant Professor
Department of Small Animal Clinical Sciences
Virginia-Maryland Regional College of Veterinary Medicine
Virginia Tech
Blacksburg, Virginia, USA
Intervertebral Disk Disease

Debbie S. Ruehlmann, DVM, MS, Diplomate ACVIM (Neurology)
Staff Neurologist
Angell Animal Medical Center
Boston, Massachusetts, USA
Myopathic Disorders

Corey F. Saba, DVM, Diplomate ACVIM (Oncology)
Instructor
Department of Small Animal Medicine and Surgery
College of Veterinary Medicine
University of Georgia
Athens, Georgia, USA
Mast Cell Tumors

Ashley B. Saunders, DVM, Diplomate ACVIM (Cardiology)
Assistant Professor
Department of Small Animal Clinical Sciences
College of Veterinary Medicine and Biomedical Sciences
Texas A&M University
College Station, Texas, USA
Cardiac Neoplasia

Krystal G. Schneider, RVT
Oncology Service Technician
Veterinary Medical Teaching Hospital
College of Veterinary Medicine and Biomedical Sciences
Texas A&M University
College Station, Texas, USA
Chemotherapy Administration

Marcia Schwassman, DVM, Diplomate ACVD
Staff Dermatologist
Veterinary Dermatology Center
Maitland, Florida, USA
How to Treat Common Parasites Safely

Andrea Valeria Scorza, MV, MS, PhD
Department of Clinical Sciences
College of Veterinary Medicine and Biomedical Sciences
Colorado State University
Fort Collins, Colorado, USA
Gastrointestinal Protozoal Infections

Nadja S. Sieber-Ruckstuhl, DrMedVet, Diplomate ACVIM, ECVIM-CA
Clinic for Small Animal Internal Medicine
Vetsuisse Faculty
University of Zurich
Zurich, Switzerland
Home Monitoring of Blood Glucose in Cats with Diabetes Mellitus

Margaret R. Slater, DVM, PhD
Senior Director of Epidemiology
Animal Health Services
ASPCA
Urbana, Illinois, USA
Understanding Population Dynamics Models: Implications for Veterinarians

Joanne R. Smith, MA, VetMB, PhD, Diplomate ACVIM
Clinical Instructor
Department of Small Animal Clinical Sciences
College of Veterinary Medicine
University of Tennessee
Knoxville, Tennessee, USA
Commercial Pet Food–Related Nephrotoxicity

Elizabeth A. Spangler, DVM, PhD, Diplomate ACVIM, ACVP (Clinical Pathology)
Assistant Professor
Department of Pathobiology
Auburn University
Auburn, Alabama, USA
Disseminated Intravascular Coagulation

Kathy Ann Spaulding, DVM, Diplomate ACVR
Clinical Professor
Department of Large Animal Clinical Sciences
College of Veterinary Medicine and Biomedical Sciences
Texas A&M University
College Station, Texas, USA
Ultrasonographic Imaging of the Gastrointestinal Tract

Jörg M. Steiner, medvet, Drmedvet, PhD, Diplomate ACVIM, ECVIM-CA
Associate Professor
Department of Small Animal Clinical Sciences
College of Veterinary Medicine and Biomedical Sciences
Texas A&M University
College Station, Texas, USA
Exocrine Pancreatic Insufficiency

Harriet M. Syme, BSc, BVetMed, PhD, Diplomate ACVIM, ECVIM-CA, MRCVS
Senior Lecturer
Department of Veterinary Clinical Sciences
The Royal Veterinary College
University of London
Hatfield, Hertfordshire, United Kingdom
Managing and Monitoring Systemic Hypertension

Ann M. Trimmer, DVM, Diplomate ACVD
Dermatologist
Animal Allergy and Dermatology Specialists
Las Vegas, Nevada, USA
Rush and Conventional Immunotherapy

Mark T. Troxel, DVM, Diplomate ACVIM (Neurology)
Staff Neurologist and Neurosurgeon
Massachusetts Veterinary Referral Hospital
Woburn, Massachusetts, USA
Brain Tumors: Clinical Spectrum

Alice Villalobos, DVM
Director
Animal Oncology Consultation Service
Woodland Hills, California, USA
Hospice "Pawspice"

Charles H. Vite, DVM, PhD, Diplomate ACVIM
Assistant Professor
Department of Clinical Studies—Philadelphia
School of Veterinary Medicine
University of Pennsylvania
Philadelphia, Pennsylvania, USA
Gene Therapy for Lysosomal Storage Diseases

Douglas J. Weiss, DVM, PhD, Diplomate ACVP
Professor
Department of Veterinary Biosciences
College of Veterinary Medicine
University of Minnesota
St. Paul, Minnesota, USA
Feline Bone Marrow Disorders

Heather M. Wilson, DVM, Diplomate ACVIM (Oncology)
Clinical Assistant Professor
Department of Small Animal Clinical Sciences
College of Veterinary Medicine and Biomedical Sciences
Texas A&M University
College Station, Texas, USA
Urinary Tract Tumors
Tumors of the Ear
Chemotherapy Administration

Zachary M. Wright, DVM, Diplomate ACVIM (Oncology)
Staff Oncologist
VCA Veterinary Care Animal Hospital and Referral Center
Albuquerque, New Mexico, USA
Facilitating Client Grief

Debra L. Zoran, DVM, PhD, Diplomate ACVIM
Associate Professor
Department of Small Animal Clinical Sciences
College of Veterinary Medicine and Biomedical Sciences
Texas A&M University
College Station, Texas, USA
Probiotics in Feline Medicine

Contents

Infectious Diseases

Julie Levy, Section Editor

CHAPTER
1 Pyothorax

Vanessa R.D. Barrs and Julia A. Beatty

Pyothorax describes an accumulation of a purulent exudate in the pleural space. Aspiration of oropharyngeal flora with subsequent colonization of the lower respiratory tract and parapneumonic spread is an important route of infection. Other organisms including gastrointestinal flora, protozoa, and fungal agents are isolated in a minority of cases, particularly in kittens. By the time they are presented, many cats are severely compromised, highlighting the importance of early recognition and stabilization. Although the disease is likely to have progressed insidiously, most patients present acutely. Rapid decompensation may follow transportation and handling. Careful handling and early consideration of stabilization, including supplemental oxygen and therapeutic thoracocentesis, are essential to avoid respiratory failure. Information gained from the analysis of appropriate diagnostic samples guides the management plan. Although initial reports were pessimistic regarding the prognosis for pyothorax, it has become clear that most cats who survive the first 48 hours from presentation can be treated successfully with aggressive medical management. Surgery may be indicated when pulmonary abscessation is identified or when medical management fails.

EPIDEMIOLOGY

Pyothorax is predominantly a disease of young cats (mean age 4 to 6 years), although cats of any age may be affected.[1-4] An increased risk for developing pyothorax has been demonstrated for cats from multiple-cat households.[3] No breed or sex predisposition has been identified. Currently, there are no data on the incidence of pyothorax. Some studies suggest a seasonal trend with more cases presenting in late summer or autumn.[3,5]

ETIOPATHOGENESIS

An understanding of the etiopathogenesis underpins recommendations for investigation, treatment, and prophylaxis. Information on mechanisms of infection of the pleural space has remained elusive, because any inciting cause is often no longer evident by the time clinical signs are observed. Pyothorax in cats most often is caused by obligate and facultative anaerobes of oropharyngeal origin (Box 1-1).[6] Oropharyngeal flora can gain access to the pleural space by aspiration, direct penetration from a bite wound, or by hematogenous spread from a distant wound. Available evidence suggests that aspiration of oropharyngeal flora, subsequent colonization of the lower respiratory tract, and direct extension is the most common route of infection of the pleural space in cats.[7] In a retrospective study, aspiration of oral flora was the most likely mechanism of pleural space infection in 78 per cent of cats in whom probable mechanisms were identified.[4] At necropsy, about 50 per cent of cats with pyothorax have pneumonia or pulmonary abscessation, supporting a pathomechanism of parapneumonic spread.[7] Aspiration of oropharyngeal flora precedes most cases of human anaerobic pyothorax and equine pleuropneumonia.[8,9] Viral upper respiratory tract (URT) infection can impair the mucociliary escalator in cats, human beings, and horses, predisposing them to pleuropneumonia.[10-12] Antecedent URT infection has been recognized as a predisposing event in up to 26 per cent of cases of feline

Box 1-1 Organisms Isolated from Feline Pyothorax

Obligate and facultative anaerobic bacteria, similar in composition to the normal feline oropharyngeal flora, are isolated most commonly. Less than 20 per cent of isolates involve nonoropharyngeal flora.[7]

OBLIGATE AND FACULTATIVE ANAEROBIC BACTERIA

Bacteroidaceae (*Bacteroides* spp., *Porphyromonas* spp., *Prevotella* spp.)
Fusobacterium spp.
Peptostreptococcus spp.
Clostridium spp.
Actinomyces spp.
Eubacterium spp.
Propionibacterium spp.
Filifactor villosus
Pasteurella multocida
Streptococcus spp.
Mycoplasma spp.

NONOROPHARYNGEAL FLORA

Staphylococcus spp., *Rhodococcus equi*, *Nocardia* spp.
Enteric gram-negative organisms: *E. coli*, *Salmonella* spp., *Klebsiella* spp., *Proteus* spp.
Nonenteric gram-negative organisms: *Pseudomonas* spp.
Protozoa: *Toxoplasma gondii*
Fungal agents: *Cryptococcus* spp., *Candida albicans*, *Blastomyces dermatitidis*

---

pyothorax.[7] The fourfold increase in risk of pyothorax in cats from multiple-cat households compared with control cats may be related to the greater risk of developing viral URT infections in this environment.[3,13]

Direct inoculation of oral flora into the thorax from a bite wound is likely to be the initiating event in some cases of pyothorax. The importance of this route may have been overemphasized, or it may have become less common, perhaps due to increased neutering and confinement.[7] Thoracic puncture wounds were identified in 4 per cent and 16 per cent of cases in recent studies.[3,4] If cat fights were a common cause of pyothorax, then free-roaming males likely would be overrepresented, whereas neither outdoor access nor gender have been identified as risk factors for the development of pyothorax. It also might be expected that the prevalence of feline immunodeficiency virus (FIV), a virus spread predominantly by biting, would be similar in cats with pyothorax to that in cats with fight wounds. Combined data on the FIV status of cats with pyothorax indicate that 5.8 per cent of 51 cats tested were seropositive.[2-4,14] The prevalence of FIV worldwide ranges from 1 to 14 per cent in asymptomatic cats, up to 44 per cent in sick cats, and recently has been shown to be 19 per cent in cats with bite wounds.[15,16] Although the data are limited, they do not support biting as a major mechanism of infection of the pleural space.

In less than 20 per cent of cases, particularly in kittens, pyothorax is caused by infectious agents other than oropharyngeal flora, emphasizing the need for pleural fluid

cytology and culture in all cases. These organisms include *Staphylococcus* spp., *Rhodococcus equi*, *Nocardia* spp., enteric gram-negative organisms (*Escherichia coli*, *Salmonella* spp., *Klebsiella* spp., *Proteus* spp.), nonenteric gram-negative organisms (*Pseudomonas* spp.), and protozoa (*Toxoplasma gondii*).[1,2,4,17-20] Fungal causes of pyothorax are rare and include *Cryptococcus* spp., *Candida albicans*, and *Blastomyces dermatitidis*.[4,21,22] Mechanisms of infection of the pleural space with nonoropharyngeal flora include penetrating thoracic trauma not associated with a cat bite. However, if environmental contamination of thoracic wounds were a common mechanism, a higher isolation rate of saprophytic bacteria such as *Nocardia* spp., *Pseudomonas* spp., and *Mycobacteria* spp. would be expected. In contrast to the situation in canine cases, *Nocardia* spp. are not commonly isolated from feline septic pleural effusions. Other routes of infection with nonoropharyngeal flora include hematogenous spread from a septic focus; perforation of the esophagus, trachea, or bronchi; or migrating plant material and parasitic migration.* Pyothorax and/or pneumonia caused by *Salmonella* spp. has been documented in cats with concurrent *Aelurostrongylus abstrusus* infestation.[19,28] Migrating lungworm or ascarid larvae can act as carriers for intestinal bacteria. Nonoropharyngeal pathogens are more likely to be isolated from kittens, perhaps because of concurrent age-related infectious or parasitic conditions.[4]

HISTORY AND CLINICAL SIGNS

Historical and physical examination findings can be attributed to the presence of a pleural effusion and/or to systemic illness. Dyspnea, inappetence, and lethargy are reported most commonly. Pleural effusion and pulmonary atelectasis cause a restrictive pattern of respiration, characterized by an increase in respiratory rate and inspiratory effort and shallow respiratory excursions. Cats typically adopt a crouched, sternally recumbent posture with elbows abducted. Poor body condition, dehydration, and abnormal lung sounds or muffled heart sounds also are common. A fluid line may be appreciated on thoracic percussion. Coughing is reported in 14 to 30 per cent of cases, reflecting pleuritis and/or concurrent pneumonia.[2,4,5,22] Pyrexia has been reported in 28 to 50 per cent of cases, although some cats in these series had received prior antibiotic treatment.[2,4] Therefore pyrexia at initial presentation may be more common than these figures suggest. Hypothermia, present in 15 per cent of cats, should alert the clinician to the possibility of severe sepsis, particularly when accompanied by bradycardia.[3,29] In the largest retrospective study of 80 cats with pyothorax, bradycardia was significantly more common in cats who were hypothermic.[3]

The duration of clinical signs prior to diagnosis typically is 1 to 2 weeks, but it may be months.[2,4,5,23] Because cats are prone to compensate for gradual onset respiratory

---

*References 2, 4, 5, 19, 23-27.

compromise by reducing activity, signs may be noted only at the acute stage or not at all by the owner. Coupled with the nonspecific nature of many of the presenting signs, many cats are presented late in the course of the disease. By the time clinical signs of respiratory compromise become obvious in feline patients, minimal respiratory reserve remains. Pyothorax should be considered as a cause of sudden death.

DIFFERENTIAL DIAGNOSIS

Pyothorax can be differentiated from other causes of pleural effusion by examination of the fluid obtained at thoracocentesis. Complete diagnostic investigation, including fluid analysis, cytological examination, and culture, should be carried out in all suspected cases of pyothorax, even when the gross characteristics are highly suggestive. This will confirm the diagnosis; identify unusual infections, nonseptic processes, or intercurrent problems (e.g., lungworm infection); and direct appropriate antimicrobial treatment.[7]

DIAGNOSIS

In most cases, the clinician will be highly suspicious of pleural effusion based on the clinical examination findings. This can be confirmed quickly and noninvasively using thoracic radiography or ultrasonography. In some cases, the presenting signs can be subtle. The absence of dyspnea does not exclude the diagnosis, supporting the use of thoracic imaging in the diagnostic investigation of cats with nonspecific signs.

STABILIZATION DURING DIAGNOSTIC INVESTIGATION

The first 48 hours from presentation is a critical time for pyothorax patients. Most nonsurvivors (60 to 100 per cent) die or are euthanized during this period. Careful handling, early stabilization, and minimally invasive diagnostic procedures are essential for any patient with pleural space disease. The additional stress imposed by transport to the hospital and examination can precipitate respiratory failure. Sepsis or the systemic inflammatory response syndrome also can contribute to these deaths.[29,30]

Assessment for, and treatment of, reduced oxygen saturation using supplemental oxygen and therapeutic thoracocentesis is of paramount importance. Oxygen should be administered immediately to cats in severe respiratory distress using a mask or chamber (Figure 1-1). Pulse oximetry can be used to monitor hemoglobin saturation noninvasively. Hemoglobin saturations of less than 90 per cent in patients breathing room air indicate severe hypoxemia and the need for oxygen supplementation. Other considerations for initial patient stabilization include identification and correction of hypothermia, hypotension, hypoglycemia, and fluid and electrolyte imbalances.

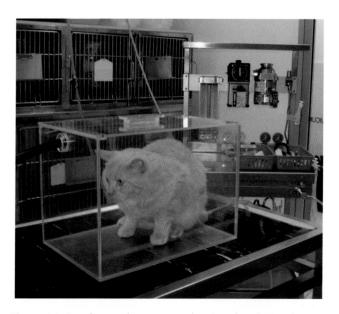

Figure 1-1 Supplemental oxygen can be given by placing the cat in a chamber.

DIAGNOSTIC IMAGING

Thoracic ultrasonography is an expedient, noninvasive technique for confirmation of a moderate to large-volume pleural effusion in the dyspneic patient. In contrast to transudates, which are anechoic, the exudate in pyothorax is hypoechoic or complex echoic. The effusion often is septate due to fibrinous or fibrous tags extending between the parietal and visceral pleura. Pulmonary abscesses and restrictive pleuritis also can be identified ultrasonographically. Effusions are bilateral in 70 to 90 per cent of cases.[2-4,17] When sonography is not available, one dorsoventral radiographic view will confirm the presence of a pleural effusion while requiring minimal restraint (Figure 1-2). Severe hypoxemia can occur if cats with large-volume effusions are placed in lateral recumbency for radiography. Horizontal beam radiography can be used to detect pleural effusion in the sternally recumbent patient. Radiographic signs of pleural effusion include retraction of the lobar borders from the thoracic wall, pulmonary atelectasis, and accentuation of lobar edges and interlobar fissures. A complete set of thoracic radiographs should be obtained after drainage of pleural effusion to assess for underlying bronchopulmonary disease.

THORACOCENTESIS

Needle thoracocentesis should be carried out early to obtain diagnostic specimens and to stabilize the patient. This will be tolerated in most cases without the need for sedation. Subcutaneous instillation of local anesthetic (e.g., 0.5 mL of 1 per cent lidocaine) at the thoracocentesis site facilitates the procedure. Diagnostic thoracocentesis should be performed, preferably under ultrasound guidance, at the ventral third of the sixth, seventh, or eighth intercostal space with the cat positioned in sternal

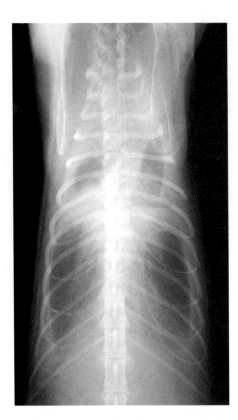

Figure 1-2 A single dorsoventral radiograph can confirm the presence of a pleural effusion. The effusion is bilateral in most cases.

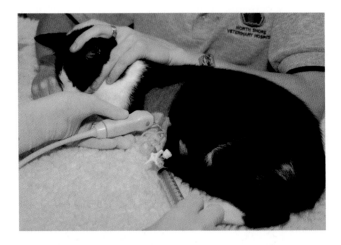

Figure 1-3 Ultrasonography can be used to confirm the presence of a pleural effusion noninvasively and to guide initial needle thoracocentesis to stabilize the patient.

recumbency (Figure 1-3). Care should be taken to avoid intercostal vessels and nerves located near the caudal rib margin. A 21- or 23-gauge butterfly needle with extension tubing and three-way tap attached to a syringe can be used for this purpose (Figure 1-4). Once a sample has been obtained for diagnostic evaluation, thoracocentesis is continued to remove as much pleural exudate as possible before general anesthesia for placement of thoracostomy tubes. Thoracocentesis should be carried out bilaterally unless imaging indicates a unilateral effusion.

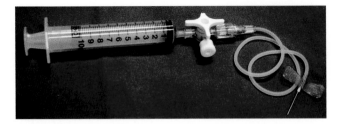

Figure 1-4 A 21- or 23-gauge butterfly needle, extension tubing, and three-way tap attached to a syringe can be used for diagnostic and therapeutic thoracocentesis.

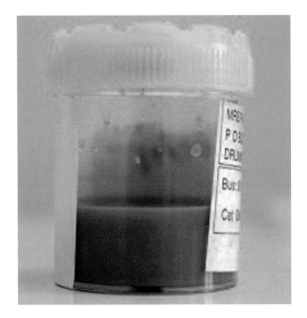

Figure 1-5 Pink-tinged, creamy exudate typical of pyothorax. This will be foul smelling unless unusual pathogens are involved.

DIAGNOSTIC SAMPLE COLLECTION

Samples of pleural fluid should be collected in ethylenediaminetetraacetic acid (EDTA) for cell counts and cytological examination, in a serum tube for biochemical analysis, and in a sterile container for aerobic culture and susceptibility testing. Commercial specimen collectors are available to facilitate reliable anaerobic culture. Susceptibility testing of obligate anaerobic bacteria is not available routinely because of time constraints, technical complexity, and the relatively low incidence of β-lactamase–producing organisms.

PLEURAL FLUID EVALUATION

The gross characteristics of the fluid usually are sufficient to direct the clinician towards a diagnosis of pyothorax. Septic exudates typically are turbid to opaque and often contain flocculent material. They usually are cream colored but can be pink, green tinged, or sanguinous (Figure 1-5). Perhaps the most compelling feature is the characteristic foul smell of the mixed anaerobic infection responsible for most cases of pyothorax. The clinician almost certainly will have experienced this odor associated with cat-fight abscesses. A lack of odor does not exclude pyothorax, but should arouse suspicion for an unusual pathogen (e.g., aerobes, yeast, or *Mycoplasma* spp.) or an alternative disease process such as feline infectious peritonitis (FIP) or a malignant effusion.

Results of laboratory analysis are consistent with an exudate, including protein greater than 3.0 g/dL, total nucleated cell count greater than 7000/μL, and specific gravity at least 1.025.[31] Neutrophils predominate in septic effusions (more than 85 per cent of total nucleated cell count). Occasionally other effusions, such as those associated with neoplasia or effusive FIP, may need to be differentiated from the septic exudate of pyothorax. The measurement of lactic dehydrogenase (LDH), glucose, and pH has been advocated to help classify feline pleural effusions. In septic effusions, LDH typically is greater than 200 IU/L, pH is equal to or less than 6.9, and glucose usually is less than 1.68 mmol/L and less than a concurrent blood glucose measurement. Neoplastic exudates typically have a normal or high pH (>7.4), low neutrophil count (<30 per cent), and low glucose (0.5 to 4.5 mmol/L).[32] In effusive FIP, the protein content is high (>3.5 g/dL), consistent with an exudative process, whereas the nucleated cell count is low, consistent with a modified transudate (<5000 cells/μL) or even a pure transudate (<1000/μL).[33]

In-house cytological examination of pleural fluid provides useful information while laboratory results are pending (Figure 1-6). On modified Wright-Giemsa–stained (e.g., "Diff-Quik," Dade Shearing) smears, polymicrobial infections of obligate anaerobes and facultative bacteria typically feature large numbers of degenerate neutrophils, a small proportion of mononuclear inflammatory cells, and large numbers of pleomorphic, intracellular, and/or extracellular bacteria. Erythrocytes, mesothelial cells, and epithelial cells also may be seen. Any combination of filamentous bacteria (e.g., *Filifactor villosus*), cocci (e.g., *Peptostreptococcus* spp.), or rods may be present. Bacterial rods may be nonenteric facultative bacteria (e.g., *Pasteurella* spp.), enteric facultative bacteria (e.g., *E. coli*), or obligate anaerobes (e.g., *Bacteroides* spp., *Prevotella* spp., *Porphyromonas* spp., or *Fusobacterium* spp.). The Gram stain is an important tool for rapid assessment of bacteria in pleural fluid. Acid-fast stains help to differentiate *Nocardia* spp. from *Actinomyces* spp. and *Filifactor* spp. because the former are partially acid-fast. In actinomycosis and *Filifactor villosus* infections, other oropharyngeal bacterial species are likely to be present.

Cytological findings should be compared with culture results to identify discrepancies. For example, when anaerobic culture is not available or appropriate specimens have not been collected, pleural fluid culture will be negative on aerobic culture of obligate anaerobic infections. Similarly, if only aerobic culture is performed, only the aerobic component of mixed infections will be cultured.

ADDITIONAL TESTING

Hematology, serum biochemistry, urinalysis, and retrovirus testing should form part of the minimum database to guide management of the patient. A neutrophilic leukocytosis with a left shift is seen in 36 to 73 per cent of cases.[2,4] Toxic changes in neutrophils are seen commonly on examination of the peripheral blood film.[34] A degenerative left shift can occur with advanced sepsis and sequestration of neutrophils in the pleural space. Mild to moderate anemia is seen in less than 20 per cent of

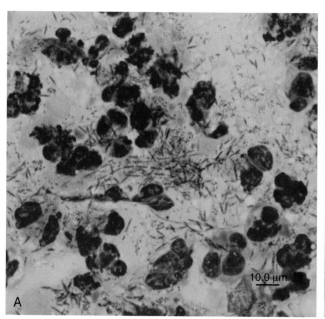
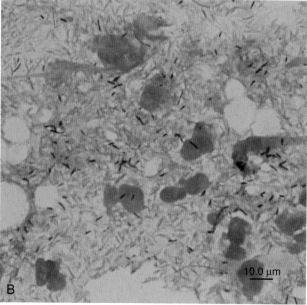

Figure 1-6 In-house cytological evaluation of smears prepared from pleural exudate is useful to guide empirical therapy while culture results are pending. A mixed population of bacteria with degenerative neutrophils, typical of most cases, is shown stained with **(A)** "Diff-Quik" (Dade Shearing) and **(B)** Gram stain.

cases.[2,4,5] The most common abnormalities on serum biochemistry are hypoalbuminemia, hyperglobulinemia, hypoglycemia or hyperglycemia, hyponatremia, hypochloremia, hypocalcemia, and mild elevations of aspartate aminotransferase and bilirubin.[2,3] Hypoalbuminemia is a common finding in sepsis, attributed to increased vascular permeability and decreased hepatic synthesis due to a shift towards synthesis of positive acute phase proteins.[29,35]

TREATMENT

Closed-tube thoracostomy, aspiration, lavage, and antimicrobial therapy can be expected to result in complete resolution of disease in most cases. Polymicrobial pyothorax is similar conceptually to a cat fight abscess, and the same basic principles of drainage, antimicrobial therapy, and supportive care apply. Although future analytical studies comparing different treatment protocols with outcomes may identify optimal treatment schedules, these basic principles are unlikely to change. We have reported a success rate of 95 per cent for cats treated using closed-tube thoracostomy.[4] The treatment recommendations outlined below are based on our findings and other available evidence as indicated.[36]

CLOSED-TUBE THORACOSTOMY

Placement of indwelling thoracostomy tubes is simple, is cost-effective, provides excellent drainage, and is well tolerated. Although there are reports of successful management of feline pyothorax using single or repeated needle thoracocentesis combined with antimicrobial therapy, mortality rates of up to 80 per cent have been reported.[3-5,17,37-39] Needle thoracocentesis can be useful when the effusion is of small volume and pneumonia is the primary problem or when euthanasia is the only other option. It is worth noting that a single ultrasound-guided pleural drainage procedure using a temporary thoracostomy tube followed by antibiotic treatment was associated with a successful outcome in 15 of 16 dogs with pyothorax.[40]

To facilitate drainage and to decrease the likelihood of mechanical complications such as kinking or obstruction, the thoracostomy tube of greatest diameter that can fit comfortably between the intercostal spaces should be used (generally 14 to 16 Fr) (Figure 1-7). Commercially available pediatric thoracic trocar catheters are inserted under general anesthesia. Mortality is reduced by using preanesthetic needle thoracocentesis and minimizing the time between diagnosis and thoracic drain insertion. The chest tube should penetrate the skin two or more intercostal spaces (ICS) caudal to where the tube enters the thoracic cavity to minimize the potential for iatrogenic pneumothorax. Preemptive analgesia can be achieved by infiltration of a local anesthetic in the ICS at a location where the drain will penetrate the body wall. The surgical site is prepared, and a small stab incision is made in the dorsal third of the 10th or 11th ICS. The trocar is advanced cranially through a subcutaneous tunnel and then

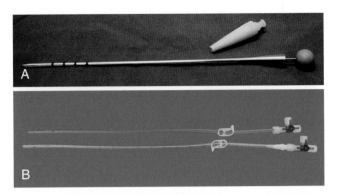

Figure 1-7   A, A fenestrated thoracic trocar catheter (16-gauge) with stylet and plastic-tube connector. **B,** Fourteen- and 16-gauge fenestrated thoracic catheters with stylets removed.

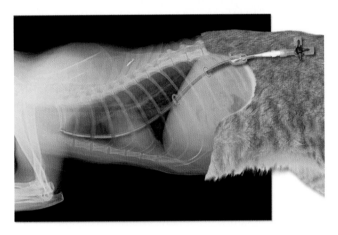

Figure 1-8 Diagram to illustrate the correct positioning of a thoracostomy tube within the pleural space. (From Barrs VR, Beatty JA: Feline pyothorax—new insights into an old problem: Part II. Treatment recommendations and prophylaxis, *Vet J* 179:171, 2009.)

driven into the pleural space through the 8th ICS. The tube is advanced over the trocar in a cranioventral direction parallel to the thoracic wall for a distance of 12 to 18 cm. The correct drain position is demonstrated in Figure 1-8. As the trocar is removed, the end of the tube is clamped to prevent pneumothorax. Alternatively, thoracostomy tubes without stylets may be placed in the same location using large hemostats to perforate the intercostal muscles.

The tube is secured to the thoracic wall by a purse-string suture to provide an airtight seal and a Chinese finger-trap suture is placed to prevent the tube from slipping. A plastic tube connector ("Christmas-tree") attached to a three-way stopcock is placed in the end of the tube, and any remaining exudate or air that entered during the procedure is evacuated and the three-way tap closed. For safety, the tube also is sealed with a G-clamp (Figure 1-9).

Placement of bilateral thoracostomy tubes is recommended unless the effusion is unilateral. Bilateral chest tubes are more likely to provide effective drainage in cases of persistent loculation of fluid or when the mediastinum is complete. Given the high mechanical complication

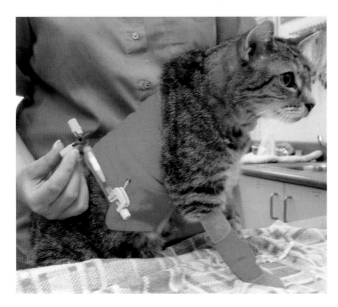

Figure 1-9 Bilateral drains should be supported with a body bandage. They are sealed with three-way stop-cocks and a G-clamp as shown.

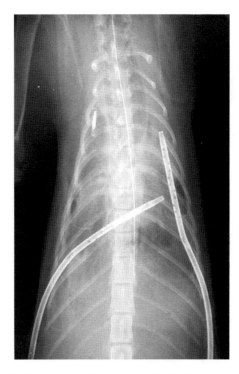

Figure 1-10 Radiographs (three views) should be taken after drain placement to ensure correct positioning. The right drain has been misplaced in this case.

rates that have been reported with thoracostomy tubes, placement of bilateral tubes reduces the likelihood of a second general anesthesia for tube replacement in case of unilateral tube failure.[4] A complete set of thoracic radiographs should be obtained after thoracostomy tube placement to assess drain position and the presence of underlying bronchopulmonary disease (Figure 1-10). If only one tube has been placed and there is minimal residual effusion, unilateral drainage may be sufficient for treatment. If effusion persists on the opposite side, a second thoracostomy tube should be placed.

MANAGEMENT OF INDWELLING THORACOSTOMY TUBES

Thoracostomy tubes can be managed effectively with intermittent suction. Continuous water seal suction is not necessary for effective pleural drainage in feline pyothorax and does not decrease the time needed to manage the condition.[2-4] While continuous suction offers maximal drainage, it is more expensive, requires continuous monitoring, and introduces the risk of leakage between the pleural cavity and water seal, which can be fatal.[41] Closed-tube thoracostomy with intermittent suction is simpler, less expensive, requires less monitoring, and achieves excellent results.[4]

Suction and lavage should be carried out q4h for the first 24 to 48 hours (Figure 1-11). Thereafter, q8h to q12h usually is adequate. Lavage maintains thoracostomy tube patency, facilitates drainage and hydraulic debridement of the pleura, and dilutes bacteria and inflammatory mediators. Hygienic precautions should be used during suction and lavage to prevent nosocomial infection. For patients managed with lavage a shorter duration of tube placement than for those managed without lavage has been reported.[2] The residual volume and gross characteristics of the fluid aspirated prior to lavage should be recorded and used to guide the frequency of the procedure. A lavage fluid of 0.9 per cent saline warmed to 38° C is suitable. A volume of 10 to 25 mL/kg can be instilled via one thoracostomy tube. The volume of fluid instilled and then aspirated should be recorded. The procedure then is repeated using the thoracostomy tube on the opposite hemithorax. Recovery of 75 per cent or more of instilled lavage solution is expected. If smaller volumes of fluid are recovered, imaging is indicated to investigate for thoracostomy tube complications or loculation of fluid due to adhesions.

The addition of fibrinolytics or antimicrobials to the thoracic lavage solution appears to offer no advantage; it is no longer recommended in treatment of human thoracic empyema.[42]

MONITORING AND ONGOING SUPPORTIVE CARE

While thoracostomy tubes are in place, analgesia can be achieved using buprenorphine (e.g., 0.02 mg/kg SQ or IV q6-8h) or morphine (e.g., 0.1 mg/kg IV q4-6h). Clinically significant opioid-induced respiratory depression is unlikely to be an issue at these doses.[43] Although intra-pleural analgesia, using bupivacaine buffered with sodium bicarbonate, can be used as an adjunct to opioid analgesia, absorption is unreliable and the potential for diaphragmatic paralysis exists in patients with poor respiratory reserve.[44] Patients with indwelling thoracostomy tubes should be monitored closely for potential complications including pneumothorax, failure of drain-

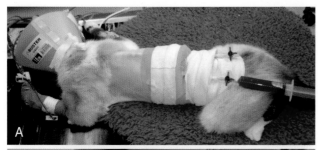

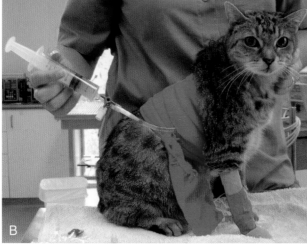

Figure 1-11 A and **B,** Lavage maintains thoracostomy tube patency, facilitates drainage and hydraulic debridement of the pleura, and dilutes bacteria and inflammatory mediators. See text for details.

age due to blockage, kinking or adhesions, subcutaneous edema, or abscesses at the site of drain insertion. Thoracic imaging should be performed q48h while chest tubes are in place to ensure early detection of drainage failure and other indications for exploratory thoracotomy.

Daily monitoring should include measurement of electrolytes, hematocrit, serum albumin, total plasma protein, volume of thoracostomy tube fluid lavaged and aspirated, and changes in bodyweight. Hypokalemia is a potential complication of lavage of the thoracic cavity.[4] Use of volumes of lavage fluid not exceeding 25 mL/kg and of a lavage solution containing potassium (e.g., Hartmann's solution [Compound Sodium Lactate]) is recommended to prevent this complication. Anorexia usually resolves within 48 hours of commencing pleural space drainage and antimicrobial therapy. Provision of early enteral nutrition through a feeding tube should be considered in cachectic or critically ill patients (see Chapter 12). Esophagostomy tubes are an appropriate choice for the short duration of nutritional support required.

Indwelling thoracostomy tubes generally are removed after 5 to 6 days when the following criteria have been met: minimal residual effusion on aspiration (arbitrarily <2 mL/kg/day), resolution of pleural effusion on thoracic imaging, and cytological resolution of infection, as indicated by absence of microorganisms, reduction of neutrophil numbers with loss of degenerate appearance, and appearance of macrophages.

Table 1-1 Parenteral Antimicrobial Agents Useful for the Treatment of Feline Pyothorax*

Antibiotic	Dosage and Frequency
Penicillin G potassium/sodium	20,000-40,000 IU/kg IV q6h
Ampicillin	20-40 mg/kg IV q6-8h
Amoxicillin	10-20 mg/kg IV q12h
Ticarcillin-clavulanic acid	40-50 mg/kg (combined) IV q6-8h
Ampicillin-sulbactam	50 mg/kg (combined) IV q8h
Amoxicillin-clavulanic acid	12-20 mg/kg (combined) SQ/IM q12h
Metronidazole	15 mg/kg IV q12h

*See text for appropriate combinations.

ANTIMICROBIAL THERAPY

Guided by in-house cytological findings, empirical therapy for most cases will involve agents effective against obligate and facultative anaerobes. The rationale for the selection of antimicrobials for empirical therapy of feline pyothorax has been described in detail elsewhere.[36] Suitable choices include penicillin G (e.g., benzylpenicillin potassium or benzylpenicillin sodium) or an aminopenicillin (e.g., ampicillin or amoxicillin), either alone or in combination with metronidazole (Table 1-1). Alternatively, monotherapy with a potentiated penicillin (e.g., amoxicillin-clavulanic acid or ticarcillin-clavulanic acid) can be used. These agents are effective against both β-lactamase–producing anaerobes and *Pasteurella* spp. Although newer methoxyfluoroquinolones such as pradofloxacin likely would be effective as a monotherapy for mixed aerobic and anaerobic infections in cats and dogs, there are concerns of increasing resistance in *Bacteroides* group isolates.[45,46]

The addition of either a fluoroquinolone or an aminoglycoside (gentamicin or amikacin) to empirical therapy for pyothorax is useful in dogs, but not necessary for cats. In dogs the facultative Gram-negative rods are often Enterobacteriaceae, particularly *E. coli*.[1,40,47] In cats, however, Enterobacteriaceae are uncommon, with *E. coli* being isolated in 0 to 7 per cent of cases of pyothorax.[1,2,4,5,48] Even when *E. coli* is isolated, resistance to fluoroquinolones can be a problem in some regions.[49-51] Of 50 *E. coli* isolates obtained from cats examined at a veterinary teaching hospital, 75 per cent were susceptible to amoxicillin-clavulanate, while only 55 per cent were susceptible to enrofloxacin.[1] Gram-negative rods seen on cytological analysis of feline pyothorax fluid are most likely to be *Pasteurella* spp.[2,48] Because *Pasteurella* spp. are susceptible to penicillin and its derivatives, the addition of a fluoroquinolone or aminoglycoside is unnecessary for empirical therapy in cats. This avoids the potential for retinotoxicity (e.g., enrofloxacin), or ototoxicity and nephrotoxicity (aminoglycosides).[52,53] Neither clindamycin nor first-generation cephalosporins have good efficacy against *Pasteurella* spp. and therefore are not recommended for initial empirical therapy of feline pyothorax.[54] Some newer generation cephalosporins, such as cefovecin, have good in-vitro activity against both *Pasteurella* spp. and obligate anaerobes.[55] Adjunctive, targeted antimicrobial therapy can be administered if indicated by the results of culture and susceptibility testing, or if gram-negative rods alone are seen on cytological examination of pleural fluid.

At least initially, the intravenous route is preferred. Preparations of amoxicillin-clavulanic acid and ampicillin with sulbactam suitable for IV use are available in some regions. Once clinical improvement is seen and the patient is eating well, oral antibiotics may be substituted. Antimicrobial therapy should be administered for 4 to 6 weeks to reduce the risk of relapse. Thoracic radiographs should be taken 1 to 2 weeks after discharge from hospital and at the completion of antimicrobial therapy to ensure complete resolution of infection.

INDICATIONS FOR SURGERY

Indications for exploratory thoracotomy include pulmonary or mediastinal abscessation, extensively loculated effusions, persistence of large-volume effusion after more than 7 days, drain obstruction, or recurrence. In the minority of cases in which medical management fails, exploratory thoracotomy is likely to be curative.[3,4] The goals of exploratory thoracotomy are to:

- Identify and remove any primary cause, such as foreign body, that may act as a nidus of infection.
- Remove isolated areas of necrotic tissue, including grossly abnormal lung lobes.
- Break down fibrinous or fibrous adhesions that may be isolating areas of the thoracic cavity.
- Ensure effective placement of bilateral thoracostomy tubes.

In dogs, isolation of *Actinomyces* spp. from pleural fluid is an indication for thoracotomy because of poor outcomes with medical therapy alone; however, this is *not* the case in cats.[36,47] While *Actinomyces* spp. are members of normal oropharyngeal flora of both dogs and cats, pyothorax in dogs has been associated with *Actinomyces* spp.–contaminated plant material. In cats, pyothorax involving *Actinomyces* spp., in combination with other oropharyngeal flora, is unlikely to be associated with grass awns and has been shown to resolve without thoracotomy.[36]

PROGNOSIS

More than 90 per cent of patients who receive aggressive medical management can be expected to survive.[36] Hypersalivation was a negative prognostic indicator in one study.[3] Information on FIV-positive cats with pyothorax is sparse, but does not support FIV infection as a predisposing factor or a negative prognostic indicator.[7] Recurrence has been reported in 5 to 14 per cent of cases managed medically.[36] In situations in which medical treatment fails and surgical intervention is required, the prognosis for resolving infection is good to excellent.

PROPHYLAXIS

Because most cases of pyothorax involve oropharyngeal flora, routine antimicrobial prophylaxis should be considered in situations in which cats are at risk of colonization of the lower respiratory tract by these organisms. These include viral upper respiratory tract infections and dental procedures under general anesthesia.

ACKNOWLEDGEMENTS

The authors thank Bozena Jantulik, Patricia Martin, and Keith Ellis for preparation of the figures.

REFERENCES

1. Walker AL, Jang SS, Hirsch DC: Bacteria associated with pyothorax of dogs and cats: 98 cases (1989-1998), *J Am Vet Med Assoc* 216:359, 2000.
2. Demetriou JL, Foale RD, Ladlow J, et al: Canine and feline pyothorax: a retrospective study of 50 cases in the UK and Ireland, *J Small Anim Pract* 43:388, 2002.
3. Waddell LS, Brady CA, Drobatz KJ: Risk factors, prognostic indicators, and outcome of pyothorax in cats: 80 cases (1986-1999), *J Am Vet Med Assoc* 221:819, 2002.
4. Barrs VR, Allan GS, Martin P, et al: Feline pyothorax: a retrospective study of 27 cases in Australia, *J Feline Med Surg* 7:211, 2005.
5. Jonas LD: Feline pyothorax: a retrospective study of twenty cases, *J Am Anim Hosp Assoc* 19:865, 1983.
6. Love DN, Malik R, Norris JM: Bacteriological warfare amongst cats: what have we learned about cat bite infections? *Vet Microbiol* 74:179, 2000.
7. Barrs VR, Beatty JA: Feline pyothorax—new insights into an old problem: Part 1. Aetiopathogenesis and diagnostic investigation, *Vet J* 179:163, 2009.
8. Racklyeft DJ, Raidal S, Love DN: Towards an understanding of equine pleuropneumonia: factors relevant for control, *Aust Vet J* 78:334, 2000.
9. Schiza S, Siafakas NM: Clinical presentation and management of empyema, lung abscess and pleural effusion, *Curr Opin Pulm Med* 12:205, 2006.
10. Carson JL, Collier AM, Hu SS: Acquired ciliary defects in nasal epithelium of children with acute viral upper respiratory infections, *N Engl J Med* 312:463, 1985.
11. Willoughby R, Ecker G, McKee S, et al: The effects of equine rhinovirus, influenza virus and herpesvirus infection on tracheal clearance rate in horses, *Can J Vet Res* 56:115, 1992.
12. Gaskell RM, Radford AD, Dawson S: Feline infectious respiratory disease. In Chandler EA, Gaskell CJ, Gaskell RM, editors: *Feline medicine and therapeutics*, ed 3, Oxford, 2004, Blackwell Publishing, p 577.
13. Binns SH, Dawson S, Speakman AJ, et al: A study of feline upper respiratory tract disease with reference to prevalence and risk factors for infection with feline calicivirus and feline herpesvirus, *J Feline Med Surg* 2:123, 2000.
14. Thompson JC, Gartrell BM, Butler S, et al: Successful treatment of feline pyothorax associated with an *Actinomyces* species and *Bacteroides melanogenicus*, *N Z Vet J* 40:73, 1992.
15. Hartmann K: Feline immunodeficiency virus infection: an overview, *Vet J* 155:123, 1998.
16. Goldkamp CE, Levy JK, Edinboro CH, et al: Seroprevalences of feline leukemia virus and feline immunodeficiency virus in cats with abscesses or bite wounds and rate of veterinarian

compliance with current guidelines for retrovirus testing, *J Am Vet Med Assoc* 232:1152, 2008.

17. Gruffydd-Jones TJ, Flecknell PA: The prognosis and treatment related to the gross appearance and laboratory characteristics of pathological thoracic fluids in the cat, *J Small Anim Pract* 19:315, 1978.

18. Sherding RG: Pyothorax in the cat, *Compend Contin Educ Pract Vet* 1:247, 1979.

19. Barrs VR, Swinney GR, Martin P, et al: Concurrent *Aelurostrongylus abstrusus* infection and Salmonellosis in a kitten, *Aust Vet J* 77:229, 1999.

20. Anfray P, Bonetti C, Fabbrini F, et al: Feline cutaneous toxoplasmosis: a case report, *Vet Dermatol* 16:131, 2005.

21. McCaw D, Franklin R, Fales W, et al: Pyothorax caused by *Candida albicans* in a cat, *J Am Vet Med Assoc* 185:311, 1984.

22. Sherding RG: Diseases of the pleural cavity. In Sherding RG, editor: *The cat: diseases and clinical management*, ed 2, New York, 1994, Churchill Livingstone, p 1053.

23. Davies C, Forrester SD: Pleural effusion in cats: 82 cases (1987 to 1995), *J Small Anim Pract* 37:217, 1996.

24. Harai BH, Johnson SE, Sherding RG: Endoscopically guided balloon dilatation of benign esophageal strictures in 6 cats and 7 dogs, *J Vet Intern Med* 9:332, 1995.

25. Pidgeon G: Feline pyothorax, *Calif Vet* (March):11, 1978.

26. Wilkinson GT: Exudative pleurisy in the cat, *Vet Rec* 68:456, 1956.

27. Hayward AHS: Thoracic effusions in the cat, *J Small Anim Pract* 9:75, 1968.

28. Foster SF, Martin P, Allan GS, et al: Lower respiratory tract infections in cats: 21 cases (1995-2000), *J Feline Med Surg* 6:167, 2004.

29. Brady CA, Otto CM, Van Winkle TJ, et al: Severe sepsis in cats: 29 cases (1986-1998), *J Am Vet Med Assoc* 217:531, 2000.

30. Purvis D, Kirby R: Systemic inflammatory response syndrome: septic shock, *Vet Clin North Am Small Anim Pract* 24:1225, 1994.

31. Greene CE, Reinero CN: Bacterial respiratory infections. In Greene CE, editor: *Infectious diseases of the dog and cat*, ed 3, Philadelphia, 2006, Saunders Elsevier, p 866.

32. Padrid P: Canine and feline pleural disease, *Vet Clin North Am Small Anim Pract* 30:1295, 2000.

33. Addie DD, Jarrett O: Feline coronavirus infections. In Greene CE, editor: *Infectious diseases of the dog and cat*, ed 3, Philadelphia, 2006, Saunders Elsevier, p 88.

34. Ottenjann M, Weingart C, Arndt G, et al: Characterization of the anemia of inflammatory disease in cats with abscesses, pyothorax, or fat necrosis, *J Vet Intern Med* 20:1143, 2006.

35. Paltrinieri S: The feline acute phase reaction, *Vet J* 177:26, 2008.

36. Barrs VR, Beatty JA: Feline pyothorax—new insights into an old problem: Part 2. Treatment recommendations and prophylaxis, *Vet J* 179:171, 2009.

37. Brodrick TW: Treatment of empyema in a cat, *Vet Rec* 112:135, 1983.

38. Anon (panel report): Management of pyothorax in the cat, *Mod Vet Pract* 55:488, 1974.

39. Bauer T: Pyothorax. In Kirk RW, editor: *Current veterinary therapy IX*, Philadelphia, 1986, WB Saunders, p 292.

40. Johnson MS, Martin MWS: Successful medical treatment for 15 dogs with pyothorax, *J Small Anim Pract* 48:12, 2007.

41. Hawkins EC, Fossum TW: Medical and surgical management of pleural effusion. In Bonagura JD, editor: *Kirk's current veterinary therapy XIII: Small animal practice*, Philadelphia, 2000, WB Saunders, p 819.

42. Anon: Managing empyema in adults, *Drug Ther Bull* 44:17, 2006.

43. Robertson SA: Managing pain in feline patients, *Vet Clin North Am Small Anim Pract* 35:129, 2005.

44. Mathews KA, Dyson DH: Analgesia and chemical restraint for the emergent patient, *Vet Clin North Am Small Anim Pract* 35:481, 2005.

45. Silley P, Stephan B, Greife H, et al: Comparative activity of pradofloxacin against anaerobic bacteria isolated from dogs and cats, *J Antimicrob Chemother* 60:999, 2007.

46. Stein EG, Goldstein EJC: Fluoroquinolones and anaerobes, *Clin Infect Dis* 42:1598, 2006.

47. Rooney MB, Monnet EM: Medical and surgical treatment of pyothorax in dogs: 26 cases (1991-2001), *J Am Vet Med Assoc* 221:86, 2002.

48. Love DN, Jones RF, Bailey M, et al: Isolation and characterisation of bacteria from pyothorax (empyema) in cats, *Vet Microbiol* 7:455, 1982.

49. Boothe DM, Boeckh A, Simpson RB, et al: Comparison of pharmacodynamic and pharmacokinetic indices of efficacy for 5 fluoroquinolones towards pathogens of dogs and cats, *J Vet Intern Med* 20:1297, 2006.

50. Clarke CR: Antimicrobial resistance, *Vet Clin North Am Small Anim Pract* 36:987, 2006.

51. Farca AM, Cavana P, Robino P, et al: In vitro antimicrobial activity of marbofloxacin and enrofloxacin against bacterial strains isolated from companion animals, *Schweiz Arch Tierheilkd* 149:265, 2007.

52. Clark CH: Toxicity of aminoglycoside antibiotics, *Mod Vet Pract* 58:594, 1977.

53. Ford MM, Dubielzig RR, Giuliano EA, et al: Ocular and systemic manifestations after oral administration of a high dose of enrofloxacin in cats, *Am J Vet Res* 68:190, 2007.

54. Goldstein EJ, Citron DM, Richwald GA: Lack of in vitro efficacy of oral forms of certain cephalosporins, erythromycin, and oxacillin against *Pasteurella multocida*, *Antimicrob Agents Chemother (Bethesda)* 32:213, 1988.

55. Stegemann MR, Passmore CA, Sherington J, et al: Antimicrobial activity and spectrum of cefovecin, a new extended-spectrum cephalosporin, against pathogens collected from dogs and cats in Europe and North America, *Antimicrob Agents Chemother (Bethesda)* 50:2286, 2006.

2 Influenza Infections

Katrin Hartmann and Julia Marschall

Influenza virus infections in cats recently have become a matter of discussion. Until 2003, feline influenza infections were not considered to be of clinical relevance: infections with influenza viruses had been described as occurring in cats, but clinical signs had never been observed. This changed, however, when highly pathogenic avian influenza virus H5N1 (HPAIV H5N1) was detected. H5N1 viruses infect not only avian species, they also can infect mammals (besides human beings, mainly felids) and can cause clinical signs in these species. Moreover, large felids and domestic cats not only can be infected by direct or indirect contact with infected birds,[1-3] but the virus additionally can be transmitted horizontally from cat to cat.[4,5] The close relationship between cats and human beings is a cause for concern because of the cat's role in the spread of H5N1, and many questions have been raised recently. Even though most feline cases have occurred in Southeast Asia, infected cats also have been found in Central Europe (Germany and Austria).[3,6]

ETIOLOGY

Influenza viruses are negative-sense, single-stranded, segmented RNA viruses that belong to the family *Orthomyxoviridae*. Influenza viruses types B and C are mainly human pathogens and are seen only rarely in animals (for example, in pigs and seals).[7] Influenza A viruses, however, act as pathogens in many mammalian species (pigs, horses, ferrets, minks, aquatic mammals), including human beings, as well as in birds.[8] Influenza A viruses are classified into distinct subtypes according to different hemagglutinin and neuraminidase glycoprotein molecules expressed on the surface. These viruses can either lead to subclinical infection or can cause serious systemic disease, depending on their pathogenicity. Among the subtypes H5 and H7, highly pathogenic variants may develop by mutation out of low-pathogenic avian influenza viruses.[9]

Older studies have shown that cats are somewhat susceptible to infection by several influenza viruses. Cats could be infected with human (H3N2), avian (H7N3), and seal (H7N7) isolates. After infection, they developed antibodies, sometimes even shed virus, but never became sick.[10] In one kitten living in close contact to a human being who suffered from influenza, virus was isolated from the kitten and antibodies were detected; however, no clinical signs were observed in the kitten.[11] In addition, presence of antibodies against human influenza viruses was demonstrated in field cats in Japan but without correlation to clinical signs.[12]

However, since the recent discovery of highly pathogenic avian influenza virus H5N1 (HPAIV H5N1), it has become obvious that cats infected with this influenza virus also can become sick and die from the infection. Highly pathogenic avian influenza virus (HPAIV) subtype H5N1 was first detected in 1996 in domestic geese in China.[13,14] After several reassortment events, this avian virus not only caused serious disease in poultry but also crossed the species barrier to infect people in Hong Kong in 1997.[14-16] During the subsequent years, different H5N1 genotypes emerged after a series of genetic changes, leading to fatal outbreaks in Asia in poultry in 2003 and 2004.[14,17] Since then, HPAIV H5N1 has spread into many countries worldwide, resulting in high mortality in poultry and fatal infections in mammalian species including human beings. Mammalian species susceptible to HPAIV H5N1 include human beings,[18,19] ferrets,[20,21] dogs,[22,23] mice,[24] stone martens,[25] pigs,[26] cynomolgus monkeys,[27,28] civets,[29] domestic cats,[4,30] tigers, and leopards.[1]

In felids, several outbreaks of infection with HPAIV H5N1 have been reported to date. The first outbreak was seen in 2003, when two tigers and two leopards suffering from high fever and respiratory distress died in a zoo in

Suphanburi, Thailand.[1] Shortly after, a clouded leopard died in a zoo in Chonburi, Thailand, from infection with influenza A H5N1. One month later, a tiger at the same zoo was found to be infected but recovered from the disease.[31] During an outbreak in a tiger zoo in Sriracha, Thailand, a total of 147 tigers died or were euthanized.[5] First evidence that domestic cats are at risk was in 2004, when three domestic cats from a household in Thailand, in which 14 cats had died, were tested positive for influenza A H5N1.[31] The virus also was detected in a domestic cat in Thailand who had died showing high fever, dyspnea, convulsions, and ataxia.[2] Experimental infection using an H5N1 virus (isolated from a fatal human case) confirmed that cats can develop severe clinical signs after intratracheal inoculation or after feeding on infected chicken.[4] The first cases of HPAIV H5N1 infection in domestic cats in Europe were detected during the outbreak of avian influenza on the German Isle of Ruegen in February 2006, during which three free-roaming cats found dead were harboring the virus.[6] At approximately the same time, three cats who did not show clinical signs tested positive by polymerase chain reaction (PCR) for influenza A H5N1 in an animal shelter in Graz, Austria, after an infected swan had been brought to the shelter.[3]

EPIDEMIOLOGY

Incidence of avian influenza in felids is associated with the occurrence of infections in poultry or wild birds in the surrounding area.[1,3,6] Phylogenetic analyses have shown that virus isolates from cats and tigers are highly similar to the virus circulating in poultry at the same time and that the viruses found in felids are of avian origin, indicating that no genetic reassortment with mammalian influenza viruses has occurred. Several point mutations have been identified that are associated with higher virulence in mammals; however, none of them seems to be essential for an infection in felids.[1,32-34]

Within the H5N1 subtype, at least two genetically and antigenically distinct lineages (clades 1 and 2) exist in nonoverlapping geographic distributions in Asia. Clade 1 was isolated mainly in Vietnam and Thailand, whereas clade 2 was found mainly in China and Indonesia. From there, the "Qinghai-like" sublineage spread westwards to the Middle East, Europe, and Africa, and was split up into three different subclusters.[34-36] All Asian cases reported in felids were caused by infections with clade 1 viruses; however, an outbreak in domestic cats in Iraq in February 2006 and the feline cases in Germany were caused by Qinghai-like clade 2 viruses ("EMA" clade 2). Therefore cats seem to be susceptible to different circulating H5N1 virus strains.[34,35]

Prevalence of infection in field cats is more or less unknown. One study in Germany showed that prevalence probably is low among pet cats at least in European countries, as neither virus excretion nor antibodies were detected in 171 cats with outdoor access in areas in which infected birds had been found at the time of investigation.[37] Also, an epidemiological study in Italy testing cats from Milan did not find any evidence of antibodies to influenza A viruses, either to subtype H5N1 or to other subtypes.[38] However, no outbreaks of avian influenza had occurred in this sampling area in Italy and thus likelihood of finding cats with antibodies there was extremely low. In contrast, 7 per cent of field cats (8/111) tested in an unpublished study of the National Institute of Animal Health in Bangkok and 20 per cent of 500 cats tested in Indonesia (unpublished study by Nidom) had antibodies to influenza A H5N1. Because the results of these Asian studies have not been evaluated scientifically and there is no reference to the applied methods, it is possible that the numbers are falsely high. It also is possible that the virus strains circulating in Asia have a higher pathogenicity in cats than the European lineage, and thus more cats were infected. Most likely, however, the difference in prevalence among cats is caused by higher risk of exposure to the virus and higher infection pressure in Asia. In contrast to the situation in Asia, only single wild birds and just a few poultry farms were affected in Europe. Additionally, cats included in the European studies were pet cats, which were fed by their owners and thus did not rely on hunting birds.

PATHOGENESIS

After transmission, the virus spreads directly to the lower respiratory tract, where it can cause severe pneumonia.[1,2,6] Predominant involvement of the lower respiratory tract and inability of the virus to attach to cells of the upper respiratory tract may be a reason why cats excrete virus at relatively low concentrations.[4,39]

Unlike other influenza viruses, which usually are restricted to the respiratory tract in mammals, HPAIV H5N1 not only replicates in respiratory tissue but also can lead to systemic infection causing severe necrosis and inflammation in many organs.[40] Two ways of virus spread to extrarespiratory tissue are discussed. The pattern of virus distribution in the body makes virus entry via viremia very likely. Alternatively, virus may enter from the intestinal lumen via nerve fibers into intestinal tissue; this hypothesis is supported by the finding of ganglioneuritis of the intestinal nervous plexi in cats who had been fed on virus-infected chicken.[40]

TRANSMISSION

Virus transmission occurs mostly through direct contact of felids with infected birds, particularly through eating infected raw poultry.[1,2,4] Both inhalation and ingestion seem to be potential routes of virus entry.[35,40] In addition, indirect virus transmission may occur after contact with contaminated bird feces; this was the suspected mode of transmission in the infected cats in Graz, Austria.[3] After experimental infection, horizontal transmission to other cats through direct contact is possible.[4] Most likely, horizontal transmission also occurred under natural circumstances in the outbreak in the Sriracha tiger zoo.[5]

Infected felids excrete virus via the respiratory, digestive, and urinary tracts, as demonstrated through virus detection in pharyngeal, nasal, and rectal swabs as well as urine and fecal samples.[2,6,35,40] Virus shedding may occur before the onset of clinical signs.[40,41] In an experimental study, virus excretion started at day 3 after infection and lasted until day 7, when the animals were euthanized.[4,40] Subclinically infected cats are assumed to excrete virus less than 2 weeks after infection.[3] So far, no case of virus transmission from cats to other species, including human beings, has been observed. Experimentally infected cats did not transmit to dogs in contact, and experimentally infected dogs did not transmit to cats.[23]

CLINICAL SIGNS

The incubation period appears to vary depending on the route of infection, and is shorter after direct experimental infection through respiratory and oral routes (1 to 2 days) than after cat-to-cat transmission (5 days).[40,41] Clinical presentations observed most commonly are disorders of the respiratory tract and the central nervous system. Clinical signs described in affected felids include fever, lethargy, labored breathing, conjunctivitis, protrusion of the third eyelid, and neurological signs such as convulsions and ataxia.[1,2,4,5] Diarrhea, described in affected poultry and also in human beings infected with HPAIV H5N1[19,42] has not been observed in affected cats. Sudden death may occur in infected cats as soon as 2 days after the onset of clinical signs.[2]

However, infection with HPAIV H5N1 also can result in subclinical infection. In Graz, three cats excreted virus after contact with an infected swan, and two cats developed antibodies to influenza A H5N1 virus, but none of them showed signs of influenza.[3] Anecdotal reports also support the existence of subclinical infections. In an unpublished study carried out by the National Institute of Animal Health in Bangkok, eight of 111 cats (7 per cent) were found to carry antibodies against influenza A H5N1. An unpublished study by Nidom suggested that 20 per cent of 500 cats tested in Indonesia had antibodies to influenza A H5N1.

Laboratory abnormalities described in tigers include severe leukopenia and thrombocytopenia and increased activities of the liver enzymes alanine aminotransferase and aspartate aminotransferase.[5] Markedly increased liver enzyme activities also have been found in diseased domestic cats.[6]

DIFFERENTIAL DIAGNOSIS

Respiratory tract disease or neurological signs are the main clinical features of influenza in cats. Thus influenza is a major differential diagnosis in cats with outdoor access in regions with endemic outbreaks in birds, where the disease presentation is characterized by acute onset and high mortality, as well as by respiratory or neurological signs, especially when combined with high fever.

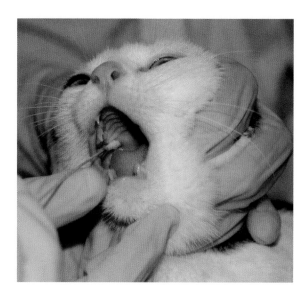

Figure 2-1 Pharyngeal swabbing in a cat suspected to be infected with highly pathogenic avian influenza virus (HPAIV) H5N1.

DIAGNOSIS

Virus detection is possible in pharyngeal, nasal, and rectal swabs, in fecal and urine samples, in organ tissues, and in pleural fluid.[2,35,40] Pharyngeal swabs seem to be most sensitive (Figure 2-1) because H5N1 has only been detected in this location in subclinically infected cats.[3] H5N1 virus RNA can be identified by real-time reverse transcriptase PCR (RRT-PCR) using primers specific for the hemagglutinin and neuraminidase genes.[1,6] Virus also can be isolated by inoculation into embryonated chicken eggs[2] or cell cultures[40] and be identified subsequently by RRT-PCR or hemagglutination and hemagglutination inhibition assays.[2] Immunohistochemistry can be used for detecting H5N1 virus antigen in affected organs.[2,40] In-house diagnostic tests designed to screen cats for infection in practice are not available commercially (e.g., the rapid test kit actim Influenza A&B [Medix Biochemica, Kauniainen, Finland] that was developed originally for the diagnosis of influenza A and B virus infections in human beings). It also is sold to veterinarians for the diagnosis of H5N1 infection in cats. However, a recent study showed that this rapid influenza antigen test is neither applicable for the diagnosis of H5N1 infection in cats, nor can it be used to help the veterinarian decide how to proceed with a suspicious cat.[43]

Antibodies to influenza A H5N1 in serum samples can be detected by a hemagglutination inhibition test.[3,44] The value of antibody detection to diagnose infection, however, is unclear to date.

TREATMENT

Not much is known about the efficacy of antiviral treatment in cats infected with HPAIV H5N1. The neuraminidase inhibitor oseltamivir (Tamiflu, Roche) has shown good antiviral activity against HPAIV H5N1 in vitro[45] as well as in experimentally infected mice and ferrets[46,47] and is recommended for treatment and prophylaxis of HPAIV H5N1 infection in people[48]; however, treatment with oseltamivir was unsuccessful in tigers during the outbreak in Sriracha tiger zoo in 2004. Oseltamivir was administered to the tigers at a dose of 75 mg/60 kg BW q12h (human dosage) for treatment and prophylaxis, but failed in symptomatic as well as asymptomatic animals. The treatment failure may have been the result of improper dosage or timing of drug administration; differences in pharmacokinetics and host metabolisms between human beings and felids, and even between large felids and domestic cats, also are likely.[5,32]

The prognosis in a cat that has been infected in the field is unclear. Subclinical infections are possible, but all domestic cats who have shown clinical signs to date have died or have been euthanized. Therefore the value of symptomatic treatment also remains unknown at this time.

MANAGEMENT

Preventive measures must be taken to minimize the risk of transmission when confronted with a cat suspected of being infected with H5N1. The cat should be isolated, and contact with the cat should be restricted to a minimum. People in contact with the cat must wear protective clothing. Uncooperative cats should be sedated before handling (Table 2-1). Surfaces should be decontaminated with standard medical disinfectant.[30]

CONTROL

Because all infections in cats so far were connected directly to the occurrence of HPAIV H5N1 in birds, contact with birds carrying the virus must be avoided to prevent infections in cats. It is advised therefore to keep cats indoors in areas with occurrence of highly pathogenic avian influenza in birds. Furthermore, cats should not be fed uncooked poultry meat.

Little is known about the actual risk for cats in the field to become infected with the virus and their role in the spread of H5N1. The risk of transmission from potentially infected cats to human beings also is unknown. One study showed, however, that there is no major risk for pet cats in areas with sporadic incidence of avian influenza in birds, because neither virus excretion nor anti-

Table 2-1 Recommendations on the Handling of Cats Suspected to Be Infected with Highly Pathogenic Avian Influenza Virus (HPAIV) H5N1[50]

RECOMMENDATIONS FOR CAT OWNERS

If HPAIV H5N1 occurs in birds, cat owners should receive information about the exact location of the outbreaks through media or internet.

Unrestricted area	Healthy indoor cat	No precautions necessary
	Outdoor cat showing respiratory signs or other clinical signs described above	Veterinarian should be consulted
Restriction zone*	Healthy cat	Cat should be kept indoors
	Cat showing acute respiratory signs or other clinical signs described above	Veterinarian should be consulted immediately and be informed of the cat's outdoor access in a restriction zone
Generally		Feeding of uncooked poultry meat should be avoided

RECOMMENDATIONS FOR VETERINARIANS

If HPAIV H5N1 occurs in birds, small animal practitioners should look for information about the exact location of the outbreaks through media or internet.

Unrestricted area	Healthy indoor cat	No further diagnostic tests
	Outdoor cat showing respiratory signs or other clinical signs described above	HPAIV H5N1 infection should be considered if no other cause for the clinical signs is found, and pharyngeal swab should be taken for viral diagnosis (preferably PCR)
Restriction zone*	Healthy indoor cat	No further diagnostic tests
	Indoor cat showing respiratory signs or other clinical signs described above	HPAIV H5N1 infection should be considered if no other cause for the clinical signs is found, and pharyngeal swab should be taken for viral diagnosis (preferably PCR)
	Healthy outdoor cat/cat with contact to poultry	HPAIV H5N1 infection should be considered, and pharyngeal swab should be taken for viral diagnosis (preferably PCR)
	Outdoor cat showing respiratory signs or other clinical signs described above	HPAIV H5N1 infection should be suspected, preventive measures should be taken when handling the cat (see text), and pharyngeal swab should be taken for viral diagnosis (preferably PCR)

*Restriction zone: area within 10-km radius around location of outbreak of avian influenza in birds for the duration of 30 days after discovery of infected birds.

bodies were detected in 171 cats with outdoor access in areas in which infected birds had been found.[37]

PREVENTION

So far, there is no licensed influenza vaccine for cats on the market. Some companies and researchers are working currently on the development of vaccines for cats, and developing an effective vaccine for cats seems indeed to be possible. After experimental vaccination with fowlpox virus expressing avian influenza virus H5 hemagglutinin gene derived from an H5N8 influenza virus, cats developed high levels of antibodies to the homologous H5N8 antigen. After administration of a second dose, antibodies were shown to cross-react with a recent HPAIV H5N1 isolate.[44] In another study, an anti-H5N1 antibody response was induced by injection of canine adenovirus expressing H5 hemagglutinin gene of a tiger isolate in one cat.[49] Whether these vaccines will appear on the market in the future is unclear. In a recent survey conducted in several European countries, veterinarians were questioned about their feelings concerning the necessity of a vaccine against influenza in cats. Most of them felt that there is neither a major need nor a big market, at least at this time.

PATHOLOGICAL FINDINGS

Respiratory signs are caused by severe pulmonary changes (consolidation, hemorrhage, edema) and pleural effusion, visible at necropsy.[1,2,5] Histological examination shows extensive inflammation and necrosis in lung tissue leading to interstitial pneumonia and diffuse alveolar damage.[2,40] Neurological signs result from cerebral and cerebellar congestion and nonsuppurative meningoencephalitis accompanied by vasculitis.[2,5] Histopathological examination of the liver shows multifocal necrotizing hepatitis, explaining the increase in liver enzyme activities and the generalized icterus that also can be seen at necropsy.[5,6,40] Multifocal hemorrhages are seen in numerous organs, including the lungs, heart, thymus, stomach, intestine, liver, tonsils, lymph nodes, kidneys, and diaphragm, as well as pancreas.[1,6,35,40]

REFERENCES

1. Keawcharoen J, Oraveerakul K, Kuiken T, et al: Avian influenza H5N1 in tigers and leopards, *Emerg Infect Dis* 10:2189, 2004.
2. Songserm T, Amonsin A, Jam-on R, et al: Avian influenza H5N1 in naturally infected domestic cat, *Emerg Infect Dis* 12:681, 2006.
3. Leschnik M, Weikel J, Möstl K, et al: Subclinical infection with avian influenza A (H5N1) virus in cats, *Emerg Infect Dis* 13:243, 2007.
4. Kuiken T, Rimmelzwaan GF, van Riel D, et al: Avian H5N1 influenza in cats, *Science* 306:241, 2004.
5. Thanawongnuwech R, Amonsin A, Tantilertcharoen R, et al: Probable tiger-to-tiger transmission of avian influenza H5N1, *Emerg Infect Dis* 11:699, 2005.
6. Klopfleisch R, Wolf PU, Uhl W, et al: Distribution of lesions and antigen of highly pathogenic avian influenza virus A/Swan/Germany/R65/06 (H5N1) in domestic cats after presumptive infection by wild birds, *Vet Pathol* 44:261, 2007.
7. Osterhaus AD, Rimmelzwaan GF, Martina BE, et al: Influenza B virus in seals, *Science* 288:1051, 2000.
8. Vahlenkamp TW, Harder TC: Influenza virus infections in mammals, *Berl Munch Tierarztl Wochenschr* 119:123, 2006.
9. Alexander DJ: A review of avian influenza in different bird species, *Vet Microbiol* 74:3, 2000.
10. Hinshaw VS, Webster RG, Easterday BC, et al: Replication of avian influenza A viruses in mammals, *Infect Immun* 34:354, 1981.
11. Paniker CK, Nair CM: Infection with A2 Hong Kong influenza virus in domestic cats, *Bull World Health Organ* 43:859, 1970.
12. Onta T, Kida H, Kawano J, et al: Distribution of antibodies against various influenza A viruses in animals, *Nippon Juigaku Zasshi* 40:451, 1978.
13. Xu X, Subbarao K, Cox, NJ, et al: Genetic characterization of the pathogenic influenza A/Goose/Guangdong/1/96 (H5N1) virus: similarity of its hemagglutinin gene to those of H5N1 viruses from the 1997 outbreaks in Hong Kong, *Virology* 261:15, 1999.
14. Li KS, Guan Y, Wang J, et al: Genesis of a highly pathogenic and potentially pandemic H5N1 influenza virus in eastern Asia, *Nature* 430:209, 2004.
15. Subbarao K, Klimov A, Katz J, et al: Characterization of an avian influenza A (H5N1) virus isolated from a child with a fatal respiratory illness, *Science* 279:393, 1998.
16. Webster RG, Guan Y, Peiris M, et al: Characterization of H5N1 influenza viruses that continue to circulate in geese in southeastern China, *J Virol* 76:118, 2002.
17. Chen H, Smith GJ, Li KS, et al: Establishment of multiple sublineages of H5N1 influenza virus in Asia: implications for pandemic control, *Proc Natl Acad Sci USA* 103:2845, 2006.
18. Claas EC, Osterhaus AD, van Beek R, et al: Human influenza A H5N1 virus related to a highly pathogenic avian influenza virus, *Lancet* 351:472, 1998.
19. Tran TH, Nguyen TL, Nguyen TD, et al: Avian influenza A (H5N1) in 10 patients in Vietnam, *N Engl J Med* 350:1179, 2004.
20. Zitzow LA, Rowe T, Morken T, et al: Pathogenesis of avian influenza A (H5N1) viruses in ferrets, *J Virol* 76:4420, 2002.
21. Govorkova EA, Rehg JE, Krauss S, et al: Lethality to ferrets of H5N1 influenza viruses isolated from humans and poultry in 2004, *J Virol* 79:2191, 2005.
22. Songserm T, Amonsin A, Jam-on R, et al: Fatal avian influenza A H5N1 in a dog, *Emerg Infect Dis* 12:1744, 2006.
23. Giese M, Harder TC, Teifke JP, et al: Experimental infection and natural contact exposure of dogs with avian influenza virus (H5N1), *Emerg Infect Dis* 14:308, 2008.
24. Gao P, Watanabe S, Ito T, et al: Biological heterogeneity, including systemic replication in mice, of H5N1 influenza A virus isolates from humans in Hong Kong, *J Virol* 73:3184, 1999.
25. Klopfleisch R, Wolf PU, Wolf C, et al: Encephalitis in a stone marten (Martes foina) after natural infection with highly pathogenic avian influenza virus subtype H5N1, *J Comp Pathol* 137:155, 2007.
26. Choi YK, Nguyen TD, Ozaki H, et al: Studies of H5N1 influenza virus infection of pigs by using viruses isolated in Vietnam and Thailand in 2004, *J Virol* 79:10821, 2005.
27. Rimmelzwaan GF, Kuiken T, Van Amerongen G, et al: Pathogenesis of influenza A (H5N1) virus infection in a primate model, *J Virol* 75:6687, 2001.
28. Kuiken T, Rimmelzwaan GF, Van Amerongen G, et al: Pathology of human influenza A (H5N1) virus infection in cyno-

molgus macaques *(Macaca fascicularis), Vet Pathol* 40:304, 2003.

29. Roberton SI, Bell DJ, Smith GJ, et al: Avian influenza H5N1 in viverrids: implications for wildlife health and conservation, *Proc Biol Sci* 273:1729, 2006.

30. Thiry E, Zicola A, Addie D, et al: Highly pathogenic avian influenza H5N1 virus in cats and other carnivores, *Vet Microbiol* 122:25, 2007.

31. Enserink M, Kaiser J: Virology. Avian flu finds new mammal hosts, *Science* 305:1385, 2004.

32. Amonsin A, Payungporn S, Theamboonlers A, et al: Genetic characterization of H5N1 influenza A viruses isolated from zoo tigers in Thailand, *Virology* 344:480, 2006.

33. Amonsin A, Songserm T, Chutinimitkul S, et al: Genetic analysis of influenza A virus (H5N1) derived from domestic cat and dog in Thailand, *Arch Virol* 152:1925, 2007.

34. Weber S, Harder T, Starick E, et al: Molecular analysis of highly pathogenic avian influenza virus of subtype H5N1 isolated from wild birds and mammals in northern Germany, *J Gen Virol* 88:554, 2007.

35. Yingst SL, Saad MD, Felt SA: Qinghai-like H5N1 from domestic cats, northern Iraq, *Emerg Infect Dis* 12:1295, 2006.

36. Salzberg SL, Kingsford C, Cattoli G, et al: Genome analysis linking recent European and African influenza (H5N1) viruses, *Emerg Infect Dis* 13:713, 2007.

37. Marschall J, Schulz B, Harder TC, et al: Prevalence of influenza A H5N1 virus in cats from areas with occurrence of highly pathogenic avian influenza in birds, *J Feline Med Surg* 10:355, 2008.

38. Paltrinieri S, Spagnolo V, Giordano A, et al: Influenza virus type A serosurvey in cats, *Emerg Infect Dis* 13:662, 2007.

39. van Riel D, Munster VJ, De Wit E, et al: H5N1 virus attachment to lower respiratory tract, *Science* 312:399, 2006.

40. Rimmelzwaan GF, Van Riel D, Baars M, et al: Influenza A virus (H5N1) infection in cats causes systemic disease with potential novel routes of virus spread within and between hosts, *Am J Pathol* 168:176, 2006.

41. Kuiken T, Fouchier RA, Rimmelzwaan GF, et al: Feline friend or potential foe? *Nature* 440:741, 2006.

42. Apisarnthanarak A, Kitphati R, Thongphubeth K, et al: Atypical avian influenza (H5N1), *Emerg Infect Dis* 10:1321, 2004.

43. Marschall J, Schulz B, Hartmann K: Evaluation of a point-of-care influenza antigen test for the detection of highly pathogenic avian influenza H5N1 virus in cats, *Transbound Emerg Dis* 55:315, 2008.

44. Karaca K, Swayne DE, Grosenbaugh D, et al: Immunogenicity of fowlpox virus expressing the avian influenza virus H5 gene (TROVAC AIV-H5) in cats, *Clin Diagn Lab Immunol* 12:1340, 2005.

45. Hurt AC, Selleck P, Komadina N, et al: Susceptibility of highly pathogenic A (H5N1) avian influenza viruses to the neuraminidase inhibitors and adamantanes, *Antiviral Res* 73:228, 2007.

46. Leneva IA, Roberts N, Govorkova EA, et al: The neuraminidase inhibitor GS4104 (oseltamivir phosphate) is efficacious against A/Hong Kong/156/97 (H5N1) and A/Hong Kong/1074/99 (H9N2) influenza viruses, *Antiviral Res* 48:101, 2000.

47. Govorkova EA, Ilyushina NA, Boltz DA, et al: Efficacy of oseltamivir therapy in ferrets inoculated with different clades of H5N1 influenza virus, *Antimicrob Agents Chemother* 51:1414, 2007.

48. Schunemann HJ, Hill SR, Kakad M, et al: WHO Rapid Advice Guidelines for pharmacological management of sporadic human infection with avian influenza A (H5N1) virus, *Lancet Infect Dis* 7:21, 2007.

49. Gao YW, Xia XZ, Wang LG, et al: Construction and experimental immunity of recombinant replication-competent canine adenovirus type 2 expressing hemagglutinin gene of H5N1 subtype tiger influenza virus, *Wei Sheng Wu Xue Bao* 46:297, 2006.

50. Marschall J, Hartmann K: Avian influenza A H5N1 infections in cats, *J Feline Med Surg* 10:359, 2008.

3   The Role of Wolbachia in Heartworm Infection

Laura Helen Kramer

Cats are considered receptive hosts for the filarial nematode *Dirofilaria immitis,* but they also seem to be more resistant to infection than dogs. Although risk of exposure to the parasite may be high in areas that are endemic for canine heartworm disease, the prevalence of patent infection in cats is low, suggesting that they are able to eliminate the parasite before it achieves maturity. There is, however, increasing evidence that even premature worms can cause respiratory problems in cats. Indeed, the cat's strong inflammatory response to the worm when it enters the pulmonary vasculature can cause significant clinical disease.

Wolbachia are gram-negative bacteria that reside within the body of many filarial nematodes, including *D. immitis.* From the moment Sironi et al[1] discovered that *D. immitis* harbors *Wolbachia,* the scientific community realized that a major discovery had been made, one that would likely change the way they looked at filarial disease. Indeed, as gram-negative bacteria, *Wolbachia* have the potential to play an important role in the pathogenesis and immune response to filarial infection. The immunopathology of filarial disease is extremely complex, and the clinical manifestations of infection are strongly dependent on the type of immune response elicited by the parasite. These bacteria are known to play a fundamental role in worm biology, reproduction, and long-term survival. Less is known about what role they may play in the pathogenesis of heartworm infection. It is likely that the proinflammatory reaction to these bacteria may exacerbate the clinical picture observed in heartworm-infected animals, including cats.

ETIOLOGY

Feline heartworm disease (FHWD) is caused by the filarial nematode *D. immitis,* which resides in the pulmonary arteries of infected cats (Figure 3-1). Female worms are approximately 15 inches in length, whereas males are shorter. They are less than 5 mm wide. Contrary to what is seen in dogs, naturally infected cats usually harbor less than six adult worms. Female worms release first-stage larvae (microfilariae) into the bloodstream and these are taken up by competent mosquito vectors. After approximately 15 days, these larvae develop into the infective third-stage larvae (L_3) and can be inoculated into a new host. Immature worms migrate first through connective tissue and then into the venous circulation, where they are carried to the pulmonary arteries. Worms are fully mature approximately 8 months after cats become infected. There is evidence that only a small portion of infective larvae reach full maturity in infected cats, likely due to a strong immune response against the immature worms. Cats also can eliminate circulating microfilariae and reduce the reproductive capacity of adult female worms.[2]

Wolbachia has been identified as an endosymbiont of many arthropods and filarial nematodes. *Wolbachia pipientis,* the only species thus far identified in the genus, are gram-negative bacteria belonging to the order Rickettsiales. They are closely related to other bacteria belonging to the same group, such as *Ehrlichia* spp. and *Anaplasma* spp., as shown in Figure 3-2.[3] Electron microscopy, histological examination, and immunohistochemistry have offered a clear description of the distribution of *Wolbachia* in *D. immitis*.[4] They are found throughout all the stages of the life cycle of the nematode, although they occur in varying proportions between individual worms and different developmental stages. In adult *D. immitis*, *Wolbachia* is found predominantly throughout the hypodermal cells of the lateral cords (Figure 3-3). In female worms, *Wolbachia* also is present in the ovaries, oocytes, and developing embryonic stages within the uteri (Figure 3-4). They have not been demonstrated in the male reproductive system, suggesting that the bacterium is maternally transmitted through the cytoplasm of the egg and not through the sperm. There are several features of the relationship between *Wolbachia* and filarial worms (including *D. immitis*) that suggest its symbiotic nature: (1) in those species of filarial worms that have been identified as harboring *Wolbachia*, all of the individuals are infected (i.e., 100 per cent prevalence); (2) the evolution of the bacteria match that of the filarial worms, as shown by phylogenic studies; (3) the bacteria are transmitted from female to offspring (thus the symbiont guarantees its own future by increasing the fitness of the host that is involved in its transmission); and (4) removal of *Wolbachia* (antibiotics/radiation) leads to sterility of female worms and eventual death of adult worms.

EPIDEMIOLOGY

Numerous studies have been carried out to determine the prevalence of exposure to *D. immitis* infection in cats from different parts of the world. Reliable results are hindered, however, by the difficulty in diagnosing patent infection in cats (see section Diagnosis). Most studies distinguish rates of mature infection (presence of at least

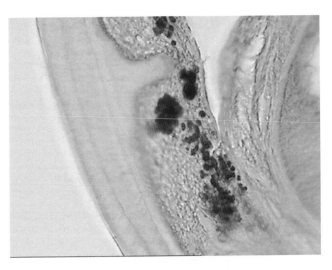

Figure 3-3 Anti–*Wolbachia* Surface Protein (WSP) immunohistochemistry. *D. immitis* female with positive staining within the lateral hypoderma chord. (ABC-HRP, 100× magnification.)

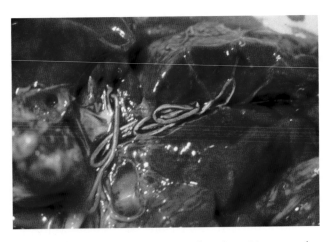

Figure 3-1 Necropsy of a heartworm-infected cat. Note several adult worms within the pulmonary arteries. (Photo courtesy Dr. Luigi Venco.)

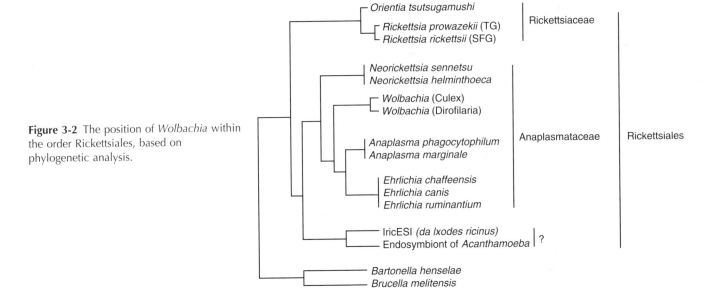

Figure 3-2 The position of *Wolbachia* within the order Rickettsiales, based on phylogenetic analysis.

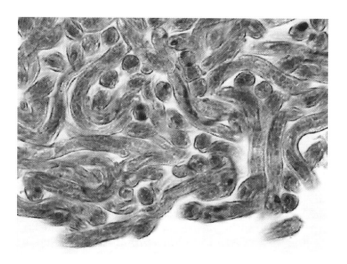

Figure 3-4 Anti-WSP immunohistochemistry. *D. immitis* female with positive staining microfilariae within the uterus. (ABC-HRP, 100× magnification.)

one adult worm in the pulmonary artery, usually at necropsy) from immature or transient infection (presence of circulating antibodies against worm antigens by serology). A large-scale study carried out on more than 2000 cats in the United States[5] reported an average rate of heartworm antibodies of 12 per cent, with peaks of more than 30 per cent in certain states like California and Florida. In a more recent study in Florida,[6] heartworms were identified at necropsy in 4.9 per cent of 640 cats in a shelter, and serological evidence of heartworm infection was present in 17 per cent. Studies from endemic areas in Europe have reported similar findings. We carried out a large study in an endemic region of Italy[7] and tested more than 1000 cats for circulating microfilariae, antigen, and antibodies against *D. immitis*. Results showed that 16 per cent of all tested cats were positive for anti–*D. immitis* antibodies, with values ranging from 9 to 27 per cent, depending on location. Of these, 3 per cent were positive on antigen testing and 4 per cent were microfilaremic (see section Diagnosis). It is generally accepted that the prevalence of heartworm infection in cats is approximately 5 to 10 per cent of the prevalence in dogs in the same geographical area.

Heartworm-infected cats show evidence of exposure to *Wolbachia*. Indeed, a varying percentage of both experimentally and naturally infected cats[8,9] present circulating antibodies against a major surface protein of *Wolbachia* (*Wolbachia* surface protein [WSP]). It is not clear at what point(s) during the infection the bacteria can leave the body of the worm and be released into the blood/tissue of the host. Because all heartworms harbor the bacteria, and because the bacteria are present in all life stages of the worm, *Wolbachia* could be released by worms during the molting process, when they shed their old cuticle to form a new one, during reproductive activity, when mature female worms release microfilariae into the bloodstream along with debris from the uterus, or following death of the worms (e.g., microfilarial turnover, spontaneous death of adults). As mentioned above, most infective larvae die before they mature to adulthood in cats.

Interestingly, it would appear that the death of infective larvae also could cause exposure to *Wolbachia* in cats. It has been shown that in experimentally infected cats, there are very high levels of anti-WSP antibodies starting at about 2 months postinfection. At this time, many L_3 and young L_4 larvae will have been eliminated by the host's immune system, and death of these larvae likely will have allowed the release of the bacteria into the surrounding tissue. These results were confirmed when another group of cats were treated with ivermectin at 2 months postinfection to induce the death of all larvae; antibody titers against *Wolbachia* were high and persistent.[9] Levy et al,[10] however, recently carried out a large-scale serological study in cats and did not report a significant correlation between infection status of cats, as determined by serology/necropsy, and the presence of anti-WSP antibodies. Clearly, there is still work to be done in determining how often cats exposed to heartworm infection also are exposed to *Wolbachia*.

PATHOGENESIS

Although live adult worms in the pulmonary arteries cause a local arteritis, some cats never manifest clinical signs. When signs are evident, they usually develop during two stages of the disease: (1) arrival of heartworms in the pulmonary vasculature and (2) death of adult heartworms. The first stage coincides with the arrival of immature adult worms in the pulmonary arteries and arterioles: approximately 3 to 4 months postinfection. These early signs are due to an acute vascular and parenchymal inflammatory response to the newly arriving worms and the subsequent death of most of these same worms. This initial phase is often misdiagnosed as asthma or allergic bronchitis, but in actuality is part of a syndrome now known as heartworm-associated respiratory disease (HARD).[11] Clinical signs associated with this acute phase subside as the worms mature, but demonstrable histopathological lesions are evident even in those cats who clear the infection. Browne et al[12] recently reported that cats with serological evidence of exposure to heartworms, including those without adult heartworms in the lungs and heart, have a greater prevalence of pulmonary arterial lesions than heartworm-negative cats without serological evidence of exposure.

The cat's response to the parasite is intense and the role of inflammation is very important, both when immature worms arrive in the lung and following the death of adult worms. The cause of the acute and often fatal crisis in the cat is lung injury resulting in respiratory distress. Frequently, this event is associated with the death of as little as one adult heartworm. The lung can become acutely edematous and cats can die from respiratory failure.

The nature of the worm antigens that cause the intense inflammatory reaction seen in cats is still not known. Immature and adult worms likely possess myriad candidate antigens and *Wolbachia* most certainly is among them. There is no evidence to date that *Wolbachia* is able to infect mammalian cells. However, in filarial infected hosts, including cats infected by *D. immitis*, the release of bacteria following worm death has been shown to be associated with the upregulation of proinflammatory cytokines, neutrophil recruitment, and an increase in specific immunoglobulins.[13] Therefore the role of *Wolbachia* in the host response to filarial infection includes interaction between bacterial molecules and the innate and adaptive immune system.

The innate immune system represents a defense mechanism against molecular structures that are conserved among a wide range of organisms. It consists of the recognition of specific "markers" (pathogen-associated molecular patterns [PAMPs]) that signal the presence of "generic" pathogens. The consequent recognition of these PAMPs by toll-like receptors (TLR) on the surface of antigen-presenting cells leads to the production of reactive oxygen species, proinflammatory cytokines, and to the upregulation of costimulatory molecules that assist in development of an adaptive immune response (Figure 3-5).

Reports of a possible role for *Wolbachia* in the immunopathogenesis of filarial infection have come from both studies in-vitro and in-vivo. Studies on the human filarial nematodes *Onchocerca volvulus* and *Brugia malayi/Wuchereria bancrofti* have demonstrated that (1) adverse reactions to filaricidal therapy (ivermectin, diethylcarbamazine) are associated with the presence of *Wolbachia* and/or its DNA in the bloodstream and peak levels of *Wolbachia* correlate with levels of proinflammatory cytokines like tumor necrosis factor alpha (TNFα)[14]; (2) *O. volvulus*–induced skin nodules feature neutrophil infiltration around adult worms and microfilariae; this inflammation subsides subsequently following antibiotic-mediated removal of *Wolbachia*[15]; interestingly, a major surface protein of *Wolbachia* from *D. immitis* has been shown to provoke chemokinesis and IL-8 production in canine neutrophils in vitro[16]; (3) filarial worm extracts stimulate cells in vitro to produce proinflammatory cytokines and this effect is abolished with antibiotic-mediated removal of *Wolbachia*[17]; and (4) chronic pathology in lymphatic filariasis (elephantiasis, hydrocele) is correlated with a strong specific humoral response to the WSP.[18]

We recently tested the hypothesis that *D. immitis*–infected dogs also come into contact with *Wolbachia* either through microfilarial turnover or natural death of adult worms.[19] In our study, intense staining for the *Wolbachia* Surface Protein was observed in various tissues from dogs who had died from natural heartworm disease. Staining for the bacterial protein was seen in lung macrophages (Figure 3-6), and in organs where microfilariae usually circulate; for example, the kidney (Figure 3-7).

There are much fewer data on the presence of *Wolbachia* or on the proinflammatory reaction to the worm in cats. In the same large-scale study mentioned above,[10] lungs and worms from infected cats were examined for the presence of the *Wolbachia* Surface Protein. All examined worms showed *Wolbachia* within the lateral chords (Figure 3-8); however, not all of the examined lungs were

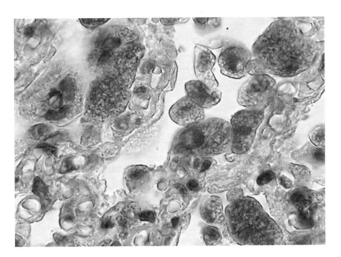

Figure 3-6 Localization of *Wolbachia* Surface Protein in lung tissue of dogs with natural *D. immitis* infection: positive staining of pulmonary macrophages. (100× magnification.)

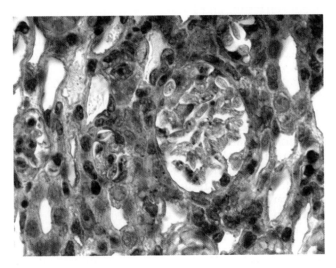

Figure 3-7 Anti-WSP immunohistochemistry. Kidney from a dog with heartworm infection. Note positive staining for the *Wolbachia* Surface Protein within microfilariae. (ABC-HRP, 60× magnification.)

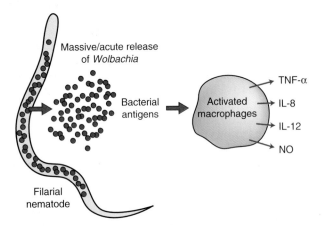

Figure 3-5 Diagram of the possible effects of *Wolbachia*-associated antigens on macrophages following the release of bacteria from a filarial worm. *IL,* Interleukin; *NO,* nitric oxide; *TNFα,* tumor necrosis factor alpha.

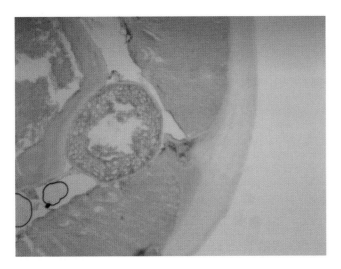

Figure 3-8 Anti-WSP immunohistochemistry. *D. immitis* female from a heartworm-infected cat. (100× magnification.)

positive for the bacterial protein, even when obvious arterial disease was present. This may be due to several reasons: the cats were all naturally infected and it was impossible to know when infection occurred. Therefore, if the main source of *Wolbachia* in heartworm-infected cats is immature larvae arriving into the pulmonary vasculature, this has already occurred in many necropsy-positive cats, provoking arterial damage. An important source of *Wolbachia* exposure in infected dogs is represented by circulating microfilariae. As mentioned previously, these are very rare in infected cats. Finally, the observed alterations in these cat lungs could have been due to other causes. The fact that many experimentally and naturally infected cats do show a specific antibody response to the bacteria, however, is highly suggestive of bacterial release from the parasite and consequent antigen recognition.

Interestingly, a recent study described the acute systemic anaphylaxis in cats who had been sensitized to *D. immitis*.[20] The study examined the reaction to repeated sensitization with worm somatic antigen (i.e., 0.5 g of a homogenate of whole male and female worms, including *Wolbachia*) followed by an intravenous challenge. In cats, the lung is the major shock organ and anaphylaxis was characterized by acute severe dyspnea. It is likely that this experiment mimics what occurs in cats following the spontaneous death of adult *D. immitis* within the pulmonary artery and may explain the acute sudden death syndrome in FHWD[21] (see section Clinical Signs).

TRANSMISSION

How at risk are our cats for heartworm infection and for all the consequences it may have? As mentioned above, the parasite can infect cats, but does so at a much lower rate than in dogs. As stated in the section Etiology, heartworms are transmitted through the bite of a mosquito that, following a blood meal on an infected host with circulating microfilariae, allows the development of the

infective L_3 larvae of *D. immitis,* which it then transmits to a new host. Therefore transmission of *D. immitis* to cats requires a mosquito species that feeds on both dogs (principal reservoir for circulating microfilariae) and cats. Several species have been identified in Europe,[22] including *Aedes caspius* and *Culex pipiens,* both of which show high dog and cat host-seeking behavior. In South America, most *Culex* and *Aedes* species also feed on cats.[23]

Cats, however, appear to be much less "attractive" for mosquitoes than dogs, possibly because of their smaller body mass. Despite earlier studies, it is now accepted that indoor and outdoor cats are equally at risk for infection, and there is no difference in prevalence between male and female cats.[21]

Population dynamics of *Wolbachia* and quantification of bacterial numbers in different developmental stages of filarial nematodes like *Brugia malayi* [24,25] have shown that the numbers of bacteria remain static in microfilariae and the mosquito-borne larval stages (L_2 and L_3). However, within the first week of infection of the mammalian host, bacterial numbers increase dramatically and the bacteria/worm ratio is the highest of all life-cycle stages. The rapid multiplication continues throughout L_4 development, so that the major period of bacterial population growth occurs within the first month of infection of the definitive host. Infection levels are then maintained in adult male worms, while in female worms, bacterial numbers increase further as the worms mature and as the ovary and embryonic larval stages become infected. The changes in the dynamics of *Wolbachia* populations throughout the life cycle therefore may illustrate the points at which the symbiotic relationship is critical and at which the feline host can come into contact with the bacteria.

CLINICAL SIGNS

The clinical picture seen in HW-infected cats ranges from no clinical signs to sudden death. Some studies have correlated certain clinical signs to seropositivity for antibodies against *D. immitis,* including respiratory and gastrointestinal disorders.[20,21] If indeed an allergic reaction is part of the pathological mechanism in cats, as has been suggested, the clinical presentation may vary and also may be very unpredictable. An initial host response of pulmonary inflammation has been reported at approximately 4 to 7 months after infection and usually is followed by a subclinical stage. As mentioned previously, however, the subsequent death of as little as one adult worm can cause acute collapse and death.

Whether any of the clinical signs of FHWD are reproducible through the sole exposure to *Wolbachia* is not known. *Wolbachia* is an abundant antigen within *D. immitis* (Figure 3-9), and its proinflammatory effects are well noted; however, the bacterium does not colonize or reproduce within the mammalian host, so we can not speak of "infection" or of a clinical picture attributable to *Wolbachia* alone. On the other hand, we can speak of a highly proinflammatory antigen, and future in-vitro and/or in-vivo studies on the effects of massive exposure to bacteria may help shed light on the role of *Wolbachia* in the clinical presentation of FHWD.

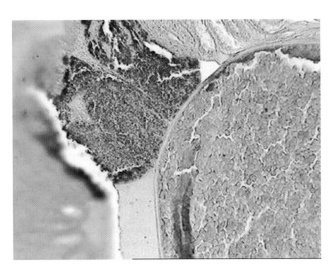

Figure 3-9 Anti-WSP immunohistochemistry. *D. immitis* female with positive staining within the lateral hypodermal chord: note the massive presence of bacteria. (100× magnification.)

DIAGNOSIS

As reported by several authors, low worm burdens and low levels of circulating antigens make diagnosis of *D. immitis* infection in cats a challenge.[21] When an antigen test is positive, or when the worm is visualized by cardiac ultrasound, active infection can be confirmed. A positive antibody test, on the other hand, is only indicative of current or previous infection and may represent either a prepatent, aborted, or past infection. Ideally, a combination of antigen and antibody testing, together with imaging, should be used when considering heartworm disease in cats.

As stated previously, infected cats can produce antibodies against the major surface protein of *Wolbachia* WSP. This has made it an interesting candidate for the serological diagnosis of heartworm infection in cats. However, preliminary results[10] would suggest that positivity for anti-WSP antibodies is neither sensitive nor specific for infection as determined by necropsy. It is necessary therefore to identify other bacterial antigens from *Wolbachia* that may perform better in order to aid diagnosis of feline infection.

TREATMENT

Currently, there is no drug available that is authorized for adulticide therapy in cats. Indeed, the drug-induced death of adult heartworms frequently leads to fatal thromboembolism in cats. Furthermore, it has been reported that the infection is self-limiting and natural attrition of adult worms usually occurs after about 2.5 years. Supportive therapy usually is recommended (see section below).

Even as the role of *Wolbachia* in the pathogenesis of feline heartworm infection remains under study, there is another promising area of research that may benefit infected cats. *Wolbachia* can be eliminated from filarial worms through antibiotic therapy of the infected host. Numerous studies have shown that various treatment protocols/dosages (tetracycline and synthetic derivatives appear to be the most effective) are able to drastically reduce if not completely remove the endosymbiont from the worm host. Such depletion of *Wolbachia* is then followed by clear antifilarial effects, including:

1. Inhibition of larval development and female worm sterility: It has been shown that antibiotic treatment of filarial-infected hosts can inhibit molting, an essential process in the maturation of worms from larvae to adults. Antibiotic treatment leads first to a reduction and then to the complete and sustained absence of microfilariae.

The detrimental effects on embryogenesis are accompanied by morphological changes within the filarial ovaries and uterus that are often empty or contain degenerating embryos. *D. immitis* adults taken from naturally infected dogs who had been treated with 20 mg/kg/day of doxycycline PO for 30 days showed morphological alterations of uterine content with a dramatic decrease in the number of microfilariae, indicating that bacteriostatic antibiotic treatment was able to block embryogenesis. Initial trials using a 6-week course of doxycycline treatment against *O. volvulus* were effective at depleting the bacteria and also resulted in a block of embryogenesis, which persisted for up to 2 years after the start of treatment. The apparent permanent block in embryogenesis was reflected in sustained reductions in skin microfilariae, the cause of onchocercal disease.[26] Depletion of *Wolbachia* by doxycycline also has been demonstrated in human lymphatic filariasis: in patients infected with *W. bancrofti*, doxycycline administered for 6 weeks at 200 mg/day resulted in a reduction of more than 95 per cent of *Wolbachia* levels compared to pretreatment levels. This treatment led to a chronic decline in microfilarial loads, followed by amicrofilaremia, which was highly significant at 12 months.[27]

These findings suggest that the mode of action of doxycycline is equivalent to that observed in animal models and human onchocerciasis—namely, a block in embryogenesis in the adult female worms when *Wolbachia* are absent or at least below a certain threshold. The implications for breaking the life cycle of these parasites are obvious.

2. Adulticide effects: This is a particularly intriguing aspect of antibiotic treatment of the filarial worm–infected host and one that merits strict attention. Langworthy et al[28] (2000) first reported potential macrofilaricide effects of doxycycline in cattle infected with *Onchocerca ochengi*. The authors showed that intermittent therapy with oxytetracycline for a 6-month period caused the death of adult worms by 9 months posttreatment. More recently, clinical trials in human filariasis have reported extremely promising results: a recent placebo-controlled trial in human beings infected with *W. bancrofti* has demonstrated a clear macrofilaricidal effect of doxycycline.[29] When administered for 8 weeks at 200 mg/day, the treatment resulted in a complete amicrofilaremia in 28 of 32 patients assessed, and an absence of scrotal worm nests (where adult worms reside) at 14 months posttreatment, as determined by ultrasonography in 21 of 27 patients. In the other patients, the number of worm nests declined.

More recent work on *D. immitis* in dogs showed nearly 80 per cent efficacy against adult worms when a combination of doxycycline and ivermectin was administered to experimentally infected animals.[30] Indeed, this treatment protocol has significant adulticide effects and is able to reduce *Wolbachia* loads more efficiently when compared to doxycycline alone. Trials are now underway in our laboratory in naturally infected dogs using 10 mg/kg of doxycycline PO daily for 30 days and bi-monthly ivermectin at prophylactic doses.

Furthermore, if we consider *Wolbachia* as a potential cause of inflammation in the course of filarial disease, depletion of the bacteria may be beneficial, independent of its effect on the worm. If indeed antibiotic treatment is able to decrease the number of bacteria within the worm, eventual proinflammatory effects following worm death may be reduced. We have reported[31] recently that when infected dogs were treated with melarsomine alone, there was an intense inflammatory reaction in the lungs and the presence of positive staining for a major surface protein of *Wolbachia*. These changes were virtually absent when adulticidal therapy was associated with the combination of doxycycline and ivermectin. These results would suggest that reducing adult worm mass and *Wolbachia* populations in *D. immitis* before adulticidal therapy could greatly improve health status of dogs treated for heartworm disease. The implications for feline infection also are potentially important. This therapeutic approach in cats with active infection may reduce the risk of sudden death syndrome associated with heartworm and merits future attention and study.

SUPPORTIVE THERAPY

Given the intense inflammatory reaction that characterizes FHWD, supportive therapy usually includes administration of corticosteroids. As noted previously, the addition of doxycycline at 10 mg/kg/day PO for 1 month could be beneficial; however, at the present time, there are no studies confirming this recommendation.

CONTROL AND PREVENTION

The American Heartworm Society has developed specific guidelines for the prevention of FHWD.[11] Numerous drugs are available for monthly preventive treatment, aimed at eliminating all immature larvae that mosquitoes have inoculated in the preceding 30 days. Therefore administration of preventives must begin at approximately 1 month after the beginning of the transmission season and end at approximately 1 month after the end of transmission. Obviously, in those areas where transmission is possible all year, preventives must be continued monthly year-round. There is no current evidence that antibiotic treatment aimed at *Wolbachia* has any prophylactic effect.

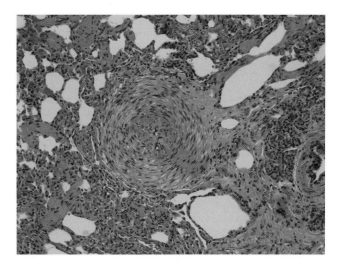

Figure 3-10 Pulmonary artery occlusive hypertrophy in a cat with heartworm disease. (Hematoxylin-eosin, 100× magnification.) (Photo courtesy Patty Dingman.)

PATHOLOGICAL FINDINGS

Browne et al[12] have observed that when cats test positive for both anti–*D. immitis* antibodies and for the presence of adult worms in the lungs, lesions include many of those observed in dogs, including proliferation of arterial endothelium, endarteritis, and fibrosis of the intima. These changes were somewhat less common in those cats with only positive antibody responses, suggesting that they are worsened in active infection with adult nematodes.

Those cats who were positive on antibody testing alone (exposed to the parasite, but no worms in the lungs) showed a degree of occlusive hypertrophy of the small pulmonary arteries that was greater than that observed in antibody-negative cats (Figure 3-10). These results would suggest that heartworm-associated respiratory disease (HARD) may develop even when adults do not reach maturity (i.e., most of the time), reiterating the need for preventive therapy to avoid even the arrival of immature worms within the pulmonary vasculature.[32]

REFERENCES

1. Sironi M, Bandi C, Sacchi L, et al: Molecular evidence for a close relative of the arthropod endosymbiont *Wolbachia* in a filarial worm, *Mol Biochem Parasitol* 74:223, 1995.
2. McCall JW, Dzimianski MT, McTier TL, et al: Biology of experimental heartworm infection in cats, Proceedings of the American Heartworm Symposium: 127, 1992.
3. Bandi C, Trees AJ, Brattig NW: *Wolbachia* in filarial nematodes: evolutionary aspects and implications for the pathogenesis and treatment of filarial diseases, *Vet Parasitol* 98:215, 2001.
4. Kramer LH, Passeri B, Corona S, et al: Immunohistochemical/immunogold detection and distribution of the endosymbiont *Wolbachia* of *Dirofilaria immitis* and *Brugia pahangi* using a polyclonal antiserum raised against WSP (*Wolbachia* surface protein), *Parasitol Res* 89:381, 2003.

5. Miller MW, Atkins CE, Stemme K, et al: Prevalence of exposure to *Dirofilaria immitis* in cats in multiple areas of the United States, Proceedings of the American Heartworm Symposium: 161, 1998.

6. Levy JK, Snyder PS, Taveres LM, et al: Prevalence and risk factors for heartworm infection in cats from northern Florida, *J Am Anim Hosp Assoc* 39:533, 2003.

7. Kramer L, Genchi C: Feline heartworm infection: serological survey of asymptomatic cats living in northern Italy, *Vet Parasitol* 104:43, 2002.

8. Bazzocchi C, Ceciliani F, McCall JW, et al: Antigenic role of the endosymbionts of filarial nematodes: IgG response against the *Wolbachia* surface protein in cats infected with *Dirofilaria immitis*, *Proc R Soc Lond B Biol Sci* 267:2511, 2000.

9. Morchón R, Ferreira AC, Martín-Pacho JR, et al: Specific IgG antibody response against antigens of *Dirofilaria immitis* and its *Wolbachia* endosymbiont bacterium in cats with natural and experimental infections, *Vet Parasitol* 125:313, 2004.

10. Levy JK, Dingman PA, Kramer LH, et al: Association of *Wolbachia* with heartworm disease in dogs and cats, Proceedings of the American Heartworm Society Symposium, Washington, DC, 2007.

11. American Heartworm Society, Feline Guidelines, 2007 at *www.americanheartwormsociety.org*

12. Browne LE, Carter TD, Levy JK, et al: Pulmonary arterial disease in cats seropositive for *Dirofilaria immitis* but lacking adult heartworms in the heart and lungs, *Am J Vet Res* 66:1544, 2005.

13. Taylor MJ, Cross HF, Ford L, et al: *Wolbachia* bacteria in filarial immunity and disease, *Parasite Immunol* 23:401, 2001.

14. Cross HF, Haarbrink M, Egerton G, et al: Severe reactions to filarial chemotherapy and release of *Wolbachia* endosymbionts into blood, *Lancet* 358:1873, 2001.

15. Brattig NW, Büttner DW, Hoerauf A, et al: Neutrophil accumulation around Onchocerca worms and chemotaxis of neutrophils are dependent on *Wolbachia* endobacteria, *Microbes Infect* 3:439, 2001.

16. Bazzocchi C, Genchi C, Paltrinieri S, et al: Immunological role of the endosymbionts of *Dirofilaria immitis:* the *Wolbachia* surface protein activates canine neutrophils with production of IL-8, *Vet Parasitol* 117:73, 2003.

17. Brattig NW, Bazzocchi C, Kirschning CJ, et al: The major surface protein of *Wolbachia* endosymbionts in filarial nematodes elicits immune responses through TLR2 and TLR4, *J Immunol* 173:437, 2004.

18. Hise AG, Gillette-Ferguson I, Pearlman E: The role of endosymbiotic *Wolbachia* bacteria in filarial disease, *Cell Microbiol* 6:97, 2004.

19. Kramer LH, Tamarozzi F, Morchón R, et al: Immune response to and tissue localization of the *Wolbachia* surface protein (WSP) in dogs with natural heartworm *(Dirofilaria immitis)* infection, *Vet Immunol Immunopathol* 106:303, 2005.

20. Litster A, Atwell RB: Physiological and haematological findings and clinical observations in a model of acute systemic anaphylaxis in *Dirofilaria immitis*–sensitised cats, *Aust Vet J* 84:151, 2006.

21. Litster AL, Atwell RB: Feline heartworm disease: a clinical review, *J Feline Med Surg* 10:137, 2008.

22. Genchi C, Di Sacco B, Cancrini G: Epizootiology of canine and feline heartworm infection in northern Italy: possible mosquito vectors. Proceedings of the American Heartworm Symposium: 39, 1992.

23. Gomes LA, Serrão ML, Duarte R, et al: Attraction of mosquitoes to domestic cats in a heartworm enzootic region, *J Feline Med Surg* 9:309, 2007.

24. McGarry HF, Egerton GL, Taylor MJ: Population dynamics of *Wolbachia* bacterial endosymbionts in *Brugia malayi, Mol Biochem Parasitol* 135:57, 2004.

25. Fenn K, Blaxter M: Quantification of *Wolbachia* bacteria in *Brugia malayi* through the nematode lifecycle, *Mol Biochem Parasitol* 137:361, 2004.

26. Hoerauf A, Mand S, Volkmann L, et al: Doxycycline in the treatment of human onchocerciasis: kinetics of *Wolbachia* endobacteria reduction and of inhibition of embryogenesis in female *Onchocerca* worms, *Microbes Infect* 5:216, 2003.

27. Hoerauf A, Mand S, Fischer K, et al: Doxycycline as a novel strategy against bancroftian filariasis: depletion of *Wolbachia* endosymbionts from *Wuchereria bancrofti* and stop of microfilaria production, *Med Microbiol Immunol* 192:211, 2003.

28. Langworthy NG, Renz A, Mackenstedt U, et al: Macrofilaricidal activity of tetracycline against the filarial nematode *Onchocerca ochengi:* elimination of *Wolbachia* precedes worm death and suggests a dependent relationship, *Proc R Soc Lond B Biol Sci* 267:1063, 2000.

29. Taylor MJ, Makunde WH, McGarry HF, et al: Macrofilaricidal activity after doxycycline treatment of *Wuchereria bancrofti:* a double-blind, randomised placebo-controlled trial, *Lancet* 365:2067, 2005.

30. Bazzocchi C, Mortarino M, Grandi G, et al: Combined ivermectin-doxycycline treatment has microfilaricidal and adulticide activity against *D. immitis* in experimentally infected dogs, *Int J Parasitol* 38:1401, 2008.

31. Kramer L, Grandi G, Leoni M, et al: *Wolbachia* and its influence on the pathology and immunology of *Dirofilaria immitis* infection, *Vet Parasitol* 158:191, 2008.

32. Dillon AR, Brawner WR Jr, Robertson-Plouch, et al: Feline heartworm disease: correlations of clinical signs, serology, and other diagnostics—results of a multi-center study, Proceedings of the American Heartworm Symposium: 153, 1998.

4 Cytauxzoon Infections

Leah A. Cohn

Feline cytauxzoonosis is an emerging infectious disease within an expanding territory. Originally recognized only in the south-central United States, the disease now can be found in a much broader geographical region. Rapid replication of the tissue phase of the causative protozoan pathogen usually results in multiple organ failure. Although cytauxzoonosis was once believed to be uniformly fatal, we now know that cats can survive the acute infection and remain parasitemic.

ETIOLOGY

Cytauxzoonosis is caused by the vector-borne hematoprotozoan parasite *Cytauxzoon felis*. Belonging to the order Piroplasmida, the organism is categorized within the family Theleriidae. Like other Theleriidae, *C. felis* exists in distinct erythrocytic and nonerythrocytic forms within the mammalian host. The organism undergoes asexual reproduction in the host's mononuclear phagocytic cells in what is termed the schizont phase of infection. Schizont-laden macrophage cells become distended (Figure 4-1), occluding vasculature to tissues and resulting in the most serious clinical manifestations of disease. Clinical disease appears to be related to the severity of schizogony. Domestic cats typically experience severe schizogony and equally severe clinical illness, while schizogony and clinical illness often are less pronounced in the bobcat reservoir host.[1,2]

Fission of the schizont within the mononuclear cells results in the formation of merozoites.[3] When merozoites are completely formed within the infected mononuclear cells, the distended cells rupture and release merozoites. Red blood cells (RBC) take up merozoites via endocytosis, producing the classic RBC piroplasms associated with infection (Figure 4-2). Piroplasms reproduce through asexual binary fission. The presence of piroplasms sometimes is associated with hemolysis during the later stages of the acute illness. However, the presence of piroplasms

is not likely a major contributor to disease. Most felidae that recover from acute infection apparently can harbor the piroplasms for months or even years without serious consequences.[4-8] Ingestion of RBC-containing piroplasms serves as the means of transmission of the parasite to the tick intermediate hosts. The tick then will be able to transmit sporozoites to the next felidae on which it feeds.

Although it is the species most relevant to the health of cats in the United States, *C. felis* is only one of several species of *Cytauxzoon* protozoal parasites.[9] A morphologically indistinguishable intraerythrocytic parasite was found after the importation of Pallas's cats *(Otocolobus manul)* from Mongolia.[10] Amplification and sequencing of the 18S ribosomal RNA gene from these cats identified a related but separate species, tentatively named *C. manul*.[11] When injected into domestic cats, this pathogen produced erythroparasitemia but no disease, and was unable to prevent virulent disease when those cats were infected subsequently with *C. felis*.[12] Another two similar but distinct pathogens have been detected in Iberian lynx *(Lynx pardinus)* from southern Spain.[13] Although the known tick vectors for *C. felis* are not found in Brazil, cytauxzoonosis has been described in cats from the region; it is unclear if this parasite is genetically identical to the *C. felis* found in the United States.[8,14]

EPIDEMIOLOGY

Cytauxzoonosis can occur in cats of any age, although most reported cases have been in young adult cats. Immune suppression is not necessary for cats to become infected, and there is no evidence that infection is more likely in retroviral-infected cats than in healthy cats. No gender or breed predilections have been identified for cytauxzoonosis. Outdoor cats are more likely to acquire this disease, presumably due to an increased exposure to the tick vectors. The greatest risk of infection seems to

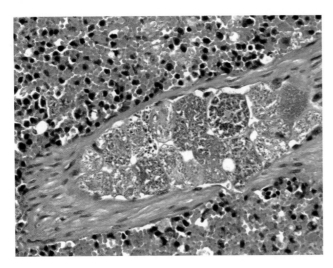

Figure 4-1 Histological section of the spleen from a cat who died from cytauxzoonosis demonstrates multiple schizont-laden mononuclear phagocytic cells. (Wright-Giemsa, 400× magnification.) (Courtesy Dr. Marlyn Whitney, University of Missouri Veterinary Medical Diagnostic Laboratory.)

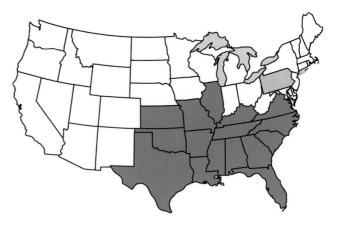

Figure 4-3 U.S. map demonstrating states from which there have been confirmed cases of *C. felis* infection in either domestic cats *(green)* or bobcats *(gold)*.

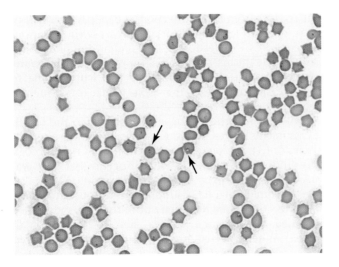

Figure 4-2 Merozoites released from schizont-distended mononuclear cells are taken up by RBC, where they form classic piroplasms, as demonstrated in this image (examples demonstrated by *black arrows*. (Wright-Giemsa stain, 1000× magnification.) (Courtesy Dr. Marlyn Whitney, University of Missouri Veterinary Medical Diagnostic Laboratory.)

occur in the spring and summer, presumably during times the tick vector is most active.[15] In Oklahoma, peak incidence occurred in May, whereas infections were identified very rarely from November through March.[15] Similarly, 75 per cent of clinical cases identified by the University of Missouri Veterinary Medical Diagnostic Laboratory over a several-year period were presented between May and July.

For many years after its original description during the mid-1970s in cats from Missouri, cytauxzoonosis was recognized only in states in the south-central United States.[16] In recent years, the geographical range of infections has expanded greatly, with infections now reported in cats throughout the southeastern, mid-Atlantic, and south-central United States (Figure 4-3).[17,18] Although not yet demonstrated in domestic cats, *C. felis* infection has been demonstrated in bobcats living as far north as Pennsylvania.[19] Because the diagnosis often is based on visualization of RBC inclusions and because necropsy diagnosis of cytauxzoonosis is even more straightforward than antemortem diagnosis, it seems unlikely that infections were simply "missed" in these areas prior to the last decade. Instead, it appears that the infection is now occurring in areas where it did not occur previously.

Because the reservoir host for the pathogen is the bobcat, infected domestic cats typically are from rural or suburban rather than urban areas. Cats living close to wooded areas or less intensely managed land are more likely to become infected.[15] It is common for multiple cats in a neighborhood or even a household to become infected within a single season, likely reflecting the presence of infected reservoir hosts in the area.

There are no large published epidemiological studies of *C. felis* infection in domestic cats. In a single study of healthy cats presented to trap-neuter-return programs in Tennessee (n = 75), Florida (n = 494), and North Carolina (n = 392), prevalence of *C. felis* as detected by polymerase chain reaction (PCR) ranged from 1.3 per cent to 0.4 per cent to 0 per cent, respectively.[5] It is likely that prevalence rates are higher in regions traditionally found to have enzootic infection; the author is aware of several colonies of cats in Missouri with prevalence rates of up to 45 per cent. Prevalence of infection in cats from Brazil with a hematoprotozoan parasite morphologically indistinguishable from *C. felis* is similarly high, up to 48.5 per cent.[8] Prevalence of infection in bobcats again depends on geography, but estimates range from 7 per cent in Pennsylvania, to 33 per cent in North Carolina, to 62 per cent in Oklahoma.[19-21] There are no published studies on incidence of infection. In a retrospective review, cytauxzoonosis accounted for approximately 1 per cent of feline submissions to the Oklahoma Animal Disease Diagnostic Laboratory, and 1.5 per cent of feline admissions to the Boren Veterinary Medical Teaching Hospital between 1995 and 2006 and 1998 and 2006, respectively.[15] Personal communications with the author suggest that veterinarians in enzootic "hot spots" see as many as five cases of cytauxzoonosis a week during the peak season, with many more veterinarians in surrounding regions reporting that they see five to 10 cases per summer.

PATHOGENESIS

The most severe manifestations of acute illness associated with cytauxzoonosis appear to be related to the schizogenous phase of infection. In the bobcat reservoir host, schizogony and clinical illness usually are self-limiting.[2] On the other hand, infection of domestic cats usually leads to massive schizogony. Mononuclear cells become greatly distended with parasites. These distended cells are found both within the lumen of venous channels and also in the interstitium of most organs; however, parasitemia can be especially severe in the lungs, liver, spleen, and other lymphoid tissues.[1,22] Vascular obstruction, anoxia, and release of damaging substances secondary to cell death and rupture all can contribute to multiple organ failure. Less virulent strains of *C. felis* might result in a more limited schizogony with less associated pathology in domestic cats. The theoretical existence of less virulent strains is supported by a regional occurrence of survivors at a greater than expected rate.[4] However, to date there has been no definitive identification of genetically identifiable strains with limited virulence.

Immunity to *C. felis* is not well understood. It is unclear why bobcats usually develop a more limited schizogenous replication than do domestic cats. We do know that erythroparasitemia acquired via transfusion of piroplasm-containing RBC (rather than erythroparasitemia that follows survival of the acute infection) does not protect domestic cats from subsequent fatal schizogony.[23,24] Experimental studies suggest that when domestic cats do survive the schizogenous phase of infection, they become immune to repeated infection and associated clinical illness.[24,25] However, the author has spoken with veterinarians in endemic regions who have observed clinical illness indistinguishable from acute cytauxzoonosis in cats known to have survived cytauxzoonosis in previous years. In none of these cats was an attempt made to identify tissue schizonts during the second illness. Therefore it can not be determined if the second illness was caused by reinfection, or if piroplasms were merely the result of infection during the first illness.

TRANSMISSION

Cytauxzoonosis is a tick-transmitted disease (Figure 4-4). A variety of ticks feed on both domestic and wild felidae, and *C. felis* has been recovered from both *Dermacentor variabilis* and *Amblyomma americanum* species ticks.[26] However, vector competence has only been investigated (and confirmed) for *D. variabilis*.[27] Other ticks also can serve as competent vectors for transmission. A parasite morphologically identical to *C. felis* is described in Brazil, where neither *D. variabilis* nor *A. americanum* are reported to occur.[8,28]

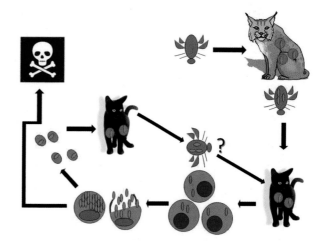

Figure 4-4 Life cycle of *C. felis*. Naïve ticks acquire the pathogen when they feed on an infected reservoir host, typically a bobcat. When the tick next feeds on a felid, it injects sporozoites that develop into schizonts in the mononuclear cells. While schizogenous asexual replication appears to be limited in the bobcat, it is profound in domestic cats. In some cases, the cat dies during schizogony and before the appearance of piroplasms in circulation. In other cases, the distended mononuclear cells rupture releasing merozoites. These merozoites are taken up by RBC, where they are known as piroplasms. Most domestic cats die soon after piroplasms are observed, but some cats apparently survive infection. These surviving cats can harbor piroplasms for months to years without obvious ill-effect. It is unknown how relevant chronically parasitemic domestic cats are to the cycle of infection, although at least experimentally, ticks can acquire the pathogen after feeding on parasitemic domestic cats.

The pathogen *C. felis* is maintained within the presumed natural reservoir host, the bobcat *(Lynx rufus rufus)*. Unlike domestic cats, when bobcats become infected they undergo a limited schizogony and typically a mild to moderate acute clinical illness (although fatal infection of bobcats has been described).[2,23,29] On recovery from illness, bobcats maintain a persistent infection with the RBC piroplasm form of the protozoan for years. Naïve ticks pick up the pathogen after feeding on these persistently infected carriers. If the tick next feeds on another bobcat, the sylvan cycle is repeated. If the tick feeds instead on a domestic cat, infection often results in massive schizogonous replication and profound illness.

Because most domestic cats die from cytauxzoonosis, they have been deemed a terminal host. In the last decade, it has become clear that domestic cats can survive acute illness due to cytauxzoonosis and can remain persistently parasitemic.[4,17,30,31] Additionally, domestic cats occasionally are identified who harbor piroplasms without any known history of clinical illness.[4,5,8] In an experimental setting, it appears that domestic cats are capable of transmitting infection through the tick vector.[32] Whether these carriers harbor an adequate parasite load to make them a reservoir host in a natural setting is unknown. If so, movement of domestic carrier cats (with their owners) might help account for the rapid expansion in the endemic geographical region for this pathogen.

Infection of domestic cats with *C. felis* in a natural setting requires a tick vector. Co-housing of ill and naïve cats is inadequate to transmit infection.[22] Transmission can be accomplished experimentally by inoculation of schizont-laden tissues, or by transfusion of blood (collected during the acute illness) that contains mononuclear cell schizonts.[22,23,33] Transfusion of blood from recovered cats, which contains only RBC piroplasms, results in chronic maintenance of the piroplasm stage of infection but does not result in schizogony or clinical illness.[23,27]

Natural infection has been either confirmed or strongly suspected in a wide variety of felid species, including captive tigers *(Panthera tigris)*, Florida panthers *(Felis concolor coryi)*, Texas cougar *(Felis concolor)*, cheetahs *(Acinonyx jubatus)*, and a caracal *(Felis caracal)*.[34-39] Extensive experimental transmission studies failed to demonstrate infection of any nonfelidae species, including immuno-deficient mice.[40]

CLINICAL SIGNS

Although historical and physical examination findings are nonspecific, an acute onset of anorexia, lethargy, and fever in cats within an endemic region (especially during spring and summer) should raise immediate suspicions for cytauxzoonosis. The onset of clinical disease occurs 1 to 3 weeks after tick-transmitted infection. Initial clinical signs are vague and typically include anorexia and lethargy. Within hours to days, illness becomes more severe and owners may notice increased vocalization, weakness, icterus, respiratory distress, obtunded mentation, or even seizures. The most consistent alteration on physical examination is pyrexia (often marked), but hypothermia is common in the moribund cat. Mucous membranes may be icteric and/or pale. Tachypnea and tachycardia are typical, with or without overt respiratory distress. Mild to moderate lymphadenomegaly may be seen, and abdominal palpation often demonstrates splenomegaly and hepatomegaly. Sometimes, muscle pain is appreciated during palpation. Cats may become comatose shortly before death. The entire disease course usually is rapid, and many cats will succumb within days of initial clinical signs.

For those cats who survive the acute illness, clinical recovery typically is complete without residual dysfunction. With the knowledge that cats can and do recover from cytauxzoonosis comes the realization that carrier cats exist. These cats can have no clinical signs of illness whatsoever. It remains unknown how many, if any, of these chronically parasitemic cats may experience delayed clinical signs such as hemolysis unassociated with the acute infection. It also is apparent that erythroparasites will only be recognized in carrier cats when blood smears are examined microscopically. Because evaluation of blood smears typically occurs only in the face of clinical illness, veterinarians will be faced with the dilemma of deciding if piroplasms are an incidental finding, or if they are in some way related to the clinical disease for which the cat has been presented.

Box 4-1 Differential Diagnosis for Feline Cytauxzoonosis

Cat bite–associated abscess
Cholangitis/cholangiohepatitis
Hepatic lipidosis
Immune-mediated hemolytic anemia
Mycoplasma haemofelis
(Candidatus) *Mycoplasma haemominutum*
Pancreatitis
Toxoplasmosis
Tularemia
Viral infection
  Feline leukemia virus
  Feline immunodeficiency virus
  Feline infectious peritonitis
  Herpesvirus
  Virulent calicivirus

DIFFERENTIAL DIAGNOSIS

Feline cytauxzoonosis has no pathognomonic, historical, or physical findings, and therefore there are many reasonable differential diagnoses (Box 4-1). Because fever is a characteristic part of the presentation, other causes of acute febrile illness are especially important differential considerations. Like cats with cytauxzoonosis, cats presenting with tularemia often are previously healthy cats with access to the outdoors and a sudden onset of lethargy/anorexia, high fever, icterus, and lymphadenomegaly/splenomegaly. Unlike cytauxzoonosis, tularemia has the potential for zoonotic transmission. Oral ulcerations or subcutaneous abscess should prompt consideration of tularemia rather than cytauxzoonosis. Although not typically associated with high fever, hematotropic mycoplasmosis is another important differential diagnosis, because both infections can result in anemia, icterus, and the observation of red cell–associated parasites. The microscopic appearance of hematotropic mycoplasmas is distinct from piroplasms of *C. felis*, however. (See Chapter 63 in the fifth volume of this series.)

DIAGNOSIS

Diagnosis of cytauxzoonosis often is straightforward and can be accomplished by identification of erythroparasitemia on peripheral blood smears in cats with compatible history and physical examination findings. A thin, well-made blood smear can be stained with either Diff-Quick or Wright's stain for identification of piroplasms. The RBC piroplasms of *C. felis* most often are shaped as 1 to 1.5 μm signet rings, but "safety pin" and tetrad forms also are observed, or rarely chains of organisms resembling cocci (Figure 4-5). Similar erythroparasites are identified in cats infected with *Babesia felis* and *C. manul*, but thus far those pathogens have not been identified as naturally occurring infections in the United States. *Mycoplasma haemofelis* might be mistaken for *C. felis* piroplasms. *M. haemofelis* occurs as epicellular, pleomorphic (cocci,

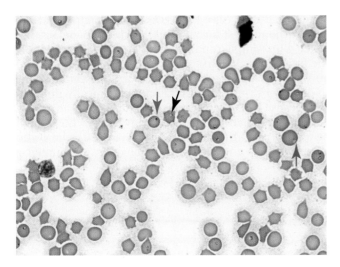

Figure 4-5 Many piroplasms of *C. felis* are seen within RBC on peripheral blood smear from an acutely ill infected cat (Wright-Giemsa stain, 1000× magnification). Caution must be exercised to avoid confusing unicellular *M. haemofelis* organisms, stain precipitate, or Howell-Jolly bodies *(red arrow)* for *C. felis* piroplasms. Round "Signet ring" *(black arrow)* and elongated "safety pin" *(green arrow)* forms are observed here and are recognized most commonly, but a variety of other morphologies are possible.

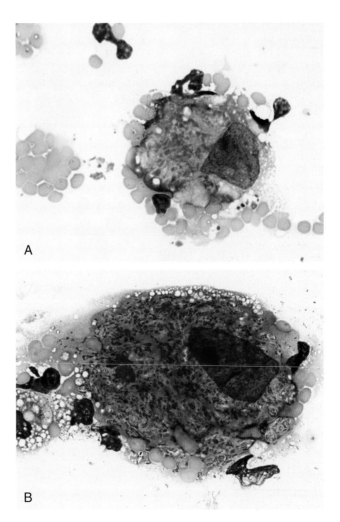

Figure 4-6 A and **B,** Mononuclear phagocytic cells distended with schizonts were detected on the feathered edge of a peripheral blood smear made from a cat with acute illness due to *C. felis.* (Wright-Giemsa stain, 1000× magnification.) The large size of the mononuclear cell can be appreciated in contrast to nearby RBC. (Courtesy Dr. Marlyn Whitney, University of Missouri Veterinary Medical Diagnostic Laboratory.)

rods, or rings) RBC pathogens. In addition to the smaller size of *M. haemofelis* (typically 0.3 to 0.8 μm), its epicellular location, frequent occurrence in pairs or short chains, and associated regenerative anemia help to distinguish it from *C. felis*. Stain precipitate found overlying RBC can be mistaken easily for piroplasms, but precipitate usually can be found unassociated with cells as well as overlying cells. Nuclear remnants known as Howell-Jolly bodies likewise can be mistaken for *C. felis* piroplasms. Identification of *C. felis* piroplasms is not a sensitive method of disease diagnosis. The feathered edge of the stained blood smear must be evaluated carefully because erythroparasite burden is often low. Even more important, piroplasms are not present in all infected cats, particularly early in the disease course. Piroplasms can be absent in up to 50 per cent of cases at the time of initial illness.[25]

Infection also can be confirmed visually by the microscopic identification of schizonts within mononuclear cells. Sometimes, careful examination of the feathered edge of a stained peripheral blood smear will demonstrate schizonts in circulating mononuclear cells (Figure 4-6). More commonly, fine-needle aspirates from parasitized tissues such as lymph node, spleen, or liver will yield samples containing schizont-laden macrophages (Figure 4-7). Tissue biopsy is rarely employed for the diagnosis of cytauxzoonosis, but infection is easily confirmed postmortem through microscopic identification of such schizont-laden cells (Figure 4-8).

Aside from identification of protozoal pathogens on blood smear, there are no specific abnormalities on routine clinicopathological testing. Pancytopenia is often found on complete blood count. Anemia typically is nor-

mocytic, normochromic, and nonregenerative due to the acute nature of illness. Erythrophagocytosis is identified on occasion, with hemolysis occurring principally in the extravascular compartment. Often, anemia is mild to moderate early in the disease course, but can become more severe later in the course of illness. A bone marrow crowded with schizont-laden macrophages can lead to neutropenia, but neutrophilia resulting from an inflammatory response to infection may be identified alternatively. Moderate to marked thrombocytopenia is believed to be related to consumptive processes, including the common complication of disseminated intravascular coagulation (DIC). Coagulation times (e.g., activated partial thromboplastin time [aPTT], one-stage prothrombin time) often are prolonged as a component of DIC. Hyperbilirubinemia is a very common finding, both as a result of intrahepatic infiltration of schizont-loaded macrophages as well as hemolysis, and liver enzymes often

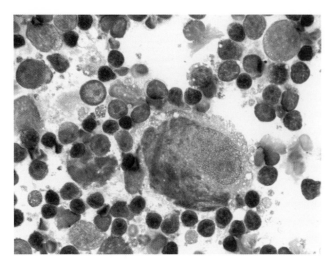

Figure 4-7 Cytological preparation made from a fine-needle aspirate of a lymph node in an acutely ill cat demonstrates a schizont-distended mononuclear phagocytic cell. (Wright-Giemsa, 1000× magnification.) Such preparations can permit rapid diagnosis in acutely ill cats who do not demonstrate piroplasms in the peripheral blood. (Courtesy Dr. Marlyn Whitney, University of Missouri Veterinary Medical Diagnostic Laboratory.)

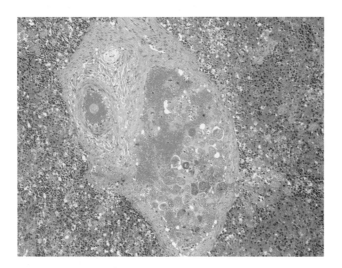

Figure 4-8 Histological image from the spleen of a cat who died of cytauxzoonosis demonstrates many readily recognizable schizont-laden mononuclear phagocytic cells. (Hematoxylin-eosin stain, 100× magnification.) Postmortem histological diagnosis of the disease is very straightforward. (Courtesy Dr. Marlyn Whitney, University of Missouri Veterinary Medical Diagnostic Laboratory.)

are increased. Prerenal azotemia, hyperglycemia, and electrolyte and acid-base disturbances are documented in many infected cats. Bilirubinuria is common, but hemoglobinuria is not observed because hemolysis is largely extravascular.

Additional diagnostic tests may be considered in ill cats. Imaging techniques do not contribute directly to the diagnosis of *C. felis* infection, but splenomegaly and hepatomegaly would be expected. A commercially available polymerase chain reaction (PCR) test can be used to confirm the presence of *C. felis* DNA (North Carolina

State University Vector Borne Disease Laboratory, Raleigh, NC). Although test turnaround time is rapid, delays associated with sample submission are important considering the brief clinical course of illness. Serological testing for antibody to *C. felis* can be used in a research setting to document prior infection, but it is clinically impractical because the infected cat may die before antibodies appear in circulation. Although convalescent titers might be used to confirm infection in surviving cats, the author is unaware of antibody tests offered on a commercial basis.

TREATMENT

Cytauxzoonosis was once described as a uniformly fatal infection; however, over the last decade there have been several reports of surviving cats. In some cases cats survived with aggressive supportive care; in other cases cats survived with supportive care plus antiprotozoal therapy. Yet others cats have been identified during the carrier piroplasm stage of infection with no known history of clinical illness. Unfortunately, no controlled prospective studies have been completed to demonstrate efficacy of any treatment regimen.

Supportive care is certainly indicated for ill cats, although there is no evidence as to which aspects of supportive care are important. It is reasonable to assume that fluid therapy is indicated to correct dehydration, preserve vascular volume, and maintain tissue perfusion. For those cats who become anemic and demonstrate tachypnea or tachycardia, provision of oxygen-carrying capacity via transfusion of whole blood, packed red blood cells, or hemoglobin-based oxygen-carrying solutions (i.e., Oxyglobin, Biopure Corporation) is indicated (see Chapter 60). Cytauxzoonosis is often accompanied by DIC; prophylactic (100 to 200 U/kg unfractionated heparin SQ q8h); therapeutic (goal, 2× prolongation of aPTT) heparin administration may prove useful. To replenish coagulation factors when treating active DIC, whole blood or plasma transfusion typically accompanies heparin therapy. Nonsteroidal antiinflammatory drugs (NSAIDs) such as meloxicam have been used to provide analgesia and reduce fever. Some veterinarians treat ill cats with low doses of prednisolone. The potential benefit of NSAIDs or corticosteroids has not been evaluated. A variety of antimicrobial drugs (e.g., sodium ampicillin, enrofloxacin, and doxycycline) have been used in infected cats alone or in combination.[30,31,41] None of these drugs has demonstrated efficacy against protozoal agents such as *C. felis*.

Definitive treatment of cytauxzoonosis would involve antiprotozoal drug administration. The antiprotozoal hydroxynapthoquinolone agents parvaquone and buparvaquone are the treatment of choice for *Theileria* spp. infection of African cattle. Despite the close relationship of *C. felis* to *Theileria* spp., these drugs demonstrate a complete lack of efficacy for treatment of cytauxzoonosis in trials to date.[24] The aromatic diamidine compounds imidocarb dipropionate (Imizol, Schering-Plough Animal Health, Kenilworth, NJ) or diminazene aceturate are used for the treatment of various protozoal agents, including

Babesia spp. and African trypanosomiasis. In a retrospective study, five of six cats treated with diminazene plus aggressive supportive care survived infection.[31] Unfortunately, diminazene is not approved for use in the United States. Although requests can be made to the Food and Drug Administration for importation of diminazene under compassionate drug use importation rules,* the time required for importation prevents its practical utility in treatment of *C. felis*, because each request must be made on behalf of a specific animal (i.e., the drug can not be stockpiled for future use). Imidocarb is readily available in the United States, and has been widely used for the treatment of cytauxzoonosis at a variety of different dose regimens (e.g., two doses at 2 mg/kg IM 7 days apart, two doses at 5 mg/kg IM 7 days apart, two doses of 5 mg/kg IM 4 days apart). Although a prospective trial evaluating the use of imidocarb at 3 to 4 mg/kg IM, twice 7 days apart is ongoing, results are not yet available. Included in a retrospective report of 18 surviving infected cats (only one of which was treated with imidocarb) was the anecdotal mention that imidocarb lacked efficacy in the treatment of experimentally induced cytauxzoonosis.[4] In the author's personal communications with veterinarians from endemic regions, some believe treatment with imidocarb results in no improvement in clinical outcome (rare survival), while others claim up to 75 per cent clinical recovery in cats treated with imidocarb and supportive care. When used, pretreatment with atropine may minimize the potential adverse cholinergic effects of imidocarb treatment. Recently, treatment has been attempted with a combination of the antiprotozoal drug atovaquone and the antibiotic azithromycin. This combination has been used successfully to treat both human and canine babesiosis.[42,43] Although a prospective clinical trial is underway, results are not yet available to either demonstrate or refute the efficacy of this combination therapy. Survival of up to 62 per cent of cats treated with this combination has been reported, although the report was not based on a controlled or comparative study.[44]

It is unclear if treatment should be administered to healthy cats with persistent erythroparasitemia. In the few cats followed for months or years, clinical disease has not occurred as a result of the piroplasm infection. However, the possibility exists that these cats may experience hemolysis at some future date. Of additional importance, it is theoretically possible that these carrier cats may infect naïve ticks that could inoculate pathogenic sporozoites when they next feed. Treatment with imidocarb apparently is not effective in eliminating parasitemia in healthy cats.[7] The combination of atovaquone and azithromycin did not cure infection uniformly, but treated cats were often cytologically and PCR-negative for parasites 8 weeks after treatment.[7]

PREVENTION

There is no vaccine currently available for the prevention of *C. felis* infection. Although apparent immunity to

*http://www.fda.gov/ora/import/ora_import_system.html.

repeated experimental infection with *C. felis* seems promising for potential vaccine development, safe and effective vaccines to prevent hematoprotozoan parasites have proven notoriously difficult to develop.[24,25,45] For now, prevention is focused on prevention of tick bites. Unfortunately, none of the currently available parasiticides for use in domestic cats prevent ticks from biting. A combination of fipronil application and indoor confinement to minimize tick exposure seems to offer the best chance of prevention in endemic regions. Prophylactic chemotherapy is used to prevent malaria in people in endemic regions. The role such prophylaxis may have in prevention of feline cytauxzoonosis remains to be determined.

PATHOLOGICAL FINDINGS

Experimental studies of *C. felis* infection have provided an extensive description of pathological findings associated with the acute illness.[1] Infected cats develop enlargement and mottling of the spleen and liver, and often develop mild to moderate lymphadenomegaly. Pulmonary edema and congestion and petechial hemorrhage on the lung surface are common. Petechial and ecchymotic hemorrhage may be detected in a variety of tissues, because DIC commonly precedes death. Venous distension can be appreciated grossly, and there can be slight swelling of the kidneys.

Histological examination readily demonstrates the tissue stage of *C. felis* infection. Schizonts occur within the cytoplasm of mononuclear phagocytes in the tissues themselves, or attached to the endothelium or within the lumen of venous channels in essentially all organs (Figure 4-9). Spleen, liver, lung, bone marrow, and lymph nodes are especially heavily parasitized. Partial or complete occlusion of venous channels by infected mononuclear cells results in marked venous congestion of tissues.

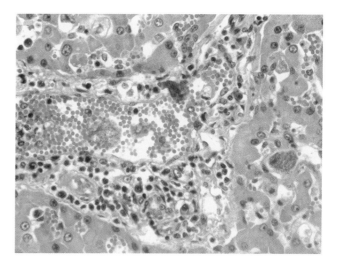

Figure 4-9 The histological image from the liver of a cat who died of cytauxzoonosis demonstrates schizont-laden mononuclear phagocytic cells within the vascular lumen. (Hematoxylin-eosin stain, 100× magnification.) (Courtesy Dr. Marlyn Whitney, University of Missouri Veterinary Medical Diagnostic Laboratory.)

REFERENCES

1. Kier AB, Wagner JE, Kinden DA: The pathology of experimental cytauxzoonosis, *J Comp Pathol* 97:415, 1987.
2. Blouin EF, Kocan AA, Kocan KM, et al: Evidence of a limited schizogonous cycle for *Cytauxzoon felis* in bobcats following exposure to infected ticks, *J Wildl Dis* 23:499, 1987.
3. Simpson CF, Harvey JW, Lawman MJ, et al: Ultrastructure of schizonts in the liver of cats with experimentally induced cytauxzoonosis, *Am J Vet Res* 46:384, 1985.
4. Meinkoth J, Kocan AA, Whitworth L, et al: Cats surviving natural infection with *Cytauxzoon felis*: 18 cases (1997-1998), *J Vet Intern Med* 14:521, 2000.
5. Haber MD, Tucker MD, Marr HS, et al: The detection of *Cytauxzoon felis* in apparently healthy free-roaming cats in the USA, *Vet Parasitol* 146:316, 2007.
6. Brown HM, Latimer KS, Erikson LE, et al: Detection of persistent *Cytauxzoon felis* infection by polymerase chain reaction in three asymptomatic domestic cats, *J Vet Diagn Invest* 20:485, 2008.
7. Cohn LA, Birkenheuer AJ, Ratcliff E: Comparison of two drug protocols for clearance of *Cytauxzoon felis* infections, *J Vet Intern Med* 22:704 (abstract), 2008.
8. Mendes-de-Almeida F, Labarthe N, Guerrero J, et al: Follow-up of the health conditions of an urban colony of free-roaming cats (*Felis catus Linnaeus*, 1758) in the city of Rio de Janeiro, Brazil, *Vet Parasitol* 147:9, 2007.
9. Criado-Fornelio A, Gonzalez-del-Rio MA, Buling-Sarana A, et al: The "expanding universe" of piroplasms, *Vet Parasitol* 119:337, 2004.
10. Ketz-Riley CJ, Reichard MV, Van den Bussche RA, et al: An intraerythrocytic small piroplasm in wild-caught Pallas's cats (*Otocolobus manul*) from Mongolia, *J Wildl Dis* 39:424, 2003.
11. Reichard MV, Van Den Bussche RA, Meinkoth JH, et al: A new species of *Cytauxzoon* from Pallas' cats caught in Mongolia and comments on the systematics and taxonomy of piroplasmids, *J Parasitol* 91:420, 2005.
12. Joyner PH, Reichard MV, Meinkoth JH, et al: Experimental infection of domestic cats (*Felis domesticus*) with Cytauxzoon manul from Pallas' cats (*Otocolobus manul*), *Vet Parasitol* 146:302, 2007.
13. Millan J, Naranjo V, Rodriguez A, et al: Prevalence of infection and 18S rRNA gene sequences of Cytauxzoon species in Iberian lynx (*Lynx pardinus*) in Spain, *Parasitology* 134:995, 2007.
14. Soares CO: Cytauxzoonose felina é diagnosticada e isolada pela primeira vez na América Latina, *Revista Clin Vet* 32:56, 2001.
15. Reichard MV, Baum KA, Cadenhead SC, et al: Temporal occurrence and environmental risk factors associated with cytauxzoonosis in domestic cats, *Vet Parasitol* 152:314, 2008.
16. Wagner JE: A fatal cytauxzoonosis-like disease in cats, *J Am Vet Med Assoc* 168:585, 1976.
17. Birkenheuer AJ, Le JA, Valenzisi AM, et al: *Cytauxzoon felis* infection in cats in the mid-Atlantic states: 34 cases (1998-2004), *J Am Vet Med Assoc* 228:568, 2006.
18. Jackson CB, Fisher T: Fatal cytauxzoonosis in a Kentucky cat (*Felis domesticus*), *Vet Parasitol* 139:192, 2006.
19. Birkenheuer AJ, Marr HS, Warren C, et al: *Cytauxzoon felis* infections are present in bobcats (*Lynx rufus*) in a region where cytauxzoonosis is not recognized in domestic cats, *Vet Parasitol* 153:126, 2008.
20. Glenn BL, Rolley RE, Kocan AA: Cytauxzoon-like piroplasms in erythrocytes of wild-trapped bobcats in Oklahoma, *J Am Vet Med Assoc* 181:1251, 1982.
21. Kocan AA, Blouin EF, Glenn BL: Hematologic and serum chemical values for free-ranging bobcats, *Felis rufus (Schreber)*, with reference to animals with natural infections of *Cytauxzoon felis* Kier, 1979, *J Wildl Dis* 21:190, 1985.
22. Wagner JE, Ferris DH, Kier AB, et al: Experimentally induced cytauxzoonosis-like disease in domestic cats, *Vet Parasitol* 6:305, 1980.
23. Glenn BL, Kocan AA, Blouin EF: Cytauxzoonosis in bobcats, *J Am Vet Med Assoc* 183:1155, 1983.
24. Motzel SL, Wagner JE: Treatment of experimentally induced cytauxzoonosis in cats with parvaquone and buparvaquone, *Vet Parasitol* 35:131, 1990.
25. Ferris DH: A progress report on the status of a new disease of American cats: cytauxzoonosis, *Comp Immunol Microbiol Infect Dis* 1:269, 1979.
26. Bondy PJ Jr, Cohn LA, Tyler JW, et al: Polymerase chain reaction detection of *Cytauxzoon felis* from field-collected ticks and sequence analysis of the small subunit and internal transcribed spacer 1 region of the ribosomal RNA gene, *J Parasitol* 91:458, 2005.
27. Blouin EF, Kocan AA, Glenn BL, et al: Transmission of *Cytauxzoon felis* Kier, 1979 from bobcats, *Felis rufus (Schreber)*, to domestic cats by *Dermacentor variabilis* (Say), *J Wildl Dis* 20:241, 1984.
28. Mendes-De-Almeida F, Faria MCF, Branco AS, et al: Sanitary conditions of a colony of urban feral cats (*Felis catus Linnaeus*, 1758) in a zoological garden of Rio de Janeiro, Brazil, *Rev Inst Med Trop Sao Paulo* 46:269, 2004.
29. Nietfeld JC, Pollock C: Fatal cytauxzoonosis in a free-ranging bobcat (*Lynx rufus*), *J Wildl Dis* 38:607, 2002.
30. Walker DB, Cowell RL: Survival of a domestic cat with naturally acquired cytauxzoonosis, *J Am Vet Med Assoc* 206:1363, 1995.
31. Greene CE, Latimer K, Hopper E, et al: Administration of diminazene aceturate or imidocarb dipropionate for treatment of cytauxzoonosis in cats, *J Am Vet Med Assoc* 215:497, 1999.
32. Kocan AA, Kocan KM, Blouin EF, et al: A redescription of schizogony of *Cytauxzoon felis* in the domestic cat, *Ann NY Acad Sci* 653:161, 1992.
33. Kier AB, Wagner JE, Morehouse LG: Experimental transmission of *Cytauxzoon felis* from bobcats (*Lynx rufus*) to domestic cats (*Felis domesticus*), *Am J Vet Res* 43:97, 1982.
34. Garner MM, Lung NP, Citino S, et al: Fatal cytauxzoonosis in a captive-reared white tiger (*Panthera tigris*), *Vet Pathol* 33:82, 1996.
35. Jakob W, Wesemeier HH: A fatal infection in a bengal tiger resembling cytauxzoonosis in domestic cats, *J Comp Pathol* 114:439, 1996.
36. Butt MT, Bowman D, Barr MC, et al: Iatrogenic transmission of *Cytauxzoon felis* from a Florida panther (*Felis concolor coryi*) to a domestic cat, *J Wildl Dis* 27:342, 1991.
37. Harvey JW, Dunbar MR, Norton TM, et al: Laboratory findings in acute *Cytauxzoon felis* infection in cougars (*Puma concolor couguar*) in Florida, *J Zoo Wildl Med* 38:285, 2007.
38. Rotstein DS, Taylor SK, Harvey JW, et al: Hematologic effects of cytauxzoonosis in Florida panthers and Texas cougars in Florida, *J Wildl Dis* 35:613, 1999.
39. Zinkl JG, McDonald SE, Kier AB, et al: Cytauxzoon-like organisms in erythrocytes of two cheetahs, *J Am Vet Med Assoc* 179:1261, 1981.
40. Kier AB, Wightman SR, Wagner JE: Interspecies transmission of *Cytauxzoon felis*, *Am J Vet Res* 43:102, 1982.
41. Hoover JP, Walker DB, Hedges JD: Cytauxzoonosis in cats: eight cases (1985-1992), *J Am Vet Med Assoc* 205:455, 1994.

42. Birkenheuer AJ, Levy MG, Breitschwerdt EB: Efficacy of combined atovaquone and azithromycin for therapy of chronic *Babesia gibsoni* (Asian genotype) infections in dogs, *J Vet Intern Med* 18:494, 2004.

43. Raju M, Salazar JC, Leopold H, et al: Atovaquone and azithromycin treatment for babesiosis in an infant, *Pediatr Infect Dis J* 26:181, 2007.

44. Birkenheuer AJ, Cohn LA, Levy MG, et al: Atovaquone and azithromycin for the treatment of *Cytauxzoon felis*, *J Vet Intern Med* 22:703 (abstract), 2008.

45. Sharma S, Pathak S: Malaria vaccine: a current perspective, *J Vector Borne Dis* 45:1, 2008.

5 Upper Respiratory Tract Aspergillosis

Vanessa R.D. Barrs and Julia A. Beatty

Although most small animal practitioners will be familiar with the clinical syndrome of canine sinonasal aspergillosis (SNA), little information has been available regarding aspergillosis affecting the upper respiratory tract (URT) of cats. Informative recent studies have highlighted major species differences that have implications for the recognition and treatment of this disease in this species. In cats, URT aspergillosis often is much more aggressive than its canine counterpart.

Although some cats present with SNA characterized by sneezing and nasal discharge, there is a propensity for the infection to extend beyond the sinonasal cavity to involve adjacent structures including the orbit, palate, nasopharynx, and cribriform plate. Therefore the first presenting signs of URT aspergillosis in cats may be referable to orbital invasion resulting in sino-orbital aspergillosis (SOA), which can be considered a progression from SNA.

Clinical signs in SOA are the result of an invasive retrobulbar fungal granuloma and include exophthalmos, prolapse of the nictitating membrane, exposure keratitis, a lesion (mass or ulcer) in the pterygopalatine fossa, and stertor.

The fungal pathogens identified in the majority of feline cases, *Neosartorya* spp., are related to, but distinct from, the major canine pathogen, *Aspergillus fumigatus*. Until more information is available on the most effective treatment for feline aspergillosis, the prognosis remains guarded, especially for SOA. Topical antifungal triazole therapy using clotrimazole infusions in combination with an oral antifungal triazole is recommended for early SNA. In all other cases, systemic antifungal therapy using combinations of triazoles, amphotericin B, and terbinafine is indicated.

ETIOLOGY

Until recently, reports of feline URT aspergillosis have been limited, describing infections in a total of 13 cats.[1-9] The affected cats presented with signs referable to sinonasal cavity infection (eight cases) or sino-orbital infection (five cases). The fungal pathogen often was not identified in these reports, because either fungal culture was negative or was not performed. In five cases in which fungal culture was positive, isolates were proposed to be *Aspergillus* spp. in four cases and *Penicillium* spp. in another.[1,2,6,8,9] Identification to species level based on morphological and cultural characteristics was performed in only two cases, in which *A. fumigatus* and *A. niger* were documented.[8,9]

In 2006 three cases of feline URT aspergillosis were diagnosed at the authors' institution. This prompted a search of our medical records, which identified only three cases in the preceding 19-year period (January 1986 to December 2005). Following publication of a description of the syndrome of SOA and a call for cases, we actively recruited 15 additional cases for prospective study between 2007 and 2008.[10] Clinicopathological data from the resulting cohort of 21 cats from Eastern Australia provide exciting new information on this disease in cats.[11] Fungal pathogens were cultured readily. Culture was attempted in all 21 cases and was positive in 20.

Sabouraud's dextrose agar was used with addition of gentamicin and chloramphenicol when bacterial contamination of diagnostic samples was suspected. Cultures were incubated at 37° C and 28° C. On the basis of colony morphology, *A. fumigatus* was the most common isolate identified in this cohort. However, it is important to understand that the correct identification of some species of fungi belonging to *Aspergillus* section *Fumigati* can not be achieved using morphological and cultural characteristics alone.[12,13] Therefore molecular diagnostics were performed on the fungal cultures and/or on formalin-fixed paraffin embedded (PE) or fresh tissues from affected cats to confirm the identity of the isolates. A panfungal polymerase chain reaction (PCR) that amplifies the internal transcribed spacer 1 (ITS1) region of the ribosomal DNA gene cluster between the 18S and 5.8S rRNA genes was used for PE or fresh tissues. A second panfungal PCR that targets a larger region of the rDNA gene cluster including the ITS1, 5.8S gene, and ITS2 regions was carried out on material obtained from fungal culture. These regions of the fungal genome were chosen because they are multicopy ($\geq$ 100 copies in the fungal genome) and because they contain highly variable regions facilitating species identification in some cases. PCR products were sequenced and compared with those in the GenBank database.[14,15]

Significantly, results of these molecular analyses indicated that the majority of feline isolates that had been identified as *A. fumigatus* based on culture morphology were actually *Neosartorya* spp. (Table 5-1). In most cases, it was not possible to classify the fungal pathogen further using the panfungal PCR because of limited sequence variation in the ITS1 region; for example, it was not possible to distinguish between *N. udagawae, N. fischeri,* and *N. aureola.* In one case, *N. pseudofischeri* was identified from PCR of both culture material and fresh tissue with 100 per cent identity to sequences in the GenBank database. In four cats, *A. fumigatus* was identified using both fungal colony morphology and PCR of culture material or tissue. In three of these cats, disease was confined to the sinonasal cavity. PCR of fungal culture material and/or tissue obtained from seven canine SNA cases also was carried out and identified *A. fumigatus* in all cases.[14] These findings suggest that *A. fumigatus* possibly may be associated with less invasive disease. Our experience has demonstrated that, unlike SNA in dogs, the most common isolates in URT aspergillosis in cats are *Neosartorya* spp. and that molecular diagnostic tests are required for the correct identification of these fungal pathogens.

CLASSIFICATION OF FUNGAL PATHOGENS

Both *Aspergillus* spp. and *Neosartorya* spp. are implicated as fungal pathogens in feline URT aspergillosis. These two genera are very closely related, and a brief review of their taxonomy is pertinent. Both are classified within *Aspergillus* section *Fumigati.* These ubiquitous, filamentous, saprophytic ascomycetes are distributed primarily in soil and decaying vegetation.[16] Confusion may arise over nomenclature because fungi can exist in different physical states corresponding to different stages of the life cycle; the anamorphic, asexual stage typically is moldlike and bears conidia (spores), whereas the teleomorphic, sexual stage is characterized by the production of fruiting bodies (cleistothecia) containing ascospores. The total organism is referred to as the *holomorph.* Some *Aspergillus* species are strictly anamorphic and therefore reproduce by asexual means only. Teleomorphic species within *Aspergillus* section *Fumigati* have been assigned to the genus *Neosartorya. Aspergillus* section *Fumigati* currently includes 9 strictly anamorphic *Aspergillus* spp. and 24 *Neosartorya* spp.[16,17] *Aspergillus fumigatus,* previously thought to be strictly anamorphic, was shown recently to have a fully functional sexual reproductive cycle that leads to the production of cleistothecia and ascospores. Its teleomorph is *Neosartorya fumigata.*[17a]

Species implicated in feline URT aspergillosis are listed in Table 5-2. *Neosartorya* spp. can exist in both anamorphic and teleomorphic states. The anamorphic states of some *Neosartorya* spp. can be mistaken for *A. fumigatus,* if identification is based on phenotypic characteristics such as thermotolerance and conidiophore morphology.[13,14] Phenotypic identification of *Neosartorya* spp. can be achieved partially from its teleomorph, including mor-

Table 5-1 Comparison of Fungal Culture Morphology versus PCR of Fungal Culture and/or Formalin-Fixed Paraffin-Embedded Tissues (PE) or Fresh Tissue for Fungus Identification (ID) in 18 Cases

Number of Cases	SOA or SNA	Fungal Culture Morphology ID	PCR of Fungal Culture ID	PCR of PE or Fresh Tissue ID
1	SNA	*A. fumigatus*	ND	*A. fumigatus*
3	SNA (2) SOA (1)	*A. fumigatus*	*A. fumigatus*	ND
1	SNA	*A. fumigatus*	*N. fischeri/ N. aureola / N. udagawae*	ND
1	SOA	Negative	ND	*A. lentulus/Neosartorya* spp.
1	SOA	*A. fumigatus*	*N. pseudofischeri*	*N. pseudofischeri*
12	SOA	*A. fumigatus*	*N. fischeri/ N. aureola / N. udagawae*	ND (n = 7) Negative (n = 2) *A. lentulus/N. fischeri* (n = 2)

phology of ascospores. However, induction of the teleomorphic state of *Neosartorya* spp. to produce these fruiting bodies can be achieved only under specific growth conditions with specialized media. Even under optimal conditions, some species may not produce fruiting bodies in the laboratory.[14] Because of these limitations for species identification using morphological criteria alone, a polyphasic taxonomic approach is recommended for identification of species within *Aspergillus* section *Fumigati*. This involves a combination of macromorphology and micromorphology, extrolite (fungal metabolite) profiles, and

Table 5-2 Species Belonging to *Aspergillus* Section *Fumigati* that Have Been Implicated in Feline Sinonasal and Sino-orbital Aspergillosis[16]

Strict Anamorphic Species	Teleomorph
Aspergillus lentulus	None
Aspergillus viridinutans	

Anamorph	Teleomorphic Species
Aspergillus aureoluteus	*Neosartorya aureola*
Aspergillus fischeranus	*Neosartorya fischeri*
Aspergillus fumigatus	*Neosartorya fumigata*
Aspergillus thermomutatus	*Neosartorya pseudofischeri*
Aspergillus udagawae	*Neosartorya udagawae*

PCR determination of gene sequences including β-tubulin, calmodulin, ITS, and actin.[16,18] The phylogenetic relatedness of species belonging to *Aspergillus* section *Fumigati*, including pathogens implicated in feline URT aspergillosis based on β-tubulin sequence data, is depicted in Figure 5-1.

EPIDEMIOLOGY AND RISK FACTORS

No age or sex predilection for feline URT aspergillosis is apparent. Disease has been reported in 15 females and 18 males; most were neutered. The median and mean age at diagnosis was 6 years, with a range from 18 months to 13 years.[1-9,11] An intriguing finding is the preponderance of brachycephalic cats affected; sixteen of 34 cases were brachycephalic, including eight Persians and six Himalayans. This contrasts starkly with canine SNA, in which dolichocephalic or mesocephalic breeds are typically affected.[19] The basis for this potential brachycephalic breed association in cats is not clear. Impaired drainage of URT secretions due to brachycephalic conformation may be important. Certainly, decreased sinus aeration and drainage of respiratory secretions secondary to infection, polyps, and allergic rhinosinusitis have been identified as risk factors for invasive SNA aspergillosis in human beings.[20] It is likely that additional risk factors are present in brachycephalic cats because brachycephalic dogs are

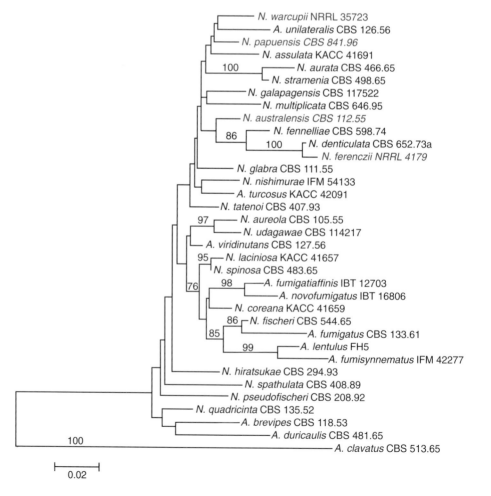

Figure 5-1 Based on β-tubulin sequence data, the phylogenetic relatedness of species belonging to *Aspergillus* section *Fumigati,* including pathogens implicated in feline upper respiratory aspergillosis is depicted.

underrepresented for SNA. These factors may include heritable defects in mucosal immunity or common environmental factors such as antecedent URT infection. Previous viral URT infection by feline calicivirus (FCV) or feline herpesvirus-1 (FHV) has been suggested as a possible risk factor for aspergillosis in cats.[7] In particular, chronic FHV infection can alter sinonasal cavity architecture severely because of turbinate lysis secondary to intense inflammation, resulting in altered local mucosal defense mechanisms. Six of 20 cats in one study had a history of chronic recurrent rhinosinusitis before aspergillosis was diagnosed, and FHV infection was confirmed by PCR in one cat.[11] Other possible risk factors identified were craniofacial trauma, diabetes mellitus, and a grass seed foreign body. There is no evidence currently of a retroviral association with feline URT aspergillosis; of 19 cats with aspergillosis tested for feline leukemia virus (FeLV) antigen, only one was positive, and all 19 cats tested for feline immunodeficiency virus (FIV) were seronegative.[3,5-9,11] Therefore it appears that URT aspergillosis in cats occurs in apparently systemically immunocompetent individuals, some of whom have identifiable breaches in local defense mechanisms.

Information on the prevalence and geographic distribution of feline URT aspergillosis is incomplete but is likely to be forthcoming now that the syndrome of SOA has been described.[10] The apparent increased prevalence at our institution is likely a consequence of increased recognition of cases. Cases have been reported most commonly in Eastern Australia (including 12 cats domiciled in New South Wales, two in Victoria, and seven in Queensland) and the United States, with individual cases from Switzerland and the United Kingdom.[1-3,5-9,11]

PATHOGENESIS

Aspergillus spp. and *Neosartorya* spp. are ubiquitous and their spores are inhaled readily. *Aspergillus* spp. can cause localized sinusitis in immunocompetent human beings or severe systemic disease as an opportunistic pathogen in immunocompromised human patients. *Neosartorya* spp. have been associated only rarely with disease; isolated cases of invasive pulmonary infection, osteomyelitis, endocarditis, peritonitis, and mycotic keratitis have been described in immunocompromised human beings.[13] The difficulty in distinguishing *A. fumigatus* from *Neosartorya* spp. using morphological criteria is likely to have resulted in underestimation of the frequency of disease caused by *Neosartorya* spp.[13]

Compared to SNA in dogs in whom fungal infection generally is confined to the sinonasal cavity, infection in cats appears to have a greater tendency to local invasion, with extension to involve the orbit. Of the 34 reported cases, 14 cats had SNA and 20 had SOA.* A brief consideration of mycotic rhinosinusitis syndromes in human beings has comparative significance because these syndromes can be either invasive or noninvasive. Invasive mycoses include acute (necrotizing) invasive fungal

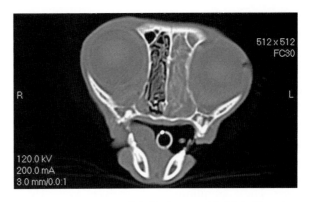

Figure 5-2 Transverse CT of skull of a cat with SOA. There is a right retrobulbar mass and diffuse opacification of the left nasal cavity. Punctate areas of lysis are visible in the right orbital lamina.

sinusitis, chronic invasive fungal sinusitis, and chronic granulomatous fungal rhinosinusitis. Noninvasive infections include fungal ball or sinus aspergilloma, allergic fungal sinusitis, and chronic erosive noninvasive fungal sinusitis.[21-24] Canine SNA bears many similarities to chronic erosive noninvasive fungal sinusitis in human patients and recently has been proposed as a model for studying the immunopathogenesis of disease in people.[24] *A. fumigatus* is the most common pathogen in dogs, although *A. niger*, *A. nidulans*, and *A. flavus* are implicated occasionally. *A. fumigatus* or *A. flavus* are isolated most commonly from human patients.[19,22,24] Neither dogs nor human beings with this type of SNA are immunocompromised systemically. Fungal hyphae do not invade the nasal mucosa and typically are present within overlying superficial necrotic plaques. There is a mixed mononuclear inflammatory response within the often ulcerated nasal mucosa that contains lymphocytes and plasma cells predominantly, with some macrophages.[19,21,22]

Like SNA in dogs, infection in cats starts almost certainly in the sinonasal cavity. It is likely that SNA and SOA in cats represent a spectrum of disease, with SOA being a manifestation of more chronic, invasive infection and progression from SNA. Progression from SNA to SOA has been documented in individual cases.[6] However, not all cases of SNA progress to SOA. Virulence factors of the fungal pathogen, including toxic secondary metabolites, are likely to be involved. Gliotoxin is considered an important virulence factor in invasive aspergillosis in human patients. All 20 cases of SOA in cats showed evidence of sinonasal cavity involvement on diagnostic imaging or at necropsy.* The orbital lamina, situated between the orbit and frontal sinus, is the most likely region where extension of infection from the sinonasal cavity to the orbit occurs. Computed tomographic (CT) examination of the skull in cases of SOA frequently identifies punctate areas of lysis in the orbital lamina (Figure 5-2). In one case of SOA, a fistula was identified at surgery in the dorsomedial aspect of the orbit, communicating with the ipsilateral frontal sinus.[11] Systemic dissemination of disease is rare. A single case of feline SOA with

---

*References 1, 2, 5, 6, 9, 11.

*References 1, 2, 5, 6, 9, 11.

concurrent pulmonary involvement has been reported. The retroviral status of that cat was unknown.[1]

SOA in cats bears a striking clinical and histological resemblance to chronic granulomatous sinusitis in people. The latter is an invasive mycosis caused by *A. flavus* or *A. fumigatus* that occurs in immunocompetent human beings subjected to hot, dry environmental conditions and poor hygiene. Most cases have been reported in Asia and Africa, predominantly in agricultural workers. The nasal cavity or sinuses invariably have been implicated as the primary site of infection following inhalation of fungal spores. A fungal granuloma forms within the sinuses. These granulomas are relatively avascular, consisting of a highly cellular inflammatory infiltrate of epithelioid macrophages ("giant cells"), histiocytes, plasma cells, and fungal hyphae. They may be necrotic or fibrotic and tend to invade contiguous structures such as the orbit or brain. Unilateral exophthalmos is common at presentation.[20,23] The histological features of URT aspergillosis in cats are not fully characterized. Both lymphoplasmacytic and suppurative noninvasive rhinitis have been described for infections confined to the sinonasal cavity.[7,8] SOA is clearly invasive, and we have found evidence of submucosal infection in the sinonasal cavity of affected cats.[11] In feline SOA, the granulomas are characterized by a necrotic center containing fungal hyphae. This is surrounded by granulation tissue that may be fibrous, infiltrated with neutrophils, lymphocytes, plasma cells, and eosinophils.[1,2,9] Commonly, we have seen retrobulbar granulomas surrounding the optic nerve. They typically feature a necrotic center containing branching septate PAS-positive fungal filaments and an inflammatory infiltrate of sheeting epithelioid macrophages with variable numbers of lymphocytes, plasma cells, and neutrophils extending into a zone of peripheral fibrosis (Figure 5-3). These fungal granulomas are well vascularized and in some cases are accompanied by heavy infiltrates of eosinophils.

HISTORY AND CLINICAL SIGNS

SINONASAL ASPERGILLOSIS

In dogs, the triad of muzzle pain, profuse mucoid to hemorrhagic chronic nasal discharge and depigmentation, and crusting or ulceration of one or both nares is highly suggestive of SNA. In cats, presenting signs of SNA are less specific. Most affected cats will have a history of sneezing and a unilateral or bilateral serous to mucopurulent nasal discharge that usually can be detected on physical examination (Figure 5-4). Intermittent epistaxis occurs in 40 per cent of cats with SNA. Interestingly, and in contrast to dogs, neither nasal depigmentation nor ulceration has been documented to date in cats with SNA. A discharging sinus or soft tissue mass may be identified overlying the frontal sinus or the nasal bone as a result of bony lysis and fungal proliferation (Figure 5-5). Facial distortion may be a feature.

Owners should be questioned specifically regarding any URT noise because this may be subtle, and the pattern of respiration should be evaluated carefully on physical examination. If it can be established that the cat has a stertor, at least part of the disease process can be localized to the caudal nasal cavity and/or nasopharynx. The stertor in SNA may result from excessive nasal secretions and/or a mass lesion in the caudal nasal cavity and/or nasopharynx (Table 5-3).

SINO-ORBITAL ASPERGILLOSIS

Although most cats with SOA have a history of sneezing or nasal discharge in the 6 months prior to presentation, it is important to note that, at the time of presentation, nasal signs may be subtle or absent. Rather, cats with SOA present typically with a constellation of clinical signs

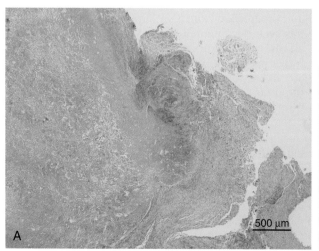
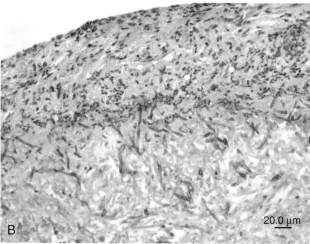

Figure 5-3 Histological examination of a retrobulbar fungal granuloma from a cat with SOA. **A,** Low magnification. **B,** High magnification. Within the necrotic center are branching, septate PAS-positive fungal filaments, surrounded by an inflammatory infiltrate of sheeting epithelioid macrophages with variable numbers of lymphocytes, plasma cells, and neutrophils, extending into a zone of peripheral fibrosis.

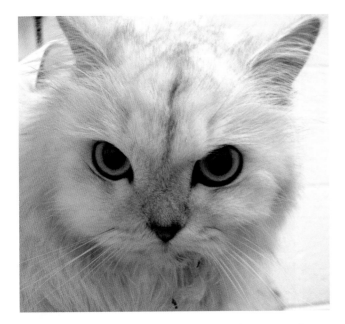

Figure 5-4 The presenting complaint in this Persian cat with SNA was sneezing and unilateral right nasal discharge.

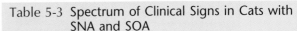

Table 5-3 Spectrum of Clinical Signs in Cats with SNA and SOA

Clinical Presentation	Clinical Signs
Sinonasal aspergillosis	Nasal discharge Discharging sinus/mass over frontal sinus or nasal bone Stertor Epistaxis
Sino-orbital aspergillosis	Exophthalmos Corneal ulceration Conjunctival hyperemia Mass or ulcer, pterygopalatine fossa Ulceration of hard palate Discharging sinus over frontal sinus Mandibular lymph node enlarged Stertor Pyrexia (temp > 39.3° C)

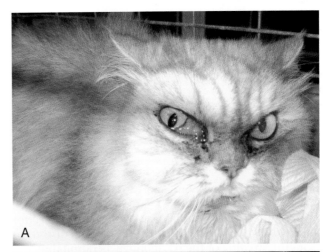

Figure 5-5 In addition to nasal discharge and sneezing, this cat with SNA had a discharging sinus over the left frontal sinus.

referable to invasive expansion of a fungal granuloma in the ventromedial orbit. These include unilateral exophthalmos with third eyelid prolapse, exposure keratitis and conjunctival hyperemia (Figure 5-6), and a mass or ulcer in the ipsilateral pterygopalatine fossa behind the last molar tooth (Figure 5-7). Stertor also is common. In the majority of affected cats, exophthalmos is unilateral, but in severe, chronic infections, bilateral exophthalmos can occur. Pain on opening the mouth typically is not present. In one cat with confirmed fungal sinusitis, marked unilateral exophthalmos resulted from retrobulbar myofasciitis rather than from a fungal granuloma.[5] Invasion

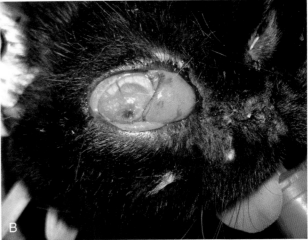

Figure 5-6 Unilateral exophthalmos with **A,** prolapse of the third eyelid, and **B,** deep corneal ulceration, in two cats with SOA.

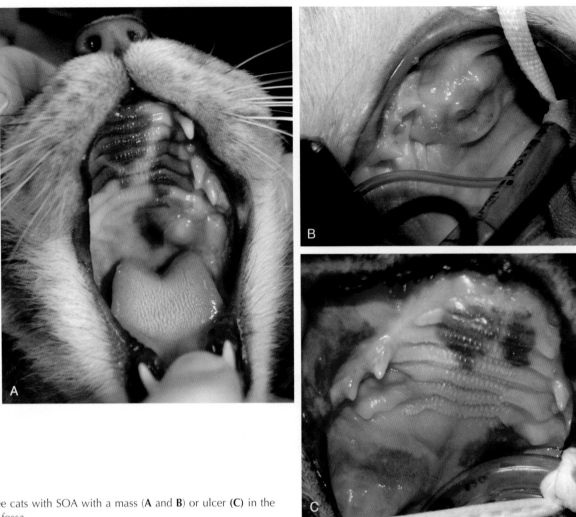

Figure 5-7 Three cats with SOA with a mass (**A** and **B**) or ulcer (**C**) in the pterygopalatine fossa.

through the palatine bone can cause ulceration of the hard palate (Figure 5-8).

In addition to exophthalmos, extension of infection outside the sinonasal cavity can result in facial distortion, including swelling of the nasal bridge, periorbital tissues, and soft tissues adjacent the maxilla (Figure 5-9). Neurological signs can develop subsequent to invasion of the central nervous system (CNS) through the cribriform plate or sphenoid sinus. One cat with intracranial extension of disease from the sphenoid sinus had hyperesthesia and blindness due to involvement of the optic chiasm.[11] Submandibular lymph node enlargement and pyrexia also are common at presentation (see Table 5-3). In contrast, cats with SNA usually are not pyrexic.

DIFFERENTIAL DIAGNOSIS

The differential diagnoses for URT aspergillosis depend on whether cats present with signs referable to sinonasal cavity infection or to orbital infection, or both. For cats presenting with chronic nasal discharge and sneezing, many infectious, inflammatory, neoplastic, and other causes are possible (Box 5-1). Consideration should be

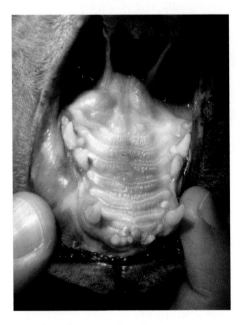

Figure 5-8 Invasion of a retrobulbar fungal granuloma through the palatine bone has resulted in ulceration of the hard palate and a mass in the left pterygopalatine fossa.

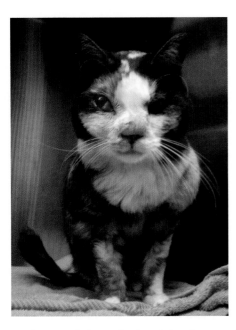

Figure 5-9 Right exophthalmos, third eyelid prolapse, and facial distortion including swelling of the nasal bridge and maxillary soft tissues in a cat with SOA.

given to the age and breed of the cat to help rank differential diagnoses. Brachycephalic conformation should increase suspicion for SNA, although these cats also are overrepresented for viral URT infections. When epistaxis is reported, ulcerative rhinitis, neoplasia, or mycotic rhinitis are more likely. Because secondary bacterial rhinitis is common, a transient response to antimicrobial therapy does not exclude mycotic rhinitis or neoplasia. Although our experience suggests that feline URT aspergillosis is more common than thought previously, cryptococcosis remains the most commonly described cause of mycotic rhinitis. For cats with stertor and suspected nasopharyngeal mass lesions, nasopharyngeal polyps and cryptococcosis are common inflammatory causes, while lymphoma is the most common neoplastic cause.[25]

The syndrome of clinical signs present in cats with SOA could occur with other expansive infectious or neoplastic processes occurring within the orbit. Inability to retropulse the exophthalmic globe enables differentiation from buphthalmos or abnormal enlargement of the globe. The differential diagnoses for retrobulbar mass lesions are listed in Box 5-2. Direct extension of any of these processes to involve the sinonasal cavity could result in concurrent nasal discharge, sneezing, and/or epistaxis. For example, orbital lymphoma may be indistinguishable clinically from SOA (Figure 5-10).

DIAGNOSIS

Definitive diagnosis of URT aspergillosis in cats is achieved by cytological or histological identification of fungal hyphae in affected tissue, together with identification of the fungal pathogen using culture and a polyphasic taxonomic approach, as described previously (see section on classification of fungal pathogens). Obtaining a definitive

---

Box 5-1 Differential Diagnoses of Sinonasal Cavity and Nasopharyngeal Disease in Cats

Neoplasia
  Lymphoma
  Carcinoma
  Other
Inflammatory
  Nasal/nasopharyngeal polyp
  Nasopharyngeal stenosis
Infectious
  Viral
    Feline herpesvirus-1
    Feline calicivirus
  Mycotic nasopharyngeal diseases
    Cryptococcosis
    Aspergillosis
    Phaeohyphomycosis
    Blastomycosis
    Histoplasmosis
    Trichosporonosis
    Sporotrichosis
  Bacterial infections (primary)
    Mycoplasma spp.
    Bordetella bronchiseptica
    Chlamydophila felis
    Mycobacteria spp.
    Actinomyces spp.
Foreign body
Congenital
  Choanal atresia
  Palatine defects
Dental disease
  Oronasal fistula
    Advanced periodontal disease
    Tooth root abscess
Accumulation of excessive nasal secretions

Box 5-2 Differential Diagnoses of Feline Retrobulbar Mass Lesions

Foreign body (e.g., grass awns)
Abscess (odontogenic, penetrating bite wound, hematogenous)
Orbital myofascitis (medial pterygoid muscle)
Zygomatic salivary gland and lacrimal gland disease
Mycotic granuloma
Phaeohyphomycosis
Cryptococcosis
Aspergillosis
Pythiosis
Orbital pseudotumor
Orbital fat prolapse
Neoplasia
Squamous cell carcinoma
Lymphoma
Adenocarcinoma/undifferentiated carcinoma
Fibrosarcoma
Melanoma
Osteoma/osteosarcoma

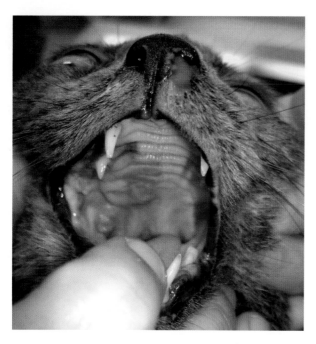

Figure 5-10 Differential diagnoses for SOA include neoplastic and infectious expansive orbital masses. This cat with right exophthalmos, purulent left nasal discharge, and an ulcerative plaque on the hard palate had orbital lymphoma.

diagnosis may require various combinations of diagnostic tests including radiography, CT, endoscopy, cytology, serology, fungal culture, and advanced mycological techniques. A stepwise diagnostic approach is recommended because there are many other differential diagnoses.

In cats with signs of sinonasal cavity disease, physical examination should include otoscopic examination to identify chronic otitis media and/or inflammatory polyps (see Chapter 30). Neurological examination is recommended because neurological sequelae such as otitis media/interna may occur with nasopharyngeal diseases and because infection can extend intracranially in cats with aspergillosis. Noninvasive investigations should be performed next, including hematology, serum biochemistries, urinalysis, serology, and thoracic radiography, to determine lower respiratory tract involvement. Retroviral serology should be performed routinely. Serological tests for aspergillosis are discussed in the next section.

A latex cryptococcal antigen agglutination test (LCAT) should be performed to exclude cryptococcal rhinitis. This test is sensitive and specific for the diagnosis of cryptococcosis. Fungal culture of superficial swabs from the rostral nasal cavity or nasal discharge is not recommended as a stand-alone test for the diagnosis of aspergillosis or cryptococcosis because these fungi may be contaminants or asymptomatic colonizers in this location.[26,27] However, isolation of *Cryptococcus* spp. in a patient with a positive LCAT or with cytological or histopathological evidence of infection is highly significant.

Bacterial culture of superficial nasal swabs rarely is rewarding due to the presence of normal flora and because bacterial rhinitis usually occurs secondary to an underlying disease. For cats with suspected viral URT infection,

confirmatory tests including virus isolation, immuno-fluorescence, enzyme-linked immunosorbent assay (ELISA), or PCR can be performed using oropharyngeal or conjunctival swabs. When enlarged local lymph nodes or facial soft tissue masses are identified, they should be aspirated for cytological examination and culture. For cats presenting with exophthalmos, diagnostic investigation should include fluorescein staining of the cornea, retinal fundic examination, and evaluation of the orbit, in addition to investigation of the sinonasal cavity. Transocular ultrasonography is an expedient tool for confirmation of a retrobulbar mass. The next step of the investigation, incorporating diagnostic imaging, endoscopic examination of the sinonasal cavity, and biopsy collection is performed with the patient anesthetized.

RESULTS OF DIAGNOSTIC INVESTIGATIONS FOR CATS WITH URT ASPERGILLOSIS

Hematology and Serum Biochemistries
Results of complete blood counts and serum biochemistry profiles usually are unremarkable or they may reflect inflammation: for example, an inflammatory leukogram and hyperglobulinemia.[6,9,11] Establishing pretreatment renal function and baseline liver enzyme values is important, because nephrotoxicity and hepatotoxicity are common with some antifungal drugs (see treatment).

Serology
Serological tests for aspergillosis include detection of serum anti-*Aspergillus* antibodies or detection of *Aspergillus* antigen. Use of the former test has been described as an adjunct to the diagnosis of SNA in dogs. Antibodies can be detected by three methods; counterimmunoelectrophoresis (CIE), agar gel immunodiffusion (AGID), or ELISA. The AGID test, based on the principle of double diffusion, is used most commonly. In recent studies using a commercially available standardized purified aspergillin composed of *A. fumigatus, A. niger,* and *A. flavus,* the sensitivity of AGID was found to be good (67 to 77 per cent) and the specificity was excellent in dogs (97 to 100 per cent).[27,28] The ELISA has the advantage of quantification of serum immunoglobulins and, using the same antigen preparation as the AGID, has good sensitivity and excellent specificity.[28] There is little information on the diagnostic utility of serum anti-*Aspergillus* antibody detection in URT aspergillosis in cats and specificity has not been evaluated. Two of three cats with SNA tested positive for serum antibodies against *A. fumigatus* using CIE, and another cat with SNA tested positive using AGID.[3,7]

Galactomannan (GM) is a water-soluble polysaccharide cell wall component of *Aspergillus* and some other fungal species that is released in variable quantities during hyphal growth in tissues. This antigen can be detected in the serum of human patients with invasive *Aspergillus* infections using a commercially available sandwich ELISA (Platelia *Aspergillus*). GM antigen levels correlate with the tissue fungal burden and can be used to monitor clinical outcome and response to therapy. Rising GM levels are often associated with treatment failures in human patients.[29] There are limitations to the use of the GM ELISA in patients with invasive aspergillosis. For example, false-positive results can occur following treatment with β-lactam antibiotics due to contamination with cell wall components of *Penicillium* spp. during drug production. The sensitivity of the GM ELISA varies considerably with immune status. In profoundly immunocompromised patients, sensitivity is greater than 90 per cent, while in less immunocompromised patients, sensitivity may be as low as 30 per cent. This is partly due to a lower fungal burden in the latter group. Further, concurrent antifungal therapy may delay detection of GM and result in lower GM levels due to decreased fungal load.[29] This same commercially available ELISA has been evaluated in dogs and was found to be unreliable for the diagnosis of SNA.[28] A GM optical density (OD) index of greater than 0.5 was considered to be positive. This is the accepted standard for diagnosis of invasive aspergillosis in human beings and the standard recommended by the manufacturer. Test results were positive in 24 per cent of dogs with SNA, 11 per cent of dogs with nasal tumors, 9 per cent of dogs with lymphoplasmacytic rhinitis, and 24 per cent of control dogs.[28] Given that SNA in dogs is noninvasive, the low sensitivity is hardly surprising. Reasons for poor specificity were not identified; concomitant use of β-lactam antimicrobials was found to have a negligible influence on results in dogs.

The use of GM assays for diagnosis and monitoring of feline aspergillosis has not been evaluated. GM was measured in six of our culture-positive cases using the Platelia *Aspergillus* assay. Using a cut-off value of 0.5, three cats with SOA were negative (GM OD index 0.11 to 0.34), one cat with SNA was positive at 20.98, and two cats with SOA were positive at 18.22 and 3.82. In the latter case, in whom combination antifungal treatment using amphotericin B, posaconazole, and terbinafine failed, the GM OD index increased subsequently to 14.83. Further studies are underway to investigate the use of GM assay in diagnosis and monitoring of therapy in cats with URT aspergillosis.

Diagnostic Imaging—Radiography, CT, and Ultrasonography

Imaging studies should be performed prior to more invasive diagnostic procedures including rhinoscopy and biopsy because any resultant inflammation or hemorrhage may obscure subtle lesions and induce imaging abnormalities. For cats presenting with exophthalmos, transocular ultrasonography is recommended to identify retrobulbar mass lesions (Figure 5-11). For further investigation of suspected sinonasal cavity or sino-orbital disease, CT is the diagnostic imaging modality of choice. Both CT and magnetic resonance imaging (MRI) have the advantage over conventional radiography of cross-sectional imaging. Other advantages of CT over conventional radiography demonstrated in dogs with SNA include increased diagnostic sensitivity, ability to adjust the contrast scale to optimize optical density and discriminate fine turbinate structures, and better evaluation of the cribriform plate using multiplanar reconstructions.[30,31] CT generally is superior to MRI for the evaluation of destructive lesions in bony structures contiguous

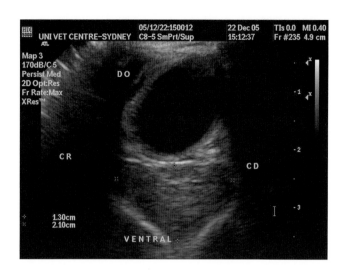

Figure 5-11 Transocular ultrasound of a cat with a retrobulbar fungal granuloma, 10 MHz linear probe.

with the sinonasal cavity. In cats with suspected intracranial extension of infection, MRI after intravenous contrast administration is superior to CT for evaluation of intracranial soft tissues.

Regardless of which imaging modality is used, the nasal cavity, nasopharynx, frontal sinuses, and tympanic bullae should be evaluated routinely. In patients with nasopharyngeal mass lesions, occlusion of the auditory tubes can result in secondary bullous effusion, which may be asymptomatic.[32] If radiography is used, views should include lateral skull, ventrodorsal skull, dorsoventral occlusal view or open-mouth ventrodorsal view, and rostrocaudal open-mouth or rostral 10° ventrocaudodorsal oblique views. Findings on radiography in cats with SNA and SOA include destructive rhinitis, lysis of paranasal bones, and focal increased soft tissue opacities.[3,7]

We have performed CT on 10 cats with URT aspergillosis, including three with SNA and seven with SOA. Our findings are summarized in Table 5-4. The most common findings were punctate lysis of the orbital lamina (see Figure 5-2), opacification of the sphenoid and frontal sinuses due to fluid or soft tissue (Figure 5-12), and a soft tissue mass in the choanae or nasopharynx. Eight of the 10 cases had punctate lysis of the orbital lamina, including two of three cases of SNA. Of the seven cases of SOA, six had an orbital mass, and in one case the CT was performed after exenteration of the orbit. There was irregular enhancement of the orbital mass in all cases after intravenous contrast administration (Figure 5-13). Orbital masses were present in the ventromedial aspect of the orbit, causing lateral and dorsal displacement of the globe. In five cats with SOA, there was a mass effect involving the soft tissues adjacent the maxilla, and four cats had soft tissue palatine masses. Punctate lysis of the cribriform plate was seen in two cases, one cat with SNA and one with SOA (Figure 5-14). Thickening of the mucosa adjacent to the inner surface of the bones of the frontal sinus, a typical finding in canine SNA, was seen in three cats, one with SNA and two with SOA (Figure

Table 5-4 Computed Tomographic Findings in 10 Cases of Feline URT Aspergillosis

Structure	Lysis	Sclerosis	Soft Tissue or Fluid Density	Thickened Mucosa	Soft Tissue Mass
Turbinates	5		3	4	
Maxilla	4				5
Palate	3				4
Cribriform plate	2				
Orbital lamina	8				
Frontal sinus and frontal bone		2	7	3	
Sphenoid sinus			7		
Septum	2				
Cribriform plate	2				
Nasopharynx/choanae					7
Orbit			1		6

Data from three cats with SNA and seven with SOA. In one case, CT was performed after exenteration of the globe.[11] Sinonasal abnormalities were unilateral in three cases and bilateral in seven cases.

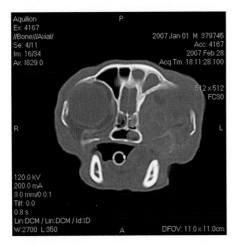

Figure 5-12 Transverse CT of skull. Opacification of the sphenoid and left frontal sinuses and nasopharyngeal mass in a cat with an expansive left orbital fungal granuloma.

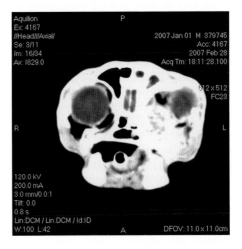

Figure 5-13 Postcontrast CT of cat in figure 5-12 showing irregular enhancement of the left orbital mass.

5-15).[30,31] There was evidence of unilateral sinonasal cavity involvement in three cases and of bilateral disease in seven affected cats. The tympanic bullae were normal in all cases. CT findings in previously reported cases (six cats with SNA and three cats with SOA) were similar, except for one case of SNA in whom a free, irregular calcified mass was present in the cranial part of the right nasal cavity.[5-9] On histological examination, the mass was identified as calcified necrotic tissue containing fungal hyphae. Concretions formed from deposition of calcium oxalate or phosphate crystals within tissues occur in human patients with sinus aspergilloma.[33]

CT findings in cats with SOA are similar to those in human beings with chronic invasive fungal sinusitis and chronic granulomatous invasive fungal sinusitis.[34] On

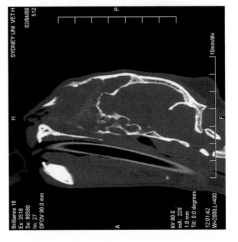

Figure 5-14 Sagittal CT skull. Punctate lysis of the cribriform plate and lysis of the nasal bone dorsally, in a cat with severe SNA.

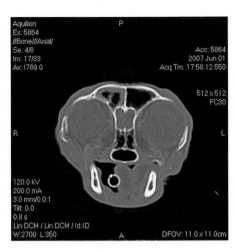

Figure 5-15 Transverse CT skull. Thickening of the mucosa adjacent to the inner surface of the bone of the left frontal sinus in a cat with SNA.

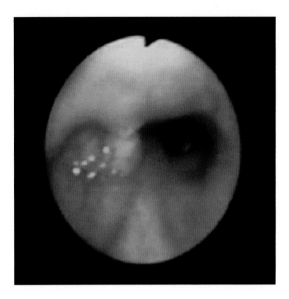

Figure 5-16 Choanal mass in a cat with SOA visualized using a retroflexed pediatric endoscope, before biopsy.

noncontrast CT in human patients, a hyperattenuating soft tissue collection, sometimes masslike, within one or more paranasal sinuses is typical. There may be destruction of sinus walls and extension into adjacent tissues. In both human beings and cats with URT aspergillosis, differentiation of invasive mycotic disease from malignant neoplasia may not be possible from imaging findings alone. On CT, destruction of maxillary turbinates is seen commonly in cats with inflammatory or neoplastic sinonasal disease.[35] Severe destruction of both maxillary turbinates and ethmoturbinates, particularly when unilateral, and/or lysis of paranasal bones have been considered more predictive of sinonasal neoplasia than of inflammatory disease.[35] However, there were no cases of mycotic rhinitis in the inflammatory disease group in that study. Many findings that were significantly associated with neoplasia are common in cats with URT aspergillosis, including unilateral lysis of ethmoturbinates, unilateral lysis of the maxilla, lysis of the vomer bone, lysis of the orbital lamina, and unilateral soft tissue or fluid within the sphenoid sinus, frontal sinus, and/or retrobulbar space.[35]

Collection of Diagnostic Biopsies

Nasopharyngoscopy and rhinoscopy are performed next to visualize the nasopharynx and nasal cavity and to obtain biopsy specimens for cytological and histological examination and culture. We freeze additional biopsy specimens routinely at this time. These samples can be retrieved for PCR if fungal hyphae are seen in tissues but fungal culture is negative. Because many cats with both SNA and SOA have granulomatous mass lesions containing fungal hyphae within the choanae or nasopharynx, retroflexed endoscopy using a pediatric bronchoscope often is rewarding (Figure 5-16). Masses in this location can be biopsied using endoscopic biopsy forceps. During nasopharyngeal endoscopy, each ventral nasal meatus is catheterized via the naris with a urinary catheter (size 5 or 6 French gauge) to check patency and to help dislodge foreign material or masses. Regional anesthesia of the pharynx with 2 per cent topical lidocaine gel and maxil-

lary nerve blocks using 0.5 per cent bupivacaine facilitates a decreased plane of general anesthesia in some cats during nasopharyngeal endoscopy.

The rostral nasal cavity can be evaluated using rigid rhinoscopy to visualize turbinate destruction and fungal plaques. Rhinoscopes with constant irrigation systems that enable biopsies to be taken during direct examination are preferred because fungal plaques could be missed during blind collection.

Nasal cavity lavage may yield larger biopsy specimens than can be acquired endoscopically. Vigorous saline flushing from the nasal cavities into the nasopharynx is useful to dislodge foreign bodies and diagnostic fragments of friable tumors such as lymphoma or granulomas. A cuffed endotracheal tube should be used. The pharynx is packed with sterile swabs to trap flushed material. A 10-mL aliquot of sterile saline is flushed briskly through one naris into the ventral nasal meatus while occluding the other naris. The procedure is repeated several times on each side. Culture of lavage fluid usually returns nonspecific results.

For cats with SOA, fine-needle biopsies of retrobulbar masses can be obtained under ultrasound guidance or via the oral cavity. CT-guided biopsies and aspirates also have been described.[9] CT is useful to identify involvement of paranasal subcutaneous soft tissues and sinuses. The former can be biopsied surgically, and the latter can be accessed via sinus trephination. When sinus involvement is identified and diagnostic biopsies can not be collected during rhinoscopy or nasopharyngeal endoscopy, sinus trephination using a Jacob chuck and intramedullary pin (3.2 to 4 mm diameter) enables endoscopic examination of the lateral compartment of the frontal sinuses and ready access to material for culture, histology, and PCR. This procedure should be performed with caution in brachycephalic cats because they have shallow sinuses in close proximity to the cranial vault.

TREATMENT AND PROGNOSIS

ANTIFUNGAL SUSCEPTIBILITY TESTING

The typical antifungal susceptibility profile of *Neosartorya* spp. isolated from cats with aspergillosis includes susceptibility to amphotericin B and posaconazole, intermediate or dose-dependent susceptibility to itraconazole and voriconazole, and resistance to 5-flucytosine, ketoconazole, and fluconazole.[11] In contrast, both voriconazole and posaconazole typically have greater activity than itraconazole in vitro against both *A. fumigatus* and other *Aspergillus* spp.[36] Interestingly, elevated minimum inhibitory concentrations (MICs) of voriconazole to *Neosartorya* spp. have been documented elsewhere.[13] However, the correlation between in vitro antifungal susceptibility test results and in vivo response to therapy is only modest at best. Other factors that influence antifungal activity in vivo include drug pharmacokinetics (e.g., stability, metabolism, drug interactions, protein binding, metabolites, tissue penetration), host factors (e.g., immune status, underlying disease), site of infection (e.g., presence of foreign body, source of infection), and virulence factors of the fungal pathogen.[37] Further, in vitro results are influenced by technical factors including the concentration of the fungal inoculum, the composition and pH of the medium, incubation temperature, and duration of incubation.

SYSTEMIC ANTIFUNGAL THERAPY

For treatment of invasive aspergillosis in human beings, voriconazole has replaced amphotericin B as the drug of choice for first-line therapy. Posaconazole is used for antifungal prophylaxis in high-risk patients and for salvage therapy. The echinocandins are reserved for salvage therapy or combination antifungal therapy for refractory invasive aspergillosis.[38] Combination antifungal therapy may provide enhanced efficacy compared to single-drug therapy for treatment of invasive aspergillosis. This concept has been controversial because in previous studies, when mice with invasive aspergillosis were treated with ketoconazole prior to amphotericin B, there was a marked decrease in the efficacy of the latter drug. It was proposed that the azole blocked the synthesis of the ergosterol target necessary for the binding of amphotericin B. Antagonism between itraconazole and amphotericin B also has been demonstrated in vitro against isolates of *A. fumigatus*.[39] However, more recently treatment of murine models of invasive aspergillosis with a triazole antifungal (voriconazole or posaconazole) and amphotericin B was not antagonistic, and treatment with liposomal amphotericin B and voriconazole in combination was significantly superior to monotherapy with either drug.[40,41]

Triazole Antifungals

Triazole antifungals, which have three nitrogen molecules in the azole ring, include fluconazole, itraconazole, voriconazole, and posaconazole. By binding to lanosterol-14α-demethylase, triazoles inhibit the synthesis of ergosterol, an essential lipid component of fungal cell walls. Fluconazole has low activity against filamentous fungi and is not recommended for treatment of aspergillosis.[42] Itraconazole has fungistatic activity against *Aspergillus,* and its pharmacological disposition has been studied in cats.[43] It is metabolized by the liver and distributed widely in body tissues other than the CNS. Oral bioavailability can be variable and is highest for capsules when administered with food and for oral solution when administered on an empty stomach. The oral solution is absorbed more effectively than capsules in cats, such that dose reduction may be necessary. Adverse effects including gastrointestinal signs and hepatotoxicity are not uncommon, are usually dose related, and resolve on cessation of therapy (Table 5-5). Voriconazole (structurally similar to fluconazole) and posaconazole (structurally similar to itraconazole) were developed as more efficacious agents for treating filamentous fungal infections and to improve on the absorption, tolerability, and drug interaction profile of itraconazole. Both voriconazole and posaconazole are fungicidal against *Aspergillus.* Their pharmacokinetics have been studied in human beings and dogs but not in cats at the time of writing.[44,45] Posaconazole is available only as a suspension for oral use. Its absorption is increased with food, especially high-fat meals, and is optimal in human patients when given as four daily divided doses. Posaconazole is metabolized in the liver by glucuronidation and is excreted primarily in bile and urine. Common adverse effects include headaches and gastrointestinal signs such as nausea, diarrhea, and vomiting. Hepatoxicity is uncommon.[42]

Posaconazole was used in the treatment of 10 cats with URT aspergillosis (see Table 5-5).[11] Inappetence and a twofold elevation in alkaline phosphatase (ALP) were seen in one cat, both of which resolved when the drug dosage was decreased. Posaconazole was well tolerated in the other nine cats and no adverse effects were recorded. Liver enzymes were within reference ranges during routine serum biochemical monitoring, which was performed at least twice in all cats. There are two other case reports describing the clinical use of posaconazole in cats for treatment of SOA and infection of the subcutis of the nose by *Mucor* species respectively. Posaconazole was well tolerated in both cases.[9,46] Voriconazole, in contrast, has 95 per cent bioavailability after oral administration in the absence of food. It is metabolized in the liver by several cytochrome P450 enzymes. In human beings, adverse effects are more common with voriconazole than with posaconazole and include visual disturbances and hepatotoxicity. Blurred vision, photophobia, and other visual changes occur in up to one third of patients treated with either IV or oral formulations. These changes often resolve in a few weeks even if therapy is continued.[42] There are no published reports of the use of oral voriconazole in cats. The authors have treated three cats with URT aspergillosis using voriconazole, two of whom showed adverse effects that resolved after drug discontinuation. One cat who had received 12 mg/kg (50 mg) daily for four doses developed anorexia and neurological

Table 5-5 Drugs Used for Treatment of Aspergillosis in Cats

Drug and Formulation	Dosage and Route of Administration	Adverse Effects
Itraconazole 100 mg capsules 10 mg/mL oral suspension (Sporanox, Janssen)	5 mg/kg PO q12h or 10 mg/kg PO q24h	Gastrointestinal—anorexia, vomiting Hepatotoxicity—increased liver enzyme activity, jaundice. Monitor ALP/ALT monthly. If hepatoxicity occurs, reduce dose to 5 mg/kg PO q24h or 10 mg/kg PO q48h
Posaconazole 40 mg/mL liquid (Noxafil, Schering-Plough)	2.5-3.75 mg/kg PO q12h	Hepatotoxicity
Voriconazole 50 mg tablets 40 mg/mL powder for oral suspension (Vfend, Pfizer)	5 mg/kg PO q24h	Neurotoxicity—blindness, ataxia, dazed
Terbinafine 250 mg tablets (Lamisil, Novartis)	30 mg/kg PO q24h	Gastrointestinal—anorexia, vomiting, diarrhea
Amphotericin B deoxycholate 50 mg vial (Fungizone, Bristol-Myers)	0.5 mg/kg of 5 mg/mL stock solution in 350 mL/cat of 0.45% NaCl + 2.5% dextrose SQ 2-3 × weekly to a cumulative dose of 10-15 mg/kg	Nephrotoxicity—pretreatment of stock solution by heating to 60° C for 5 minutes reduces nephrotoxicity. Monitor urea/creatinine every 2 weeks. Discontinue for 2-3 weeks if azotemia
Liposomal Amphotericin (AmBisome, Gilead)	1-1.5 mg/kg IV q48h to a cumulative dose of 12-15 mg/kg Given as a 1-2 mg/mL solution in 5% dextrose by IV infusion over 1-2 h	Azotemia

signs including altered mental status, dilated pupils, and hind limb ataxia. Another cat treated with 5 mg/kg daily developed behavioral changes and apparent visual impairment. A third cat was treated with 6 mg/kg daily (25 mg) for 10 days with no adverse effects.

Polyenes

Amphotericin B is a polyene macrolide antibiotic derived from the actinomycete *Streptomyces nodosus* with fungicidal activity against *Aspergillus*. Preferential binding to ergosterol in the fungal cell membrane results in altered permeability, leakage of cell components, and cell death. Amphotericin B deoxycholate must be administered parenterally, either intravenously or as a subcutaneous infusion (see Table 5-5). The major toxicity in all species is nephrotoxicity. The development of lipid formulations of amphotericin B, which are less toxic than amphotericin B deoxycholate (AMB-D), has resulted in enhanced antifungal activity because increased doses of amphotericin B can be administered with improved delivery of active drug to sites of infection. Lipid formulations of amphotericin B are concentrated in the reticuloendothelial system, and liposomal amphotericin B attains high concentrations in brain tissue. The authors have used liposomal amphotericin B (AMB-L) in cats with aspergillosis at a dosage of 1 to 1.5 mg/kg IV q48h (see Table 5-5). Although AMB-L is much less nephrotoxic than AMB-D, nephrotoxicity still can occur, and renal function should be monitored during the treatment period. AMB-D has been administered directly into the retrobulbar space in isolated cases of invasive SOA in human beings as an adjunct to surgical debridement when maximal drug doses have been given systemically.[47] In vitro and in vivo resistance to amphotericin B has been reported in one case of feline SOA.[9] In vitro resistance to amphotericin B (MIC > 2 mg/L) is rare and arises because of a mutation in the ergosterol biosynthesis pathway resulting in production of ergosterol-like compounds that have reduced binding affinity for amphotericin B.[48]

Terbinafine

Terbinafine is an allylamine antifungal. It inhibits fungal ergosterol synthesis via inhibition of the enzyme squalene mono-oxygenase, which converts squalene to ergosterol. Synergy between antifungal triazoles and terbinafine has been demonstrated against filamentous fungi in vitro.[49] To date, the main indication for terbinafine in cats has been in the treatment of dermatophytosis.[50]

Echinocandins

The echinocandins, including caspofungin, micafungin, and anidulafungin, inhibit 1,3-β-D-glucan synthesis, an essential polysaccharide cell wall component of many fungal species. The echinocandins are the most recently developed class of antifungal drug and are characterized by low toxicity and rapid fungicidal activity. They have additive or synergistic activity with amphotericin B and triazoles against filamentous fungi, including *Aspergillus*.[51] Because the oral bioavailability of echinocandins is very low, they must be administered parenterally. In human beings, they are eliminated primarily as metabolites in the urine and in the feces following degradation in the liver via nonoxidative pathways. Metabolism is thought to be independent of the cytochrome system and does not inhibit cytochrome P450 isoenzymes. The pharmacology and pharmacokinetics of echinocandins have not been studied in cats, and there are no reports of their use in this species.

THERAPEUTIC APPROACH TO SNA AND SOA IN CATS

Because of its more invasive nature, URT aspergillosis in cats is more difficult to treat than SNA in dogs. In general, treatment carries a better prognosis for SNA than SOA. The prognosis for resolution of SOA is poor.

SNA—Topical Clotrimazole Infusions

The technique of single topical sinonasal clotrimazole infusions, which has good efficacy for treatment of SNA in dogs, has been reported in three cats.[6-8] In one cat, infection was confined to the sinonasal cavity and treatment with oral itraconazole and a 1 per cent clotrimazole infusion was successful.[7] In two other cats with SOA, a clotrimazole infusion was part of a multimodal therapeutic approach. One cat was euthanized because of suspected progression of infection despite treatment with itraconazole and radical surgical debridement of the orbit, including exenteration of the globe.[6] In another cat with SOA, treatment with itraconazole, topical clotrimazole, and AMB-D did not resolve infection. However, the cat was cured after treatment with oral posaconazole administered for 16 weeks.[9] Our current recommendation is to restrict the use of topical 1 per cent clotrimazole infusions to the treatment of cats with SNA in whom there is an intact cribriform plate, no evidence of orbital involvement on CT, and no histological evidence of submucosal fungal invasion. Commercial preparations of 1 per cent clotrimazole in a polyethylene glycol base are available. Formulations that contain propylene glycol or isopropyl alcohol should be avoided because of greater potential for pharyngeal edema, as reported in dogs.[52] Concomitant systemic antifungal therapy with itraconazole or posaconazole also is recommended.

SNA—Systemic Antifungal Therapy

Antifungal triazole drugs are the mainstay of therapy and can be given alone or in combination with terbinafine or amphotericin B (see Table 5-5). Itraconazole or posaconazole are the triazoles of choice. When concurrent topical azole therapy is administered (i.e., topical clotrimazole infusion) and disease is mild, amphotericin B administration may not be necessary. Also, it should be noted that treatment with itraconazole alone has been successful occasionally in resolving SNA.[8] For cases of severe SNA in which there is evidence of lysis of the orbital lamina or cribriform plate and risk of extension of infection beyond the sinonasal cavity, we recommend concurrent administration of amphotericin B (see Table 5-5). When the course of amphotericin B is completed, therapy can be continued with the oral triazole and terbinafine. The duration of treatment necessary to resolve SNA varies depending on the severity of infection, but usually is 4 to 6 months.[7]

SOA—Systemic Antifungal Therapy

The optimal treatment regimen for SOA in cats has not been identified. Of 20 reported cases, treatment was attempted in 14 and infection resolved in only four patients.[9,11] Of the cases treated successfully, three were treated with medical therapy alone, including one that resolved after posaconazole administration for 16 weeks.[9] Infection resolved in one cat treated for 7 months with combination therapy using itraconazole, AMB-D (cumulative dose 11 mg/kg), and terbinafine. A third cat responded well to 8 months of therapy with itraconazole and AMB-D (cumulative dose 14 mg/kg). Exophthalmos improved dramatically in this patient after 7 days of treatment with itraconazole and AMB-D (cumulative dose 14 mg/kg). However, clinical and CT evidence of infection recurred 3 weeks after itraconazole was stopped and after 8 months of treatment. Treatment was reinstituted with combination therapy using terbinafine and posaconazole for 4 months, followed by posaconazole alone for a further 3 months. Signs resolved and the cat remained asymptomatic 1 year later. The third case was treated with surgical debridement of the frontal sinuses during diagnostic investigation followed by AMB-D (cumulative dose 10 mg/kg) and itraconazole for 7 months. Clinical signs of infection resolved and the cat was asymptomatic 2 years later. Treatment failures occurred in four cats who were treated with medical therapy alone, and in six patients treated with combination antifungal medical therapy and radical surgical debridement of orbital granulomas, including exenteration in five cases.[11]

It is clear that the factors that determine whether a cat with SOA will respond to treatment have yet to be identified. Consideration should be given to surgical debridement of large fungal granulomas within the retrobulbar space, although evidence for efficacy of this approach in cats currently is lacking. Treatment of immunocompetent human beings with chronic granulomatous sinusitis involves aggressive surgical debridement and chronic antifungal therapy.[52] Current recommendations for medical therapy in cats with SOA are the same as for cats with severe SNA (see Table 5-5).

SUMMARY

URT aspergillosis can cause a spectrum of disease in cats ranging from noninvasive sinonasal cavity infection to severe invasive sino-orbital disease. *Aspergillus fumigatus* is the cause of some infections, but a closely related species, *Neosartorya*, is implicated more commonly. Identification of *Neosartorya* infection requires a polyphasic taxonomic approach, including fungal colony cultural characteristics and PCR. Aspergillosis should be included in the differential diagnosis of retrobulbar disease, and diagnostic investigations should include imaging of the sinonasal cavity. More work needs to be done to identify the optimal therapeutic approach to treatment of upper respiratory aspergillosis in cats.

ACKNOWLEDGMENTS

This work represents a tremendous team effort. The authors sincerely thank Dr. Catriona Halliday and Sue Sleiman from the Centre for Infectious Diseases at Westmead Hospital, Dr. Patricia Martin from the University of Sydney Veterinary Pathology Diagnostic Laboratory, and the many other colleagues and dedicated cat owners who made this work possible.

REFERENCES

1. Peiffer RL, Belkin PV, Janke BH: Orbital cellulitis, sinusitis, and pneumonitis caused by *Penicillium* sp in a cat, *J Am Vet Med Assoc* 176:449, 1980.
2. Wilkinson GT, Sutton RH, Grono LR: *Aspergillus* spp infection associated with orbital cellulitis and sinusitis in a cat, *J Small Anim Pract* 23:127, 1982.
3. Goodall SA, Lane JG, Warnock DW: The diagnosis and treatment of a case of nasal aspergillosis in a cat, *J Small Anim Pract* 25:627, 1984.
4. Davies C, Troy GC: Deep mycotic infections in cats, *J Am Anim Hosp Assoc* 32:380, 1996.
5. Halenda RM, Reed AL: Ultrasound computed tomography diagnosis—fungal sinusitis and retrobulbar myofascitis in a cat, *Vet Radiol Ultrasound* 38:208, 1997.
6. Hamilton HL, Whitley RD, McLaughlin SA: Exophthalmos secondary to aspergillosis in a cat, *J Am Anim Hosp Assoc* 36:343, 2000.
7. Tomsa K, Glaus TM, Zimmer C, et al: Fungal rhinitis and sinusitis in three cats, *J Am Vet Med Assoc* 222:1380, 2003.
8. Whitney BL, Broussard J, Stefanacci JD: Four cats with fungal rhinitis, *J Feline Med Surg* 7:53, 2005.
9. McLellan GJ, Aquino SM, Mason DR, et al: Use of posaconazole in the management of invasive orbital aspergillosis in a cat, *J Am Anim Hosp Assoc* 42:302, 2006.
10. Barrs VR, Beatty JA, Lingard AE, et al: Feline sino-orbital aspergillosis: an emerging clinical syndrome, *Aust Vet J* 85:N23, 2007.
11. Barrs VR et al: Feline upper respiratory aspergillosis: 21 cases; manuscript in preparation, 2009.
12. Balajee SA, Gribskov JL, Hanley E, et al: *Aspergillus lentulus* sp. nov., a new sibling species of *A. fumigatus*, *Eukaryot Cell* 4:625, 2005.
13. Balajee SA, Gribskov J, Brandt M, et al: Mistaken identity: *Neosartorya pseudofischeri* and its anamorph masquerading as *Aspergillus fumigatus*, *J Clin Microbiol* 43:5996, 2005.
14. Barrs VR, Martin P, Beatty JA, et al: Feline sino-orbital aspergillosis: an emerging clinical syndrome? *J Vet Intern Med* 21:579, 2007.
15. Lau A, Chen S, Sorrell T, et al: Development and clinical application of a panfungal PCR assay to detect and identify fungal DNA in tissue specimens, *J Clin Microbiol* 45:380, 2007.
16. Samson RA, Hong S, Peterson SW, et al: Polyphasic taxonomy of Aspergillus section Fumigati and its teleomorph *Neosartorya*, *Stud Mycol* 59:147, 2007.
17. Geiser DM, Klich MA, Frisvad JC, et al: The current status of species recognition and identification in *Aspergillus*, *Stud Mycol* 59:1, 2007.
17a. O'Gorman CM, Fuller HT, Dyer PS: Discovery of a sexual cycle in the opportunistic fungal pathogen *Aspergillus fumigatus*, *Nature* 457:471, 2008.
18. Peeters D, Clercx C: Update on canine sinonasal aspergillosis, *Vet Clin North Am Small Anim Pract* 37:901, 2007.
19. Siddiqui AA, Shah AA, Bashir SH: Craniocerebral aspergillosis of sinonasal origin in immunocompetent patients: clinical spectrum and outcome in 25 cases, *Neurosurgery* 55:602, 2004.
20. Uri N, Cohen-Kerem R, Elmalah I, et al: Classification of fungal sinusitis in immunocompetent patients, *Otolaryngol Head Neck Surg* 129:372, 2003.
21. Panda NK, Balaji P, Chakrabarti A, et al: Paranasal sinus aspergillosis: its categorization to develop a treatment protocol, *Mycoses* 47:277, 2004.
22. Hope WW, Walsh TJ, Denning DW: The invasive and saprophytic syndromes due to *Aspergillus* spp, *Med Mycol* 43:S207, 2005.
23. Day MJ: Canine sino-nasal aspergillosis: parallels with human disease, *Med Mycol* 26:1, 2008.
24. Allen HS, Broussard J, Noone K: Nasopharyngeal diseases in cats: a retrospective study of 53 cases (1991-1998), *J Am Anim Hosp Assoc* 35:457, 1999.
25. Malik R, Wigney DI, Muir DB, et al: Asymptomatic carriage of *Cryptococcus neoformans* in the nasal cavity of dogs and cats, *Med Mycol* 35:27, 1997.
26. Pomrantz JS, Johnson LR, Nelson RW, et al: Comparison of serologic evaluation via agar gel immunodiffusion and fungal culture of tissue for diagnosis of nasal aspergillosis in dogs, *J Am Vet Med Assoc* 230:1319, 2007.
27. Billen F, Peeters D, Peters IR, et al: Comparison of the value of measurement of serum galactomannan and *Aspergillus*-specific antibodies in the diagnosis of canine sino-nasal aspergillosis, *Vet Microbiol* 133:358, 2009.
28. Husain S, Kwak EJ, Obman A, et al: Prospective assessment of Platelia *Aspergillus* galactomannan antigen for the diagnosis of invasive aspergillosis in lung transplant recipients, *Am J Transplant* 4:796, 2004.
29. Saunders JH, Zonderland JL, Clercx C, et al: Computed tomographic findings in 35 dogs with nasal aspergillosis, *Vet Radiol Ultrasound* 43:5, 2002.
30. Saunders JH, Van Bree H: Comparison of radiography and computed tomography for the diagnosis of canine nasal aspergillosis, *Vet Radiol Ultrasound* 44:414, 2003.
31. Detweiler DA, Johnson LR, Kass PH, et al: Computed tomographic evidence of bulla effusion in cats with sinonasal disease: 2001-2004, *J Vet Intern Med* 20:1080, 2006.
32. Connor SE, Hussain S, Woo EK-F: Sinonasal imaging, *Imaging* 19:39, 2007.
33. Aribandi M, McCoy VA, Bazaan C: Imaging features of invasive and noninvasive fungal sinusitis: a review, *Radiographics* 27:1283, 2007.
34. Tromblee TC, Jones JC, Etue AE, et al: Association between clinical characteristics, computed tomography characteristics, and histologic diagnosis for cats with sinonasal disease, *Vet Radiol Ultrasound* 47:241, 2006.
35. Arikan S, Sancak B, Alp S, et al: Comparative in vitro activities of posaconazole, voriconazole, itraconazole, and amphotericin B against *Aspergillus* and *Rhizopus*, and synergy testing for *Rhizopus*, *Med Mycol* 46:567, 2008.
36. Perea S, Patterson TF: The role of antifungal susceptibility testing in the management of patients with invasive mycoses, *Rev Iberoam Micol* 16:180, 1999.
37. Patterson TF: Treatment of invasive aspergillosis; polyenes, echinocandins, or azoles? *Med Mycol* 44:S357, 2006.
38. Kontoyiannis DP, Lewis RE, Sagar N, et al: Itraconazole-amphotericin B antagonism in *Aspergillus fumigatus*: an E-test-based strategy, *Antimicrob Agents Chemother* 44:2915, 2000.
39. Navjar LK, Cacciapuoti A, Hernandez S, et al: Activity of posaconazole combined with amphotericin B against *Aspergillus flavus* infection in mice: comparative studies in two laboratories, *Antimicrob Agents Chemother* 48:758, 2004.

40. Clemons KV, Espiritu M, Parmar R, et al: Comparative efficacies of conventional amphotericin B, liposomal amphotericin B (AmBisome), caspofungin, micafungin, and voriconazole alone and in combination against experimental murine central nervous system aspergillosis, *Antimicrob Agents Chemother* 49:4867, 2005.

41. Zonios DI, Bennett JE: Update on azole antifungals, *Semin Respir Crit Care Med* 29:198, 2008.

42. Boothe DM, Herring I, Calvin J, et al: Itraconazole disposition after single oral and intravenous and multiple oral dosing in healthy cats, *Am J Vet Res* 58:872, 1997.

43. Nomier AA, Kumari P, Hilvert MJ, et al: Pharmacokinetics of SCH 5692, a new azole broad-spectrum antifungal agent, in mice, rats, rabbits, dogs, and cynomolgus monkeys, *Antimicrob Agents Chemother* 44:727, 2000.

44. Roffey SJ, Cole S, Comby P, et al: The disposition of voriconazole in mouse, rat, rabbit, guinea pig, dog, and human, *Drug Metab Dispos* 31:731-741, 2003.

45. Wray JD, Sparkes AH, Johnson EM: Infection of the subcutis of the nose in a cat caused by *Mucor* species: successful treatment using posaconazole, *J Feline Med Surg* 10:523, 2008.

46. Wakabayashi T, Oda H, Kinoshita N, et al: Retrobulbar amphotericin B injections for treatment of invasive sino-orbital aspergillosis, *Jpn J Ophthalmol* 51:309, 2007.

47. Ellis D: Amphotericin B: spectrum and resistance, *J Antimicrob Chemother* 49(Suppl 1):7, 2002.

48. Howden BP, Slavin MA, Schwarer AP, et al: Successful control of disseminated *Scedosporium prolificans* infection with a combination of voriconazole and terbinafine, *Eur J Clin Microbiol Infect Dis* 22:111, 2003.

49. Kotnik T: Drug efficacy of terbinafine hydrochloride (Lamisil) during oral treatment of cats, experimentally infected with *Microsporum canis*, *J Vet Med B Infect Dis Vet Public Health* 49:120, 2002.

50. Letscher-Bru V, Herbrecht R: Caspofungin: the first representative of a new antifungal class, *J Antimicrob Chemoth* 51:513, 2003.

51. Caulkett N, Lew L, Fries C: Upper-airway obstruction and prolonged recovery from anesthesia following intranasal clotrimazole administration, *J Am Anim Hosp Assoc* 33:264, 1997.

52. Walsh TJ, Anaissie EJ, Denning DW, et al: Treatment of aspergillosis: clinical practice guidelines of the Infectious Diseases Society of America, *Clin Infect Dis* 46:327, 2008.

6 Progress on Diagnosis of Retroviral Infections

Cynda Crawford

Retroviral infection is one of the most common infectious diseases in cats in the United States and worldwide. The true prevalence of feline leukemia virus (FeLV) and feline immunodeficiency virus (FIV) infections is unknown because testing is voluntary, results are not reported to a central database, and most screening test results are not confirmed by another technology. Although characteristics such as gender, age, lifestyle, and health status can be used to assess the likely risk of retroviral infections, most cats have some degree of infection risk. Accurate diagnosis of retroviral infections is important for both uninfected and infected cats. Failure to identify infected cats may lead to inadvertent exposure and transmission to uninfected cats. Misdiagnosis of infection in uninfected cats may lead to inappropriate changes in lifestyle or even euthanasia.

Retroviral infections are lifelong and have significant impact on the health and welfare of infected cats. To prevent new infections and optimize health care for infected cats, the American Association of Feline Practitioners (AAFP) believes that the retroviral status of all cats should be known, and recommends testing cats for retrovirus infection when they are newly acquired, sick, prior to vaccination for FeLV or FIV, or when exposed to potentially infected cats.[1] Although point-of-care testing for FeLV and FIV infection is readily available, relatively inexpensive, and easily performed, less than 25 per cent of cats in the United States have ever been tested.[2]

The objective of this chapter is to present new information on diagnostic testing for retroviral infections and on progress toward overcoming challenges that still hinder accurate diagnosis. The chapter reviews epidemiological and pathogenetic factors pertinent to the diagnosis of FeLV and FIV, discusses strengths and weaknesses of current testing methodologies, identifies challenges to the development of future test strategies, and summarizes the recent AAFP recommendations for retroviral testing of pet cats and cats in shelters.

FELINE LEUKEMIA VIRUS

EPIDEMIOLOGY AND PATHOGENESIS

Household clusters of lymphoma and lymphocytic leukemia led to the discovery of FeLV more than 40 years ago.[3] Although FeLV is one of the most common infectious diseases of cats around the world, the prevalence of infection has been decreasing since the 1980s.[4-6] The decline most likely is a result of widespread test and removal/segregation programs and availability of FeLV vaccines. In the United States, recent studies report prevalences of FeLV infection ranging from less than 2 per cent for healthy cats up to 15 per cent for high-risk cats and cats tested during illness.[2,4-6] In a recent survey of more than 18,000 North American pet and feral cats tested in veterinary clinics and animal shelters,[5] the overall prevalence was 2.3 per cent. Infection rates were higher in pet cats than in shelter cats, and lower in healthy feral cats compared with healthy outdoor pet cats (Table 6-1). Risk factors for infection included male gender, adulthood, illness, and outdoor access. Infection rates were highest among sick feral cats, followed by sick pet cats allowed access to the outdoors.

FeLV contains a single-stranded RNA genome that encodes several major protein groups: *gag* (group-specific antigens), *pol* (reverse transcriptase), and *env* (envelope). Once the viral RNA genome is reverse-transcribed into

Table 6-1   Prevalence of FeLV and FIV Infection in 18,038 Cats*

		Number Tested	Prevalence (%) FeLV	Prevalence (%) FIV
Test site	Animal shelter	8068	1.5	1.7
	Veterinary clinic	9970	2.9	3.1
Source	Clinic (indoors only)	3613	1.5	0.9
	Shelter (stray/ relinquished)	7359	1.6	1.5
	Shelter (feral)	709	1.7	3.9
	Clinic (outdoor access)	6357	3.6	4.3
Age	Juvenile	9556	1.4	1.0
	Adult	8482	3.3	4.1
Sex	Intact female	2611	1.7	1.2
	Spayed female	6588	1.9	1.7
	Intact male	5855	2.5	3.3
	Neutered male	2984	2.9	4.3
Health status	Healthy	15312	1.6	1.8
	Sick	2726	6.3	6.1

*Cats in 345 veterinary clinics and 145 animal shelters in North America were tested from August to November 2004 with a single point-of-care ELISA screening test for FeLV antigen and FIV antibody (SNAP® FeLV/FIV Combo Test, IDEXX Laboratories). Confirmatory tests were not performed. From Levy JK, Scott HM, Lachtara JL, et al: Seroprevalence of feline leukemia virus and feline immunodeficiency virus infection among cats in North America and risk factors for seropositivity, *J Am Vet Med Assoc* 228:371, 2006.

Table 6-2   Infection Outcomes for Cats Exposed to FeLV*

Blood Tests	Progressive Infection	Regressive Infection
p27 antigen	Positive	Negative
Viral RNA	Positive	Variable
Proviral DNA	Positive	Positive
Virus culture	Positive	Negative
Virus shedding	Yes	No
FeLV-associated disease	Likely	Unlikely

*The FeLV status of the cats was determined by soluble antigen testing, IFA testing for intracellular antigen, virus culture, and real-time PCR analysis.
Modified from Levy J, Crawford C, Hartmann K, et al: 2008 American Association of Feline Practitioners' feline retrovirus management guidelines, *J Feline Med Surg* 10:300, 2008.

DNA within infected cells, the DNA copies are inserted randomly into the host genome, and the integrated provirus is retained during cellular division. Natural FeLV infection primarily is a concern for cats who socialize with other cats and for kittens who acquire infection from their mothers. In addition to prepartum and postpartum transmission, the virus is transmitted commonly between cats via the oronasal route and by bite wounds. The prevalence of FeLV in cats with bite wound abscesses is very high (8.8 per cent).[2]

Much of the knowledge regarding FeLV pathogenesis has been provided by studies of experimental infections. Based on virus culture and antigen testing, it was generally believed for many years that approximately one-third of infected cats remain persistently infected, whereas up to two-thirds develop an effective immune response with eventual recovery from infection. However, recent studies utilizing highly sensitive real-time polymerase chain reaction (PCR) techniques have redefined the outcomes of FeLV infection and suggest that cats most likely remain infected for life.[8-14] FeLV proviral DNA and viral RNA transcripts are detectable by PCR in circulating lymphocytes and monocytes within 1 week of infection, even if viral antigen is not.[8,11-14] Regardless of the eventual outcome of infection, all cats appear to develop similar proviral and plasma viral RNA loads during the early phase.[8-14]

In *progressive infection*, insufficient FeLV-specific immunity results in extensive virus replication that occurs first in the lymphoid tissues and then in the bone marrow.[15,16] Spread to mucosal and glandular tissues and excretion of infectious virus in various secretions (saliva, feces, urine, milk) occur at about the same time as bone marrow infection. Bone marrow infection results in a secondary viremia in which all leukocyte subsets and platelets contain high proviral DNA and RNA loads.[14] These cats are persistently viremic and antigenemic, and succumb to FeLV-associated diseases within a few years (Table 6-2).

In *regressive infection* an effective immune response limits virus replication prior to bone marrow infection.[15,16] FeLV antigen and infectious virus usually are detectable in peripheral blood for 2 to 3 weeks after virus exposure, but then disappear 2 to 8 weeks later or, in rare cases, after many months. However, these cats have not cleared the infection. PCR assays have shown that circulating lymphocytes contain low amounts of proviral DNA and RNA transcripts (see Table 6-2).[10-14] The clinical relevance of regressive infections is not yet clear. Cats with regressive infection do not shed virus and are unlikely to develop FeLV-associated diseases.[13,14] Even though viral shedding does not occur, it is possible that cats with regressive infection can still transmit FeLV via blood and tissue donation, because the proviral DNA might be infectious. In addition, recurrence of viremia and subsequent clinical disease have been observed in some cats.[10,11] Research on the possible outcomes for FeLV exposure is ongoing and controversial, but underpins new recommendations for diagnostic testing. As more information emerges, the outcomes likely will continue to evolve and be refined, along with diagnostic approaches.

DIAGNOSIS

The FeLV p27 *gag* protein is abundant in the plasma and cytoplasm of infected cells during the acute phase of infection and in progressively infected cats. Detection of circulating p27 protein is the basis for rapid-screening test kits used with serum, plasma, and whole blood. These kits are available in enzyme-linked immunosorbent assay (ELISA) and membrane immunochromatography formats for use in veterinary clinics, animal shelters, and diagnostic laboratories. The soluble antigen screening tests usually are positive within 30 days of viral exposure, but development of antigenemia is variable, especially in cats with regressive infection. Kittens may be tested at any time because passively acquired maternal antibody to FeLV does not interfere with testing for viral antigen. However, kittens infected as a result of maternal transmission may not test positive for weeks to months after birth.[17]

Recent studies[18-20] have found acceptable diagnostic accuracy for several commercially available screening tests for soluble FeLV p27 antigen; sensitivities (proportion of positive results for infected cats) range from 92 to 94 per cent, and specificities (proportion of negative results for uninfected cats) range from 92 per cent to greater than 99 per cent. Negative screening test results are reliable because of the high sensitivity of the tests and low prevalence of infection (negative predictive value >99 per cent). If the results of soluble antigen testing are negative but recent exposure can not be ruled out, antigen testing should be repeated a minimum of 30 days after the last potential exposure. However, a negative soluble antigen test result does not rule out the possibility that a cat has regressive infection. Detection of regressively infected cats requires testing a blood sample for FeLV DNA using a PCR assay (see the following). Recent studies using real-time PCR have shown that 5 to 10 per cent of cats with negative results on soluble antigen tests were positive for FeLV provirus by PCR.[7,21]

The positive predictive value (probability that a cat with a positive result is truly infected) of currently available screening tests for FeLV p27 is low (<90 per cent), especially in low-risk and asymptomatic patients.[18,19] Importantly, the two most widely used point-of-care tests in the United States, Witness FeLV Test (SynBiotics Corporation, Kansas City, MO) and SNAP FeLV/FIV Combo Test (IDEXX Laboratories, Westbrook, ME), have a positive predictive value of only 74 per cent.[18,19] Therefore confirmatory testing of positive screening test results is recommended. Multiple options exist for confirmation of a positive screening test result. Initially, antigen testing can be repeated, preferably using a test from a different manufacturer.[7-19] In a recent comparative study,[19] testing samples with a combination of soluble antigen tests from different manufacturers improved the positive predictive value to nearly 90 per cent. Another option for verification of positive screening tests is performance of an immunofluorescent antibody (IFA) test on blood or bone marrow smears. The IFA test detects viral p27 antigen within infected leukocytes and platelets subsequent to bone marrow infection in cats with progressive infection. False-negative IFA results can occur when neutropenia or thrombocytopenia is present. In general soluble antigen tests are considered to be slightly more sensitive (fewer false-negatives), and the IFA test to be slightly more specific (fewer false-positives).

Discordant test results may occur when results of soluble antigen screening tests and confirmatory IFA tests do not agree, making determination of the true FeLV status difficult. The most common scenario occurs when the soluble antigen test is positive and the IFA test for intracellular antigen is negative. Cats can have discordant results if they are tested during the acute phase of infection before the virus spreads to the bone marrow. Similarly cats with regressive infection may be transiently positive on soluble antigen tests, but negative by IFA. In contrast to progressively infected cats, these cats eventually revert to negative status on any antigen detection test. Cats with discordant antigen test results are best considered potential sources of infection for other cats until their status is clarified. The true infection status eventually may be resolved by repeating both the soluble antigen test and IFA test in 2 months and annually thereafter until the test results agree. Alternatively, blood samples can be tested for FeLV proviral DNA using PCR (see the following). Cats with either progressive or regressive infection should have detectable proviral DNA in circulating cells.

Virus isolation generally has been accepted as the reference test or gold standard for confirmation of FeLV antigen screening tests. This assay detects replication-competent infectious virus and therefore usually agrees with antigen screening test results. In one recent study,[20] about 25 per cent of cats tested by antigen detection assays and virus isolation had discordant results. Cats who tested positive for p27 antigen but negative by virus isolation were retested using a real-time PCR assay for FeLV proviral DNA. About 50 per cent of these cats were FeLV-positive by PCR, suggesting the possibility of regressive infections. The other 50 per cent who tested negative for FeLV DNA may have been falsely positive on the antigen test because these latter tests for FeLV have a lower positive predictive value.

PCR is a highly sensitive test for FeLV DNA, but also is highly susceptible to technical errors, contamination during sample collection and handling, and poor quality control, any of which reduce the accuracy of results. At this time, there are no reports comparing the reliability and accuracy of FeLV PCR tests offered by different commercial laboratories. When performed under optimal conditions, real-time PCR is the most sensitive test methodology for detection of FeLV DNA (detection limit of five to 10 copies) and can help to resolve the status of patients with discordant antigen test results or when infection is suspected but not confirmed by antigen testing. PCR can be performed on blood, bone marrow, and tissues. In addition PCR testing of saliva has been shown to have high correlation with blood antigen tests.[21] Because cats with regressive infection can transmit FeLV proviral DNA that may be infectious, all feline blood and tissue donors should be tested for FeLV antigen by serology and for provirus by real-time PCR.

Because FeLV tests are based on detection of antigen or DNA and not antibodies, vaccination against FeLV generally does not interfere with testing. However, blood collected immediately following vaccination may contain detectable FeLV vaccine strain antigens or DNA.[9-11] The extent and duration of vaccine interference with testing is unknown, but diagnostic samples should be collected prior to starting the vaccination series. Cats also should be tested before vaccination because administration of FeLV vaccines to infected cats is not believed to have any value. With the advent of highly sensitive PCR testing, some vaccinated cats have been identified as infected after viral exposure. These cats had regressive infection demonstrated by PCR detection of circulating proviral DNA and plasma viral RNA, in the absence of antigenemia or viremia.[9-11]

Adherence to AAFP recommendations to test all cats for FeLV is likely to result in the identification of many asymptomatic cats with positive test results. Early identification of cats who test positive permits actions to prevent the spread of infection through segregation and to optimize the health care of infected cats. The recommendation to use PCR testing to confirm the FeLV status for antigen-discordant patients, suspect cases who are antigen-negative, and blood and tissue donors may create a new dilemma regarding the appropriate management of cats. Although cats with regressive infection do not shed detectable replication-competent virus, the FeLV provirus present in circulating lymphocytes is potentially infectious if inoculated into other cats.

FELINE IMMUNODEFICIENCY VIRUS

EPIDEMIOLOGY AND PATHOGENESIS

First reported more than 20 years ago,[22] FIV has a worldwide distribution in domestic cats, with infection rates approaching one third of the cat population in some locations. Similar to FeLV, studies have shown that the prevalence of FIV is highly variable, dependent on age, gender, lifestyle, physical condition, and geographic location. In the recent serosurvey of more than 18,000 cats in North American veterinary clinics and animal shelters,[5] the overall prevalence of FIV seropositivity was 2.5 per cent. Prevalence was higher in cats tested at veterinary clinics than in animal shelters, in healthy feral cats and pet cats with outdoor access, in adults, in males, and in cats who were sick at the time of testing (see Table 6-1). FIV infection is mainly a concern for cats who are "unfriendly" with other cats, and the risk is highest for sexually intact males whose fighting and biting behavior is believed to be the main source of transmission. Cat-bite abscesses are associated with a very high prevalence (12.7 per cent) of FIV infection.[2] FIV is transmitted most commonly between cats by biting; vertical transmission from queen to kittens can occur but is uncommon.

Similar to other lentiviruses such as HIV, FIV has a high intrinsic mutation rate in the envelope (env) and capsid (gag) genes. There are five well-characterized subtypes of FIV (A to E) based on genetic divergence in the env and gag genes.[23-25] Sequence divergence in these genes ranges up to 26 per cent within a subtype and between subtypes. Cats in the United States are infected most commonly with A, B, and occasionally C subtypes. Cats may be infected with one subtype only or co-infected with different subtypes.[26] Genetic recombination events can occur between different co-infecting subtypes to create novel inter-subtype recombinants.[26,27] Recently, A/B and A/C inter-subtype recombinants were identified in FIV-infected cats in Canada.[27]

The FIV genome is single-stranded RNA that is reverse-transcribed to DNA in infected cells. The DNA copies are integrated randomly into the host genome and the proviral sequences are retained during cellular division. FIV infection is lifelong. High concentrations of virus can be detected in circulating lymphocytes and monocytes by culture and PCR within 2 weeks of infection. Infected cells carry the virus to other organs, but lymphoid tissues remain the primary site of viral replication. After 2 months, the circulating viral load decreases concomitant with vigorous cell-mediated and humoral immune responses. Following acute infection, FIV-infected cats enter a prolonged asymptomatic stage during which progressive dysfunction of the immune system occurs.

DIAGNOSIS

Cats infected with FIV have low levels of viral antigens in their blood; this has prevented use of screening assays based on antigen detection as is used in diagnosis of FeLV. However, FIV-infected cats produce high levels of circulating antiviral antibodies.[22,28] Detection of antiviral antibody is the basis for rapid-screening test kits used with serum, plasma, and whole blood. The kits are available in ELISA format worldwide, and in the immunochromatography format in Europe. Most cats produce antibodies to FIV within 2 months of exposure, but a detectable antibody response may be delayed in some cats.[22,28]

Recent studies[18-20] have found that the diagnostic accuracy for several commercially available screening tests for FIV antibody is very high, with sensitivities (proportion of positive results for infected cats) of 93 to 100 per cent, and specificities (proportion of negative results for uninfected cats) of 99 to 100 per cent. Negative screening test results are highly reliable because of the high sensitivity of the tests and the low prevalence of infection (negative predictive value >99 per cent). False-negative results are possible when cats have not yet seroconverted after recent exposure to FIV or when the concentration of FIV antibodies is less than the detection limit. If the initial screening test is negative but there is clinical or historical suspicion of virus exposure, the test should be repeated at least 2 months later to allow for seroconversion. Occasionally cats with end-stage infection revert to a seronegative status and test false-negative on antibody-based diagnostic tests.

The positive predictive value (probability that a cat with a positive result is truly infected) of currently available screening tests for FIV is high (91 to 100 per cent).[18-20] The two most widely used point-of-care tests in the United States and Europe, Witness FeLV/FIV Combi (SynBiotics Corporation) and SNAP FeLV/FIV Combo (IDEXX Laboratories), have a positive predictive value of 95 per cent.[18,19] The microtiter plate ELISAs manufactured by SynBiotics (Virachek FIV) and IDEXX (Pet Chek FIV) and used by diagnostic laboratories for testing of large numbers of samples have positive predictive values of 98 to 100 per cent.[18,19] However, the AAFP recommends confirmation of positive screening test results, especially in low-risk and asymptomatic patients in whom the possibility of a false-positive result is higher. False-positive results occur more frequently when whole blood is used.[18] Antibody detection by Western blot or IFA has long been recommended for confirmatory testing; however, contrary to expectations, these tests are less accurate than the point-of-care screening tests.[29] Confirmatory testing can be achieved by submission of the sample to a diagnostic laboratory for testing in the microtiter plate ELISAs. One diagnostic laboratory (New York State Animal Health Diagnostic Center, Cornell University, Ithaca, NY) offers a kinetic ELISA (KELA) that claims to provide clear separation of negative or positive reactions from equivocal reactions caused by extremely low levels of FIV antibodies or nonspecific reactivity in the cat's serum. In one study,[30] some cats had discordant results for the point-of-care tests, Western blot, and KELA; the true FIV status of these cats could not be determined by serological tests.

Positive FIV antibody tests in kittens less than 6 months old are unreliable. Passively acquired antiviral antibodies from FIV-infected queens often persist past the age of 8 weeks when many kittens are adopted and first tested for retroviral infection. Because the risk of acquiring FIV infection from infected mothers is low, most kittens who test positive for FIV antibodies are not truly infected and will revert eventually to a seronegative status. Kittens who are seropositive after 4 to 6 months of age most likely are infected.

The diagnosis of FIV infection based on antibody detection has been confounded by availability of an FIV vaccine (Fel-O-Vax FIV, Fort Dodge Animal Health, Fort Dodge, IA).[29-33] This vaccine is a dual-subtype whole-virus vaccine containing formalin-inactivated subtype A and subtype D virions, virus-infected cells, and an adjuvant.[28,34] Because the vaccine contains whole virus, cats respond to immunization by producing antibodies that are indistinguishable from those produced during natural infection.[28-30,34] In a recent study,[29] antibodies were detected by ELISA, Western blot, and IFA tests as early as 2 weeks after administration of the first vaccine dose, and vaccine interference persisted for at least 1 year (Table 6-3). Some cats have been reported to have positive FIV antibody tests for more than 4 years after their last FIV vaccination.[1] Kittens born to FIV-vaccinated queens absorbed colostral FIV antibodies that were detected at 2 days of age.[35] A majority of kittens still tested positive for FIV at 8 weeks of age; however, all of these kittens had negative test results by 12 weeks of age. Thus FIV vaccination of queens results in passively acquired FIV antibodies in kittens that frequently persist past the age of weaning when many kittens are tested for FIV prior to adoption.

The advent of FIV vaccination has created a diagnostic dilemma for FIV testing; it is now difficult to determine whether a positive FIV antibody test means the cat is truly infected with FIV, is vaccinated against FIV but not infected, or is a vaccinated cat who has become infected.[31-33] With the promise of more FIV vaccines on the horizon, the development of a DIVA (differentiation of infected from vaccinated animals) strategy is greatly warranted. Recently an ELISA technique was developed

Table 6-3 Diagnostic Performance of Different Commercially Available Serological Assays for Detection of FIV Antibodies*

Assay	Sensitivity (%)	Specificity (%) Unvaccinated Cats	Specificity (%) Vaccinated Cats
Point-of-care ELISA	100	100	0
Microtiter plate ELISA	100	100	0
Western blot	98	98	54
IFA	100	90	22

*Uninfected (n = 42), FIV-infected (n = 41), and FIV-vaccinated (n = 41) cats were tested for FIV antibodies using a panel of commercially available serology assays.
Sensitivity is the percentage of FIV-infected cats identified correctly as infected. Specificity is the percentage of uninfected cats identified correctly as negative for infection. False-positive reactions were very high in uninfected cats who were vaccinated.
From Levy JK, Crawford PC, Slater MR: Effect of vaccination against feline immunodeficiency virus on results of serologic testing in cats, *J Am Vet Med Assoc* 225:1558, 2004.

in Japan that differentiates uninfected from infected cats regardless of FIV vaccination history.[36] This technique is based on measurement of antibody reactivity (absorbance values) to two FIV antigens: formalin-fixed whole virus and a synthetic transmembrane (TM) peptide. In plots of antibody reactivity to whole virus versus antibody reactivity to the TM peptide, a line can be determined that discriminates between uninfected and infected cats based on the antibody reactivity of negative and positive controls. The diagnostic accuracy of this discriminant ELISA was 97 per cent when validated with samples from cats with known vaccination and infection status.[36] In a follow-up study, the discriminant ELISA was used to test in a blinded fashion a large number of defined samples from uninfected, FIV-infected, FIV-vaccinated, and FIV-vaccinated and infected cats.[37] The sensitivity of the test was 97 per cent and the specificity was 100 per cent. All uninfected cats were identified correctly regardless of their vaccination status (Figure 6-1). The discriminant ELISA also identified FIV infection in cats who were vaccinated.[36,37] This result has important clinical relevance in that some infected cats may be immunized subsequently against FIV, while others may become infected after they have been vaccinated. The exceptional accuracy of the discriminant ELISA conforms to criteria for a DIVA test. If the discriminant ELISA was available commercially, the best diagnostic strategy for FIV testing would include initial screening with a point-of-care ELISA and confirmation of positive results by the discriminant ELISA. If the discriminant ELISA is negative, the cat most likely is vaccinated against FIV. If the discriminant ELISA is positive, the cat most likely is infected, regardless of its FIV vaccination history. Unfortunately, the discriminant ELISA is not available commercially at this time.

PCR for virus-specific DNA in infected blood lymphocytes is another methodology that may be suitable as a

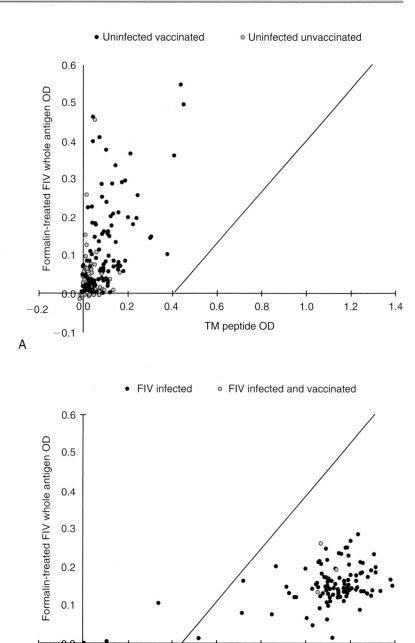

Figure 6-1 The discriminant ELISA for identification of uninfected and FIV-infected cats based on antibody measurement. Serum samples from uninfected cats, FIV-infected cats, FIV-vaccinated cats, and FIV-vaccinated cats that were infected were tested for antibodies to formalin-inactivated whole virus and a synthetic transmembrane (TM) peptide. The optical density values representing relative amounts of antibody to whole virus (y-axis) were plotted against the optical densities for reactivity to the TM peptide (x-axis). A discriminant line separating negative antibody reactivity from positive antibody reactivity was determined based on a panel of negative and positive control sera. **A,** All of the uninfected cats, whether vaccinated (black dots) or not (orange dots), were identified correctly to the left of the discriminant line. **B,** Except for three cats, all of the FIV-infected cats (black dots) were identified correctly to the right of the discriminant line, including three cats who were both vaccinated and infected (orange dots). (From Levy JK, Crawford PC, Kusuhara K, et al: Differentiation of feline immunodeficiency virus vaccination, infection, or vaccination and infection in cats, *J Vet Intern Med* 22:330, 2008.)

DIVA test to differentiate between FIV-infected and FIV-vaccinated cats. However, the marked genetic diversity among FIV strains poses a high potential for PCR primer mismatches and failure to detect diverse isolates in infected cats. Recent studies comparing the diagnostic accuracy of FIV PCR assays offered by research and diagnostic laboratories in North America have shown widely variable results. In one study using blinded samples from a defined population of uninfected, FIV-infected, and FIV-vaccinated cats,[38] test sensitivities ranged from 41 to 93 per cent and test specificities ranged from 81 to 100 per cent (Table 6-4). An unexpected and unexplained finding was that false-positive results were higher in FIV-vaccinated cats than in unvaccinated cats. Another study

found that assay specificity was improved by sequence analysis of PCR products to eliminate false-positive reactions.[30] Attempts are underway to improve the diagnostic accuracy of FIV PCR tests for verification of the infection status in antibody-positive cats and in cats with discordant serological test results; however, the genetic diversity of the virus makes this a daunting and ongoing challenge.

At the time of this writing, there are no routinely available diagnostic tests in the United States that can differentiate FIV-infected cats from vaccinated cats accurately. Although virus culture can determine the infection status of seropositive cats reliably,[33,38] it is too technical, expensive, and slow for diagnostic laboratories to offer as a

Table 6-4 Diagnostic Performance of Different Commercially Available PCR Assays for Detection of FIV DNA*

Assay	Overall Accuracy (%)	Sensitivity (%)	Specificity (%)	
			Unvaccinated Cats	Vaccinated Cats
PCR1	90	76	100	95
PCR2	80	93	81	66
PCR3	59	51	81	44
PCR4	58	41	81	51

*Whole blood samples from uninfected (n = 42), FIV-infected (n = 41), and FIV-vaccinated (n = 42) cats were tested for FIV DNA by PCR assays offered by four different laboratories.
The overall accuracy of each PCR assay is the percentage of correct results for all tested cats. Sensitivity is the percentage of FIV-infected cats identified correctly as infected. Specificity is the percentage of uninfected cats identified correctly as negative for infection. False-positive results were common in uninfected cats who were vaccinated.
From Crawford PC, Slater MR, Levy JK: Accuracy of polymerase chain reaction assays for diagnosis of feline immunodeficiency virus infection in cats, *J Am Vet Med Assoc* 226:1503, 2005.

routine confirmatory test for FIV. Until more accurate testing methodologies that satisfy the DIVA principle become readily available, the best approach for confirming the infection status of cats testing seropositive in the FIV point-of-care ELISA is to first submit a serum sample to a diagnostic laboratory for testing in the microtiter plate ELISA or kinetic ELISA. If these tests are still positive, then whole blood can be submitted to a diagnostic laboratory that performs real-time PCR for FIV or a conventional PCR assay with sequence analysis of PCR products to rule out false-positive reactions. Cats with indeterminate status should be isolated indoors to protect other cats from possible infection and to reduce their risk of contracting other infectious diseases.

AMERICAN ASSOCIATION OF FELINE PRACTITIONERS' RECOMMENDATIONS FOR RETROVIRAL DIAGNOSIS

The retroviral status of all cats should be known to prevent transmission of new infections and to optimize the health care program for infected cats.[1] All cats have some degree of risk for exposure to retroviruses and may require testing at different times in their lives. Infection rates vary for kittens in litters and cats from the same household, so pooling samples from multiple cats for testing as one sample reduces test sensitivity and should not be performed. Similarly test results for one kitten or cat can not be extrapolated accurately to others in the litter or household. Testing records should identify each cat individually and should accurately reflect the actual testing procedures performed. Storage of test kits and test procedures must be performed as indicated by the manufacturer to maintain accuracy.

No test is 100 per cent accurate at all times under all conditions; therefore retrovirus test results should be interpreted while considering the patient's health and risk factors. Retroviral tests only diagnose infection, not clinical disease, and cats infected with FeLV or FIV may live for many years (Box 6-1). A decision for euthanasia should never be based solely on whether or not the cat is infected with a retrovirus.

RETROVIRAL DIAGNOSTIC TESTING IN ANIMAL SHELTERS

Although the prevalence of retrovirus infections in animal shelters is low,[5] all cats entering shelters should be considered potentially infected, regardless of age and the environment from which they originated. Ideally all cats should be tested at admission using a screening test, preferably with serum instead of whole blood. This testing includes unweaned orphaned kittens, who may have been infected by the queen or another cat prior to admission, and cats who are returned to the shelter following a failed adoption because it is not possible to determine the risks encountered outside the shelter. Cats who test negative on their initial test should be retested 2 months later because of the possibility of recent exposure prior to admission.

When resources are inadequate to test all cats, shelters may prioritize testing cats selected for adoption, high-risk cats, or sick cats. Testing one cat as a proxy for another, or pooling samples from multiple cats for testing, is inaccurate and inappropriate. Each cat should be tested individually. Testing is optional for cats who are housed singly. Adopted cats or cats transferred to a foster home should be kept separate from other cats pending testing, preferably until a second test is performed 2 months later. Resident cats in adoptive homes or foster homes also should be tested before being exposed to new cats.

Only cats who are retrovirus negative should be considered for group housing in shelters and sanctuaries. Ideally, cats should be tested twice over a 2-month period before introduction into the group. Group housing of cats from unknown backgrounds constitutes a higher risk for retrovirus exposure, and because diagnostic tests are not 100 per cent accurate, annual retesting is advisable for all cats housed in this manner.

Trap-neuter-return (TNR) programs for feral cats represent a special situation in which cost-benefit considerations favor allocation of all resources to sterilization instead of diversion to retrovirus testing.[39,40] This philosophy is supported by the fact that sterilization is more effective in reducing the transmission modes for FeLV (reproduction) and FIV (fighting) than test-and-cull

Box 6-1 The 2008 AAFP Recommendations for Retrovirus Testing

1. All cats and kittens should be tested for FeLV and FIV when first acquired.
   a. Although the importance of testing new cats before introduction into a household with other cats is obvious, cats who will be living alone also should be tested for the following reasons:
      i. Impact of retroviral infection on health
      ii. Possibility that other cats may be added to the household
      iii. Possibility that indoor cats may escape and be exposed to other cats
   b. Initial testing can be performed with a screening test.
      i. Negative test results are reliable if there has been no exposure to infected cats or to cats of unknown retroviral status.
      ii. Positive test results should be confirmed by repeating the screening testing with a different brand, or submitting a blood sample to a diagnostic laboratory for FeLV IFA, FeLV PCR, FIV microwell or kinetic ELISA, or FIV PCR.
   c. Kittens less than 6 months old with positive FIV antibody test results
      i. Because of the possibility of false-positive results from maternal antibody, these kittens should be segregated from other cats and retested monthly.
      ii. If seropositivity persists beyond 6 months of age, the kitten most likely is infected.
2. Cats with known exposure to infected cats or to cats with unknown retrovirus status should be tested regardless of previous test results.
   a. Immediate testing with a screening test is recommended.
      i. FeLV-exposed cats with negative results should be retested 1 month later.
      ii. FIV-exposed cats with negative results should be retested 2 months later.
      iii. If the type of retrovirus exposure is unknown, then retesting for both viruses 2 months later is most practical.
   b. To identify cats with regressive infection, FeLV PCR testing should be considered for cats with strong suspicion of FeLV infection but negative serological test results.
3. Cats with bite wounds, abscesses, or other illness should be tested regardless of previous test results. Testing should be conducted as outlined for cats exposed to retrovirus-infected cats (see entry 2).
4. Cats with high-risk lifestyles, including outdoor access and a history of fighting and cat-bite abscesses, should be tested on a regular basis.
5. Cats living in households with retrovirus-infected cats should be tested annually unless they are segregated effectively.
6. Cats should be tested prior to initial vaccination against FeLV or FIV.
7. Cats who participate in a blood or tissue donation program should have negative serological tests for FeLV and FIV, and a negative real-time PCR test for FeLV.
8. Cats with confirmed negative infection status do not need intermittent retesting unless they have an opportunity for retrovirus exposure or become ill.

Data from Levy J, Crawford C, Hartmann K, et al: 2008 American Association of Feline Practitioners' feline retrovirus management guidelines, *J Feline Med Surg* 10:300, 2008.

approaches. In addition, healthy feral cats have low infection rates (one to four per 100 cats),[5,41,42] so testing of all cats to identify the few infected ones is very costly.

REFERENCES

1. Levy J, Crawford C, Hartmann K, et al: 2008 American Association of Feline Practitioners' feline retrovirus management guidelines, *J Feline Med Surg* 10:300, 2008.
2. Goldkamp CE, Levy JK, Edinboro CH, et al: Seroprevalences of feline leukemia virus and feline immunodeficiency virus in cats with abscesses or bite wounds and rate of veterinarian compliance with current guidelines for retrovirus testing, *J Am Vet Med Assoc* 232:1152, 2008.
3. Jarrett WF, Crawford EM, Martin WB, et al: A virus like particle associated with leukemia (lymphosarcoma), *Nature* 202:567, 1964.
4. Crawford PC, Levy JK, Bicknell JM, et al: FeLV, FIV, and FIP: epidemiology and clinical disease syndromes, *J Vet Intern Med* 15:276, 2001.
5. Levy JK, Scott HM, Lachtara JL, et al: Seroprevalence of feline leukemia virus and feline immunodeficiency virus infection among cats in North America and risk factors for seropositivity, *J Am Vet Med Assoc* 228:371, 2006.
6. Moore GE, Ward MP, Dhariwal J, et al: Use of a primary care veterinary medical database for surveillance of syndromes and diseases in dogs and cats, *J Vet Intern Med* 18:386, 2004.
7. Hofmann-Lehmann R, Huder JB, Gruber S, et al: Feline leukaemia provirus load during the course of experimental infection and in naturally infected cats, *J Gen Virol* 82:1589, 2001.
8. Torres AN, Mathiason CK, Hoover EA, et al: Re-examination of feline leukemia virus: host relationships using real-time PCR, *Virology* 332:272, 2005.
9. Hofmann-Lehmann R, Tandon R, Boretti FS, et al: Reassessment of feline leukaemia virus (FeLV) vaccines with novel sensitive molecular assays, *Vaccine* 24:1087, 2006.
10. Hofmann-Lehmann R, Cattori V, Tandon R, et al: Vaccination against the feline leukaemia virus: outcome and response categories and long-term follow-up, *Vaccine* 25:5531, 2007.
11. Hofmann-Lehmann R, Cattori V, Tandon R, et al: How molecular methods change our views of FeLV infection and vaccination, *Vet Immunol Immunopathol* 123:119, 2008.
12. Torres AN, O'Halloran KP, Larson LJ, et al: Development and application of a quantitative real-time PCR assay to detect feline leukemia virus RNA, *Vet Immunol Immunopathol* 123:81, 2008.

13. Cattori V, Tandon R, Pepin A, et al: Rapid detection of feline leukemia virus provirus integration into feline genomic DNA, *Mol Cell Probes* 20:172, 2006.

14. Cattori V, Pepin AC, Tandon R, et al: Real-time investigation of feline leukemia virus proviral and viral RNA loads in leukocyte subsets, *Vet Immunol Immunopathol* 123:124, 2008.

15. Flynn JN, Hanlon L, Jarrett O: Feline leukaemia virus: protective immunity is mediated by virus-specific cytotoxic T lymphocytes, *Immunology* 101:120, 2000.

16. Flynn JN, Dunham SP, Watson V, et al: Longitudinal analysis of feline leukemia virus-specific cytotoxic T lymphocytes: correlation with recovery from infection, *J Virol* 76:2306, 2002.

17. Levy JK, Crawford PC: Feline leukemia virus. In Ettinger SJ, Feldman EC, editors: *Textbook of veterinary internal medicine*, ed 6, Philadelphia, 2005, Saunders, p 653.

18. Hartmann K, Werner RM, Egberink H, et al: Comparison of six in-house tests for the rapid diagnosis of feline immunodeficiency and feline leukaemia virus infections, *Vet Rec* 149:317, 2001.

19. Hartmann K, Griessmayr P, Schulz B, et al: Quality of different in-clinic test systems for feline immunodeficiency virus and feline leukaemia virus infection, *J Feline Med Surg* 9:439, 2007.

20. Pinches MDG, Diesel G, Helps CR, et al: An update on FIV and FeLV test performance using a Bayesian statistical approach, *Vet Clin Pathol* 36:141, 2007.

21. Gomes-Keller MA, Gonczi E, Tandon R, et al: Detection of feline leukemia virus RNA in saliva from naturally infected cats and correlation of PCR results with those of current diagnostic methods, *J Clin Microbiol* 44:916, 2006.

22. Yamamoto JK, Hansen H, Ho EW, et al: Epidemiologic and clinical aspects of feline immunodeficiency virus infection of cats from the continental United States and Canada and possible mode of transmission, *J Am Vet Med Assoc* 194:213, 1989.

23. Maki N, Miyazawa T, Fukasawa M, et al: Molecular characterization and heterogeneity of feline immunodeficiency virus isolates, *Arch Virol* 123:29, 1992.

24. Rigby MA, Holmes EC, Pistello M, et al: Evolution of structural proteins of feline immunodeficiency virus: molecular epidemiology and evidence of selection for change, *J Gen Virol* 74:425, 1993.

25. Hohdatsu T, Motokawa K, Usami M, et al: Genetic subtyping and epidemiological study of feline immunodeficiency virus by nested polymerase chain reaction restriction fragment length polymorphism analysis of the gag gene, *J Virol Methods* 70:107, 1998.

26. Bachmann MH, Mathiason-Rubard C, Learn GH, et al: Genetic diversity of feline immunodeficiency virus: dual infection, recombination, and distinct evolutionary rates among envelope sequence clades, *J Virol* 71:4241, 1997.

27. Reggeti F, Bienzle D: Feline immunodeficiency virus subtypes A, B, and C and intersubtype recombinants in Ontario, Canada, *J Gen Virol* 85:1843, 2004.

28. Yamamoto JK, Pu R, Sato E, et al: Feline immunodeficiency virus pathogenesis and development of a dual-subtype feline-immunodeficiency-virus vaccine, *AIDS* 21:547, 2007.

29. Levy JK, Crawford PC, Slater MR: Effect of vaccination against feline immunodeficiency virus on results of serologic testing in cats, *J Am Vet Med Assoc* 225:1558, 2004.

30. Bienzle D, Reggeti F, Wen X, et al: The variability of serological and molecular diagnosis of feline immunodeficiency virus infection, *Can Vet J* 45:753, 2004.

31. Richards JR: Feline immunodeficiency virus vaccine: implications for diagnostic testing and disease management, *Biologicals* 33:215, 2005.

32. Little S: Feline immunodeficiency virus: complications of testing and vaccination, *Adv Small Anim Med Surg* 19:1, 2006.

33. Crawford PC, Levy JK: New challenges for the diagnosis of feline immunodeficiency virus infection, *Vet Clin North Am Small Anim Pract* 37:335, 2007.

34. Uhl EW, Heaton-Jones TG, Pu R, et al: FIV vaccine development and its importance to veterinary and human medicine: a review. FIV vaccine 2002 update and review, *Vet Immunol Immunopathol* 90:113, 2002.

35. MacDonald K, Levy JK, Tucker SJ, et al: Effects of passive transfer of immunity on results of diagnostic tests for antibodies against feline immunodeficiency virus in kittens born to vaccinated queens, *J Am Vet Med Assoc* 225:1554, 2004.

36. Kusuhara H, Hohdatsu T, Seta T, et al: Serological differentiation of FIV-infected cats from dual-subtype feline immunodeficiency virus vaccine (Fel-O-Vax FIV) inoculated cats, *Vet Microbiol* 120:217, 2007.

37. Levy JK, Crawford PC, Kusuhara K, et al: Differentiation of feline immunodeficiency virus vaccination, infection, or vaccination and infection in cats, *J Vet Intern Med* 22:330, 2008.

38. Crawford PC, Slater MR, Levy JK: Accuracy of polymerase chain reaction assays for diagnosis of feline immunodeficiency virus infection in cats, *J Am Vet Med Assoc* 226:1503, 2005.

39. Levy JK, Crawford PC: Humane strategies for controlling feral cat populations, *J Am Vet Med Assoc* 225:1354, 2004.

40. Wallace JL, Levy JK: Population characteristics of feral cats admitted to seven trap-neuter-return programs in the United States, *J Feline Med Surg* 8:279, 2006.

41. Lee IT, Levy JK, Gorman SP, et al: Prevalence of feline leukemia virus infection and serum antibodies against feline immunodeficiency virus in unowned free-roaming cats, *J Am Vet Med Assoc* 220:620, 2002.

42. Luria BJ, Levy JK, Lappin MR, et al: Prevalence of infectious diseases in feral cats in northern Florida, *J Feline Med Surg* 6:287, 2004.

7 Diagnosis and Treatment of Feline Infectious Peritonitis

Katrin Hartmann

Feline infectious peritonitis (FIP) is an immune-mediated disease, triggered by infection with a feline coronavirus (FCoV). FIP is a major challenge to every veterinarian treating cats, because it is (1) very frequent, (2) sometimes very difficult to diagnose, (3) almost impossible to prevent, at least in multiple-cat environments, and (4) almost inevitably fatal within a short period of time. FIP is seen by primary veterinarians as often as by specialists. Approximately one of every 200 new feline cases presented to American veterinary teaching hospitals are cats with FIP.[1] FIP is one of the most—if not the most—important reasons for death by infection in cats at this time.

FCoV belongs to the family Coronaviridae of the Order Nidovirales, a group of large, spherical, enveloped, positive-sense, single-stranded ribonucleic acid (RNA) viruses that are found very frequently in cats. With a genome of 27 to 32 kb, encoding for an approximately 750 kDa polyprotein, four structural proteins, and up to five accessory nonstructural proteins, coronaviruses are the largest RNA viruses known to date. FCoV can be subdivided into two types. Type I virus is the most prevalent in the field; type II virus is less common and results from recombination between type I FCoV and canine coronavirus involving the spike gene.[2] Both types of viruses can induce FIP.

FCoV is transmitted fecal-orally between felids but is not infectious to other species (including human beings).

Coronavirus-specific antibodies are present in up to 90 per cent of cats in catteries and in up to 50 per cent of cats in single cat households; however, only about 5 per cent of FCoV-infected cats will develop FIP in multiple-cat households.[3]

Initially it was hypothesized that FCoV strains causing FIP are different from avirulent enteric FCoV strains, and FCoV strains had been subdivided into two distinct "biotypes," *feline enteric coronavirus* (FECV) and *feline infectious peritonitis virus* (FIPV). However, it is now known that all FCoV types may induce systemic infection as demonstrated by reverse-transcriptase polymerase chain reaction (RT-PCR) studies and that those "biotypes" are not two different virus species, but only represent virulence variants of the same virus.[4]

The precise process by which FIP develops is unclear, but there are two main hypotheses.[5] The first hypothesis, the so-called internal mutation theory, is based on the fact that a mutation is necessary that favors viral replication in macrophages.[6-9] In this case, cats are infected with the primarily avirulent FCoV, which replicates in enterocytes. In some instances, however, a mutation occurs in a certain region of the FCoV genome that confers to a new phenotype, leading to the ability of the mutated virus to replicate within macrophages. Although called internal mutation theory, no consistent mutation has been identified to date. In support of this hypothesis

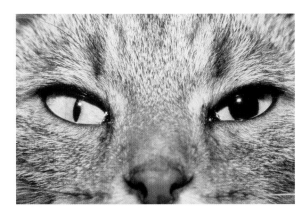

Figure 7-1 Cat with neurological signs including anisocoria due to granulomatous changes in the central nervous system caused by FIP.

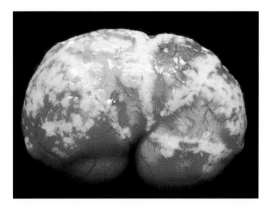

Figure 7-3 Granulomatous lesions in the kidneys at necropsy in a cat with FIP. (Courtesy Prof. Reinacher, Giessen, Germany.)

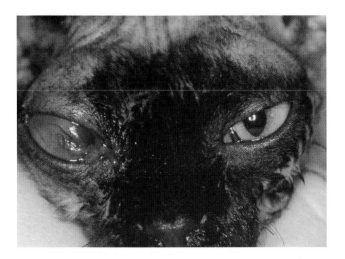

Figure 7-2 Cat with uveitis caused by FIP.

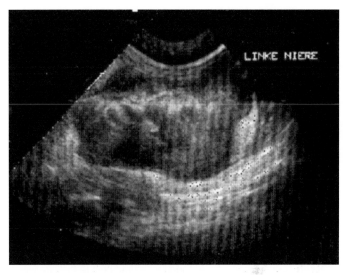

Figure 7-4 Granulomatous lesions in the kidneys visualized at abdominal ultrasound in a cat with FIP.

is the presence of highly virulent strains of FCoV that are capable of inducing FIP consistently, albeit under experimental conditions.[10] The second hypothesis for the development of FIP is that any FCoV can cause FIP but that viral load and the cat's immune response determine whether FIP will develop.[9-14] It is likely that both factors, namely viral genetics and host immunity, play a role in the development of FIP. In both hypotheses, the key pathogenic event in the development of FIP is the massive replication of FCoV in macrophages. If the cat fails to eliminate the macrophages infected with the replication-competent virus early in infection, the presence of the virus within macrophages initiates an ultimately fatal Arthus-type immune-mediated reaction that defines FIP.

Affected cats will develop signs caused by (1) granulomatous lesions in target organs, including central nervous system (Figure 7-1), eyes (Figure 7-2), and parenchymatous organs (Figure 7-3), that usually are small and only in exceptional cases visible by diagnostic imaging methods (Figure 7-4); and (2) vasculitis leading to fluid redistribution into second spaces with fluid accumulation in body cavities manifesting as ascites (Figures 7-5 to 7-7)

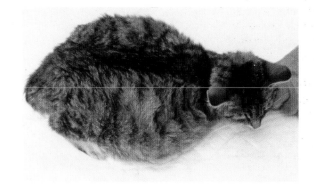

Figure 7-5 Six-month-old cat with massive ascites caused by FIP.

and thoracic (Figures 7-8 to 7-10) as well as other effusions (e.g., pericardial effusion, scrotal effusion). A rare nodular enteric form (Figure 7-11), seen in young cats with diarrhea and vomiting, is associated with intestinal granulomatous lesions.[15] In addition to the well-known clinical presentations, some unusual pictures have been

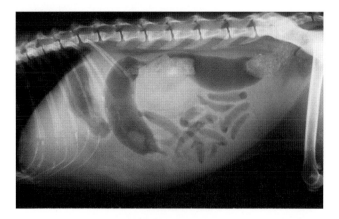

Figure 7-6 Abdominal radiograph (lateral view) of a cat with ascites caused by FIP.

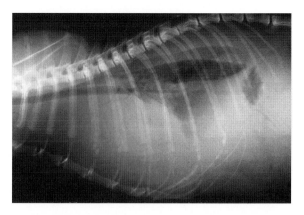

Figure 7-9 Thoracic radiograph (lateral view) of a cat with thoracic effusion caused by FIP.

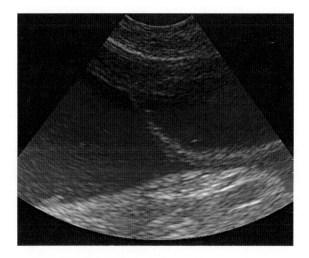

Figure 7-7 Abdominal ultrasound with fluid next to the urinary bladder in a cat with ascites caused by FIP.

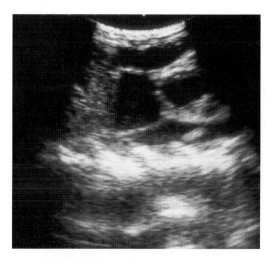

Figure 7-10 Thoracic ultrasound with fluid next to the heart in a cat with thoracic effusion caused by FIP.

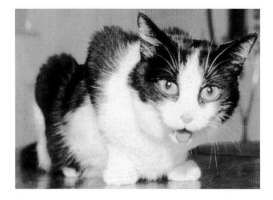

Figure 7-8 Sixteen-year-old cat with dyspnea and open mouth breathing caused by thoracic effusion due to FIP.

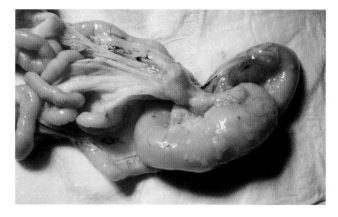

Figure 7-11 Granulomatous lesions in the intestines at necropsy in a cat with FIP presented for chronic diarrhea. (Courtesy Dr. Unterer, Munich, Germany.)

described. Skin fragility syndrome was found in a cat with FIP,[16] and other skin lesions (e.g., nodular skin lesion, papular skin lesions, pododermatitis) may be present as well.[17,18] One cat presented with priapism, and FCoV antigen was demonstrated immunohistochemically in its penile tissue.[19]

DIAGNOSIS

Because FIP is not only common but also deadly and no effective long-term management is available at this time, a reliable and rapid diagnosis is extremely important. Definitively diagnosing FIP in vivo, however, is extremely challenging. Difficulties in diagnosing this disease definitively arise from absence of noninvasive confirmatory tests in cats without obvious effusion. Presence of effusion should be excluded first, because obtaining and analyzing effusion is minimally invasive and much more sensitive than diagnostic tests using blood. In cats with no effusion, several parameters, including background of the cat, history, clinical signs, laboratory changes, and level of antibody titers should be taken into consideration to help to make the decision for invasive confirmative diagnostic methods.

HEMATOLOGY AND SERUM BIOCHEMISTRY EVALUATION

Hematology results often are abnormal in cats with FIP, but the changes are not pathognomonic. White blood cell counts can be decreased or increased. Lymphopenia commonly is present, mainly caused by apoptosis of uninfected T cells, primarily CD8+ T cells, as a result of high tumor necrosis factor-α (TNFα) concentrations produced by virus-infected macrophages.[20] However, lymphopenia in combination with neutrophilia generally is common in cats as a stress leukogram, is not typical for FIP, and can occur in many severe diseases in cats. A mild to moderate nonregenerative anemia also is a common finding in cats with FIP, but is another nonspecific laboratory abnormality that may occur in almost any chronic disease in cats.

The most common laboratory abnormality in cats with FIP is an increase in total serum protein concentration caused by increased globulins, mainly γ-globulins.[21,22] In one study, hyperproteinemia was present in about 50 per cent of cats with effusion and in 70 per cent of cats without effusion.[23] After experimental induction of FIP, an early increase of α_2-globulins is present, while γ-globulins and antibody titers increase only just before appearance of clinical signs.[24,25] The characteristically high levels of γ-globulins and the increased antibody titers invite the conclusion that hypergammaglobulinemia is due to a specific anti-FCoV immune response. Antibody titers and hypergammaglobulinemia show a linear correlation, but the wide variation in anti-FCoV titers at a given concentration of γ-globulins indicates that additional (autoimmune) reactions play a major role in the pathogenesis of FIP. It has been discussed that stimulation of B cells by interleukin-6, which is produced as part of the disease process, contributes to the increase in γ-globulins.[26] Thus, total protein in cats with FIP can reach very high concentrations of up to 120 g/L (12 g/dL) and higher. Albumin-to-globulin ratio, however, has a significantly higher diagnostic value to differentiate FIP from other diseases than total serum protein or γ-globulin concentrations, because a decrease in serum albumin also may occur through a decrease in production in association with liver failure or protein loss.[27,28] Protein loss in cats with FIP is caused by glomerulopathy secondary to immune complex deposition, by loss of protein due to exudative enteropathy in the case of granulomatous changes in the intestines, or by extravasation of protein-rich fluid during vasculitis.[28] An optimal cut-off

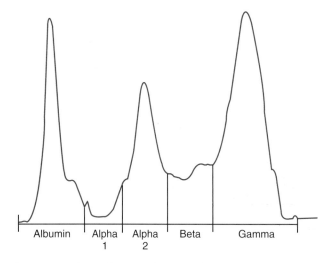

Figure 7-12 Electrophoresis of a cat with hypergammaglobulinemia caused by FIP.

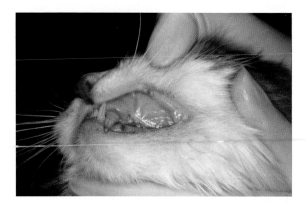

Figure 7-13 Yellow mucous membranes in a cat with liver insufficiency and hepatic icterus due to FIP.

value of 0.8 was determined for the albumin-to-globulin ratio.[28]

Serum protein electrophoresis also is often performed in cats suspected to have FIP (Figure 7-12); the main rationale behind the test is to distinguish a polyclonal from a monoclonal hypergammaglobulinemia in order to differentiate FIP (and other chronic infections) from tumors such as multiple myelomas or other plasma cell tumors (see Chapter 65). However, in cats with FIP, both polyclonal and monoclonal hypergammaglobulinemia can occur, and the same is found in tumors. Therefore the value of electrophoresis is limited.

Other laboratory parameters, including liver enzymes, bilirubin, blood urea nitrogen, and creatinine, can be elevated variably depending on the degree and localization of organ damage but are not helpful in establishing an etiological diagnosis. Hyperbilirubinemia and icterus (Figure 7-13) often are observed and frequently are a reflection of hepatic necrosis. Sometimes bilirubin concentration is increased in cats with FIP without evidence of hemolysis, liver disease, or cholestasis; this unusual finding is otherwise observed only in septic animals. Bilirubin metabolism and excretion into the biliary system is compromised in these cats, likely due to high

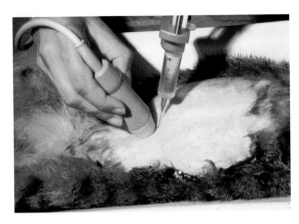

Figure 7-14 Ultrasound-guided puncture to obtain ascites for diagnostic tests in a cat with FIP.

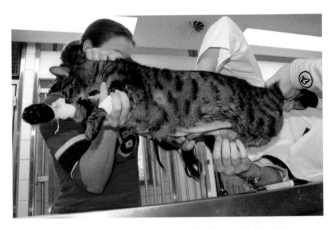

Figure 7-15 "Flying cat technique" to obtain ascites without ultrasound by puncturing at the lowest point of the "flying" cat.

levels of TNFα that inhibit transmembrane transport. Thus, high bilirubin in the absence of hemolysis and elevation of liver enzyme activity should raise the suspicion of FIP.[28]

Recent research has focused on the diagnostic value of acute-phase reaction parameters including α1-acid glycoprotein (AGP), a serum acute phase protein that is elevated in cats with FIP.[29,30] AGP is not only overexpressed in cats with FIP but also undergoes several modifications in the sialic acid content, including decreased expression of both α(2,6)-linked and α(2,3)-linked sialic acid.[31] High serum AGP levels (>3 mg/mL) can support the diagnosis of FIP,[32] but levels also rise in other inflammatory conditions, and thus these changes are not specific. Additionally, AGP also may be high in asymptomatic cats infected with FCoV, especially in households in which FCoV is endemic.[33]

EFFUSION FLUID EXAMINATION

If there is effusion, the most important diagnostic step is to get a fluid sample because tests on effusion have a much higher diagnostic value than tests that can be performed on blood. Fluid can be obtained through ultrasound-guided fine-needle aspiration (Figure 7-14) or using the "flying cat technique" in case of ascites (Figure 7-15). Only about one half of all cats who are presented with effusion have FIP.[34] Thus, although effusions of clear yellow color (Figure 7-16) and sticky consistency often are called "typical," the presence of this type of fluid in body cavities alone is not diagnostic. Sometimes the fluid caused by FIP has a totally different appearance, and even some cases with pure chylous effusion have been reported.[35] Usually, the effusion's protein content is very high (>3.5 g/dL) and consistent with an exudate, whereas the cellular content is low (<5000 nucleated cells/mL) and resembles more that of a modified transudate or even pure transudate.

Major differential diagnoses for these effusions include inflammatory liver disease, lymphoma, heart failure, and bacterial peritonitis or pleuritis. Lactate dehydrogenase (LDH) activity typically is high (>300 IU/L) in effusions due to FIP as it is released from inflammatory cells. Cyto-

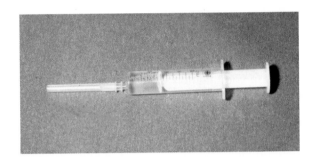

Figure 7-16 "Typical" effusion of clear yellow color and sticky consistency obtained from a cat with FIP.

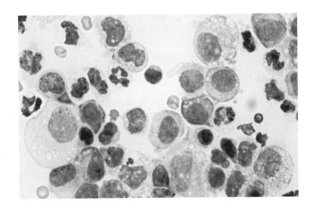

Figure 7-17 Cytological examination of the effusion with predominance of macrophages and neutrophils in a modified transudate of a cat with FIP.

logical examination of the effusion in cats with FIP shows a variable picture, but often consists predominantly of macrophages and neutrophils (Figure 7-17). Cytological changes may appear similar in cats with bacterial serositis or sometimes with lymphoma; these effusions, however, usually can be differentiated by the presence of malignant cells or intracellular bacteria in cytological specimens and by bacterial growth on culture, respectively. Electrophoresis on effusion fluid is a diagnostic tool with a relatively high positive predictive value (if albumin-

To perform the Rivalta's test, a transparent reagent tube (volume 10 mL) is filled with approximately 8 mL distilled water, to which 1 drop of acetic acid (highly concentrated vinegar, 98 per cent) is added and mixed thoroughly. On the surface of this solution, 1 drop of the effusion fluid is carefully layered. If the drop disappears and the solution remains clear, the Rivalta's test is defined as negative. If the drop retains its shape, stays attached to the surface, or floats slowly down to the bottom of the tube (droplike or jellyfish-like), the Rivalta's test is defined as positive.

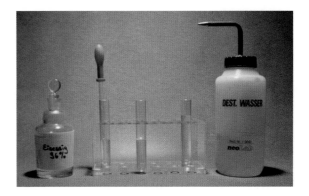

Figure 7-18 Reagents necessary to perform the "Rivalta's test" including a transparent reagent tube (volume 10 mL), distilled water, acetic acid (highly concentrated vinegar, 98 per cent).

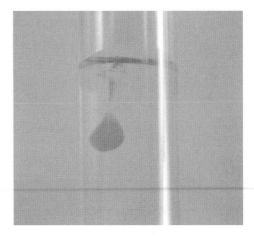

Figure 7-19 Positive "Rivalta's test" with a drop retaining its shape and staying attached to the surface. Performed with the effusion of a cat with FIP.

globulin ratio is <0.4) and a relatively high negative predictive value (if the ratio is >0.8).

"Rivalta's test" is a very simple, inexpensive method that does not require special laboratory equipment and can be performed easily in private practice. This test was developed originally by an Italian researcher (named "Rivalta") around 1900 and was used to differentiate transudates and exudates in human patients. However, other methods have replaced this test in human medicine. It is not diagnostically helpful in dogs with effusion. However, this test is very useful in cats to differentiate between effusions due to FIP and effusions caused by other diseases.[28] The high protein content and high concentrations of fibrin and inflammatory mediators lead to a positive reaction (Box 7-1). To perform this test (Figure 7-18), a transparent reagent tube (volume 10 mL) is filled with approximately 8 mL distilled water, to which one drop of acetic acid (highly concentrated vinegar, 98 per cent) is added and mixed thoroughly. On the surface of this solution, one drop of the effusion fluid is layered carefully. If the drop disappears and the solution remains clear, the Rivalta's test is defined as negative. If the drop retains its shape, stays attached to the surface, or floats slowly down to the bottom of the tube (droplike or jellyfish-like), the Rivalta's test is defined as positive (Figure 7-19). The Rivalta's test had a high positive predictive value (86 per cent) and a very high negative predictive value for FIP (96 per cent) in a study in which cats who presented with effusion were investigated (prevalence of FIP 51 per cent).[28] Positive Rivalta's test results sometimes can occur in cats with bacterial peritonitis or lymphoma. Those effusions, however, usually are easy to differentiate through macroscopic and cytological examinations, and/or bacterial culture.

CEREBROSPINAL FLUID EXAMINATION

Analysis of cerebrospinal fluid (CSF) from cats with neurological signs due to FIP lesions may reveal elevated protein (50 to 350 mg/dL with a normal value of less than 25 mg/dL) and pleocytosis (100 to 10,000 nucleated cells/mL) containing mainly neutrophils, lymphocytes, and macrophages.[36-38] This is, however, a relatively nonspecific finding. Many cats with neurological signs caused by FIP have normal CSF.

MEASUREMENT OF ANTIBODIES

Antibody titers measured in serum are an extensively used diagnostic tool. However, a high percentage of healthy cats are FCoV antibody–positive, and most of those cats will never develop FIP. There is no "FIP antibody test"; all that can be measured is antibodies against FCoV. Thus, antibody titers must be interpreted extremely cautiously; the inadequacies and pitfalls of this test have been the topic of continuous discussions and controversies, and it has been assumed that more cats have died of misleading FCoV antibody test results than of FIP.[39] Although criticized frequently, antibody testing still has a certain role in the diagnosis and, more importantly, in the management of FIP, when done by appropriate methodologies and when results are interpreted properly. However, antibody testing can only be useful if the laboratory is reliable and consistent, because methodologies and antibody titer results may vary significantly. A single serum sample, divided and sent to five different laboratories in the United States, yielded five different results.[40]

It is important to understand that the presence of antibodies does not indicate FIP and the absence of antibodies does not exclude FIP. Low or medium titers have no diagnostic value.[28] It has been shown that in cats with fulminant FIP, titers decrease terminally,[39] and approximately 10 per cent of cats with clinically manifest FIP have negative results.[28] This is either because large amounts of virus in the cat's body bind to antibodies and render them unavailable to bind the antigen in the antibody test, or because the antibodies are lost into the effusion when protein is translocated during vasculitis. If interpreted carefully, very high titers can be of certain diagnostic value.

It also has been shown that the height of the antibody titer correlates directly with the amount of virus that is shed in the feces: cats with high antibody titers are more likely to shed FCoV and to shed more consistently higher amounts of the virus.[41] Therefore the height of the titer is correlated directly with virus replication rate and the amount of virus in the intestines.

Antibody measurement also may be important for the common situation in practice, in which a cat is presented because it had been in contact with a cat with FIP or a suspected or known virus excreter. Either the owner wants to know the prognosis for the exposed cat, or the owner wishes to obtain another cat and needs to know whether the exposed cat is shedding FCoV. Also, cat breeders may request testing with the goal of creating a FCoV-free cattery. Screening a cattery for the presence of FCoV or screening a cat before introduction into a FCoV-free cattery also are important indications.

Measuring antibodies in fluids (e.g., effusion, CSF) other than blood has been investigated. Presence of antibodies in effusion is correlated with the presence of antibodies in blood,[42] and thus, antibody titers in effusions also are not very helpful. Cats in a recent study had medium antibody titers irrespective of whether they had FIP or not.[43] One study looking into the diagnostic value of antibody detection in CSF found a very good correlation to the presence of FIP when compared to histopathological examination[44]; however, two recent studies of a large number of cats presented to veterinary teaching hospitals revealed no significant difference in antibody titers in CSF from cats with neurological signs due to FIP compared to cats with other neurological diseases confirmed by histopathological examination.[45,46]

FCoV REVERSE-TRANSCRIPTASE POLYMERASE CHAIN REACTION (RT-PCR)

FCoV RT-PCR in blood is used with increasing frequency as diagnostic tool for the diagnosis of FIP. However, so far, no PCR has been developed that can diagnose FIP definitively. Although FIP-causing viruses are, according to the internal mutation theory, genetic mutants of harmless enteric FCoV, numerous sites exist in the 3C and 7B genes that can be mutated or deleted and confer on the virus the capability to infect and replicate within macrophages. Sometimes the change can be a single RNA base. As a result, PCR primers to discriminate between FIP-causing viruses and harmless enteric FCoV can not be designed, and it is not possible to distinguish between a mutated and a nonmutated virus by PCR.[47] Additionally, PCR results are not easy to interpret. PCR can provide

false-negative results (e.g., because the assay requires reverse transcription of viral RNA to deoxyribonucleic acid [DNA] prior to amplification of DNA, and degradation of RNA can be a potential problem because ribonucleases [RNases] are virtually ubiquitous), or false-positive results (e.g., the assay does not distinguish between "virulent" and "avirulent" FCoV strains, nor will it discriminate FCoV from coronaviruses from other species).

Furthermore, several studies support the hypothesis that viremia occurs not only in cats with FIP but also in healthy carriers. FCoV RNA could be detected in the blood of cats with FIP but also in healthy cats that do not develop FIP for a period of up to 70 months.[48,49] It was even shown that in households in which FCoV is endemic, cats can be viremic irrespective of their health status and that the presence of viremia does not predispose the cats to the development of FIP.[50]

Another approach is to measure messenger RNA (mRNA) by RT-PCR in blood, with the rationale that levels of mRNA may correlate with the level of replication of FCoV and thus be correlated with the presence of FIP. However, the validity of this test is unclear at the moment, and 5 to 50 per cent of healthy cats were positive in that test.[51] An additional problem is that the test currently is not available in Europe or the United States.

Therefore the results of PCR tests in general must be interpreted carefully, and PCR can not be used as a tool for diagnosing FIP definitively. There may be a difference in serum virus load in cats with FIP versus cats with viremia in "harmless" FCoV infection,[13] but further studies are necessary to support this hypothesis. PCR in effusion or CSF also has been discussed as a diagnostic tool. However, data on the usefulness of these approaches are not yet available.

For another strategy, PCR has been used to detect FCoV in fecal samples and is sensitive and useful for documenting that a cat is shedding FCoV in feces. The strength of the PCR signal in feces correlates with the amount of virus present in the intestines,[41] and these results can be useful in detecting cats who shed high virus loads chronically and thus pose a high risk in multiple-cat households.

ANTIBODY ANTIGEN COMPLEX DETECTION

Because FIP is an immune-mediated disease and antibody antigen complexes play an important role in the pathogenesis, it has been suggested to look for circulating immune complexes in serum and effusions. Coronavirus-specific antibody antigen complex detection can be performed using a competitive enzyme-linked immunosorbent assay (ELISA). Usefulness, however, is limited, and the positive predictive value of this test was not very high (67 per cent) in one study evaluating a high number of patients with FIP and control cats.[28]

IMMUNOSTAINING OF FCoV ANTIGEN IN MACROPHAGES

Other methods to detect the virus include detection of the presence of FCoV antigen in macrophages using immunofluorescence (in effusion macrophages) (Figure 7-20) or immunohistochemistry (in tissue macrophages) (Figure 7-21). Immunostaining can not differentiate between the "harmless" FCoV and FIP-causing FCoV, but only FIP-causing virus is able to replicate in sufficiently large amounts in macrophages to result in a positive staining. Although FCoV may be present systemically in cats without FIP, only in FIP will there be a sufficiently large amount of virus in macrophages required to obtain a positive staining. In a recent study in which a large number of cats with confirmed FIP and controls with other (confirmed) diseases were investigated (n = 171, prevalence of FIP 64 per cent), positive immunofluorescence staining of intracellular FCoV antigen in macrophages of the effusion was 100 per cent predictive of FIP.[28] Unfortunately, the negative predictive value of the test is not very high (57 per cent), which can be explained mainly by low numbers of macrophages on effusion smears (even for cats with FIP), resulting in negative staining.[28]

Immunohistochemistry can be used to detect the expression of FCoV antigen in tissue, and it also proved to be 100 per cent predictive of FIP if positive.[52,53] However, invasive methods (e.g., laparotomy or laparoscopy) usually are necessary to obtain appropriate tissue samples. When the diagnostic sensitivity between true-cut biopsy (TCB) and fine-needle aspiration (FNA) of liver and kidney tissue obtained at necropsy was compared, the sensitivity of FNA was similar to TCB; however, a higher sensitivity in the liver versus kidneys was observed.[54] The value of ultrasound-guided FNA to diagnose FIP in vivo, however, still has to be investigated in further studies.

Therefore there are two diagnostic strategies to obtain a definitive diagnosis of FIP. The first step in the diagnostic process always is to look for effusion (Figure 7-22). If there is effusion, immunofluorescence staining of FCoV antigen in effusion macrophages can diagnose FIP. If there is no effusion, tissue samples of altered organs have to be obtained for a definitive diagnosis. Either histological examination itself is confirmatory, or immunohisto-

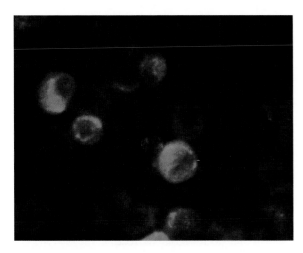

Figure 7-20 Positive immunofluorescence staining of FCoV antigen in macrophages in the effusion of a cat with FIP.

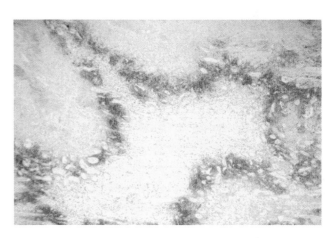

Figure 7-21 Positive immunohistochemistry staining of FCoV antigen in macrophages in granulomatous lesions in the kidney of a cat with FIP.

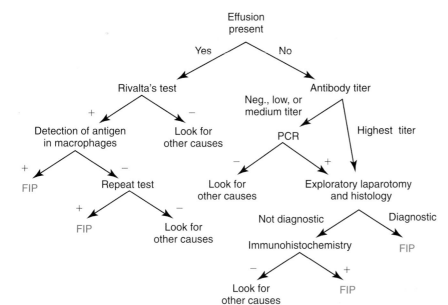

Figure 7-22 Diagnostic algorithm to obtain a definitive diagnosis.

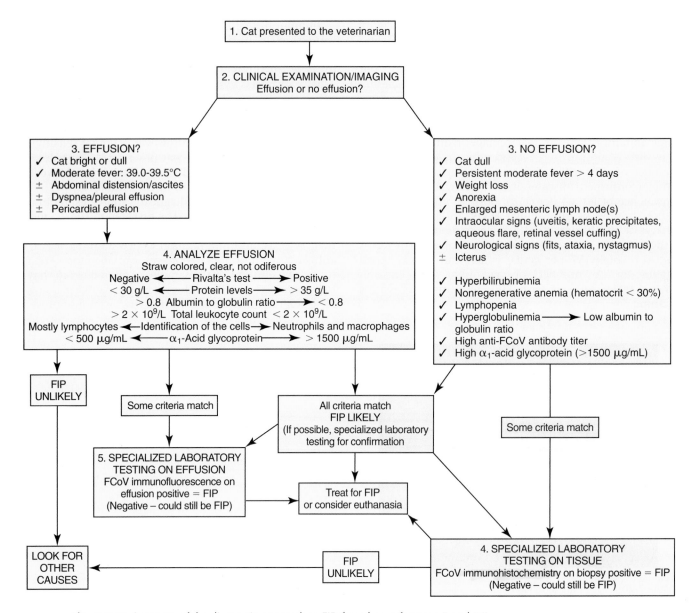

Figure 7-23 Summary of the diagnostic approach to FIP (based on references 5 and 74).

chemistry staining of FCoV antigen in tissue macrophages can be used to diagnose FIP. A summary of the diagnostic approach to FIP is provided in Figure 7-23.

TREATMENT

To date, treatment of cats with FIP remains frustrating and has to be limited to the few patients who respond favorably within the first few days. Virtually every cat with FIP dies. There are occasional reports of cats surviving with treatment for up to several months after diagnosis of FIP who enjoyed a reasonable quality of life. It is not clear whether this "long-term" survival is actually caused by treatment. There even have been some rare reports of cats who have "recovered" from FIP; however,

a definitive diagnosis of FIP has not been obtained in these patients. Once clinical signs become debilitating and weight and appetite decline, the owners must be prepared for the reality that their cat is dying.[55] Treatment (or euthanasia) should only be considered after every effort has been made to obtain a definitive diagnosis. Treatment options are summarized in Table 7-1.

PROGNOSIS

The prognosis for a cat with FIP is very poor. In a prospective study including 43 cats with confirmed FIP, the median survival after the definitive diagnosis was 9 days. Some cats, however, live for several months[56]; one cat who lived 200 days after definitive diagnosis has been documented.[57] Factors that indicate a bad prognosis and

Table 7-1 Drugs that Have Been Used to Treat Cats with FIP, Including Author's Recommendation and Evidence-Based Medicine (EBM) Level

	Comment	Author's Recommendation	EBM Level
Ribavirin	Works in vitro but toxic in cats	Not recommended	2
Vidarabine	Works in vitro, but toxic in cats	Not recommended	4
Human interferon-α SQ high dose	Although human interferon-α is effective in vitro against FCoV, SQ treatment did not work in an experimental trial	Ineffective	2
Human interferon-α PO low dose	No trials Only acts as immune stimulant if given orally Immune stimulation should be avoided in cats with FIP	Contraindicated	4
Feline interferon-ω	One placebo-controlled double-blind field study	Ineffective	1
Prednisolone/dexamethasone (immunosuppressive doses)	No controlled studies; some cats have improved during treatment and survived for several months, but does not cure FIP	Currently supportive treatment of choice If effusion is present, dexamethasone IT or IP may be helpful	3
Pentoxifylline	Aimed at treating the vasculitis Some veterinarians in practice have tried, but there are no published studies or case reports	Requires studies	4
Ozagrel hydrochloride	Thromboxane synthesis inhibitor aimed at treating the inflammatory response, only used in 2 cases with beneficial effect	May have some beneficial effect, controlled studies needed	3
Cyclosporine A	Aimed to immunosuppress (lower the corticosteroid dose) No published studies	Not recommended because more directed against cellular immunity than humoral (lack of data)	4
Cyclophosphamide	Aimed to immunosuppress (lower the corticosteroid dose) No published studies	Might be considered in combination with glucocorticoids	4
Chlorambucil	Aimed to immunosuppress (lower the corticosteroid dose) No published studies	Might be considered in combination with glucocorticoids	4
Azathioprine	Toxic in cats Aimed to immunosuppress (lower the corticosteroid dose) No published studies	Not recommended	4
Acetylsalicylic acid, platelet inhibitory dosage	Aimed at treating the inflammatory response as well as the vasculitis No published studies	May have some beneficial effect, but side effects possible if used in combination with high-dose glucocorticoids	4

EBM level 1, Confirmed by placebo-controlled double-blind field study; EBM level 2, shown in a controlled experimental study; EBM level 3, supported by case series; EBM level 4, only based on expert opinion; IP, intraperitoneal; IT, intrathoracic.

a short survival time are a low Karnofsky's score (index for quality of life),[58] thrombocytopenia, lymphopenia, hyperbilirubinemia, and a large amount of effusion.[56] Seizures also have to be considered an unfavorable prognostic sign because they are significantly more frequent in patients with marked extension of the inflammatory lesions to the forebrain.[59] Cats who show no improvement within 3 days after treatment initiation are unlikely to show any benefit from therapy, and euthanasia should be considered.

SYMPTOMATIC TREATMENT

Because FIP is caused by inflammatory and inappropriate immune responses to FCoV, supportive treatment is aimed at suppressing this immune overreaction, usually using corticosteroids. There are, however, no controlled studies that indicate whether corticosteroids have any beneficial effects. Occasional patients treated with corticosteroids have shown improvement for up to several months, but these are only anecdotal reports. Immune-suppressive drugs such as prednisone (2 to 4 mg/kg PO q24h) or cyclophosphamide (2 to 4 mg/kg PO q48h) have been recommended.[60] Some cats with effusion benefit from tapping and removal of the fluid and injection of dexamethasone into the abdominal or thoracic cavity (1 mg/kg q24h until no further effusion is present).

Cats with FIP also should be treated with broad-spectrum antibiotics and supportive therapy (subcutaneous fluids) in addition. A thromboxane synthetase inhibitor (ozagrel hydrochloride) that inhibits platelet aggregation has been used in a small number of affected cats and has led to some improvement of clinical signs.[61]

IMMUNE MODULATORS

Some veterinarians use immune modulators (e.g., *Propionibacterium acnes,* acemannan) to treat cats with FIP with no documented controlled evidence of efficacy. It has been suggested that these agents may benefit infected animals by restoring compromised immune function, thereby allowing the patient to control the viral burden and recover from clinical signs. However, a nonspecific stimulation of the immune system actually seems to be contraindicated because clinical signs develop and progress as a result of an immune-mediated response.

Some old reports are published in which the immune-modulator tylosin was used. Tylosin belongs to the macrolide class of antibiotics but, like other macrolides, also has immune-modulatory effects. Using tylosin at a dose of 22 mg/kg/day, a "temporary remission" was achieved in 10 cats; however, FIP was not confirmed in these cases. Three cats suspected of having FIP were treated with tylosin (starting at 88 mg/kg PO q12h) and prednisolone (starting at 4 mg/kg/day PO) as well as supportive treatment with fluids and vitamins. One cat died after 42 days, the others were still alive and healthy after 180 and 210 days, respectively. The diagnosis of FIP, however, also was not confirmed in these cats. One cat suspected to have FIP was treated with tylosin orally (50 mg/cat PO q8h) as well as prednisolone (10 mg/cat) and tylosin (200 mg/cat intraperitoneally) after each of several abdominocenteses. This cat recovered within 2 months; however, several other cats treated in a similar manner died.[60]

The immune modulator promodulin was used in 52 cats suspected to have FIP who responded favorably to treatment; a rapid remission of clinical signs (anorexia, fever, effusion) was observed. However, once again FIP was not confirmed in these cats, and there were no control group or long-term follow-up evaluations included in the study.[60]

In one study, 29 cats suspected to have FIP were treated in five groups over 6 weeks, and received either ampicillin (100 mg/kg/day), prednisolone (4 mg/kg/day), and cyclophosphamide (4 mg/kg/day); dexamethasone (2 mg/kg at day 1 and day 5) and ampicillin (20 mg/kg q8h for 10 days); human interferon-α (6 × 10^5 IU/cat 5 days a week for 3 weeks); a paraimmunity inducer (0.5 mL/cat/week for 6 weeks); or nothing. Between 29 per cent and 80 per cent (depending on the group) of the cats died within 3 years. However, FIP was not confirmed in these cats either, and inclusion criteria remain unclear.[62]

ANTIVIRAL CHEMOTHERAPY

To date, search for an effective antiviral treatment for cats with FIP, unfortunately, has not been very successful, although a number of studies have been performed. However, objective assessment of these studies is hampered by the lack of well-controlled clinical trials in which new treatments are compared against a standard care or placebo. In most studies, presence of FIP was not even confirmed before treatment was initiated, making an assessment of the outcome very difficult. Currently, no treatment has been proved effective in curing FIP.[60]

The antiviral drug ribavirin (16.5 mg/kg q24h for 10 to 14 days PO, IM, or IV) was administered to specific pathogen-free kittens 18 hours after experimental challenge with an FIP-causing virus. Ribavirin, a nucleoside analogue, prevents formation of viral proteins, most likely by interfering with capping of viral mRNA. All kittens, including ribavirin-treated and untreated kittens, succumbed to FIP. Clinical signs of disease were even more severe in the ribavirin-treated kittens, and their mean survival times were shortened. Although active against FCoV in vitro,[63,64] ribavirin was not an effective treatment for cats with FIP because of its severe side effects.[65] An attempt to decrease the toxicity of ribavirin by incorporating it into lecithin-containing liposomes and giving it at lower dosage (5 mg/kg) intravenously to cats challenged with a FIP-causing virus also failed.[66]

One 3-year-old male cat who was feline leukemia virus–positive and suspected to have FIP was treated with melphalan, an alkylating agent of the nitrogen mustard group that interacts irreversibly with DNA. The cat received melphalan (starting at 1 mg/kg q72h for 9 months), prednisone (10 mg/kg q12h, that was reduced after 3 weeks over the next 6 weeks to 5 mg/kg q48h), ampicillin (10 mg/kg q8h for 10 days), and streptokinase (10^4 IU/cat intraperitoneally after abdominocenteses q12h for 4 days). Additionally, vitamins and minerals were administered. The cat responded well to treatment for 9 months, then developed a myeloproliferative disorder and died. The diagnosis of FIP was not confirmed in this case either; on histopathological examination, there was no evidence of FIP.[60]

Interferons have been used frequently in cats with FIP. Human interferon-α has a direct antiviral effect by inducing a general "antiviral state" of interferon-α–containing cells that prevent virus replication. In vitro, antiviral efficacy of human interferon-α was demonstrated against an FIP-causing FCoV strain. In a controlled treatment study including 74 specific pathogen-free cats (52 treated, 22 controls) in whom FIP was induced experimentally, cats received human interferon-α, feline interferon-β, *Propionibacterium acnes* (an immune-modulatory compound), a combination, or placebo. Neither the prophylactic nor the therapeutic administration of high doses (10^4 or 10^6 IU/kg) of interferon-α, feline interferon-β (10^3 IU/kg), or *Propionibacterium acnes* (0.4 mg/cat or 4 mg/cat) reduced mortality significantly in treated versus untreated cats. Only in cats treated with 10^6 IU/kg interferon-α in combination with *Propionibacterium acnes* was the mean survival time significantly prolonged (for about 3 weeks). This is one of the few published studies in which the diagnosis of FIP was confirmed (artificial infection, histopathological examination at the end of the study) and in which a control group was included.[67]

Recently, feline interferon-ω was licensed for use in veterinary medicine in some European countries and Japan. Interferons are species-specific, and cats can be treated parenterally over long periods of time without developing antibodies. FCoV replication is inhibited by feline interferon-ω in vitro.[68] Promising results were obtained in one uncontrolled trial, but FIP was not confirmed in these cases.[69] In a recently performed randomized placebo-controlled double-blind treatment trial, 37 cats with FIP were treated with interferon-ω or placebo. In all cats, FIP was confirmed by immunofluorescence staining or immunohistochemical staining of FCoV antigen in effusion or tissue macrophages. All cats received corticosteroids, either as dexamethasone in case of effusion (1 mg/kg intrathoracic or intraperitoneal injection q24h) or prednisolone (2 mg/kg PO q24h). In addition, cats received either interferon-ω (10^6 U/kg SQ q24h for 8 days and subsequently once every week) or placebo. There was no statistically significant difference in the mean survival time of cats treated with interferon-ω versus placebo. Cats survived for a period of 3 to 200 days.[57] (See Chapter 36 for a discussion on the use of interferon-ω in feline skin diseases.)

CONTROL OF INFECTION

MANAGEMENT OF CATS AFTER CONTACT WITH A CAT WITH FIP

Often the question will arise whether it is dangerous to bring a cat with diagnosed FIP back into a household with other cats. When a cat in a household develops FIP, all in-contact cats will have been exposed already to the same FCoV. It has remained a matter of discussion whether the FIP-causing virus may be excreted and, as a result, whether FIP could be transmitted between cats. This seems generally not to be the case under natural circumstances. Studies to detect the mutated virus (referring to the internal mutation theory) in secretions or excretions of cats with FIP have failed. After FIP has developed, a cat will shed less "harmless" FCoV than it did before the development of FIP. However, under experimental conditions, it has been possible to transmit FIP-causing virus from a cat with FIP to in-contact cats. Recently, the genomic RNA sequence of a field FCoV strain isolated postmortem from the jejunum and liver of a cat with FIP was determined, and comparisons of the enteric (jejunum)–derived and nonenteric (liver)–derived viral RNA sequences revealed 100 per cent nucleotide identity, a finding that challenges the "internal mutation theory."[14] Based on current understanding, the advice seems appropriate that it is relatively safe to take the cat with FIP back into the household with the cats who already have been in contact with the FCoV strain, because these cats will have a certain immunity to that specific strain. It is, however, not recommended to allow contact of a cat with FIP with any new "naïve" cat.[5]

If a cat has been euthanized or has died due to FIP, and there are no remaining cats, the owner should wait about 3 months before obtaining another cat, because FCoV can stay infectious for at least 7 weeks in the environment. If there are other cats in that household, they are most likely infected with FCoV and are shedding FCoV. In "natural circumstances," cats go outside to defecate and bury their feces, in which case the virus remains infectious hours to days (slightly longer in freezing conditions). However, domesticated cats have been introduced to litter boxes in which FCoV may survive for several days and possibly up to 7 weeks in desiccated feces. Therefore cats who had contact with FCoV-shedding cats most likely have a better chance of eliminating the virus if allowed to go outside (optimal situation is in a fenced garden).

It is very common that a cat is presented to the veterinarian because it was in contact with a cat with FIP or with a suspected or known virus excreter. The owner may want to know the prognosis for the exposed cat, or may want to obtain another cat and needs to know whether the exposed cat is shedding FCoV. It is very likely that this cat will be antibody-positive because 95 to 100 per cent of cats exposed to FCoV become infected and develop antibodies approximately 2 to 3 weeks after exposure. There are very few cats, however, who may be resistant to FCoV infection. It has been shown that some cats in FCoV-endemic multiple-cat households remain antibody-negative continuously.[70] The mechanism of action for this resistance is still unknown.

The owner should be advised that cats in contact most likely will have antibodies and should be reassured that this is not associated necessarily with a poor prognosis. Most cats infected with FCoV will not develop FIP, and many cats in single-cat or two-cat households eventually will clear their infection and become antibody-negative in a few months to years (usually about 6 months). Ideally, the owner should be advised to wait until antibody titers of all cats are negative or until fecal PCR tests are negative before obtaining a new cat. (If four fecal samples obtained within a period of 2 weeks are negative by PCR, the cat is very unlikely to harbor FCoV.) If antibody testing is used, cats should be retested (using the same laboratory) every 6 to 12 months until the antibody test is negative. Some cats, however, will remain antibody-positive for years.

MANAGEMENT OF MULTIPLE-CAT HOUSEHOLDS WITH FIP

In most multiple-cat households, FCoVs are endemic, and thus FIP will occur almost inevitably. Ideally, multiple-cat households should be free of FCoV. This, however, is not realistic. Households of fewer than five cats may become FCoV-free spontaneously and naturally, but this is almost impossible in households with more than 10 cats, because the virus will pass from one cat to another maintaining the infection.[71] This holds true for virtually all multiple-cat environments, such as breeding catteries, shelters, foster homes, and other multiple-cat homes. In these FCoV-endemic environments, there is virtually nothing to prevent FIP. Vaccination in any FCoV-endemic environment or in a household with known cases of FIP is not effective.[72]

Various strategies have been used to eliminate FCoV from an endemic cattery. Reducing the number of cats (especially kittens less than 12 months old) and keeping possibly FCoV-contaminated surfaces clean can minimize population loads of FCoV. Serum antibody or fecal PCR testing and segregating should be performed to stop exposure. Approximately one third of antibody-positive cats excrete virus[3]; therefore every antibody-positive cat has to be considered infectious. After 3 to 6 months, antibody titers can be retested to determine whether cats become seronegative. Alternatively, PCR testing of (several) fecal samples can be performed to detect chronic FCoV carriers so that those cats can be removed. In large multiple-cat environments, 40 to 60 per cent of cats shed virus in their feces at any given time. About 20 per cent will shed virus persistently, whereas 20 per cent will be immune and not shed virus. If a cat remains persistently PCR-positive for more than 6 weeks, it should be eliminated from the household and placed in a single-cat environment.[71]

More than any other factor, the management of kittens determines whether they become infected with FCoV. Kittens of FCoV-shedding queens should be protected from infection by maternally derived antibodies until they are 5 to 6 weeks old. An early weaning protocol for the prevention of FCoV infection in kittens has been proposed, consisting of isolation of queens 2 weeks prior to parturition, strict quarantine of queen and kittens, and early weaning at 5 weeks of age.[40] Early removal of kittens from the queen and prevention of infection from other cats may succeed in raising these kittens free of infection. For early weaning to be most effective, kittens should be taken to a new home (with no other cats) at 5 weeks of age. Although straightforward in concept, isolation of queens and early weaning is not simple. The procedure requires quarantine rooms and procedures that absolutely ensure that new virus does not enter. In addition, special care must be taken during the 2- to 7-weeks-of-age period to socialize these kittens. The success of early weaning and isolation depends on effective quarantine and low numbers of cats (< 5) in the household. If both are not possible, performing early weaning becomes questionable. Also, time and money involved with early weaning procedures, as well as space to keep queens and litters under quarantine, may be a problem in large multiple-cat households. In a study in large catteries in Switzerland in which the above-described early weaning protocol was followed, the procedure failed, and viral infection of kittens as young as 2 weeks old was demonstrated.[41]

Following another approach, it has been proposed that heritable resistance to FIP in breeding catteries should be maximized. Genetic predisposition plays a role, but is not understood completely. Full-sibling littermates of kittens with FIP have a higher likelihood of developing the disease than other cats in the same environment. If a cat has two or more litters in which kittens develop FIP, that cat should not be bred again. Particular attention should be paid to pedigrees of tomcats in which FIP is overrepresented. As line breeding often uses valuable tomcats extensively, eliminating such animals may have an effect on improving overall resistance.[71]

In a shelter, prevention of FIP is virtually impossible unless cats are kept strictly in separate cages and handled only through sterile handling devices (comparable to isolation units). Isolation often is not effective because FCoV is transported easily on clothes, shoes, dust, and cats. Comparison of shelters with different types of handling procedures revealed significant correlation between an increase in the number of handling events outside the cages and an increase in the percentage of antibody-positive cats. In a study in which feral cats were tested at the time they were brought into local shelters (in which multiple cats were kept together) and at 1- to 2-week intervals thereafter, only a low number of cats had antibodies at the time of entering; however, the percentage of seropositive cats increased rapidly until virtually all cats in the shelters were infected with FCoV.[73] Shelters should have written information sheets or contracts informing adopters about FCoV and FIP. Shelter personnel should understand that FCoV is unavoidable in multiple-cat environments and that FIP is an unavoidable consequence of endemic FCoV. Shelters need to optimize facilities and husbandry, so they can be cleaned easily and at least minimize virus spread. It is essential to decrease viral load and also stress levels in such an environment.[71] (See Chapter 74 for more information about disease control in shelters.)

REFERENCES

1. Rohrbach BW, Legendre AM, Baldwin CA, et al: Epidemiology of feline infectious peritonitis among cats examined at veterinary medical teaching hospitals, *J Am Vet Med Assoc* 218:1111, 2001.
2. Herrewegh AA, Smeenk I, Horzinek MC, et al: Feline coronavirus type II strains 79-1683 and 79-1146 originate from a double recombination between feline coronavirus type I and canine coronavirus, *J Virol* 72:4508, 1998.
3. Addie DD, Toth S, Murray GD, et al: Risk of feline infectious peritonitis in cats naturally infected with feline coronavirus, *Am J Vet Res* 56:429, 1995.
4. Herrewegh AA, Vennema H, Horzinek MC, et al: The molecular genetics of feline coronaviruses: comparative sequence analysis of the ORF7a/7b transcription unit of different biotypes, *Virology* 212:622, 1995.
5. European Advisory Board on Cat Diseases: Feline infectious peritonitis. Guidelines of The European Advisory Board on Cat Diseases. [WWW page]. http://www.abcd-vets.org/guidelines/index.asp, 2009.
6. Vennema H, Poland A, Foley J, et al: Feline infectious peritonitis viruses arise by mutation from endemic feline enteric coronaviruses, *Virology* 243:150, 1998.
7. Haijema BJ, Volders H, Rottier PJ: Live, attenuated coronavirus vaccines through the directed deletion of group-specific genes provide protection against feline infectious peritonitis, *J Virol* 78:3863, 2004.
8. Rottier PJ, Nakamura K, Schellen P, et al: Acquisition of macrophage tropism during the pathogenesis of feline infectious peritonitis is determined by mutations in the feline coronavirus spike protein, *J Virol* 79:14122, 2005.
9. Cornelissen E, Dewerchin HL, Van Hamme E, et al: Absence of surface expression of feline infectious peritonitis virus (FIPV) antigens on infected cells isolated from cats with FIP, *Vet Microbiol* 121:131, 2007.

10. Poland AM, Vennema H, Foley JE, et al: Two related strains of feline infectious peritonitis virus isolated from immuno-compromised cats infected with a feline enteric coronavirus, *J Clin Microbiol* 34:3180, 1996.

11. Addie DD, Toth S, Murray GD, et al: The risk of typical and antibody enhanced feline infectious peritonitis among cats from feline coronavirus endemic households, *Feline Practice* 23:24, 1995.

12. Meli M, Kipar A, Müller C, et al: High viral loads despite absence of clinical and pathological findings in cats experimentally infected with feline coronavirus (FCoV) type I and in naturally FCoV-infected cats, *J Feline Med Surg* 6:69, 2004.

13. Kipar A, Baptiste K, Barth A, et al: Natural FCoV infection: cats with FIP exhibit significantly higher viral loads than healthy infected cats, *J Feline Med Surg* 8:69, 2006.

14. Dye C, Siddell SG: Genomic RNA sequence of feline coronavirus strain FCoV C1Je, *J Feline Med Surg* 9:202, 2007.

15. Harvey CJ, Lopez JW, Hendrick MJ: An uncommon intestinal manifestation of feline infectious peritonitis: 26 cases (1986-1993), *J Am Vet Med Assoc* 209:1117, 1996.

16. Trotman TK, Mauldin E, Hoffmann V, et al: Skin fragility syndrome in a cat with feline infectious peritonitis and hepatic lipidosis, *Vet Dermatol* 18:365, 2007.

17. Cannon MJ, Silkstone MA, Kipar AM: Cutaneous lesions associated with coronavirus-induced vasculitis in a cat with feline infectious peritonitis and concurrent feline immunodeficiency virus infection, *J Feline Med Surg* 7:233, 2005.

18. Declercq J, De Bosschere H, Schwarzkopf I, et al: Papular cutaneous lesions in a cat associated with feline infectious peritonitis, *Vet Dermatol* 19:255, 2008.

19. Rota A, Paltrinieri S, Jussich S, et al: Priapism in a castrated cat associated with feline infectious peritonitis, *J Feline Med Surg* 10:181, 2008.

20. Takano T, Hohdatsu T, Toda A, et al: TNF-alpha, produced by feline infectious peritonitis virus (FIPV)-infected macrophages, upregulates expression of type II FIPV receptor feline aminopeptidase N in feline macrophages, *Virology* 364:64, 2007.

21. Paltrinieri S, Grieco V, Comazzi S, et al: Laboratory profiles in cats with different pathological and immunohistochemical findings due to feline infectious peritonitis (FIP), *J Feline Med Surg* 3:149, 2001.

22. Paltrinieri S, Comazzi S, Spagnolo V, et al: Laboratory changes consistent with feline infectious peritonitis in cats from multicat environments, *J Vet Med A Physiol Pathol Clin Med* 49:503, 2002.

23. Sparkes AH, Gruffydd-Jones TJ, Harbour DA: An appraisal of the value of laboratory tests in the diagnosis of feline infectious peritonitis, *J Am Anim Hosp Assoc* 30:345, 1994.

24. Gunn-Moore DA, Caney SM, Gruffydd-Jones TJ, et al: Antibody and cytokine responses in kittens during the development of feline infectious peritonitis (FIP), *Vet Immunol Immunopathol* 65:221, 1998.

25. Pedersen NC: The history and interpretation of feline coronavirus serology, *Feline Pract* 23:46, 1995.

26. Goitsuka R, Ohashi T, Ono K, et al: IL-6 activity in feline infectious peritonitis, *J Immunol* 144:2599, 1990.

27. Rohrer C, Suter PF, Lutz H: The diagnosis of feline infectious peritonitis (FIP): retrospective and prospective study, *Eur J Comp Anim Pract* 4:23, 1994.

28. Hartmann K, Binder C, Hirschberger J, et al: Comparison of different tests to diagnose feline infectious peritonitis, *J Vet Intern Med* 17:781, 2003.

29. Duthie S, Eckersall PD, Addie DD, et al: Value of alpha-1-acid glycoprotein in the diagnosis of feline infectious peritonitis, *Vet Rec* 141:299, 1997.

30. Paltrinieri S: The feline acute phase reaction, *Vet J* 177:26, 2008.

31. Ceciliani F, Grossi C, Giordano A, et al: Decreased sialylation of the acute phase protein alpha-1-acid glycoprotein in feline infectious peritonitis (FIP), *Vet Immunol Immunopathol* 99:229, 2004.

32. Saverio P, Alessia G, Vito T, et al: Critical assessment of the diagnostic value of feline alpha1-acid glycoprotein for feline infectious peritonitis using the likelihood ratios approach, *J Vet Diagn Invest* 19:266, 2007.

33. Paltrinieri S, Metzger C, Battilani M, et al: Serum alpha1-acid glycoprotein (AGP) concentration in non-symptomatic cats with feline coronavirus (FCoV) infection, *J Feline Med Surg* 9:271, 2007.

34. Hirschberger J, Hartmann K, Wilhelm N, et al: Clinical symptoms and diagnosis of feline infectious peritonitis, *Tierärztl Prax* 23:92, 1995.

35. Savary KC, Sellon RK, Law JM: Chylous abdominal effusion in a cat with feline infectious peritonitis, *J Am Anim Hosp Assoc* 37:35, 2001.

36. Singh M, Foster DJ, Child G, et al: Inflammatory cerebrospinal fluid analysis in cats: clinical diagnosis and outcome, *J Feline Med Surg* 7:77, 2005.

37. Rand JS, Parent J, Percy D, et al: Clinical, cerebrospinal fluid, and histological data from twenty-seven cats with primary inflammatory disease of the central nervous system, *Can Vet J* 35:103, 1994.

38. Foley JE, Rand C, Leutenegger C: Inflammation and changes in cytokine levels in neurological feline infectious peritonitis, *J Feline Med Surg* 5:313, 2003.

39. Pedersen NC: An overview of feline enteric coronavirus and infectious peritonitis virus infection, *Feline Practice* 23:7, 1995.

40. Addie DD, Jarrett O: Feline coronavirus infections. In Greene CE, editor: *Infectious Diseases of the Dog and Cat*, ed 3, St. Louis, 2006, Elsevier Saunders, p 88.

41. Lutz H, Gut M, Leutenegger CM, et al: Kinetics of FCoV infection in kittens born in catteries of high risk for FIP under different rearing conditions. Second International Feline Coronavirus/Feline Infectious Peritonitis Symposium, Glasgow, Scotland, 2002.

42. Soma T, Ishii H: Detection of feline coronavirus antibody, feline immunodeficiency virus antibody, and feline leukemia virus antigen in ascites from cats with effusive feline infectious peritonitis, *J Vet Med Sci* 66:89, 2004.

43. Kennedy MA, Brenneman K, Millsaps RK, et al: Correlation of genomic detection of feline coronavirus with various diagnostic assays for feline infectious peritonitis, *J Vet Diag Invest* 10:93, 1998.

44. Foley JE, Lapointe JM, Koblik P, et al: Diagnostic features of clinical neurologic feline infectious peritonitis, *J Vet Intern Med* 12:415, 1998.

45. Boettcher IC, Steinberg T, Matiasek K, et al: Use of anti-coronaviral antibody testing of cerebrospinal fluid for diagnosis of feline infectious peritonitis involving the central nervous system in cats, *J Am Vet Med Assoc* 230:199, 2007.

46. Steinberg TA, Boettcher IC, Matiasek K, et al: Use of albumin quotient and IgG index to differentiate blood- vs brain-derived proteins in the cerebrospinal fluid of cats with feline infectious peritonitis, *Vet Clin Pathol* 37:207, 2008.

47. Fehr D, Bolla S, Herrewegh A, et al: Detection of feline coronavirus using RT-PCR: basis for the study of the pathogenesis of feline infectious peritonitis (FIP), *Schweiz Arch Tierheilkd* 138:74, 1996.

48. Gamble DA, Lobbiani A, Gramegna M, et al: Development of a nested PCR assay for detection of feline infectious peritonitis virus in clinical specimens, *J Clin Microbiol* 35:673, 1997.

49. Herrewegh AA, Mahler M, Hedrich HJ, et al: Persistence and evolution of feline coronavirus in a closed cat-breeding colony, *Virology* 234:349, 1997.

50. Gunn-Moore DA, Gruffydd-Jones TJ, Harbour DA: Detection of feline coronaviruses by culture and reverse transcriptase-polymerase chain reaction of blood samples from healthy cats and cats with clinical feline infectious peritonitis, *Vet Microbiol* 62:193, 1998.

51. Simons FA, Vennema H, Rofina JE, et al: A mRNA PCR for the diagnosis of feline infectious peritonitis, *J Virol Methods* 124:111, 2005.

52. Tammer R, Evensen O, Lutz H, et al: Immunohistological demonstration of feline infectious peritonitis virus antigen in paraffin-embedded tissues using feline ascites or murine monoclonal antibodies, *Vet Immunol Immunopathol* 49:177, 1995.

53. Kipar A, Bellmann S, Kremendahl J, et al: Cellular composition, coronavirus antigen expression and production of specific antibodies in lesions in feline infectious peritonitis, *Vet Immunol Immunopathol* 65:243, 1998.

54. Giordano A, Paltrinieri S, Bertazzolo W, et al: Sensitivity of tru-cut and fine needle aspiration biopsies of liver and kidney for diagnosis of feline infectious peritonitis, *Vet Clin Pathol* 34:368, 2005.

55. Hartmann K: Feline infectious peritonitis, *Vet Clin North Am Small Anim Pract* 35:39, 2005.

56. Ritz SJ, Hartmann K: Prognostic parameters to predict survival time of cats with feline infectious peritonitis, *J Feline Med Surg*, in press 2009

57. Ritz SJ, Egberink H, Hartmann K: Influence of feline interferon-omega on the survival time and quality of life of cats with feline infectious peritonitis, *J Vet Intern Med* 21:1193, 2007.

58. Hartmann K, Kuffer M: Karnofsky's score modified for cats, *Eur J Med Res* 3:95, 1998.

59. Timmann D, Cizinauskas S, Tomek A, et al: Retrospective analysis of seizures associated with feline infectious peritonitis in cats, *J Feline Med Surg* 10:9, 2008.

60. Hartmann K, Ritz S: Treatment of cats with feline infectious peritonitis, *Vet Immunol Immunopathol* 123:172, 2008.

61. Watari T, Kaneshima T, Tsujimoto H, et al: Effect of thromboxane synthetase inhibitor on feline infectious peritonitis in cats, *J Vet Med Sci* 60:657, 1998.

62. Bolcskei A, Bilkei G: Langzeitstudie über behandelte FIP-verdächtige Katzen. Die Auswirkung verschiedener Therapieversuche auf das Überleben FIP-verdächtiger Katzen, *Tieraerztl Umschau* 50:21, 1995.

63. Weiss RC, Oostrom-Ram T: Inhibitory effects of ribavirin alone or combined with human alpha interferon on feline infectious peritonitis virus replication in vitro, *Vet Microbiol* 20:255, 1989.

64. Barlough JE, Scott FW: Effectiveness of three antiviral agents against FIP virus in vitro, *Vet Rec* 126:556, 1990.

65. Weiss RC, Cox NR, Boudreaux MK: Toxicologic effects of ribavirin in cats, *J Vet Pharmacol Ther* 16:301, 1993.

66. Weiss RC, Cox NR, Martinez ML: Evaluation of free or liposome-encapsulated ribavirin for antiviral therapy of experimentally induced feline infectious peritonitis, *Res Vet Sci* 55:162, 1993.

67. Weiss RC, Cox NR, Oostrom-Ram T: Effect of interferon or *Propionibacterium acnes* on the course of experimentally induced feline infectious peritonitis in specific-pathogen-free and random-source cats, *Am J Vet Res* 51:726, 1990.

68. Mochizuki M, Nakatani H, Yoshida M: Inhibitory effects of recombinant feline interferon on the replication of feline enteropathogenic viruses in vitro, *Vet Microbiol* 39:145, 1994.

69. Ishida T, Shibanai A, Tanaka S, et al: Use of recombinant feline interferon and glucocorticoid in the treatment of feline infectious peritonitis, *J Feline Med Surg* 6:107, 2004.

70. Addie DD, Schaap I, Nicolson L, et al: The persistence and transmission of type I feline coronavirus in natural infections. Abstract. Second International Feline Coronavirus/Feline Infectious Peritonitis Symposium, Glasgow, Great Britain, 2002.

71. Addie DD, Paltrinieri S, Pedersen NC: Second international feline coronavirus/feline infectious peritonitis symposium. Recommendations from workshops of the second international feline coronavirus/feline infectious peritonitis symposium, *J Feline Med Surg* 6:125, 2004.

72. Richards JR, Elston TH, Ford RB, et al: The 2006 American Association of Feline Practitioners feline vaccine advisory panel report, *J Am Vet Med Assoc* 229:1405, 2006.

73. Pedersen NC, Sato R, Foley JE, et al: Common virus infections in cats, before and after being placed in shelters, with emphasis on feline enteric coronavirus, *J Feline Med Surg* 6:83, 2004.

74. Addie DD: Feline Infectious Peritonitis and Coronavirus Website. [WWW page]. www.catvirus.com, 2007.

SECTION

II

Nutrition in Health and Disease

Debra L. Zoran, Section Editor

CHAPTER

8   Dietary Therapy of Chronic Diarrhea

Dorothy P. Laflamme

Management of diarrhea depends on identifying and correcting the underlying cause. Until the primary cause is corrected, dietary management in cats with diarrhea is predominantly symptomatic. As such, the goal of management is to provide the patient with all of its essential nutrients in an available form that is acceptable to the cat, while minimizing the adverse signs associated with gastrointestinal (GI) disease. It also is important to support the various functions of the GI tract to promote recovery and to optimize ongoing GI function. To ensure that these goals are met, the specific compromises in GI function, as well as the anticipated duration, must be considered when selecting a nutritional approach. There is no single diet or nutrient profile that is appropriate for all cats with chronic diarrhea. Therefore this chapter will review pertinent aspects of key nutrients, then will address common types of chronic diarrhea and suggest dietary approaches.

KEY NUTRIENTS IN GASTROINTESTINAL HEALTH AND DISEASE

PROTEINS AND AMINO ACIDS

The layer of epithelial cells that lines the intestines forms a continuous sheet throughout the intestine. These cells are renewed continuously from stem cells in the crypts such that intestinal epithelial cells are replaced about every three days. This rapid regeneration helps the intestine to heal quickly following an injury, but the continuous turnover of cells exerts a high demand for nutrients. These cells use between 10 and 20 per cent of total energy expenditure and approximately 50 per cent of ingested

protein, with more than 90 per cent of the aspartate, glutamate, and glutamine used by the intestinal tissues.[1] Therefore the GI tract is highly sensitive to protein or amino acid deficiency.

Inadequate intake of dietary protein or essential amino acids can cause GI tract atrophy with a decrease in absorptive cells, alterations in digestive enzymes, reduction in immunoglobulins and immune cells in the intestine, and an increased risk for colonization and translocation of pathogenic microorganisms.[2-5] Dietary protein deficiency also can lead to atrophy of the pancreas and a reduction in digestive enzymes. Correction of the protein deficit before the condition reaches an irreversible stage restores normal function.

The amino acids glutamine and glutamate are critical for the health of the GI tract, where they serve as key energy sources. In addition, glutamine promotes the natural barrier function of the intestinal mucosa.[6] Glutamine often is cited as a "conditionally essential" amino acid because inadequate quantities may be produced under certain conditions, such as with limited food intake.[7] If dietary glutamine is excluded following intestinal injury, the intestinal mucosa atrophies and bacterial translocation from the intestinal lumen can occur. However, glutamine is found abundantly in meat and other proteins and normally is made in the body from other amino acids. As long as dietary protein intake is sufficient, additional glutamine is not of benefit.

Adequate protein and amino acid intake is critical to promote intestinal healing, and protein does not appear to contribute to diarrhea. Cats are unique in requiring a much greater intake of dietary protein compared with dogs and most other species. When preservation of lean body mass in healthy cats was used as the criterion for protein adequacy, about 5 g/protein per kg body weight, or about 9 g/100 kcal metabolizable energy, was needed daily.[8] Additional protein may be of benefit in situations of low calorie intake, dietary malabsorption, or protein-losing enteropathy (PLE).

Dietary protein increases the rate of gastric emptying in other species, but this does not appear to be true for cats. In cats, a high-protein meal actually slowed gastric emptying time, and gastric emptying was faster with a high-fat diet.[9] Therefore a high-protein diet may be of benefit in cats with diarrhea by slowing the rate at which the compromised GI tract must process the incoming nutrients.

On the other hand, proteins are implicated in food allergy–induced diarrhea. Not all adverse reactions to food are true allergies. Animals (and human beings) can have idiosyncratic reactions to any food component independent of an immunological response. Thus food intolerance includes both immunological (allergic) and nonimmunological (idiosyncratic) responses. Food allergies are caused by an abnormal immunological response to normal proteins in the intestine. Most often, these appear to be dietary proteins, but bacterial proteins also have been implicated. This will be addressed in more detail in the section on food allergy.

FATS

Compared to protein and carbohydrate, fat digestion is more complex. The stages include intraluminal digestion; micellar solubilization; permeation from the lumen to the cell; intracellular re-esterification; chylomicron formation; and transport via the lymphatic circulation. For complete digestion, this requires lipase, colipase, and phospholipase A_2 from the pancreas, as well as bile acids that are produced by the liver, then stored and released from the gall bladder. Once inside the enterocyte, fatty acids and monoglycerides must be reformed into triglycerides. This is an active, energy-expending process, resulting in production of chylomicrons, which then enter into the intestinal lacteals and are transported via the lymphatic system to the systemic bloodstream. This differs from other nutrients, which are transported directly to the liver via the portal blood.

Despite the complexity, fat digestion is highly efficient so that most ingested fat is absorbed in healthy subjects. Yet, because of the complexity, fat digestion is compromised easily. When fat digestion is incomplete, bacteria in the colon can ferment the undigested fat, producing potent secretagogues and proinflammatory compounds. This results in a secretory diarrhea as well as intestinal inflammation. Thus, low-fat diets have long been recommended for animals with GI disease and diarrhea. However, cats appear to respond differently to fat compared with dogs and other species. In most species, fat is thought to slow the rate of gastric emptying, leading to an increased risk for vomiting and delayed gastric emptying. In cats, fat appears to have an opposite effect and cats fed a high-fat diet actually had faster gastric emptying.[9] Dietary fat also appears less important in the management of some types of chronic diarrhea in cats. In a double-blinded clinical trial evaluating the effect of high-fat versus low-fat diets in cats with diarrhea, there were no differences between the diets in terms of clinical response.[10]

CARBOHYDRATES

There is an often repeated, yet incorrect, perception that cats do not digest carbohydrates well. Cats, like dogs, do not have salivary amylase, but intestinal digestion of starches is initiated by pancreatic amylase, and completed by enzymes at the intestinal brush border. The brush border enzymes include sucrase, maltase, isomaltase, and lactase. Although some reports indicate low levels of enzyme activity in cats, others have demonstrated that the activity of these brush border enzymes, especially sucrase and maltase, is greater in cats than in dogs.[11] Cats may not handle large amounts of simple sugars well, but they are able to digest starches and other carbohydrates efficiently.[11,12] Even lactose is not an issue for normal cats, despite the perception that many cats are lactose intolerant. Relatively recent research showed that 10 per cent dietary lactose (1.2 g/kg body weight) in normal cats did not affect stool quality.[13]

With intestinal disease, however, carbohydrate digestion may decrease. The disaccharidases that complete the digestion of carbohydrates are located in the small intestinal brush border, which may be damaged due to disease. Increased carbohydrate fermentation, indicative of carbohydrate malabsorption, has been confirmed by breath hydrogen testing in cats with inflammatory bowel disease (IBD).[14] Carbohydrate malabsorption may occur in IBD if inflammation inhibits production of digestive enzymes, or if inflammatory infiltrates compromise nutrient absorption.[14]

When carbohydrate malabsorption does occur, it can contribute to osmotic diarrhea, as well as bacterial overgrowth and other problems. In such cases, avoidance of carbohydrates may help manage the clinical signs of diarrhea. One clinical study indicated that about 58 per cent of cats with chronic diarrhea improved when fed a low-carbohydrate (15 per cent dry matter) dry diet.[15]

DIETARY FIBER

Although dietary fibers are carbohydrates, their physiological effect is very different from digestible carbohydrates. Dietary fibers are structurally similar to starches and other digestible carbohydrates in that they are composed of strings of sugar molecules bound together. However, unlike digestible carbohydrates, which are linked with an alpha linkage that is cleaved easily by mammalian alpha-amylase, the sugars in dietary fiber are linked by a beta linkage. Beta links between sugar molecules are not digestible by mammalian digestive enzymes, but are cleaved by bacterial enzymes, so these substrates remain intact until digested (fermented) by bacteria.

Dietary fibers can be classified in many different ways, although the most common are based on the water solubility of the fiber or the fermentability by microorganisms. Although there are exceptions, it is generally recognized that more soluble fibers tend to be more fermentable. The functionality of dietary fibers is related to these two characteristics. Soluble fibers tend to form viscous gels, which can slow gastric emptying and GI transit. Insoluble fibers tend to adsorb water and increase fecal bulk, which can help normalize GI motility. Highly soluble fibers are found in pectins, gums, psyllium, and oligofructoses. Cellulose and most brans are examples of insoluble fibers. Many fibrous ingredients in foods and pet foods contain differing degrees of both soluble and insoluble fiber (Table 8-1). Likewise, the fermentability of fibers in pet foods varies. Cellulose undergoes little fermentation, pea fiber and soybean hulls are moderately fermented, while beet pulp can be highly fermentable.

Insoluble fibers tend to adsorb water and add bulk to intestinal contents and feces. This provides several benefits for GI health. The bulk stimulates GI motility and peristaltic movements, preventing gut stasis and promoting regular bowel habits. The spongelike effect of adsorbing water helps soften stool to aid in passage. Also, the bulk provides a dilutional effect for any endogenous or exogenous toxins that might be present in the bowel, reducing the likelihood of adverse effects.

Soluble, fermentable fibers serve as a substrate for the intestinal microflora to produce short chain fatty acids (SCFAs): acetate, butyrate, and propionate. SCFAs provide an energy source for colonocytes, stimulate colonic blood flow, promote water absorption, and promote growth and cellular turnover in the lower intestine. In addition, SCFAs help lower the pH of intestinal contents, which inhibits the growth of pathogenic bacteria. The lower pH also can reduce the absorption of some toxins, including ammonia. Dietary fibers, especially fermentable fibers, also can modulate properties of the immune system, likely through their effects on intestinal microflora.[16] Due to the various effects of both soluble and insoluble dietary fibers, they may be of benefit in the management of GI disease, especially diseases of the large bowel. Excessive soluble fiber, however, will cause loose, watery stools, and can cause the production of excess gas, while excess insoluble fiber can contribute to excessive stool volume, and may reduce absorption of some essential nutrients.

A subset of fermentable fibers includes *prebiotics*. By definition, these fibers are fermented selectively by health-promoting bacteria, especially strains of *Lactobacillus* and *Bifidobacteria*.[17,18] This results in their ability to increase the number or percentage of these organisms, while decreasing the prevalence of potential pathogens, such as *Salmonella*, *Clostridia*, or *E. coli*. Prebiotics also produce some of the health benefits generally associated with dietary fibers, such as reducing blood lipids and cholesterol, reducing constipation, and aiding in various types of diarrhea and inflammatory conditions of the GI tract, as well as being a substrate for SCFA production.[17-19] Among the many fibers available for use as prebiotic supplements are beta-glucans; pectin; resistant starch; various oligosaccharides, such as inulin, fructooligosaccharide (FOS), and mannanoligosaccharides (MOS); and others.[19-21]

PROBIOTICS

Although not a nutrient, probiotics are potential dietary components that may be of value for GI health. Probiotics are live microorganisms, consumed in food or supplements, that affect the host beneficially by improving its microbial balance and by interacting with the gut-associated lymphoid tissue (GALT). The GALT is the largest immunological organ in the body as it contains all of the lymphoid tissue, nodules, Peyer's patches, and

Table 8-1 Characteristics of Some Fibrous Ingredients Used in Pet Foods or Supplements

Fiber Source	g/100 g Ingredient				Fermentability
	Crude Fiber	Total Dietary Fiber	Soluble Fiber	Insoluble Fiber	
Beet pulp	17.6	50.5	11.2	39.3	+++
Cellulose	66.4	96.8	1.2	95.6	−
Corn bran	16.1	79.3	78.8	0.6	+
Oat fiber	52.3	90.0	NA	NA	+
Pea fiber	33.2	58.5	4.6	54.0	++
Psyllium	27.9	80.0	71.0	9.0	NA
Oat fiber	30.7	76.9	<0.5	76.9	+
Rice bran	7.6	21.3	1.9	19.5	−
Soy fiber	12.3	77.4	6.8	70.6	+
Soybean hulls	34.8	67.9	5.1	62.7	++
Vegetable gums	0.3	87.8	87.3	0.5	+
Wheat bran	11.7	44.4	2.7	41.4	+++

NA, Information not available.

Fermentability: −, Nonfermentable; +, modestly fermentable; ++, moderately fermentable; +++, highly fermentable.

individual lymphocytes found in the intestinal walls. About 70 to 80 per cent of the immunoglobulin-producing cells of the body are located in the GI tract.[20] Stimulation of the immune system within the GI tract also can result in effects throughout the body. Activated plasma cells migrate to the bloodstream and to other parts of the body. Therefore antigen priming at one surface area (the intestinal mucosa) can result in antibodies being synthesized and secondary responses occurring at other sites. Through this mechanism, probiotics interacting with the GALT can influence GI and systemic health and immune function.

Some of the most commonly fed probiotics include *Lactobacillus* species, *Bacillus subtilis,* and *Enterococcus faecium* SF68.[22] Multiple meta-analyses of clinical trials in human beings have confirmed the benefit of probiotics in the control of antibiotic-associated diarrhea.[23,24] Probiotics have proven beneficial in the management of acute diarrhea, viral and bacterial diarrhea, and IBDs, reducing either the duration, severity, or both.[25-28] In a murine model of sepsis, probiotics were able to prevent the breakdown in colonic barrier function and reduce bacterial translocation and liver injury.[29] Such data are not yet available for cats, but probiotics have been evaluated in a number of animal studies.

In dogs, the probiotic *Enterococcus faecium* SF68 provides several documented benefits, including enhanced response to vaccination and increased intestinal IgA.[30] In piglets, this probiotic reduced the development of diarrhea, decreased mortality, and enhanced growth performance.[31,32] In kittens, this same probiotic increased fecal bifidobacteria and decreased *C. perfringens,* increased serum IgA concentrations, and reduced the severity and incidence of diarrhea significantly during a natural outbreak in the colony.[22] The probiotic *Lactobacillus acidophilus* also was confirmed to beneficially alter fecal microflora and markers of immune function in healthy cats,[33] and a probiotic containing both *Lactobacillus* and *E. faecium* enhanced fecal quality effectively in captive cheetahs prone to diarrhea.[34] (See Chapter 11 for a complete discussion on probiotics.)

VITAMINS

A deficiency of any one of several B vitamins can result in compromised GI function, although this has not been recognized clinically in cats. An exception to this is cobalamin, or vitamin B_{12}. In two studies involving a total of 85 cats with chronic diarrhea, 16 per cent had low serum cobalamin.[10,35] A deficiency of cobalamin can result in GI mucosal atrophy and reduced GI function; however, the cause of cobalamin deficiency most often is itself GI disease.

Normal uptake of cobalamin requires a binding factor (intrinsic factor), which is secreted from the pancreas of cats, followed by a receptor-mediated uptake in the ileum. These receptors are located on the brush border of ileal enterocytes. A compromise in either pancreatic or ileal function can lead to cobalamin deficiency in cats (see Chapter 20). In dogs, intestinal bacterial overgrowth also

may contribute to cobalamin deficiency. IBD, lymphoma, cholangiohepatitis or cholangitis, and pancreatic inflammation have been associated with cobalamin deficiency in cats.[36] Weight loss, diarrhea, anorexia, and vomiting were the most common signs in cats with low serum cobalamin levels.[36] Older cats with GI disease seem to be more predisposed to cobalamin deficiency than younger cats.[37]

Because cobalamin functions as a co-factor in many processes involved in cellular turnover, a deficiency in cobalamin can lead to atrophy of the rapidly dividing cells of the intestinal mucosa, further decreasing function and compromising recovery. A recent study by the author suggested that cats with diarrhea and low serum cobalamin levels are less likely to respond to dietary therapy alone, whereas diarrhea improved with diet change alone in more than 75 per cent of cats with normal cobalamin concentrations.[35] Correcting a cobalamin deficiency via parenteral supplementation (250 μg subcutaneously, once weekly for 4 weeks) resulted in clinical improvement in one study of cats with GI disease and low cobalamin levels.[38] (The reader is referred to Chapter 13 in the fifth volume of this series for a complete discussion of the role of cobalamin in the diagnosis and management of GI disease.)

Serum folate is another B vitamin that may be abnormal in GI disease. An increase in serum folate may be caused by an overgrowth of bacteria in the small intestine, although this has not been documented in cats. Low serum folate, however, appears to be associated with disease of the proximal small intestine. A retrospective survey of cats with GI disease for which serum folate and cobalamin levels were analyzed indicated that 39 per cent of these cats had low folate levels.[39] In that study, cats with both low folate and cobalamin levels were more likely to be underweight and have a low body condition, compared to other cats in the study. Whether the low folate is simply a marker secondary to disease, or a contributor towards ongoing disease, has not been determined.

In conditions in which fat digestion or absorption are compromised, there exists the likelihood for a deficiency of fat-soluble vitamins. This includes cats with pancreatic exocrine insufficiency, and some old cats, in addition to cats with primary GI disease. Although such deficiencies have been reported only rarely in cats, supplementation might be worth considering if diarrhea is prolonged. Vitamin K deficiency has been reported in cats with IBD, while deficiencies in vitamins A and E have been described in human beings with IBD.[40] Absorption of vitamin E also is compromised in aging cats expressing fat malabsorption.[41]

APPLYING NUTRITIONAL CONCEPTS TO MANAGEMENT OF DIARRHEA

The GI tract functions to digest and absorb essential nutrients, including water. It also provides nonimmunological barriers and immunological defenses against bacteria and toxins attempting to enter the body. Cats with diarrhea have an obvious breakdown in one of these functions—that of absorbing water. What may not be as obvious is the potential breakdown in other functions of the GI tract. Therapeutic and dietary options, based on appropriate diagnostic procedures, should target restoration of both digestive and protective functions afforded by the GI tract.

Given the extent of the GI tract's responsibilities, it is not surprising that the digestive system contains some of the most metabolically active tissues in the body. The stomach, intestines, pancreas, and spleen together account for less than 6 per cent of body weight, yet account for about 20 per cent of energy expenditure and 50 per cent of the whole-body protein turnover.[1,42] Intestinal cells derive much of their nutrition from the intestinal lumen which is necessary for proper healing. Without adequate nutrition to the GI cells themselves, atrophy of the mucosa and breakdown of the GI tract's protective systems can occur. Therefore withholding of food should be avoided or minimized. Provision of oral or enteral nutrition can preserve the integrity of the GI tract and aid in recovery.

The choice of what to feed cats with chronic diarrhea is dependent on the cause and clinical signs (Table 8-2). There are many causes of infectious colitis and enteritis. Evaluation and/or treatment for Giardia, tritrichomonosis and other intestinal parasites should be completed

before pursuing other diagnoses (see Chapter 18). If IBD or food "allergy" is suspected, additional dietary guidelines might be appropriate. Otherwise, dietary management is symptomatic and should consider the following principles.

SMALL BOWEL CHRONIC DIARRHEA

Small intestinal disease often is associated with mucosal compromise, hence a reduced ability to digest and absorb nutrients. Feeding a highly digestible diet can help to compensate for this adverse effect. Generally, this is defined as a low-fiber diet, and qualified commercial diets should have an apparent digestibility well above 80 per cent. Small, frequent meals also may be of benefit.

Poor intake or poor absorption of nutrients can lead to energy deficiency and weight loss. A target for calorie intake should be established based on maintenance energy requirements (50 to 60 kcal/kg ideal body weight), and actual intake should be monitored. Body weight and body condition should be assessed and monitored for changes. When poor intake is an issue, offering different brands, flavors, and textures of diet with suitable nutritional characteristics may enhance intake.

A dietary change, regardless of specific diets involved, may be of benefit in cats with chronic diarrhea. Any change in diet has the potential to induce changes in both GI mucosa and microflora. Approximately 75 per cent of cats with nonspecific, chronic diarrhea improved when changed from their previous diet to a highly digestible, experimental diet.[35] Cats with chronic diarrhea, unlike other species, do not appear sensitive to dietary fat. In one study, cats with nonspecific chronic diarrhea were equally responsive to highly digestible diets regardless of fat content.[10] Whether or not this also applies to cats with pancreatitis remains to be determined. Although clinical studies evaluating diets in cats with a confirmed diagnosis of pancreatitis have not been completed, the previously mentioned study included a number of cats with elevated feline trypsin-like immunoreactivity (fTLI). Among these cats, those fed the high-fat diet did at least as well as those fed a low-fat diet. Low-carbohydrate diets have been recommended for cats with small intestinal disease. In disease-induced carbohydrate malassimilation, poorly digested or poorly absorbed carbohydrates can contribute to osmotic diarrhea, reduced protein assimilation, and alterations in GI microflora. In a study of cats with chronic diarrhea, more than half responded positively to a low-carbohydrate diet.[15]

Hypocobalaminemia is not uncommon in cats with GI disease. Low cobalamin levels may recover on their own in cats following resolution of diarrhea. However, cats with low serum cobalamin are at greater risk for nonresponsive diarrhea.[35] In this situation, correction of hypocobalaminemia with parenteral cobalamin injections is necessary. Administer 250 µg of cobalamin SQ weekly for 6 weeks, followed by similar doses every 2 weeks for an additional 6 weeks. Unless the intestinal disease has resolved, monthly injections will be needed to maintain serum cobalamin within normal levels.

Table 8-2   Summary of Typical Diets Used in Common GI Diseases

Condition	Nutrient Modifications
Chronic small bowel diarrhea	Highly digestible diet. Consider low carbohydrate. Consider probiotics. Feed small, frequent meals.
Chronic large bowel diarrhea	Include mix of soluble and insoluble dietary fiber. Consider hypoallergenic (hydrolyzed protein/novel protein) diet. Consider probiotics.
Food-allergic diarrhea	Hypoallergenic (hydrolyzed protein). Novel protein
Inflammatory bowel disease	Highly digestible diet. Consider hypoallergenic (hydrolyzed protein/novel protein) diet. Include source of fermentable dietary fiber. Consider probiotics. Consider dry diet.
Protein-losing enteropathy	Highly digestible diet. Increased protein content. Consider hydrolyzed protein diets. Consider parenteral vitamin supplementation.
Exocrine pancreatic insufficiency	Highly digestible diet. Consider hydrolyzed protein. Consider parenteral vitamin supplementation. Treat secondary bacterial overgrowth and consider probiotics.
Pancreatitis	Highly digestible diet initially. High fiber, low fat if weight loss needed.

LARGE BOWEL CHRONIC DIARRHEA

Dietary fiber provides multiple benefits for patients with large bowel disease. Dietary fibers with gelling properties, such as psyllium, can adsorb water and enhance the appearance of stools. It also helps to normalize gut motility. Fermentable fibers provide SCFAs that can aid water absorption as well as provide an energy source for colonocytes. SCFAs also stimulate colonic smooth muscle fibers, which should help to normalize GI transit during diarrhea. Fiber need not be excessive however, and diets containing 5 to 10 per cent total dietary fiber (TDF) may be sufficient. Note that TDF is not the same as crude fiber, the assay required to be used on pet food labels. As a general rule, TDF will be two to four times greater than crude fiber in complete foods. Additional fiber can be added at a rate of 2.5 to 5.0 g (0.5 to 1.0 teaspoons) daily, divided and added to meals.

Prebiotics, fermentable fibers, and probiotics may help normalize disrupted GI microflora (see Chapter 11). A number of probiotics have proven beneficial in the management of diarrhea in human patients. A commercially available probiotic, *Enterocccus faecium* SF68, reduced the severity of diarrhea in adult cats, and reduced the incidence as well as required treatment days for diarrhea when provided to a group of kittens subsequently exposed to infectious diarrhea.[22]

FOOD-RESPONSIVE DIARRHEA

Antigens, or foreign proteins, can trigger a food-sensitivity reaction resulting in vomiting or diarrhea. Between 15 and 29 per cent of cats with chronic diarrhea may be food-sensitive.[43,44] Intestinal antigenic exposure that may be altered with a dietary change can include food proteins, bacteria, and other foreign proteins or organisms. Although not all food sensitivities are true allergies, many are believed to have an immunological component. Dietary allergies are due to an inappropriate immunological reaction to a normal food protein.

The epithelial lining over each Peyer's patch contains specialized antigen-presenting cells, called M cells (microfold cells), that play a role in development of food tolerance. Antigens taken up into M cells are presented directly to lymphocytes within the Peyer's patches. This allows the immune system to develop an appropriate recognition and response to that particular antigen, either to develop a tolerance to a food protein or to mount a defense against an invading organism. Errors in this process can result in development of allergies or infections. Stimulation of the immune system within the GI tract can have systemic effects, as activated plasma cells migrate via the bloodstream to other parts of the body. Through this mechanism, food allergies can cause systemic effects, such as dermatological lesions. Therefore cats with food allergy may have GI signs, dermatological signs, or both. Cats with both diarrhea and pruritus have a twofold to threefold greater likelihood of being food-sensitive, compared to those with only pruritus or GI signs.[43]

If food allergy is suspected as a cause of diarrhea, a food trial should be conducted using an appropriate elimination diet. Several options are available for an elimination trial, with the goal being to remove potential dietary antigens. Because essentially all dietary antigens are proteins, the focus is on minimizing the number of antigens, especially those to which the cat may have had prior exposure, while still ensuring complete nutrition. Highly digestible diets are typically recommended, on the assumption that this reduces the intact antigens reaching the Peyer's patches. Options include novel protein diets or hydrolyzed protein diets.

Novel protein diets can be prepared commercially or homemade. In either case, the goal is to feed only proteins to which the patient has not been exposed previously. Consideration should be for the primary protein sources, as well as the proteins contained in grains and other dietary components. Minimizing the number of proteins in the diet, as well as selecting proteins to which that cat has not had prior exposure, reduces the likelihood that the cat will be allergic to components of the trial diet. However, novel protein diets are not inherently less allergenic than other diets. Therefore some cats with allergies may continue to show signs when fed these diets or may even develop new allergies to these diets.

Hydrolyzed protein diets minimize allergenic exposure by breaking down the dietary proteins to a size below that required to trigger cross-linking of immunoglobulins—a necessary step in allergic reactions. If all the sources of protein in the diet are sufficiently hydrolyzed, the allergenic potential of such diets is greatly reduced compared to intact proteins, minimizing (although not completely eliminating) the likelihood of an allergic response.

The GI tract responds more quickly to removal of antigenic stimulation compared to skin, so clinical response should be noted within 2 to 4 weeks unless secondary complications are present.[35,43] Food allergy is confirmed if the clinical signs recur upon re-exposure to the prior diet. Complete and balanced hydrolyzed or novel protein diets can be fed long-term. However, if the specific allergens to which the cat is sensitive can be identified, most cats can be fed commercial diets that omit the identified allergens.

Cats may respond to a dietary change, yet not recrudesce when challenged with the original diet. In this case, the cat is not likely to have an allergy. In these patients, the improvement may be related to a change in GI microflora or other changes in the intestinal environment. Although less than 30 per cent of cats with diarrhea are likely to have a food allergy, up to 75 per cent of cats with chronic diarrhea may improve simply by changing the diet to a highly digestible diet.[35]

INFLAMMATORY BOWEL DISEASE

IBD is associated with immune dysregulation and an inappropriate immunological reaction to various stimuli. The reaction may be to dietary allergens; therefore food allergy diarrhea may be considered a subset of IBD. Other potential stimuli include intestinal parasites and intestinal microflora. An improper immune response to the GI microflora may be a component of IBD, but recent studies suggest that the resident GI microflora in cats with IBD is altered.

In addition to beneficial direct effects on the host's immune system, the resident microflora can have additional direct and indirect protective effects. The flora of the digestive tract normally acts competitively against potential pathogens by preventing them from attaching to the GI epithelium. The GI microflora can stimulate expression of specific epithelial glycoconjugates on luminal surfaces, which can serve as receptors for bacterial attachment.[45] The specificity of these receptors influences which bacteria can bind to that cell. In addition, the GI microflora influence the mucus layer that overlays the epithelial cells of the intestines.[46] As such, the defensive capacity of the mucus, which lies partly in its ability to entrap pathogenic bacteria, can be altered. For example, certain strains of *Lactobacillus* can induce increased expression of the MUC2 and MUC3 genes that promote mucus secretion in the colon and inhibit the attachment of pathogenic *E. coli*.[46] Thus, maintenance of normal microflora is important to GI health. When the natural flora of the intestine is eliminated or its composition changed dramatically, such as from the use of antibiotics, an overgrowth of potentially pathogenic bacteria can occur, leading to severe colitis.[47]

Identification of intestinal microflora has been limited by the ability to culture the different organisms. Newer methods that do not rely on culture, such as denaturing gradient gel electrophoresis (DGGE) and fluorescence in situ hybridization, can identify many more of the bacterial species. Based on these newer methods, it has been confirmed that cats with IBD have very different patterns of GI microflora, compared with normal cats.[48-50] Among other changes, there was a decrease in diversity among different species of bacteria. The beneficial bacteria, *Bifidobacterium* and *Bacteroides*, appeared to be reduced in cats with IBD, compared with healthy cats.[49] Increases in mucosal-adherent Enterobacteriaceae, *E. coli* and *Clostridium* spp were associated with abnormalities in mucosal architecture, increased inflammatory mediators, and with clinical signs in cats with IBD.[50] Cats with IBD also had significant numbers of *Desulfovibrio* spp., a bacterium known to produce toxic sulphide metabolites.[49]

Probiotics and prebiotics can be used to correct imbalances in GI microflora. In human patients with IBD, as well as animal models of IBD, the use of probiotics appears to be beneficial. To date, however, no studies have been published evaluating probiotics in cats with IBD.

In addition to prebiotics and probiotics, alterations in diet will cause changes in GI microflora. Protein and dietary fiber have been well-documented to alter fecal microflora.[51] Diet type (commercial canned versus dry diets) also will alter microflora. Fecal *Clostridia* are increased, and *Lactobacillus* or *Bifidobacteria* are decreased, in animals fed meat or canned commercial diets, compared with those fed commercial dry foods.[51-53] In healthy dogs, consumption of dry food decreased putrefactive or odor-causing compounds (fecal indole, sulphide, and ammonia), and reduced enzymes (e.g., β-glucosidase, β-glucuronidase, and nitroreductase) linked with produc-

tion of toxic and mutagenic compounds.[52] Unfortunately, fecal microflora is quite different from small intestinal microflora, and there is limited information about the effects of diet on small intestinal microflora of cats or dogs.

Carbohydrate malabsorption appears to be common in cats with IBD.[14] Measurement of hydrogen in exhaled breath is used as an indicator of carbohydrate malassimilation (see Chapter 15). Nondigested carbohydrates are fermented by intestinal microflora, producing hydrogen gas, whereas carbohydrates that have been fully digested and absorbed are unavailable for bacterial fermentation. Cats with IBD have an increase in breath hydrogen, compared with healthy cats.[14] Whether the increase in breath hydrogen in IBD is due exclusively to carbohydrate maldigestion or in part due to adverse changes in bacterial populations has not been fully evaluated. However, both of these factors can be influenced by diet. Different forms of food can affect breath hydrogen tests differentially in normal cats. Despite the lower carbohydrate content of canned cat foods, cats fed these diets had significantly greater breath hydrogen than when they were fed dry, extruded cat foods.[54] Some of the hydrogen may be from fermentation of undigested proteins, which suggests the potential for residual dietary and microbial antigens to remain in the intestines of cats fed the canned diets.[54] Given these findings, there may be an advantage to using highly digestible dry foods for cats with intestinal disease, especially IBD.

Dietary recommendations for cats with IBD are mostly empirical. Use of an elimination diet (novel or hydrolyzed protein diet) is a reasonable approach to first exclude food-responsive diarrhea. However, a large number of cats can be expected to respond to a dietary change but not recrudesce upon challenge. It is likely that the response observed in these cats is due to alterations in their GI microflora. Some cats may respond to added dietary fiber, especially those showing evidence of large bowel involvement. A mix of soluble/fermentable fiber and insoluble fiber can help normalize GI transit, absorb excess fecal water, and promote alterations in the GI microflora. Administration of probiotics also may be of benefit to patients with IBD. Cats with protein-losing enteropathy secondary to IBD may benefit from increased dietary protein. Use of a highly digestible protein, or a hydrolyzed protein source, may help with absorption.

SUMMARY

Dietary management in cats with diarrhea predominantly is symptomatic. Highly digestible diets appear to be of benefit for many cats with chronic diarrhea. When an allergic component is suspected, a novel protein or hydrolyzed protein diet can be helpful. For most cats with chronic diarrhea, dietary fat restriction does not appear to be important, whereas some cats may benefit from a high-protein, low-carbohydrate diet. If an improvement is not seen within a few weeks, the cat is unlikely to respond to dietary management alone, and further diagnostic tests and therapeutic options should be pursued. Cats with subnormal serum cobalamin levels may be less responsive to therapy until normal serum cobalamin levels are restored with parenteral supplementation. Although additional research is necessary, it appears that probiotics may be of benefit for cats with some types of chronic diarrhea. (The reader is referred to Chapter 22 for a discussion of other therapeutic strategies for patients with chronic diarrhea.)

REFERENCES

1. Van der Schoor SRD, Reeds PJ, Stoll B, et al: The high metabolic cost of a functional gut, *Gastroenterology* 123:1931, 2002.
2. Manhart N, Vierlinger K, Bergmeister H, et al: Influence of short-term protein malnutrition of mice on the phenotype and costimulatory signals of lymphocytes from spleen and Peyer's patches, *Nutrition* 16:197, 2000.
3. Rana SV, Gupta D, Katyal R, et al: Mild-to-moderate malnutrition alters glutathione, gamma-glutamyl-transpeptidase and glycine uptake in small intestinal brush-border vesicles of rhesus monkeys, *Ann Nutr Metab* 45:143, 2001.
4. Cuoto JL, Ferreira HS, da Rocha DB, et al: Structural changes in the jejunal mucosa of mice infected with *Schistosoma mansoni,* fed low or high protein diets, *Rev Soc Bras Med Trop* 35:607, 2003.
5. Takahashi K, Kita E, Konishi M, et al: Translocation model of *Candida albicans* in DBA-2/J mice with protein calorie malnutrition mimics hematogenous candidiasis in humans, *Microb Pathog* 35:179, 2003.
6. Li N, Demarco VG, West CM, et al: Glutamine supports recovery from loss of transepithelial resistance and increase of permeability induced by media change in caco-2 cells, *J Nutr Biochem* 14:401, 2003.
7. Andrews FJ, Griffiths RD: Glutamine: essential for immune function in the critically ill, *Br J Nutr* 87(Suppl):S3, 2002.
8. Hannah SS, Laflamme DP: Effect of dietary protein on nitrogen balance and lean body mass in cats, *Vet Clin Nutr* 3:30 (Abstr), 1996.
9. Foster LA, Hoskinson JJ, Goggin JM, et al: Gastric emptying of diets varying in macronutrient composition in cats, *Compend Contin Educ Pract Vet* 21(Suppl):61 (Abstr), 1999.
10. Laflamme DP, Xu H, Long GL: Do cats with chronic diarrhea benefit from a low fat diet? *J Vet Intern Med* 21:611 (Abstr), 2007.
11. Morris JG, Rogers QR: Comparative aspects of nutrition and metabolism in dogs and cats. In Burger IH, Rivers JPW, editors: *Nutrition of the dog and cat.* Waltham Symposium Number 7, Cambridge, 1989, Cambridge University Press, p 35.
12. De-Oliveira LD, Carciofi AC, Oliveira MC, et al: Effects of six carbohydrate sources on cat diet digestibility and postprandial glucose and insulin response, *J Anim Sci* 86:2237, 2008.
13. Beynen AC, Yu S: Magnesium balance in adult cats fed a dry food rich in lactose, *J Anim Physiol Anim Nutr* 87:245, 2003.
14. Ugarte C, Guilford WG, Markwell P, et al: Carbohydrate malabsorption is a feature of feline inflammatory bowel disease but does not increase clinical gastrointestinal signs, *J Nutr* 134:2068S, 2004.
15. Laflamme DP, Long GM: Evaluation of two diets in the nutritional management of cats with naturally occurring chronic diarrhea, *Vet Ther* 5:43, 2004.
16. Schley PD, Field CJ: The immune enhancing effects of dietary fibers and prebiotics, *Br J Nutr* 87(Suppl 2):221S, 2002.
17. Roberfroid M, Slavin J: Nondigestible oligosaccharides, *Crit Rev Food Sci Nutr* 40:461, 2000.
18. Duggan C, Gannon J, Walker WA: Protective nutrients and functional foods for the gastrointestinal tract, *Am J Clin Nutr* 75:789, 2002.
19. Flickinger EQ, Van Loo J, Fahey GC: Nutritional responses to the presence of inulin and oligofructose in the diets of domesticated animals: a review, *Crit Rev Food Sci Nutr* 43:19, 2003.
20. Bengmark S: Gut microbial ecology in critical illness: is there a role for prebiotics, probiotics and synbiotics? *Curr Opin Crit Care* 8:145, 2002.
21. Swanson KS, Grieshop CM, Flickinger EA, et al: Supplemental fructooligosaccharides and mannanoligosaccharides influence immune function, ileal and total tract nutrient digestibilities, microbial populations and concentrations of protein catabolites in the large bowel of dogs, *J Nutr* 132:980, 2002.
22. Czarnecki-Maulden GL: Effect of dietary modulation of intestinal microbiota on reproduction and early growth, *Theriogenology* 70:286, 2008.
23. D'Souza AL, Rajkumar C, Cooke J, et al: Probiotics in prevention of antibiotic associated diarrhea: meta-analysis, *Brit Med J* 324:1361, 2002.
24. Johnston BC, Supina AL, Vohra S: Probiotics for pediatric antibiotic-associated diarrhea: a meta-analysis of randomized placebo-controlled trials, *Can Med Assoc J* 175:377, 2006.
25. Buydens P, Debeuckelaere S: Efficacy of SF68 in the treatment of acute diarrhea. A placebo-controlled trial, *Scand J Gastroenterol* 31:887, 1996.
26. Chandra RK: Effect of *Lactobacillus* on the incidence and severity of acute rotavirus diarrhea in infants. A prospective placebo-controlled double-blind study, *Nutr Res* 22:65, 2002.
27. Devrese M, Marteau PR: Probiotics and prebiotics: effects on diarrhea, *J Nutr* 137:803S, 2007.
28. Sheil B, Shanahan F, O'Mahony L: Probiotic effects on inflammatory bowel disease, *J Nutr* 137:819S, 2007.
29. Ewaschuk J, Endersby R, Thiel D, et al: Probiotic bacteria prevent hepatic damage and maintain colonic barrier function in a mouse model of sepsis, *Hepatology* 46:841, 2007.
30. Benyacoub J, Czarnecki-Maulden GL, Cavadine C, et al: Supplementation of food with *Enterococcus faecium* (SF68) stimulates immune function in young dogs, *J Nutr* 133:1158, 2003.
31. Taras D, Vahjen W, Macha M, et al: Performance, diarrhea incidence, and occurrence of *Escherichia coli* virulence genes during long-term administration of a probiotic *Enterococcus faecium* strain to sows and piglets, *J Anim Sci* 84:608, 2006.
32. Zeyner A, Boldt E: Effects of a probiotic *Enterococcus faecium* strain supplemented from birth to weaning on diarrhea patterns and performance in piglets, *J Anim Physiol Anim Nutr* 90:25, 2006.
33. Marshall-Jones Z, Baillon MLA, Croft JM, et al: Effects of *Lactobacillus acidophilus* DSM13241 as a probiotic in healthy adult cats, *Am J Vet Res* 67:1005, 2006.
34. Koeppel KN, Bertschinger H, van Vuuren M, et al: The use of a probiotic in captive cheetahs (*Acinonyx jubatus*), *J S Afr Vet Assoc* 77:127, 2006.
35. Laflamme DP: Feline diarrhea, unpublished data 2007.
36. Simpson KW, Fyfe J, Cornetta A, et al: Subnormal concentrations of serum cobalamin (vitamin B12) in cats with gastrointestinal disease, *J Vet Intern Med* 15:26, 2001.
37. Williams DA, Steiner JM, Ruaux CG: Older cats with gastrointestinal disease are more likely to be cobalamin deficient, *Compend Contin Educ Pract Vet* 26(Suppl):62 (Abstr), 2004.
38. Ruaux CG, Steiner JM, Williams DA: Early biochemical and clinical responses to cobalamin supplementation in cats with signs of gastrointestinal disease and severe hypocobalaminemia, *J Vet Intern Med* 19:155, 2005.

39. Reed N, Gunn-Moore D, Simpson K: Cobalamin, folate and inorganic phosphate abnormalities in ill cats, *J Feline Med Surg* 9:278, 2007.

40. Cave NJ, Marks SL: Mechanisms and clinical applications of nutrition in inflammatory bowel disease, *Compend Contin Educ Pract Vet* 26(Suppl 2A):51, 2004.

41. Perez-Camargo G, Young L: Nutrient digestibility in old versus young cats, *Compend Contin Educ Pract Vet* 27(Suppl 3A):84, 2005.

42. Cant JP, Mcbride BW, Croom WJ: The regulation of intestinal metabolism and its impact on whole animal energetics, *J Anim Sci* 74:2541, 1996.

43. Guilford WG, Markwell PJ, Jones BR, et al: Prevalence and causes of food sensitivity in cats with chronic pruritus, vomiting or diarrhea, *J Nutr* 128:2790S, 1998.

44. Guilford WG, Jones BR, Markwell PJ, et al: Food sensitivity in cats with chronic idiopathic gastrointestinal problems, *J Vet Intern Med* 15:7, 2001.

45. Salminen S, Bouley C, Boutron-Ruault MC, et al: Functional food science and gastrointestinal physiology and function, *Br J Nutr* 80(Suppl 1):S147, 1998.

46. Deplancke B, Gaskins HR: Microbial modulation of innate defense: goblet cells and the intestinal mucus layer, *Am J Clin Nutr* 73(Suppl):1131S, 2001.

47. Tizard IR: *Veterinary immunology: an introduction,* ed 6, Philadelphia, 2000, WB Saunders.

48. Burke KF, Steiner JM, Broussard JD, et al: Evaluation of fecal bacterial diversity in healthy cats and cats with inflammatory bowel disease or gastrointestinal neoplasia, *J Vet Intern Med* 20:788 (Abstr), 2006.

49. Inness VL, Mccartney AL, Khoo C, et al: Molecular characterization of the gut microflora of healthy and inflammatory bowel disease cats using fluorescence in situ hybridization with special reference to *Desulfovibrio* spp, *J Anim Physiol Anim Nutr* 91:48, 2007.

50. Janeczko S, Atwater D, Bogel E, et al: The relationship of mucosal bacteria to duodenal histopathology, cytokine mrna, and clinical disease activity in cats with inflammatory bowel disease, *Vet Microbiol* 128:178, 2008.

51. Zentek J, Marquart B, Pietrzak T, et al: Dietary effects on bifidobacteria and *Clostridium perfringens* in the canine intestinal tract, *J Anim Physiol Anim Nutr* 87:397, 2003.

52. Martineau B, Laflamme DP, Jones W, et al: Effect of diet on markers of intestinal health in dogs, *Res Vet Sci* 72:223, 2002.

53. Patil AR, Rayner L, Carrion PA: Effect of diet type on fecal microflora in cats, *Compend Contin Educ Pract Vet* 26(Suppl):72 (Abstr), 2004.

54. Backus RC, Puryear LM, Crouse BA, et al: Breath hydrogen concentrations of cats given commercial canned and extruded diets indicate gastrointestinal microbial activity vary with diet type, *J Nutr* 132:1763S, 2002.

CHAPTER

9 Dietary Therapy of Diseases of the Lower Urinary Tract

Joseph W. Bartges and Claudia A. Kirk

INCIDENCE

Lower urinary tract disease occurs commonly in cats. Previous estimates of the incidence in the United States and United Kingdom were 0.85 to 1.0 per cent per year.[1,2] These estimates were based on presence of clinical signs only and therefore did not consider actual diagnoses. The proportional morbidity rate, defined as the frequency with which cases are seen at veterinary hospitals, has been reported to be 10 per cent[3]; although 1 to 6 per cent is reported more commonly.[3,4] In a cross-sectional study of 15,226 cats examined at 52 private practices, cats were likely to be examined because of renal disease, cystitis, feline urologic syndrome, and inappetence.[5]

FELINE LOWER URINARY TRACT DISEASE

Any disorder of the lower urinary tract may cause signs of lower urinary tract disease. In two prospective studies, one of 143 cats[6] and one of 109 cats[7] with lower urinary tract disease, idiopathic cystitis was diagnosed most commonly (Figure 9-1). In a retrospective study performed at the University of Georgia and the University of Tennessee, of 110 cats more than 10 years of age with lower urinary tract disease, bacterial cystitis was diagnosed most commonly.[8] Thus, causes of lower urinary tract disease

appear to be different in different-aged cats, although clinical signs are similar.

IDIOPATHIC CYSTITIS

The most common cause of lower urinary tract disease in cats less than 10 years of age is idiopathic cystitis. Idiopathic cystitis is characterized by signs of lower urinary tract disease (hematuria, stranguria, pollakiuria, and inappropriate urination) without identifiable cause(s). Often the clinical signs resolve in 3 to 7 days; however, recurrence is variable and unpredictable. Because no specific cause has been identified, no specific treatment is available that works consistently in all cats.

The role of canned diet in managing cats with idiopathic cystitis has been evaluated in two studies. In one nonrandomized, prospective study of cats with idiopathic cystitis, recurrence of clinical signs occurred in 11 per cent of cats consuming a canned food and in 39 per cent of cats consuming a dry food.[9] The diets evaluated in this study were acidifying and formulated to prevent struvite crystalluria and urolithiasis. In another study, clinical improvement and decreased recurrence of clinical signs in cats with idiopathic cystitis were associated with the owners feeding canned foods.[10] The outcomes of these studies have resulted in the recommendation to feed canned food to cats with idiopathic cystitis; however,

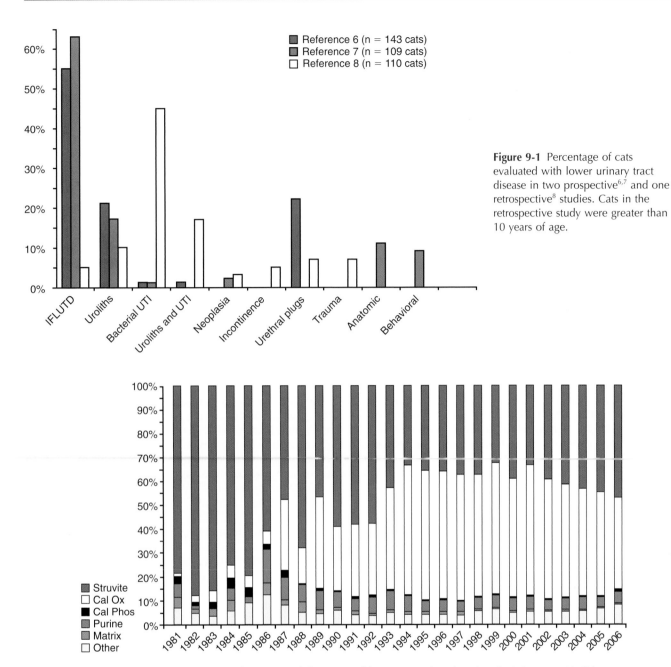

Figure 9-1 Percentage of cats evaluated with lower urinary tract disease in two prospective[6,7] and one retrospective[8] studies. Cats in the retrospective study were greater than 10 years of age.

Figure 9-2 Mineral composition of 55,418 uroliths retrieved from cats and analyzed at the Minnesota Urolith Center between 1981 and 2006.[61] *Cal Ox,* Calcium oxalate, monohydrate, and/or dihydrate; *Cal Phos,* calcium phosphate.

these studies were not randomized, controlled trials. Furthermore, specific dietary ingredients have not been evaluated in cats with idiopathic cystitis.

CRYSTAL-RELATED LOWER URINARY TRACT DISEASE

Of the various causes of feline lower urinary tract disease, crystal-related disease accounts for 15 to 45 per cent of cases. There are many minerals that may precipitate in the urinary tract to form crystals and stones; however, more than 90 per cent of uroliths from cats are composed either of struvite (magnesium ammonium phosphate

hexahydrate) or of calcium oxalate monohydrate or dihydrate (Figure 9-2). Struvite is the most common mineral observed to occur in matrix-crystalline urethral plugs (Figure 9-3).

Urolith and matrix-crystalline plug formation involves complex physiochemical processes. Major factors include (1) urine supersaturation resulting in crystal formation (nucleation); (2) effect of inhibitors of mineral nucleation, crystal aggregation, and crystal growth; (3) crystalloid complexors; (4) effects of promoters of crystal aggregation and growth; (5) effects of noncrystalline matrix; and (6) urine retention or slowed transit for the process to occur.[11,12] Urethral matrix-crystalline plugs have only been identified in male cats and may represent

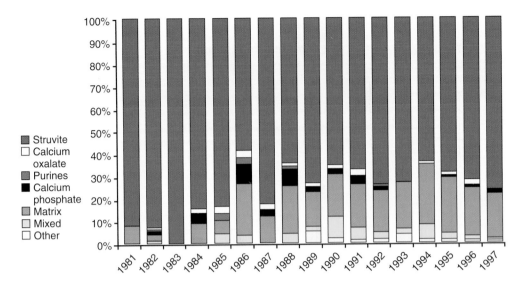

Figure 9-3 Mineral composition of 1901 matrix-crystalline urethral plugs retrieved from male cats and analyzed at the Minnesota Urolith Center between 1981 and 1997.[57]

an intermediate phase between lower urinary tract inflammation without crystals and urolith formation.[13] The most important driving force behind urolith formation is urinary supersaturation with calculogenic substances[14]; however, as mentioned before, other factors are important. The goal of treatment of urinary crystal-related disease is to promote a reduced state of urinary saturation.

Urolithiasis

Calcium Oxalate

Calcium oxalate urolith formation occurs when urine is oversaturated with calcium and oxalate.[14] In addition to these alterations in activities of ions, high-molecular-weight proteins occurring in urine, such as nephrocalcin, uropontin, and Tamm-Horsfall mucoprotein, influence calcium oxalate formation.[15] We have a limited understanding of the role of these macromolecular and ionic inhibitors of calcium oxalate formation in cats. Certain metabolic factors are known to increase risk of calcium oxalate urolith formation in several species, including cats. Medical and nutritional strategies for stone prevention have focused on amelioration of these factors.

Hypercalcemia is associated with increased risk of calcium oxalate urolith formation. In cats with calcium oxalate uroliths, hypercalcemia was observed in 35 per cent of the cases.[16] Conversely, uroliths developed in 35 per cent of cats with idiopathic hypercalcemia.[17] Hypercalcemia, when severe, results in increased calcium fractional excretion and hypercalciuria.

Hypercalciuria is a significant risk factor but not necessarily the cause of calcium oxalate urolith formation in human beings, dogs, and cats.[18] Hypercalciuria can result from excessive intestinal absorption of calcium (gastrointestinal hyperabsorption), impaired renal reabsorption of calcium (renal leak), and/or excessive skeletal mobilization of calcium (resorptive).[12] In Miniature Schnauzers, gastrointestinal hyperabsorption appears to occur most commonly, although renal leak hypercalciuria also has

been observed.[19] Hypercalciuria has not been well defined in normocalcemic cats with calcium oxalate uroliths but is thought to occur.

Metabolic acidosis promotes hypercalciuria by promoting bone turnover (release of calcium with buffers from bone), increasing serum ionized calcium concentration (resulting in increased urinary calcium excretion), and decreasing renal tubular reabsorption of calcium. In cats consumption of diets supplemented with the urinary acidifier ammonium chloride has been associated with increased urinary calcium excretion.[20] Significant aciduria (urine pH < 6.2) may represent a risk factor for calcium oxalate formation because of acidemia and hypercalciuria. In addition, acidic urine alters function and concentration of crystal inhibitors. Low urine pH decreases urinary citrate concentration by increasing renal proximal tubular citrate reabsorption. Acidic urine is known to impair function of macromolecular protein inhibitors.

Inhibitors, such as citrate, magnesium, and pyrophosphate, form soluble salts with calcium or oxalic acid and reduce availability of calcium or oxalic acid for precipitation. Other inhibitors, such as Tamm-Horsfall glycoprotein and nephrocalcin, interfere with the ability of calcium and oxalic acid to combine, thereby minimizing crystal formation, aggregation, and growth.

Oxalic acid is a metabolic end product of ascorbic acid (vitamin C) and several amino acids, such as glycine and serine, derived from dietary sources. Oxalic acid forms soluble salts with sodium and potassium ions but a relatively insoluble salt with calcium ions. Therefore any increased urinary concentration of oxalic acid may promote calcium oxalate formation. Dietary increases of oxalate and vitamin B_6 deficiency are known factors increasing urinary oxalate. Hyperoxaluria has been observed experimentally in kittens consuming vitamin B_6–deficient diets[11] but has not been associated with naturally occurring calcium oxalate urolith formation. Genetic anomalies also may increase urine oxalic acid concentration. Hyperoxaluria also has been recognized in a group of related cats with reduced quantities of hepatic D-glycerate dehydrogenase, an enzyme involved in metabolism of oxalic acid precursors (primary hyperoxaluria type II).[21] Hyperoxaluria also has been associated with defective peroxisomal alanine/glyoxylate aminotransferase activity (primary hyperoxaluria type I) and intestinal disease in human beings (enteric hyperoxaluria). These abnormalities have not been evaluated in cats.

Decreased urine volume results in increased calcium and oxalic acid saturation and an increased risk for urolith formation. Cats can achieve urine specific gravities in excess of 1.065, indicating a marked ability to produce concentrated urine. Many cats affected with calcium oxalate uroliths have a urine specific gravity greater than 1.040 unless there is some impairment of renal function or urine-concentrating ability.[18]

Detection of calcium oxalate crystals indicates that urine is supersaturated with calcium oxalate and, if persistent, represents an increased risk for calcium oxalate urolith formation. However, calcium oxalate crystalluria is present in less than 50 per cent of feline cases at time of diagnosis of calcium oxalate urolithiasis.[18]

Medical protocols that will promote dissolution of calcium oxalate uroliths currently are not available; therefore uroliths must be removed physically, either surgically or by voiding urohydropropulsion[22] (see Chapter 52).

Nutritional and/or medical protocols should be considered to minimize urolith recurrence or to prevent further growth of uroliths remaining in the urinary tract. A significant number of cats will develop recurrent uroliths within 2 years of their initial episode if prevention protocols are not initiated.[23] If possible, metabolic factors known to increase calcium oxalate risk should be corrected or minimized. Goals of dietary prevention include (1) reducing urine calcium and oxalate concentration, (2) promoting high concentrations and activity of urolith inhibitors, (3) reducing urine acidity (increase urine pH), and (4) promoting dilute urine.

Increasing urine volume is a mainstay of preventive therapy for calcium oxalate urolithiasis in human beings. By increasing water intake, urinary concentrations of calculogenic minerals are reduced. In addition, larger urine volumes typically increase urine transit time and voiding frequency, thereby reducing retention time for crystal formation and growth. Feeding cats a canned food is the most practical means of increasing water intake and lowering calcium oxalate urine saturation. The goal is to dilute urine to a specific gravity of less than 1.030.[24] Flavoring water, enhancing water access, and adding water to dry foods may be helpful for cats who refuse to eat canned foods. Sodium chloride should not be added routinely to the diet to stimulate thirst. Although cats will increase water intake and dilute urine in response to salt, the consequence of high-sodium foods in cats prone to oxalate uroliths is unknown. Increased dietary sodium may increase urinary calcium excretion in at-risk cats and can contribute to ongoing renal damage in cats with marginal renal function.[24]

The solubility of calcium oxalate in urine is influenced minimally by pH; however, epidemiological studies consistently identify acidifying diets among the most prominent risk factors for calcium oxalate urolithiasis.[25-27] Persistent aciduria may be associated with low-grade metabolic acidosis, which promotes bone mobilization and increases urinary calcium excretion. In a case series of five cats with hypercalcemia and calcium oxalate uroliths, discontinuation of acidifying diets or urinary acidifiers was associated with normalization of serum calcium concentration.[26] Furthermore, aciduria promotes hypocitraturia and functional impairment of endogenous urolith inhibitors. Thus, feeding an acidifying diet or administering urinary acidifiers to cats at risk for calcium oxalate is contraindicated. A target urine pH of 6.6 to 7.5 is suggested in cats at risk for calcium oxalate urolith recurrence.[24]

Although reduction of urine calcium and oxalic acid concentrations by restriction of dietary calcium and oxalic acid appears logical, it is not without risk. Reducing consumption of only one of these constituents may increase availability and intestinal absorption of the other, resulting in increased urinary excretion. Conversely, increasing dietary calcium levels in normal cats contributes directly to increased urine calcium concentration. Because epidemiological data in cats suggest that marked dietary calcium restriction increases urolith risk, moderate levels of dietary calcium are advised in nonhypercalcemic cats.[24]

Urinary oxalate is derived from endogenous metabolism of oxalate precursors (i.e., glycine and ascorbic acid) and dietary oxalic acid. Most pet food ingredients are low in oxalic acid, with the exception of vegetables, legumes, and several vegetable-based fermentable fibers (e.g., beet pulp and soybean fiber). Dietary oxalic acid concentrations in foods for cats should be reduced to the lowest possible level. Suggested levels are less than 20 mg oxalic acid/100g of food (dry matter basis).[25]

Excess intake of vitamin C, a metabolic oxalate precursor, similarly should be avoided.[24] Although normal dietary vitamin C levels are not considered a risk in human beings, very small increases in urinary oxalate are a concern in urolith formers. Because cats do not have a dietary vitamin C requirement, supplementation should be avoided in foods fed to cats at risk for calcium oxalate uroliths. Cranberry concentrate tablets also are contraindicated. They provide mild acidification and are high in oxalate, as well as vitamin C.[28]

Potassium citrate often is included in diets designed for calcium oxalate prevention. In urine, citric acid combines with calcium to form soluble complexes, thereby reducing ionic calcium concentration. Citric acid also inhibits nucleation of calcium and oxalate crystals directly. When oxidized within the tricarboxylic acid cycle, supplemental citrate results in urine alkalinization due to production of bicarbonate. The metabolic alkalinization increases endogenous renal citrate excretion and reduces calcium absorption and urinary excretion.[24] Commercial products that add citrate but continue to acidify the urine (pH < 6.5) negate the benefit of citrate therapy.

Consumption of high levels of sodium may augment renal calcium excretion in human beings. Recent studies in healthy cats did not find increased urine calcium excretion in response to high dietary salt intake.[24] In cats with marginal renal function and increased calciuria, sodium exacerbated calcium excretion. No studies have evaluated the effect of sodium in cats prone to calcium oxalate stones. Epidemiological evidence suggests that low dietary sodium levels in cat foods increase the risk for calcium oxalate urolithiasis.[29] Nonetheless, when fed a food lower in sodium, cats with naturally occurring calcium oxalate uroliths excreted less urine calcium.[23] Until further data are available, treatments for diuresis that include orally administered sodium chloride or loop diuretics, which promote renal sodium excretion, should be used cautiously and with careful monitoring because they may increase risk of calcium oxalate urolith formation in some patients. Recommended levels of sodium in foods for cats predisposed to calcium oxalate formation is between 0.3 and 0.5 per cent sodium on a dry matter basis.

Dietary phosphorus should not be restricted in cats with calcium oxalate urolithiasis. Low dietary phosphorus is a risk factor for calcium oxalate urolith formation in cats.[29] Reduction in dietary phosphorus may be associated with activation of vitamin D, which in turn promotes intestinal calcium absorption and hypercalciuria. Additionally, phosphate status determines pyrophosphate urinary concentrations, an inhibitor of calcium oxalate urolith formation in human beings and rodents. If calcium oxalate urolithiasis is associated with hypophosphatemia and normal calcium concentration, oral phosphorus supplementation may be considered. Caution should be used, however, because excessive dietary phosphorus may predispose to formation of calcium phosphate uroliths. Whether this occurs in cats is unknown. Phosphorus levels in the foods for cats predisposed to calcium oxalate formation should not be excessive. Levels from 0.5 to 0.8 per cent have been recommended.[24]

Urinary magnesium forms complexes with oxalic acid, reducing the amount of oxalic acid available to form calcium oxalate. Studies in cats associate low dietary magnesium with calcium oxalate risk.[26,27,29-32] In human beings, supplemental magnesium has been used to minimize recurrence of calcium oxalate uroliths; however, supplemental magnesium may increase the risk of struvite formation in cats. At this time, because the risks and benefits of magnesium supplementation to cats with calcium oxalate urolithiasis have not been evaluated, it is not advised. It appears logical that magnesium should not be highly restricted in diets that are consumed by cats with calcium oxalate urolithiasis. Many diets that claim to benefit feline "urinary tract health" are reduced in magnesium and promote urinary acidification. These foods are designed for struvite prevention and are not appropriate for cats at risk for calcium oxalate urolithiasis. Prudent levels of dietary magnesium are from 0.08 to 0.10 per cent dry matter, or approximately 20 mg magnesium/100 kcal.[24,29]

Consumption of high amounts of animal protein by human beings is associated with an increased risk of calcium oxalate formation. Dietary protein of animal origin may increase urinary calcium and oxalic acid excretion, decrease urinary citrate excretion, and promote bone mobilization in order to buffer the acid intake from metabolism of animal proteins. However, a case control study showed that higher protein concentration in cat foods appeared protective against calcium oxalate uroliths.[29] Protein levels between 8 and 9 g protein/100 kcal appeared most protective. Although several coassociations (e.g., higher protein in canned foods) might explain this finding, cats are obligatory carnivores, and dietary protein restriction in the management of calcium oxalate urolithiasis is not advised.

Excessive levels of vitamin D (which promotes intestinal absorption of calcium) and vitamin C (which is a precursor of oxalic acid) should be avoided. Diets with vitamin D between 500 to 2000 IU/kg should suffice. As discussed above, vitamin C is an oxalate precursor, as well as a weak urinary acidifier. Both features may increase likelihood of urolith recurrence.

The diet should be adequately fortified with vitamin B_6, because vitamin B_6 deficiency promotes endogenous production and subsequent urinary excretion of oxalic acid.[33] There is no evidence that providing increased vitamin B_6 beyond meeting the nutritional requirement provides a benefit in cats. Because most commercial diets designed for cats are well fortified with vitamin B_6, it is unlikely that additional supplementation will be beneficial, except in homemade diets. Regardless, vitamin B_6 is reasonably safe and sometimes is provided to cats with persistent calcium oxalate crystalluria or frequent recurrences.

Increased dietary fiber intake is associated with decreased risk of calcium oxalate recurrence in some human beings, but not in cats unless they are hypercalcemic. Certain types of fiber (soy or rice bran) decrease calcium absorption from the gastrointestinal tract, which may decrease urinary calcium excretion. Also, higher-fiber diets tend to be less acidifying. In five cats with idiopathic hypercalcemia and calcium oxalate uroliths, feeding a high-fiber diet with supplemental potassium citrate resulted in normalization of serum calcium concentrations[34]; however, efficacy of increased fiber intake is unproved at this time.

Although the relationship of obesity to urolith formation is not understood, it remains a consistent risk factor in all studies to date. Restricting food intake to obtain an ideal weight and body condition is encouraged.

Cats who are meal fed have on average a more alkaline urinary pH, better controlled food intake for obesity prevention, and a lower risk of calcium oxalate urolith formation. This method of feeding also is the preferred choice for canned foods. This is a relatively simple step that owners can take to improve preventive measures.

At the time of writing, four therapeutic foods are formulated and marketed for the prevention of calcium oxalate uroliths in cats (Table 9-1). These diets either contain potassium citrate (as an alkalinizing agent and as a source of citrate) and are designed to induce a higher urine pH than standard foods and limit mineral intake, or they are designed to promote significant increases in water intake. Consumption of Prescription Diet Feline c/d Multicare (Hill's Pet Nutrition, Inc., Topeka, KS) and Urinary SO (Royal Canin, St. Charles, MO) by healthy cats results in low urine saturation with calcium oxalate. Clinical trials using the predecessor to c/d Multicare (Prescription Diet Feline x/d) in cats with naturally occurring

Table 9-1 Comparison of Diets Formulated for Prevention of Calcium Oxalate Urolithiasis in Cats

Component	Multicare Dry*	Multicare Canned*	pH/O Dry[†]	pH/O Canned[†]	S/O Dry[‡]	S/O Canned[‡]
MOISTURE						
As fed (%)	8	76	10	78	7	79
PROTEIN						
As fed (%)	31.3	10.5	32.4	10.6	32.2	8.5
Dry matter (%)	34.0	42.9	36.0	48.3	34.6	40.5
g/100 kcal ME	8.3	8.8	7.7	9.2	7.8	8.3
FAT						
As fed (%)	15.3	4.8	16.5	6.9	17.5	9.1
Dry matter (%)	16.6	19.6	18.3	31.2	18.0	43.1
g/100 kcal ME	4.1	4.0	3.9	5.9	4.2	8.8
FIBER						
As fed (%)	0.8	0.6	1.7	0.2	3.0	0.51
Dry matter (%)	0.9	2.4	1.9	1.0	3.2	2.4
g/100 kcal ME	0.2	0.5	0.4	0.2	0.7	0.5
SODIUM						
As fed (%)	0.33	0.09	0.44	0.11	1.3	0.2
Dry matter (%)	0.36	0.37	0.49	0.5	1.4	1.0
g/100 kcal ME	0.09	0.08	0.10	0.10	0.32	0.20
CALCIUM						
As fed (%)	0.70	0.17	1.01	0.27	1.0	0.21
Dry matter (%)	0.76	0.69	1.12	1.23	1.1	1.0
g/100 kcal ME	0.19	0.14	0.24	0.23	0.24	0.20
PHOSPHORUS						
As fed (%)	0.61	0.13	0.87	0.20	0.8	0.28
Dry matter (%)	0.66	0.53	0.97	0.91	0.86	1.33
g/100 kcal ME	0.16	0.11	0.21	0.17	0.19	0.27
MAGNESIUM						
As fed (%)	0.07	0.02	0.08	0.02	0.07	0.02
Dry matter (%)	0.08	0.08	0.09	0.14	0.08	0.09
g/100 kcal ME	0.02	0.02	0.02	0.02	0.02	0.02

Dry matter (%), percentage of nutrient in product after moisture is removed; *g/100 kcal ME,* nutrient intake for every 100 kcal of metabolizable energy consumed.

*Prescription Diet Feline c/d Multicare. Nutrient information for diets as of November 2004; manufactured by Hill's Pet Nutrition, Inc, Topeka, KS.

[†]Moderate pH/O/Feline. Nutrient information for diets as of July 2003; manufactured by Iams Company, Dayton, OH.

[‡]Urinary S/O. Nutrient information for diets as of November 2004; manufactured by Royal Canin, St. Charles, MO.

calcium oxalate urolithiasis reduced calcium oxalate supersaturation by 59 per cent.[23] The reduction in calcium oxalate formation product appeared to be a function of its ability to lower urine calcium. We have had some success in reducing mild hypercalcemia in certain calcium oxalate urolith–forming cats by feeding a high-fiber diet (Prescription Diet Feline w/d; Hill's Pet Nutrition Inc., Topeka, KS) and by administering potassium citrate.

Struvite

Struvite is another term for crystals or uroliths composed of magnesium ammonium phosphate hexahydrate. The chemical composition of struvite is $Mg^{2+}NH_4^+PO_4^{3-}\cdot6H_2O$.

In order for uroliths to form, urine must be oversaturated with respect to the minerals that precipitate to form that type of urolith. In order for struvite uroliths to form, urine must be oversaturated with magnesium, ammonium, and phosphate ions. Urinary oversaturation with struvite may occur as a consequence of a urinary tract infection with a urease-producing microbe (infection-induced struvite) or without the presence of a urinary tract infection (sterile struvite) in cats.[35]

Sterile Struvite In cats sterile struvite uroliths typically form between 1 and 10 years of age. Risk for struvite urolith formation decreases after approximately 6 to 8 years of age.[32] They occur with equal frequency in male and female cats. Sterile struvite uroliths form because of dietary composition as well as innate risks for urolith formation. Experimentally, magnesium phosphate and struvite uroliths formed in healthy cats consuming calculogenic diets containing 0.15 to 1.0 per cent magnesium (dry matter basis).[36-38] These data are difficult to interpret, however, because the amount of magnesium consumption by cats in these studies may be different than by cats who form sterile struvite uroliths spontaneously while consuming commercial diets, which may differ from calculogenic diets in caloric density, palatability, and digestibility.[39] The influence of magnesium on struvite formation depends on urine pH[40] and influence of ions, minerals, and other components in urine.[41] Alkaluria is associated with increased risk for struvite formation.[42,43] In a clinical study including 20 cats with naturally occurring struvite urocystoliths and no detectable bacterial urinary tract infection, the mean urinary pH at the time of diagnosis was 6.9 ± 0.4.[35] An additional factor is water intake and urine volume. Consumption of increased quantities of water may result in lowering concentrations of calculogenic substances in urine, thus decreasing risk of urolith formation.[44] Consumption of small quantities of food frequently, rather than one or two large meals per day, is associated with production of more acidic urine and a lesser degree of struvite crystalluria by cats.[45,46]

Sterile struvite uroliths can be dissolved by feeding a diet that is restricted in magnesium, phosphorus, and protein and that induces aciduria relative to maintenance adult cat foods.[35] In a clinical study including 22 cats with sterile struvite urocystoliths, urocystoliths dissolved in 20 cats in a mean of 36.2 ± 26.6 days (range, 14 to 141 days).[35] The cats were fed a high-moisture (canned), calorically dense diet containing 0.058 per cent magnesium (dry matter basis) and increased sodium chloride (0.79 per cent dry matter basis). The diet (Prescription Diet Feline s/d, Hill's Pet Nutrition, Inc.) induced a urine pH of approximately 6.0.

Prevention of sterile struvite uroliths involves inducing a urine pH less than approximately 6.8, increasing urine volume, and decreasing excretion of magnesium, ammonium, and phosphorus. There are many diets available that are formulated to be "struvite preventive."

Infection-Induced Struvite Infection-induced struvite uroliths occur more commonly in cats less than 1 year and greater than 10 years of age. There is no published information on gender predilection for infection-induced struvite uroliths in cats. Infection-induced struvite uroliths form because of an infection by a urease-producing microbe in a fashion similar to that in dogs and human beings.[38] In this situation, dietary composition is not important, because the production of the enzyme urease by the microbial organism is the driving force behind struvite urolith formation.

Infection-induced struvite uroliths can be dissolved by feeding a "struvite dissolution" diet and administering an appropriate antimicrobial agent based on bacteriological culture and sensitivity. Average dissolution time for infection-induced struvite uroliths was 79 days (range, 64 to 92 days) in three cats reported in a study.[35] It is important that the cat receive an appropriate antimicrobial agent during the entire time of medical dissolution because bacteria become trapped in the matrix of the urolith and bacteria are released into urine as the urolith dissolves. If therapeutic levels of an appropriate antimicrobial agent are not present in urine, an infection will recur, and dissolution will cease.

Prevention of infection-induced struvite does not require feeding a special diet. Because the infection causes these struvite uroliths to form, prevention involves ensuring that a bacterial urinary tract infection does not recur and treating bacterial infections as they arise. Dietary manipulation will not prevent infection-induced struvite uroliths from recurring because diet will not prevent recurrence of a bacterial urinary tract infection.

Purines

Uric acid is one of several biodegradation products of purine nucleotide metabolism.[47] In most dogs and cats, allantoin is the major metabolic end product; it is the most soluble of the purine metabolic products excreted in urine. Purine accounted for approximately 5 to 8 per cent of feline uroliths submitted to the Minnesota Urolith Center from 1981 to 2002; 64 (0.14 per cent) were composed of xanthine and the rest were composed of urate (see Chapter 50). Ammonium urate is the monobasic ammonium salt of uric acid, and it is the most common form of naturally occurring purine uroliths observed to occur in dogs and cats.[48] Other naturally occurring purine uroliths include sodium urate, sodium calcium urate, potassium urate, uric acid dihydrate, and xanthine.

Urate Urate uroliths have been observed in several breeds of cats; males appear to be affected as frequently as females. Most urate uroliths occur before 4 years of age. Urate uroliths may occur as a consequence of liver disease, specifically a portovascular anomaly, or without the presence of liver disease, a condition termed *idiopathic urate urolithiasis*. Urate uroliths occurring in association with portovascular anomalies most commonly are composed of ammonium urate and often are diagnosed before 1 year of age.

There have been few studies of the biological behavior of ammonium urate uroliths in dogs with portovascular anomalies[49-52] and none in cats. It is logical to hypothesize that elimination of hyperuricuria and reduction of urine ammonium concentration following surgical correction of anomalous shunts would result in spontaneous dissolution of uroliths composed primarily of ammonium urate. Appropriate clinical studies are needed to prove or disprove this hypothesis. We occasionally have been successful in medically dissolving urate uroliths in dogs with portovascular anomalies but have not attempted dissolution in cats with ammonium urate uroliths and portovascular anomalies. Additional clinical studies are needed to evaluate the relative value of calculolytic diets, allopurinol, and/or alkalinization of urine in dissolving ammonium urate uroliths in cats with portovascular anomalies. The pharmacokinetics and efficacy of allopurinol may be altered in cats with portovascular anomalies because biotransformation of this drug, which has a very short half-life, to oxypurinol, which has a longer half-life, requires adequate hepatic function. Xanthine uroliths have been observed to form in dogs with portovascular anomalies given allopurinol; therefore allopurinol has an effect on xanthine oxidase conversion of xanthine to uric acid.

Although no studies have been performed evaluating the efficacy or safety of medical dissolution of urate uroliths in cats with idiopathic urate urolithiasis, we have dissolved urate uroliths successfully in cats using a low-protein diet (Prescription Diet k/d, Hill's Pet Products, Topeka, KS) and allopurinol (7.5 mg/kg PO q12h). Until further studies are performed to confirm the safety and efficacy of medical dissolution, surgical removal remains the treatment of choice for urate uroliths in cats. Prevention of urate urolith recurrence in cats has been greater than 90 per cent when using a protein-restricted, alkalinizing diet (Prescription Diet k/d, Hill's Pet Products, Topeka, KS).

Xanthine Xanthine uroliths retrieved and analyzed from cats contain pure xanthine, although a few contain small quantities of uric acid. In one report, of 64 cats who formed xanthine uroliths,[53] none had been treated with the xanthine oxidase inhibitor allopurinol. Sixty-one xanthine uroliths were obtained from the lower urinary tract, while xanthine uroliths from three cats came from the upper urinary tract. Xanthine uroliths occurred in 30 neutered and eight nonneutered males and 25 neutered females (the gender of one cat was not specified). Mean age of cats at time of diagnosis of xanthine uroliths was 2.8 ± 2.3 years (range = 4 months to 10 years). Eight of the 64 cats were less than 1 year old. Urinary uric acid excretion was similar between eight xanthine urolith-forming cats and healthy cats (2.09 ± 0.8 mg/kg/d vs. 1.46 ± 0.56 mg/kg/d); however, urinary xanthine excretion (2.46 ± 1.17 mg/kg/d) and urinary hypoxanthine excretion (0.65 ± 0.17 mg/kg/d) were higher (neither is detectable in urine from healthy cats).

No medical dissolution protocol exists for feline xanthine uroliths. Prevention involves feeding a protein-restricted, alkalinizing diet. Without preventive measures, xanthine uroliths often recur within 3 to 12 months following removal. In 10 cats consuming the protein-restricted alkalinizing diet and followed for at least 2 years, only one has had recurrence.

Cystine

Cystine accounts for less than 1 per cent of feline uroliths. They occur with equal frequency in male and female cats. The mean age of diagnosis of cats with cystine uroliths is 4.1 years (range, 10 months to 11 years).[39] Most cats affected with cystine uroliths are domestic shorthair.

Cystine uroliths occur when urine is oversaturated with cystine. Cystine is a disulfide-containing amino acid that is normally filtered and reabsorbed by proximal renal tubular cells. Therefore cystinuria occurs when there is a defect in proximal renal tubular absorption and must be present for cystine uroliths to form. Evaluation of urine amino acid profiles from four cats with cystine uroliths revealed increased concentrations of the amino acids cystine, arginine, lysine, and ornithine.[39,54]

Medical protocols exist for dissolution of cystine uroliths in dogs utilizing thiol-containing drugs, such as N-(2-mercaptopropionyl)-glycine (2-MPG), with or without dietary modification[55] or urinary alkalinization. Reducing dietary protein has the potential of minimizing formation of cystine uroliths by decreasing intake and excretion of sulfur-containing amino acids and by decreasing renal medullary tonicity and thus increasing urine volume. Many feline protein-restricted diets are formulated for use by cats with renal failure and have an added advantage of containing a urinary alkalinizing agent. Solubility of cystine increases exponentially when the urine pH is greater than 7.2.[56] If necessary, or if dietary modification can not be done, potassium citrate may be administered to induce alkaluria. Although thiol-containing drugs are used in dogs and human beings, their use has not been evaluated adequately in cats.

Matrix-Crystalline Urethral Plugs

Urethral matrix-crystalline plugs occur in approximately 20 per cent of male cats under 10 years of age who present with obstructive lower urinary tract disease.[6] Urethral plugs have only been observed to occur in male cats. They are composed of at least 45 to 50 per cent matrix and variable amounts of mineral; they may be composed entirely of matrix.[57] Struvite is the most common mineral found in urethral plugs. Multiple factors are thought to be associated with urethral plug formation. If a mineral is present in the urethral plug, risk factors associated with that crystal formation, as discussed previously, are involved, at least in part. Compared with uroliths, urethral plugs contain large quantities of matrix. Components of matrix that may be important in urethral plug formation include Tamm-Horsfall mucoprotein, serum proteins, cellular debris, and virus-like particles.[13,58]

Management of urethral matrix-crystalline plugs involves relieving the obstructive uropathy.[59] Modifying urine composition by feeding a therapeutic diet may be beneficial if mineral is present in the urethral plug. Increasing urine volume may help to decrease the concentration of minerals and matrix components in urine. Successful prevention of recurrent urethral obstruction utilizing diets designed to reduce urine pH and urine magnesium and phosphorus concentrations has been reported.[60] Perineal urethrostomy may be considered in cats with recurrent urethral plug formation; however, it is associated with complications including recurrent bacterial urinary tract infections and lower urinary tract disease.[60]

SUMMARY

Not all feline urinary tract disorders are associated with dietary factors; however, most benefit from nutritional management. It is important to understand the pathophysiology of feline lower urinary tract disease and the physiological effects of foods and feeding in order to formulate the best nutritional and treatment plan.

REFERENCES

1. Lawler DF, Sjolin DW, Collins JE: Incidence rates of feline lower urinary tract disease in the United States, *Feline Pract* 15:13, 1985.

2. Willeberg P: Epidemiology of naturally occurring feline urologic syndrome, *Vet Clin North Am Small Anim Pract* 14:455, 1984.

3. Foster SJ: The "urolithiasis" syndrome in male cats: a statistical analysis of the problems, with clinical observations, *J Small Anim Pract* 8:207, 1967.

4. Osborne CA, Kruger JM, Johnston GR, et al: Feline lower urinary tract disorders. In Ettinger SJ, editor: *Textbook of veterinary internal medicine*, ed 3, Philadelphia, 1989, WB Saunders, pp 2057.

5. Lund EM, Armstrong PJ, Kirk CA, et al: Health status and population characteristics of dogs and cats examined at private veterinary practices in the United States, *J Am Vet Med Assoc* 214:1336, 1999.

6. Kruger JM, Osborne CA, Goyal SM, et al: Clinical evaluation of cats with lower urinary tract disease, *J Am Vet Med Assoc* 199:211, 1991.

7. Buffington CA, Chew DJ, Kendall MS, et al: Clinical evaluation of cats with nonobstructive urinary tract diseases, *J Am Vet Med Assoc* 210:46, 1997.

8. Bartges JW: Lower urinary tract disease in older cats: what's common, what's not? Health and Nutrition of Geriatric Cats and Dogs, 1996.

9. Markwell PJ, Buffington CA, Chew DJ, et al: Clinical evaluation of commercially available urinary acidification diets in the management of idiopathic cystitis in cats, *J Am Vet Med Assoc* 214:361, 1999.

10. Gunn-Moore DA, Shenoy CM: Oral glucosamine and the management of feline idiopathic cystitis, *J Feline Med Surg* 6:219, 2004.

11. Brown C, Purich D: Physical-chemical processes in kidney stone formation. In Coe F, Favus M, editors: *Disorders of bone and mineral metabolism*, New York, 1992, Raven Press, p 613.

12. Coe FL, Parks JH, Asplin JR: The pathogenesis and treatment of kidney stones, *N Engl J Med* 327:1141, 1992.

13. Osborne CA, Lulich JP, Kruger JM, et al: Feline urethral plugs. Etiology and pathophysiology, *Vet Clin North Am Small Anim Pract* 26:233, 1996.

14. Bartges JW, Osborne CA, Lulich JP, et al: Methods for evaluating treatment of uroliths, *Vet Clin North Am Small Anim Pract* 29:45, 1999.

15. Balaji KC, Menon M: Mechanism of stone formation, *Urol Clin North Am* 24:1, 1997.

16. Bartges JW: Calcium oxalate urolithiasis. In August JR, editor: *Consultations in feline internal medicine*, vol 4, Philadelphia, 2001, WB Saunders, p 352.

17. Midkiff AM, Chew DJ, Randolph JF, et al: Idiopathic hypercalcemia in cats, *J Vet Intern Med* 14:619, 2000.

18. Bartges JW, Kirk C, Lane IF: Update: Management of calcium oxalate uroliths in dogs and cats, *Vet Clin North Am Small Anim Pract* 34:969, 2004.

19. Lulich JP, Osborne CA, Nagode LA, et al: Evaluation of urine and serum metabolites in miniature schnauzers with calcium oxalate urolithiasis, *Am J Vet Res* 52:1583, 1991.

20. Ching SV, Fettman MJ, Hamar DW, et al: The effect of chronic dietary acidification using ammonium chloride on acid-base and mineral metabolism in the adult cat, *J Nutr* 119:902, 1989.

21. McKerrell RE, Blakemore WF, Heath MF, et al: Primary hyperoxaluria (L-glyceric aciduria) in the cat: a newly recognised inherited disease, *Vet Rec* 125:31, 1989.

22. Lulich JP, Osborne CA, Sanderson SL, et al: Voiding urohydropropulsion: lessons from 5 years of experience, *Vet Clin North Am Small Anim Pract* 29:283, 1999.

23. Lulich JP, Osborne CA, Lekcharoensuk C, et al: Effects of diet on urine composition of cats with calcium oxalate urolithiasis, *J Am Anim Hosp Assoc* 40:185, 2004.

24. Kirk CA, Ling GV, Osborne CA, et al: Clinical guidelines for managing calcium oxalate uroliths in cats: medical therapy, hydration, and dietary therapy. *Managing urolithiasis in cats: recent updates and practice guidelines*, Topeka, KS, 2003, Hill's Pet Nutrition, p 10.

25. Kirk CA, Ling GV, Franti CE, et al: Evaluation of factors associated with development of calcium oxalate urolithiasis in cats, *J Am Vet Med Assoc* 207:1429, 1995.

26. Thumchai R, Lulich J, Osborne CA, et al: Epizootiologic evaluation of urolithiasis in cats: 3,498 cases (1982-1992), *J Am Vet Med Assoc* 208:547, 1996.

27. Lekcharoensuk C, Lulich JP, Osborne CA, et al: Association between patient-related factors and risk of calcium oxalate and magnesium ammonium phosphate urolithiasis in cats, *J Am Vet Med Assoc* 217:520, 2000.

28. Terris MK, Issa MM, Tacker JR: Dietary supplementation with cranberry concentrate tablets may increase the risk of nephrolithiasis, *Urology* 57:26, 2001.

29. Lekcharoensuk C, Osborne CA, Lulich JP, et al: Association between dietary factors and calcium oxalate and magnesium ammonium phosphate urolithiasis in cats, *J Am Vet Med Assoc* 219:1228, 2001.

30. Robertson WG: Urinary calculi. In Nordin BEC, Need AG, Morris HA, editors: *Metabolic bone and stone disease*, Edinburgh, 1993, Churchill Livingstone, p 249.

31. Lulich JP, Osborne CA, Bartges JW, et al: Canine lower urinary tract disorders. In Ettinger SJ, Feldman EC, editors: *Textbook of veterinary internal medicine*, ed 5, Philadelphia, 1999, WB Saunders, pp 1747.

32. Smith BHE, Moodie SJ, Wensley S, et al: Differences in urinary pH and relative supersaturation values between senior and young adult cats. Proceedings of the 15th ACVIM Forum: 674, 1997.

33. Bai SC, Sampson DA, Morris JG, et al: Vitamin B6 requirement of growing kittens, *J Nutr* 119:1020, 1989.

34. McClain HM, Barsanti JA, Bartges JW: Hypercalcemia and calcium oxalate urolithiasis in cats: a report of five cases, *J Am Anim Hosp Assoc* 35:297, 1999.

35. Osborne CA, Lulich JP, Kruger JM, et al: Medical dissolution of feline struvite urocystoliths, *J Am Vet Med Assoc* 196:1053, 1990.

36. Buffington T: Struvite urolithiasis in cats, *J Am Vet Med Assoc* 194:7, 1989.

37. Finco DR, Barsanti JA, Crowell WA: Characterization of magnesium-induced urinary disease in the cat and comparison with feline urologic syndrome, *Am J Vet Res* 46:391, 1985.

38. Osborne CA, Polzin DJ, Abdullahi SU, et al: Struvite urolithiasis in animals and man: formation, detection, and dissolution, *Adv Vet Sci Comp Med* 29:1, 1985.

39. Osborne CA, Kruger JM, Lulich JP, et al: Feline lower urinary tract diseases. In Ettinger SJ, Feldman EC, editors: *Textbook of veterinary internal medicine*, ed 5, Philadelphia, 1999, WB Saunders, p 1710.

40. Buffington CA, Rogers QR, Morris, JG: Effect of diet on struvite activity product in feline urine, *Am J Vet Res* 51:2025, 1990.

41. Buffington CA, Blaisdell JL, Sako T: Effects of Tamm-Horsfall glycoprotein and albumin on struvite crystal growth in urine of cats, *Am J Vet Res* 55:965, 1994.

42. Tarttelin MF: Feline struvite urolithiasis: factors affecting urine pH may be more important than magnesium levels in food, *Vet Rec* 121:227, 1987.

43. Bartges JW, Tarver SL, Schneider C: Comparison of struvite activity product ratios and relative supersaturations in urine collected from healthy cats consuming four struvite management diets. Proceedings of the Ralston Purina Nutrition Symposium, 1998.

44. Smith BH, Stevenson AE, Markwell PJ: Urinary relative supersaturations of calcium oxalate and struvite in cats are influenced by diet, *J Nutr* 128:2763S, 1998.

45. Finke MD, Litzenberger BA: Effect of food intake on urine pH in cats, *J Small Anim Pract* 33:261, 1992.

46. Tarttelin MF: Feline struvite urolithiasis: fasting reduced the effectiveness of a urinary acidifier (ammonium chloride) and increased the intake of a low magnesium diet, *Vet Rec* 121:245, 1987.

47. Bartges JW, Osborne CA, Lulich JP, et al: Canine urate urolithiasis. Etiopathogenesis, diagnosis, and management, *Vet Clin North Am Small Anim Pract* 29:161, 1999.

48. Osborne CA, Bartges JW, Lulich JP, et al: Canine urolithiasis. In Hand MS, Thatcher CD, Remillard RL, et al, editors: *Small animal clinical nutrition*, ed 4, Marceline, MO, 2000, Wadsworth Publishing, pp 605.

49. Marretta SM, Pask AJ, Greene RW, et al: Urinary calculi associated with portosystemic shunts in six dogs, *J Am Vet Med Assoc* 178:133, 1981.

50. Hardy RM, Klausner JS: Urate calculi associated with portal vascular anomalies. In Kirk RW, editor: *Current veterinary therapy VIII*, Philadelphia, 1983, WB Saunders, p 1073.

51. Brain PH: Portosystemic shunts—urate calculi as a guide to diagnosis, *Aust Vet Pract* 18:3, 1988.

52. Johnson CA, Armstrong PJ, Hauptman JG: Congenital portosystemic shunts in dogs: 46 cases (1979-1986), *J Am Vet Med Assoc* 19:1478, 1987.

53. Osborne CA, Bartges JW, Lulich JP: Feline xanthine urolithiasis: a newly recognized cause of urinary tract disease, *Urol Res* 32:171 (Abstract), 2004.

54. DiBartola SP, Chew DJ, Horton ML: Cystinuria in a cat, *J Am Vet Med Assoc* 198:102, 1991.

55. Osborne CA, Sanderson SL, Lulich JP, et al: Canine cystine urolithiasis. Cause, detection, treatment, and prevention, *Vet Clin North Am Small Anim Pract* 29:193, 1999.

56. Milliner DS: Cystinuria, *Endocrinol Metab Clin North Am* 19:889, 1990.

57. Osborne CA, Lulich JP, Albasan H, et al: Mineral composition of feline uroliths and urethral plugs: current status. In Davis CA, editor: *Proceedings of managing urolithiasis in cats: recent updates and practice guidelines 2003*, Topeka, KS, 2003, Hill's Pet Nutrition, p 26.

58. Kruger JM, Osborne CA: The role of viruses in feline lower urinary tract disease, *J Vet Intern Med* 4:71, 1990.

59. Osborne CA, Kruger JM, Lulich JP, et al: Medical management of feline urethral obstruction, *Vet Clin North Am Small Anim Pract* 26:483, 1996.

60. Osborne CA, Caywood DD, Johnston GR, et al: Perineal urethrostomy versus dietary management in prevention of recurrent lower urinary tract disease, *J Small Anim Pract* 32:296, 1991.

61. Lulich JP, Osborne CA: Why study the past: shifting urolith types, Proceedings of the ACVIM Forum, Seattle, 2007.

10 Metabolism, Diet, and Obesity

Margarethe Hoenig

Feline obesity has increased dramatically in the past two to three decades and rivals the increase seen in human beings. Simply stated, obesity occurs when energy input is greater than energy output. One might assume in today's society that cats should not have any weight problems. Because cats are kept mostly indoors, they do not have access to external food sources; thus owners control the amount of food available to them. The fact that obesity now is a pandemic in cats indicates that many factors play a role in this trend. One likely factor is that owners do not perceive obesity as a disease and may actually like their cats to be obese. Cats often are more relaxed when they are obese than when they are lean.

Many obese cats are healthy, and owners may not understand the veterinary concern about the increase in weight. Not all obese cats develop diseases that have been associated with obesity such as arthritis, cardiovascular disease, respiratory conditions, dermatopathies, urinary tract disease, and cancer.[1,2]

About 20 per cent of obese people develop diabetes,[3] and although a similar assessment has not been made in cats, it is likely that obese cats also are at high risk to develop the disease, as well as other diseases associated with obesity in human beings.[4] The veterinarian therefore has an important role in educating cat owners about the dangers of obesity. Veterinarians must assess a cat's body condition at each practice visit and educate owners about the importance of monitoring their pet's weight. Unfortunately, this is a difficult topic to discuss with owners, many of whom also suffer from weight problems.

DEFINITION

Obesity is a condition in which there is an excessive amount of body fat or adipose tissue in relation to lean body mass. It is the most common nutritional disorder in cats in the United States, affecting about one third of the cat population.[1,2]

Well-defined, objective parameters to distinguish between a cat with normal weight, one that is overweight, and one that is grossly obese do not exist. Obesity can be assessed subjectively using the body scoring system developed by Laflamme.[5] However, it can be difficult to use in cats, especially in those who have lost weight recently or who have long hair.

Objective ways to judge obesity in cats do exist. Body mass index (BMI) is well known from human medicine, where it is used to assess adiposity. It can be calculated in cats according to the following formula[6]:

$$\textbf{BMI} = \textbf{Body weight}\,(\textbf{kg})/(\textbf{Body length}\ [\textbf{m}] \times \textbf{Height}\ [\textbf{m}])$$

where height is the distance from the point of the shoulder through the point of the elbow to the proximal boundary of the metacarpal pad, and length is the distance from the point of the shoulder to the tuber ischium. Obesity also can be assessed by measuring the girth circumference immediately caudal to the last rib.[7] Both girth and BMI measurements do not need any specialized equipment. Highly sophisticated evaluations of adiposity include dual energy x-ray absorptiometry (DEXA) and magnetic resonance imaging.[8,9] The latter modality allows the exact localization of fat depots in the body, which is not possible with DEXA. We have found that BMI and girth correlate well with DEXA results and are excellent objective markers of adiposity that could be used by clinicians. When cats become obese, both abdominal subcutaneous and visceral fat mass increase to the same extent, and both are associated with insulin resistance.[8] This contrasts with human subjects in whom obesity usually is associated with a larger increase in abdominal visceral than abdominal subcutaneous obesity, and it is the former that correlates negatively with insulin sensitivity.[10]

PATHOGENESIS

Obesity is a sign of energy excess. Cats used to be hunters, whereas now they are typically fed a high-energy diet but have a sedentary lifestyle. As is the case in the human population, cats' energy output often is much less than their energy input, which tilts their weight maintenance balance towards fat storage. Overnutrition leads to myriad changes that threaten to overwhelm the body's adaptive mechanisms. We are just starting to accumulate basic knowledge of normal metabolism in cats, which will help us to detect aberrations of the obese and design strategies for treatment.

HORMONAL AND METABOLIC CHANGES

Insulin is one of the primary regulators of energy metabolism. In obesity, two major changes develop in cats. There is a qualitative and quantitative change in the secretion of insulin, and there is change in the tissue responsiveness to insulin called *insulin resistance*. In fact, it has been shown that each kilogram increase in body weight in cats is associated with a 30 per cent decrease in insulin sensitivity.[8,11]

Glucose is the primary physiological stimulus of insulin secretion in most species. Insulin secretion in healthy subjects follows any increase in blood glucose very tightly, thereby ensuring that blood glucose is maintained within a very narrow range even after food intake. The secretion occurs in a biphasic manner and consists of an acute first phase and a delayed second, or maintenance, phase[12] (Figure 10-1). Insulin resistance primarily affects the second phase of insulin secretion. A marked hypersecretion is seen in obese cats during that phase (Figure 10-2). This is a physiological response to lower tissue uptake of glucose caused by a lower expression of the insulin-sensitive glucose transporter GLUT4 in muscle and adipose tissue.[13] Short term, the pancreas is able to secrete more insulin to overcome this tissue resistance. However, maintaining hypersecretion of insulin long term is only possible if the pancreatic mass and function can adapt to the increase in demand. If it fails, overt diabetes ensues. As stated above, this adaptation fails in 20 per cent of obese people and in a large percentage of obese cats.

Obesity in cats also is associated with a change in the secretion of proinsulin, which is cleaved to insulin and C-peptide in the beta cell secretory granules.[14] The ratio of proinsulin to insulin in the secretory granule repre-

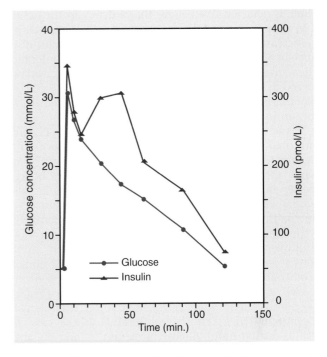

Figure 10-1 Mean plasma and insulin concentration in eight cats after intravenous administration of glucose (1 g/kg).[12]

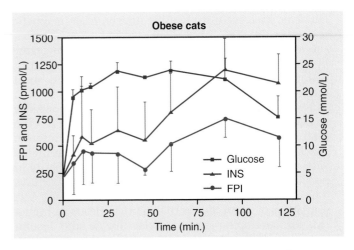

Figure 10-2 Intravenous glucose tolerance testing in six obese cats with determination of serum feline proinsulin (FPI), insulin (INS), and glucose serum concentrations (mean + SD).[14]

sents an estimate for the efficiency of this conversion process, which becomes abnormal with progressive failure of beta cells. Obese cats show an initial increased proinsulin/insulin ratio when stimulated with glucose; however, this reverses during the later phase, indicating that the cellular machinery responsible for cleavage of proinsulin to insulin can respond in a delayed fashion to a strong stimulus (see Figure 10-2). There are no data about proinsulin during the progression to diabetes and in newly diagnosed diabetic cats.

It is not known if a defect in insulin secretion in obesity develops before a change in insulin sensitivity of liver and of peripheral tissues, such as muscle and adipose tissue, is detected. We believe that a defect in the action of insulin occurs first in cats, because we have identified an increase in insulin secretion indicative of insulin resistance in a group of lean cats showing glucose intolerance when made obese; however, the same increase was not observed in lean cats who maintained normal glucose tolerance when they became obese during a 6-month ad libitum food intake period.[7]

It is well known that many signaling pathways become abnormal with the development of obesity, not only leading to changes in glucose transport but affecting many other metabolic functions. In human beings, obesity is one of the characteristics of metabolic syndrome, as is the coexistence of insulin resistance (or glucose intolerance) with hypertension and atherogenic dyslipidemia, among other risk factors for diabetes and cardiovascular disease.[15] The lipid and lipoprotein alterations seen in obese individuals include elevated cholesterol, triglycerides, and apolipoprotein B concentrations, as well as higher very-low-density lipoprotein (VLDL), low-density lipoprotein (LDL), and lower high-density lipoprotein (HDL) cholesterol levels.[16] Obese cats are insulin resistant and glucose intolerant,[8,17] and yet they do not show atherosclerosis and hypertension. We hypothesized that this was because even in long-term obese and insulin-resistant cats, fasting and postprandial lipid and lipoprotein concentrations would not show similarities to those found in obese human beings. However, in a recent study using novel nuclear magnetic resonance (NMR) technology, we were able to show that cats with long-term obesity develop many of the same lipid changes that are seen in obese people, whereas this is not the case for cats who have been obese only short term.[18]

NMR technology has greatly expanded our knowledge of plasma lipid subclasses. It is now known that not the total concentration of a lipoprotein but the lipoprotein subclass concentration and particle size correlate highly with the development of the comorbidities of obesity in people. For example, increases in large VLDL particles have been associated with coronary artery disease. The formation of small, dense HDL particles leads to higher risk for developing cardiovascular disease and insulin resistance.[19,20] Small, dense LDL particles are more susceptible to oxidative modification than large particles, and thus more likely to do damage to the endothelium, which leads to atherosclerosis.[21]

The development of obesity in cats is associated with an increase in plasma triglycerides, nonesterified fatty acids, and VLDL. The overproduction of VLDL in cats is associated with an increase in the VLDL large and medium-size particles that, in people, have been associated with cardiovascular disease.[22] Despite the high VLDL concentrations, chronically obese cats show no change in baseline LDL concentrations; however, obese cats have an almost threefold higher concentration of very small and medium small LDL particles than of large particles. Increased levels of small, dense LDL particles have been shown to be strongly associated with coronary artery disease risk in people. Small HDL particles also have been associated with cardiovascular disease in human beings and are significantly higher in obese cats (Figure 10-3). It

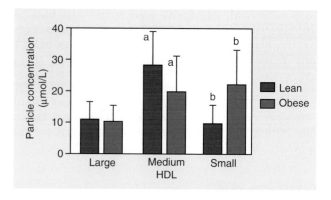

Figure 10-3 Nuclear magnetic resonance–determined HDL particle concentrations (mmol/L) in lean (L) and obese (OB) cats (n = 24, 12 L and 12 OB). (a) and (b) denote significant difference (p < 0.01) between L and OB particle concentrations.

is interesting that despite all of the similarities between cats and human beings with metabolic syndrome, atherosclerosis and cardiovascular disease are not features of obesity and diabetes in cats. This suggests that additional factors present in obese people, but not in obese cats, are important in their pathogenesis.

Other similarities and differences exist between feline and human fat metabolism. In a recent study comparing obese to lean cats, lipoprotein lipase (LPL) plasma and fat activity, as well as fat mRNA levels, were significantly lower (50 per cent, 80 per cent, and 50 per cent, respectively) in obese cats, whereas the muscle/fat ratio of LPL was significantly higher, favoring a partitioning of fatty acids away from adipose to muscle tissue.[23] Indeed, increased myocellular lipids were found in obese cats.[7] Free fatty acid uptake inhibits insulin-stimulated glucose transport, and increases in lipid deposition in muscle tissue have been associated with insulin resistance.[24]

Major regulators of lipid and glucose metabolism are a group of ligand-activated transcription factors called peroxisome proliferator-activated receptors (PPARs). They belong to the nuclear receptor superfamily that also includes steroid hormones and thyroid hormone. Three members, α, γ, and β/δ, share significant homologies. PPARα regulates genes that are involved in lipid and lipoprotein metabolism. PPARγ regulates genes involved in adipocyte cell differentiation, and serves an important role as an insulin sensitizer. Finally, PPARδ stimulates fatty acid oxidation and suppresses inflammation that is thought to occur in response to an increase in fat cell size. The PPARs, among several other transcription factors, are targets for the transcriptional coactivator PGC1A, an important regulator of mitochondrial metabolism. The PGC1A gene is highly inducible by any physiological condition that requires increased mitochondrial energy production, such as fasting and increased exercise.[25] It is well known that obesity and insulin resistance are associated with disturbed mitochondrial energy metabolism and a lower mitochondrial–to–nuclear DNA ratio. As expected, PPARs and PGC1A are all down-regulated in muscle and fat tissue of obese cats[26] (Figure 10-4).

Obesity does not lead only to changes in insulin sensitivity. The development of obesity in the cat is associ-

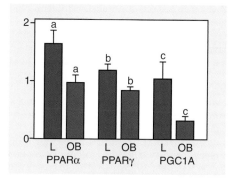

Figure 10-4 PPARα, PPARγ, and PGC1A expression in fat tissue from eight lean (L) and eight obese (OB) cats. The data are expressed as arbitrary units obtained after normalization by feline beta actin. Values with the same transcript letter differ significantly.

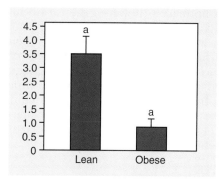

Figure 10-5 Adiponectin expression in fat from eight lean and eight obese cats. The data are expressed as arbitrary units obtained after normalization by feline beta actin. Values with the same transcript letter differ significantly.

ated with a significant increase in free thyroxine (T_4) within the physiological range, a change that correlates with the increase in plasma nonesterified fatty acid (NEFA) concentrations. It is believed that the primary effect of obesity on free T_4 concentrations in cats is the elevation of NEFAs, which increase the free T_4 fraction significantly in vitro.[27] In long-term obese cats, an increase in total T_4 also is seen.[28]

Fat itself is now considered an important endocrine organ secreting several hormones and cytokines involved in the regulation of metabolism. Adiponectin, leptin, and tumor necrosis factor alpha (TNFα) have been studied in cats.[8,23,29,30] Adiponectin inhibits hepatic gluconeogenesis and stimulates fatty acid oxidation, glucose uptake, and lactate production. It also increases insulin sensitivity in muscle and liver by enhancing insulin signaling.[31] Expression (Figure 10-5) and plasma concentrations of adiponectin are low in obese cats,[8] and they normalize with weight loss.[8] The hormone leptin stimulates energy expenditure and decreases food intake in lean subjects. Obese human beings and cats are resistant to the effect of leptin. Similar to adiponectin, its levels normalize with weight loss.[8] TNFα regulates adiposity through suppression of lipoprotein lipase and induction of apoptosis of fat cells.[32] Obese cats have higher expression of TNFα than lean cats and lower lipoprotein lipase expression and activity in fat but not muscle tissue, as discussed above. The resultant partitioning of fatty acids away from fat to muscle tissue may be a physiological response to limit the increasing fat cell size that occurs with excess energy intake, and to provide fatty acids to muscle where the uptake of the fuel glucose has decreased (Figure 10-6).

Obesity also has been linked to impaired immunity in several species,[33-36] and it has been suggested that obese dogs and cats[37] have decreased immune function; however, specific studies assessing their immune function have not been performed until recently. In a study of newly obese cats, a strong innate immune and adaptive immune response was elicited in cats irrespective of diet or body condition, and there was no correlation between body condition, diet, and any of the quantitative and

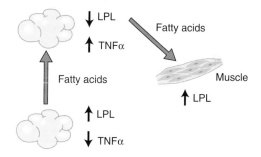

Figure 10-6 Schematic of changes in LPL activity expression in fat and muscle and expression of TNFα in fat leading to a partitioning of fatty acids to muscle.

qualitative responses of the immune system.[38] Further studies are needed to determine if this is also the case in cats who have been obese for several years.

TREATMENT

The aim of treatment of primary obesity is to increase energy expenditure and to decrease energy intake. This is accomplished through management of diet and lifestyle. The diet should be high in protein, which increases loss of fat mass and preserves lean body mass.[8,39,40] It also was shown that a high-protein–low-carbohydrate diet causes a higher heat production than a low-protein–high-carbohydrate diet.[8] Neutered cats need less calories than intact cats because they have a lower basal metabolic rate.[41] They are at greater risk to develop obesity because neutering also has been shown to increase appetite.[42] Energy restriction should proceed slowly in order to avoid the development of hepatic lipidosis in cats. A 1 to 1.5 per cent weight loss per week has been reported to be safe. Several commercial weight-loss diets are available to cat owners and provide the necessary nutrients despite reduced caloric intake. In addition, special computer programs have been designed to aid owners in their quest to have a slimmer pet.

Obesity leads to many metabolic and hormonal changes. Most changes can be reversed completely when the cat regains its normal lean weight.[8] Insulin sensitivity returns to normal. If, however, the cat's beta cell mass becomes too small to compensate for peripheral insulin resistance, irreversible alterations occur. Therefore it is important for the veterinarian to recognize obesity and educate the client about the energy balance equation. For the owner, the challenge is to become innovative in increasing the pet's exercise and strict in controlling its food intake. The reader is referred to Chapter 19 in the fifth volume of this series for a detailed discussion on the management of feline obesity.

REFERENCES

1. Scarlett JM, Donoghue S, Saidla J, et al: Overweight cats: prevalence and risk factors, *Int J Obes Relat Metab Disord* 18(Suppl 1):S22, 1994.
2. Lund EM, Armstrong J, Kirk CA, et al: Prevalence and risk factors for obesity in adult cats from private US veterinary practices, *Int J Appl Res Vet Med* 3:88, 2005.
3. Wolfson W: Leapin' lizards: amylin targets diabetes and obesity via incretins, *Chem Biol* 14:235, 2007.
4. Prahl A, Guptill L, Glickman NW, et al: Time trends and risk factors for diabetes mellitus in cats presented to veterinary teaching hospitals, *J Feline Med Surg* 9:351, 2007.
5. Laflamme D: Development and validation of a body condition score system for cats: a clinical tool, *Feline Pract* 25:13, 1997.
6. Nelson RW, Himsel CA, Feldman EC, et al: Glucose tolerance and insulin response in normal-weight and obese cats, *Am J Vet Res* 51:1357, 1990.
7. Wilkins C, Long RC, Waldron M, et al: Assessment of the influence of fatty acids on indices of insulin sensitivity and myocellular lipid content by use of magnetic resonance spectroscopy in cats, *Am J Vet Res* 65:1090, 2004.
8. Hoenig M, Thomaseth K, Waldron M, et al: Insulin sensitivity, fat distribution, and adipocytokine response to different diets in lean and obese cats before and after weight loss, *Am J Physiol* 292:R227, 2007.
9. Speakman JR, Booles D, Butterwick R: Validation of dual energy X-ray absorptiometry (DXA) by comparison with chemical analysis of dogs and cats, *Int J Obes* 25:439, 2001.
10. Wagenknecht LE, Langefeld CD, Scherzinger AL, et al: Insulin sensitivity, insulin secretion, and abdominal fat. The Insulin Resistance Atherosclerosis Study (IRAS) Family Study, *Diabetes* 52:2490, 2003.
11. Hoenig M, Thomaseth K, Brandao J, et al: Assessment and mathematical modeling of glucose turnover and insulin sensitivity in lean and obese cats, *Domest Anim Endocrinol* 31:573, 2006.
12. Hoenig M, Hall G, Ferguson D, et al: A feline model of experimentally induced islet amyloidosis, *Am J Pathol* 157:2143, 2000.
13. Brennan CL, Hoenig M, Ferguson DC: GLUT4 but not GLUT1 expression decreases early in the development of feline obesity, *Domest Anim Endocrinol* 26:291, 2004.
14. Kley S, Caffall Z, Tittle E, et al: Development of a feline proinsulin immunoradiometric assay and a feline proinsulin enzyme-linked immunosorbent assay (ELISA): a novel application to examine beta cell function in cats, *Domest Anim Endocrinol* 34:311, 2008.
15. Eckel RH, Grundy SM, Zimmet PZ: The metabolic syndrome, *Lancet* 365:1415, 2005.
16. Griffin BA: Lipoprotein atherogenicity: an overview of current mechanisms, *Proc Nutr Soc* 58:163, 1999.
17. Hoenig M, Alexander S, Holson J, et al: Influence of glucose dosage on interpretation of intravenous glucose tolerance tests in lean and obese cats, *J Vet Intern Med* 16:529, 2002.
18. Jordan E, Kley S, Le N-A, et al: Dyslipidemia in obese cats, *Domest Anim Endocrinol* 35:290, 2008.
19. Mackey RH, Kuller LH, Sutton-Tyrrell K, et al: Lipoprotein subclasses and coronary artery calcium in postmenopausal women from the healthy women study, *Am J Cardiol* 90:71, 2002.
20. Garvey WT, Kwon S, Zheng D, et al: Effects of insulin resistance and type 2 diabetes on lipoprotein subclass particle size and concentration determined by nuclear magnetic resonance, *Diabetes* 52:453, 2003.
21. Berliner JA, Navab M, Fogelman AM, et al: Atherosclerosis: basic mechanisms. Oxidation, inflammation, and genetics, *Circulation* 91:2488, 1995.
22. Freedman DS, Otvos JD, Jeyarajah EJ, et al: Relation of lipoprotein subclasses as measured by proton nuclear magnetic resonance spectroscopy to coronary artery disease, *Arterioscler Thromb Vasc Biol* 18:1046, 1998.
23. Hoenig M, McGoldrick JB, DeBeer M, et al: Activity and tissue-specific expression of lipases and tumor-necrosis factor α in lean and obese cats, *Domest Anim Endocrinol* 30:333, 2006.
24. Shulman GI: Cellular mechanisms of insulin resistance, *J Clin Invest* 106:171, 2000.
25. Chiarelli F, Di Marzio D: Peroxisome proliferator-activated receptor-gamma agonists and diabetes: current evidence and future perspectives, *Vasc Health Risk Manag* 4:297, 2008.
26. Hoenig M, Caffall Z, Ferguson DC: Triiodothyronine differentially regulates key metabolic factors in lean and obese cats, *Domest Anim Endocrinol* 34:229, 2008.
27. Hoenig M, Caffall Z, Ferguson DC: Obesity increases free thyroxine proportionally to nonesterified fatty acid concentrations in adult neutered female cats, *J Endocrinol* 194:267, 2007.
28. Kley S, Glushka J, Jin E, et al: Impact of obesity, gender and diet on hepatic glucose production in cats, *Am J Physiol Regul Integr Comp Physiol* 296:R936, 2009.
29. Backus RC, Havel PJ, Gingerich RL, et al: Relationship between serum leptin immunoreactivity and body fat mass as estimated by use of a novel gas-phase Fourier transform infrared spectroscopy deuterium dilution method in cats, *Am J Vet Res* 61:796, 2000.
30. Appleton DJ, Rand JS, Sunvold GD: Plasma leptin concentrations in cats: reference range, effect of weight gain and relationship with adiposity as measured by dual energy X-ray absorptiometry, *J Feline Med Surg* 2:83, 2002.
31. Gil-Camposa M, Canete R, Gil A: Adiponectin, the missing link in insulin resistance and obesity, *Clin Nutr* 23:963, 2004.
32. Kern PA, Saghizadeh M, Ong JM, et al: The expression of tumor necrosis factor in human adipose tissue. Regulation by obesity, weight loss, and relationship to lipoprotein lipase, *J Clin Invest* 95:2111, 1995.
33. Dovio A, Caramello V, Masera RG, et al: Natural killer cell activity and sensitivity to positive and negative modulation in uncomplicated obese subjects: relationships to leptin and diet composition, *Int J Obes Relat Metab Disord* 28:894, 2004.
34. Moriguchi S, Kato M, Sakai K, et al: Exercise training restores decreased cellular immune functions in obese Zucker rats, *J Appl Physiol* 84:311, 1998.
35. Moriguchi S, Oonishi K, Kato M, et al: Obesity is a risk factor for deteriorating cellular immune functions decreased with aging, *Nutr Res* 15:151, 1995.
36. Nieman DC, Henson DA, Nehlsen-Cannarella SL, et al: Influence of obesity on immune function, *J Am Diet Assoc* 99:294, 1999.
37. German AJ: The growing problem of obesity in dogs and cats, *J Nutr* 136:1940S, 2006.

38. Jaso-Friedmann L, Leary JH 3rd, Praveen K, et al: The effects of obesity and fatty acids on the feline immune system, *Vet Immunol Immunopathol* 122:146, 2008.

39. Szabo J, Ibrahim WH, Sunvold GD, et al: Influence of dietary protein and lipid on weight loss in obese ovariohysterectomized cats, *Am J Vet Res* 61:559, 2000.

40. Laflamme DP, Hannah SS: Increased dietary protein promotes fat loss and reduces loss of lean body mass during weight loss in cats, *Intern J Appl Res Vet Med* 3:62, 2005.

41. Hoenig M, Ferguson DC: Effects of neutering on hormonal concentrations and energy requirements in male and female cats, *Am J Vet Res* 63:634, 2002.

42. Fettman MJ, Stanton CA, Banks LL, et al: Effects of neutering on body weight, metabolic rate and glucose tolerance of domestic cats, *Res Vet Sci* 62:131, 1997.

11 Probiotics in Feline Medicine

Stanley L. Marks and Debra L. Zoran

The mammalian intestinal tract contains a complex, dynamic, and diverse society of pathogenic and non-pathogenic bacteria. Researchers have estimated that the human body contains 10^{14} cells, only 10 per cent of which are not bacteria and belong to the human body proper.[1] There has been extensive research on the mechanisms by which pathogenic bacteria influence intestinal function and induce disease; however, recent attention has focused on the indigenous nonpathogenic microorganisms and the ways by which they may benefit the host. Initial colonization of the sterile newborn intestine occurs with maternal vaginal and fecal bacterial flora. The first colonizers, which have a high reductive potential, include species such as *Enterobacter, Streptococcus,* and *Staphylococcus.* These bacteria metabolize oxygen, favoring the growth of anaerobic bacteria such as *Lactobacillus* species and *Bifidobacterium* species. Colonization with these bacteria is delayed significantly in cesarean deliveries,[2] leading to delayed activation of the efferent limb of the mucosal immune response.[3] The detrimental effects of not developing a normal bacterial flora are seen in germ-free mice, whose small intestines weigh less than those of their healthy counterparts. This is partly an effect of lymphoid constituent underdevelopment—in particular, of an absence of plasma cells in the lamina propria and Peyer's patches and subsequent reduction in immunoglobulin (Ig) A expression. Exposure to bacteria results in a reversal of this phenomenon within 28 days of exposure.[4]

HISTORY OF PROBIOTIC HEALTH CLAIMS

Documentation of the health benefits of bacteria in food dates back to as early as the Persian version of the Old Testament (Genesis 18:8), which states that "Abraham owed his longevity to the consumption of sour milk." Plinius, a Roman historian in 76 BC, recommended the use of fermented milk products for the treatment of gastroenteritis.[5] One-hundred years ago, the Nobel Prize–winning Russian scientist Elie Metchnikoff suggested that the ingestion of *Lactobacillus*-containing yogurt decreased the number of toxin-producing bacteria in the intestine, contributing to the longevity of Bulgarian peasants.[6] These observations led to the concept of a "probiotic" (from the Greek, meaning "for life"). The term *probiotic* was first used in 1965 to define "substances secreted by one microorganism that stimulate the growth of another" and was thus contrasted with the term *antibiotic*.[7] The meaning of the word subsequently has evolved to apply to bacteria that "contribute to intestinal balance." The current and more complete definition of a probiotic refers to "a preparation of or a product containing viable, defined microorganisms in sufficient numbers, which alter the microflora in a compartment of the host and by that exert beneficial health effects on the host."[8]

Different strains of probiotic bacteria may exert different effects based on specific capabilities and enzymatic activities, even within one species.[9,10] Different microorganisms express habitat preferences that may differ in various host species. *Lactobacillus* species are among the indigenous flora colonizing the chicken's crop, the stomach of mice and rats, and the lower ileum in human beings. Bacteria colonizing such high-transit-rate sites must adhere firmly to the mucosal epithelium and adapt to the milieu of this adhesion site.[11] The competition for adhesion receptors between probiotic and pathogenic microorganisms therefore depends on such habitat specifics. Four microhabitats in the gastrointestinal tract were outlined by Freter (1992) as follows[12]: (1) the surface of epithelial cells; (2) the crypts of the ileum, cecum, and colon; (3) the mucus gel that overlays the epithelium; and (4) the lumen of the intestine. The luminal content of bacteria depends greatly on bowel transit, resulting in a relatively low microbial density in the small bowel. It should be emphasized that a proven probiotic effect found in one strain or species can not be transferred to other strains or species because of differences in strain characteristics and habitat preferences.

Because of these multiple mechanisms of action, many different probiotics have potential applications to various diseases. Those in most widespread use, and which have undergone the most clinical testing, include *Lactobacillus* species (such as *L. acidophilus*, *L. rhamnosus*, *L. bulgaricus*, *L. reuteri*, and *L. casei*); *Bifidobacterium* species; and *Saccharomyces boulardii*, which is a nonpathogenic yeast. Despite the explosion of interest and publications on probiotics in recent years, their clinical application has been limited by the paucity of well-designed and mechanistically based laboratory, translational, and clinical studies.

MECHANISMS OF PROBIOTIC ACTION

PROBIOTICS BLOCK INTESTINAL PATHOGENIC BACTERIAL EFFECTS

Probiotics have been shown to mediate maintenance of the gastrointestinal microbial balance via two mechanisms: production of antibacterial substances and competitive inhibition of pathogen and toxin adherence to the intestinal epithelium.[13-16]

Probiotic-Derived Antibacterial Substances

Probiotics exert direct antibacterial effects on pathogens through production of antibacterial substances, including bacteriocins and acid.[13,14] The primary mechanism of bacteriocin action is to form pores in the cytoplasmic membrane of sensitive bacteria, but they also can interfere with essential enzyme activities in sensitive species. The two-component lantibiotics, a class of bacteriocins produced by gram-positive bacteria such as *Lactococcus lactis*, are small antimicrobial peptides.[13] These peptides

have been found to be active at nanomolar concentrations to inhibit multidrug-resistant pathogens by targeting the lipid II component of the bacterial cell wall.[17] Other non–lanthionine-containing bacteriocins are small antimicrobial peptides produced by *Lactobacillus* species. These peptides have a relatively narrow spectrum of activity and are mostly toxic to gram-positive bacteria, including *Lactococcus*, *Streptococcus*, *Staphylococcus*, *Listeria*, and *Mycobacteria*. Several strains of *Bifidobacterium* have been found to produce bacteriocin-like compounds toxic to both gram-positive and gram-negative bacteria.[18] Probiotic bacteria, especially strains of *Lactobacillus*, produce acetic, lactic, and propionic acids that lower the local pH, leading to inhibited growth of a wide range of gram-negative pathogenic bacteria.[19]

Competitive Inhibition of Pathogen and Toxin Adherence to the Intestinal Epithelium

Several strains of *Lactobacillus* and *Bifidobacterium* are able to decrease adhesion of both pathogens and their toxins to the intestinal epithelium, and they can displace pathogenic bacteria even if the pathogens have attached to intestinal epithelial cells prior to probiotic treatment.[15,16] However, specific probiotics or probiotic combinations should be selected based on their ability to inhibit or displace a specific pathogen. One of the mechanisms by which pathogenic bacteria bind to intestinal epithelial cells is the interaction between bacterial lectins and carbohydrate moieties of glycoconjugate receptor molecules on the cell surface. Studies have confirmed that probiotic inhibition of pathogen adherence to intestinal cells is mediated in part by competition for lectin-binding sites on glycoconjugate receptors on the cell surface.[20,21] Blockade of bacterial enterotoxin binding also has been demonstrated as a mechanism with therapeutic potential.[21a]

PROBIOTICS REGULATE MUCOSAL IMMUNE RESPONSES

Both in vitro and in vivo studies show effects of probiotics on host immune functions: up-regulation of immune function may improve the ability to fight infections or inhibit tumor formation; down-regulation may prevent the onset of allergy or intestinal inflammation. One mechanism of probiotics regulating immunomodulatory functions is activation of toll-like receptors (TLRs).[22,23]

Enhancing Host Innate Immunity

Probiotics have the potential to stimulate innate immune responses against microorganisms and dietary antigens newly encountered by the host through several mechanisms. Intestinal dendritic cells can retain commensal bacteria by activating B lymphocytes selectively to produce IgA to reduce mucosal penetration by bacteria. The dendritic cells carrying commensals are restricted to the intestinal mucosal lymphoid tissues and thus avoid potential systemic immune responses.[24] Treatment of mice with nonviable *Lactobacillus* GG (LGG) results in a significant elevation of fecal sIgA and enhanced secretion of interleukin (IL)–6, which augments IgA antibody responses at the mucosal surface.[25] Importantly, LGG stimulates only moderate expression of costimulatory molecules, low production of tumor necrosis factor (TNF) and CCL20, and no production of IL-2, IL-12, IL-23, and IL-27 in dendritic cells compared with vigorous Th-1 type responses to pathogenic *Streptococcus pyogenes*. This phenomenon underscores the differential modulation of dendritic cells to pathogenic and nonpathogenic probiotic bacteria.[26]

Modulation of Pathogen-Induced Inflammatory Responses

The host innate defenses must modulate responses appropriate to the level of threat provided by a given pathogen. If the response is too weak, the infection may not be cleared, leaving the host susceptible to systemic infection. However, if it is too strong, the result may be excess tissue damage. Probiotics can protect against pathogen-induced injury and inflammation by modulating the balance of proinflammatory and antiinflammatory cytokine production.

Increasing Antiinflammatory Cytokine Production

Probiotics can induce dendritic cells to produce antiinflammatory cytokines, including IL-10, which suppress the Th1 response.[27] However, the role of IL-10 production in probiotic prevention of Th1 responses is controversial and may be through both IL-10–dependent and IL-10–independent mechanisms.

Suppressing Proinflammatory Cytokine Production

Probiotics such as LGG have been shown to inhibit lipopolysaccharide (LPS)– and *Helicobacter pylori*–stimulated TNF production by murine macrophages.[28] In addition, LGG-conditioned cell culture media decreases TNF production in macrophages, indicating that soluble molecules derived from LGG exert this immunoregulatory role.[28] Inhibition of *Escherichia coli* or LPS-induced TNF production also occurs secondary to increased production of granulocyte colony-stimulating factor (G-CSF) production from macrophages. Probiotics such as LGG, *L. rhamnosus* GR-1, and their cell culture supernatants induce high levels of G-CSF production from macrophages, facilitating decreased production of TNF.[29] The suppression of TNF production by G-CSF is mediated through STAT3 and subsequent inhibition of c-Jun N-terminal kinases (JNKs).[29]

Up-Regulation of Host Immune Responses to Defend Against Infection

Probiotics and commensal microflora may regulate a balance between proinflammatory and antiinflammatory mucosal responses, leading to intestinal homeostasis. Probiotics facilitate this important function by stimulating host immunological functions, including Th1 responses, through dendritic cell–directed T-cell activation. During colonization of mice with *B. fragilis*, dendritic cells take up and retain a bacterial polysaccharide that promotes maturation of dendritic cells, Th1-type cytokine production including IL-4, IL-12, and interferon (IFN)–γ, and subsequent CD4+ T-cell expansion.[30]

Regulation of Immune Responses by Probiotic DNA

There have been a number of intriguing studies documenting the beneficial immunomodulatory properties of probiotic DNA in people and murine models. DNA isolated from the probiotic VSL#3 mixture decreases LPS-activated IL-8 production and TNF and IFN release in vivo and in vitro. VSL#3 DNA also inhibits p38 MAP kinase and delays NF-κB activation.[31] The unmethylated CpG dinucleotides, found commonly in bacterial and other nonmammalian genomes, activate innate immunity through TLR9. Administration of *E. coli*–derived DNA protects against injury in the dextran sulfate sodium (DSS) model of colitis in a TLR-dependent manner.[22] The specificity of TLR9 response was confirmed following the loss of CpG protection in a TLR9-knockout model.[22] Of equal importance, the study by Rachmilewitz et al showed a therapeutic effect of *E.coli*–derived DNA when given subcutaneously to mice with experimentally induced colitis. These pivotal studies prove that the protective effects of probiotics are mediated by their own DNA rather than by their metabolites or by their ability to colonize the colon. TLR9 signaling is essential in mediating the antiinflammatory effect of probiotics, and live microorganisms are not required to attenuate experimental colitis because nonviable probiotics are equally effective.

Differential Activation of TLRs by Probiotics in Immune Cells

Different probiotic bacteria stimulate distinct TLRs on host cells, an essential consideration in designing any therapeutic trials. Probiotic bacteria possess molecular recognition patterns similar to pathogenic bacteria; however, the probiotic organisms do not normally initiate pathogenic inflammatory responses. The probiotic *E. coli* Nissle 1917 expresses increased levels of both TLR2 and TLR4,[23] whereas the probiotic VSL#3 mixture mediates its immunostimulatory response via TLR9 signaling.[22] It appears that probiotics exert both up-regulatory and down-regulatory effects on immune responses, and TLR-regulated signaling pathways appear to be one of the mechanisms for these immunoregulatory actions. There clearly is a need to define the mechanism(s) for observed differences among the signals induced by probiotics and pathogens, which use similar receptors to induce divergent responses.

PROBIOTICS REGULATE INTESTINAL EPITHELIAL CELL FUNCTIONS

Substantial evidence indicates that probiotic bacteria stimulate intestinal epithelial cell responses, including restitution of damaged epithelial barrier,[32] production of antibacterial substances and cell-protective proteins,[33] and prevention of cytokine-induced intestinal epithelial cell apoptosis.[34] Many of these responses result from probiotic stimulation of specific intracellular signaling pathways in the intestinal epithelial cells.

CURRENT APPLICATIONS AND USES OF PROBIOTICS IN HUMAN BEINGS

One important characteristic of probiotics is their ability to suppress the proliferation and virulence of pathogenic organisms; this is an increasingly well-documented role of probiotic bacteria in the gastrointestinal and genitourinary tracts. However, it is becoming increasingly clear that probiotic microbiota have direct effects on human physiology and immunity, including allergic disease (e.g., asthma, hay fever), autoimmune diseases (e.g., multiple sclerosis and type 1 diabetes), diseases of the oral cavity (e.g., periodontal disease and caries), and diseases of the nervous system (e.g., autism and depression).[35] This section will review our current understanding of the multiple, systemic effects of probiotics in human beings, dogs, and cats.

PROBIOTICS AND ORAL HEALTH

Oral disorders in people, in particular dental caries, periodontal disease, oral *Candida albicans* infection, and halitosis, are associated with an alteration or imbalance in the oral microbial flora that potentially can be manipulated or restored with the introduction of probiotics.[36] These probiotics must adhere to and colonize the specific surfaces of the oral cavity to confer their long-term health benefits. Although this is possible with individual strains of bacteria, the best effects appear to be the coordinated application of multiple strains that coaggregate and generate beneficial biofilms—a process that has been difficult to duplicate with many probiotics used individually. The first colonizers of the human oral cavity are *Lactobacillus* species, followed by Viridans group *Streptococci*. However, *Streptococcus mutans*, the primary agent of dental caries, is not present in the mouth until the eruption of the first teeth, because it requires solid surfaces for attachment and proliferation.[37] These bacteria have highly developed mechanisms for carbohydrate metabolism that allow them to convert carbohydrates to exopolysaccharides, which promote bacterial attachment to dental surfaces and enhance accumulation of oral microbes in plaque to form biofilms.[38] Thus the potential role of probiotics is to interfere in several steps of oral biofilm formation, modify the development of oral microecology, and reduce the proliferation of plaque-inducing microorganisms in saliva. Unfortunately, permanent oral colonization by established probiotics has not been reported when exogenous strains (*Lactobacillus* species or *Bifidobacterium* species) have been administered to human subjects.[39,40] Therefore, although multiple studies show beneficial reductions of dental caries and reduction of oral *Streptococci* in both in vitro studies and in clinical trials, further work is needed to find optimal combinations of bacteria that can develop permanent colonization and show long-term benefit.[41-43] There has been only one randomized,

controlled trial performed to date evaluating probiotics for management and prevention of oral *Candida* infections and periodontal disease.[44] In vitro studies demonstrate that *Lactobacillus* species and other probiotic bacteria inhibit the growth of oral pathogens involved in periodontal disease, such as *Porphyromonas gingivalis, Prevotella intermedia,* and *Bacteroides* spp., as well as the invasive yeast *Candida albicans,* an organism that commonly affects elderly, immunocompromised human beings or individuals with xerostomia.[44-46] As a result, probiotic applications in oral biology continue to be an area of significant research and clinical interest.

PROBIOTICS IN GASTROINTESTINAL DISEASE

Of the potential benefits of probiotics, their role in prevention or treatment of gastrointestinal disease in human beings and animals has drawn the most interest. Human and experimental studies with probiotics have targeted specific health benefits associated with three functional areas of the gut microbiota: metabolic effects, protective effects, and trophic effects.[47] Probiotics have metabolic effects on digestion, particularly of lactose and other disaccharides, and on the production of intestinal gas, a significant problem in patients with irritable bowel syndrome (IBS).

In one study the addition of probiotics such as *Lactobacillus* and *Streptococcus* (which are present as starter cultures in yogurt) to the diet of lactose-intolerant individuals resulted in improved lactose digestion and fewer clinical symptoms due to the presence of β-galactosidase, which hydrolyzes lactose, in these bacteria.[48] The effect of probiotics in reducing bloating and gas production in patients with IBS has been well documented in randomized clinical trials. Colonic bacteria ferment ingesta to produce short-chain fatty acids, hydrogen, carbon dioxide, water, and other gases. Some microbial species produce large amounts of gas; other species consume gas, particularly hydrogen. The balance between gas-consuming and gas-producing microbes determines the amount, frequency, and odor of intestinal gas production. To date, it appears that *Bifidobacterium* species have the highest rates of therapeutic benefit in adults with IBS.[49] However, in a study in colicky infants, a *Lactobacillus* strain resulted in the greatest reduction in intestinal bloating and gas.[50] These different responses highlight the complexity of interactions between the microflora in each unique ecological habitat and emphasize the need to be cautious in predicting specific responses in individual subjects.

The protective effects of probiotics on the gastrointestinal tract include the prevention and treatment of acute diarrhea, the eradication of *H. pylori* infection, and prevention of systemic infections (septicemia) from bacterial translocation.[47] Acute diarrhea due to antibiotics, nosocomial infections, community-acquired infectious enteritis, and traveler's diarrhea are common disorders that have been managed with a variety of probiotic formulations. There have been a plethora of clinical trials studying the efficacy of probiotics in the treatment of acute diarrhea in adults (infectious diarrhea, traveler's diarrhea); however, the evidence is most compelling for the administration of probiotics to decrease morbidity in people with antibiotic-associated diarrhea. In placebo-controlled studies, antibiotic-induced diarrhea occurred in 15 to 27 per cent of adults receiving placebo, but in only 3 to 7 per cent of adults receiving the probiotic.[51] It is important to recognize that many different strains or combinations of strains were tested in multiple studies (e.g., *L. rhamnosus* GG, *L. acidophilus*, *L. casei*, *Bacillus clausii*), so specific recommendations are difficult. Nevertheless, meta-analyses of controlled trials and the Cochrane Systematic review concluded that some probiotics can be used to prevent antibiotic-associated diarrhea in children and adults.[52-55]

Prevention and management of *Clostridium difficile* infection in human beings secondary to prolonged antibiotic administration is a significant concern due to the morbidity associated with this infection and the difficulty in treatment. There have been few randomized controlled studies evaluating the efficacy of probiotics for management of *C. difficile* infection, and most have utilized the yeast organism *Saccharomyces boulardii* in this capacity. However, in one nonrandomized clinical study of a group of seven dialysis patients in a nephrology ward who developed *C. difficile* infection unresponsive to standard antibiotic therapy, *S. boulardii* administration was associated with complete resolution of the diarrhea in 75 per cent (5) of patients.[56] Probiotic therapy with *S. boulardii* also was associated with a significant reduction in recurrent episodes of *C. difficile* infection (17 per cent of patients), versus 50 per cent of patients receiving placebo.[57] The efficacy data of probiotics for prevention of community-acquired diarrhea and traveler's diarrhea are more unclear; however, most studies suggest that probiotic therapy is beneficial. In a recent meta-analysis, probiotic therapy was more effective in preventing traveler's diarrhea (7 per cent of people developed diarrhea) than a placebo group in which 31 per cent of people developed diarrhea.[58]

Another area of intense interest is the role of probiotics in preventing or inhibiting the colonization of the gastric mucosa by *H. pylori*. Some strains of *Lactobacillus* are known to inhibit the growth of *Helicobacter* in vitro; however, when these bacteria were added to yogurt in a clinical trial, they were not effective in eradicating the infection.[59] A recent meta-analysis of 14 randomized trials evaluating the efficacy of probiotic therapy in combination with standard triple or quadruple antibiotic therapy showed that probiotic supplementation resulted in a higher incidence of *Helicobacter* infection eradication and a decreased incidence of antibiotic-associated diarrhea.[60]

Probiotics currently are being evaluated for their ability to reduce bacterial translocation and to prevent development of systemic infection (sepsis). This is a common, and potentially fatal, complication of a variety of pathological conditions resulting in mucosal barrier disruption (e.g., postoperative patients, and people with severe pancreatitis, multisystem organ failure, or necrotizing enterocolitis). Current recommendations for the implementation of probiotics in this group of patients are considered preliminary because of the paucity of large, randomized trials in this area. However, in a group of liver transplant patients who were given either antibiotic therapy for bowel decontamination, live probiotic (a *Lactobacillus*), or dead probiotic (same organism), the results were striking: infections occurred in 48 per cent of the antibiotic group, 13 per cent of the live probiotic group, and 34 per cent of the dead probiotic group.[61] Additional randomized trials are needed to make confident predictions and recommendations for the administration of probiotics in postsurgical patients; however, the general consensus is that probiotics appear to be beneficial.[47] Conversely, use of probiotic therapy in critically ill patients has not been generally recommended because additional evidence is still needed to support safety and effectiveness in that setting.

The third important area of probiotic influence in the gastrointestinal tract is its trophic effects on mucosal immunity and epithelial cell growth. There are three specific focus areas under this umbrella: IBD, food allergy, and colon cancer. Although the etiology of IBD in human beings (e.g., Crohn's disease and ulcerative colitis) is unknown, substantial experimental and clinical evidence suggests that the mucosal immune system displays an aberrant response towards luminal antigens, most probably commensal bacteria, in genetically susceptible people.[62] It is well known that certain bacteria activate proinflammatory mucosal responses, while others downregulate intestinal inflammation. Thus it has been hypothesized that creating a favorable local microecology may restore homeostasis of the local immune response and thus resolve the intestinal inflammation.[47] Multiple randomized clinical trials have been performed combining standard drug therapy with different strains of probiotic (*Lactobacillus*, *E. coli*, *Bifidobacterium*) and one combination probiotic product (VSL#3: three *Bifidobacterium* spp., four *Lactobacillus* spp., and *S. salivarius*).[63-65] In these trials, addition of probiotics to the therapeutic regimen resulted in longer relapse-free remission times in patients with ulcerative colitis in some studies, but not in others; however in Crohn's disease, the results were uniformly equivocal. The best evidence for use of probiotics in human beings with IBD is in chronic relapsing pouchitis, in which administration of VSL#3 was associated with a relapse in only three of 20 patients in the 4-month test period, compared to all of the patients relapsing in the placebo group.[66] These results underscore the importance of cautiously interpreting studies utilizing probiotics in patients with IBD, because the dysbiosis (dysregulated bacterial ecosystem) varies in each form of IBD, necessitating careful selection of specific bacteria for different intestinal disorders.

In summary, in people evidence for the benefit of using probiotics to treat certain gastrointestinal disorders is increasing as more randomized trials are completed. At this time, there is level 1 evidence (i.e., data from either high-quality, randomized controlled trials with statistically significant results and few design limitations or from systematic reviews of trials) for effectiveness of probiotics in treating lactose intolerance/maldigestion, treating acute infectious or nosocomial diarrhea in children, preventing or treating antibiotic-associated diarrhea, preventing and maintaining remission of pouchitis in adult human beings, and maintaining remission of ulcerative colitis in adults.[47] In addition, there is level 2 evidence (evidence obtained from randomized trials that have limitations in methodology or results that have wide confidence intervals) for using of probiotics to treat traveler's diarrhea, prevent sepsis secondary to severe acute pancreatitis, and prevent infections in postoperative patients.[47] As improved tools for investigation of gut colonization and microbial communities are developed, a more complete picture of the role of commensal microbes and the interactions of these microflora in inducing or controlling inflammation will be gained, facilitating better selection of probiotics and improved outcomes in the patients with gastrointestinal disease.

PROBIOTICS AND GENITOURINARY DISEASES

There is increasing evidence to support the use of probiotics for prevention or treatment of many different diseases of the urogenital tract, including urinary tract infections (UTI), yeast vaginitis, urolithiasis, bacterial vaginosis, and bladder or cervical cancer.[67,68] Despite the lack of evidence for clinical effectiveness based on randomized trials, there is some rationale for using probiotics to prevent sexually transmitted diseases such as human immunodeficiency virus and Herpes, Group B streptococcal infection in pregnancy, prostatitis, and interstitial cystitis.[67,68] In the early 1980s, *Lactobacillus* species were selected as the best probiotic for human urogenital tract health, primarily because they were the most common species associated with a normal urinary tract and they were effective in inhibiting the growth and adhesion of pathogens.[69] Since that time, a variety of *Lactobacillus* strains (*L. rhamnosus, L. reuteri, L. jensenii,* and *L. crispatus*) have shown effectiveness in preventing infection or augmenting the effectiveness of antibiotics for a wide spectrum of urogenital diseases.[67] Current research also is evaluating nonvirulent strains of *E. coli* that have been shown recently to effectively colonize the urinary bladder and to prevent infection in trials of patients with spinal cord injury or in patients prone to recurrent UTI.[70] Although probiotics are not likely to replace antibiotic therapy in the immediate future, probiotic strains currently in use appear to augment antimicrobial effectiveness as well as reduce the adverse effects of antibiotic therapy on morbidity and quality of life.

PROBIOTICS IN ALLERGY AND AUTOIMMUNE DISEASE

There has been an increasing incidence of allergic and autoimmune diseases (e.g., type 1 diabetes, multiple sclerosis) in human beings from Western countries.[71] There are many potential reasons for this change, but a common theory is the "hygiene" hypothesis, which attributes the failure to decreased exposure to organisms that promote immunoregulation. In Western cultures a much smaller portion of the population is now exposed to intestinal parasites such as helminths due to their eradication in

people. Also, injudicious antibiotic administration in human beings may play a role in the higher incidence of childhood allergies (there is direct evidence that these individuals have fewer *Lactobacillus* species in the gut microbiota).[72-75] The hygiene hypothesis is based on the concept that exposure to these organisms drives the development of immunoregulatory mechanisms of tolerance. Interestingly, the validity of these arguments is supported by clinical trials and experimental models in which parasites and microorganisms that are depleted from the environment in Western countries have been shown to treat allergy,[76,77] autoimmunity,[78] or intestinal inflammation.[79] For example, individuals infected by helminths are less likely to have allergic sensitization or allergic disorders, and treatment of helminth infections tends to increase allergic sensitization.[80] The concept that modulating the intestinal microbiota can modulate chronic inflammatory disorders has a long history, beginning with studies in rats in the mid 1980s showing that susceptibility of these animals to adjuvant arthritis was dependent on their gut microbiota.[81] There are a variety of clinical studies of probiotics used in human beings with allergic rhinitis, cow's milk allergy, cedar pollinosis, and autoimmune diseases such as rheumatoid arthritis or type 1 diabetes; however, there is no overall agreement about the strength of the evidence for efficacy of probiotics in allergy or autoimmune diseases.[72]

There is clear agreement that the immunological principles behind the use of probiotics for therapy is convincing; however, there are several important criteria that must be evaluated critically to facilitate addressing this malady. Consistent selection of the appropriate probiotic strain in an antiinflammatory strategy for assessment, as well as careful screening and recruitment of appropriate patients with inclusion and exclusion criteria, is warranted.[72]

PROBIOTIC THERAPY IN DOGS

To date, only a relatively small number of studies have been published evaluating the effects of probiotics in dogs, and most of these have focused on the intestinal microflora in apparently healthy dogs. Specifically, probiotic strains of human or canine origin (*Lactobacillus, Bifidobacterium,* and *Enterococcus*) were used in healthy adult dogs to assess their effects on intestinal microbial populations, their ability to reduce specific pathogens in feces, and effectiveness as immunomodulators.[82-88] In many of these studies, probiotics added to the food in healthy dogs had an equivocal effect on fecal microflora and pathogens.[86,89] However, it is important to note that most of these studies were not randomized, controlled trials, and the strains of probiotic varied from study to study, making interpretation of findings more challenging. In addition, many studies focused on fecal isolation and quantitative cultures of putative pathogenic bacteria such as *C. perfringens,* rather than on the evaluation of more meaningful end points such as shifts in the microbial flora, mucosal immunopathology, and alterations in intestinal integrity. Only two studies addressing the role of probiotics in management of dietary sensitivity and food-responsive diarrhea have been published to date, with overall positive results.[83,85] Only one of these studies was a randomized, placebo-controlled clinical trial (Sauter), and the results of that study, although clinically positive (all of the dogs in the study improved when they were placed on the elimination diet) showed no specific changes in the inflammatory cytokine patterns or a specific benefit of the probiotic.[83] The immunomodulatory effects of *Enterococcus faecium* SF68 have been studied in dogs, and the probiotic was associated with increased fecal IgA concentrations and increased vaccine-specific circulating IgG and IgA concentrations.[90] Although increased immune globulins may suggest enhanced immune response, the clinical relevance of this finding is not known. Additional studies are warranted in dogs to further assess the immunomodulatory effects of probiotics and to evaluate their safety. The latter issue is particularly important given the recent finding of increased intestinal adhesion of *Campylobacter jejuni* in an in vitro model of canine intestinal mucus following incubation with *E. faecium*.[91] It should be noted that this *E. faecium* strain is different from the *E. faecium* SF68 strain available commercially; moreover, to date there has been no clinical or anecdotal evidence of *Campylobacter*-associated diarrhea in dogs.

Despite the paucity of prospective, randomized, placebo-controlled clinical trials in dogs, tremendous interest has been shown among commercial pet food companies who are marketing probiotics for use in dogs or cats. Unfortunately, most of the evidence surrounding the use of probiotics in puppies or adult dogs with stress colitis or antibiotic-responsive diarrhea is anecdotal, with no prospective, randomized, placebo-controlled studies in these disorders published to date.

PROBIOTIC THERAPY IN CATS

Unfortunately, there is little published information pertaining to probiotic use in cats, and there are no clinical studies reporting a beneficial effect of probiotic therapy for any feline disease.[92] One study evaluating the effect of dietary supplementation with the probiotic strain of *L. acidophilus* DSM 13241 (2×10^8 CFU/d for 4.5 weeks) administered to 15 healthy adult cats demonstrated that recovery of the probiotic from the feces of the cats was associated with a significant reduction in *Clostridium* spp. and *Enterococcus faecalis*.[93] However, the immunomodulatory effects were reported based on decreased lymphocyte and increased eosinophil populations and increased activities of peripheral blood phagocytes. The relevance of these findings is unclear, because this study was not a randomized trial and the changes reported in the populations of peripheral blood cells can not be extrapolated into evidence of systemic health benefits. Evaluation of the effect of supplementation with *E. faecium* strain SF68 on immune function responses following administration of a multivalent vaccine was evaluated in specific pathogen-free kittens.[94] This prospective, randomized, placebo-controlled study resulted in the recovery of *E. faecium* SF68 from the feces of seven of nine cats treated with the probiotic, and a nonsignificant increase in feline herpes-

virus 1–specific serum IgG levels. Concentrations of total IgG and IgA in serum were similar in the probiotic and placebo groups, and the percentage of CD4+ lymphocytes was increased significantly only in kittens at 27 weeks and not at any other time points.

Probiotics also have been evaluated in juvenile captive cheetahs, a population with a relatively high incidence of bacteria-associated enteritis. Administration of a species-specific probiotic containing *Lactobacillus* Group 2 and *E. faecium* to 27 juvenile cheetahs was associated with a significantly increased body weight in the treatment group, with no increase in the control group.[95] In addition, administration of the probiotic was associated with improved fecal quality in the probiotic group.

It should be emphasized that all studies were performed in healthy kittens or cats, and there are no published studies to date evaluating the use of probiotics in cats with gastrointestinal disorders such as bacterial or parasitic-associated diarrhea, food allergy, antibiotic-associated diarrhea, or IBD.

REGULATORY ISSUES

The term *probiotic* remains undefined legally in many countries, and regulatory approaches differ among countries worldwide. The guidelines for what is required for a product to be called a probiotic, published by the Food and Agriculture Organization of the United Nations (FAO) and the World Health Organization (WHO), require that strains be designated individually, speciated appropriately, and retain a viable count at the end of their shelf life in the designated product formulation that confers a proven clinical end point.[96] The fact that some products continue to be of dubious quality and carry unsupported health claims suggests that many national regulatory authorities are not participating in the recommended process. This problem is compounded by the diverse categories that encompass probiotic products, including food, functional food, novel food, natural remedy (Denmark, Sweden, and Finland), natural health product (Canada), dietetic food (Italy), dietary supplement (United States), and biotherapeutics and pharmaceuticals (probiotic pharmaceuticals are available in Canada, China, and a number of European countries).

The definition of a probiotic requires that the term only be applied to live microbes having a substantiated beneficial effect. Thus microbes administered live are considered probiotics regardless of their ability to survive intestinal transit. Although a preparation of nonviable bacteria may mediate a physiological benefit, they are not considered to be "probiotics" under the present definition. Furthermore, any strains that do not confer clinically established physiological effects should not be referred to as probiotics. In vitro tests to establish mechanisms of action are insufficient substantiation for the use of the term. The basis for a microbe being termed a probiotic should be proven efficacy and safety under the recommended conditions of use, with considerations given to target population, route of administration, and dose applied.[96] Box 11-1 contains a list of criteria to which all probiotics should adhere.

Box 11-1 Optimal Criteria for Probiotics

A probiotic should:
- Be of animal or human host origin (the attachment to ECs is very host-specific, which in practical terms means that a strain that is suitable for development in one animal species may not be active in another)
- Be nonpathogenic
- Be resistant to destruction by technical processing
- Be resistant to destruction by gastric acid and bile
- Adhere to intestinal epithelial tissue
- Colonize the gastrointestinal tract, if even for a short time
- Produce antimicrobial substances
- Modulate immune responses
- Influence gut metabolic activities (e.g., cholesterol assimilation)

From Teitelbaum JE, Walker WA: Nutritional impact of pre- and probiotics as protective gastrointestinal organisms, *Annu Rev Nutr* 22:107, 2002.

In the United States, the Food, Drug, and Cosmetic Act (FDCA) lays out the legal framework that governs a wide array of products, the specific categorization of which determines the role that the Food and Drug Administration (FDA) will play in the regulation of the product. Probiotics can be categorized in one of four regulatory categories, depending on their intended use: (1) food or food ingredient, (2) medical food, (3) dietary supplement, or (4) drug or biological product.[97] A probiotic is categorized as a *medical food* if it is "intended for enteral use in the dietary management of disease for which distinctive nutritional requirements have been established by medical evaluation, and is to be administered under the supervision of a physician" (FDCA, U.S. code 21, section 360 [ee]). A *dietary supplement* is not conventional food and is intended to "supplement the diet" or contain a "dietary ingredient" and thus can be added to food (e.g., added to dry dog food) or given as a supplement that is mixed with food (U.S. code 21, section 321 [ff]). A probiotic is categorized as a *drug* if it is intended for the cure, mitigation, treatment, diagnosis, or prevention of disease (U.S. code 21, section 321 [g][1][B]). A probiotic is categorized as a *biological product* if it contains a virus, serum, or toxin that is applicable to the prevention, treatment, or cure of a disease or condition (U.S. code 21, section 262 [a]). A probiotic that is categorized as a *food* or *food ingredient* is regulated by the FDA as either a food additive subject to premarket clearance or as a GRAS (generally recognized as safe) food ingredient subject to regulation under the postmarket controls that govern the adulteration of food.[97] The concept of GRAS is unique to the United States, which does not have a novel food category. Further, the key focus of the FDA in this process is safety—not benefits of the product. GRAS status indicates that the probiotic is exempt from the food additive definition and places it in the element of "common knowledge." Obtaining a GRAS designation requires that the information supporting the determination be in widely known publication and generally accepted as common knowledge by the scientific community.[98] Conversely, any pro-

biotic designated as a food additive falls under a "technical elements" category and thus is evaluated more rigorously during the required premarket approval process. The premarket approval process must contain the following information (published in the Federal Register): identity and composition of the additive, proposed use, amount to be added to food, data establishing its effect, quantitative detection methods in food, full toxicological reports, proposed tolerances, and environmental information.[98] If a probiotic is categorized as a dietary supplement, no premarket approval is required for the dietary ingredients; however, notification requirements apply that limit the claims a manufacturer can make concerning a product's benefits and effects. Any claim must be able to be supported by appropriate materials, should the FDA challenge its propriety. The most common claims in the marketing of human probiotics in the United States are those of structure/function, because the FDA has not approved health claims for probiotics to date.[99] This primarily is because most clinical trials of probiotics are conducted under the category of probiotics as food, which leads to a health claim, rather than the category of probiotics as biologicals, which leads to a therapeutic claim.[100]

PROPER LABELING

Despite the prolonged marketing of "probiotic" products, there is little or no enforced worldwide regulation regarding labeling for quality or efficacy. A relatively large number of products are mislabeled—with inaccurate use of nomenclature for genus and species, inaccurate cell count, or unsubstantiated structure/function statements—yet continue to be sold worldwide.[101] From a scientific perspective, a suitable description of a probiotic, printed on the product label, should include the following information[101a]:

- Genus and species identification, with nomenclature consistent with current scientifically recognized names
- Strain designation
- Viable count of each strain at the end of shelf life
- Recommended storage conditions
- Safety under the conditions of recommended use
- Recommended dose
- An accurate description of the physiological effect (as far as is allowable by law)
- Contact information for postmarket surveillance

SAFETY

Probiotic preparations labeled for use in dogs or cats are classified as nutritional supplements, not pharmaceutical products. As a result, they are poorly regulated, and specific product labeling and demonstration of efficacy are not required. This important point is best illustrated by a recent study by Weese et al, in which 19 commercially available canine and feline diets purporting to contain probiotics were evaluated bacteriologically.[101] Quantitative bacterial cultures were performed on all products, and the labeling claim of each product was compared to the qualitative and quantitative culture results. None of the products contained all of the claimed organisms, and nine of the 19 (47 per cent) products did not contain any of the organisms listed on their labels. Eleven diets contained additional, related products, and five (26 per cent) diets did not contain any relevant growth. The diets tested contained between 0.0 and 1.8×10^5 CFU/g. Of equal concern, no dose-response trials appear to have been carried out for any of these products in human beings or animals, leaving the question of what constitutes a minimum effective dose of a particular probiotic unanswered.

SAFETY OF PROBIOTICS IN HEALTHY OR IMMUNOCOMPROMISED PEOPLE

Cases of infection due to *Lactobacillus* species and *Bifidobacterium* species are extremely rare and are estimated to represent 0.05 to 0.4 per cent of cases of infective endocarditis and bacteremia.[102] Importantly, increasing consumption of probiotic *Lactobacillus* species and *Bifidobacterium* species has not led to an increase in such opportunistic infections in healthy consumers.[103] Rare cases of *Saccharomyces boulardii* fungemia have been reported in immunocompromised human patients, and contamination of the air, environmental surfaces, and hands following the opening of a packet of the yeast probiotic suggests that catheter contamination may have been a source of infection.[104] Only rare cases of local or systemic infections, including septicemia and endocarditis due to *Lactobacillus* species, *Bifidobacterium* species, or other lactic acid bacteria, have been reported in immunocompromised people or patients with abnormal heart valves.[105,106] The ability of certain lactic acid bacteria to interfere with the adhesion of selected canine and zoonotic pathogens to immobilized mucus isolated from canine jejunal chyme in vitro was investigated.[107] Adhesion of *Clostridium perfringens* was reduced significantly by all tested LAB strains; however, two *E. faecium* strains tested enhanced the adhesion of *C. jejuni* significantly. Further studies are warranted to determine whether *E. faecium* may favor the adhesion and colonization of *C. jejuni* in the canine intestine, making it a potential carrier and possibly a source for human infection.

ANTIBIOTIC RESISTANCE AND PROBIOTICS

Antibiotic resistance screening has shown that the spontaneous mutation rate to antibiotic resistance among *Lactobacillus* species can be quite high, on the order of 2×10^5, depending on the strain.[108] Among 45 strains of *Lactobacillus fermentum* originating from human feces, most showed a low-level penicillin resistance with minimal inhibitory concentrations (MIC) of 0.03 to 0.44 IU/mL.[109] Several animal isolates of *L. acidophilus* and *L. reuteri* were tested for antibiotic resistance, and all 16 *L. reuteri* strains were resistant to vancomycin and polymyxin B irrespective of their source, while only four of 30 *L. acidophilus* strains were vancomycin resistant and seven were chloramphenicol resistant.[110] Antibiotic resistance in plasmids

from *Lactobacillus* species have been detected in a number of studies. Curing techniques have been applied to study the strain-dependent resistance to macrolides, tetracycline, and chloramphenicol in *L. acidophilus* and *L. reuteri* of animal origin.[111] Although enterococci are normal inhabitants of the gastrointestinal tract and are used widely as both human and animal probiotics, in vivo conjugative transfer of antibiotic resistance plasmids from *L. reuteri* to *E. faecalis* has been demonstrated in germ-free mice.[112] In most cases, antibiotic resistance to LAB is not of the transmissible type but represents an intrinsic species-specific or genus-specific characteristic of the organism. Knowledge of the ability of a proposed probiotic strain to act as a donor of conjugative antibiotic resistance genes is a prudent precaution. Although the enterococcal transmissible vancomycin resistance poses an important issue, there is no evidence of this occurring in clinical cases to date.

FUTURE CONSIDERATIONS

The potential benefits and specific indications for probiotics in feline medicine have yet to be defined, and our understanding of the nature and diversity of the feline intestinal microflora during health and disease is expanding slowly. Separating these intestinal bacteria into "good" or "bad" bacteria, a marketing strategy often used in the commercial industry, is a gross oversimplification and takes no account of host differences as a contributing factor. Furthermore, the diverse microbial content of the intestinal tract is not reflected adequately by fecal analysis, which has been the predominant sample analyzed to date. Applying either polymerase chain reaction (PCR)–Denaturing Gradient Gel Electrophoresis or Terminal Restriction Fragment Length Polymorphisms (TRF) and high-throughput sequencing of 16S rRNA libraries to the study of gastrointestinal tract microbial ecology should facilitate the identification of major culturable and nonculturable populations and provide a tool for studying shifts in these populations over time and under different conditions. In cats, defining a role for probiotics will require completion of prospective, randomized, placebo-controlled studies that rely on clinically relevant end points related to a particular physiological or pathological condition.

Further studies are warranted to determine the need for probiotics to be live microorganisms following the provocative studies of Rachmilewitz et al, which documented that live bacteria are unnecessary because the beneficial effects of probiotics are mediated by their DNA.[22] Another study, which documented the beneficial mucosal immunomodulatory effects of parenterally administered bacterial DNA in a murine colitis model, suggests that the oral administration of probiotics may not be mandatory.[113] The key unanswered question is whether deliberate manipulation of the bacterial microflora in the gut can confer clinical benefit. Probiotics do appear to have a potential role in the prevention and treatment of various gastrointestinal illnesses, but it is likely that benefits achieved are specific to the bacterial species used and to the underlying disease context.

REFERENCES

1. Savage DC: Microbial ecology of the human gastrointestinal tract, *Annu Rev Microbiol* 31:10, 1977.
2. Gronlund MM, Lehtonen OP, Eerola E, et al: Fecal microflora in healthy infants born by different methods of delivery: permanent changes in intestinal flora after cesarean delivery, *J Pediatr Gastroenterol Nutr* 28:19, 1999.
3. Insoft RM, Sanderson IR, Walker WA: Development of immune function in the intestine and its role in neonatal diseases, *Pediatr Clin North Am* 43:551, 1996.
4. McCraken VJ, Lorenz RG: The gastrointestinal ecosystem: a precarious alliance among epithelium, immunity and microbiota, *Cell Microbiol* 3:1, 2001.
5. Bottazzi V: Food and feed production with microorganisms, *Biotechnology* 5:315, 1983.
6. Metchnikoff E: *The prolongation of life. Optimistic studies*, London, 1907, Butterworth-Heinemann.
7. Lilly DM, Stillwell RH: Probiotics. Growth promoting factors produced by micro-organisms, *Science* 147:747, 1965.
8. Schrezenmeir J, deVrese M: Probiotics, prebiotics, and synbiotics—approaching a definition, *Am J Clin Nutr* 73:361S, 2001.
9. Ouwehand AC, Kirjavainen PV, Grönlund M-M, et al: Adhesion of probiotic micro-organisms to intestinal mucus, *Int Dairy J* 9:623, 1999.
10. Bernet MF, Brassart D, Neeser JR, et al: Adhesion of human bifidobacterial strains to cultured human intestinal epithelial cells and inhibition of enteropathogen-cell interactions, *Appl Environ Microbiol* 59:4121, 1993.
11. Savage DC: Associations and physiological interactions of indigenous microorganisms and gastrointestinal epithelia, *Am J Clin Nutr* 25:1372, 1972.
12. Freter R: Factors affecting the microecology of the gut. In Fuller R, editor: *Probiotics, the scientific basis*, London, 1992, Chapman & Hall, p 111.
13. Cotter PD, Hill C, Ross RP: Bacteriocins: developing innate immunity for food, *Nat Rev Microbiol* 3:777, 2005.
14. Servin AL: Antagonistic activities of lactobacilli and bifidobacteria against microbial pathogens, *FEMS Microbiol Rev* 28:405, 2004.
15. Collado MC, Meriluoto J, Salminen S: Role of commercial probiotic strains against human pathogen adhesion to intestinal mucus, *Lett Appl Microbiol* 45:454, 2007.
16. Candela M, Seibold G, Vitali B, et al: Real-time PCR quantification of bacterial adhesion to Caco-2 cells: competition between bifidobacteria and enteropathogens, *Res Microbiol* 156:887, 2005.
17. Morgan SM, O'Connor PM, Cotter PD, et al: Sequential actions of the two component peptides of the lantibiotic lacticin 3147 explain its antimicrobial activity at nanomolar concentrations, *Antimicrob Agents Chemother* 49:2606, 2005.
18. Collado MC, Hernandez M, Sanz Y: Production of bacteriocin-like inhibitory compounds by human fecal *Bifidobacterium* strains, *J Food Prot* 68:1034, 2005.
19. Makras L, Triantafyllou V, Fayol-Messaoudi D, et al: Kinetic analysis of the antibacterial activity of probiotic lactobacilli towards *Salmonella enterica* serovar *Typhimurium* reveals a role for lactic acid and other inhibitory compounds, *Res Microbiol* 157:241, 2006.
20. Mukai T, Kaneko S, Matsumoto M, et al: Binding of *Bifidobacterium bifidum* and *Lactobacillus reuteri* to the carbohydrate moieties of intestinal glycolipids recognized by peanut agglutinin, *Int J Food Microbiol* 90:357, 2004.

21. Sun J, Le GW, Shi YH, et al: Factors involved in binding of *Lactobacillus plantarum* Lp6 to rat small intestinal mucus, *Lett Appl Microbiol* 44:79, 2007.
21a. Focareta, Paton JC, Morona R, et al: A recombinant probiotic for treatment and prevention of cholera, *Gastroenterology* 128:1219, 2005.
22. Rachmilewitz D, Katakura K, Karmeli F, et al: Toll-like receptor 9 signaling mediates the anti-inflammatory effects of probiotics in murine experimental colitis, *Gastroenterology* 126:520, 2004.
23. Grabig A, Paclik D, Guzy C, et al: *Escherichia coli* strain Nissle 1917 ameliorates experimental colitis via toll-like receptor 2- and toll-like receptor 4-dependent pathways, *Infect Immun* 74:4075, 2006.
24. Macpherson AJ, Uhr T: Induction of protective IgA by intestinal dendritic cells carrying commensal bacteria, *Science* 303:1662, 2004.
25. He F, Morita H, Kubota A, et al: Effect of orally administered non-viable *Lactobacillus* cells on murine humoral immune responses, *Microbiol Immunol* 49:993, 2005.
26. Veckman V, Miettinen M, Pirhonen J, et al: *Streptococcus pyogenes* and *Lactobacillus rhamnosus* differentially induce maturation and production of Th1-type cytokines and chemokines in human monocyte-derived dendritic cells, *J Leukoc Biol* 75:764, 2004.
27. Hart AL, Lammers K, Brigidi P, et al: Modulation of human dendritic cell phenotype and function by probiotic bacteria, *Gut* 53:1602, 2004.
28. Pena JA, Versalovic J: *Lactobacillus rhamnosus* GG decreases TNF-α production in lipopolysaccharide-activated murine macrophages by a contact-independent mechanism, *Cell Microbiol* 5:277, 2003.
29. Kim SO, Sheikh HI, Ha SD, et al: G-CSF-mediated inhibition of JNK is a key mechanism for *Lactobacillus rhamnosus*-induced suppression of TNF production in macrophages, *Cell Microbiol* 8:1958, 2006.
30. Mazmanian SK, Liu CH, Tzianabos AO, et al: An immunomodulatory molecule of symbiotic bacteria directs maturation of the host immune system, *Cell* 122:107, 2005.
31. Jijon H, Backer J, Diaz H, et al: DNA from probiotic bacteria modulates murine and human epithelial and immune function, *Gastroenterology* 126:1358, 2004.
32. Zyrek AA, Cichon C, Helms S, et al: Molecular mechanisms underlying the probiotic effects of *Escherichia coli* Nissle 1917 involve ZO-2 and PKCzeta redistribution resulting in tight junction and epithelial barrier repair, *Cell Microbiol* 9:804, 2007.
33. Tao Y, Drabik KA, Waypa TS, et al: Soluble factors from *Lactobacillus* GG activate MAPKs and induce cytoprotective heat shock proteins in intestinal epithelial cells, *Am J Physiol Cell Physiol* 290:C1018, 2006.
34. Yan F, Polk DB: Probiotic bacterium prevents cytokine-induced apoptosis in intestinal epithelial cells, *J Biol Chem* 277:50959, 2002.
35. Spinler JK, Versalovic J: Probiotics in human medicine: Overview. In Versalovic J, Wilson M, editors: *Therapeutic microbiology: probiotics and related strategies*, Washington DC, 2008, ASM Press, p 225.
36. Meurman JH, Stamatova I: Probiotics: contributions to oral health, *Oral Dis* 13:443, 2007.
37. Meurman JH: Probiotics in oral biology and dentistry. In Versalovic J, Wilson M, editors: *Therapeutic microbiology: probiotics and related strategies*, Washington DC, 2008, ASM Press, p 249.
38. Kolenbrander PE: Oral microbial communities: biofilms, interactions, and genetic systems, *Annu Rev Microbiol* 54:413, 2000.

39. Meurman JH, Antila H, Salminen S: Recovery of *Lactobacillus* strain GG (ATCC 53103) from saliva of healthy volunteers after consumption of yoghurt prepared with the bacterium, *Microb Ecol Health Dis* 7:295, 1994.

40. Yli-Knuuttila H, Snall J, Kari K, et al: Colonization of *Lactobacillus rhamnosus* GG in the oral cavity, *Oral Microbiol Immunol* 21:129, 2006.

41. Busscher HJ, Mulder AF, van der Mei CH: In vitro adhesion to enamel and in vivo colonization of tooth surfaces by lactobacilli from a bio-yoghurt, *Caries Res* 33:403, 1999.

42. Näse L, Hatakka K, Savilahti E, et al: Effect of long term consumption of a probiotic bacterium, *Lactobacillus rhamnosus* GG, in milk on dental caries and caries risk in children, *Caries Res* 35:412, 2001.

43. Caglar E, Cilder SK, Ergeneli S, et al: Salivary mutans streptococci and lactobacilli levels after ingestion of the probiotic bacterium *Lactobacilli reuteri* ATCC 55739 by straws or tablets, *Acta Odontol Scand* 64:314, 2007.

44. Hatakka K, Ahola AJ, Yli-Knuuttila H, et al: Probiotics reduce the prevalence of oral Candida in the elderly—a randomized controlled trial, *J Dent Res* 86:125, 2007.

45. Koll-Klais P, Mandar R, Leibur E, et al: Oral lactobacilli in chronic periodontitis and periodontal health: species composition and antimicrobial activity, *Oral Microbiol Immunol* 20:354, 2005.

46. Elahi S, Pang G, Clancy A, et al: Enhanced clearance of *Candida albicans* from the oral cavities of mice following oral administration of *Lactobacillus acidophilus*, *Clin Exp Immunol* 141:29, 2005.

47. Guarner F: Probiotics in gastrointestinal diseases. In Versalovic J, Wilson M, editors: *Therapeutic microbiology: probiotics and related strategies*, Washington DC, 2008, ASM Press, p 255.

48. de Vrese M, Stegelmann A, Richter B, et al: Probiotics—compensation for lactase deficiency, *Am J Clin Nutr* 73(suppl):421S, 2001.

49. Guyonnet D, Chassany O, Ducrotte P, et al: Effect of a fermented milk containing *Bifidobacterium animalis* DN-173010 on the health-related quality of life and symptoms in irritable bowel syndrome in adults in primary care: a multi-center, randomized, double-blind, controlled trial, *Aliment Pharmacol Ther* 26:475, 2007.

50. Savino F, Pelle E, Palumeri E, et al: *Lactobacillus reuteri* (American Type Culture Collection Strain 55730) versus simethicone in the treatment of infantile colic: a prospective randomized study, *Pediatrics* 119:e124, 2007.

51. Sullivan A, Nord CE: Probiotics and gastrointestinal diseases, *J Intern Med* 257:78, 2005.

52. Cremonini F, DiCaro S, Nista EC, et al: Meta-analysis: the effect of probiotic administration on antibiotic-associated diarrhea, *Aliment Pharmacol Ther* 16:1461, 2002.

53. D'Souza AI, Rajkumar C, Cooke J, et al: Probiotics in prevention of antibiotic associated diarrhea, *Brit Med J* 324:1361, 2002.

54. Szajewska H, Mrukowwicz J: Meta-analysis: non-pathogenic yeast *Saccharomyces boulardii* in the prevention of antibiotic-associated diarrhea, *Aliment Pharmacol Ther* 22:365, 2005.

55. Johnston BC, Supina AI, Ospina M, et al: Probiotics for the prevention of pediatric antibiotic-associated diarrhea, *Cochrane Database Syst Rev* 2:CD004827, 2007.

56. Popoola J, Swann A, Warwick G: *Clostridium difficile* in patients with renal failure: management of an outbreak using biotherapy, *Nephrol Dial Transplant* 15:571, 2000.

57. Surawicz CM, McFarland IV, Greenherg RN, et al: The search for a better treatment for recurrent *Clostridium difficile* disease: use of high dose vancomycin combined with Saccharomyces boulardii, *Clin Infect Dis* 31:1012, 2000.

58. McFarland LV: Meta-analysis of probiotics for the prevention of traveler's diarrhea, *Travel Med Infect Dis* 5:97, 2007.

59. Wendakoon CN, Thomson AB, Ozimeki I: Lack of therapeutic effect of a specially designed yogurt for the eradication of *Helicobacter pylori* infection, *Digestion* 65:16, 2002.

60. Tong JL, Ran ZH, Shen J, et al: Meta-analysis: the effect of supplementation with probiotics on eradication rates and adverse events during *Helicobacter pylori* eradication therapy, *Aliment Pharmacol Ther* 25:155, 2007.

61. Rayes N, Seehofer D, Hansen S, et al: Early enteral supply of lactobacillus and fiber versus selective bowel decontamination: a controlled trial in liver transplant recipients, *Transplantation* 74:123, 2002.

62. Sartor RB: Therapeutic manipulation of the enteric microflora in inflammatory bowel diseases: antibiotics, probiotics, and prebiotics, *Gastroenterology* 126:1620, 2004.

63. Ishikawa H, Akedo I, Umesaki Y, et al: Randomized, controlled trial of the effect of bifidobacteria-fermented milk on ulcerative colitis, *J Am Coll Nutr* 22:56, 2003.

64. Kruis W, Rfic P, Pokrotnicks J, et al: Maintaining remission of ulcerative colitis with the probiotic *Escherichia coli* Nissle 1917 is as effective as with standard mesalazine, *Gut* 53:1617, 2004.

65. Zocco MA, dal Verme LZ, Cremonini F, et al: Efficacy of *Lactobacillus* GG in maintaining remission of ulcerative colitis, *Aliment Pharmacol Ther* 23:1567, 2006.

66. Gionchetti P, Rizzello F, Venturi A, et al: Oral bacteriotherapy as maintenance treatment in patients with chronic pouchitis: a double-blind, placebo-controlled trial, *Gastroenterology* 119:305, 2003.

67. Reid G: Probiotics and diseases of the genitourinary tract. In Versalovic J, Wilson M, editors: *Therapeutic microbiology: probiotics and related strategies*, Washington DC, 2008, ASM Press, p 271.

68. Lenoir-Wijnkoop I, Sanders ME, Cabana MD, et al: Probiotic and prebiotic influence beyond the intestinal tract, *Nutr Rev* 65:469, 2007.

69. Chan RC, Redi G, Irvin RT, et al: Competitive exclusion of uropathogens from uroepithelial cells by *Lactobacillus* whole cells and cell wall fragments, *Infect Immunol* 47:84, 1985.

70. Darouiche RO, Thornby JI, Cerra-Stewart C, et al: Bacterial interference for prevention of urinary tract infection: a prospective, randomized, placebo-controlled double-blind pilot trial, *Clin Infect Dis* 41:1531, 2005.

71. Bach JF: The effect of infections on susceptibility to autoimmune and allergic diseases, *N Engl J Med* 347:911, 2002.

72. Rook GAW, Witt N: Probiotics and other organisms in allergy and autoimmune diseases. In Versalovic J, Wilson M, editors: *Therapeutic microbiology: probiotics and related strategies*, Washington, DC, 2008, ASM Press, p 231.

73. Flohr C, Tuyen IN, Lewis S, et al: Poor sanitation and helminth infection protect against skin sensitization in Vietnamese children: a cross-sectional study, *J Allergy Clin Immunol* 118:1305, 2006.

74. Reidler J, Braun-Fahrlander C, Eder W, et al: Exposure to farming in early life and development of asthma and allergy: a cross-sectional survey, *Lancet* 358:1129, 2001.

75. Farooqi IS, Hopkin JM: Early childhood infection and atopic disorder, *Thorax* 53:927, 1998.

76. Wilson MS, Taylor MD, Balic A, et al: Suppression of allergic airway inflammation by helminth-induced regulatory T cells, *J Exp Med* 202:1199, 2005.

77. Ricklin-Gutzwiller ME, Reist M, Peel JE, et al: Intradermal injection of heat-killed *Mycobacterium vaccae* in dogs with atopic dermatitis: a multicenter, pilot study, *Vet Dermatol* 18:87, 2007.

78. Zaccone P, Fehervari Z, Jones FM, et al: Schistosoma mansoni antigens modulate the activity of the innate immune response and prevent onset of type I diabetes, *Eur J Immunol* 33:1439, 2003.

79. Di Giacinto C, Marinaro M, Sanchez M, et al: Probiotics ameliorate recurrent Th1-mediated murine colitis by inducing IL-10 and IL-10 dependent TGF-β bearing regulatory cells, *J Immunol* 174:3237, 2005.

80. Yazdanbakhsh M, Kremsner PG, van Ree R: Allergy, parasites, and the hygiene hypothesis: regulating the immune system? *Science* 296:490, 2002.

81. Kohashi O, Kohashi Y, Takahashi T, et al: Reverse effect of gram-positive bacteria vs. gram-negative bacteria on adjuvant-induced arthritis in germfree rats, *Microbiol Immunol* 29:487, 1985.

82. Stromptova V, Laukova A, Ouwehand AC: Lactobacilli and enterococci-potential probiotics for dogs, *Folia Microbiol (Praha)* 49:203, 2004.

83. Sauter SN, Benyacoub J, Allenspach K, et al: Effects of probiotic bacteria in dogs with food responsive diarrhea treated with an elimination diet, *J Anim Physiol Anim Nutr* 90:269, 2006.

84. Perelmuter K, Fraga M, Zunino P: In vitro activity of potential probiotic *Lactobacillus murinus* isolated from the dog, *J Appl Microbiol* 104:1718, 2008.

85. Pascher M, Hellweg P, Khol-Parisini A, et al: Effects of a probiotic *Lactobacillus acidophilus* strain on feed tolerance in dogs with non-specific dietary sensitivity, *Arch Anim Nutr* 62:107, 2008.

86. Vahjen W, Manner K: The effect of a probiotic *Enterococcus faecium* product in diets of healthy dogs on bacteriological counts of *Salmonella*, *Campylobacter*, and *Clostridium* in feces, *Arch Anim Nutr* 57:229, 2003.

87. Swanson KS, Grieshop CM, Flickinger EA, et al: Fructooligosaccharides and *Lactobacillus acidophilus* modify gut microbial populations, total tract nutrient digestibilities and fecal protein catabolite concentrations in healthy adult dogs, *J Nutr* 132:3721, 2002.

88. Biagi G, Cipollini I, Pompei A, et al: Effect of a *Lactobacillus animalis* strain on composition and metabolism of the intestinal microflora in adult dogs, *Vet Microbiol* 124:160, 2007.

89. Baillon MLA, Marshall-Jones ZV, Butterwisk RF: Effects of probiotic *Lactobacillus acidophilus* strain DSM 13241 in healthy adult dogs, *Am J Vet Res* 65:338, 2004.

90. Benyacoub J, Czarnecki-Maulden GI, Cavadini C, et al: Supplementation of food with *Enterococcus faecium* SF68 stimulates immune functions in young dogs, *J Nutr* 133:1158, 2003.

91. Rinkinen M, Jalava K, Westermarck E, et al: Interaction between probiotic lactic acid bacteria and canine enteric pathogens: a risk factor for intestinal *Enterococcus faecium* colonization? *Vet Microbiol* 92:111, 2003.

92. Weese JS, Sharif S, Rodriguez-Palacios A: Probiotics in veterinary medicine. In Versalovic J, Wilson M, editors: *Therapeutic microbiology: probiotics and related strategies*, Washington DC, 2008, ASM Press, p 341.

93. Marshall-Jones ZV, Baillon MI, Croft JM, et al: Effects of *Lactobacillus acidophilus* dSM 13241 as a probiotic in healthy adult cats, *Am J Vet Res* 67:1005, 2006.

94. Veir JK, Knorr R, Cavadini D, et al: Effect of supplementation with *Enterococcus faecium* (SF68) on immune function in cats, *Vet Ther* 8:229, 2007.

95. Koeppel KN, Bertschinger H, van Vuuren M, et al: The use of a probiotic in captive cheetahs (*Acinonyx jubatus*), *J S Afr Vet Assoc* 77:127, 2006.

96. FAO/WHO. Guidelines for the evaluation of probiotics in food. In: Joint FAO/WHO Working Group Report on Drafting Guidelines for the Evaluation of Probiotics in Food, 2002.

97. Degnan FH: The US Food and Drug Administration and Probiotics: Regulatory Categorization, *Clin Infect Dis* 46:133S, 2008.

98. Mattia A, Merker R: Regulation of probiotic substances as ingredients in foods: Premarket approval or "generally recognized as safe" notification, *Clin Infect Dis* 46:115S, 2008.

99. Saldanha LG: US Food and Drug Administration regulations governing label claims for food products, including probiotics, *Clin Infect Dis* 46:119S, 2008.

100. Hibberd PI, Davidson L: Probiotic foods and drugs: impact of US regulatory status on design of clinical trials, *Clin Infect Dis* 46:137S, 2008.

101. Weese JS, Arroyo L: Bacteriological evaluation of dog and cat diets that claim to contain probiotics, *Can Vet J* 44:212, 2003.

101a. Reid G, Sanders ME, Gaskins HR, et al: New scientific paradigms for probiotics and prebiotics, *J Clin Gastroenterol* 37:105, 2003.

102. Saxelin M, Chuang NH, Chassy B, et al: Lactobacilli and bacteremia in southern Finland, 1989-1992, *Clin Infect Dis* 22:564, 1996.

103. Borriello SP, Hammes WP, Holzapfel W, et al: Safety of probiotics that contain Lactobacilli or Bifidobacteria, *Clin Infect Dis* 36:775, 2003.

104. Hennequin C, Kauffmann-Lacroix C, Jobert A, et al: Possible role of catheters in *Saccharomyces boulardii* fungemia, *Eur J Clin Microbiol Infect Dis* 19:16, 2000.

105. Horwitch CA, Furseth HA, Larson AM, et al: Lactobacillemia in three patients with AIDS, *Clin Infect Dis* 21:1460, 1995.

106. Husni RN, Gordon SM, Washington JA, et al: *Lactobacillus* bacteremia and endocarditis: review of 45 cases, *Clin Infect Dis* 25:1048, 1997.

107. Rinkinen M, Jalava K, Westermarch E, et al: Interaction between probiotic lactic acid bacteria and canine enteric pathogens: a risk factor for intestinal *Enterococcus faecium* colonization? *Vet Microbiol* 92:111, 2003.

108. Curragh HJ, Collins MA: High levels of spontaneous drug resistance in *Lactobacillus*, *J Appl Bacteriol* 73:31, 1992.

109. Yokokura T, Mutai M: Penicillin resistance and its elimination by treatment with acriflavine in *Lactobacillus fermentum*, *Jap J Microbiol* 20:241, 1976.

110. Sarra PG, Vescovo M, Morelli L, et al: Antibiotic resistance in *L. acidophilus* and *L. reuteri* from animal gut, *Ann Microbiol Enzymol* 32:71, 1982.

111. Vescovo M, Morelli L, Bottazzi V: Drug resistance plasmids in *Lactobacillus reuteri* and *Lactobacillus acidophilus*, *Appl Environ Microbiol* 43:50, 1982.

112. Morelli L, Sarra PG, Bottazzi V: In vivo transfer of pAMß1 from *Lactobacillus reuteri* to *Enterococcus faecalis*, *J Appl Bacteriol* 65:371, 1988.

113. Sheil B, McCarthy J, O'Mahony L, et al: Is the mucosal route of administration essential for probiotics function? Subcutaneous administration is associated with attenuation of murine colitis and arthritis, *Gut* 53:694, 2004.

CHAPTER

12 Critical Care Nutrition

Daniel L. Chan

IMPORTANCE OF NUTRITION DURING CRITICAL ILLNESS

Compared to other animal species, cats have several metabolic adaptations that impact their ability to maintain homeostasis in the face of injury, disease, and food deprivation. For example, cats have a higher requirement for protein and certain amino acids than most other species.[1] Critical illness induces further metabolic alterations in cats that put them at even higher risk for developing malnutrition and experiencing its deleterious effects. Similar to other species, the body of a diseased cat responds differently to inadequate nutritional intake than does the body of a healthy cat. During periods of nutrient deprivation, a healthy animal will lose glycogen and fat primarily (simple starvation). However, sick or traumatized patients will catabolize lean body mass when they are not provided with sufficient calories (stressed starvation). During the initial stages of fasting in the healthy state, glycogen stores are used as the primary source of energy. Within days, a metabolic shift occurs towards the preferential use of stored fat deposits, sparing catabolic effects on lean muscle tissue. In diseased states, the inflammatory response triggers alterations in cytokines and hormone concentrations and shifts metabolism rapidly towards a catabolic state.[2,3]

There are alterations in lipid, carbohydrate, and protein metabolism that can affect the animal's nutritional status and the outcome of the condition. The metabolic changes documented in critically ill cats include lower circulating concentration of insulin and higher concentrations of glucose, lactate, cortisol, glucagon, norepinephrine, and nonesterified fatty acids.[4,5] Glycogen stores are depleted quickly, especially in strict carnivores such as cats, and this leads to an early mobilization of amino acids from muscle stores (up-regulation of proteolysis). As cats undergo continuous gluconeogenesis, the mobilization of amino acids from muscles is more pronounced than

that observed in other species. Unlike other species, cats do not down-regulate gluconeogenesis or proteolysis in the face of low protein intake.[6] With continued lack of food intake, energy is derived almost completely from accelerated proteolysis, which in itself is an energy-consuming process. Therefore these animals may preserve fat deposits in the face of lean muscle tissue losses. These shifts in metabolism commonly result in significant negative nitrogen and energy balance. The consequences of continued lean body mass losses include negative effects on wound healing, immune function, strength (both skeletal and respiratory), and ultimately on overall prognosis.[7] The metabolic derangements that occur in critically ill cats and the deleterious effects of malnutrition make the provision of nutritional support to hospitalized cats an essential and vital part of the therapeutic approach.

INDICATIONS FOR NUTRITIONAL SUPPORT

In cats, inadequate calorie intake commonly is due to a loss of appetite (hyporexia), an inability to eat, or from persistent vomiting that accompanies many disease processes. Appetite suppression may be instigated directly by inflammatory cytokines (e.g., IL-1β, IL-6, TNFα) or secondarily by pathological processes (e.g., nausea, pyrexia, pain, ileus).[8] Because malnutrition can occur quickly in these patients, it is important to provide nutritional support by either enteral or parenteral nutrition if oral intake is not adequate. Identification of overt malnutrition in cats can be challenging because there are no established criteria of malnutrition in companion animals. Because detectable impairment of immune function (e.g., decreased lymphocyte counts, reduced CD4+/CD8+ ratio can be demonstrated in healthy cats subjected to acute starvation by day 4, nutritional support should

116

be considered in any ill cat with inadequate food intake for more than 3 days.[9] The need to implement a nutritional intervention becomes more urgent when a cat has not eaten for more than 5 days.

There are many goals of nutritional support, but two important objectives are to treat malnutrition when it is present and to prevent malnutrition in animals at risk. Whenever possible, the enteral route should be used because it is the safest, most convenient, and most physiologically sound method of nutritional support.[10] However, when patients are unable to tolerate enteral feeding (e.g., because of vomiting or diarrhea, cramping, nausea, discomfort from feeding) or unable to utilize nutrients administered enterally (e.g., because of severe inflammatory bowel syndrome, intestinal lymphoma), parenteral nutrition should be considered. Ensuring the successful nutritional management of critically ill patients involves selecting the right patient, making an appropriate nutritional assessment, and implementing a feasible nutritional plan.

NUTRITIONAL ASSESSMENT

As with any medical intervention, there are risks of complications when initiating nutritional interventions. Minimizing such risks depends on patient selection and patient assessment. The first step in designing a nutritional strategy is to conduct a *nutritional assessment,* which involves making a systematic evaluation of the patient. Nutritional assessment identifies malnourished patients who require immediate nutritional support, as well as patients who require nutritional support because they are at high risk for developing malnutrition.[11]

Purported indicators of overt malnutrition include recent weight loss of at least 10 per cent of body weight, poor haircoat quality, muscle wasting, signs of poor wound healing, hypoalbuminemia, lymphopenia, and coagulopathies (vitamin K deficiency).[12] However, these abnormalities are not specific to malnutrition and are not present early in the process. In addition, fluid shifts may mask weight loss in critically ill patients. Factors that predispose a patient to malnutrition include anorexia lasting longer than 3 days, serious underlying disease (e.g., trauma, sepsis, peritonitis, pancreatitis, and gastrointestinal surgery), and large protein losses (e.g., resulting from protracted vomiting, diarrhea, or draining wounds).[12,13] Nutritional assessment also identifies factors that can impact the nutritional plan, such as cardiovascular instability, electrolyte abnormalities, hyperglycemia, and hypertriglyceridemia, or concurrent conditions, such as renal or hepatic disease, that will impact the nutritional plan. Because a main priority of nutritional support is to avoid metabolic complications, identification of abnormalities via nutritional assessment may prompt alterations to the nutritional plan. For example, cats with uremia may not tolerate high-protein diets. Appropriate laboratory analysis should be performed in all patients to assess these parameters. Before any nutritional plan is implemented, the patient must have a stable cardiovascular system, with major electrolyte, fluid, and acid-base abnormalities corrected.

GOALS OF NUTRITIONAL SUPPORT

Even in patients with severe malnutrition, the immediate goals of therapy should focus on fluid resuscitation, cardiovascular stabilization, and identification of the primary disease process. As steps are taken to address the primary disease, formulation of a nutritional plan should strive to prevent (or correct) overt nutritional deficiencies and imbalances. Once the body is provided with adequate energy substrates, protein, essential fatty acids, and micronutrients, it can support wound healing, immune function, and tissue repair. A major goal of nutritional support is to minimize metabolic derangements and catabolism of lean body tissue. During hospitalization, restoring body weight is not a priority; this will occur only when the patient has recovered from a state of critical illness. The ultimate goal of nutritional support is to have the cat eating adequate amounts of food in its own environment.

NUTRITIONAL PLAN

Proper diagnosis and treatment of the underlying disease is the key to the success of nutritional support. Based on the nutritional assessment, a plan is formulated to meet energy and other nutritional requirements of the patient and, at the same time, address any concurrent conditions requiring adjustments to the nutritional plan. The anticipated duration of nutritional support should be determined and factored into the plan. This will depend largely on clinical familiarity with the specific disease process and sound clinical judgment. For example, a cat diagnosed with idiopathic hepatic lipidosis is likely to require long-term nutritional support (several weeks) and benefit from tube feeding. Conversely, cats with minor injuries are unlikely to require feeding tubes for nutritional management.

For each patient, the clinician should determine the appropriate route of nutrition—either enteral or parenteral. This decision should be based on the underlying disease and the patient's clinical signs. Important factors to consider include the urgency of commencing nutritional support (e.g., cat shows overt signs of malnutrition, is at high risk of developing malnutrition, or has serious underlying disease with an expected recovery time of several weeks) and contraindications to a particular mode of nutritional support (e.g., cats with protracted vomiting will not tolerate oral or esophageal feeding, cats with oral or pharyngeal disease may benefit from gastric tube feeding). Whenever possible, the enteral route should be considered as the first choice. If enteral feedings are not tolerated or the gastrointestinal tract or parts of the gastrointestinal tract must be bypassed, parenteral nutrition should be instituted. When only a portion of the cat's nutritional needs can be met enterally (e.g., minimal tolerance to small volumes of enteral feeding), supplemental parenteral nutrition has been demonstrated to be beneficial.[14] The various alterations in metabolic pathways that occur following injury and food deprivation suggest that nutritional support should be introduced gradually and reach target levels in 48 to 72 hours.[4,5]

CALCULATING NUTRITIONAL REQUIREMENTS

The patient's resting energy requirement (RER) is the number of calories required for maintaining homeostasis while the animal rests quietly. The RER is calculated using the following formula:

$$RER = 70 \times (body\ weight\ in\ kg)^{0.75}$$

For animals weighing between 2 and 30 kg, the following linear formula gives a good approximation of energy needs:

$$RER = (30 \times body\ weight\ in\ kg) + 70$$

Traditionally, the RER was multiplied by an illness factor between 1.0 to 2.0 to account for increases in metabolism associated with different conditions and injuries. Recently, there has been less emphasis on these subjective illness factors, and current recommendations are to use more conservative energy estimates to avoid overfeeding.[10,12] Overfeeding can result in metabolic and gastrointestinal complications, hepatic dysfunction, increased carbon dioxide production, and weakened respiratory muscles. Of the metabolic complications, the development of hyperglycemia is most common and possibly the most detrimental. In two recent studies evaluating parenteral nutrition in cats, the application of illness factors above 1.0 was associated with higher complication rates and perhaps with higher mortality rates.[15,16]

Currently, the RER is used as an initial estimate of a critically ill patient's energy requirements. It should be emphasized that these general guidelines should be used as starting points, and animals receiving nutritional support should be monitored closely for tolerance of nutritional interventions. Continual decline in body weight or body condition should prompt the clinician to reassess and perhaps modify the nutritional plan (e.g., increase the number of calories provided by 25 per cent). No published studies are available that determine energy expenditure in clinically ill cats; however, based on extrapolation from other species, conditions such as burns and peritonitis may be associated with increased caloric requirements.

Although definitive studies determining the actual nutritional requirements of critically ill cats have not been performed, general recommendations can be made. Currently, it is generally accepted that cats should be supported with 6 or more grams of protein/100 kcal (25 to 35 per cent of total energy requirements). Commercial diets formulated for recovery or recrudescence, which tend to have relatively high fat and protein contents, are typically used to meet this requirement. Patients with protein intolerance (e.g., those with hepatic encephalopathy or severe azotemia) should receive reduced amounts of protein (i.e., 4 grams protein/100 kcal).[12] Similarly, patients with hyperglycemia or hyperlipidemia also may require decreased amounts of these nutrients, especially cats receiving parenteral nutrition.

Specific guidelines for instituting insulin therapy in nondiabetic cats receiving parenteral nutrition have not been published. However, administration of insulin to nondiabetic cats receiving parenteral nutrition has been reported.[17] In one study evaluating the use of parenteral nutrition in cats, hyperglycemia was noted in 66 per cent of cats treated, and 75 per cent of these cats were treated with insulin.[17] More recent studies have reported decreased use of insulin therapy for parenteral nutrition-related hyperglycemia, perhaps reflecting the trend of not applying illness factors in energy estimation in cats.[16] In the event of cats developing hyperglycemia or hyperlipidemia, the author decreases the rate of infusion transiently by 50 per cent and reassesses response after 6 hours. If these abnormalities persist, the author reformulates the parenteral admixture to include reduced amounts of dextrose or lipids. Other nutritional requirements will depend on the patient's underlying disease, clinical signs, and laboratory parameters.

ENTERAL NUTRITION

The enteral route of nutritional support is the preferable approach, primarily because it is safer and less expensive than parenteral nutrition and helps to maintain intestinal structure and function. Even with the use of feeding tubes, patients can be discharged easily for home care with good owner compliance. The majority of complications with feeding tubes include tube occlusion and localized irritation at the tube exit site. Occasionally, more serious complications can occur, including infection at the exit site or, rarely, complete tube dislodgment that could result in peritonitis if a gastrostomy or jejunostomy tube was used. Complications can be avoided by using the appropriate tube, selecting the proper food and preparing it correctly, monitoring the patient carefully, and educating the owner about food choice and preparation.

Although the enteral route should be utilized if at all possible, it is contraindicated in cats who are vomiting persistently, have severe malabsorptive conditions, or are comatose. If the enteral route is chosen for nutritional support, the next step is selecting the type of feeding tube to be used (Table 12-1). Feeding tubes used commonly in cats include nasoesophageal, esophagostomy, gastrostomy, and jejunostomy tubes. In non–surgically placed feeding tubes such as nasoesophageal or esophagostomy tubes, confirmation of correct placement via radiology or fluoroscopy is recommended. Alternatively, proper placement of these feeding tubes within the esophagus can be confirmed by use of an end-tidal carbon dioxide (CO_2) monitor that detects CO_2 if the tube is placed incorrectly in the trachea (Figure 12-1).

An appropriate diet should be selected based on the type of feeding tube chosen and the disease process being treated. For most critically ill cats, an energy-dense, high-protein, and high-fat commercial feline diet is preferred. However, the choice of diet also can depend on the animal's clinical parameters and laboratory results. Diets

Table 12-1 Types of Feeding Tubes

Feeding Tube	Duration	Advantages	Disadvantages
Nasoesophageal	Short term (<5 days)	Inexpensive Easy to place No anesthesia required	Requires liquid diet Some animals will not eat voluntarily with tube in place
Esophagostomy	Long term	Inexpensive Easy to place Can use calorically dense diets	Requires anesthesia (short term) Cellulitis is major complication seen
Gastrostomy	Long term	Can use calorically dense diets	Requires anesthesia and/or surgery or endoscopy to place PEG Tube displacement may result in peritonitis
Jejunostomy	Long term	Bypasses stomach and duodenum Can be used in patients with pancreatitis	Requires anesthesia and laparotomy For in-hospital use Requires continuous rate infusion Requires liquid diet

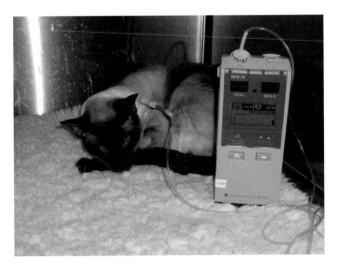

Figure 12-1 End-tidal CO_2 monitor being used to confirm proper placement of esophagostomy tube within the esophagus.

designed for other species (e.g., dogs, human beings) are not suitable for cats because they often do not meet the unique nutritional needs of cats.

The amount of food then is calculated and a specific feeding plan devised (Box 12-1). Generally, feedings are administered every 4 to 6 hours and feeding tubes should be flushed with five to 10 mL of water after each feeding to minimize clogging of the tube. By the time of discharge, however, the number of feedings should be reduced to three to four per day to facilitate owner compliance. Commercially available veterinary liquid diets should be used for nasoesophageal and jejunostomy tube feedings due to the small bore sizes of these catheters (typically <5 Fr). Typical recovery diets usually are unsuitable for small bore tubes because of their tendency to clog these tubes. Jejunostomy tubes primarily are for in-hospital use because they require administration of a liquid diet by continuous rate infusion, and this technique also requires more vigilant monitoring. Esophagostomy and gastrostomy tubes generally are larger (>14 Fr) and allow for more calorically dense, blenderized diets to be admin-

istered. This decreases the volume of food necessary for each feeding. These tubes can be used for long-term enteral feeding. In the author's opinion, mastering the placement of esophagostomy feeding tubes is essential in the management of critically ill animals, and this technique should be adopted in almost all practices. Placement of esophagostomy tubes requires minimal equipment, is a straightforward technique, and enables effective nutritional support. Complications associated with esophagostomy are minimal, and client compliance and satisfaction are very good. Detailed stepwise instructions are listed in Box 12-2.

The maximum safe volume of food to administer per feeding to a cat likely depends on a combination of factors including underlying disease and individual variation. A volume of 5 to 10 mL/kg per individual feeding generally is well tolerated, but this may vary with the individual patient. In cats who are generally healthy but can not consume food orally (e.g., symphyseal jaw fractures), larger volumes of food per feeding (15 to 20 mL/kg) may be tolerated; however, this volume must be given slowly over 15 to 20 minutes to allow gastric accommodation, or vomiting will occur. Because enteral diets are composed mostly of water (most canned food is already >75 per cent water), the amount of fluids administered parenterally should be adjusted accordingly to avoid volume overload. Premature removal of tubes by the patients can be prevented by using an Elizabethan collar and by wrapping the tube securely. Care should be taken to avoid wrapping too tightly because this could lead to patient discomfort and even compromise proper ventilation.

PARENTERAL NUTRITION

Parenteral nutrition is more expensive than enteral nutrition and is recommended only for in-hospital use. Indications for parenteral nutrition include intractable vomiting, severe malabsorptive disorders, and severe ileus. Examples of patients who may require parenteral nutrition include cats with severe inflammatory bowel disease,

---

Box 12-1 Formulating an Enteral Nutritional Plan

1. Calculate patient's RER (Resting Energy Requirements)

   RER = $70 \times$ (body weight)$^{0.75}$
   Or, if weight is between 2 kg and 30 kg,
   = $30 \times$ (body weight) + 70
   = _____ **kcal to feed per day**

2. Select diet to use based on type of tube used (see below).

   For nasoesophageal tubes: Use liquid diets designed for cats (typically 1 kcal/mL)

   For esophageal tubes: Tube ≥14 Fr can use blenderized diets

   For gastrostomy tubes: Blenderized diets

   For jejunostomy tubes: Use liquid diets designed for cats

3. Product selected: _____
   Contains _____ kcal/mL

4. Total amount to be administered per day:

   kcal required per day ÷ kcal per mL in diet =
   _____ mL of diet mixture/day

5. Feeding schedule:

½ of total requirement on Day 1	= _____ mL/day
Total requirement on Day 2	= _____ mL/day
Divide total daily amounts into 4 to 6 feedings	= _____ feedings/day

6. Calculate volume per feeding:

Total mL/day ÷ Number of feedings/day	= _____ mL/feeding (Day 1)
	_____ = _____ mL/feeding (Day 2)

   DIET OPTIONS
   Esophagostomy and Gastrostomy Tubes
   Eukanuba Maximum Calorie canned
       Supplies 2.1 kcal/mL straight from can, but needs to be diluted further for feeding tubes
       1 can + 50 mL water = 1.6 kcal/mL
       1 can + 25 mL water = 1.8 kcal/mL
   Hill's a/d canned
       Supplies 1.3 kcal/mL straight from can but needs to be diluted further for feeding tubes
       1 can + 50 mL water = 1.0 kcal/mL
       1 can + 25 mL water = 1.1 kcal/mL
   Royal Canin Canine/Feline Recovery RS
       Supplies 1 kcal/mL straight from can, but needs to be diluted further for feeding tubes
       1 can + 25 mL water = 0.9 kcal/mL
   Nasoesophageal and Jejunostomy Tubes
   Veterinary liquid diets
   CliniCare Canine/Feline Liquid diet (1 kcal/mL) (Abbott Animal Health)
   CliniCare RF Feline Liquid diet (1 kcal/mL) (Abbott Animal Health)

---

diffuse intestinal lymphoma, and acute necrotizing (surgical) pancreatitis. In the initial management stages of these disorders, therapies directed at the underlying etiology may take time to have an effect; parenteral nutrition allows nutrient delivery until gastrointestinal function normalizes.

The terminology of parenteral nutrition can be confusing and therefore this chapter utilizes the most commonly used terms encountered in the veterinary literature: total parenteral nutrition (TPN) and partial or peripheral parenteral nutrition (PPN).[10] TPN typically is delivered via a central venous (jugular) catheter and provides for all energy and the three major types of nutrient (protein, lipid, and carbohydrate) requirements of the patient. Technically, cats do not have a carbohydrate requirement, but meeting all of a cat's energy requirements with lipid and protein alone without exceeding recommended limits of protein and lipids would be difficult. As a result of this high glucose concentration, cats on TPN become hyperglycemic and may require insulin therapy. Due to the high osmolarity of the TPN solution (usually 1100 to 1500 mOsm/L), it must be administered through a central venous (jugular) catheter. PPN is formulated so that it can be administered through a peripheral catheter; however, because it is more dilute, it can provide only a portion of the patient's energy requirements (40 to 70 per cent). The lower osmolarity of the solution means that it can be administered through a large peripheral vein such as the femoral vein in cats, which is more feasible in practice. Because PPN only provides a portion of the patient's requirements, it is intended only for short-term use in a nondebilitated patient with average nutritional requirements.

Regardless of the exact form of parenteral nutrition, intravenous nutrition requires a dedicated catheter that is placed using aseptic technique. Long catheters composed of silicone, polyurethane, or tetrafluoroethylene are recommended for use with parenteral nutrition to reduce the risk of thrombophlebitis. Multi-lumen catheters (Figure 12-2) are often recommended for parenteral nutrition because they can remain in place for longer periods of time as compared to normal jugular catheters and they provide other ports for blood sampling and administering additional fluids and IV medications. Most parenteral nutrition solutions are composed of a carbohydrate source (dextrose), a protein source (amino acids), and a fat source (lipids). Vitamins and trace metals also can be added.

Formulation of TPN and PPN solutions can be individualized to each patient according to the worksheets in

Box 12-2 Stepwise Instructions for Placement of Esophagostomy Tubes in Cats

1. Proper placement of an esophagostomy feeding tube requires the distal tip to be placed in the distal esophagus at the level no further than the 9th intercostal space. This may require premeasuring the tube. Rather than cutting the distal tip and creating a sharp edge, the exit hole should be elongated using a small blade.

2. The patient should be anesthetized and preferably intubated. While in right lateral recumbency, the left side of the neck should be clipped, and a routine surgical scrub should be performed.

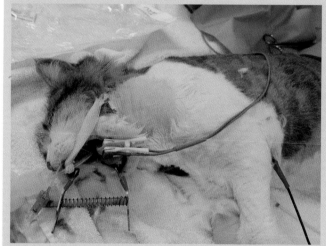

Placement of esophagostomy tube. Cat is anesthetized and placed in right lateral recumbency; the neck is clipped and prepared aseptically.

3. A curved Rochester Carmalt clamp is placed into the mouth and down the esophagus to the midcervical region. The jugular vein should be identified and avoided.

4. The tip of the Carmalt clamp then is pushed dorsally, elevating the esophagus towards the skin.

5. The tip of the Carmalt clamp is palpated over the skin to confirm its location and an incision is made through the skin onto the tip of the Carmalt clamp in the esophagus. The mucosa of the esophagus is relatively more difficult to incise than the skin.

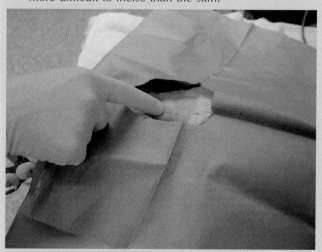

A Rochester Carmalt clamp is placed within the esophagus and the tip of the instrument is palpated through the skin.

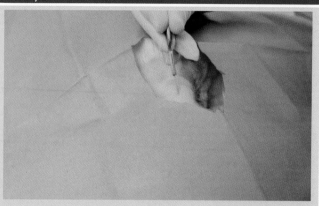

An incision is made directly over the palpated tip of the instrument until the tip of the clamp comes through the incision.

6. The tip of the instrument then is forced through the incision, which can be enlarged slightly with the blade to allow opening of the tip of the Carmalt clamp and placement of the esophagostomy tube within the tips.

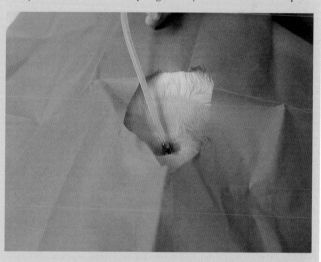

The tip of the esophagostomy tube is clamped with the Rochester Carmalt.

7. The Carmalt clamp then is clamped closed and pulled from the oral cavity.

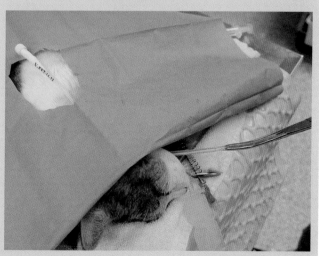

The clamped tube is pulled through the mouth.   *Continued*

Box 12-2 Stepwise Instructions for Placement of Esophagostomy Tubes in Cats—cont'd

8. Disengage the tips of the Carmalt clamp and curl the tip of the esophagostomy tube back into the mouth and feed it into the esophagus. As the curled tube is pushed into the esophagus, the proximal end is pulled gently. This will result in subtle "flip" as the tube is redirected within the esophagus. The tube should slide back and forth easily a few millimeters, confirming that the tube has straightened.

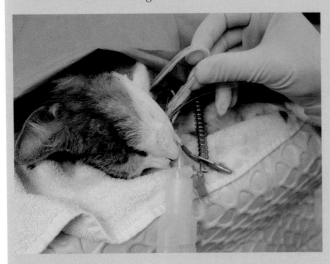

The tube is curled back into the pharynx.

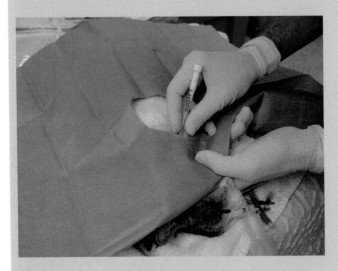

The curled tube is pushed back into the pharynx while slightly pulling at the distal end to straighten the tube within the esophagus.

9. Visually inspect the oropharynx to confirm that the tube is no longer present within the oropharynx.
10. The incision site should be rescrubbed briefly before a purse-string suture is placed, followed by a "Chinese finger trap," further securing the tube in place.

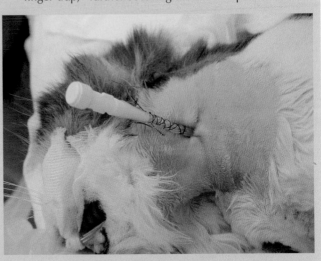

A purse-string suture is placed around the incision and a Chinese–finger trap suture is applied to the tube.

11. A light wrap is applied to the neck.
12. Correct placement should be confirmed with either radiography or fluoroscopy.

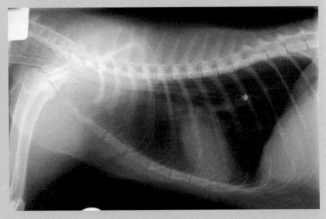

Radiograph of cat with esophagostomy tube in place, demonstrating ideal placement of tube within the esophagus.

Boxes 12-3 and 12-4. TPN and PPN must be mixed in a sterile manner; in most cases, it is easiest to have a local human hospital or human home health care company formulate the solutions.

Alternatively, commercial ready-to-use preparations of glucose and amino acids are available for peripheral use; however, these products provide less than 50 per cent of required calories (when administered at maintenance fluid rate) and should be used only for short-term or interim nutritional support. As with enteral nutrition, parenteral nutrition should be instituted gradually over 48 to 72 hours. With both TPN and PPN, the patient's catheter and lines must be handled with aseptic technique to avoid complications. To avoid volume overload,

Box 12-3 Calculation of Total Parenteral Nutrition in Cats

1. Calculate resting energy requirement (RER)

   RER = 70 × (current body weight
   in kg)$^{0.75}$
   or for animals weighing between
   2 and 30 kg:
   RER = (30 × current body weight   RER = _____ kcal/day
   in kg) + 70

2. Protein requirements for cats

	(g/100 kcal)
*Standard	6
*Reduced (hepatic/renal disease)	3 to 4
*Increased (excessive protein losses)	6 to 8

   $(RER \div 100) \times \dfrac{\text{g/100 kcal}}{\text{protein required}} =$
   _____ g protein required/day

3. Volume of nutrient solutions required
   a. 8.5 per cent amino acid solution = 0.085 g
      protein/mL

      _____ g protein required/day   = _____ mL/day of
      ÷ 0.085 g/mL   amino acids

   b. Nonprotein calories:

      The calories supplied by protein (4 kcal/g) are
      subtracted from the RER to get total nonprotein
      calories needed.
      _____ g protein required/day   = _____ kcal provided
      × 4 kcal/g   by protein
      RER − kcal provided by   = _____ total nonprotein
      protein   kcal/day required

   c. Nonprotein calories are usually provided as a 50:50
      mixture of lipid and dextrose.

      *20% lipid solution = 2 kcal/mL
      To supply 50% of nonprotein calories
      _____ lipid kcal required ÷   = _____ mL of lipid
      2 kcal/mL

      *50% of dextrose solution = 1.7 kcal/mL
      To supply 50% of nonprotein calories
      _____ dextrose kcal required ÷   = _____ mL of dextrose
      1.7 kcal/mL

4. Total daily requirements
   _____ mL of 8.5% amino acid solution
   _____ mL of 20% lipid
   _____ mL of 50% dextrose
   _____ total of TPN solution to be administered over 24
   hours

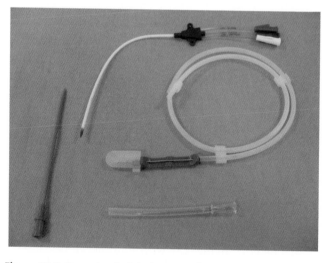

Figure 12-2 Example of triple-lumen catheter that can be used for administration of parenteral nutrition.

adjust other intravenous fluids accordingly for the amount of fluid being administered in the parenteral nutrition.

MONITORING AND REASSESSMENT

Body weight should be monitored daily in any hospitalized cat, but especially in those patients receiving enteral or parenteral nutrition. However, the clinician should take into account fluid shifts in evaluating changes in body weight. For this reason, body condition scoring is important as well, especially in determining those cats who have muscle wasting. The use of the RER as the patient's caloric requirement is merely a starting point. The number of calories provided may need to be increased, typically by 25 per cent if nutritional support is well tolerated, to keep up with the patient's changing needs. In patients unable to tolerate the prescribed amounts, the clinician should consider reducing amounts of enteral feedings and supplementing the nutritional plan with PPN.

Metabolic complications of enteral nutritional support include electrolyte disturbances, hyperglycemia, volume overload, and gastrointestinal signs (e.g., vomiting, diarrhea, cramping, bloating). In most cases, severe hypophosphatemia results in muscle weakness and hemolysis. However, it also can result in severe neurological impairment, hypoventilation, cardiac failure, and even death.[18,19]

Rarely, feeding a chronically debilitated and severely malnourished cat results in a condition known as *refeeding syndrome*. The major shifts in electrolytes observed in refeeding syndrome relate to the resurgence of insulin following administration of carbohydrates. In severe malnourished states, insulin levels are extremely low and adenosine triphosphate (ATP) synthesis is minimal. Following administration of carbohydrates, insulin instigates electrolyte shifts and cellular processes such as synthesis of ATP until phosphorus is depleted, resulting

---

Box 12-4 Calculation of Partial Parenteral Nutrition in Cats

1. Calculate resting energy requirement (RER)

   RER = 70 × (current body weight
   in kg)$^{0.75}$
   or for animals weighing between
   2 and 30 kg:
   RER = (30 × current body weight   RER = _____ kcal/day
   in kg) + 70

2. Calculate the partial energy requirement (PER)
   Plan to supply 50% of the animal's RER with PPN:

   PER = RER × 0.50 = _____ kcal/day

3. Proportion of nutrient requirements according to body
   weight:

   (Note: for animals ≤3 kg, the formulation will exceed
   maintenance fluid requirements.)

   a. Cats (3 to 5 kg):
      PER × 0.20 = _____ kcal/day carbohydrate required
      PER × 0.20 = _____ kcal/day protein required
      PER × 0.60 = _____ kcal/day lipid required

   b. Cats (6 to 10 kg):
      PER × 0.25 = _____ kcal/day carbohydrate required
      PER × 0.25 = _____ kcal/day protein required
      PER × 0.50 = _____ kcal/day lipid required

4. Volumes of nutrient solutions required:
   a. 5% dextrose solution = 0.17 kcal/mL
      _____ kcal carbohydrate   = _____ mL/day dextrose
      required/day ÷
      0.17 kcal/mL

   b. 8.5% amino acid solution = 0.34 kcal/mL
      _____ kcal protein required/   = _____ mL/day amino
      day ÷ 0.34 kcal/mL   acids

   c. 20% lipid solution = 2 kcal/mL
      _____ kcal lipid required/   = _____ mL/day lipid
      day ÷ 2 kcal/mL

                                     = _____ total mL of PPN
                                       to be administered
                                       over 24 hrs

---

in the clinical manifestations of refeeding syndrome.[19] Strategies to decrease risk of the development of refeeding syndrome include very gradual and conservative provision of nutrition and very low amounts of carbohydrates.[19] Correction of fluid and electrolyte imbalances should take priority over nutritional support in such extreme malnourished cases.

Monitoring parameters for patients receiving enteral nutrition include body weight, serum electrolytes, tube patency, appearance of tube exit site, gastrointestinal signs (e.g., vomiting, regurgitation, diarrhea), and signs of volume overload or aspiration pneumonia.

Possible complications with parenteral nutrition include sepsis, mechanical complications of the catheter and lines, thrombophlebitis, and metabolic disturbances such as hyperglycemia, electrolyte shifts, hyperammonemia, and hypertriglyceridemia. Avoiding serious consequences of complications associated with parenteral nutrition requires early identification of problems and prompt action. Frequent monitoring of vital signs, catheter exit sites, and routine serum biochemistry panels can alert the clinician to evolving problems. The development of persistent hyperglycemia during nutritional support may require adjustment of the nutritional plan (e.g., decreasing dextrose content in parenteral nutrition) or administration of regular insulin. This obviously necessitates more vigilant monitoring. Preventing hyperglycemia in critically ill cats may be prudent because there is growing evidence that the development of this abnormality may be detrimental in feline patients.[15,16]

With continual reassessment, the clinician can determine when to transition the patient from assisted feeding to voluntary consumption of food. The discontinuation of nutritional support should begin only when the cat can consume approximately its RER without much coaxing. In patients receiving TPN, transitioning to enteral nutrition should occur over the course of at least 12 to 24 hours, depending on patient tolerance of enteral nutrition.

PHARMACOLOGICAL AGENTS IN NUTRITIONAL SUPPORT

Because critically ill animals often are hyporexic or anorexic, the temptation exists to use appetite stimulants to increase food intake. Unfortunately, appetite stimulants generally are unreliable and seldom result in adequate food intake in critically ill cats.[20] Pharmacological stimulation of appetite often is short-lived and only delays true nutritional support. Loss of appetite is simply a clinical sign and not a disease process itself; therefore the use of pharmacological agents to treat this sign without addressing the underlying condition is illadvised. The author does not believe in the use of appetite stimulants in hospitalized patients when more effective measures of nutritional support, such as placement of feeding tubes, are more appropriate. For example, an inappetent, uremic cat with chronic kidney disease should be treated with fluid therapy and antacids rather than with appetite stimulants. An argument could be made that such a patient could be treated for its uremia for a few days and reassessed for the need of further nutritional interventions (i.e., placement of feeding tube). Appetite stimulants may be considered in cats who are treated as out-patients (i.e., not sick enough to be hospitalized) or in recovering animals because the primary reason for loss of appetite ideally should have been reversed by this time. As with many drugs, appetite stimulants also have negative side effects, such as behavioral changes associated with cyproheptadine and sedation associated with diazepam (oral diazepam also can lead to severe hepatotoxicity), and therefore should be used with caution or avoided completely.

Recently, there has been interest in the use of mirtazapine as an appetite stimulant in cats. There is very limited information regarding the use of this agent in cats. Mirtazapine is a tetracyclic antidepressant that appears to have some antiemetic and appetite-stimulating effects.[21] Mirtazapine also relies on glucuronidation for clearance; therefore this agent should be used with caution in cats with hepatic disease. Moreover, side effects associated with mirtazapine include sedation and hypotension.[21]

FUTURE DIRECTION IN CRITICAL CARE NUTRITION

In its current state, veterinary critical care nutrition focuses on proper recognition of animals requiring nutritional support and the implementation of strategies to best provide nutritional therapies. Important areas needing further evaluation in critically ill cats include how to determine the optimal composition and caloric target of nutritional support and what strategies to use to minimize complications and optimize outcome. Recent studies implicating poor clinical outcome in the development of hyperglycemia in critically ill people have led to more vigilant monitoring and stricter control of blood glucose, with obvious implications for nutritional support. Evidence of a similar relationship in cats is mounting; however, further studies are warranted.[15,16] Until studies demonstrate otherwise, efforts to reduce the incidence of hyperglycemia in critically ill cats, especially those being administered nutritional support, should be pursued strongly.

Other exciting initiatives in clinical nutrition in critical care include the use of special nutrients that possess immunomodulatory properties, such as glutamine, arginine, n-3 fatty acids, and antioxidants. In specific patient populations, these nutrients, used singly or in combination, have shown promising results.[22] However, the response has not been consistent, and ongoing trials continue to evaluate their efficacy. Limited information is available on using these nutrients to modulate disease, specifically in clinically affected animals. The only study using enteral glutamine in cats did not show any benefit.[23] Future studies should focus on whether manipulating these nutrients offers any benefits in critically ill cats.

Further developments in veterinary critical care nutrition may transform nutrition management from a strictly supportive measure to an integral part of treating disease and improving outcomes. Despite the lack of concrete results, many diets have been developed already for critically ill cats that contain increased levels of glutamine, arginine, omega-3 fatty acids, and antioxidants. It is unknown if the amounts of such nutrients found in these diets are adequate to confer pharmacological benefits; however, they are unlikely to lead to any detriment. Because the majority of veterinary patients are hospitalized only for a short term (a relatively low percentage are hospitalized for more than 10 days), the pharmacological effects of nutrients will be difficult to discern.

SUMMARY

Given their more pressing problems, critically ill cats often are not regarded as being in urgent need of nutritional support; however, the severity of their injuries, their altered metabolic condition, and necessity of frequent fasting (e.g., for diagnostic or surgical procedures) all place these patients at high risk for becoming malnourished during their hospitalization. The metabolic peculiarities of cats make them particularly prone to energy and protein catabolism, and nutritional support in this species may be more important during critical illness than it is for other animals. Proper identification of patients in need of nutritional support and careful planning and execution of a nutrition plan can be key factors in the successful recovery of these patients. In the future, the use of immune-modulating nutrients may play a larger role in modulating disease in critically ill cats.

REFERENCES

1. MacDonald ML, Rogers QR, Morris JG: Nutrition of the domestic cat, a mammalian carnivore, *Annu Rev Nutr* 4:521, 1984.
2. Mitchel KE: Nitrogen metabolism in critical care patients, *Vet Clin Nutr* (Suppl):20, 1998.
3. Sakurai Y, Zhang X, Wolfe RR: Short-term effects of tumor necrosis factor on energy and substrate metabolism in dogs, *J Clin Invest* 91:2437, 1993.
4. Brown B, Mauldin GE, Armstrong J, et al: Metabolic and hormonal alterations in cats with hepatic lipidosis, *J Vet Intern Med* 14:20, 2000.
5. Chan DL, Freeman LM, Rozanski EA, et al: Alterations in carbohydrate metabolism in critically ill cats, *J Vet Emerg Crit Care* 16:S7, 2006.
6. Rogers QR, Morris JG, Freedland RA: Lack of hepatic enzymatic adaptation to low and high levels of dietary protein in the adult cat, *Enzyme* 22:348, 1977.
7. Remillard RL: Nutritional support in critical care patients, *Vet Clin North Am Small Anim Pract* 32:1145, 2002.
8. Perbone S, Inui A: Anorexia in cancer: role of feeding-regulatory peptides, *Philos Trans R Soc Lond B Biol Sci* 361:1281, 2006.
9. Freitag KA, Saker KE, Thomas E, et al: Acute starvation and subsequent refeeding affect lymphocyte subsets and proliferation in cats, *J Nutr* 130:2444, 2000.
10. Freeman LM, Chan DL: Total parenteral nutrition. In DiBartola SP, editor: *Fluid, electrolyte, and acid-base disorders in small animal practice*, ed 3, St. Louis, 2006, Elsevier, p 584.
11. Buffington T, Holloway C, Abood A: Nutritional assessment. In Buffington T, Holloway C, Abood S, editors: *Manual of veterinary dietetics*. St. Louis, 2004, WB Saunders, p 1.
12. Chan DL: Nutritional requirements of the critically ill patient, *Clin Tech Small Anim Pract* 19:1, 2004.
13. Thatcher CD: Nutritional needs of critically ill patients, *Compend Contin Educ Pract Vet* 18:1303, 1996.
14. Chan DL, Freeman LM, Labato MA, et al: Retrospective evaluation of partial parenteral nutrition in dogs and cats, *J Vet Intern Med* 16:440, 2002.
15. Pyle SC, Marks SL, Kass PH: Evaluation of complications and prognostic factors associated with administration of total parenteral nutrition in cats: 75 cases (1994-2001), *J Am Vet Med Assoc* 255:242, 2004.

16. Crabb SE, Chan DL, Freeman LM: Retrospective evaluation of total parenteral nutrition in cats: 40 cases (1991-2003), *J Vet Emerg Crit Care* 16:S21, 2006.

17. Lippert AC, Fulton RB, Parr AM: A retrospective study of the use of total parenteral nutrition in dogs and cats, *J Vet Intern Med* 7:52, 1993.

18. Justin RB, Hohenhaus AE: Hypophosphatemia associated with enteral alimentation in cats, *J Vet Intern Med* 9:228, 1995.

19. Armitage-Chan EA, O'Toole T, Chan DL: Management of prolonged food deprivation, hypothermia and refeeding syndrome in a cat, *J Vet Emerg Crit Care* 16:S41, 2006.

20. Delaney SJ: Management of anorexia in dogs and cats, *Vet Clin Small Anim* 36:1243, 2006.

21. Plumb DC: *Plumb's veterinary drug handbook*, ed 6, Ames, Iowa, 2008, Blackwell Publishing Professional.

22. Chan DL: The role of nutrients in modulating disease, *J Small Anim Pract* 49:266, 2008.

23. Marks SL, Cook AK, Reader R, et al: Effects of glutamine supplementation of an amino acid-based purified diet on intestinal mucosal integrity in cats with methotrexate-induced enteritis, *Am J Vet Res* 60:755, 1999.

CHAPTER
13 Unconventional Diets

Jennifer A. Larsen and Sally C. Perea

Unconventional diets are defined as those that fall outside of the usual categories of commercially available cat foods. The term applies not only to commercial niche diets that contain ingredients that are organic, human grade, natural, vegetarian/vegan, or raw, but also to a wide variety of home-prepared diets. Owners choose to pursue unconventional foods and feeding practices for a wide variety of reasons. Distrust of specific brands, categories of foods, or of commercially available diets in general drives some decisions in this area. Pet foods marketing can be convincing and even aggressive, persuading some owners to switch brands or to try a different strategy. Additionally, owners seek advice from many sources, including Internet websites, books, friends and family, or their veterinarian. Nutritional management advice from veterinarians is highly variable, and depends not only on veterinary school training and continuing education activities, but also on clinical experience, client interests, and compliance issues. Some veterinarians advise owners to switch brands or types of cat foods or to offer home-prepared diets both on general principle and to address specific disease processes, while others only advise a change in the face of a specific problem.

Some facets of consumer behavior have been influenced by an increased general awareness of environmental and/or socioeconomic issues. This has informed choices of products and food items not only for the family but also for the family pets. The focus in this area has been on organic and locally grown foods, as well as on foods produced and harvested using sustainable and low-impact methods. The market share of products that serve consumers who have concerns relative to these issues has not been predominant to date, but this segment is growing.

A recent article published in the trade publication *Petfood Industry* reported a survey showing that 8 to 27 per cent of pet owners are considering a switch to a different brand of pet food.[1] Many of these pet owners are making the switch to alternative pet foods labeled as "natural, organic, raw/frozen, refrigerated, homemade, 100 per cent U.S. sourced, locally grown," as well as to other small-batch pet foods. Another survey conducted in May 2007 reported that 69 per cent of pet specialty retailers had seen increased sales of natural and organic pet food, while 21 per cent of pet-specialty retailers had seen a decline in sales of traditional pet food.[1] This same survey also reported that sales of fresh and/or raw pet foods had increased by more than one third. With this movement toward alternative diets, the challenge for veterinarians and pet owners is to interpret and understand the terms and claims used to describe these unconventional pet foods.

REGULATORY DEFINITIONS

There is frequent confusion regarding the marketing terms and the regulatory purview they may fall under. Terms used in product promotional materials or on labels, such as *natural, organic, human grade, premium, gourmet,* and *holistic* often do not have officially recognized definitions (Box 13-1). Consumers (and veterinarians) often are left with the impression that any such language is standardized or regulated in some way, but that is not always the case.

The Association of American Feed Control Officials (AAFCO) defines a *natural* feed or ingredient as one that is:

> derived solely from plant, animal or mined sources, either in its unprocessed state or having been subject to physical processing, heat processing, rendering, purification, extraction, hydrolysis, enzymolysis or fermentation, but not having been produced by or subject to a chemically synthetic process and not containing any additives or processing aids that are chemically synthetic except in amounts as might occur unavoidably in good manufacturing practices.[2]

The term *natural* should be used only to describe products for which all of the ingredients and components of ingredients meet this definition. An exception is made to allow the use of chemically synthesized vitamins, minerals, or other trace nutrients; however, a disclaimer must be present to inform the consumer that these supplemented nutrients are not natural.

The term *organic* refers to the conditions under which the ingredients used in products, and the product itself, were produced, and must be consistent with regulations developed by the United States Department of Agriculture (USDA). Current regulations covering organic products do not apply to pet foods; however, the USDA is developing regulations for organic labeling of pet foods. The USDA Organic Pet Food Task Force issued a report in 2006 outlining some of their proposed regulatory changes.[3] The Task Force recommended that product composition requirements for organic pet food be similar to those for livestock, but that labeling categories be the same as for processed human food. These require a minimum of 70 per cent organic ingredients for the use of the claim "made with organic," and at least 95 per cent organic content for the use of the claim "organic." All products labeled as "made with organic ingredients" or "organic" must exclude ingredients that are genetically engineered, are produced using sludge or irradiation, or contain synthetic substances not on the National List of Allowed and Prohibited Substances as defined by the National Organic Standards Board (advisory to the federal Secretary of Agriculture). They also can not contain sulfites, nitrates or nitrites, or organic and nonorganic forms of the same ingredients. In addition, products labeled "organic" can not contain nonorganic ingredients when organic sources are available.

Another term that is gaining use is *human grade.* Currently, there is no official definition or regulation regarding the use of this term. According to AAFCO, this means that the term is not allowed.[4] However, there is no legal prohibition, and the term continues to be applied widely to a variety of pet foods. In 2007, one pet food company was denied the right to sell their product in the state of Ohio due to the use of the term *human food grade.*[5] The Ohio State Department of Agriculture argued that the term was misleading and refused to grant a license to the company. The company followed with a lawsuit, which eventually sided in their favor due to the argument that the company had the constitutional right to make truthful statements about the quality of its pet food product on the label. So, despite the unclear and likely variable and inconsistent interpretation of the term, its use is gaining popularity as more pet owners are selecting foods with improved safety and quality, whether these qualities are true or perceived.

Other descriptors used commonly include *premium, super premium, gourmet,* and *holistic.* These terms are used solely as marketing tools, and have no official definitions. Products labeled as such can have widely variable nutritional profiles, micronutrient concentrations, and ingredient types. They are not required to be of superior quality in any way or to contain different nutrient levels than other products. The term *holistic* often has been used to describe various commercially available and home-cooked diets, but appears to be used primarily as a marketing term, as the philosophical concept of holism is not only linked intrinsically to the individual as a whole, but also is descriptive of a manner of thinking or approach to a problem, rather than being applicable to substances. The application of classical holism becomes imprecise when applied to populations with varied characteristics. Nutritional science, while often observational, involves hierarchical theories and relies on the testing of hypotheses, precise measurements, and linear logistical constructs. Some aspects of the science of nutrition are based on the application of concepts established in small numbers of animals to the study or treatment of a population, while other facets, especially clinical nutrition, involve the consideration of the individual animal's needs, comorbid conditions, lifestyle, and many other individual factors. Because most diets are formulated to satisfy average or expected needs within a particular population, only individual nutritional management plans that are part of a larger and more cohesive medical prevention and treatment strategy, rather than the diets themselves, can be considered truly holistic in nature.

HOME-PREPARED DIETS

Home-prepared diets for cats have become increasingly popular. The reasons owners want or need to prepare their cat's food are many and varied. Cat owners often will express concerns regarding the use of commercial diets for their healthy cats. In addition, owners of cats with health problems may wish to participate in the management of their pet's condition by providing a home-prepared diet, even if a commercially available diet would be appropriate. These owners may believe that a home-prepared diet is safer, more natural, or more healthful than a commercially available diet. They may wish to avoid certain ingredients (such as grains, chemical preservatives, or by-products) or to include certain ingredients (such as specific protein or fat sources). Other owners wish to feed their cats according to their own philosophical views, and choose home-prepared diets that are vegetarian, organic, natural, or raw. Another reason owners may feed home-prepared diets is that their cat refuses commercially available diets. In some patients, this is a learned behavior, while in others it may be the result of a food aversion secondary to a disease condition (such as chronic kidney disease). Finally, a patient may have a particular combination of diseases for which no suitable commercial diet exists. In these cases, a home-prepared diet can be an appropriate solution.

Although many of the reasons owners wish to avoid traditional commercial diets are the result of misinformation and myths, most owners want to provide healthful diets on which their pets thrive and purposefully do not feed inadequate diets that do not meet basic requirements or that are potentially harmful. Recognizing this, the veterinarian should play an active role in the nutritional management of all patients, even if they are healthy. Encouraging dialogue regarding nutritional needs for individual pets is an opportunity to educate clients regarding commercial pet foods (including testing procedures, ingredient definitions, and marketing strategies) and any issues specific to their pet, as well as the impact of nutrition on any potential disease processes. Animals eating home-prepared diets should be assessed on a regular basis, and the general clinical evaluation should include discussion with the owner regarding fecal quality, appetite, presence of vomiting, and any other abnormalities that have been noted. Every patient also should have a thorough diet history collected at each visit, in addition to a complete physical examination, including skin and coat evaluation, body weight, and body condition score. This helps ensure that potential problems are identified and addressed early. This is particularly important when a home-cooked diet is being fed because the recipe will often "drift." Drift can occur when supplements are omitted or altered frequently, which may be a result of inconvenience or a lack of understanding regarding the importance of these ingredients. Also, properly formulated home-prepared diets will be more expensive than most commercially available diets, and this can result in recipe changes. Sometimes, owners will substitute ingredients in the original recipe, which can change the nutritional profile substantially. Even a small difference in ingredients can change the nutritional profile of the diet.

Although many recipes for home-prepared cat foods are available on the Internet and in books, the majority of these diets are inadequate when compared to updated recommendations for nutrient intakes using modern ingredient databases and formulation methods. The recipes also tend to have vague instructions, contain errors or omissions in formulation, incorporate potentially problematic ingredients, or feature outdated or otherwise inappropriate strategies for addressing specific disease conditions. One study evaluated recipes available in popular books and compared the analyses to nutrient-intake recommendations established by AAFCO and the National Research Council. Many of these widely available recipes were found to provide less-than-recommended amounts of multiple essential nutrients, including taurine, minerals, and vitamins.[6] Another issue is that some owners do not follow any particular recipe, do not provide nutritional supplements, or feed their cats solely items that are palatable or convenient. Also, because certain feeding styles have become popular (such as raw diets), additional concerns must be addressed.

Nutritional adequacy is a major concern in regard to home-prepared diets. Providing appropriate levels of essential nutrients is crucial to optimize health and longevity, the foremost goals of individualized nutritional management (Table 13-1). Formulations are inherently imperfect at providing accurate levels of essential nutrients to the individual animal due to limitations in nutrient database information, variation in the nutritional profiles and preparation of the ingredients, limitations of the formulation methodology and/or software, limitations of the current understanding of the nutrient requirements of individual animals, and the inability to assess customized diets for appropriate digestibility and bioavailability of the nutrients. One study that evaluated the nutritional adequacy of home-prepared dog foods by laboratory analysis demonstrated that 35 different diets were below AAFCO recommendations for calcium, vitamins A and E, zinc, copper, and potassium.[7] Another study utilized computer analysis to assess home-prepared diets that were recommended for the diagnosis and/or treatment of adverse reactions to foods in dogs and cats.[8] Compared to nutrient intake recommendations at the time, most recipes that were recommended for long-term feeding of adult cats were too low in calcium, iron, taurine, and thiamin, and some also provided inadequate levels of potassium, phosphorus, and sodium. Owners should understand the limitations of any diet they choose to feed, and they should have the tools and guidance available to evaluate resources and recipes effectively, so that informed decisions can be made regarding an appropriate diet for individual animals. This is particularly important when feeding cats with one or more diseases amenable to nutritional management because disease progression or other changes in the clinical picture may warrant changes in the feeding plan.

Home-prepared diet recipes must be evaluated with a critical eye. For healthy adult pets, basic qualitative assessment of the proposed/current home-prepared diet recipe can be done during the course of the clinic visit (Table 13-2). If raw animal products are included, concerns regarding pathogenic contamination should be discussed with the owner, particularly if vulnerable human populations are potentially exposed (infants, elderly, immunocompromised). This potential problem should not be minimized and is discussed in more detail below.

Additionally, any other potentially dangerous ingredients (including supplements) should be identified, such as grapes/raisins, garlic/onions, or bones (Table 13-3). Next, the diet recipe should provide a source of protein

Table 13-1 Clinical Signs of Vitamin and Mineral Deficiency and Toxicity, Diagnostic Tests, and Dietary Sources*

Nutrient	Clinical Signs of Deficiency	Clinical Signs of Toxicity	Diagnostic Tests for Status Assessment	Dietary Source
FAT-SOLUBLE VITAMINS				
Vitamin A	Anorexia, weight loss, ataxia, xerophthalmia, conjunctivitis, corneal opacity and ulceration, skin lesions, metaplasia of the bronchiolar epithelium, pneumonitis, and increased susceptibility to infections	Extensive osseocartilaginous hyperplasia of the first three cervical vertebrae, poor bone growth, gingivitis, tooth loss, fetal malformations, cleft palates	Serum or liver retinol concentrations	Liver, meat, poultry
Vitamin D	Rickets	Lethargy, anorexia, vomiting, polydipsia	Radiographic imaging of skeletal bones, serum 25-hydroxyvitamin D	Fish, fish oil
Vitamin E	Muscle weakness, reproductive failure, nodular adipose tissue (associated with steatitis)	Growth depression, decreased bone growth, increased prothrombin time (associated with vitamins D and K antagonism)	Plasma alpha-tocopherol	Nuts, oils
Vitamin K	Excessive bleeding, prolonged clotting times	None reported in cats	Prothrombin times, PIKA (Proteins induced by vitamin K antagonism)	Green leafy vegetables, some vegetable oils (olive, soybean, canola)
WATER-SOLUBLE VITAMINS				
Thiamin	Inappetence, weight loss, coprophagia, muscle weakness, ataxia, paraparesis, torticollis, circling, tonic-clonic convulsions, ventroflexion, death	None reported in cats	Plasma concentration of thiamin-phosphorylated esters, erythrocyte transketolase saturation	Yeast, wheat germ, kidney, liver, legume seeds, egg yolk
Riboflavin	Anorexia, weight loss, periauricular alopecia, epidermal atrophy, cataracts, fatty liver	None reported in cats	Erythrocyte glutathione reductase activity coefficient	Meat, milk, eggs, liver, kidney, heart
Pyridoxine (vitamin B_6)	Anorexia, microcytic hypochromic anemia, convulsions, enhanced oxalate excretion (cats)	None reported in cats	Pyridoxal blood concentration, aminotransferase activity, kynureninase activity	Liver, yeast, cereals, wheat, and corn
Niacin	Black tongue, stomatitis, 4 Ds = dermatitis, diarrhea, dementia, and death	None reported in cats. High doses reported to cause bloody feces, convulsions, and death in dogs.	Nicotinamide loading test; urine N'-methylnicotinamide concentration	Meat, liver
Folic acid	Macrocytic hypochromic anemia	None reported in cats	Serum folic acid concentration	Green leafy vegetables, lima beans, citrus fruit, meats (particularly liver and kidneys)
Vitamin B_{12}	Macrocytic hypochromic anemia	None reported in cats	Serum vitamin B_{12} concentration	Animal products
Pantothenic acid	Dermal lesions (dermatitis and alopecia), anorexia, diarrhea, locomotive incoordination, ketoacidosis	None reported in cats	Urinary output of pantothenate	Widespread distribution in foods, yeast, egg yolk, liver, kidney, beef, milk, whole grains

Table 13-1 Clinical Signs of Vitamin and Mineral Deficiency and Toxicity, Diagnostic Tests, and Dietary Sources—cont'd

Nutrient	Clinical Signs of Deficiency	Clinical Signs of Toxicity	Diagnostic Tests for Status Assessment	Dietary Source
Biotin	Alopecia, dermatitis, metabolic acidosis	None reported in cats	Serum biotin concentration, acetyl CoA carboxylase and propionyl CoA carboxylase activities	Liver, kidney, egg yolk, peanuts, whole grain, yeast
VITAMIN-LIKE COMPOUNDS				
Choline	Fatty liver	None reported in cats	Serum alanine aminotransferase activity (rises approximately 1 week after feeding a choline-deficient diet)	Lecithin found in dietary fats; choline equivalents may be provided by other methyl donors such as methionine or betaine
MACROMINERALS				
Calcium	Reluctance to move, posterior lameness, uncoordinated gait and painful enlarged joints, rickets, osteoporosis, spontaneous fractures	Inappetence, poor growth	Radiographic imaging of skeleton, parathyroid hormone levels, serum ionized calcium concentration	Most foods poor source, whole prey (including skeleton), milk products (generally not sufficient)
Phosphorus	Hemolytic anemia, locomotor disturbances, metabolic acidosis	Depression, dehydration, metabolic acidosis	Plasma concentration (not a good assessment of body stores)	Meat, bone meal
Potassium	Depression, ventroflexion of neck, weight loss	None reported in cats	Plasma concentration (not a good assessment of body stores)	Plants, vegetables
Sodium	Inappetence, polyuria/polydipsia in kittens	None reported in cats	Increased plasma and urine aldosterone concentration (serum levels not a reliable indicator of nutritional deficiency)	Processed foods, mineral supplements
Chloride	Deficiency leads to excess potassium excretion in the kidneys; therefore, clinical signs of potassium deficiency may occur	None reported in cats	Plasma concentration (not a good assessment of body stores)	Limited in most foods, generally requires supplementation
Magnesium	Tetany, tremors, hyperexcitability, tachycardia, and seizures	Struvite urolithiasis	Ionized serum magnesium concentration	Meat, bone meal, corn products, soybean meal
TRACE MINERALS				
Iron	Pale mucous membranes, lethargy, weakness, weight loss or lack of weight gain, hematuria, melena	Vomiting (acute toxicity)	Total serum iron binding capacity, serum iron concentration	Meat, organ meats, beet pulp, peanut hulls
Zinc	Decreased appetite, parakeratosis, reproductive failure, decreased wound healing	No reports in cats In dogs—acute gastroenteritis, hemolytic anemia, and lethargy	Plasma or whole blood zinc concentration (may not be a reliable indicator of zinc stores), liver biopsy	Red meat, milk, gelatin, egg yolks, shellfish, beans, peas, liver, whole grains, lentils, rice, and potatoes
Manganese	Retarded bone growth, lameness, enlarged joints, poor locomotor function	None reported in cats	Lymphocyte manganese concentration	Cereal grains, meats, poultry, seafood

Continued

Table 13-1 Clinical Signs of Vitamin and Mineral Deficiency and Toxicity, Diagnostic Tests, and Dietary Sources—cont'd

Nutrient	Clinical Signs of Deficiency	Clinical Signs of Toxicity	Diagnostic Tests for Status Assessment	Dietary Source
Copper	Neurological signs, anemia	None reported in cats	Liver biopsy, erythrocyte copper/zinc SOD activity	Shellfish, liver, kidney, heart, meat, nuts, mushrooms, cereals, legumes
Iodine	Goiter, alopecia, dry sparse overall hair coat, weight gain	Excessive lacrimation, salivation, nasal discharge, a flaky and dry skin and hair coat	Urine iodine excretion, thyroid hormone levels	Kelp, thyroid tissue, iodized salts
Selenium	Anorexia, depression, dyspnea, "white muscle disease"	None reported in cats	Plasma concentration of selenium and activity of glutathione peroxidase (GPX) in whole blood	Red meat, poultry, fish, shellfish, grains, eggs, and plant foods

SOD, Superoxide dismutase.
*National Research Council: *Nutrient requirements of dogs and cats,* Washington, DC, 2006, The National Academies Press.

Table 13-2 Home-Prepared Diet Checklist

Ingredient	Purpose
Protein source	Provides amino acids, nitrogen, energy, palatability using animal-source proteins
Fat source	Provides fatty acids, energy, palatability, energy density
Carbohydrate source	Provides micronutrients, fiber, energy
SUPPLEMENTS	
Calcium source	Provides calcium, sometimes also phosphorus and other minerals
Salt source(s)	Provides sodium, chloride, potassium, iodine
Other multimineral source	Provides zinc, copper, many other minerals
Vitamin source	Provides fat-soluble and water-soluble vitamins

Table 13-3 Partial List of Ingredients to Avoid in Feline Diets

Ingredient	Concern
Onions and garlic	Erythrocyte oxidation and Heinz body anemia[25]
Lipoic acid	Hepatocellular toxicity[26]
Kelp	Arsenic toxicity[27,28]
Bone meal	Lead toxicity[29]
Vitamin C	Increased urinary oxalate excretion[30]
Grapes and raisins	Nephrotoxicity[31]

and fat. One common problem in many home-prepared diets is the lack of an appropriate vegetable oil, such as corn oil or canola oil, to provide specific essential omega-6 fatty acids. Some protein and carbohydrate sources will provide these fatty acids, but many do not. Some owners wish to feed specific fat and oil products that provide health benefits for people, such as olive oil; however, these usually should be considered only as a source of fat calories because they are often poor sources of essential fatty acids. Also to be noted are the sources of calcium, taurine, and many other micronutrients.

The form of supplementation for minerals and vitamins is important. Many recipes recommend the inclusion of a "multivitamin"; however, this is not an adequate descriptor. There is a wide range of multivitamin/multimineral products available for both human beings and animals, and very few provide essential nutrients in

appropriate amounts and proportions for balancing home-prepared diets. Most supplements marketed for pets are designed to be safe when added to a balanced, commercially available diet. They do not contain essential nutrients in high enough amounts to be adequate for supplementing home-prepared diets. Other multinutrient supplements provide individual nutrients at inappropriately high, possibly toxic, concentrations. Finally, preparation instructions should be reviewed for specificity. For example, the nutrient profile of the final diet will be affected by cooking method—for example, whether fat is drained or retained when cooking meats.

Beyond the basic and preliminary evaluation described above, the diet recipe also must undergo quantitative assessment for nutritional adequacy. Multiple resources are available to assist veterinarians with diet assessment and other services (Box 13-2). Further evaluation of the diet recipe is necessary to ensure that the base ingredients, with additional supplements, supply adequate amounts of essential nutrients for long-term feeding of the specific patient. The provision of all essential nutrients, plus any necessary safety factors or adjustments based on individual animal factors, must be considered. The quantitative assessment is best done by computer, and interpretation and application of nuances in evalua-

Box 13-2 Nutrition Resources

INSTITUTIONS WITH CLINICAL NUTRITION FACULTY AND RESIDENTS AVAILABLE FOR CONSULTATION

University of California, Davis
http://www.vetmed.ucdavis.edu/vmth/small_animal/
nutrition/default.cfm
530-752-1387

University of Missouri
http://www.vmth.missouri.edu
573-882-7821

University of Tennessee
http://www.vet.utk.edu/clinical/sacs/nutrition.php
865-974-8387

HOME-COOKED DIET FORMULATIONS

Veterinary Nutritional Consultations
http://www.petdiets.com
800-649-2043
508-429-2043

Davis Veterinary Medical Consulting, Inc.
http://www.dvmconsulting.com
http://www.balanceit.com
530-756-3862
888-346-6362

University of California, Davis
http://www.vetmed.ucdavis.edu/vmth/small_animal/
nutrition/default.cfm
530-752-1387

The UCVMC-SD Clinical Nutrition Program
http://www.ucvmc-sd.vetmed.ucdavis.edu/nutrition.cfm
858-875-7505

Tufts Cummings School of Veterinary Medicine
http://www.tufts.edu/vet
508-839-5395 x 84696

VETERINARY NUTRITION ORGANIZATIONS

American College of Veterinary Nutrition
http://www.acvn.org

American Academy of Veterinary Nutrition
http://www.aavn.org

HUMAN FOODS NUTRIENT CONTENT INFORMATION

USDA Nutrient Database
http://www.nal.usda.gov/fnic/foodcomp/search/

COMMERCIAL PET FOOD REGULATION AND INGREDIENT DEFINITIONS

Association of American Feed Control Officials
http://aafco.org/

tion and formulation require experience. This is particularly important when a home-prepared diet is being proposed for cats with one or more diseases. Customized nutritional management plans for individual animals are indicated to address comorbid conditions, whether this involves commercial or home-prepared diets. Further, home-prepared diets are not well suited for the needs of the growing kitten or reproducing queen. The small margin of error and the real limitations of these diets as described above are factors that increase the risk of using

such diets for life stages beyond adult maintenance. Another situation in which home-prepared diets are of limited usefulness is for the management of the obese or overweight patient. Because most of these diets are energy dense, typically quite palatable, and can not always provide precisely determined micronutrient concentrations reliably, home-prepared diets are not suited for safe weight loss programs, and they are often not successful. Clients should be encouraged to work with a veterinary nutritionist if they wish to attempt safe weight loss in their cat using a home-prepared diet.

However, home-prepared diets offer advantages for the management of many patients. They can be formulated to allow for restricted levels of fat (and/or protein) while meeting essential fatty acid (and/or amino acid) requirements, allow for inclusion of specific ingredients, and ensure appropriate supplementation of required micronutrients. For example, cats with chronic kidney disease and inflammatory bowel disease may benefit from the use of a home-prepared diet with modifications for kidney disease that is formulated with specific novel/tolerated ingredients. For some cats, particularly if there are fixed flavor or texture preferences, the transition to a home-prepared diet can be challenging. Adjusting the protein and fat levels, if possible, in addition to alternating the moisture content, can help increase the palatability and acceptance of a home-prepared diet. Other techniques such as warming food, trying a very gradual transition, and using broths, meat purees, and other flavorings, at least temporarily, also can be useful. These diets can be excellent options for many pets, but due to the common problems discussed above, proper formulation and careful introduction is crucial to the success of the dietary management plan that includes a home-prepared diet.

RAW FOOD FEEDING: ADDITIONAL CONSIDERATIONS

In addition to the concerns regarding the nutritional inadequacy or imbalances of both commercially available and home-prepared raw diets, additional risks that may come with the feeding of raw food include pathogenic bacterial infection and/or environmental contamination, as well as potential gastrointestinal obstruction by bones. Food-borne illness in people is a serious problem, and the contamination of raw pet foods with pathogenic bacteria has been well documented.[9-13] Although the number of pets who develop illness when feeding raw food is unknown, clinical cases have been documented in the scientific literature.

One report described salmonellosis in two cats from the same household fed a raw beef–based diet.[12] The first cat from this household (a 14-year-old, intact male, exotic shorthair) was deceased on presentation, and clinical signs prior to death included weight loss, soft stools, and anorexia of one week's duration. Tissue cultures taken at necropsy from the lung, liver, spleen, and kidney were shown to be positive for *S. typhimurium*. Unfortunately, samples from this cat's diet were not available for culture. The second cat (a 10-week-old, intact male, exotic shorthair kitten) presented 9 months later. The kitten was moribund on presentation, and euthanasia was performed at the owner's request. Necropsy revealed suppurative pneumonia and enteritis with villous blunting and erosion. Tissue cultures and subtyping revealed *Bordetella bronchiseptica* in the lung, and *Salmonella newport* in both lung and small intestine samples. Samples of the raw ground beef fed to this kitten were shown subsequently to be positive for *S. newport,* confirming the raw meat as the source of infection.

In addition to raw meat, raw bones also can introduce pathogenic bacteria, and large bone pieces can lead to esophageal and gastrointestinal obstructions. Raw bones may be less likely to splinter than cooked bones; however, sharp bone fragments can still occur, putting the cat at risk for intestinal perforation. The use of a bone grinder can help to reduce the risk of obstruction and perforation by grinding the bone to smaller pieces. However, there is little known about the bioavailability of calcium from these bone pieces. The presence of undigested bone pieces in the feces of cats fed raw bones is not uncommon and raises the concern that calcium needs are not being met. Finally, the use of bone and bone meal for calcium supplementation has fallen out of favor due to the risk of lead contamination.[14] Therefore supplementation with a safer calcium source, such as calcium carbonate or dicalcium phosphate, is preferred.

Pets who do not develop clinical illness when fed contaminated raw meat products still introduce a risk to human beings and other pets in the environment through shedding of organisms in the feces and contamination of feeding bowls and surrounding feeding environment.[15,16] Children, seniors, and immunocompromised individuals are at the greatest risk of environmental contamination. In response to public health concerns, the Food and Drug Administration (FDA) provides guidelines for pet owners on the proper handling of raw pet foods to help minimize the risk of cross contamination of pathogens.[17] The guidelines state, "The FDA does not advocate a raw meat, poultry or seafood diet for pets, but is stepping up its efforts to minimize the risk such foods pose to animal and human health because we understand that some people prefer to feed these types of diets to their pets." This educational approach also should be implemented by veterinarians when discussing raw pet foods with clients. Discussing both risk to the pet and zoonotic risks is important to ensure that owners are well educated regarding their feeding choice. After discussing these risks with the owner, alternative feeding options that will improve safety can be offered. Many commercially available cooked pet foods offer caloric distributions similar to those of raw foods and incorporate similar feeding philosophies such as avoidance of grains, the use of vegetables, and the use of natural preservatives and ingredients. For pet owners who prefer to prepare the food at home, a complete and balanced home-cooked diet also can be suggested as an alternative.

VEGETARIAN AND VEGAN FEEDING

The feeding of vegetarian or vegan diets generally reflects the pet owner's philosophies and dietary choices. Unlike raw-food feeders whose motivations may be to feed what is "natural" for the pet, pet owners feeding vegetarian or vegan foods may be motivated for ethical reasons.[18] Because cats are obligate carnivores, feeding vegan or vegetarian foods to cats raises some concerns relative to the ability to provide adequate amounts of some essential nutrients. It is well known that cats have a higher protein requirement than dogs, but additional nutrients such as arachidonic acid, niacin, cobalamin, pyroxidine, vitamin A, and vitamin D, as well as some amino acids such as taurine, arginine, methionine, and lysine, can be limiting in vegan and vegetarian ingredients, making it difficult to meet cats' minimum requirements for these nutrients.[19] One study using laboratory analysis to evaluate two commercially available feline vegan diets found multiple nutrient deficiencies in the two diets, including total protein, methionine, taurine, lysine, arginine, arachidonic acid, calcium, phosphorus, vitamin A, pyridoxine, niacin, and cobalamin.[20] This study reinforced the concerns that had been raised about feeding cats vegan or vegetarian foods, and cat owners should be alerted to these risks when electing to feed these types of foods.

It is best to encourage cat owners to feed an appropriate meat-based cat food, and educate them about the health risks associated with vegan and vegetarian feeding. Vegan foods are more difficult than vegetarian foods to properly balance for the cat's unique nutrient requirements, so redirecting clients to vegetarian foods that provide egg or dairy protein and fat sources is an alternative that can be considered for cat owners who strongly oppose meat-based diets. In these situations, in which the owner objects strongly to a meat-based food, monitoring of the cat's whole blood and plasma amino acid levels should be recommended. Monitoring amino acid levels can help to identify potential protein or amino acid deficiencies prior to the development of clinical problems. More regular veterinary exams (at least every 4 to 6 months) also should be recommended to help to identify potential nutrient deficiencies.

SUPPLEMENTS AND NUTRACEUTICALS

A wide variety of supplements and other nutritional products are available for human and veterinary use. Some supplements are strictly functional and are meant to supply specific nutrients, while others include herbs and other bioactive compounds or nutraceuticals. Many herbal preparations and other plant-based products contain dozens of different compounds, both identified and unidentified. The exact biological effects of each of these compounds in a particular product are unknown, and their safety and efficacy have not been evaluated in most species. The possibility of nutrient and drug interactions also is of concern. Many herbal products are associated with cautions regarding the adverse effects on micronutrient bioavailability due to an effect on absorption. For example, in people black catechu has been reported not only to work synergistically with antihypertensive medications, but also to decrease the absorption of dietary zinc; likewise, hawthorn and marshmallow may decrease the absorption of dietary iron.[21] It is recommended to consult with an experienced veterinary herbologist when managing patients taking herbal products with conventional pharmaceuticals.

Some people are of the opinion that whole foods diets are more desirable and beneficial than those that include supplements. While this is an appealing concept, achieving a balanced diet without the use of concentrated supplements in practice is exceedingly difficult. The addition of a specific food to supply a particular micronutrient also adds calories and many other nutrients that affect the overall diet. For an average-sized cat, this could require more than two dozen different "whole food" ingredients, all in very small amounts, to supply the target energy level. Even if this were possible, it may not be beneficial or desirable due to the complexity, expense, and increased dietary variability with the use of multiple ingredients. For human beings, the approach that has been most successful in achieving significant reductions in important deficiency syndromes has been the enrichment of certain staple foods with specific micronutrients, as with the fortification of breakfast cereals, rice, table salt, and milk. Conditions such as osteoporosis and iron deficiency are still treated commonly with targeted nutrient supplementation.[22,23] Similarly, whole foods are not relied on to supply folic acid for pregnant women.[24]

The bioavailability of micronutrients from whole foods is variable and in many cases is much lower than in purified forms. For example, phosphorus from plant sources often is found in the form of phytate, an organic complex that is poorly available for nonruminant species. Nutrient bioavailability also depends on the food source, processing methods and conditions, and animal factors. For animal products, overall and relative micronutrient content will reflect the nutritional status of those species, as well as potential degradation secondary to storage and/or cooking. Of course, the nutritional profile also will vary with the specific animal product, as even skeletal muscle will differ relative to the "cut." Similarly, organ meats and other by-products vary widely in nutrient content. Additionally, the variability in nutrient profile of different foods grown in different climates, with different soil conditions, and under different storage and preparation conditions, is likely to have a much greater impact on the final profile of the overall diet than it is with purified supplements. Regardless of life stage or disease process, the primary goals of implementing a nutritional management plan for either a population or for a specific individual should be to provide adequate amounts of energy and levels of all essential nutrients. There is no guarantee that a varied diet will provide "balance over time," and no evidence is available to suggest that a diet supplying essential micronutrients from whole foods is superior in any way to a diet that relies on supplement products to provide essential nutrients.

With the growing use of alternative diets among cat owners, it is important to maintain good communication regarding dietary choices with clients. Understanding the motives that drive selection of alternative foods can help veterinarians guide clients to dietary options that balance client concerns with the nutritional needs of their pet. Educating owners regarding potential risks and safe alternatives will help ensure that an appropriate and safe diet is fed.

REFERENCES

1. Petfood Industry: *Product safety and alternative petfoods report released* (web page): http://www.petfoodindustry.com/viewnews.aspx?id=14364&terms=ALTERNATIVE+PET+FOODS.
2. Association of American Feed Control Officials: *Official feed terms. Official publication of the Association of American Feed Control Officials*, Oxford, IN, 2008, AAFCO, p 246.
3. Interim Report of the National Organic Program, *Organic Pet Food Task Force* (web page): http://www.ams.usda.gov/nosb/meetings/OrgPetFood.pdf.
4. Association of American Feed Control Officials: *Pet food label claims*. In *AAFCO pet food and specialty pet food labeling guide*, Oxford, IN, 2007, AAFCO, p 74.
5. Petfood Industry. *"Human food grade" to stay on petfood* (web page): http://www.petfoodindustry.com/ViewContent.aspx?id=19032.
6. Lauten SD, Smith TM, Kirk CA, et al: Computer analysis of nutrient sufficiency of published home-cooked diets for dogs and cats [abstract], *J Vet Intern Med* 19:476, 2005.
7. Streiff EL, Zwischenberger B, Butterwick RF, et al: A comparison of the nutritional adequacy of home-prepared and commercial diets for dogs, *J Nutr* 132(6 Suppl 2):1698S, 2002.
8. Roudebush P, Cowell CS: Results of a hypoallergenic diet survey of veterinarians in North America with a nutritional evaluation of homemade diet prescriptions, *Vet Dermatol* 3:23, 2002.
9. Weese JS: Bacterial evaluation of commercial canine and feline raw diets, *Can Vet J* 46:513, 2005.
10. Strohmeyer RA, Morley PS, Hyatt DR, et al: Evaluation of bacterial and protozoal contamination of commercially available raw meat diets for dogs, *J Am Vet Med Assoc* 228:537, 2006.
11. Chengappa MM, Staats J, Oberst RD, et al: Prevalence of *Salmonella* in raw meat used in diets of racing greyhounds, *J Vet Diagn Invest* 5:372, 1993.
12. Stiver SL, Frazier KS, Mauel MJ, et al: Septicemic salmonellosis in two cats fed a raw-meat diet, *J Am Anim Hosp Assoc* 39:538, 2003.
13. Morley PS, Strohmeyer RA, Tankson JD, et al: Evaluation of the association between feeding raw meat and *Salmonella enterica* infections at a Greyhound breeding facility, *J Am Vet Med Assoc* 228:1524, 2006.
14. Scelfo GM, Flegal AR: Lead in calcium supplements, *Environ Health Perspect* 108:309, 2000.
15. Finely R, Ribble C, Aramini J, et al: The risk of salmonellae shedding by dogs fed *Salmonella*-contaminated commercial raw food, *Can Vet J* 48:69, 2007.
16. Finley R, Reid-Smith R, Weese JS: Human health implications of *Salmonella*-contaminated natural pet treats and raw pet food, *Clin Infect Dis* 42:686, 2006.
17. FDA, Center for Veterinary Medicine. FDA tips for preventing foodborne illness associated with pet food and pet treats. *Center for Veterinary Medicine* (website): http://www.fda.gov/cvm/foodbornetips.htm.
18. Wakefield LA, Shofer FS, Michel KE: Evaluation of cats fed vegetarian diets and the attitudes of their caregivers, *J Am Vet Med Assoc* 229:70, 2006.
19. MacDonald ML, Rogers QR, Morris JG: Nutrition of the domestic cat, a mammalian carnivore, *Annu Rev Nutr* 4:521, 1984.
20. Gray CM, Sellon RK, Freeman LM: Nutritional adequacy of two vegan diets for cats, *J Am Vet Med Assoc* 225:1670, 2004.

21. Skidmore-Roth L: *Mosby's handbook of herbs and natural supplements*, ed 2, St. Louis, 2004, Mosby.

22. Lanham-New SA: Importance of calcium, vitamin D and vitamin K for osteoporosis prevention and treatment, *Proc Nutr Soc* 67:163, 2008.

23. Makrides M, Crowther CA, Gibson RA, et al: Efficacy and tolerability of low-dose iron supplements during pregnancy: a randomized controlled trial, *Am J Clin Nutr* 78:145, 2003.

24. Ryan-Harshman M, Aldoori W: Folic acid and prevention of neural tube defects, *Can Fam Physician* 54:36, 2008.

25. Robertson JE, Christopher MM, Rogers QR: Heinz body formation in cats fed baby food containing onion powder, *J Am Vet Med Assoc* 212:1260, 1998.

26. Hill AS, Werner JA, Rogers QR, et al: Lipoic acid is 10 times more toxic in cats than reported in humans, dogs or rats, *J Anim Physiol Anim Nutr (Berl)* 88:150, 2004.

27. Walkiw O, Douglas DE: Health food supplements prepared from kelp—a source of elevated urinary arsenic, *Clin Toxicol* 8:325, 1975.

28. Amster E, Tiwary A, Schenker MB: Case report: potential arsenic toxicosis secondary to herbal kelp supplement, *Environ Health Perspect* 115:606, 2007.

29. Ross EA, Szabo NJ, Tebbett IR: Lead content of calcium supplements, *JAMA* 284:1425, 2000.

30. Taylor EN, Curhan GC: Determinants of 24-hour urinary oxalate excretion, *Clin J Am Soc Nephrol* 3:1453, 2008.

31. Stokes JE, Forrester SD: New and unusual causes of acute renal failure in dogs and cats, *Vet Clin North Am Small Anim Pract* 34:909, 2004.

14 Nutritional Management of Chronic Kidney Disease

Denise A. Elliott

Chronic kidney disease (CKD) has been reported to affect one in three cats over the age of 12 years.[1] A study by Jepson et al reported that within 12 months, one in three cats aged 9 years or older developed biochemical evidence of azotemia.[2] Although CKD is a leading cause of death in cats, progression to an end stage is not inevitable in all cases. Indeed, recent research continues to elucidate key risk factors for progression, and to identify therapies designed to slow disease progression.

Dietary therapy has remained at the forefront of the management of CKD for decades. There are two fundamental approaches of nutrition in CKD: the first is the essential role that certain nutrients have in altering disease progression, and the second is the role of nutrition in controlling clinical signs of uremia and improving the quality of life. Nutritional therapy introduced in Stages II and III of CKD is aimed at factors that delay progression; whereas once late stage III/IV has been reached, clinical signs of the uremic syndrome are evident and dietary treatment is designed more to improve the quality of life of the patient than to slow disease progression (see Chapter 47). Regular monitoring to ensure that dietary and medical management remains optimal for the needs of the patient is crucial for the long-term successful treatment of the patient with CKD.

ENERGY

Sufficient energy needs to be provided to prevent endogenous protein catabolism that will result in malnutrition and exacerbation of azotemia. The energy requirements of cats have been reported to be 50 to 60 kcal/kg/day, although there is a 25 per cent variation in individual energy requirements. Age, activity level, and the effect of neutering (spay or castration) can affect the energy requirements of any individual cat significantly. This starting point should be adjusted based on serial determinations of body weight and body condition score. Carbohydrate and fat provide the nonprotein sources of energy in the diet. Fat provides approximately twice the energy per gram than carbohydrate. Therefore fat increases the energy density of the diet, which allows the patient to obtain its nutritional requirements from a smaller volume of food. A smaller volume of food minimizes gastric distension, which reduces the likelihood of nausea and vomiting. Traditionally the level of fat in the diet designed for cats with CKD is between 30 and 50 per cent metabolizable energy (ME). The level of carbohydrate is determined by the level of protein restriction (see the following). There have not been any studies to evaluate the type of carbohydrate; however, highly digestible

Table 14-1 Therapeutic Agents That Can Be Used to Stimulate the Appetite

Agent*	Conventional Dose	Contraindications
Cyproheptadine†	2-4 mg/cat PO q12h	Antiserotoninergic; can cause sedation or paradoxical excitability, aggression and vomiting
Oxazepam	2 mg/cat PO q12h	Contraindicated in hepatic disease
Diazepam†	0.2 mg/kg IV	
Mianserin chlorohydrate	2-4 mg/kg PO q24h	Excitability, aggression, vomiting
Mirtazapine	⅛ to ¼ of a 15-mg tablet PO q72h	Excitability, aggression, vomiting

*Most of these drugs have not been approved for use in the cat.
†Agent undergoes renal excretion and the dosage must be adjusted accordingly to prevent toxicity.

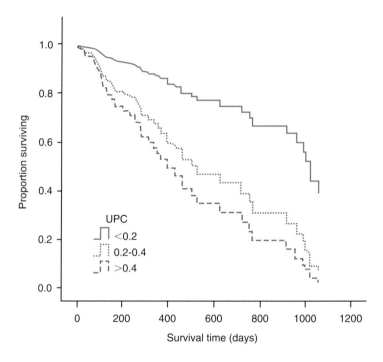

Figure 14-1 Survival curves of 126 cats with chronic kidney disease, stratified according to the urine protein:creatinine ratio.

carbohydrate sources such as rice would appear to be logical choices, given the effect that uremia can have on gastrointestinal health.

Cats with CKD often are anorexic or have reduced appetites. However, the efficiency of nutritional therapy depends on the diet being fed consistently and exclusively. Therefore the diet must be palatable enough to avoid any risk of refusal. Practical measures to improve intake include the use of highly odorous foods, warming the foods prior to feeding, and stimulating eating by positive reinforcement with petting and stroking behavior. Appetite stimulants such as the benzodiazepam derivatives or serotonin antagonists (Table 14-1) may be administered judiciously to cats who are hyporexic or show decreased interest in food; however, in many of these cases, more aggressive therapy such as esophagostomy or gastrostomy tube feeding is clinically indicated (see Chapter 12).

In human beings, and most likely cats, uremia affects the sense of taste and smell, and coupled with food aversion these factors can contribute to food refusal or inappetence. In this regard it is not advisable to institute dietary changes when cats are hospitalized. Rather the renal support diet should be instituted in the home environment when the cat is stable.

PROTEIN

PROTEINURIA

Studies by Syme et al suggested that the upper limit of the reference range for the urine protein:creatinine ratio (UPC) for healthy aged cats is 0.4.[3] Recent evidence suggests that the UPC is an independent risk factor for all-cause mortality of cats with CKD,[3,4] with systemic hypertension,[5] and with uremic crisis[6] (see Chapter 49). Plasma creatinine concentration and blood pressure are risk factors associated with proteinuria. Age, plasma creatinine, and proteinuria are significant and independent risk factors associated with reduced survival time of cats with CKD.[3] Indeed cats with a UPC greater than 0.4 have a four times higher risk of death compared with cats with a UPC less than 0.2 (Figure 14-1).

Glomerular capillary hypertension, hyperfiltration, and mild proteinuria have been reported in cats following renal mass reduction.[7] This leakage of protein into the glomerular filtrate has been implicated in causing renal pathology. Excessive leakage of protein appears to overwhelm the normal reuptake process of the proximal tubule cells. As a consequence the proximal tubule cells are stimulated to secrete several inflammatory cytokines including endothelin-1, monocyte chemoattractant protein-1 (MCP-1), and RANTES (Regulated upon Activation, Normal T Cell Expressed, and Secreted). These agents contribute to interstitial inflammation and fibrosis, which then leads to development of tubular dysfunction and eventually reduced ability to concentrate urine.[8]

Because proteinuria is a significant risk factor for reduced survival in cats with CKD, therapeutic strategies should be employed to minimize the proteinuria. Specific treatment should be instituted when the UPC is greater than 0.4 in cats without concurrent evidence of inflammatory or infectious lower urinary tract signs that could cause proteinuria. Angiotensin converting enzyme inhibitor therapy has been shown to reduce glomerular capillary pressure and to lower the UPC.[4,9]

The effect of dietary protein restriction on proteinuria in cats with stage II/III disease is not clear. Initial studies in feline remnant kidney models suggested a beneficial effect of protein restriction on the development of glomerular lesions.[10,11] However, the results of these studies were confounded by alterations in both protein and energy intake. A subsequent study by Finco et al failed to demonstrate a benefit of protein restriction on renal lesions.[12] The cats in Finco's study developed borderline proteinuria (UPC 0.24 to 0.27); however, no significant difference in UPC was noted between any of the groups of cats. Based on studies in other species, it seems logical that restricting protein intake would limit feeding-related hyperfiltration. The patients most likely to benefit are those with UPC greater than 0.4. It is clear that further studies are required to evaluate the effect of protein restriction on proteinuria and disease progression in cats with naturally occurring CKD.

UREMIA

Every cat who is symptomatic for Stage III/IV CKD should benefit from a protein-restricted diet. At this stage of disease, the buildup of nitrogenous waste products reaches a level at which appetite is affected and irritation of the mucosal membranes with nausea and vomiting occurs. Controlled reduction of nonessential protein results in decreased production of nitrogenous wastes with consequent amelioration or elimination of clinical signs, even though renal function may remain essentially unchanged. The minimal dietary protein requirements for cats with CKD are not known, but are presumed to be similar to the minimal protein requirements of normal cats (i.e., 3.97 to 4.96 g/kg/day). However, this degree of restriction is necessary only in cats with profound uremia. For cats with documented azotemia and clinical signs, dietary protein should be reduced to approximately 20 to 25 per cent protein on a metabolizable energy (ME) basis.

The dietary protein then should be adjusted to minimize excesses in azotemia while simultaneously avoiding excessive restriction because of the risk of protein malnutrition. Laboratory indicators of malnutrition include hypoalbuminemia, decreased blood urea nitrogen, hypocholesterolemia, anemia, and lymphopenia. However, alterations of these common laboratory indicators of malnutrition often are indistinguishable from those that can occur with CKD and/or concurrent disease. Furthermore, significant and often irreversible protein malnutrition has occurred prior to alterations in laboratory indicators. Clearly the dietary history and physical examination including body weight, body condition score, and cachexia score are more appropriate and sensitive indicators of protein malnutrition. The initial loss of lean body mass can be subtle and usually is first noted in the epaxial, gluteal, scapular, or temporal muscles. A subjective cachexia scoring system will facilitate the identification of those patients either with cachexia or at risk of impending cachexia (Table 14-2). If evidence of protein malnutrition occurs, dietary protein should be increased gradually until these abnormalities are corrected.

PHOSPHATE

Phosphate retention and hyperphosphatemia occur early in CKD,[13] and play a primary role in the genesis and progression of renal secondary hyperparathyroidism, renal osteodystrophy, and relative or absolute deficiency of 1,25-dihydroxyvitamin D. Soft-tissue calcification and nephrocalcinosis may contribute to progression of renal injury. By minimizing hyperphosphatemia, secondary hyperparathyroidism and its sequelae can be prevented.[14] A recent retrospective case review of 211 cats with naturally occurring CKD reported that for each 1 U increase in the phosphorus level at the time of diagnosis, there is an 11.8 per cent increase in the risk of death.[15] Reduction of dietary phosphate intake was associated with reduced mineralization and fibrosis in feline renal model studies.[16] Furthermore, control of phosphate concentrations has been associated with a reduction in all-cause mortality in cats with naturally occurring CKD.[17]

The International Renal Interest Society recommends that the serum phosphate concentration should be

Table 14-2 Cachexia Scoring System

Cachexia Score	Description
0	Good muscle tone with no evidence of muscle wasting
1	Early, mild muscle wasting, especially in the hindquarters and lumbar region
2	Moderate muscle wasting apparent in all muscle groups
3	Marked muscle wasting as evidenced by atrophy of all muscle groups
4	Severe muscle wasting

maintained at 2.7 to 4.5 mg/dL for stage II; less than 5 mg/dL for stage III, and less than 6 mg/dL for stage IV disease. This may be achieved in the first instance by limiting dietary phosphate intake. If normophosphatemia can not be accomplished within 2 to 4 weeks of implementing dietary phosphate restriction, intestinal phosphate binders should be added to the treatment plan. The phosphate binders must be mixed with the food. Adequate hydration also is important to facilitate renal phosphate excretion (see the following).

FLUID BALANCE

Osmotic polyuria and compensatory polydipsia are fundamental consequences of CKD. To guarantee adequate hydration status, it is necessary to ensure that the cat has ready access to fresh water at all times. However, some patients will fail to consume sufficient water and will become dehydrated. A retrospective case study by Boyd et al reported that 30 per cent (19 of 64 cats) with stage IV CKD had prerenal azotemia.[15] Dehydration and volume depletion have several adverse consequences including the risk of precipitating acute-on-chronic kidney disease. Methods to encourage water intake include providing bowls in several locations, using bowls with a wide surface area so that the cat's sensitive whiskers do not touch the side of the bowl, keeping the bowl full of fresh water, providing a variety of water types (e.g., distilled, bottled, warm, cool), providing a running source of water (e.g., water fountains), and keeping the bowls away from the litter box areas. Water intake also can be increased by feeding a wet compared to a dry diet, providing a highly digestible diet, and offering multiple small meals, because water intake in cats has been shown to increase significantly by increasing meal frequency.

When the above methods are inadequate to maintain fluid balance, fluid supplementation is necessary. Subcutaneous fluid supplementation with maintenance fluids (e.g., plasmalyte 56, plasmalyte M, Normosol M) has long been the traditional standard of care. Chronic administration of replacement fluids (e.g., lactated Ringer's solution, 0.9 per cent sodium chloride) is not recommended because these fluids may contribute to hypernatremia as they do not provide sufficient free water. Conversely, 5% dextrose in water also is not recommended for subcutaneous administration because of its hypotonicity. Enteral feeding devices (e.g., esophagostomy or gastrostomy tubes) provide an effective solution to not only facilitate dietary intake, but also to allow for the administration of water and maintenance of euvolemia (see Chapter 12).

ELECTROLYTES

SODIUM

Sodium restriction has been recommended historically for cats with CKD. The rationale was based on the reduced ability of the remaining nephrons to excrete sodium, and the concern that whole body sodium accumulation would contribute to the development of hypertension. Hypertension is indeed common in cats with CKD and has been implicated with progression of kidney disease (see Chapter 49). Approximately 20 per cent of cats with naturally occurring CKD have arterial blood pressures that place them at severe risk of target organ (kidney, eye, brain, heart) damage secondary to hypertension. However, blood pressure is not higher in cats with more severe CKD.[18] Furthermore, blood pressure increases gradually over time in cats with naturally occurring CKD, but this is not associated with a decline in kidney function.[19]

There have not been any reported studies demonstrating that sodium restriction will alleviate hypertension or slow disease progression. Syme[19] reported that systolic blood pressure did not change following the introduction of a sodium-restricted renal care diet to cats with naturally occurring CKD.[19] The plasma aldosterone concentration and plasma renin activity were higher when the cats were consuming the sodium-restricted renal diet. A recent study in cats with surgically induced kidney disease reported that sodium restriction (0.5 g/1000 kcal) activated the renin-angiotensin-aldosterone system, significantly lowered plasma potassium concentration, and had no effect on arterial blood pressure.[20] Therefore the ideal dietary sodium concentrations for cats with CKD have not been defined clearly, and it is not known if reducing sodium intake will limit the increases in blood pressure that occur over time in cats with CKD.

POTASSIUM

Hypokalemia occurs in about 20 per cent of cats with CKD, although this number may underestimate the true prevalence of whole body potassium depletion.[21] Furthermore, an association between CKD and hypokalemia has been reported in cats.[22,23] Dow et al hypothesized that potassium depletion may lead to a self-perpetuating cycle of renal damage and further potassium loss.[24] However, the causal relationship between whole body potassium deficit and progressive renal injury remains to be proved.

Hypokalemia can occur at any stage of disease. Elliott et al reported hypokalemia in 14.3 per cent of cats with stage II, 25 per cent of cats with stage III, and 30 per cent of cats in stage IV disease.[25] Hypokalemia typically is mild, and is not associated with overt clinical signs; however, the clinician should not wait for clinical signs before treating for hypokalemia. Clinical improvement in appetite and activity level has been noted following potassium supplementation. Hypokalemia also appears to be associated with an increased risk of systemic hypertension in cats with CKD.[18] However, a randomized controlled clinical trial failed to identify any beneficial effect of potassium gluconate supplementation on blood pressure or kidney function in cats with naturally occurring CKD.[25]

Not all cats with CKD are hypokalemic. One study reported 13 per cent of 116 cats with CKD were hyperkalemic,[26] emphasizing the need to monitor potassium status and adjust intake with oral potassium gluconate on an individual basis.

ACID-BASE BALANCE

The kidneys excrete metabolically derived nonvolatile acid (sulfates, hydrogen ions) and hence are central to maintenance of acid-base balance. As renal function is lost, the capacity to excrete hydrogen ions and reabsorb bicarbonate ions is lost and metabolic acidosis ensues. Metabolic acidosis results in increased renal ammoniagenesis, which has been associated with activation of complement, culminating in the progression of renal failure. In addition, metabolic acidosis increases catabolism and degradation of skeletal muscle protein, disrupts intracellular metabolism, and promotes dissolution of bone mineral, thus exacerbating azotemia, loss of lean body mass, and renal osteodystrophy. Metabolic acidosis exacerbates the likelihood of hypokalemia occurring because potassium moves out of the cells in response to metabolic acidosis and is lost in urine. Dietary protein restriction results in the consumption of reduced quantities of protein-derived acid precursors; however, this alone is rarely adequate to prevent metabolic acidosis.

Metabolic acidosis typically is evident in cats by late stage III (prevalence 15 per cent) and stage IV (prevalence 52.6 per cent) CKD.[27] At these stages, supplementation with alkalinizing agents such as sodium bicarbonate, calcium carbonate, or potassium citrate is required to maintain bicarbonate levels between 18 to 24 mmol/L. Whether providing alkali supplementation prior to the detection of metabolic acidosis would be beneficial remains to be determined. The choice of alkalinizing agent is determined by patient factors, including palatability when added to the diet, the presence of hypokalemia (when potassium salts will be chosen), and the presence of hyperphosphatemia (calcium salts may be considered because of their phosphate-binding capabilities, as long as hypercalcemia does not occur).

MISCELLANEOUS NUTRIENTS

Long-chain omega-3 fatty acids (eicosapentaenoic acid [EPA] and docosahexaenoic acid [DHA]) compete with arachidonic acid and alter eicosanoid production. Preliminary renal model studies in other species have reported that supplementation with long chain n-3 fatty acids lowered glomerular capillary pressure, reduced proteinuria, and slowed progressive decline in glomerular filtration rate.[28] Omega-6 fatty acids (safflower oil) appeared to be detrimental to renal disease.[29] Some commercially available diets have an adjusted omega-6:omega-3 ratio of 5:1; however, the ideal ratio for diets has yet to be determined. Rather than focusing on ratios, the absolute concentrations of specific omega-3 fatty acids would be more appropriate. Polyunsaturated fatty acid metabolism is unique in cats because they lack delta-6 desaturase. Although studies of the effect of variation in dietary fatty acid composition in cats with CKD have not been performed, providing EPA and DHA derived from fish oil probably is important. Studies are clearly needed to evaluate the effect of n-3 fatty acid supplementation on proteinuria and disease progression in cats with CKD.

Fermentable fiber is a recent addition to the nutritional management of CKD. It is hypothesized that the fermentable fiber provides a source of carbohydrate nutrition for gastrointestinal bacteria, which then utilize blood urea as a source of nitrogen for growth, increasing fecal nitrogen excretion in the bacterial cell mass, decreasing urinary nitrogen excretion, and thereby reducing the need for protein restriction. However, the major concern with this concept is that unlike blood urea nitrogen, the classical uremic toxins (middle-molecules) are too large in molecular size to cross membrane barriers readily. As a consequence, it is highly unlikely that these toxins are reduced by bacterial utilization of ammonia. Furthermore, studies to document these changes have not been reported. As a consequence, widespread application of fermentable fiber as a nitrogen trap can not be recommended at this time.

Fiber may be beneficial, however, for modulating gastrointestinal health in patients with CKD. Constipation can occur in cats with CKD. The causes are numerous and include dehydration, reduced gastrointestinal motility, high doses of phosphate binders, and as a side effect of other therapeutic agents such as calcium channel blockers used to manage hypertension. Therefore the addition of mixed fibers to increase fecal bulk, and ensure the production of soft but formed feces, is beneficial for cats with CKD.

Endothelial cell dysfunction is thought to contribute to systemic hypertension, glomerular pathology, progressive proteinuria, and tubular interstitial inflammation and fibrosis in human and animal models of kidney disease. There are several proposed mechanisms of action by which endothelial cell dysfunction arises in renal disease. These include a reduction in the renal synthesis of L-arginine, the precursor of nitric oxide; oxidative stress, which reduces nitric oxide release from the endothelium and stimulates the production of profibrotic mediators from the endothelium; and the accumulation of asymmetric dimethylarginine (ADMA), an inhibitor of endothelial nitric oxide synthase. Jepson et al reported that ADMA accumulates in stages II, III, and IV of CKD, and the plasma concentration of ADMA correlated with the serum creatinine concentration.[30]

There have not been any studies to date to evaluate the effect of nutrients on endothelial cell dysfunction in cats with CKD. However, several strategies may be considered, including supplementation with L-arginine; flavonols; and antioxidants such as vitamin E, vitamin C, taurine, lutein, lycopene, or β-carotene. L-arginine may increase the production of nitric oxide and counteract the inhibition induced by ADMA. Flavonols increase the endothelial production of nitric oxide, are effective antioxidants that trap free radicals generated by circulatory disorders within the glomeruli that occur in CKD, and have an antihypertensive action.[31]

CLINICAL EFFICACY

The effect of a modified protein, low-phosphate diet on the outcome of 50 cats with stable, naturally occurring stage II/III CKD has been reported by Elliott et al.[17]

Table 14-3 Nutritional Recommendations Based on the Stage of Chronic Kidney Disease

	Stage I	Stage II	Stage III	Stage IV
Hydration	Fresh water at all times	Fresh water at all times	Fresh water at all times	Fresh water at all times
Control phosphate		2.7-4.5 mg/dL	<5 mg/dL	<6 mg/dL
Protein modification	UPC >0.4	UPC >0.4	Appropriate dietary protein reduction to decrease phosphorus concentration, minimize uremia	Appropriate dietary protein reduction to decrease phosphorus concentration, minimize uremia
Control acidosis			Maintain bicarbonate 18-24 mmol/L	Maintain bicarbonate 18-24 mmol/L
Control potassium		Maintain potassium >3.5 mmol/L	Maintain potassium >3.5 mmol/L	Maintain potassium >3.5 mmol/L
Control blood pressure		Maintain systolic arterial blood pressure <175 mm Hg	Maintain systolic arterial blood pressure <175 mm Hg	Maintain systolic arterial blood pressure <175 mm Hg
Prevent protein calorie malnutrition		Monitor food intake, body weight, body condition score, cachexia score	Monitor food intake, body weight, body condition score, cachexia score	Feeding tube intervention

Twenty-nine of the 50 cats received a modified protein, low-phosphate diet, while the other 21 cats remained on their normal diets. The median survival time of the cats fed the modified protein, low-phosphate diet was significantly greater than the cats fed the normal diet (633 days versus 264 days, $p < 0.0036$). Cats fed a renal diet had a median survival time that was 2.4 times longer than cats fed a maintenance diet. The results of this study suggest that feeding a renal diet to cats with CKD will double their life expectancy.

Ross et al, using a randomized controlled masked clinical trial, evaluated the effect of a renal diet on time to uremic crisis or renal death in cats with naturally occurring stage II/III CKD.[32] The renal diet was associated with a significantly lower number of uremic crises and renal-related deaths compared to a maintenance diet.

Both renal diets used in the above clinical studies included a combination of nutrient alterations compared to maintenance diets; therefore it is not possible to hypothesize which of the nutrient alterations was responsible for the improved clinical outcome for the cats with CKD. Nevertheless, the evidence from these clinical studies indicates that nutritional intervention is clearly warranted for cats with naturally occurring CKD (Table 14-3).

SUMMARY

Diet plays an important role in the management of cats with CKD. Implementation of nutritional therapy at stages II and III will improve survival and limit uremic crises. Phosphorus restriction clearly is indicated to slow disease progression. Protein restriction is indicated in patients with marked proteinuria (UPC > 0.4). Potassium and alkali supplementation are necessary only in patients who are hypokalemic or acidotic, respectively. Nutri-

tional therapy for cats with stage III and IV disease is designed to improve the quality of life and minimize the clinical signs associated with uremia. Regardless of the stage of the disease, the diet must be tailored to the individual needs of the patient, and adjustments are to be expected through the course of treatment. Clinical studies have clearly demonstrated that dietary therapy can make a significant difference on disease progression and outcome in cats with naturally occurring CKD.

REFERENCES

1. Lulich JP, Osborne CA, O'Brien TD, et al: Feline renal failure: questions, answers, questions, *Compend Contin Educ Pract Vet* 14:127, 1992.
2. Jepson RE, Syme HM, Vallance C, et al: Proteinuria, albuminuria, creatinine concentration and urine specific gravity as prospective predictors for the development of azotemia in cats, *J Vet Intern Med* 21:598, 2007.
3. Syme HM, Markwell PJ, Pfeiffer DU, et al: Survival of cats with naturally occurring chronic renal failure is related to severity of proteinuria, *J Vet Intern Med* 20:528, 2006.
4. King JN, Gunn-Moore DA, Tasker S, et al: Benazepril in renal insufficiency in cats study group: tolerability and efficacy of benazepril in cats with chronic kidney disease, *J Vet Intern Med* 20:1054, 2006.
5. Jepson RE, Elliott J, Brodbelt D, et al: Evaluation of the effects of control of systolic blood pressure on survival in cats with systemic hypertension, *J Vet Intern Med* 3:402, 2007.
6. Kuwahara Y, Ohba Y, Kitih K, et al: Association of laboratory data and death within one month in cats with chronic renal failure, *J Small Anim Pract* 47:446, 2006.
7. Brown SA, Brown CA: Single-nephron adaptations to partial renal ablation in cats, *Am J Physiol* 269:R1002, 1995.
8. Remuzzi G, Bertani T: Pathophysiology of progressive nephropathies, *N Engl J Med* 339:1448, 1998.
9. Brown SA, Brown CA, Jacobs G, et al: Effects of the angiotensin converting enzyme inhibitor benazepril in cats with induced renal insufficiency, *Am J Vet Res* 62:375, 2001.

10. Adams LG, Polzin DJ, Osborne CA, et al: Effects of dietary protein and calorie restriction in clinically normal cats and in cats with surgically induced chronic renal failure, *Am J Vet Res* 54:1653, 1993.

11. Adams LG, Polzin DJ, Osborne CA, et al: Influence of dietary protein/calorie intake on renal morphology and function in cats with 5/6 nephrectomy, *Lab Invest* 70:347, 1994.

12. Finco DR, Brown SA, Brown CA, et al: Protein and calorie effects on progression of induced chronic renal failure in cats, *Am J Vet Res* 59:575, 1998.

13. Barber PJ, Elliott J: Feline chronic renal failure: calcium homeostasis in 80 cases diagnosed between 1992 and 1995, *J Small Anim Pract* 39:108, 1998.

14. Barber PJ, Rawlings JM, Markwell PJ, et al: Effect of dietary phosphate restriction on secondary renal hyperparathyroidism in the cat, *J Small Anim Pract* 40:62, 1999.

15. Boyd LM, Langston C, Thompson K, et al: Survival in cats with naturally occurring chronic kidney disease (2000-2002), *J Vet Intern Med* 22:1111, 2008.

16. Ross LA, Finco DR, Crowell WA, et al: Effect of dietary phosphorus restriction on the kidneys of cats with reduced renal mass, *Am J Vet Res* 43:1023, 1982.

17. Elliott J, Rawlings JM, Markwell PJ, et al: Survival of cats with naturally occurring renal failure: effect of conventional dietary management, *J Small Anim Pract* 41:235, 2000.

18. Syme HM, Barber PJ, Rawlings JM, et al: Incidence of hypertension in cats with naturally occurring chronic renal failure, *J Am Vet Med Assoc* 220:1799, 2002.

19. Syme HM: *Studies of the epidemiology and aetiology of hypertension in the cat*. PhD thesis, 2003, University of London.

20. Buranakarl C, Mathur S, Brown SA: Effects of dietary sodium chloride intake on renal function and blood pressure in cats with normal and reduced renal function, *Am J Vet Res* 65:620, 2004.

21. Theisen SK, DiBartola SP, Radin J, et al: Muscle potassium and potassium gluconate supplementation in normokalemic cats with naturally occurring chronic renal failure, *J Vet Intern Med* 11:212, 1997.

22. DiBartola SP, Rutgers HC, Zack PM, et al: Clinicopathologic findings associated with chronic renal disease in cats: 74 cases (1973-1984), *J Am Vet Med Assoc* 190:1196, 1987.

23. Elliott J, Barber PJ: Feline chronic renal failure: clinical findings in 80 cases diagnosed between 1992 and 1995, *J Small Anim Pract* 39:78, 1998.

24. Dow SW, Fettman MJ: Chronic renal disease and potassium depletion in cats, *Semin Vet Med Surg (Small Anim)* 7:198, 1992.

25. Elliott J, Syme HM: Response of cats with chronic renal failure to dietary potassium supplementation, *J Vet Intern Med* 17:418, 2003.

26. Dow SW, Fettman MJ, Curtis CR, et al: Hypokalemia in cats: 136 cases (1984-1987), *J Am Vet Med Assoc* 194:1604, 1989.

27. Elliott J, Syme HM, Reubens E, et al: Assessment of acid-base status of cats with naturally occurring chronic renal failure, *J Small Anim Pract* 44:65, 2003.

28. Brown SA, Brown CA, Crowell WA, et al: Beneficial effects of chronic administration of dietary omega-3 polyunsaturated fatty acids in dogs with renal insufficiency, *J Lab Clin Med* 13:447, 1998.

29. Brown SA, Brown CA, Crowell WA, et al: Effects of dietary polyunsaturated fatty acid supplementation in early renal insufficiency in dogs, *J Lab Clin Med* 135:275, 2000.

30. Jepson RE, Elliott J, Syme HM: Evaluation of plasma asymmetric dimethylarginine (ADMA), symmetric dimethylarginine (SDMA) and l-arginine in cats with renal disease, *J Vet Intern Med* 22:317, 2008.

31. Jouad H, Lacaille-Dubois MA, Lyoussi B, et al: Effects of the flavonoids extracted from *Spergularia purpurea* Pers. on arterial blood pressure and renal function in normal and hypertensive rats, *J Ethnopharmacol* 76:159, 2001.

32. Ross SJ, Osborne CA, Kirk CA, et al: Clinical evaluation of dietary modification for treatment of spontaneous chronic kidney disease in cats, *J Am Vet Med Assoc* 229:949, 2006.

SECTION
III

Gastrointestinal System

Jörg M. Steiner, Section Editor

CHAPTER

15 Gastrointestinal Function Testing

Audrey K. Cook

The overall purpose of the gastrointestinal (GI) system is the assimilation of nutrients and calories. This necessitates the movement, digestion, and absorption of food, and requires the support of the liver, exocrine pancreas, and autonomic nervous system. Selective permeability also is essential, allowing the entry of digested particles without the loss of valuable molecules and fluid into the intestinal lumen. In addition, the GI tract must detect and eliminate toxins and pathogens, while maintaining immunological tolerance towards food antigens.

Patients with GI disease present with signs reflecting compromise to one or more of these functions (Table 15-1). Although our ability to assess GI function is limited, it is sometimes useful to evaluate patients critically from this perspective and also serves as a reminder of the complexity of the GI system.

THE ROLE OF GI FUNCTION TESTS

The investigation of cats with GI disease can be challenging because clinical signs often are nonspecific and the initial patient evaluation (Table 15-2) frequently is unremarkable. Therefore it is essential to investigate GI function systematically before considering more invasive diagnostic tests or therapeutic trials. Function tests may provide a definitive answer, but more often the results confirm or localize GI disease and complement other

clinical findings (e.g., imaging studies, histopathological findings) (Box 15-1). Ideal function tests have high positive and negative predictive values, good accuracy (defined by both a high sensitivity and high specificity), involve minimal patient risk or discomfort, and have a low cost/benefit ratio. The positive and negative predictive values of a test provide an indication of the reliability of the result (either positive or negative) in a given patient. However, they are difficult to determine and most studies therefore only report the sensitivity and specificity of the test in question. These parameters are inferior to positive and negative predictive values because they do not address the prevalence of disease in a certain patient population. This chapter will review both established and novel GI function tests (Table 15-3) and describe their indications and limitations.

MOTILITY

A healthy GI tract moves food from the mouth to the distal colon, allowing adequate time for digestion and absorption. Waste products then are stored in the rectum until they are voided voluntarily. Normal GI motility is controlled principally by the intrinsic enteric nervous system, with additional input from the central nervous system. Derangements in motility may be primary or secondary, and may lead to regurgitation, vomiting, diarrhea, obstipation, or constipation.

147

Table 15-1 Summary of Gastrointestinal Functions and Signs of Compromise

Function	Signs of Compromise
Motility	Anorexia, regurgitation, vomiting, constipation, diarrhea
Digestion	Diarrhea, weight loss, polyphagia
Absorption	Diarrhea, weight loss
Permeability	Diarrhea, weight loss
Immunological responses	Anorexia, diarrhea, vomiting, weight loss

Table 15-2 Minimum Database for a Cat with Suspected Gastrointestinal Disease

Data	Comments
History	Include information on diet and food intake
Physical examination	Assess weight loss, body condition, and hydration status
Complete blood count	Including blood smear examination
Chemistry profile	Including electrolytes
Urine analysis	Including sediment examination
Thyroid evaluation	Indicated in any cat over 5 years of age
Retroviral testing (FeLV and FIV)	Indicated in any cat if >12 months since last test
Fecal examination	Flotation and direct examination; PCR test for *Tritrichomonas foetus*, especially in young cats

FeLV, Feline leukemia virus; *FIV,* feline immunodeficiency virus; *PCR,* polymerase chain reaction.

Box 15-1 Clinical Applications of Gastrointestinal Function Testing

- Identify patients with occult gastrointestinal disease/dysfunction.
- Localize gastrointestinal disease/dysfunction.
- Guide therapeutic decisions.
- Monitor response to therapy.
- Monitor disease progression.
- Complement information gained from other diagnostic tests.

PRIMARY MOTILITY DISORDERS

Primary motility disorders arise from pathological processes directly affecting the smooth muscle or its innervation. Examples include cricopharyngeal dysphagia, idiopathic megaesophagus, idiopathic megacolon, and feline dysautonomia.

Table 15-3 Gastrointestinal Function Tests

Function	Function Tests
Motility	Radiographic studies—fluoroscopy, barium, BIPS* Scintigraphy ^{13}C-octanoic acid breath and blood tests[†] Ultrasonography[†] Breath hydrogen testing[†]
Digestion	Trypsin-like immunoreactivity (fTLI) Fecal proteolytic activity Fecal sudan stains Serum folate concentration
Absorption	Serum folate concentration Serum cobalamin concentration Breath hydrogen testing[†]
Permeability	Sugar probes—rhamnose/lactulose[†] ^{51}Cr-EDTA[†] Fecal feline alpha$_1$-proteinase inhibitor
Immunological responses	Retroviral testing (FIV, FeLV) Macroscopic food-sensitivity testing[†] Antigen-specific IgE measurement[†]

*Barium-impregnated radiopaque markers.

[†]No data reported for cats with spontaneous GI disease.

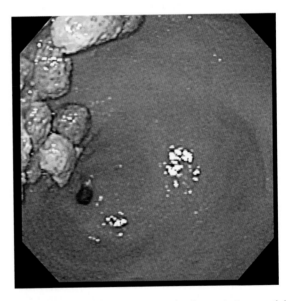

Figure 15-1 Delayed gastric emptying. Endoscopic image of the gastric antrum of a cat with infiltrative gastric disease. Retained food is noted, despite withholding food for 14 hours, indicating delayed gastric emptying. (Courtesy Dr. Michael D. Willard, Texas A&M University.)

SECONDARY MOTILITY DISORDERS

Changes in GI motility can occur in many cats with inflammatory or infiltrative bowel disease. For example, retained food is noted commonly during endoscopy in cats with GI disease and is a reliable indication of delayed gastric emptying (Figure 15-1). The mechanisms behind secondary motility disorders are not well understood, but, most likely, locally produced inflammatory mediators (e.g., cytokines) disrupt the intrinsic enteric nervous system.[1] Functional/paralytic ileus (with global impairment of normal contractility) sometimes is noted in cats with severe enteritis, although other causes (e.g., peritonitis, opioid administration) are more common.

ASSESSMENT OF PHARYNGEAL AND ESOPHAGEAL MOTILITY

Fluoroscopic Contrast Studies

Pharyngeal and esophageal motility disorders are best appreciated with fluoroscopic contrast studies, although still images also may provide a diagnosis.[2] The patient should be conscious because sedation limits the cat's ability to protect the airway from aspiration and may affect the swallowing response. In general, 5 mL of a liquid barium sulfate suspension (45 to 85 per cent w/w) should be administered and images collected immediately. If this study is unremarkable, food impregnated with barium should be given and further images collected.

ASSESSMENT OF GASTRIC MOTILITY

Radiographic Contrast Studies

Contrast radiographic studies are a simple and readily available method to assess gastric emptying.[3] However, results are influenced by patient anxiety, the use of sedation, and the physical and biochemical properties of the mixture administered. In general, a barium-water slurry usually leaves the stomach within an hour, whereas food generally is cleared by 4 to 12 hours.[4] A high fat content may slow gastric emptying substantially, and longer times (up to 16 hours) have been reported for healthy cats. Misleading results can be obtained if the barium separates from the food and leaves the stomach before the ingested material.

Barium-impregnated radiopaque markers (BIPS, Med I.D. Systems) can be used (Figure 15-2) instead of food mixed with a liquid contrast agent. BIPS also may provide information about transit through the small intestine and colon.[5] A mixture of small (1.5-mm diameter) and large (5-mm diameter) spheres is given with specific foods (listed in the package insert), and two to four radiographs are taken over the next 6 to 24 hours. The transit patterns of the two differently sized spheres are thought to mimic liquid-phase and solid-phase gastric emptying. Normal gastric clearance and intestinal transit curves are provided by the manufacturer for comparison. However, gastric emptying times determined using BIPS do not correlate well with scintigraphical studies, and it has been suggested that the 1.5-mm spheres may exceed the threshold size for liquid-phase passage through the feline pylorus.[6]

Nuclear Scintigraphy

Scintigraphy generally is regarded as the gold standard for assessment of gastric emptying. A radio-labeled marker (e.g., technetium or indium) is mixed with food, and the

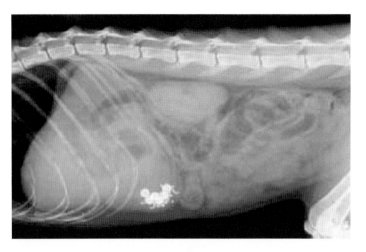

Figure 15-2 Delayed gastric emptying. Lateral abdominal radiograph of a cat taken 8 hours after administration of barium-impregnated radiopaque markers (BIPS, Med I.D. Systems). All the BIPS have settled in the antrum, indicating delayed gastric emptying. (Courtesy Med I.D. Systems.)

gastric area is scanned at timed intervals using a gamma camera. The activity measured then is converted into a graph depicting the rate of passage of ingesta from the stomach. If two markers are used, the same test can evaluate emptying times simultaneously for both liquid and solid materials. This test is performed routinely in human beings, and advanced data collection and analysis provides additional information about the frequency and velocity of gastric contractions.[7]

Nuclear scintigraphy has the advantage of being reliable and repeatable, with minimal patient stress and discomfort. However, animals and staff are exposed to ionizing radiation, and special training and equipment are required.

^{13}C-Octanoic Acid Breath or Blood Tests

These tests are simpler than scintigraphy and avoid the technical complications associated with the use of radioactive materials. Instead, the metabolism of a foodstuff labeled with a stable carbon isotope is used to indicate gastric emptying.[8] A ^{13}C-labeled medium chain triglyceride (octanoic acid) is mixed with a test meal, and serial breath or blood samples are collected at regular intervals over the next several hours. After the labeled fatty acid leaves the stomach, it is absorbed immediately in the duodenum and then transported via the portal vein to the liver. Hepatic metabolism releases the ^{13}C, which is oxidized to carbon dioxide (CO_2), which is transported to the lungs and excreted subsequently across the alveoli. Thus a rise of $^{13}CO_2$ in a gas sample extracted from blood, or in a sample of exhaled air, corresponds with duodenal filling. Breath samples can be collected with a face mask or chamber system and stored at room temperature for several months before analysis using fractional mass spectrometry, or with laser or infrared spectroscopy. Various data points, including the lag time, half excretion time, and latency phase then are calculated and compared to established normal ranges.

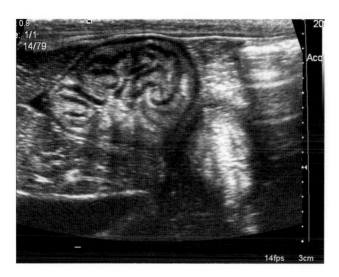

Figure 15-3 Ultrasonographic image of the gastric fundus. Note the distinct rugal folds.

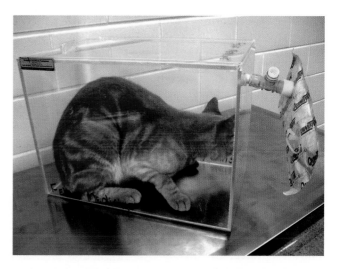

Figure 15-4 Breath collection. System for collection of exhaled breath samples in feline patients. Room air enters the chamber through a one-way valve and exhaled air is collected in the reservoir bag.

[13]C-octanoic acid testing has been described in research cats, but findings in cats with clinical disease have not been reported.[9]

Ultrasonography

Ultrasonographic assessment of gastric size may provide reliable information about emptying time and has been shown to correlate well with the results of scintigraphy in human beings.[10] Serial measurements of a standardized cross-sectional image of the antrum are collected following ingestion of a test meal, until emptying appears complete (Figure 15-3). Operator skill is required for the data to be reliable and consistent, and image collection may be compromised by excessive gas within the gastric lumen.

ASSESSMENT OF SMALL INTESTINAL MOTILITY

Radiographic Studies

Generalized ileus of the small intestine may be identified on plain radiographs as a homogeneous soft-tissue opacity or as a mixed air/fluid pattern within the bowel lumen. However, radiographic findings in patients with functional ileus may mimic those seen with distal intestinal obstructions, and contrast studies or ultrasound examination may be necessary to rule out an underlying disorder.

Breath Hydrogen Testing

Serial determination of the hydrogen concentration in exhaled air can be used to measure orocecal transit time in cats.[11] Test subjects are given meals containing a fermentable sugar (e.g., lactulose), which is metabolized by colonic bacteria. Hydrogen is released as a by-product, enters the blood stream, and is excreted across the lungs. The rise in breath hydrogen concentration therefore indicates the time at which ingested material leaves the ileum. Breath samples are collected using a chamber or face mask (Figure 15-4) and can be stored for several days

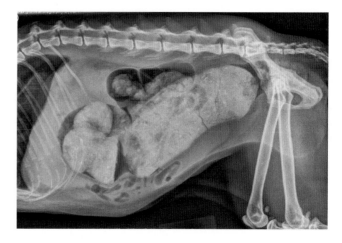

Figure 15-5 Feline megacolon. Lateral abdominal radiograph of a cat with fecal impaction and megacolon. Stool is evident within the distended colon and rectum.

prior to analysis. Bench-top analyzers are available and provide results in less than a minute. However, no commercial laboratories currently measure hydrogen breath concentrations. Transit times have been shown to be faster in kittens, but findings in cats with signs of GI disease have not been described.[12]

ASSESSMENT OF COLONIC MOTILITY

Radiographic Studies

Inadequate colonic motility results in constipation. This usually is apparent on plain abdominal radiographs (Figure 15-5). Barium-impregnated radiopaque markers may be helpful in questionable cases, and barium enemas may help rule out occult obstructions (e.g., mass or stricture).

DIGESTION

Digestion describes the breakdown of complex molecules into smaller particles, in preparation for absorption by the intestinal mucosa. Digestion begins in the mouth when saliva contacts food and then continues in the stomach and small intestine.

The majority of digestion occurs in the proximal small intestine, as enzymes are released in response to the arrival of chyme from the stomach. The exocrine pancreas is the primary site of digestive enzyme production, although the gastric mucosa (e.g., gastric lipase, pepsin, and chymosin) and brush border–associated enzymes of the intestinal mucosa (e.g., peptidases, disaccharidases) also contribute.

Although bile acids do not directly digest macronutrients, they play a crucial role in the assimilation of dietary fats through emulsification. This process converts large fat globules into microscopic particles, permitting interaction with pancreatic lipase and colipase. In addition, bile acids solubilize lipids and cholesterols, which keeps these particles in suspension in an aqueous environment. Bile acids are synthesized by hepatocytes from cholesterol, are stored in the gall bladder, and secreted into the duodenum after a meal.

MALDIGESTION DISORDERS

Because pancreatic enzymes play a central role in macronutrient digestion, exocrine pancreatic insufficiency (EPI) (see Chapter 20) is an important cause of maldigestion.

Selective enzyme deficiencies, such as lactase deficiency, are observed commonly in human patients but have not been demonstrated conclusively in cats. Lactase is a brush-border enzyme and as such is synthesized by the enterocytes. Although most human beings produce adequate amounts of this enzyme at birth, some people have an inherited tendency to lose this ability as they age.[13] Ingestion of lactose-containing foods triggers diarrhea, bloating, and flatulence. Many adult cats appear to be lactose intolerant, with diarrhea reported after the ingestion of milk or yoghurt. Avoidance of milk-based foodstuffs eliminates clinical signs in affected individuals.

Severe diffuse mucosal disorders have been shown to affect brush-border enzyme synthesis globally in human beings, and it is logical to assume that similar inflammatory intestinal processes in cats also affect brush-border enzyme production.[14] Lack of these enzymes may contribute to patient cachexia, and the osmotic effect of undigested food may exacerbate diarrhea in affected cats.

ASSESSMENT OF DIGESTIVE FUNCTION

Serum Feline Trypsin-Like Immunoreactivity (fTLI)

This test uses immunoassays to determine serum concentrations of trypsinogen and trypsin. Under physiological conditions, small amounts of trypsinogen (the inactive precursor of trypsin) enter the blood stream after synthesis by pancreatic acinar cells. In patients with loss of acinar cells (either by destruction or atrophy), trypsinogen synthesis is decreased markedly, leading to decreased serum fTLI concentrations. Subnormal serum fTLI concentration therefore serves as a specific marker for EPI.[15] Food should be withheld for 12 hours prior to serum collection; failure to do so may affect the sensitivity of the test and some affected cats may be overlooked.

Serum Feline Pancreatic Lipase Immunoreactivity (fPLI)

Many cell types within the body synthesize lipases. These enzymes hydrolyze triglycerides into more polar products that can then permeate cell membranes. Pancreatic lipase is produced exclusively by pancreatic acinar cells and can be measured by species-specific immunoassays. Similar to serum fTLI concentration, serum fPLI concentration is decreased in cats with loss of exocrine pancreatic function. However, serum fTLI is superior for the diagnosis of EPI, and assays for measurement of serum fPLI therefore have been optimized to focus on the upper portion of the working range. This has led to an assay that is highly sensitive and specific for feline pancreatitis. In one study, serum fPLI concentration was 100 per cent specific when assessed in healthy and symptomatic (i.e., cats with anorexia, vomiting, diarrhea, weight loss) cats with normal pancreatic histology.[16] The assay was 100 per cent sensitive for moderate to severe pancreatitis, and 67 per cent sensitive for all grades of pancreatitis in this patient population. The assay presently is available through the Gastrointestinal Laboratory at Texas A&M University and through certain commercial veterinary laboratories as the Spec fPL test.

Fecal Proteolytic Activity

Prior to the advent of the fTLI assay, fecal proteolytic activity (FPA) was used to assess exocrine pancreatic function. In simple terms, FPA quantifies the amount of proteolytic enzymes in the feces. Because the primary source of these enzymes is the exocrine pancreas, subnormal FPA strongly suggests EPI.[17]

In rare cases, an obstruction to the pancreatic duct by tumor or fibrosis results in inadequate release of enzymes despite normal production. These patients have normal serum TLI concentrations despite a total lack of pancreatic enzymes in the small intestine and a very low FPA; they show clinical improvement following pancreatic enzyme supplementation. FPA can be determined by radial enzyme diffusion methods using either casein or albumin as a substrate. At least three stool samples from consecutive days should be evaluated to maximize accuracy. Test results should be interpreted cautiously in patients with suspected protein-losing enteropathy because plasma antiproteinases lost into the intestinal lumen will decrease fecal proteolytic activity, resulting in an incorrect diagnosis of EPI.[18]

Fecal Sudan Staining

Fat maldigestion results in steatorrhea (Figure 15-6), which can be confirmed with Sudan staining of fecal specimens. However, this test does not differentiate maldigestive from malabsorptive disorders and rarely provides useful information in clinical cases.

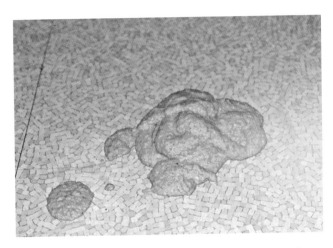

Figure 15-6 Steatorrhea. Stool from a cat with fat malassimilation due to exocrine pancreatic insufficiency. Note the greasy appearance and mustard color.

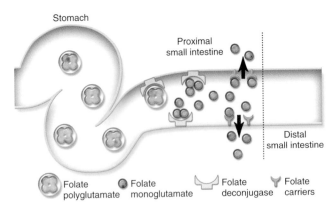

Figure 15-7 Physiology of folate absorption. Dietary folate is predominantly in the polyglutamate form. Folate deconjugase, a brush-border enzyme in the proximal small intestine, deconjugates the folate polyglutamate to folate monoglutamate. Specific folate carriers present on the luminal surface of enterocytes located in the proximal small intestine subsequently absorb folate monoglutamate. Both the deconjugase and folate carrier molecules are restricted to the cranial small intestine. There is no appreciable absorption of folate in the distal small intestine or colon. (Reproduced with permission; Suchodolski JS, Steiner JM: Laboratory assessment of gastrointestinal function, *Clin Tech Small Anim Pract* 18:203, 2003.)

Brush-Border Enzyme Activity

Human studies have reported extensively on changes in brush-border enzyme production in patients with chronic intestinal conditions such as celiac disease. However, complex diagnostic procedures (e.g., immunohistochemistry, tissue culture) are required to identify these changes and are not available currently for routine use. Also, enzyme activities may vary with patient age, dietary history, and sampling site.

Although studies directly evaluating brush-border enzymes in cats have not been reported, serum folate (vitamin B_9) concentrations provide some indication of enzyme synthesis by jejunal enterocytes. Folate occurs in the diet in a polyglutamate form, which must be broken down by folate deconjugase prior to absorption in the proximal small intestine (Figure 15-7). Because dietary folate deficiency is very unlikely in cats fed commercial diets, subnormal serum folate concentrations suggest either a change in jejunal brush-border enzyme production or compromised absorption (see below).

ABSORPTION

Absorption is the movement of micronutrients, such as fatty acids, amino acids, and simple sugars, from the intestinal lumen into the blood or lymphatic system. This process may occur by active, passive, or facilitated methods and may require uptake by specific receptors. The absorptive capacity of the intestine is influenced therefore by several factors, namely the available surface area, mucosal blood flow, the function of the intestinal lacteals, and the number and activity of enterocyte surface receptors.

MALABSORPTIVE DISORDERS

Any disease that results in the loss of enterocyte surface area (e.g., villous blunting) has a profound effect on the absorptive capacity of the intestine. Inflammatory or infiltrative disease also will affect absorptive function, due to compromised attachment to receptors and/or transport between or through enterocytes.[19] In addition, the absence or dysfunction of a specific receptor type in an otherwise healthy intestine can impact micronutrient uptake without affecting absorption globally. A good example of this scenario is the inherited defect of the receptor responsible for absorption of the cobalamin-intrinsic factor complex described in Giant Schnauzers.[20] Similar disorders have not been reported in cats to date.

ASSESSMENT OF ABSORPTIVE FUNCTION

Sugar Probe Studies

Sugar probe studies have been used for many years to investigate intestinal function in human beings, laboratory animals, and dogs. Few studies are available for cats, and these show little promise for the clinical utility of sugar absorption testing in this species.[21]

Folate

Folate is a water-soluble vitamin (B_9). Serum folate concentrations are influenced by dietary intake, brush-border folate deconjugase activity, and the number and function of specific carriers in the proximal small intestine (see Figure 15-7). As dietary deficiency of this vitamin is extremely uncommon, subnormal serum folate concentrations therefore suggest proximal small intestinal mucosal disease, with loss of the necessary brush-border enzyme and/or compromise of the transport carriers. It is important to remember that hemolysis causes the release of folate from red blood cells. Therefore poor sample handling can result in spuriously high serum folate concentrations.

Elevated serum folate concentrations in human beings are strongly associated with stagnant loop syndrome. These patients have a section of by-passed intestine in which the microflora can flourish. These bacteria produce folate, which then is absorbed into the systemic circulation. Small studies in both healthy cats and cats with GI disease have not found an association between bacterial activity (both type and absolute numbers) and serum folate concentrations.[22] Increased serum folate concentrations were reported in 10 of 27 cats (37 per cent) with low-grade intestinal lymphoma; however, no explanation was provided for this finding.[23]

Cobalamin

Cobalamin (vitamin B_{12}) also is a water-soluble vitamin. It can be synthesized only by certain bacteria; therefore carnivores, such as cats, are dependent on dietary sources (namely animal proteins). After ingestion, cobalamin is released through digestion of these proteins by pepsin and hydrochloric acid. Cobalamin then is bound to salivary and gastric R-protein, which in turn is digested in the small intestine by pancreatic proteinases. In the duodenum, cobalamin binds to intrinsic factor (Figure 15-8).

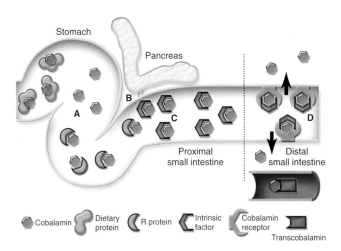

Figure 15-8 Physiology of cobalamin absorption. Cobalamin in the diet is bound to dietary protein. **A,** In the stomach, pepsin and hydrochloric acid digest the dietary protein, releasing the cobalamin. The cobalamin is bound immediately by R-protein, which is produced by the gastric mucosa and is transported in this form to the duodenum. In the duodenum, pancreatic proteinases digest the R-protein, releasing the cobalamin. **B,** Free cobalamin in the duodenum is bound by intrinsic factor. In the cat, only the pancreas produces intrinsic factor. **C,** Cobalamin remains bound to intrinsic factor during passage through the proximal small intestine. **D,** In the distal small intestine, the cobalamin/intrinsic factor complexes are taken up by specific receptors found only on the luminal surface of enterocytes in the ileum. The enterocytes process the intrinsic factor/cobalamin complex and release cobalamin into circulation, where a final set of binding proteins (i.e., transcobalamins) bind the vitamin and carry it to the cells. (Reproduced with permission; Suchodolski JS, Steiner JM: Laboratory assessment of gastrointestinal function, *Clin Tech Small Anim Pract* 18:203, 2003.)

In cats, the exocrine pancreas is the only source of this essential protein, so EPI results in profound hypocobalaminemia. In cats with normal pancreatic function, the cobalamin-intrinsic factor complex attaches subsequently to specific receptors in the ileum. Consequently, in patients who do not have EPI, subnormal serum cobalamin concentrations suggest mucosal disease in the distal small intestine.[24] However, it is important to note that certain bacterial populations, particularly *Clostridium* spp. and *Bacteroides* spp., utilize cobalamin and thereby limit its availability within the intestine. Hypocobalaminemia in human beings also is associated with increased small intestinal bacterial populations (e.g., stagnant loop syndrome). However, this connection has not been demonstrated in cats.

Breath Hydrogen Testing

The rate of hydrogen production by intestinal bacteria is influenced by the microbial population (i.e., species and number of bacteria) and by the availability of suitable substrates (i.e., unassimilated carbohydrates). Increased breath hydrogen concentrations therefore reflect compromised carbohydrate digestion or absorption. If a simple inert sugar, such as xylose, is administered prior to serial breath hydrogen measurement, conclusions can be made about the absorptive function of the small intestine. Although data from healthy cats have been reported, similar studies in cats with GI disease are lacking.[25]

PERMEABILITY TESTING

One of the more complex functions of a healthy intestine is the maintenance of selective permeability. This is an intricate balance, in which the inward movement of desired solutes is permitted but potentially harmful substances are excluded and valuable extracellular fluid components are retained. The tight junctions between enterocytes play a crucial role because they limit the passage of large molecules both to and from the intestinal lumen. Disruption of these intercellular junctions is thought to be a primary mechanism leading to increased intestinal permeability.

PERMEABILITY DISORDERS

Increased intestinal permeability may be the cause or consequence of inflammatory or infiltrative disorders. The damaged mucosal membrane is unable therefore to exclude foreign antigens, which may stimulate further inflammation. As a result, infectious agents and bacterial endotoxins may enter the deeper tissues and eventually reach the blood stream. Simultaneous loss of plasma constituents (e.g., albumin and antithrombin III) may occur, with resultant cachexia, metabolic compromise, and hypercoagulability.

Increased permeability also may occur in the absence of mucosal inflammation. Any disease that limits flow in the intestinal lymphatics (the lacteals) will increase the hydrostatic pressure in those vessels, resulting in leakage of fluid and protein into the intestinal lumen.[26] The classic pattern of idiopathic intestinal lymphangiectasia seen in dogs has not been described in cats; however, congestive heart failure or infiltration of the mesenteric lymph nodes may produce the same effect.

The consequences of increased permeability are profound, and include loss of oral tolerance, translocation of intestinal microorganisms, and hypoalbuminemia.

ASSESSMENT OF INTESTINAL PERMEABILITY

Increased permeability is confirmed in one of two ways: either an orally administered substrate is shown to enter the blood stream inappropriately or a blood constituent is demonstrated to be present in the stool.

Sugar Probe Studies: Lactulose and Rhamnose

Studies using sugar probes of different sizes are a standard way to evaluate the permeability of the intestinal epithelium to luminal contents in human beings and have been used successfully in dogs. Rhamnose is a small molecule that is thought to traverse the intestinal epithelial cells passively via small pores on the mucosal surface (transcellular transport), whereas lactulose is much larger and enters the body through the tight junctions (paracellular transport). Damage to these junctions will facilitate the uptake of lactulose, causing an increase in the ratio of recovered lactulose to rhamnose. However, an elevated ratio also is consistent with a reduction in the intestinal surface area because rhamnose absorption will be limited. Normal ranges have been established for cats, but useful studies looking at these parameters in cats with intestinal disease have not been reported.[27]

[51]Chromium-Ethylenediaminetetraacetic Acid (^{51}Cr-EDTA) Uptake

Radio-labeled EDTA is presumed to move through the mucosal barrier via the tight junctions and may be used in place of lactulose. This molecule may be a superior marker because it is not subject to bacterial degradation. However, special handling and safety precautions are necessary.

Fecal Alpha₁-Proteinase Inhibitor Concentration

Intestinal protein loss is best documented by measurement of fecal alpha$_1$-proteinase inhibitor concentration.[28] This plasma protein is approximately the same size as albumin but resists digestion within the intestinal lumen. Its presence in feces therefore is a useful marker for GI protein loss. Freshly voided fecal samples must be collected for 3 consecutive days. Special tubes and handling are required (http://www.cvm.tamu.edu/gilab/assays). The test presently available is validated only for adult cats. Fecal concentrations in kittens are highly variable and are not a reliable indicator of GI protein loss.

IMMUNOLOGICAL RESPONSES

A healthy GI immune system must tolerate ingested food antigens and the harmless commensal microflora, but respond quickly and appropriately to pathogens and toxic agents. Therefore a complex balance between activation and suppression of the immune response is necessary to maintain optimal function.[29]

GI immune responses can be classified as *innate* or *adaptive*. Innate responses generally have limited specificity and are designed to shield the intestinal mucosa from pathogen attachment and invasion. Numerous sensor and effector molecules have been identified, each with a specific role. One example are defensins, which are peptides that are secreted by many cells, including enterocytes, and cause disruption of bacterial cell membranes and subsequent cell death.[30]

Adaptive immune responses require immunological priming (i.e., sensitization) but provide a more targeted approach. The process starts with macrophages and dendritic cells, which sample luminal antigens and transport them across the epithelial barrier into the lymphoid tissue for processing and presentation. The second step involves the proliferation and migration of immunoglobulin A–committed antigen-specific B-lymphocytes. Lymphocyte activation triggers the release of proinflammatory cytokines and the recruitment of further immune effector cells.

IMMUNOLOGICAL DISORDERS

Abnormal GI immune responses may be due to immunodeficiency (either innate or adaptive) or aberrant immunological activity. Either scenario may result in GI dysfunction and disease.

Retroviral Infection

Both feline immunodeficiency virus (FIV) and feline leukemia virus (FeLV) infections can cause substantial immunocompromise. FIV affects T-lymphocyte populations and results in an inversion of the usual CD4+/CD8+ ratio. Infected cats are predisposed to clinical illness from opportunistic infections, although the prevalence of GI pathogens, such as *Cryptosporidium parvum* and *Giardia* spp., apparently reflects that of the general feline population.[31] It is interesting to note that chronic diarrhea was reported in 10 cats infected experimentally with FIV. Comprehensive evaluation of GI status and function failed to identify the cause of the diarrhea, and intestinal biopsy specimens were unremarkable.[32]

FeLV infection may impact the bone marrow directly, with subsequent severe immunocompromise. In addition, the oncogenic effects of the virus may result in lymphoma, further impacting systemic immune function.

Immune-Mediated Disorders

Aberrant or exaggerated immune responses play an important role in the development of chronic GI disease in many species. For example, inflammatory bowel disease (IBD) in dogs and cats and Crohn's disease and ulcerative colitis in human beings appear to have an immunological basis. Immunohistochemical studies have shown increased major histocompatibility complex class II expression by leukocytes in the duodenal lamina propria in cats with IBD, along with higher numbers of immunoglobulin (Ig) M–positive plasma cells when compared to clinically healthy specific-pathogen free (SPF) cats. The T cell distribution and subset balance were the same for both groups.[33]

The underlying etiology of IBD in human beings and animals is uncertain, but it seems likely that a combination of factors (i.e., genetic predisposition, environmental and dietary triggers, and the intestinal microflora) is required to produce clinical disease.[34]

An inappropriate immunological response to dietary antigens may play a role in the development of feline IBD. Food sensitivity has been reported in 29 per cent of cats with IBD, and many patients show clinical improvement with novel antigen or hydrolyzed protein diets.[35] However, it is important to remember that a positive response to dietary change does not prove a diagnosis of food hypersensitivity conclusively. At present, the factors affecting oral tolerance are not well understood. In fact, serological studies suggest that a robust IgG and IgA response to ingested antigens may occur routinely.[36]

The impact of mucosa-associated bacteria on the development of IBD remains unclear. Although significant differences in bacterial populations have been reported between normal cats and those patients with chronic intestinal disease, direct causal relationships have not been demonstrated.[37,38] However, the recent identification of invasive, intracellular *Escherichia coli* isolates in Boxer dogs with granulomatous colitis raises the possibility that other disorders presently regarded as idiopathic IBD may have a bacterial cause.[39]

ASSESSMENT OF INTESTINAL IMMUNE FUNCTION AND RESPONSE

Retroviral Testing

Any cat with an opportunistic or persistent GI infection should be tested for FeLV and FIV. As the current tests for FIV detect circulating antibodies, positive test results are expected in vaccinated cats and do not necessarily indicate infection (see Chapter 6).

Macroscopic Food-Sensitivity Testing

Gastroscopic food-sensitivity tests (FST) have been used in dogs to identify allergens associated with adverse reactions to foods. A small amount of the test food is dripped onto the stomach lining using an endoscope, and the mucosa is evaluated visually for signs of inflammation (e.g., swelling, erythema, and hyperperistalsis). In dogs with atopy, a positive reaction to test antigens has been shown to correlate with results of oral food challenge.[40] The nature of the response to gastric FST indicates a type 1 hypersensitivity reaction, most likely mediated by IgE. These tests therefore may fail to identify patients with delayed reactions and do not provide any information about events in the small intestine. In fact, the sensitivity of gastric FST was shown to be poor in a group of dogs with GI disease and presumed dietary intolerance. In that study, many of the dogs with negative test results still improved on a hypoallergenic diet.[41] In addition, poor correlation between FST results and clinical response to dietary antigen challenge was reported in a group of dogs

with confirmed protein-losing enteropathy. Only 19 per cent of adverse reactions noted during oral provocation were supported by a positive reaction when the antigen was applied directly to the gastric mucosa.[42]

Colonoscopic FST (also called *allergen provocation*) may be a more useful tool in the diagnosis of IgE-mediated food allergies. In a recent study, this procedure identified 73 per cent of 23 dogs with known food allergies, and negative results were reported in all control dogs.[43] At the present time, there are no published reports describing either gastroscopic or colonoscopic FST in cats.

Antigen-Specific IgE Measurement

Serological assays for food-specific IgE are performed routinely in animals with atopic skin disease and have been evaluated in patients with GI disease. In a group of dogs with food hypersensitivity, the onset of clinical signs (i.e., diarrhea and pruritus) was associated with increased serum allergen-specific IgE concentrations.[44] Changes in fecal IgE also may indicate an abnormal response to dietary allergens in affected patients.

Although serum IgE concentrations have been investigated in cats with inhalant allergies, studies in cats with dietary-responsive GI disease have not been reported.

SUMMARY

The clinical manifestations of GI disease are a reflection of an underlying dysfunction. Although our ability to evaluate GI function objectively is limited, approaching patients from this perspective may mitigate our current reliance on histopathological findings. More clinically applicable function tests are certainly needed, so that diseases can be defined more precisely and therapeutic responses measured objectively.

REFERENCES

1. Cheng L, Cao W, Behar J, et al: Inflammation induced changes in arachidonic acid metabolism in cat LES circular muscle, *Am J Physiol Gastrointest Liver Physiol* 288:G787, 2005.
2. Moses L, Harpster NK, Beck KA, et al: Esophageal motility dysfunction in cats: a study of 44 cases, *J Am Anim Hosp Assoc* 36:309, 2000.
3. Wyse CA, McLellan J, Dickie AM, et al: A review of methods for assessment of the rate of gastric emptying in the dog and cat: 1898-2002, *J Vet Intern Med* 17:609, 2003.
4. Steyn PF, Twedt DC: Gastric emptying in the normal cat: a radiographic study, *J Am Anim Hosp Assoc* 30:78, 1994.
5. Chandler ML, Guilford WG, Lawoko CRO: Radiopaque markers to evaluate gastric emptying and small intestinal transit time in healthy cats, *J Vet Intern Med* 11:361, 1997.
6. Goggin JM, Hoskinson JJ, Kirk CA, et al: Comparison of gastric emptying times in healthy cats simultaneously evaluated with radiopaque markers and nuclear scintigraphy, *Vet Radiol Ultrasound* 40:890, 1999.
7. Maurer AH, Parkman HP: Update on gastrointestinal scintigraphy, *Semin Nucl Med* 36:110, 2006.
8. Wyse CA, Preston T, Yam PS, et al: Current and future uses of breath analysis as a diagnostic tool, *Vet Rec* 154:353, 2004.

9. Peachey SE, Dawson JM, Harper EJ: Gastrointestinal transit times in young and old cats, *Comp Biochem Physiol A Mol Integr Physiol* 126:85, 2000.

10. Benini L, Sembenini C, Heading RC, et al: Simultaneous measurement of gastric emptying of a solid meal by ultrasound and by scintigraphy, *Am J Gastroenterol* 94:2861, 1999.

11. Sparkes AH, Papasouliotis K, Viner J, et al: Assessment of orocaecal transit time in cats by the breath hydrogen method: the effects of sedation and a comparison of definitions, *Res Vet Sci* 60:243, 1996.

12. Papasouliotis K, Sparkes AH, Gruffydd-Jones TJ, et al: Use of the breath hydrogen test to assess the effect of age on orocecal transit time and carbohydrate assimilation in cats, *Am J Vet Res* 59:1299, 1998.

13. Grand RJ, Montgomery RK, Chitkara DK, et al: Changing genes; losing lactase, *Gut* 52:617, 2003.

14. Mercer J, Eagles ME, Talbot IC: Brush border enzymes in coeliac disease: histochemical evaluation, *J Clin Pathol* 43:307, 1990.

15. Steiner JM, Williams DA: Trypsin-like immunoreactivity (fTLI) in cats with exocrine pancreatic insufficiency (EPI), *J Vet Intern Med* 14:627, 2000.

16. Forman MA, Marks SL, De Cock HEV, et al: Evaluation of serum feline pancreatic lipase immunoreactivity and helical computed tomography versus conventional testing for the diagnosis of feline pancreatitis, *J Vet Intern Med* 18:807, 2004.

17. Williams DA, Reed SD, Perry L: Fecal proteolytic activity in clinically normal cats and in a cat with exocrine pancreatic insufficiency, *J Am Vet Med Assoc* 197:210, 1990.

18. Ruaux CF, Steiner JM, Williams DA: Protein-losing enteropathy in dogs is associated with decreased fecal proteolytic activity, *Vet Clin Pathol* 33:20, 2004.

19. Ugarte CE, Guilford WG, Markwell PJ: Carbohydrate malabsorption is a feature of feline inflammatory bowel disease but does not increase clinical gastrointestinal signs, *J Nutr* 134:2068S, 2004.

20. Fyfe JC, Giger U, Hall CA, et al: Inherited selective intestinal cobalamin malabsorption and cobalamin deficiency in dogs, *Pediatr Res* 29:24, 1991.

21. Johnston KL, Ballèvre OP, Batt RM: Use of an orally administered combined sugar food-sensitivity tests (FST) solution to evaluate intestinal absorption and permeability in cats, *Am J Vet Res* 62:111, 2001.

22. Johnston KL, Swift NC, Forster-van Hijfte M, et al: Comparison of the bacterial flora of the duodenum in healthy cats and cats with signs of gastrointestinal tract disease, *J Am Vet Med Assoc* 218:48, 2001.

23. Kiselow MA, Rassnick KM, McDonough SP, et al: Outcome of cats with low-grade lymphocytic lymphoma: 41 cases (1995-2005), *J Am Vet Med Assoc* 232:405, 2008.

24. Simpson KW, Fyfe J, Cornetta A, et al: Subnormal concentrations of serum cobalamin (vitamin B12) in cats with gastrointestinal disease, *J Vet Intern Med* 15:26, 2001.

25. Muir P, Papasouliotis K, Gruffydd-Jones TJ, et al: Evaluation of carbohydrate malassimilation and intestinal transit time in cats by measurement of breath hydrogen excretion, *Am J Vet Res* 52:1104, 1991.

26. Kull PA, Hess RS, Craig LE, et al: Clinical, clinicopathologic, radiographic, and ultrasonographic characteristics of intestinal lymphangiectasia in dogs: 17 cases (1996-1998), *J Am Vet Med Assoc* 219:197, 2001.

27. Randel SC, Hill RC, Scott KC, et al: Intestinal permeability testing using lactulose and rhamnose: a comparison between clinically normal cats and dogs and between dogs of different breeds, *Res Vet Sci* 7:45, 2001.

28. Fetz K, Ruaux CG, Steiner JM, et al: Purification and partial characterization of feline alpha₁-proteinase inhibitor and the development and validation of a radioimmunoassay for the measurement of alpha₁-PI in serum, *Biochimie* 86:67, 2004.

29. Stokes CR, Waly NE: Mucosal defence along the gastrointestinal tract of cats and dogs, *Vet Res* 37:281, 2006.

30. Linde A, Ross CR, Davis EG, et al: Innate immunity and host defense peptides in veterinary medicine, *J Vet Intern Med* 22:247, 2008.

31. Hill SJ, Cheney JM, Taton-Allen GF, et al: Prevalence of enteric zoonotic organisms in cats, *J Am Vet Med Assoc* 216:687, 2000.

32. Papasouliotis K, Gruffydd-Jones TJ, Werrett G, et al: Assessment of intestinal function in cats with chronic diarrhea after infection with feline immunodeficiency virus, *Am J Vet Res* 59:569, 1998.

33. Waly NE, Stokes CR, Gruffydd-Jones TJ, et al: Immune cell populations in the duodenal mucosa of cats with inflammatory bowel disease, *J Vet Intern Med* 18:813, 2004.

34. Jergens AE: Inflammatory bowel disease: current perspectives, *Vet Clin North Am Small Anim Pract* 29:501, 1999.

35. Guilford WG, Jones BR, Markwell PJ, et al: Food sensitivity in cats with chronic idiopathic gastrointestinal problems, *J Vet Intern Med* 15:7, 2001.

36. Cave NJ, Marks SL: Evaluation of the immunogenicity of dietary proteins in cats and the influence of the canning process, *Am J Vet Res* 65:1427, 2004.

37. Janeczko S, Atwater D, Bogel L, et al: The relationship of mucosal bacteria to duodenal histopathology, cytokine mRNA, and clinical disease activity in cats with inflammatory bowel disease, *Vet Microbiol* 128:178, 2008.

38. Inness VL, McCartney AL, Khoo C, et al: Molecular characterization of the gut microflora of healthy and inflammatory bowel disease cats using fluorescence in situ hybridization with special reference to *Desulfovibrio* spp, *J Appl Physiol Anim Nutr (Berl)* 91:48, 2007.

39. Simpson KW, Dogan B, Rishnew M, et al: Adherent and invasive *Escherichia coli* is associated with granulomatous colitis in boxer dogs, *Infect Immun* 74:4778, 2006.

40. Guilford WG, Strombeck DR, Rogers Q, et al: Development of gastroscopic food sensitivity testing in dogs, *J Vet Intern Med* 8:414, 1994.

41. Elwood CE, Rutgers HC, Batt RM: Gastroscopic food sensitivity testing in 17 dogs, *J Small Anim Pract* 35:199, 1994.

42. Vaden SL, Hammerberg B, Davenport DJ, et al: Food hypersensitivity reactions in Soft Coated Wheaten Terriers with protein-losing enteropathy or protein-losing nephropathy or both: gastroscopic food sensitivity testing, dietary provocation, and fecal immunoglobulin E, *J Vet Intern Med* 14:60, 2000.

43. Allenspach K, Vaden SL, Harris TS: Evaluation of colonoscopic allergen provocation as a diagnostic tool in dogs with proven food hypersensitivity reactions, *J Small Anim Pract* 47:21, 2006.

44. Jackson HA, Hammerberg B: Evaluation of a spontaneous canine model of immunoglobulin E-mediated food hypersensitivity: dynamic changes in serum and fecal allergen-specific immunoglobulin E values relative to dietary change, *Comp Med* 52:316, 2004.

CHAPTER

16 Ultrasonographic Imaging of the Gastrointestinal Tract

Kathy Ann Spaulding

CHAPTER OUTLINE

Ultrasound imaging has become widely accepted as an important diagnostic tool for imaging the gastrointestinal tract in veterinary patients. Initially it was thought that artifacts created by gas and ingested material would significantly limit or exclude the use of ultrasound for examining the gastrointestinal tract. However, experience has shown that these artifacts, although present and at times obstructive, rarely interfere significantly with a thorough ultrasonographic examination. The technology has continued to improve. Higher resolution (12 to 18 MHz and higher) transducers and more affordable equipment—along with the availability of Doppler ultrasound—have made it possible to image the gastrointestinal tract more thoroughly, enhancing the ability to evaluate and understand changes produced by diseases affecting that organ.[1]

Ultrasound uses sound reflected from the tissue boundaries within the body to form an image that we can recognize and interpret. At diagnostic frequencies (1 to 25 MHz) it is noninvasive and does not pose any known significant biological risk. It is particularly useful in evaluating the intestinal wall, the luminal contents, and function evidenced by peristalsis. It also can interrogate the surrounding organs such as the peritoneum, pancreas, liver, and lymph nodes. Ultrasound can guide needle placement for either an aspirate or biopsy of a detected abnormality. Intestinal ultrasound provides additional and complementary information to other diagnostic modalities (e.g., survey radiographs, computed tomography, nuclear medicine, magnetic resonance imaging, and contrast radiography).

Ultrasound imaging now has become so integral to the diagnostic evaluation of small animals with gastrointestinal signs that there has been a marked reduction in radiographic contrast procedures. Ultrasound is faster, is more cost-effective, and often provides as much or more information than these other diagnostic modalities. However, these improvements also have raised questions about the significance of some findings, and a great deal remains to be learned regarding the feline intestinal tract. One example is differentiating the various etiological causes for the appearance of the thickened muscular layer of the small intestine. It is especially important to correlate ultrasound findings with the history, clinical findings, laboratory results, and ultimately cytological and histopathological findings.

METHOD OF EVALUATION

It is preferred, but not always necessary, that the patient be held off food before the ultrasonographic examination. Withholding food for 8 to 12 hours can reduce interference from gas and ingested contents. This is especially helpful when examining the patient for suspected foreign bodies within the intestinal lumen and when evaluating intestinal walls. An enema is not recommended or usually needed because this introduces gas into the colon, which may interfere with the examination. Gas within the lumen often is manifested by reverberation, comet tails, and acoustic shadowing artifacts. A *comet-tail artifact* is a streaklike or cone-shaped reverberation phenomenon, typically occurring deep to metallic objects. A *ring-down artifact* is a streaklike reverberation phenomenon, typically occurring deep to a fluid-gas interface. It has the appearance of vertical hyperechoic

157

lines extending from the first encounter with the surface of the air interface to deep within the image. These artifacts can obscure normal or diseased tissue and also can mimic disease. Feces within the colon or barium contrast material anywhere in the intestinal tract can attenuate the sound beam (Figure 16-1). This often obscures the far wall of the intestine and limits the ability to evaluate that section of intestine. Survey radiographs can be helpful in providing an overall view of the abdomen and to confirm or identify sonographic findings.

If possible, the ultrasound examination should be performed before an upper gastrointestinal study with barium or before administration of oral medications, especially those that contain bismuth. If a diagnostic procedure requires administration of food, such as for measurement of postprandial serum bile acid concentrations, or the patient is diabetic and needs to be fed regularly, the ultrasound examination should be performed before any food is given.

Feces within the colon typically are not a problem during evaluation of the small intestine. However, if artifacts from the feces interfere with colonic evaluation or with the evaluation of an adjacent area that needs to be examined, varying the pressure applied to the transducer or imaging from a different window can be helpful. If an important region is obscured from evaluation, providing a tray with cat litter to encourage defecation or repeating the examination the day after a fast may be warranted.

To achieve the best image quality, hair should be shaved in the area that needs to be imaged using a surgical clipping blade. The shaved area usually is rectangular, extending from the epaxial muscles in the dorsocranial

abdomen (usually eighth to ninth rib) to the caudal abdomen just in front of the pelvic limbs and ventrally to the midline on both sides of the cat. An attempt should be made to keep the margins of the clipped area straight because the area's appearance is often noticed and important to the owner. Mammary papillae obscured by surrounding hair may be at risk for trauma from the clipper blades when the patient is shaved by an inexperienced individual. The area to be clipped will be more extensive when the patient is imaged from a lateral position than it will be for a patient in a dorsal recumbent position. If the animal has thin hair, it can be moistened with water and alcohol in lieu of cutting the hair. Commercially available water-soluble ultrasound gel is used as an interface between the skin and the transducer. Alcohol also may be used to clean dry, dirty, or scaly skin. This application of alcohol often reduces the amount of gel needed and also improves image quality.

The method of positioning the cat for examination often varies depending on the experience and training of the individual performing the examination. Usually either a lateral imaging plane (i.e., left or right lateral recumbency) or a dorsal recumbency imaging plane is used. Each sonologist should establish a consistent scanning protocol. A routine examination includes an attempt to identify and image each section of the intestine. If the standard viewing window does not provide an adequate image, the sonologist can change the position of the transducer as necessary to complete the evaluation. For the challenging patient, changing the position of the cat relative to the transducer can help in avoiding troublesome gas pockets. The author typically examines each

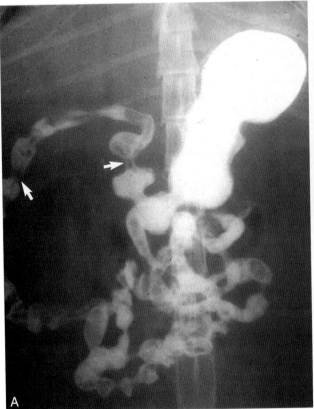

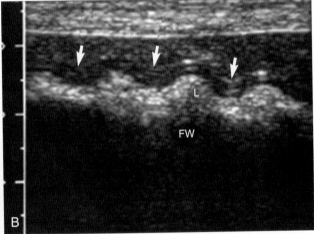

Figure 16-1 Normal feline duodenum. This figure shows a radiographic contrast study (**A**) and an ultrasound image (**B**) of the duodenum in a normal cat. Both imaging studies show multiple dynamic segmental contractions *(arrows)* within the duodenum and to a lesser extent within the jejunum. These segmental contractions sometimes are referred to as a "string of pearls." In this patient, the ultrasound examination was performed after the contrast study. The barium in the duodenum has caused a hyperechoic appearance of the luminal contents *(L)* in the near field with attenuation of the sound and shadowing, leading to a loss of visualization of the far wall *(FW)* and any structures that are deeper than the duodenum.

patient in both recumbent lateral positions. Positional studies, such as the recumbent ventrodorsal or standing positions, can be used to afford an acoustic window not otherwise available in a specific patient.

The highest MHz transducer available should always be used. To image the layers of intestinal walls, a minimum of a 7-MHz transducer should be used. A 5-MHz transducer will allow visualization of the intestinal tract; however, the detail required to assess the intestinal wall often is not adequate. A 10- to 18-MHz transducer will allow better imaging of the intestinal wall layers. Endosonography uses a specialized intracavitary transesophageal/transcolonic transducer to image from within the lumen of the intestine. These high-resolution transducers are especially helpful in evaluating the individual wall layers of the intestine for changes secondary to neoplasia and inflammatory bowel disease. Some are equipped with endoscopic biopsy instruments. More than one transducer may be required to image the entire intestinal tract at different depths. A linear probe provides better imaging of the superficial intestinal tract. The pie-shaped image afforded by a sector transducer provides a limited view of a segment of the intestinal tract in the near field. Because each machine type is different, it is often necessary to experiment with one's own machine for the optimal imaging transducer. Both transverse and longitudinal views of gastrointestinal segments are needed to assess both the intestinal wall and lumen. Measurements of the wall can be made from longitudinal views, but reports indicate that measurements are most accurate when made from the transverse image to avoid oblique sections through the wall. The luminal axis of the intestinal segment evaluated, and not the plane through the patient's body, determines the plane of the image seen on the screen (i.e., longitudinal, transverse, or oblique). Color Doppler and/or pulse wave Doppler are useful aids to assess blood flow to certain segments of the intestinal tract.

NORMAL ANATOMY

Ultrasonographic study of the abdomen includes interrogation of each region of the gastrointestinal tract (i.e., esophagus, stomach, duodenum, jejunum, ileum, and colon), noting the wall thickness, distinction of the wall layers, luminal contents, motility, and vascular integrity.

In the cat abdominal visceral detail usually is good for both ultrasonographic and radiographic imaging. A significant amount of heterogeneous and mildly hyperechoic omental and falciform fat often is present, but usually does not affect image quality negatively.

Some appearances and features of the intestinal tract are found in both cats and dogs. However, there also are unique features of the feline intestinal tract. In the cat only the cervical part of the esophagus and a small segment of abdominal esophagus (between the cardia of the stomach and the diaphragm) are accessible for sonographic evaluation. The cervical portion of the esophagus can be imaged lateral to the trachea, from the larynx to the thoracic inlet. The abdominal esophagus is best seen from a right dorsal imaging window. The esophagus is seen ventral to the aorta and dorsal to the caudal vena cava as it traverses the diaphragm and courses to the cardia of the stomach. The majority of the esophagus can be imaged best with radiography and a radiographic contrast study (i.e., esophagogram).

The stomach (the fundus to the pylorus), duodenum, jejunum, ileum, and colon all can be identified separately in the cat. The stomach is located in the left cranial abdomen just caudal to the liver, craniomedial to the head of the spleen, and cranial to the left kidney (Figure 16-2). The wall may be mildly thickened and contain a hyperechoic submucosal layer from adipose tissue, especially in overweight cats (Figure 16-3). The pylorus is located on the midline, as opposed to the right of midline as in dogs. During an abdominal ultrasound examination the stomach usually is empty and typically has a rosette or wagon-wheel appearance. It shows a characteristic pattern with its size, shape, and prominent rugal folds.

The duodenum courses in a straight superficial path from the pylorus along the right body wall for approximately two-thirds the length of the abdomen. From there it curves medially at the caudal flexure and then courses craniomedially. The sphincter of Oddi, the entrance of the conjoined bile duct and pancreatic duct, is located in the proximal flexure of the duodenum just distal to the

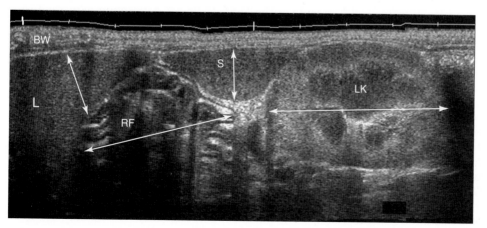

Figure 16-2 Panoramic abdominal ultrasonographic view of a normal cat. This figure shows a panoramic dorsal view of the left cranial abdomen of a normal cat. The left liver lobe *(L)* is cranial and adjacent to the body wall *(BW)* in the left part of the image. The rugal folds *(RF)* of the stomach are located caudal to the liver and craniomedial to the spleen *(S)*. The spleen is lying along the cranial border of the left kidney *(LK)* in this normal patient.

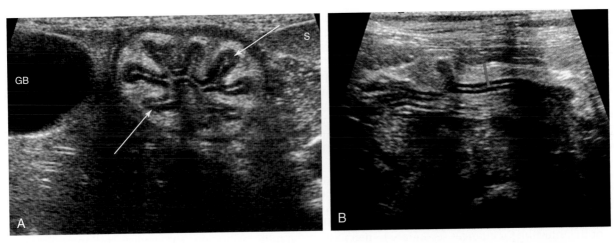

Figure 16-3 Empty stomach. **A,** Short-axis view of the collapsed stomach. The stomach in the cat is often empty during ultrasonographic examination and the rugal folds appear as spokes on a wagon wheel radiating towards the center *(arrows)*. Cats with an overabundance of body wall fat may have a hyperechoic submucosal layer due to fat accumulation. This often results in a widened and hyperechoic submucosal layer. The spleen *(S)* and the gall bladder *(GB)* are seen caudal and cranial to the stomach on this image. **B,** Longitudinal view of the stomach. The increased fat in the wall can be seen and represents a hyperechoic submucosal wall layer *(red line)*.

pylorus. The pancreatic duct and bile duct join before entering the duodenum at the cistern of Vater. Approximately 90 per cent of cats have only the primary pancreatic papilla; the rest also have a minor duodenal papilla. The Peyer's patches (lymphoid aggregates), which can be seen on the antimesenteric surface of the duodenum in dogs, are usually not seen in cats. The duodenum, and sometimes parts of the jejunum, can show segmental contractions resulting in a "string of pearls" appearance as opposed to the stripping peristaltic activity seen in dogs (Figure 16-4). The jejunum is identified as a long intestinal segment between the duodenum and the shorter ileum. The ileum is a small section of intestine that can be identified by its characteristic appearance (often contracted, with a "wagon wheel" appearance) and its position at the entrance into the colon. The ileum has a prominent hyperechoic submucosal layer and a corresponding undulating mucosal layer.

The ileum and/or the cecum can be seen connecting to the larger section of intestine, the colon. The cecum is a cul de sac. It enters the colon adjacent to the ileocolic junction, which is best identified from the right side in the midabdomen. The wall of the tip of the cecum often is thickened and hypoechoic with a reduction in wall layering. Left colic lymph nodes usually are seen in cats near the ileocolic junction, in addition to the mesenteric (jejunal) lymph nodes located at the root of the mesentery. In a recent paper, at least two colic lymph nodes were identified in all of 31 normal cats evaluated.[2] The diameter of these lymph nodes ranged from 1.9 to 5.2 mm. In this study, at least one, and usually both, normal medial iliac lymph nodes were found. In interrogations of the intestinal tract, the pericolic and jejunal lymph nodes are especially useful to image and measure because they drain the intestinal tract and can be used as a sentinel reflecting an abnormality within it.

In contrast to the small intestine, the colon is recognized by its larger size, thinner wall, location (extending dorsal to the bladder through the pelvic inlet), and appearance (with sound attenuation and shadowing caused by luminal contents [feces] or reverberations by a gas-distended lumen) (Figure 16-5). The ascending, transverse, and descending colon can be followed. It is easiest to trace the short ascending segment from the right side and the descending segment from the left side of the abdomen. If it is unclear whether a loop of intestine is an abnormal segment of small intestine or colon, it is helpful to follow the loop to see if it courses through the pelvic canal or to trace a segment of bowel known to be colon to the area in question. Small intestine has a thicker wall and does not have the dilated lumen with shadowing contents seen in the colon.

The wall layers of the intestinal tract are similar to the appearance described in human beings and dogs.[3] Depending on the section of intestine examined, the wall layer thickness and appearance varies. The wall layers identified sonographically are formed by the interface of specific histological components of the layers of the intestine, which generate different acoustic impedance values between the layers, and by internal reflecting margins within tissue layers. The ultrasound measurements of the apparent layers correspond with the histological measurements but are affected by the axial resolution of the transducer used and the speed of sound in the different tissue layers. The higher the resolution of the transducer, the better the corresponding morphological correlation. The mucosa layer is most apparent in the duodenum and jejunum and less apparent in other segments of the intestine (i.e., colon and ileum), likely because of the change in function and role in the absorptive process. The wall of the intestine includes five layers with an alternating hyperechoic and hypoechoic appearance. The three hyperechoic layers (the S layers) are serosa, submucosa, and the surface of the mucosa; the two hypoechoic layers (the M layers) are the muscularis and the mucosal layers (Figure 16-6).

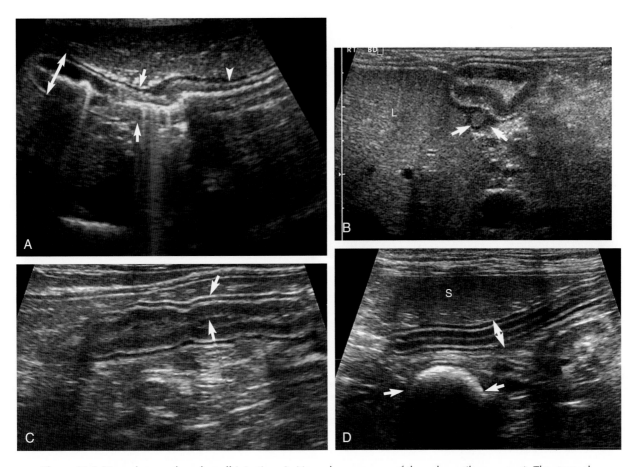

Figure 16-4 Normal stomach and small intestine. **A,** Normal appearance of the pylorus *(long arrows)*. The stomach is to the right *(arrowhead)* and the pylorus is to the left. Note that the layers are not as distinct and the hypoechoic mucosal layer seen in the duodenum is not evident. **B,** Cross section of the duodenum at the proximal duodenal flexure. The caudate liver lobe *(L)* is adjacent and cranial to the duodenum. The small nodule *(arrows)* along the medial surface of the duodenum represents the sphincter of Oddi. The bile duct and pancreatic duct enter the duodenum through this sphincter. **C,** Longitudinal view of the duodenum. The thickness of the intestinal wall is seen *(arrows)*. **D,** Jejunum as it is viewed from the left side. The spleen *(S)* can be seen in the near field and the colon *(arrows)* in the far field in relation to the jejunum *(double arrows)*. The five layers of the wall of the intestine can be seen in each of the segments of intestine and form the surface of the mucosa, mucosa, submucosa, muscularis, and serosa (from the center of the *double arrows* outwards in both directions).

The wall thickness in part is related to the degree of distension of the loop of intestine and gets mildly thinner the more distended it becomes (Figure 16-7). Contraction during normal peristaltic activity does affect the width of the intestinal wall although the width of specific layers can change momentarily with contractions. Because the intestinal tract is dynamic, contractions shorten the loop of intestine in the contracted area and increase the width of the muscular and mucosal layers compared to adjacent dilated segments. It is important to be consistent in placing the cursors for wall measurements. The stomach wall thickness varies from 1.7 to 2.8 mm. It is important to avoid measurement of rugal folds or oblique cuts to prevent erroneously thickened measurements. It is easiest and most accurate to measure the wall when a small amount of fluid is present within the gastric lumen. This may require administering water orally if there is any question about the wall thickness. The thickness of the duodenum and jejunum usually is between 2.3 and 2.8 mm. It is more difficult to measure the wall thickness

of the ileum accurately due to its "wagon wheel" appearance. The ileum has a prominent hyperechoic submucosa due to fat and lymphatics, and a hypoechoic muscularis layer. Ileal wall thickness may measure between 2.4 and 2.8 mm. The colonic wall is thinner (usually 1.4 to 2.3 mm), and the wall layers are less distinct.[4,5] The far wall of the colon often is obscured by shadowing artifacts due to absorption of sound by fecal material. In general, intestinal wall thickness in cats is fairly consistent at 2.3 to 2.8 mm; it is regarded as abnormally thick when wall thickness is greater than 3 mm or the appearance of individual wall layers changes.

The appearance of luminal contents varies depending on the ingested material. Gas, fluid, mucus, food, and feces are normal contents observed. Ring down, comet tail, and sometimes attenuation and shadowing artifacts are observed frequently due to the sound interacting with the luminal contents. The luminal contents often contain mucus mixed with tiny gas bubbles, fluid, and/or ingesta. In fact, fluid (with minimal gas bubbles) may be given by

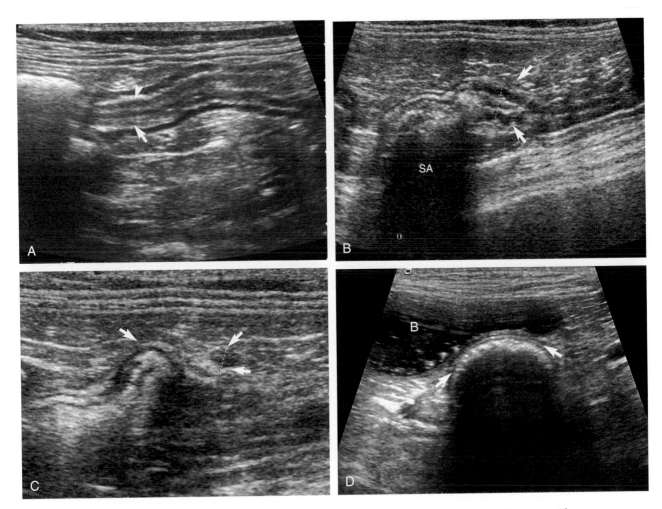

Figure 16-5 Normal ileum and colon. **A,** Ileum *(arrow)* entering the colon on the left side of the image. The submucosal layer *(arrowhead)* often is hyperechoic due to fat and lymphatics. **B,** Cecum *(two arrows)* entering the colon. The shadowing artifact *(SA)* is due to absorption of the sound by feces within the colon. The wall of the cecum at the tip often is thickened and hypoechoic. **C,** Small pericolic lymph node *(two arrows)* next to the colon, which can be seen to the left *(arrow)*. **D,** Transverse section of the colon *(two arrows)* at the level of the urinary bladder *(B)*. There is significant shadowing deep to the near wall of the colon due to fecal material inside the lumen obscuring the far wall of the colon.

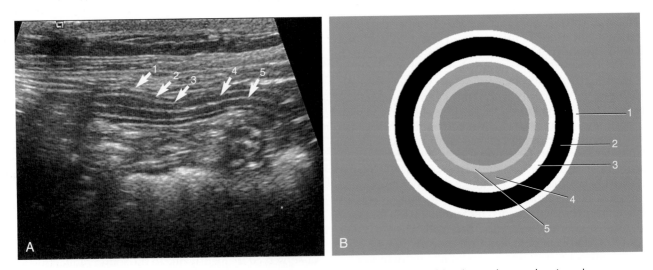

Figure 16-6 Normal layering of the intestinal wall. The intestinal wall consists of five layers that can be viewed as distinct layers on an ultrasound image (*1,* serosal layer; *2,* muscularis layer; *3,* submucosal layer; *4,* mucosal layer; *5,* surface of the mucosa). The muscularis and mucosal layers (two M layers) are hypoechoic, and the three S layers are hyperechoic.

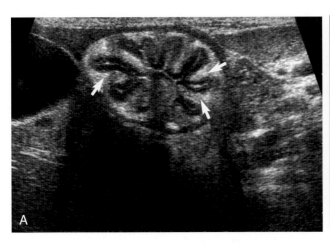 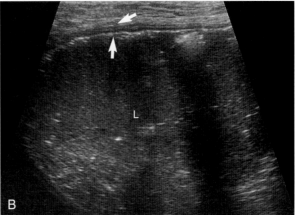

Figure 16-7 Gastric wall thickness. The thickness of the wall of the gastrointestinal tract varies depending on the degree of distension. **A,** Stomach is empty and contracted. The rugal folds are very prominent making the thickness of the wall difficult to measure *(arrows)*. **B,** Stomach is distended due to obstruction of the pylorus. The wall *(arrows)* is stretched and is thinner due to the distension of the lumen *(L)*. However, wall layering is maintained. Mild fluid distension of the gastrointestinal lumen is ideal for ultrasonographic imaging because it allows easier and more accurate measurement of the wall thickness.

mouth to accentuate imaging of the wall and the lumen of the proximal gastrointestinal tract.

Normal motility can be observed with real-time ultrasound. Four to five contractions per minute is normal in the stomach and duodenum; one to three is normal in the remainder of the small intestine. It is not common to see contractions in the colon.

The entire intestinal tract, including each segment of intestine, should be identified. Different methods for locating the intestinal segments can be employed. The abdomen can be divided into four quadrants. Each quadrant is scanned individually, with specific segments of intestine identified within that quadrant. No attempt is made to follow each bowel segment. Another method is to look for, and follow, specific segments such as the stomach, duodenum, or ileum separately, using their normal location in the abdomen and characteristic appearance as guides, and then to scan the remainder of the gastrointestinal tract systematically by imaging the quadrants without following every section of the intestinal tract. If an abnormality is detected, a known segment of bowel can be followed proximal and distal to the abnormality. Another method is to follow the entire gastrointestinal tube from proximal (i.e., stomach) to distal (i.e., colon). However, this approach is more time consuming and difficult due to patient movement and skill needed.

IMAGING OF SPECIFIC GASTROINTESTINAL DISORDERS

Disorders involving the gastrointestinal tract may be divided into those involving the lumen or the wall, or those arising outside the intestinal wall. A final diagnosis or differential diagnosis involves correlating the abnormal sonographic findings to history, clinical presentation, and laboratory results. The final diagnosis also may

require an aspirate or biopsy for cytological and/or histopathological confirmation.

LUMINAL CHANGES

The normal ultrasonographic size of the lumen and the appearance of the contents vary with the segment of intestine and the type of material ingested. The stomach and the small intestine often are empty or contain only a small amount of gas, fluid, or food material. The colon often is partially distended with formed shadowing feces. Luminal abnormalities seen typically are an increased volume of contents with distension of the bowel proximal to the area of an obstruction, and the obstructing material itself (e.g., an intraluminal foreign body, an intussusception, or a mural mass). This distension of the intestine also can be uniform, consistent with a mechanical obstruction downstream (aborad) from the point of imaging. In other instances the dilation can be combined with specific wall patterns or mural changes that indicate gathering from a linear foreign body or an infiltrated area or mass secondary to neoplasia or fungal disease. A dilated intestine is not always the result of a mechanical obstruction: it may be associated with diminished motility secondary to effects of drugs or metabolic, neurological, or inflammatory disorders. The luminal contents obviously should remain within the lumen. Gas within the intestinal wall or peritoneal cavity or contents (i.e., gas, fluid, or ingesta) outside the lumen are surgical emergencies.

Obstruction

Ultrasound is a useful diagnostic modality to determine if a gastrointestinal obstruction is caused by an intraluminal foreign body, stricture, mural mass, or an extramural mass. A gas-distended gastrointestinal tract on a radiographic study does not preclude the use of abdominal ultrasound in identifying the cause for the abnormality. A distended stomach may be due to a recent meal, a motility problem, or a gastric outflow obstruction. To determine the significance of a distended gastric lumen or the small intestinal lumen, the clinician should ask the owner when the last meal was ingested or whether gastrointestinal signs are present. If the patient has eaten recently or if a question remains regarding the clinical significance of the gastric distension, food should be withheld from the patient for 12 hours and the study repeated to ascertain whether the material is still present. In a vomiting patient or a fasted patient with a distended stomach, a careful evaluation of the wall and lumen of the antrum, pylorus, and the proximal duodenum is warranted.

The cause of the obstruction can be intraluminal, mural, or (less often) extramural. In an intraluminal obstruction, the intestinal tract often will be distended with motile, hypoechoic fluid, and possibly gas or food, orad to the point of the obstruction. The fluid may be propelled ineffectively aborad by peristaltic waves and may move back and forth. In a patient with an acute obstruction peristalsis often is increased, but intestinal smooth muscle also may be hypomotile if the obstruction is chronic. If the high obstruction is very proximal within the duodenum, vomiting and thus periodic removal of some of the contents may decrease distension of the lumen. Distension of the intestine due to an obstruction of the distal small intestine may vary depending on the obstruction's duration and scope (i.e., partial or complete). Segments of small intestine distal to the obstruction usually are of normal size. When a dilated segment of intestine is observed, it is useful to determine the section of intestine involved. To accomplish this, the dilated segment is followed in each direction to the point of the obstruction. By following the segment in each direction, the orad and aborad course of the intestine can

be determined. The lumen and wall at the point of the change in diameter of the intestine is examined critically to determine if there is any evidence of a luminal or mural obstruction (Figures 16-8 and 16-9). The lumen is evaluated critically for a focal change in appearance of the contents. This may be manifested by a change in echogenicity, amount of sound attenuated by the contents, or by the shape, size, or margin definition observed. The wall is interrogated for a change in thickness (increased or focally decreased), for a change in echogenicity and visibility of separate wall layers, for gas in the wall, and for plication (Figure 16-10). The adjacent peritoneal cavity also is evaluated for fluid, free air, and hyperechoic omentum, which may be adhered to the serosal wall, consistent with inflammation and possibly intestinal leakage.

As discussed previously, a stricture may cause a distended intestinal lumen orad to the site of obstruction with a normal luminal size distal to the obstruction, and with minimal to no apparent change in the wall thickness at the site of the obstruction. This narrowed area should be monitored for several minutes to rule out the possibility of focal temporary narrowing due to a peristaltic wave. If an obstruction occurs within the ileum, the entire small intestine may be distended. Locating the ileum in the right midabdomen as it enters the colon is useful to make sure that the luminal distension is due to an obstructive process and not due to functional ileus. With exocrine pancreatic insufficiency, malabsorption, feline dysautonomia, or some inflammatory diseases, the intestine may be distended markedly throughout its length without any normal-sized small intestine detected. If the entire small intestine and the colon are dilated and if there is no mass or intussusception at the ileocolic junction, it is unlikely that the luminal dilation was caused by surgery or a mechanical obstruction. In this case a medical cause should be investigated. An exception

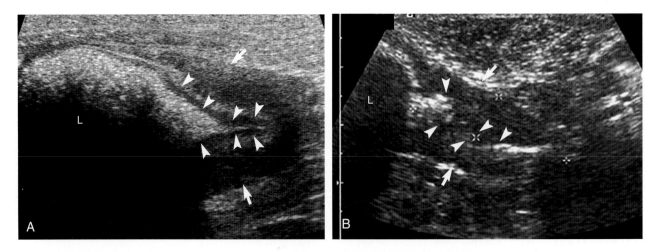

Figure 16-8 Intestinal obstruction. Obstruction of the intestine may be due to a foreign object within the lumen or a stricture or mural mass narrowing and occluding the lumen. **A** and **B,** Mural masses that have obstructed the small intestinal lumen. The *arrows* point to the serosal surface of the intestinal wall. The dilated proximal segment of intestine can be seen to the left on each image. The *arrowheads* point to the narrowing of the lumen and the thickened wall. **A,** The mucosal surface of the intestine is smooth, suggesting a lymphosarcoma. **B,** The mucosal surface of the intestine is very irregular, suggesting a carcinoma. However, a biopsy is required for definitive diagnosis.

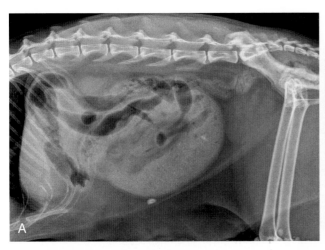
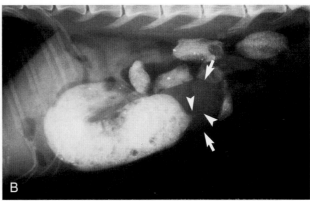

Figure 16-9 Intestinal obstruction. Complete or partial obstruction of the intestine often results in dilation of the intestine proximal to the point of obstruction (mechanical or obstructive ileus). **A,** Large segment of small intestine that is distended and filled with heterogeneous material. **B,** Barium in the dilated segment of bowel. The lumen *(arrowheads)* at the point of obstruction is narrowed. Visible borders *(arrows)* help distinguish the obstructing mass, which was diagnosed as an adenocarcinoma.

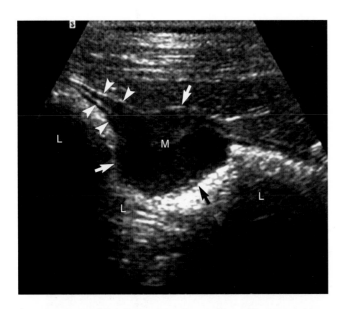

Figure 16-10 Mural colonic mass. A mural mass in the colonic wall extends into the lumen *(L, arrows)*. On both sides of the mass *(M)* more normal wall can be seen. The wall layers are normal at the left side of the image but then are gradually lost. The wall is expanded and becomes confluent with the mass *(arrowheads)*. The mass is hypoechoic and extends into the lumen. The hyperechoic contents of the lumen are displaced by this focal wall tumor.

would be the presence of a volvulus/torsion of the colon and the small intestine at the root of the mesentery. In this situation, which often is accompanied by markedly gas-distended intestinal loops, the patient usually is in critical condition with marked vascular compromise of the intestine.

Foreign Bodies

Foreign bodies are a frequent cause of a luminal obstruction in feline patients. Correlating the ultrasound findings with abdominal radiographs can help identify the significance of an ingested foreign body. Determining the location, the type of foreign body, and the impact it has had on the intestine and surrounding tissues is important in the diagnostic evaluation of the patient. Using ultrasound to identify and locate the foreign object in multiple planes can be beneficial in deciding whether endoscopy or surgery would be appropriate for removing the foreign body. The sonographic appearance of a foreign body will vary relative to its physical and mechanical makeup. Luminal fluid often surrounds and outlines the margin of the foreign object. This highlights the contour or shape and can help the sonologist recognize a characteristic shape (Figure 16-11). Some foreign bodies, such as a ball, are easy to identify. Others, such as cloth, plastic, or rubber products, are highly attenuating, can have a hyperechoic surface, and involve multiple or long sections of intestine (Figure 16-12).[6] These are more difficult to image and identify.

Not all foreign objects incite a clinical problem in the patient, and grass, hair, food, or other ingested materials may be identified incidentally during the ultrasound examination. Determining if foreign objects are incidental is important for the management of the patient and can be accomplished by examining the relevant historical signs of intestinal disease and determining if the foreign object is causing a change of the luminal size, shape, or wall thickness. Intraluminal nematodes, such as ascarids (i.e., *Toxocara cati*), may be identified as double-walled, tubular, undulating, often tangled foreign objects within the intestinal lumen (Figure 16-13). Occasionally, they may cause an obstruction due to focal accumulation of the worms.

Foreign bodies such as hair balls (gastric or enteric trichobezoars) often have an irregular, poorly defined margin, are heterogeneous and space occupying, and have a hyperechoic surface with significant attenuation and shadowing (Figure 16-14). They are often found in

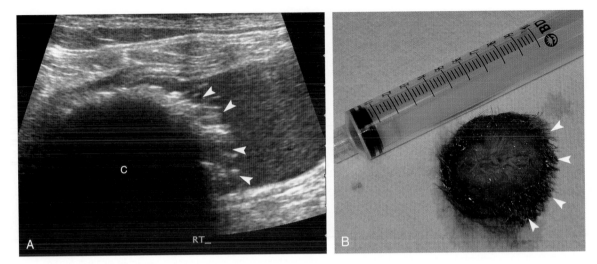

Figure 16-11 Gastric foreign body. **A,** Foreign body obstructing the pylorus of the stomach. The center of the circular mass is highly attenuating and causes a significant shadow distal to the object *(C)*. The border of the foreign object shows linear projections into the lumen that are mobile in the surrounding fluid *(arrowheads)*. The appearance of the object on the ultrasound image is understandable when compared to the appearance of the toy **(B)** removed from the stomach.

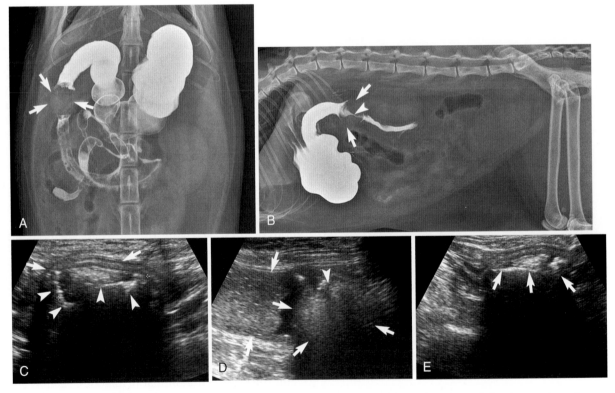

Figure 16-12 Intestinal foreign body. This foreign object was within the lumen of the proximal duodenum. **A,** and **B,** Barium outlines the proximal margin and partially outlines the outer border of the foreign object *(arrows)*. It is also able to pass though the small center of the foreign object *(arrowhead)*. **C,** The stomach and duodenum proximal to the obstruction are dilated. The stomach *(arrows)* also contains some foreign objects *(arrowheads)*. **D** and **E,** The ultrasound image. The lumen of the duodenum is dilated *(arrows)* with fluid outlining the irregular margins of this shadowing foreign object *(arrowhead)*, which was a piece of plastic. The object was effectively obstructing the lumen.

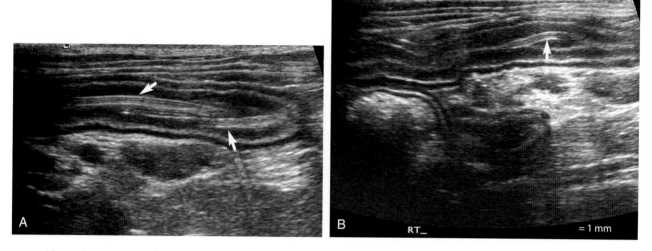

Figure 16-13 Intestinal nematodes. This ultrasound image shows linear double-walled foreign objects *(arrows)* that represent Ascarids *(Toxocara cati)* in the lumen of the jejunum. Roundworms often are linear, but may fold back on themselves. Other foreign objects such as straw or plant material also can have this tubular appearance. These live worms can move independently of the peristaltic activity of the intestine.

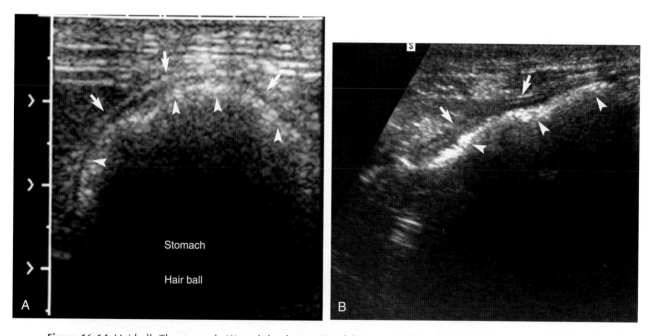

Figure 16-14 Hairball. The stomach **(A)** and duodenum **(B)** of this cat are distended, with contents that shadow and have a hyperechoic surface *(arrowheads)*. The mildly irregular surface often is not sharply margined, and the luminal contents are partially outlined by fluid in the lumen. It may completely or partially fill the lumen of the stomach or small intestine. This appearance is consistent with a hairball or possibly cloth or some type of plastic. If any question remains whether the material could be food, food should be withheld and a repeat examination performed after 8 to 12 hours. *Arrows* point to the gastric wall **(A)** and duodenal wall **(B)**.

the stomach, but also may be found obstructing the small intestine. A suspicious accumulation of hair in the stomach may or may not be clinically relevant: Some types of food or incidental accumulations of hair can mimic a clinically relevant hairball. Correlating the findings with an appropriate history and repeating the exam after withholding food for 12 hours may be warranted in a patient prior to anesthesia for surgery or endoscopy to ascertain that the material is still present.

Some foreign objects have sharp margins and may penetrate or irritate the wall, resulting in peritonitis or vascular compromise. The shape of the object, the contact with the wall, the reaction of the adjacent wall, vascular compromise, and evidence of perforation are important parameters to examine. Determining the kind of foreign body present often is challenging.

Linear Foreign Body

Like other foreign bodies, linear objects within the intestinal lumen may be clinically relevant or incidental. Linear foreign objects may be ingested material such as hair or grass. Such material is not embedded in the intestinal wall, has ends that are free in the lumen (not anchored in the stomach), does not have a taut (i.e., anchored) appearance, and is not on the mesenteric side of the small intestine. The adjacent intestine appears normal (not plicated or gathered).

The appearance of a true linear foreign body will depend on the type of material present (e.g., string vs. cloth). Linear foreign bodies have a place of secured attachment such as around the tongue, trapped within the stomach, or, less frequently, bound in multiple areas of the small intestine (Figure 16-15). The remainder progresses downstream. Peristalsis and segmental contractions cause the string to become embedded in the wall of the intestine, which results in gathering or plication of the intestine as the bowel shortens. Typically, the foreign body is located eccentrically on the mesenteric (short)

side of the bowel. The ends of the string are not free or seen within the lumen because they are anchored, resulting in a taut or stretched appearance (Figure 16-16). Both a transverse and a longitudinal view should be obtained. The longitudinal view helps the sonologist recognize the plication pattern evidenced over the length of the intestine and see the string progress and cross multiple undulating segments of intestine in a straight line. The transverse view displays the taut object embedded in the wall on the mesenteric side of the intestinal loops and the potential impact on the surrounding tissue. Echogenic peritoneal fluid may be present, which is consistent with an exudate and peritonitis. Free air in the peritoneal cavity often indicates perforation from erosion through the wall.

Pantyhose, clothlike material, plastic, or rubber products all have a different appearance than a simple string. They often will attenuate the beam, occupy more of the lumen, and show shadowing similar to that of colonic feces. There may be a focal accumulation of clothlike material in one section of intestine and then a string connecting it to a more distal focal accumulation. The section of intestine between the two focal accumulations of foreign material may be plicated. This pattern can be

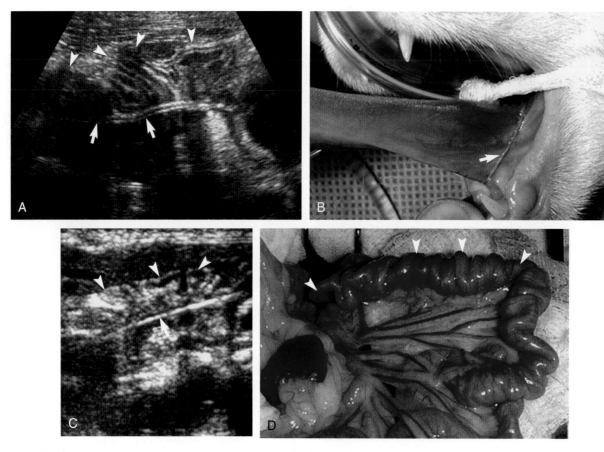

Figure 16-15 Linear foreign bodies. **A,** Linear foreign bodies usually are anchored proximal in the gastrointestinal tract, often under the tongue **(B)** or in the stomach *(arrow)*. The remainder of the string progresses downstream. The intestine may "climb" up on the string, giving a plicated or gathered appearance. **C,** The ultrasound images show the linear foreign object in the center of the intestine *(arrows)* and the corresponding intestinal loops gathered on the string *(arrowheads)*. **D,** The gross specimen shows the gathered pattern of the intestine *(arrowheads),* which helps identify this as a linear foreign body during imaging.

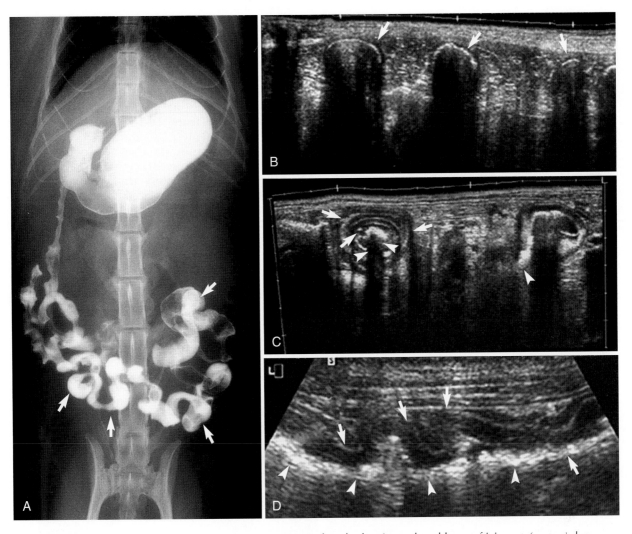

Figure 16-16 Linear foreign body. **A,** Upper gastrointestinal study showing gathered loops of jejunum *(arrows)* due to a linear foreign body anchored in the stomach in this cat. **B,** Ultrasound study on a different patient also shows multiple loops of end-on segments of the gathered small intestine. The long normal segments can not be seen. **C,** An intussusception imaged in a cross section shows a hyperechoic shadowing object *(arrowheads)* within the lumen. **D,** Plications are visible on this section of duodenum, and the lumen contains a hyperechoic linear object that extends throughout the gathered segment of intestine. A linear foreign body was identified that resulted in an intussusception in this patient.

more challenging to identify compared to a simple string such as dental floss because some of the material, due to its size and attenuating properties, can appear to represent feces. Making sure that the segment of intestine in question is the small intestine and not the colon also is important. As mentioned previously, the colon should have a thinner wall, have the smaller ileum entering into it, and exit through the pelvic canal. If necessary, the colon can be located and identified as it courses through the pelvic canal. It then can be followed orad to determine if it communicates with the questionable segment of intestine. The stomach and the pylorus also should be evaluated for any evidence of the foreign body passing through its lumen. When a linear foreign body is identified, the wall should be examined closely for any thickening, ulceration, or perforation. Intussusceptions can occur in conjunction with a linear foreign object due to the

abnormal motility and constriction caused by the plicated segment of intestine.

Intussusception

An *intussusception* occurs when one segment of the gastrointestinal tract is invaginated into an adjacent segment. Gastroesophageal and duodenogastric intussusceptions have the more distal end enter the proximal segment. However, ileocolic intussusceptions are the most frequently encountered. The ultrasonographic appearance of an intussusception is unique, and the diagnosis typically is straightforward. There usually is a fluid distension of the intestine orad to the location of the intussusception, indicating the presence of a mechanical obstruction. The intussusception is made up of the outer intussuscipiens and the inner loop of invaginated intestine, the intussusceptum.

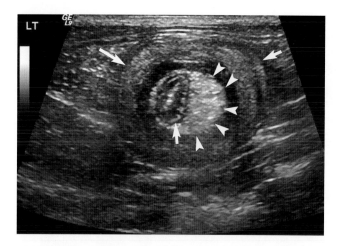

Figure 16-17 A typical transverse ultrasonographic image of an intussusception. The mesentery within the intussusception *(arrowheads)* is hyperechoic. The inner bowel segment *(long arrow),* or intussusceptum, is located eccentrically due to the adjacent mesentery. An outer wall of the double-walled intussuscipiens *(short arrows)* also can be seen.

The classic sonographic image is generated via a transverse plane through the intussusception (Figure 16-17). Concentric hypoechoic rings form the thicker double outer wall, which surrounds a central hyperechoic core (mesentery) and the eccentrically located collapsed small intestine. The intussusceptum usually appears as a normal empty loop of intestine pushed to one side within the intussuscipiens (Figure 16-18). The adjacent trapped hyperechoic mesentery is attached to the mesenteric border of the intussuscepted segment of intestine and is pulled into the intussusception with its segment of intestine. Because the mesentery acts as a mass, its attached segment of intestine is displaced to the opposite wall. The intussuscepted mesentery should appear uniform, except for small mesenteric vessels. Rarely fluid is present within or around the invaginated mesentery as a result of hemorrhage or cystic formations caused by lymphatic obstruction or vascular compromise. These changes are seen in cases of chronic intussusception (Figure 16-19). Interrogation of the blood flow within the bowel loops may help to determine the viability of the intestine. The longitudinal plane through the intussusception shows one bowel segment telescoped into the other. The entrance and the

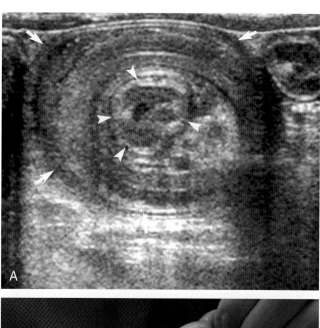

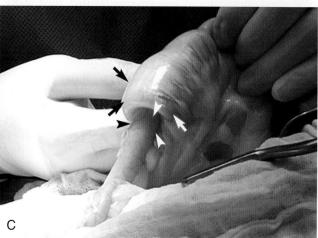

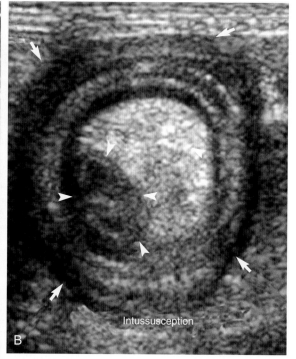

Figure 16-18 Intestinal intussusception. **A** and **B,** Typical transverse ultrasonographic views of an intussusception. The intussuscipiens is double-walled and appears thickened *(arrows).* The invaginated loop of intestine is located eccentrically, with the hyperechoic mesentery *(arrowheads)* displacing the loop of intestine to the side. **C,** On exploratory laparotomy a piece of small intestine was invaginated into the lumen of another segment of small intestine.

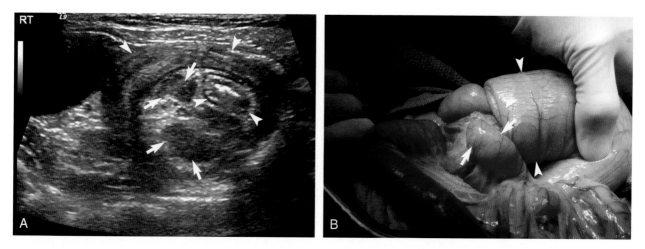

Figure 16-19 Intestinal intussusception. **A,** Transverse ultrasonographic view through an intussusception that showed multiple masses in the mesentery *(arrows)* that were pulled into the intussusception with the mesentery. The *arrowheads* point to the segments of intestine involved in the intussusception. **B,** On exploratory laparotomy these masses were identified as enlarged, infiltrated lymph nodes secondary to a carcinoma at the ileocolic junction *(arrows)*.

extent of involvement can be seen on this view. The leading edge of the intussusceptum can be identified because it is surrounded by focal fluid at the aborad (distal) portion of the intussusception. The intussusceptum should be empty of luminal contents. However, a hyperechoic internal structure may indicate a linear foreign body as the inciting cause. Such a structure can be followed beyond the intussusception, where the plicated intestine is found.

Enlarged lymph nodes or a thickened gastrointestinal wall may be seen near or within the mesentery in patients with an intussusception. This can help identify the initiating cause of the intussusception as an intestinal tumor, granuloma, or infiltrated lymph node. In one report of 20 cats with an intussusception, lymphoma was found in association with the intussusception in seven cases.[7]

MURAL CHANGES

Diagnosing the underlying cause of mural changes often is complicated by an incomplete understanding of specific changes associated with different diseases, the varying severity of changes associated with a specific disease, similar pathological changes seen in different disease processes, and the limitations of current technology. These factors lead to overlapping and nonspecific findings and point to the work needed to clarify this area. Infiltrative disease, regardless of the underlying cause, affects the sonographic appearance of the intestinal wall because it leads to thickening (focal or diffuse) of one or all of the layers (Figure 16-20). The layers also can be disrupted, with loss of distinction of one or more layers. In these situations ultrasonographic findings need to be combined with information derived from the history, laboratory data, and abnormalities affecting other organs to determine the underlying disease process. Some diseases associated with unique or specific changes may be easier to diagnose. It is crucial to realize that an ultrasonographic appearance does not provide a histological diagnosis; however, through pattern recognition of typical changes associated with specific diseases, it can yield a reasonable list of differential diagnoses for most patients. Serum concentrations of folate and cobalamin can be assessed in combination with other laboratory results and correlated with the history and ultrasound findings to help determine the significance of the sonographic findings and rank the differential diagnoses.[8] An aspiration or biopsy (endoscopic, transabdominal, or surgical) may be necessary for determining the definitive diagnosis.

Diseases that affect the wall of the intestines are divided into inflammatory or neoplastic conditions. Thickening (focal or diffuse) of the wall, presence or absence of distinct wall layers (one or multiple), and echogenicity are useful aids in evaluating the gastrointestinal wall. Intestinal wall thickening is the most consistent sonographic finding in an infiltrative disease process. All wall layers may be involved uniformly, or only specific layers may be affected. A change in the hypoechoic layers (i.e., muscular and mucosal layers) may be easier to appreciate sonographically (Figure 16-21). The detection of diffuse changes or a focal change has been reported to be helpful in ranking the list of differential diagnoses.[12,29,32,34] Generalized thickening often is seen with inflammatory disorders, but also sometimes with intestinal lymphoma. Localized and asymmetrical thickening with disruption of wall layering often indicates a potentially serious infiltrative process and neoplasia. In general, the more aggressive the lesion appears—and the more involved the intestine and surrounding area or adjacent organs—the more likely it is that the underlying disease process is neoplastic. Unfortunately, the severity of intestinal thickening is not always a parameter that can be used to distinguish an inflammatory disease from a neoplastic process (see Chapter 17).

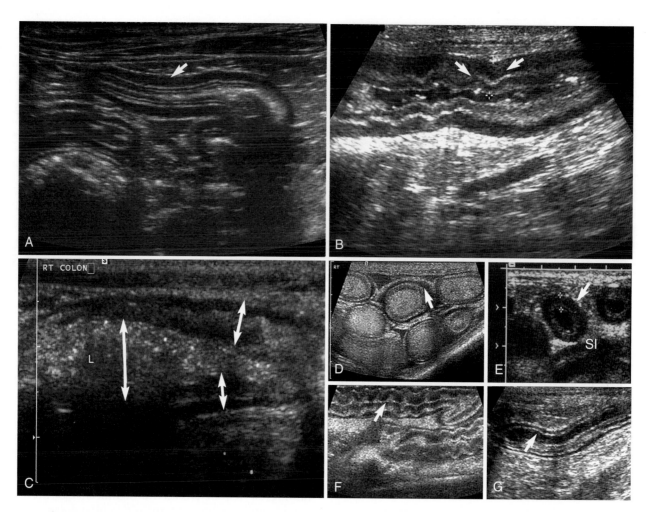

Figure 16-20 Intestinal infiltrative lesions. **A,** Thickened muscular layer *(arrow)*. The other layers appear normal. This patient was diagnosed with an intestinal lymphosarcoma. **B,** The intestinal muscularis layer *(arrows)* also is thickened and layering is intact, but there is a change in the thickness, smoothness, and echogenicity of the layers. These ultrasonographic findings were secondary to histoplasmosis. **C,** The intestinal wall becomes gradually thicker *(double-ended small arrows)* and obstructs the lumen of the bowel *(L)*. The wall layers are less distinct than normal. This patient had an inflammatory infiltrate in the colon. **D,** There are multiple loops of intestine, which are dilated. Increased motility could be appreciated during the ultrasound study. One segment of intestine *(arrow)* shows mild thickening compared to the remaining loops. Peritoneal effusion also is present. This patient had an intestinal lymphosarcoma. **E,** Thickening, change in echogenicity, and loss of wall layer distinction *(arrow)* due to toxoplasmosis. **F,** The bowel wall *(arrow)* is spastic due to an irritated segment of intestine, which was suspected to be due to ischemia. **G,** One layer of the intestinal wall is thickened on one side *(arrow)*, which was determined to be due to an intestinal lymphosarcoma.

Inflammatory Diseases

Many diseases are associated with an inflammatory infiltration of the intestinal wall. Possible causes include dietary allergens, protein-losing enteropathy, lymphocytic-plasmacytic enteritis, eosinophilic enteritis, bacterial enteritis, viral enteritis, fungal disease, and protozoal or helminthic infestation.[9,10] Inflammatory intestinal disease, such as lymphocytic-plasmacytic enteritis, is a frequent problem in cats (Figure 16-22).[11] Some of these conditions cause minimal ultrasonographic mural changes, while others result in diffuse or focal thickening or erosive changes of the mucosal surface. Differentiation of a specific infiltrative disease often is difficult because disease indications frequently overlap and there are few

specific ultrasonographic features to differentiate among these types of lesions.[12,13]

Ultrasound often is used to locate the affected bowel segment, to determine the extent of disease, and to further classify or describe the effect on the wall's thickness and the specific appearance of its layers. Sonographic changes that indicate inflammatory disease may be absent, minimal, moderate, or severe, in regard to thickening of the bowel wall and alteration of bowel wall layering. In general, the distinction of the wall layers is retained. Wall thickening primarily may affect the mucosa, the submucosa, or the muscular layer. There may be pinpoint hyperechoic foci in the mucosa or an echogenic band in the area of the mucosa. The latter often is

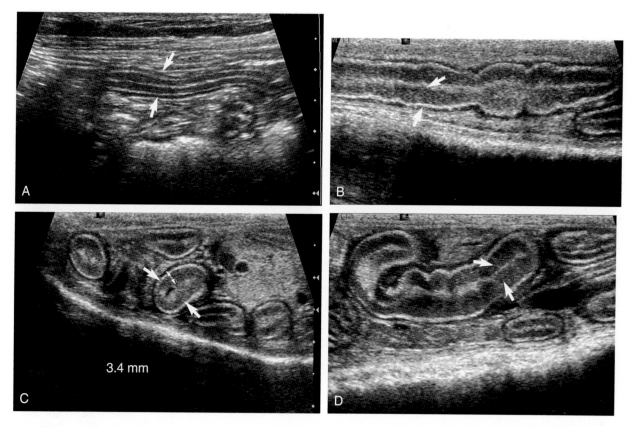

Figure 16-21 Inflammatory bowel disease. Ultrasonographic findings in a patient with inflammatory bowel disease. **A,** Normal segment of duodenum showing the normal intestinal wall layering *(arrows).* **B** to **D,** Various intestinal segments that show **(B)** a thickened wall (3.4 mm), **(C)** a thickened mucosa, and **(D)** an increased echogenicity of the bowel wall *(arrows).*

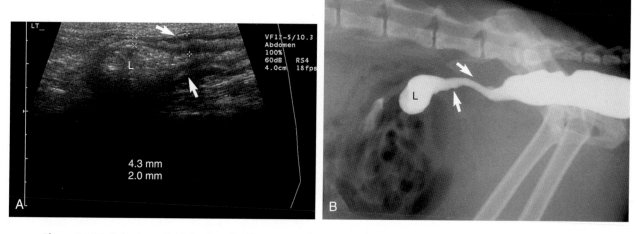

Figure 16-22 Colonic wall thickening. **A,** Ultrasonographic image of a patient with focal colonic thickening (4.3 mm vs. 2.0 mm in the normal wall) of the distal descending colon. The thickened wall is restricting and partially obstructing the lumen *(L).* **B,** Barium enema in the same patient, showing the normal lumen *(L)* to the left and the focally narrowed lumen *(arrows)* in the center of the image. These findings were due to inflammatory colitis.

easier to recognize in dogs with infiltrative lesions because the intestinal wall is thicker in this species. In dogs, the linear hyperechoic areas, which appear either as bands or striations aligned perpendicular to the lumen of the bowel, have been reported in patients with protein-losing enteropathy and dilated lacteals from lymphangiectasia.

Loss of wall layer integrity may occur with severe ulcerative enteritis or inflammatory diseases caused by *Histoplasma capsulatum* or *Mycobacterium* spp. Inflammatory disease of the pancreas, liver, and the intestinal tract has been reported to occur concurrently in cats.[14] Therefore it is helpful to examine the liver and the pancreas

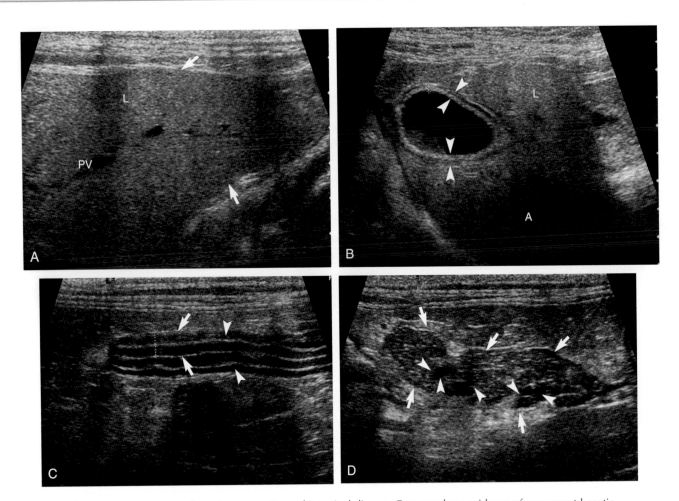

Figure 16-23 Concurrent hepatic, pancreatic, and intestinal disease. Cats can show evidence of concurrent hepatic lipidosis, cholangitis/cholangiohepatitis, pancreatitis, and inflammatory bowel disease. **A,** Enlarged hyperechoic attenuating liver *(L),* suggesting hepatic lipidosis.[15,56] The hypoechoic structure is a hepatic vessel *(PV).* **B,** The gall bladder has a double wall *(arrowheads),* the liver is hyperechoic *(L),* and there is attenuation of the sound in the distal liver *(A),* suggesting cholangiohepatitis. **C,** The wall of the intestine appears thickened overall *(arrows)* and the muscular layer is specifically thickened *(arrowheads).* These findings can be associated with inflammatory bowel disease. **D,** Pancreas shows hypoechoic areas *(arrowheads)* and is enlarged *(arrows),* which is consistent with pancreatitis.

routinely for evidence of pancreatitis and/or cholangitis/cholangiohepatitis (Figure 16-23). In one study, 80 per cent of cats with cholangiohepatitis had inflammatory bowel disease and 50 per cent had pancreatitis.[15]

Thickening of the intestinal muscularis layer appears to have been detected more frequently in recent years— or possibly recognized more frequently as imaging tools improve. Reports indicate that the thickening often is due to smooth muscle hypertrophy (Figure 16-24). Intestinal muscular hypertrophy has been reported in a variety of species.[16] The pathogenesis is poorly understood in any species. There are two major forms, with more than one pathophysiological mechanism leading to its formation. One form is viewed as a compensatory mechanism, but the second form is less well understood and is classified as idiopathic. The compensatory form has been associated with chronic enteritis or secondary to chronic obstruction cranial to an area of an intestinal stenosis. One report speculated that the pathogenesis of muscular hypertrophy in horses could be associated with tapeworm

infestation *(Anoplocephala perfoliata),* irritation from accumulated ingested sand, or chronic intestinal distension.[17] Rabbits with experimentally induced partial intestinal stenosis initially had intestinal dilation followed by muscular hypertrophy 8 to 10 days following the induction of the stenosis. Dogs, rats, and guinea pigs also developed muscular hypertrophy 3 to 5 weeks after induction of an intestinal stenosis.[18-20] In these reports, both the circular and longitudinal layers of the muscularis were hypertrophied.

The pathogenesis of the idiopathic form of muscular hypertrophy is not well understood. Possible factors include autonomic imbalance producing uncontrolled peristalsis, or prolonged spastic contractions associated with neurogenic abnormalities, mucosal inflammation, and stagnation of intestinal contents.[21,22] There is speculation that chemical mediators associated with parasitism, as seen in rat and guinea pig models, also may be a factor. When parasite-free foals were infected with *Parascaris equorum,* they developed hyperplasia of the muscu-

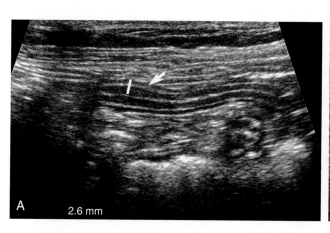
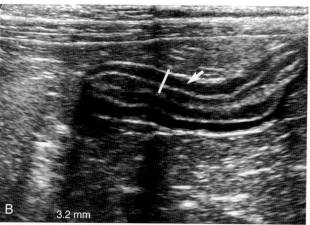

Figure 16-24 Smooth muscle hypertrophy. **A,** Segment of intestine with a normal wall thickness of 2.6 mm *(bar)* and normal muscular layer *(arrow)*. **B,** The intestinal wall is thickened (3.2 mm; *bar*) and the muscular layer is hypoechoic *(arrow)* and thickened, consistent with smooth muscle hypertrophy seen in patients with inflammatory bowel disease.

laris 80 days postinfection.[23] Four cats with confirmed intestinal smooth muscle hypertrophy have been reported.[24] One case was associated with stenosis due to adjacent alimentary lymphoma, one with a foreign body, and two with chronic enteritis. It is important to be aware that the ultrasonographic appearance of small cell lymphoma can be similar to that of idiopathic muscular hypertrophy (see Chapter 17). There is speculation that cats with this ultrasonographic change may develop lymphoma later or that this condition represents an early phase of the disease. Therefore, when a uniform thickening of the muscularis layer is observed, it may be useful to obtain a full-thickness biopsy to differentiate small cell lymphoma from idiopathic muscular hypertrophy. It also may be of benefit to follow these patients to identify the underlying cause and to determine if there is an association with developing lymphoma later. An ultrasound-guided transabdominal aspirate of the affected wall does not provide enough unique cells to distinguish between the two conditions. In cats with inflammatory bowel disease, the regional lymph nodes often are only mildly enlarged (2 to 4 mm in width), mildly rounded, and hypoechoic. Attempts can be made to aspirate these lymph nodes, but this may be challenging. When aspirating these lymph nodes, the clinician must take care to avoid penetrating the mesenteric veins and arteries sandwiched between them. Often the mesenteric lymph nodes are quite mobile and move away from the needle.

Specific infectious agents can cause inflammatory changes and may cause mild to moderate wall thickening secondarily in the intestine. Examples include granulomatous diseases due to *Histoplasma capsulatum, Mycobacterium* spp., *Toxoplasma gondii,* or other infectious agents.[25,26] A subtle loss of wall layering may be observed. Often the adjacent regional lymph nodes are mildly to moderately enlarged and rounded. Other fungal diseases (e.g., mucormycosis) can result in significant thickening of the wall with loss of wall layering. This can be observed more frequently in dogs than in cats. Endoparasites,

including *Toxocara cati,* also may result in minimal to mild thickening of the wall. Infrequently, there may be focal wall thickening from hemorrhage associated with trauma or focal intramural bleeding from warfarin toxicity, or from adjacent inflamed tissue secondary to pancreatitis.

Ingestion of noxious or corrosive material may damage the intestinal wall and cause erosive gastritis and/or enteritis. Transient colonic wall thickening has been observed in some cats secondary to repeated enemas. Also, hydrogen peroxide often is given to induce vomiting; however, because it is an oxidizing agent, it also can induce erosive gastritis and/or enteritis in some cats (Figure 16-25). Furthermore, embolization of air from hydrogen peroxide has been reported to result in brain and spinal cord infarction in human beings, but this has not been reported in cats. Sloughing of the mucosal surface or erosive enteritis may be seen with a corrosive material, severe bacterial enteritis such as clostridial enteritis, or in a segment of intestine that shows vascular compromise due to severe bowel ischemia. Patients with these signs may display defects of the mucosa, air within the intestinal wall, ulcers, or a pseudomembrane in the lumen (Figure 16-26). These patients also often show poor intestinal motility and mild fluid distension of the lumen. Focal air in the wall of the intestine occasionally may be found incidentally, due to a foreign object that has partially penetrated the wall. However, focal air also may be present secondary to a severe ulceration, tumor necrosis, or vascular compromise of the intestinal wall (Figure 16-27). The adjacent wall and the lumen should be examined closely for any evidence of a potential cause, as well as the surrounding tissue for any evidence of a communication with the peritoneal cavity.[27]

Feline infectious peritonitis (FIP) can present sonographically with a diffusely thickened wall, loss of layering, focal masses, and also with effaced, enlarged, hypoechoic lymph nodes. In a study that reviewed records of cats with FIP, 26 of 156 cats (16.7 per cent) with a histological diagnosis of FIP had apparently

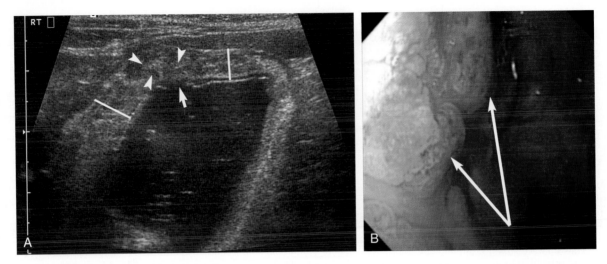

Figure 16-25 Gastric lesions due to hydrogen peroxide. **A,** Ultrasonographic image of this stomach shows a greatly thickened wall *(bars)*. The wall layers *(arrowheads)* are indistinct and patchy. The mucosal surface has areas that are denuded *(large arrow)*. **B,** On the endoscopic image the surface of the gastric mucosa shows ulcerated and edematous areas *(arrows)*. These lesions were secondary to the caustic changes due to hydrogen peroxide.

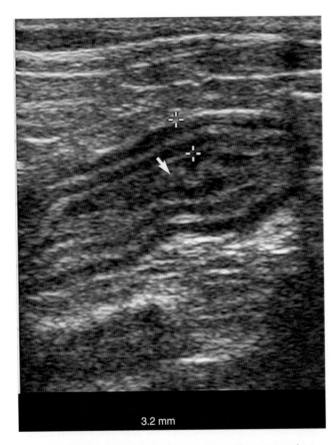

Figure 16-26 Pseudomembrane. Ultrasonographic image of a pseudomembrane *(arrow)* in the lumen of this intestine, resulting from sloughing of the mucosa due to severe enteritis and vascular compromise. The wall of the intestine is thickened at 3.2 mm.

solitary mural intestinal lesions (Figure 16-28). All of the affected cats had lesions in the colon or involving the ileocecocolic junction that initially were thought to be neoplastic. The affected intestine was markedly thickened, nodular, and firm with multifocal pyogranulomas extending throughout the wall of the bowel. Associated lymph nodes were enlarged.[28] In such cases aspiration of affected intestinal wall and lymph nodes may be necessary to determine that the underlying disease process is pyogranulomatous and to rule out additional types of enteritis or neoplasia[29] (see Chapter 71).

Bowel sections also can have a spastic or "thumbprinting" appearance. This corrugation of the intestine appears as an undulating longitudinal segment of intestine. This is a nonspecific finding that indicates an irritated segment of intestine, which could be due to enteritis, pancreatitis, peritonitis, neoplasia, or vascular compromise. When seen, the surrounding tissue should be examined carefully for evidence of peritonitis, focal inflammation from pancreatitis, or rupture of the urinary bladder, gall bladder, or possibly the intestinal tract. Also, the vasculature of the affected segment of intestine should be examined for patency and for evidence of high resistance to flow (Figures 16-29 and 16-30). Echogenic peritoneal fluid is consistent with an exudate, which may be due to inflammation or hemorrhage. An aspirate of the fluid may be useful in determining the underlying cause and if surgery is warranted.

Neoplastic Diseases

Neoplasia in the gastrointestinal tract of cats is relatively common, with lymphoma being the most common type identified. Intestinal lymphoma can be divided further into large cell lymphoma and small cell lymphoma (see Chapter 17). Other types of round cell tumors that can be identified in the intestinal tract of cats include mast cell tumor, plasma cell tumor, and histiocytic neopla-

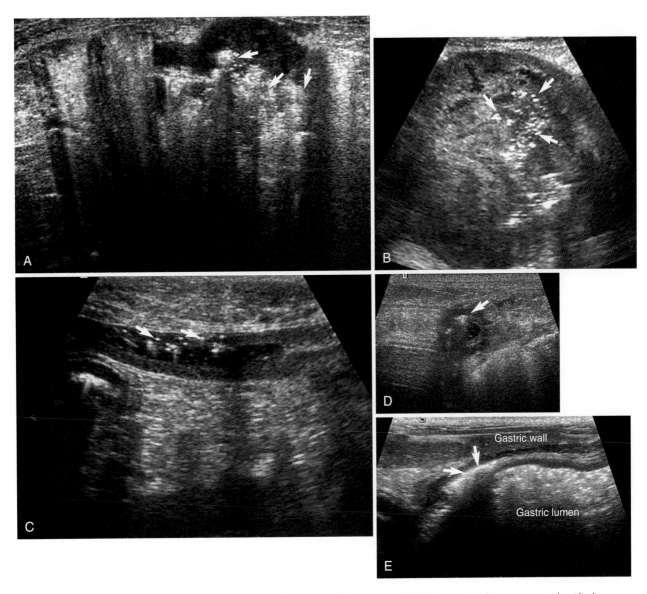

Figure 16-27 Intestinal tumor. **A,** Focal intestinal mass containing gas and fluid *(arrows)*. This mass was identified as an intestinal tumor with breakdown of the wall and subsequent abscess formation. **B,** Large cecal tumor with gas in the center and visible hyperechoic foci *(arrows)*. **C,** Hyperechoic foci in the wall of the intestine. The layers are also indistinct and hypoechoic *(arrows)*. This patient had severe enteritis. **D,** Focal gas can be seen in the wall of the intestine *(arrow)* due to a perforated duodenal ulcer from a mast cell tumor in the spleen. Air and fluid also are present in the peritoneal cavity due to septic peritonitis. **E,** Focal air *(arrows)* can be seen in the wall of the stomach. A straight foreign body (not seen in the image) was present in the lumen of the stomach and was suspected to have partially penetrated the wall of the stomach with migration of air into the wall. An exploratory surgery the following day showed resolution of the gas in the wall but focal gas in the adjacent liver. There was straw or plant material in the stomach.

sia[30,31] (see Chapters 65 and 67). Carcinomas (i.e., adenocarcinoma, carcinoma, or undifferentiated carcinoma) also can affect any section of the gastrointestinal tract; however, it has been reported that there is an increased frequency of occurrence in the ileocolic region, especially in Siamese cats.[32,33] Less frequent tumors include leiomyosarcomas or benign polyps (Figure 16-31).[34-38]

Ultrasonographic evaluation in patients with gastrointestinal neoplasia often is useful to help determine the site and extent of the disease. Asymmetric wall thickening with loss of the layering is typical of an aggressive process, such as neoplasia, abscess, or fungal disease (Figure 16-32). Most neoplasias lead to hypoechoic mass effects associated with a disruption of the wall layering. Also, disruption of the mucosal surface often denotes an aggressive process. A focal infiltrative disease may distort the wall and protrude into the lumen and compromise it, but it also may extend beyond the serosal surface. The

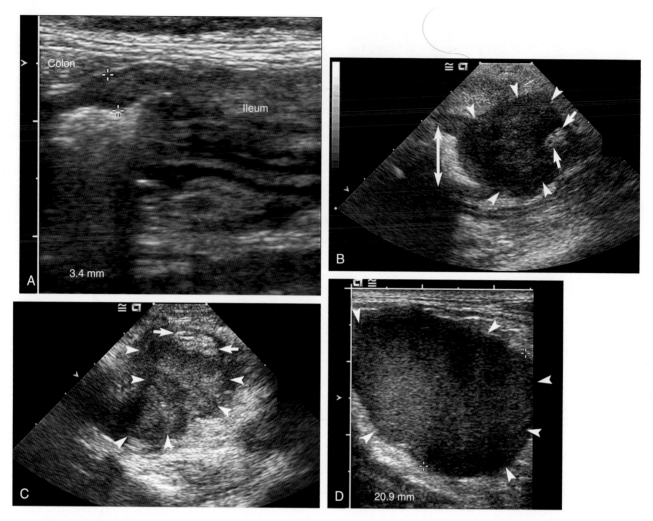

Figure 16-28 Feline infectious peritonitis (FIP). FIP can result in a thickened intestinal wall and enlarged lymph nodes. **A,** In this patient the wall of the colon is focally thickened (3.4 mm). **B,** The wall of the ileum also is greatly thickened. The lumen *(arrows)* can be seen, as well as the thickened eccentric wall infiltrate adjacent to it *(arrowheads)*. The lumen of the intestine adjacent to this area is dilated *(double arrow)*. **C,** A segment of jejunum is infiltrated and a mass *(arrowheads)* can be seen. The remaining intestine is depicted by the *arrows.* **D,** An enlarged (20.9 mm diameter) lymph node near the ileocolic junction *(arrowheads)*. The appearance of FIP can mimic that of intestinal neoplasia.

appearance will vary depending on the stage of advancement of disease. As a general rule round cell tumors (e.g., lymphoma, mast cell, plasma cell, and histiocytic tumors) have a similar ultrasonographic appearance (Figure 16-33). Gastrointestinal large cell lymphoma has been reported to result in the disruption of wall layering.[39] Often, there is a transmural lesion with symmetric thickening of the intestine. The infiltrated area often is homogeneous with smooth walls. Gastric lymphoma may be associated with asymmetric thickening (wall thickness 0.5 to 5 cm). Regional lymphadenopathy also is often observed. Small cell lymphoma can be challenging to identify and can not be differentiated from intestinal inflammation definitively through ultrasonographic examination (Figure 16-34).[40] Small cell lymphoma may cause a thickening of the muscular layer, may cause only minor increases in wall thickness, or may not be associated with any apparent ultrasonographic changes. (See

Chapter 17 for a discussion of low-grade alimentary lymphoma.)

Hypereosinophilic paraneoplastic syndrome is associated with peripheral eosinophilia, eosinophilic infiltration of the intestinal mucosa, and organ dysfunction and is classified as idiopathic, neoplastic, or paraneoplastic. Paraneoplastic hypereosinophilic syndrome has been used as a marker for systemic or intestinal mast cell neoplasia. It also has been documented in cats with T-cell lymphosarcoma.[41-45]

Carcinomas usually present as a large localized mass. They often have a more heterogeneous asymmetric appearance with an irregular contour and can lead to obstruction of the lumen. There often is transmural thickening. A communication with the gastrointestinal lumen may be seen anytime there is a disruption of the mucosal surface. Obstruction from the mural mass also can be present. Ulcers identified as gas-filled craters surrounding

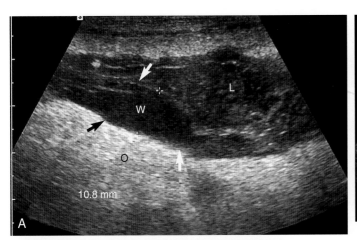

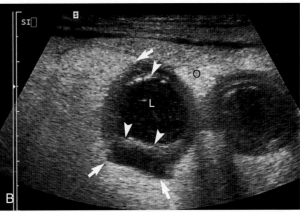

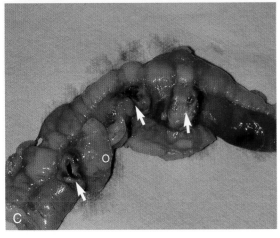

Figure 16-29 Focal intestinal necrosis. Ultrasonographic changes in a patient with focal necrosis and penetrating ulcers. **A,** Longitudinal view of the affected intestine. **B,** Short axis view of the same section of intestine. The intestinal wall shows focal thickening and hypoechoic areas. Gas is present in the wall and also in the area adjacent to it *(arrowheads)*. The omentum *(O)* is adhered to the serosal surface of the wall. **C,** The gross specimen shows the multiple perforated ulcers *(arrows)* and the omentum *(O)*, which is adhered to the surface of the intestine. The cause for the focal necrosis and ulceration in this patient was not determined.

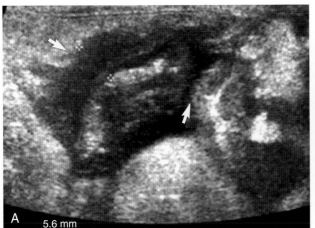

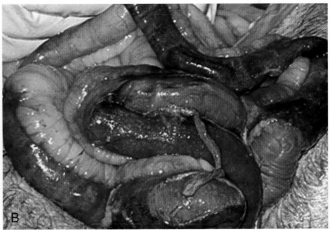

Figure 16-30 Vascular compromise and ischemia. **A,** Wall of the intestine is thickened (3.6 mm) and wall layers are indistinct, with some adhesions to adjacent loops of intestine and omentum *(arrows)*. No blood flow was detected by Doppler. **B,** Necrosis of the wall resulted from vascular compromise to this segment of intestine and led to the death of this patient.

a thickened wall also have been reported to be associated with tumors, but they also can be seen secondary to effects of a tumor elsewhere, such as a mast cell tumor or the administration of nonsteroidal antiinflammatory drugs (Figure 16-35). Rigidity of the infiltrated wall may be determined by evaluating peristaltic waves that progress though a specific wall segment. Wall thickness (either symmetric or asymmetric) and extent of disease (localized or generalized) can help to identify an infiltrated area and to form a list of differential diagnoses. However, an aspirate and/or a biopsy is needed to ascertain the cell type.[46-50]

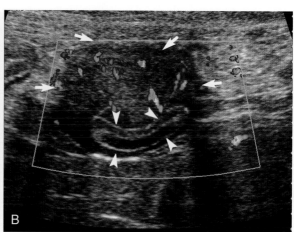

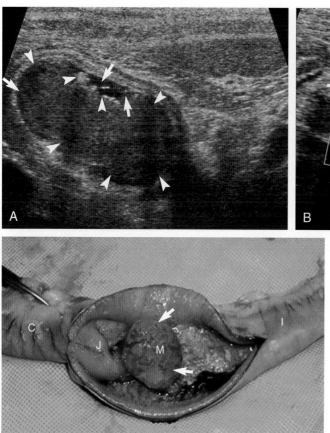

Figure 16-31 Intestinal neoplasia. Masses can extend into the lumen or be external to the wall. **A,** Ultrasonographic image of a carcinoma that has invaded the lumen of the stomach. A small amount of fluid *(arrows)* surrounds and partially outlines the large mass *(arrowheads)* within the gastric lumen. **B,** Ultrasonographic image of a vascular (note the color Doppler depicting the vessels in the mass), eccentrically located mass *(arrows)* along the wall of the intestine *(arrowheads),* which was identified as a mast cell tumor. **C,** An open ileum *(I)* near the colon *(C)* at the ileocolic junction *(J).* The intraluminal mass *(arrows, M)* was identified as a leiomyoma or polyp.

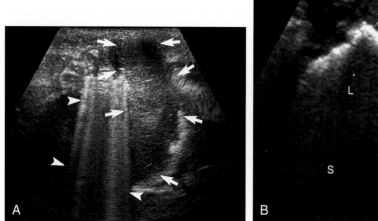

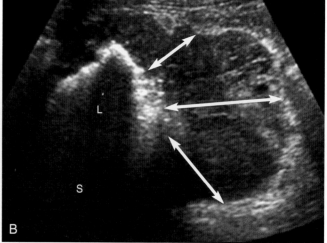

Figure 16-32 Gastric and intestinal neoplasia. Ultrasonographic examinations showing thickened and irregular wall with loss of wall layering (secondary to gastric or intestinal neoplasia). **A,** A gastric carcinoma. The mass is located in the area of the greater curvature *(arrows).* There is a reverberation artifact from gas present in the remaining lumen of the stomach *(arrowheads).* **B,** This patient had a lymphosarcoma of the stomach. The lumen *(L)* has a hyperechoic surface and shadowing *(S)* from the luminal contents. The gastric wall *(double arrows)* is irregular and greatly thickened. The wall layers are lost and the appearance of the wall is heterogeneous.

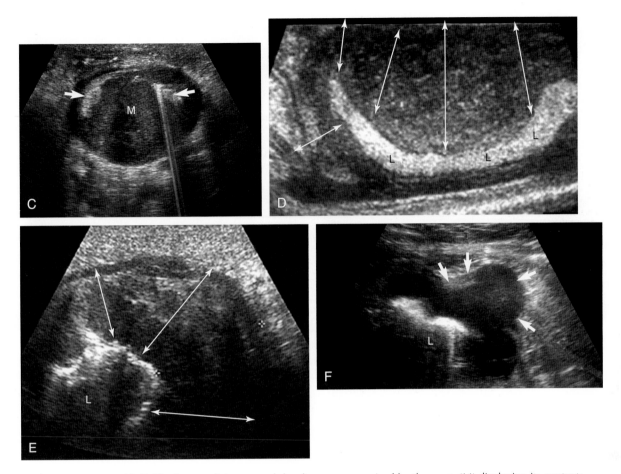

Figure 16-32, cont'd C, The lumen of the stomach has been compromised by the mass *(M)* displacing its contents. The mass was identified as a carcinoma. Note the markedly reduced size of the lumen remaining *(arrows).* **D,** A C-shaped hyperechoic area represents the lumen *(L)* of a segment of small intestine. The lumen is located eccentrically and compressed by the infiltrated wall of the intestine *(double arrows),* which was identified as a mast cell tumor. **E,** The wall of the intestine is markedly thickened and heterogeneous *(double arrows),* and the lumen *(L)* is surrounded by the mast cell tumor. **F,** The serosal surface of the intestinal wall mass (carcinoma) is markedly irregular, with extension and growth of the tumor onto the serosal surface *(arrows).* The lumen *(L)* is partially distended with hyperechoic contents.

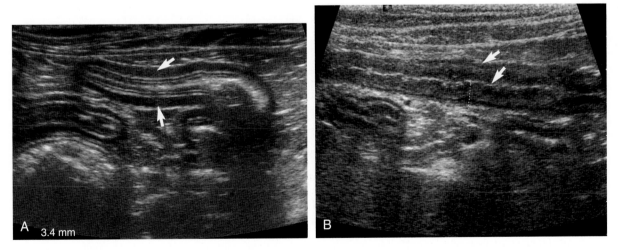

Figure 16-33 Round cell tumors. The appearance of various types of round cell tumors is diverse and may mimic inflammatory bowel disease. **A,** Thickening of the muscular layer and **(B)** the thickened wall and loss of layering with increased echogenicity to the mucosal layer secondary to inflammatory bowel disease and mucosal hypertrophy of the wall *(arrows).*

Continued

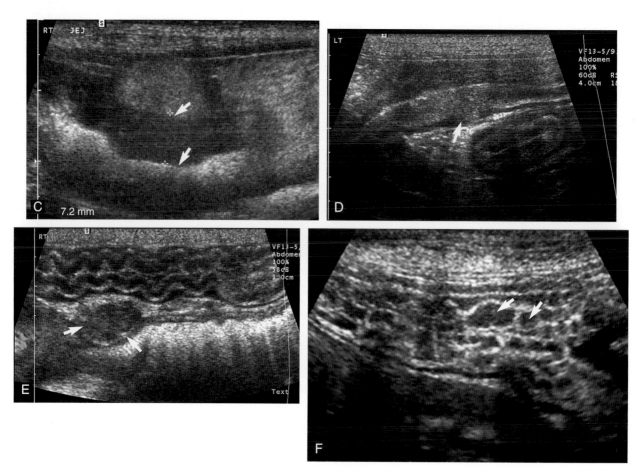

Figure 16-33, cont'd C, The greatly thickened wall with loss of wall definition *(arrows)* due to mast cell tumor. **D,** Focal thickening of the wall *(arrow)* due to a lymphosarcoma. **E and F,** The focal nodules and irregular contour *(arrows)* were due to a plasma cell tumor. Because of the variety of change that can be evidenced, cytological and/ or histopathological examinations are needed for a definitive diagnosis.

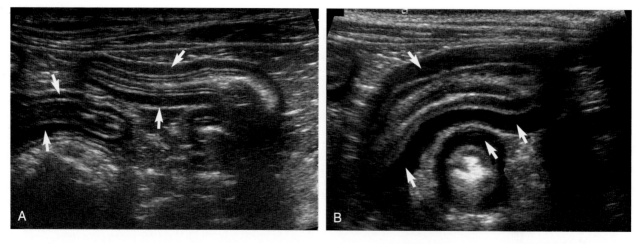

Figure 16-34 Muscular hypertrophy. Thickening of the muscularis layer of the intestinal wall. **A,** Thickening *(arrows)* due to muscular hypertrophy likely associated with inflammatory bowel disease. **B,** Muscular wall layer thickening due to lymphosarcoma *(arrows)*.

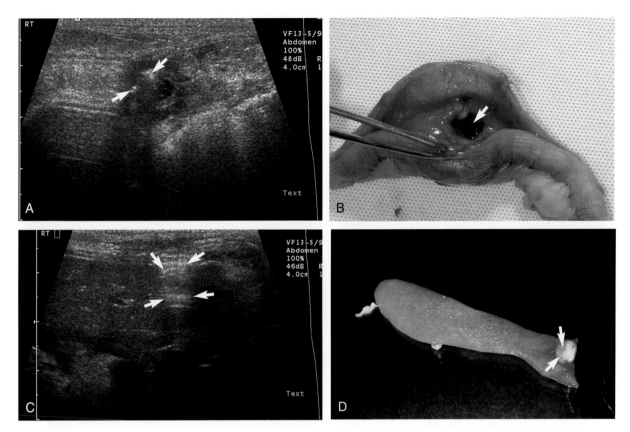

Figure 16-35 Mast cell tumor. A mast cell tumor in the spleen of this patient resulted in a perforated duodenal ulcer. **A,** Gas within the duodenal wall *(arrows)*. **B,** Perforating ulcer in the duodenum *(arrow)*. **C,** Free air can be seen in the peritoneal cavity *(arrows)*. **D,** Mast cell tumor in the spleen *(arrows)*. Histamine released by the mast cell tumor was suspected to have resulted in the perforating ulcer in the duodenum.

The neoplastic infiltrate may extend from the serosal layer to the root of the mesentery, especially with round cell tumors. Therefore evaluation of the corresponding mesenteric veins for vascular flow, vascular invasion, or evidence for effusion is warranted (Figures 16-36 and 16-37). Noting the extent of vascular involvement is important. Vascular involvement can be used as a negative prognostic indicator because these lesions often are nonresectable and can result in fatal vascular compromise of the intestine.

DISPLACEMENT OF INTESTINE

The intestinal tract is highly mobile and sometimes can be pushed through an opening in the body wall (Figure 16-38). Displaced intestinal loops may be seen secondary to a space-occupying lesion and can provide useful information about the source and extent of the mass. The intestine also can be displaced due to trauma and/or loss of integrity of the body wall or diaphragm. Ultrasound is helpful in identifying a hernia containing intestinal loops. It also can provide additional information about the integrity of the intestinal wall, obstruction of the lumen, and viability of the intestine based on vascular compromise noted by color Doppler.

RUPTURE

Dehiscence and rupture or perforation of the intestinal tract, which can be a life-threatening situation, can occur secondary to a surgical enterotomy or a primary intestinal disease. Often, an echogenic peritoneal effusion, consistent with a cellular fluid from an exudate, can be observed during the ultrasound examination. Such fluid accumulation can be focal and walled-off or diffuse. The omentum often is hyperechoic because steatitis with saponification of the mesenteric fat may occur secondary to the peritonitis. If the steatitis is focal, segments of intestine in the same region need to be examined carefully. Often there will be focal thickening of the wall of the offending loop of intestine and the omentum will be attached with minimal fluid between them. The mucosal surface may be irregular and gas may be seen in the intestinal wall, or the wall may appear very thin.

Occasionally, communication of the intestinal lumen with the peritoneal cavity is documented. The omentum may be adhered to the surface of the offending loop of intestine and adhesions between that segment and surrounding structures may be present. There may be corrugation and a spastic appearance to the surrounding intestine. Gas outside the intestinal wall also may be present. The use of gravity to search for free air often is

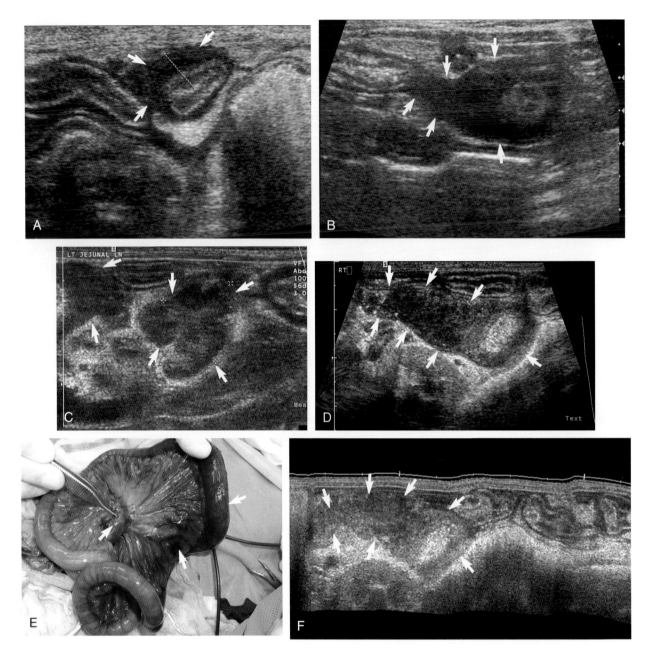

Figure 16-36 Intestinal lymphosarcoma. Lymphosarcoma in the wall of the intestine with extension beyond the serosal surface, following the lymphatics to the root of the mesentery. **A,** Thickened intestinal wall with loss of distinction of the layers of a section of small intestine *(arrows)*. **B,** The infiltrated wall extends beyond the serosal surface because there is extension along the lymphatics. **C,** Adjacent lymph nodes are enlarged and heterogeneous and show loss of the normal shape. These findings are consistent with regional lymph node infiltration. **D** and **F** show the tumor extending from the wall of the intestine into the adjacent mesentery to its root. **E,** Infiltration extending to the root of the mesentery with involvement of the vessels, which led to vascular compromise of the jejunal arteries and veins and vascular compromise to the segment of intestine.

useful. Air may be trapped next to the loop of intestine or free within the abdomen. However, similar changes may be seen postoperatively after an enterotomy. It may be necessary to aspirate peritoneal fluid to look for intracellular bacteria and to correlate these findings with the clinical picture in those cats in whom it is unclear if the changes seen are due to a recent enterotomy or due to intestinal leakage.[51-53]

ASPIRATION

Ultrasound-guided percutaneous fine-needle aspirates of the intestinal tract are a routine and relatively safe procedure. A 22- or 20-gauge needle typically is used. If other organs appear abnormal, such as the spleen or liver, aspirates from those organs are obtained at the same time. Aspiration of a gastrointestinal wall that is only mildly

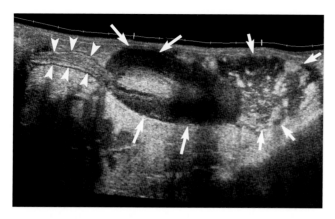

Figure 16-37 Ileal lymphosarcoma. The ileum of this patient is focally infiltrated by a round cell tumor (lymphosarcoma, *long arrows*). The more normal portion of the ileum *(arrowheads)* enters the colon on the left side of the image. There is an infiltrate into the surrounding mesentery to the right of the ileal mass *(short arrows)*. The tumor also is invading the adjacent lymphatics.

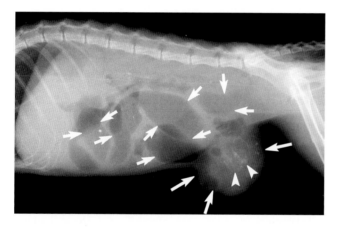

Figure 16-38 Abdominal hernia. Radiographic view of a caudal ventral abdominal traumatic hernia. An incarcerated obstructed intestine *(long arrows)* is seen within the hernia and severely dilated small intestinal loops in the abdominal cavity *(small arrows)*. Radiopaque material within the hernia that does not appear to be totally confined within loops of intestine *(arrowheads)* was due to rupture of the herniated intestine. The loss of detail in the abdomen is due to lack of abdominal fat and peritoneal effusion.

thickened may be unrewarding; exfoliation of cells usually is more successful when the wall is significantly thickened or masses are large (>2 cm).[54] However, some tumors, even when large (e.g., leiomyosarcomas), will not exfoliate adequately. Aspiration of a regional enlarged, rounded, hypoechoic lymph node can help support a diagnosis. However, mildly enlarged jejunal lymph nodes are difficult to aspirate. The cytopathologist often has difficulty in distinguishing the normal or reactive population of lymphocytes from cells from a small round cell tumor (see Chapter 71). The diagnostic yield from aspiration of more destructive and diffuse lesions usually is higher. In one study of six dogs and seven cats, aspiration

of a diagnostic sample was achieved in 83 per cent of the cases. Also, the diagnostic yield improved with larger masses (>2 cm) and with lymphosarcoma.[55]

REFERENCES

1. Gaschen L, Kircher P, Lang J: Endoscopic ultrasound instrumentation, applications in humans, and potential veterinary applications, *Vet Radiol Ultrasound* 44:665, 2003.
2. Schreurs E, Vermote K, Barberet V: Ultrasonographic anatomy of abdominal lymph nodes in the normal cat, *Vet Radiol Ultrasound* 49:68, 2008.
3. Penninck D, Nyland T, Fisher P, et al: Ultrasonography of the normal canine gastrointestinal tract, *Vet Radiol Ultrasound* 30:272, 1989.
4. Groggin JM, Biller DS, Debey BM, et al: Ultrasonographic measurement of gastrointestinal wall thickness and the ultrasonographic appearance of the ileocolic region in healthy cats, *J Am Anim Hosp Assoc* 36:224, 2000.
5. Delaney F, O'Brien RT, Walker K: Ultrasound evaluation of small bowel thickness compared to weight in normal dogs, *Vet Radiol Ultrasound* 44:577, 2003.
6. Tidwell A, Penninck D: Ultrasonography of gastrointestinal foreign bodies, *Vet Radiol Ultrasound* 33:160, 1992.
7. Burkitt JM, Drobatz KJ, Hess RS, et al: Intestinal intussusception in twenty cats, *J Vet Intern Med (abstract)* 15:313, 2001.
8. Simpson KW, Fyfe J, Cornetta A, et al: Subnormal concentrations of serum cobalamin (vitamin B-12) in cats with gastrointestinal disease, *J Vet Intern Med* 15:26, 2001.
9. Jergens AE: Inflammatory bowel disease—current perspectives, *Vet Clin North Am Small Anim Pract* 29:501, 1999.
10. Graham JP, Newell SM, Roberts GD, et al: Ultrasonographic features of canine gastrointestinal pythiosis, *Vet Radiol Ultrasound* 41:273, 2000.
11. Guilford WG, Jones BR, Markwell PJ, et al: Food hypersensitivity in cats with chronic idiopathic gastrointestinal problems, *J Vet Intern Med* 15:7, 2001.
12. Baez JL, Hendrick MJ, Walker LM, et al: Radiographic, ultrasonographic, and endoscopic findings in cats with inflammatory bowel disease of the stomach and small intestine: 33 cases (1990-1997), *J Am Vet Med Assoc* 215:349, 1999.
13. Kircher PR, Spaulding KA, Vaden S, et al: Doppler ultrasonographic evaluation of gastrointestinal hemodynamics in food hypersensitivities: a canine model, *J Vet Intern Med* 18:605, 2004.
14. Newell SM, Selcer BA, Girard E, et al: Correlations between ultrasonographic findings and specific hepatic diseases in cats: 72 cases (1985-1997), *J Am Vet Med Assoc* 213:94, 1998.
15. Weiss DJ, Gagne JM, Armstrong PJ: Relationship between inflammatory hepatic disease and inflammatory bowel disease, pancreatitis, and nephritis in cats, *J Am Vet Med Assoc* 209:1114, 1996.
16. Diana A, Pietra M, Guglielmini C, et al: Ultrasonographic and pathologic features of intestinal smooth muscle hypertrophy in four cats, *Vet Radiol Ultrasound* 44:566, 2003.
17. Chaffin MK, Fuenteabla IC, Schumacher J, et al: Idiopathic muscular hypertrophy of the equine small intestine: 11 cases (1980-1991), *Equine Vet J* 24:372, 1992.
18. Okada A, Okamoto E: Myenteric plexus in hypertrophied intestine, *J Neurovisc Relat* 32:75, 1971.
19. Gabella G, Lond J: Hypertrophy of smooth muscle, *J Physiol* 249:183, 1975.
20. Enochsson L, Hellstrom PM, Nylander G: Myoelectric motility patterns during mechanical obstruction and paralysis of the small intestine in the rat, *Scand J Gastroenterol* 22:969, 1987.

21. Robertson JT: Idiopathic diseases. In Colahan PT, Mayhew JG, Merritt AM, et al, editors: *Equine medicine and surgery,* ed 4, Goleta, Calif, 1991, American Veterinary Publications, p 623.

22. Robertson JT: Diseases of the small intestine. In White NA, editor: *The equine acute abdomen,* Malvern, PA, 1990, Lea & Febiger, p 347.

23. Srihakim, S, Swerczek TW: Pathologic changes and pathogenesis of *Parascaris equorum* infection in parasite-free pony foals, *Am J Vet Res* 39:1155, 1978.

24. Alessia D, Pietra M, Uglielmidnvi C, et al: Ultrasonographic and pathologic features of intestinal smooth muscle hypertrophy in four cats, *Vet Radiol Ultrasound* 44:566, 2003.

25. Cooper DM, Gebhart CJ: Comparative aspects of proliferative enteritis, *J Am Vet Med Assoc* 212:1446, 1998.

26. Bright RM, Jenkins C, DeNovo R, et al: Chronic diarrhea in a dog with regional granulomatous enteritis, *J Small Anim Pract* 35:423, 1994.

27. Van der Gaag I, Happe RP, Wolvekanp WTC: Eosinophilic enteritis complicated by partial ruptures and a perforation of the small intestine in a dog, *J Small Anim Pract* 24:575, 1983.

28. Harvey CJ, Lopez JW, Hendrick MJ: An uncommon intestinal manifestation of feline infectious peritonitis: 26 cases (1986-1993), *J Am Vet Med Assoc* 209:117, 1996.

29. Regnier A, Delverdier M, Dossin O: Segmental eosinophilic enteritis mimicking intestinal tumors in a dog, *Canine Pract* 21:25, 1996.

30. Alroy J, Leav I, DeLellis RA, et al: Distinctive intestinal mast cell neoplasms of domestic cats, *Lab Invest* 33:159, 1975.

31. Turk MA, Gallina AM, Russell TS: Nonhematopoietic gastrointestinal neoplasia in cats: a retrospective study of 44 cases, *Vet Pathol* 18:614, 1981.

32. Cribb AE: Feline gastrointestinal adenocarcinoma: a review and retrospective study, *Can Vet J* 29:709, 1988.

33. Kosovsky JE, Matthiesen DT, Patnaik AK: Small intestinal adenocarcinoma in cats: 32 cases (1978-1985), *J Am Vet Med Assoc* 192:233, 1988.

34. Penninck D, Smyers B, Webster CR, et al: Diagnostic value of ultrasonography in differentiating enteritis from intestinal neoplasia in dogs, *Vet Radiol Ultrasound* 44:570, 2003.

35. Rivers BJ, Walter PA, Feeney DA, et al: Ultrasonographic features of intestinal adenocarcinoma in five cats, *Vet Radiol Ultrasound* 38:300, 1997.

36. MacDonald JM, Mullen HS, Moroff SD: Adenomatous polyps of the duodenum in 18 cats (1985-1990), *J Am Vet Med Assoc* 202:647, 1993.

37. Brody RS: Alimentary tract neoplasms in the cat: a clinicopathologic survey of 46 cases, *Am J Vet Res* 27:74, 1966.

38. Barrand KR, Scudamore CL: Intestinal leiomyosarcoma in a cat, *J Small Anim Pract* 40:216, 1999.

39. Darbes J, Majzoub M, Breuer M, et al: Large granular lymphocyte leukemia/lymphoma in six cats, *Vet Pathol* 35:370, 1998.

40. Roccabianca P, Woo JC, Moore PF: Characterization of the diffuse mucosal associated lymphoid tissue of feline small intestine, *Vet Immunol Immunopathol* 75:27, 2000.

41. Barrs VR, Beatty JA, McCandish IA, et al: Hypereosinophilic paraneoplastic syndrome in a cat with intestinal T-cell lymphosarcoma, *J Small Anim Pract* 43:401, 2002.

42. Gabor LJ, Malik R, Canfield PJ: Clinical and anatomical features of lymphosarcoma in 118 cats, *Aust Vet J* 76:725, 1998.

43. Fondacaro JV, Richter KP, Carpenter JL, et al: Feline gastrointestinal lymphoma: 67 cases (1988-1996), *Eur J Comp Gastroenterol* 4:5, 1999.

44. Hittmair K, Krebitz-Gressl E, Kubber-Heiss A, et al: Feline alimentary lymphosarcoma: radiographical, ultrasonographical, histological and virological findings, *Eur J Compan Anim Pract* 11:119, 2001.

45. Mahony OM, Moore AS, Cotter SM, et al: Alimentary lymphoma in cats: 28 cases (1988-1993), *J Am Vet Med Assoc* 207:1593, 1995.

46. Penninck DG, Nyland T, Kerr L, et al: Ultrasonographic evaluation of gastrointestinal diseases in small animals, *Vet Radiol Ultrasound* 31:134, 1990.

47. Penninck DG, Moore AS, Tidewell AS, et al: Ultrasonography of alimentary lymphosarcoma in the cat, *Vet Radiol Ultrasound* 35:299, 1994.

48. Rivers BJ, Walter PA, Feeney DA, et al: Ultrasonographic features of intestinal adenocarcinoma in five cats, *Vet Radiol Ultrasound* 38:300, 1997.

49. Grooters AM, Biller DS, Ward H, et al: Ultrasonographic appearance of feline alimentary lymphoma, *Vet Radiol Ultrasound* 35:468, 1994.

50. Penninck DG: Characterization of gastrointestinal tumors, *Vet Clin North Am Small Anim Pract* 28:777, 1998.

51. Hinton LE, McLoughlin MA, Johnson SE, et al: Spontaneous gastroduodenal perforation in 16 dogs and seven cats (1982-1999), *J Am Anim Hosp Assoc* 38:176, 2002.

52. Liptak JM, Hunt GB, Barrs VDR, et al: Gastroduodenal ulceration in cats: eight cases and a review of the literature, *J Feline Med Surg* 4:27, 2002.

53. Stanton ME, Bright RM: Gastroduodenal ulceration in dogs. Retrospective study of 43 cases and literature review, *J Vet Intern Med* 3:238, 1989.

54. Penninck DG, Crystal MA, Matz ME, et al: The technique of percutaneous ultrasound guided fine-needle aspiration biopsy and automated microcore biopsy in small animal gastrointestinal diseases, *Vet Radiol Ultrasound* 34:433, 1993.

55. Crystal MA, Penninck DG, Matz ME, et al: Use of ultrasound-guided fine needle aspiration biopsy and automated core biopsy for the diagnosis of gastrointestinal diseases in small animals, *Vet Radiol Ultrasound* 34:438, 1993.

56. Akol KG, Washabau RJ, Saunders HM, et al: Acute pancreatitis in cats with hepatic lipidosis, *J Vet Intern Med* 7:205, 1993.

17 Diagnosis and Treatment of Low-Grade Alimentary Lymphoma

Vanessa R.D. Barrs and Julia A. Beatty

Low-grade alimentary lymphoma (LGAL) is a recently described clinical entity affecting middle-aged and older cats. Emerging evidence indicates that LGAL is likely to be a common problem. The major presenting signs are weight loss with chronic vomiting and/or diarrhea. Abnormal abdominal palpation, characterized by diffusely thickened intestinal loops or a mass lesion, is a frequent finding. In cats with consistent clinical signs, LGAL needs to be differentiated from other primary and secondary gastrointestinal diseases. The clinical presentation of LGAL in some cats is indistinguishable from lymphocytic-plasmacytic inflammatory bowel disease (IBD). Abdominal ultrasonography is valuable in the diagnostic investigation. Histopathological examination of multiple small intestinal biopsies is required for definitive diagnosis. The prognosis with treatment and supportive care is good to excellent.

CLASSIFICATION OF ALIMENTARY LYMPHOMA

Feline lymphoma can be classified broadly according to anatomical location, histological grade, or immunophenotype. The traditional anatomical classification recognizes mediastinal, multicentric, alimentary, and extranodal forms. Alimentary lymphoma is characterized by infiltration of the gastrointestinal tract with neoplastic lymphocytes, with or without mesenteric lymph node involvement.[1-3] Feline alimentary lymphoma can be classified according to histological criteria using the National Cancer Institute Working Formulation (NCIWF) into high-grade, intermediate-grade, or low-grade forms (Table 17-1).[4-8] Low-grade alimentary lymphoma (LGAL) has been recognized increasingly in cats over the last 10 years.[6,9-12] Synonyms of LGAL include well-differentiated, lymphocytic, and small cell alimentary lymphoma. Most LGALs are of the small lymphocytic lymphoma subtype (see Table 17-1).[9,10,12] A separate histological subclassification of alimentary lymphoma, that of large granular lymphocytic lymphoma, also is recognized.[13,14] The majority of LGAL and large granular lymphocytic lymphomas are of the T-cell immunophenotype, whereas intermediate- or high-grade lymphomas in the gastrointestinal tract typically are of B-cell origin.[5-10,13-16] LGAL and high-grade alimentary lymphoma (HGAL) in cats differ markedly in clinical presentation, as well as in techniques required for diagnosis, treatment, and prognosis (Table 17-2). The two forms should be considered as distinct clinical entities.

Table 17-1 Histological Classification of Feline Lymphoproliferative Disease as Applied to Feline Lymphoma or Lymphoid Leukemia[7]

	Tumor Type	Acronym
Low Grade	Chronic lymphocytic leukemia	CLL
	Small lymphocytic lymphoma	SLL
	Small lymphocytic intermediate lymphoma	SLLI
	Small lymphocytic plasmacytoid/ plasmacytoma	SLLP
	Follicular small cleaved-cell lymphoma	FSC
	Follicular mixed-cell lymphoma	FM
Intermediate Grade	Follicular large-cell lymphoma	FL
	Small cleaved-cell lymphoma	SCC
	Mixed-cell lymphoma	MC
	Large-cell lymphoma	LC
	Large cleaved-cell lymphoma	LCC
High Grade	Acute lymphocytic leukemia	ALL
	Immunoblastic lymphoma	IB
	Immunoblastic small-cell lymphoma	IBS
	Immunoblastic polymorphous lymphoma	IBP
	Small noncleaved-cell lymphoma	SNC
	Lymphoblastic lymphoma	LB
	Lymphoblastic convoluted-cell lymphoma	LBC

Table 17-2 Comparison of Clinically Relevant Features of High-Grade and Low-Grade Alimentary Lymphoma in Cats

	High Grade	Low Grade
Median age at presentation	12 years	13 years
FeLV antigen status	>70% negative	>99% negative
Gross appearance	Usually focal or segmental intestinal involvement	Usually diffuse intestinal involvement
Immunophenotype	B cell	T cell
Recommended chemotherapy protocol	Multiagent CHOP	Prednisolone and chlorambucil
Major route of chemotherapy administration	Intravenous	Oral
Complete remission (CR)	38-87%	56-76%
Median survival time (for cats achieving CR)	8 months	19-29 months

EPIDEMIOLOGY

Alimentary lymphoma is the most common anatomical form of lymphoma in cats identified in most studies.[1,17-20] The declining influence of feline leukemia virus (FeLV) worldwide has resulted in an increase in the prevalence of alimentary lymphoma relative to other anatomical forms because alimentary lymphoma has the weakest association with FeLV antigenemia. Some studies suggest that the incidence of lymphoma, particularly alimentary lymphoma, is increasing.[19] At one institution, cases of retrovirus-negative lymphoma increased by 78 per cent in the period of 1994 to 2003, when compared to the period of 1984 to 1994.[19] This could not be accounted for by the coincident increase in the feline caseload, which was 29 per cent for the same period. However, whether this trend reflects a true increase in the incidence of alimentary lymphoma or an increased demand for further investigation of feline disorders is unclear.

Low-grade lymphomas constitute 10 to 13 per cent of all feline lymphomas.[5,7,10] The relative incidence of the different histological subtypes of alimentary lymphoma in the general population is unknown. However, LGAL is common among referral feline populations, comprising 45 per cent and 75 per cent of all cases of alimentary lymphoma.[6,12] At our institution, the proportion of alimentary lymphomas that were classified as LGAL increased from 11 per cent in 1999 to 45 per cent in 2008.[5,12] We consider the most likely reason for this increase to be a greater awareness of low-grade disease. Another contributing factor could be that the diagnosis of intermediate- or high-grade alimentary lymphoma is often obtained with less invasive diagnostic tests, such as cytological examination of fine-needle aspirates, resulting in less frequent referral.

RISK FACTORS

FeLV, a directly oncogenic retrovirus, has a strong association with mediastinal and multicentric T-cell lymphoma in young cats. FeLV antigenemia confers a sixtyfold increased risk for lymphoma development compared to antigen-negative status.[21] The ability to detect FeLV provirus may shed more light on the potential role of this virus in lymphomagenesis in exposed but antigen-negative cats.[22] Feline immunodeficiency virus (FIV) infection also increases the risk of lymphomagenesis, but to a lesser degree (fivefold compared to seronegative cats) than that associated with FeLV infection.[21] An indirect role is favored for FIV in the development of extranodal B-cell neoplasms.[23] There currently is no evidence of a retroviral association with LGAL. Of 76 cats with LGAL tested for FeLV antigen, all were negative, and only one of 77 cats tested for FIV antibody was seropositive.[6,9,10,12]

It has been suggested that chronic intestinal inflammation is a risk factor for the development of LGAL in cats, but definitive proof is lacking. The phenomenon of inflammation-associated neoplasia is well established and the mechanisms involved are being elucidated.[24] Celiac disease in human beings is an inflammatory intestinal disease associated with gluten sensitivity. In genetically predisposed individuals, celiac disease increases the risk of intestinal malignancies, including enteropathy-associated T-cell lymphoma.[25] The histological features of the latter are very similar to those of LGAL in cats, to the extent that some veterinary pathologists refer to LGAL as enteropathy-associated T-cell lymphoma.[11,26] Differentiation of neoplastic from inflammatory populations of lymphocytes in the intestine can be extremely difficult using morphological features alone. Immunophenotyping and clonality testing may be required for a definitive differentiation. It has been proposed that lymphocytic-plasmacytic inflammatory bowel disease (IBD) may be a precursor to lymphoid malignancy of the intestinal tract in some cats.* Consistent with this theory, concurrent lymphocytic-plasmacytic IBD has been identified in other regions of the alimentary tract in up to 20 per cent of cats with LGAL.[9,12] There are other examples of the apparent progression of chronic inflammation to neoplasia in cats, including injection-associated sarcomas and posttraumatic ocular sarcomas (see Chapter 70), suggesting that this species may be predisposed to inflammation-associated neoplasia.[28,29]

SIGNALMENT

LGAL typically affects middle-aged to older domestic crossbred cats. The median age at diagnosis is 13 years, with a range of 5 to 18 years. No breed or gender predilection has been identified.[6,9,10,12]

HISTORY AND CLINICAL SIGNS

The most common clinical signs in cats with LGAL are weight loss (≥ 80 per cent), vomiting (≥ 70 per cent), diarrhea (≥ 60 per cent), and partial or complete anorexia (≥ 50 per cent). In our experience, the diarrhea usually is small bowel in origin. The patient's appetite may be normal, although polyphagia is noted occasionally. Less frequently reported signs include lethargy and polydipsia.[6,9,10,12,30] In the majority of cases, clinical signs are chronic (i.e., present for more than one month).[9,12,30] Abdominal palpation is clinically useful because it is often abnormal in cats with LGAL. Diffusely thickened intestinal loops are detected in one third to more than one half of affected cats (Figure 17-1). An abdominal mass is palpable in 20 to 30 per cent of cases, attributable to either mesenteric lymph node enlargement or, less commonly, to a focal intestinal mass.[6,9,12] Because abdominal palpation can be unremarkable in cats with LGAL, the diagnosis can not be excluded on the basis of normal findings during palpation alone.

*References 1, 11, 14, 19, 26, 27.

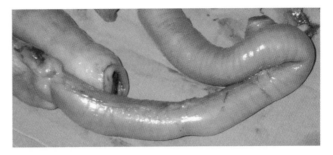

Figure 17-1 Intestinal thickening. Diffusely thickened small intestine at necropsy from a cat with severe LGAL.

DIFFERENTIAL DIAGNOSIS

The presenting signs of LGAL are common to many primary and secondary gastrointestinal diseases. Inflammatory bowel disease is a major differential diagnosis. In one study comparing cats with IBD and LGAL, there was no correlation between the clinical findings and the final diagnosis.[30] In older cats with chronic weight loss, vomiting, and/or diarrhea, the exclusion of secondary gastrointestinal diseases can be accomplished by performance of a complete blood count (CBC), biochemistry profile, urinalysis, thoracic radiographs, total serum thyroxine concentration, and retrovirus testing. Measurement of serum trypsin-like immunoreactivity (TLI) and feline pancreatic lipase immunoreactivity (fPLI; now measured as Spec fPL) also may be indicated.

Primary gastrointestinal disorders that may cause this constellation of clinical signs are listed in Box 17-1. Tests for intestinal parasitism should include direct fecal microscopy and zinc sulfate centrifugation flotation. Fecal immunoassays, direct fluorescent antigen tests, or polymerase chain reaction (PCR)–based assays facilitate the detection of *Giardia* spp., *Cryptosporidium* spp., *Campylobacter* spp., and enteropathogenic bacterial toxins. Even when test results are negative, routine treatment for endoparasites with fenbendazole is warranted early during the investigation. For cats with mixed or large bowel diarrhea, further testing for *Tritrichomonas foetus* by fecal smear examination, culture, or PCR is warranted.[31] In cats with bloody diarrhea, especially if accompanied by pyrexia and hematological findings consistent with sepsis, fecal culture for enteropathogenic bacteria, such as *Salmonella* spp., *Clostridium* spp., and *Campylobacter* spp., should be considered. The results should be interpreted with caution because of high carriage rates of these organisms in healthy cats.[32] (See Chapters 5 and 15 in the fifth volume of this series for further discussion of these tests.) Dietary elimination trials, using single novel protein and carbohydrate sources or hydrolyzed protein diets, are an important diagnostic tool for suspected adverse food reactions (see Chapter 8). Serum cobalamin and folate concentrations should be measured in all cats with suspected small intestinal disease (see Chapter 15).

The finding of a palpable intestinal or lymph node mass in an older cat with chronic weight loss, vomiting, and/or diarrhea might suggest HGAL. In these patients,

Box 17-1 Primary Gastrointestinal Diseases Associated with Chronic Weight Loss, Vomiting, and/or Diarrhea

INFLAMMATORY
Adverse food reaction
IBD
  Lymphocytic-plasmacytic
  Eosinophilic
  Neutrophilic
Gastrointestinal ulceration

INFECTIOUS
Viral
  Granulomatous enterocolitis (FIP)
  Chronic feline enteric coronavirus infection
Bacterial
  Salmonella spp.
  Campylobacter spp.
  Clostridium perfringens
  Clostridium difficile
  Mycobacterium spp.
  Small intestinal bacterial overgrowth
Fungal
  Histoplasma spp.
  Aspergillus spp.
  Pythium insidiosum

PARASITIC
Protozoal
  Giardia spp.

Cryptosporidium spp.
Toxoplasma gondii
Tritrichomonas foetus
Helminths
  Gastric
    Physaloptera spp.
    Ollulanus tricuspis
  Intestinal
    Ascarids
    Hookworms
    Strongyloides spp.

NEOPLASTIC
Lymphoma
Adenocarcinoma
Mast cell neoplasia

OBSTRUCTIVE
Pyloric stenosis
Foreign body
Intussusception
Polyp

MOTILITY DISORDERS
Ileus
Megacolon

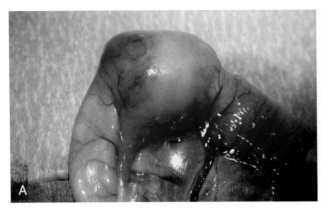
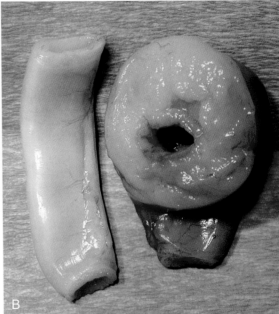

Figure 17-2 High-grade alimentary lymphoma. **A,** Focal intestinal wall mass from a cat with HGAL. **B,** Note the normal intestinal wall thickness for comparison.

segmental, often eccentric, mural thickening and/or mesenteric lymphadenomegaly is common (Figure 17-2). Epithelial or mast cell neoplasia also should be considered. It is important that LGAL is included on the list of differential diagnoses when an abdominal mass is identified. The latter generally carries a more favorable prognosis with treatment.

Laboratory investigations are likely to be informative rather than diagnostic in many cats with these signs, and abdominal ultrasonography usually is indicated. As outlined below, normal sonographic findings do not exclude a diagnosis of LGAL, and histological examination of gastrointestinal biopsies is required for reaching a definitive diagnosis.

DIAGNOSIS

ROUTINE LABORATORY TESTING

Hematological abnormalities in cats with LGAL can include mild anemia from chronic disease or gastrointestinal blood loss, monocytosis, and/or neutrophilic leukocytosis.[9,12] On serum biochemistry analysis, hypoalbuminemia may be present, but this occurs less commonly in LGAL (0 to 49 per cent of cases) than with intermediate-grade alimentary lymphoma or HGAL (50 to 75 per cent of cases).[6,12,20] Hypoalbuminemia occurs from loss of albumin into the intestinal lumen when the intestinal wall is compromised, but also when the capacity of the liver to synthesize albumin is exceeded. Hypoalbuminemia is less common in cats with LGAL because the integrity of the intestinal wall usually can be maintained until late in the disease process. Increases of serum liver enzyme activities also can occur and may indicate concurrent hepatic involvement.[9,12,30]

Up to 80 per cent of cats with LGAL are hypocobalaminemic.[10] This finding is not unexpected: cobalamin is absorbed through the ileum, and the ileum and jejunum are the most common sites for LGAL. Additionally, utilization of cobalamin by a proliferating intestinal microflora in the proximal intestine can decrease cobalamin available for absorption.[33] (See Chapter 13 in the fifth volume of this series for a discussion on the role of cobalamin in the diagnosis and treatment of gastrointestinal disease.) Serum folate concentrations may be low, normal, or high in cats with LGAL.[9,10] Folate deconjugase (a brush border enzyme) and a carrier protein required for folate absorption are located only in the proximal small intestine. Therefore, low serum folate concentrations occur with proximal small intestinal disease due to reduced mucosal absorption. High serum folate concentrations can occur due to proliferation of the intestinal microflora that synthesizes folate.[33] In one study, serum folate concentrations were decreased in 5 per cent and increased in 40 per cent of cats with LGAL.[10]

ABDOMINAL ULTRASONOGRAPHY

Abdominal ultrasonography facilitates evaluation of the gastrointestinal tract by assessment of wall thickness, layering, motility, and luminal content. Intestinal wall thickening can be characterized further by symmetry and anatomical location, as well as by whether the thickening is focal, multifocal, or diffuse. The normal intestinal wall appears as a five-layered image with alternating hyperechoic and hypoechoic layers, corresponding to the luminal surface, mucosa, submucosa, muscularis, and serosa (Figure 17-3). Using ultrasonography, the normal duodenal and jejunal wall thickness is less than or equal to 2.8 mm, the ileal wall thickness is less than or equal to 3.2 mm, and the mesenteric lymph node diameter is less than or equal to 5 mm.[34,35]

Ultrasonographic features of LGAL contrast to those of HGAL. The latter include transmural intestinal thickening with disruption of normal wall layering, reduced wall

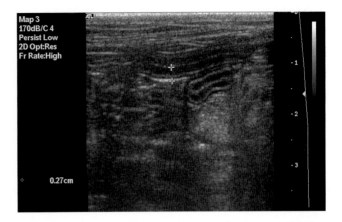

Figure 17-3 Normal intestinal wall. Ultrasonographic appearance of a normal section of small intestine in longitudinal section and cross-section. The pattern of normal intestinal layering can be seen as alternating hyperechoic and hypoechoic layers corresponding to the luminal surface *(upper +)*, mucosa, submucosa, muscularis, and serosa *(lower +)*.

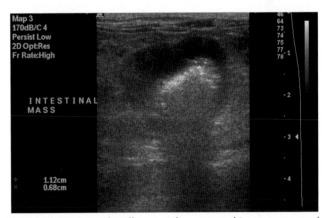

Figure 17-4 Intestinal wall mass. Ultrasonographic appearance of a focal intestinal wall mass in a cat with HGAL. Thickening of the wall and loss of wall layering can be appreciated.

echogenicity, localized hypomotility, and abdominal lymphadenomegaly. Loss of intestinal wall layering occurs due to infiltration of the intestinal wall with neoplastic or inflammatory cells, as well as to secondary necrosis, edema, and/or hemorrhage (Figure 17-4).[36,37] In patients with LGAL, the ultrasonographic appearance of the affected region(s) of intestine is very different: the intestinal wall thickness may be normal or increased, and layering usually is preserved (Figure 17-5, *A*). The mean wall thickness of cats with LGAL and diffuse small intestinal wall thickening in one study was 4.3 mm (median 4.5 mm; range 3.4 to 5.0 mm).[12] Mesenteric lymph node enlargement also is a common finding on abdominal ultrasonography (Figure 17-5, *B*). In the same study mentioned above, the mean lymph node diameter of 11 of 17 cats with LGAL and mesenteric lymph node enlargement was 1.59 cm (median 1 cm; range 0.65 to 3.0 cm). In general, ultrasonographic features of LGAL are not sufficient to distinguish it from IBD. However, in one recent study, thickening of the muscularis layer of the intestine on ultrasonography was associated with LGAL

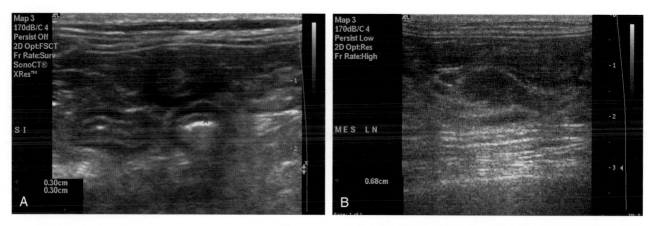

Figure 17-5 Low-grade alimentary lymphoma. **A,** Ultrasonographic appearance of a section of thickened small intestine in a cat with diffuse LGAL. Note that the wall layering is preserved. **B,** Enlarged mesenteric lymph node from the same cat.

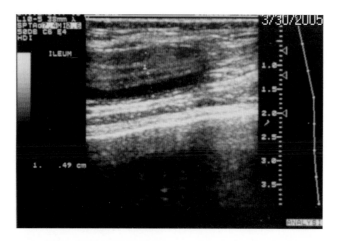

Figure 17-6 Low-grade alimentary lymphoma. Ultrasonographic appearance of a diffusely thickened section of ileum in a cat with LGAL. Note the preservation of intestinal wall layering and a prominent muscularis layer.

but not with IBD or a normal small intestine (Figure 17-6).[38] Less common findings in cats with LGAL on abdominal ultrasound include a focal intestinal mass or intussusception.[9,12] Diffuse infiltration of the liver may be present histologically, but usually is not readily identifiable on ultrasonographic examination.[12] (The reader is referred to Chapter 16 for a discussion of imaging of the gastrointestinal tract.)

CYTOLOGICAL EXAMINATION OF ULTRASOUND-GUIDED FINE-NEEDLE ASPIRATES

Fine-needle aspiration of diffusely thickened intestinal walls can be technically difficult and usually is nondiagnostic. Similarly, cytological examination of enlarged mesenteric lymph nodes is not helpful in establishing a diagnosis of LGAL because it is not possible to distinguish well-differentiated neoplastic lymphocytes, characteristic

of low-grade disease, from benign lymphoid hyperplasia.[12] A tissue biopsy of the affected lymph node is required for histological demonstration of disruption of the normal lymph node architecture by the neoplastic infiltrate. This contrasts with the diagnosis of HGAL, which often can be made on the basis of cytological evaluation of a fine-needle aspirate of a focal intestinal wall lesion or enlarged mesenteric lymph nodes. This often can be achieved successfully because the greater degree of intestinal thickening facilitates aspiration and because the morphology of the neoplastic infiltrate (large lymphoblastic cells) is easier to differentiate cytologically from the background population of lymphocytes.

PROCUREMENT OF INTESTINAL BIOPSIES

Histological evaluation of intestinal biopsies is warranted when intestinal wall thickening or mesenteric lymphadenomegaly is detected during abdominal ultrasonography because these changes are observed commonly in patients with either LGAL or IBD.[30] It should be emphasized that the finding of a normal intestinal wall thickness and normal mesenteric lymph nodes on abdominal ultrasonography does not exclude a diagnosis of LGAL and should not preclude histological evaluation of intestinal biopsies. We currently use full-thickness intestinal biopsy samples (FTB) to diagnose LGAL. These can be obtained at exploratory celiotomy or laparoscopically, while partial thickness biopsy specimens can be obtained endoscopically (EB). A comparison of the utility of these techniques is presented in Table 17-3.

LGAL typically is a diffuse or multifocal disease affecting more than one region of the gastrointestinal tract. Similar to enteropathy-associated T-cell lymphoma in human beings, dogs, pigs, and horses, there is a predilection for the jejunum and ileum.[1,12,25,30] Duodenal involvement is almost as common but may be less severe.[11,12,30] Few studies have reported on the evaluation of all gastrointestinal regions concurrently. In one report, neoplastic infiltration of more than one anatomical region of the gastrointestinal tract was found in 16 of 17 cats, while in

Table 17-3   Comparison Between Full-Thickness Intestinal Biopsies (FTB) and Partial-Thickness Endoscopically Derived Intestinal Biopsies (EB) for Diagnosis of LGAL in Cats

	FTB (Laparotomy, Laparoscopy)	EB (Endoscopy)
Intestinal wall layers sampled	Mucosa, submucosa, muscularis, serosa	Mucosa and submucosa only
Assessment of abdominal organs	Inspection of serosal surface of entire gastrointestinal tract and all other abdominal organs	Inspection of luminal surface of partial gastrointestinal tract only
Degree of invasiveness	Higher: usually longer hospital stays required	Lower: usually shorter hospital stays required
Gastrointestinal regions accessed	All	Stomach, duodenum (gastroduodenoscopy) Colon, ileum (colonoscopy) Jejunum is not accessible
Requirements for waiting time for chemotherapy	Required because of risk of intestinal dehiscence during postoperative wound healing (7 days)	No delay required
Operator skill	Advanced training not required for celiotomy Advanced training required for laparoscopy	Advanced training required to access duodenum reliably and obtain diagnostic-quality biopsies.
Pathologist skill and interpretation	FTB are more likely to be oriented in the correct plane than EB, aiding interpretation; FTB less subject to artifact	Poor-quality EB hampers pathologist's interpretation Greater level of pathologist expertise required for correct interpretation of poor-quality EB

one cat, lymphoma was restricted to the jejunum.[12] Gastric involvement occurs in 25 to 40 per cent of cases.[6,12,30] Too few cases have been evaluated to determine the frequency of large intestinal involvement—colonic involvement was reported in one of five cats with LGAL from whom colonic biopsies were taken.[12]

HISTOLOGICAL FEATURES OF LGAL

A histological diagnosis of LGAL of the small lymphocytic type is not straightforward because neoplastic infiltrates of small lymphocytes are often morphologically indistinguishable from those present in the gastrointestinal mucosa of healthy cats and cats with lymphocytic-plasmacytic IBD. Mitotic figures are seen infrequently in patients with LGAL. Histological differentiation of LGAL from IBD can be particularly challenging, especially in the early stages of the disease.

Histopathological standards for characterizing the nature and severity of changes to the feline gastrointestinal mucosa in inflammatory disease have been developed by the Gastrointestinal Standardization Group of the World Small Animal Veterinary Association.[39] These criteria facilitate the assessment of the severity of morphological and inflammatory changes and are particularly pertinent to the evaluation of endoscopic biopsies. International application of these standards will reduce variation in interpretation between pathologists, facilitate comparisons between different published studies, and help to standardize differences between lymphocytic-plasmacytic IBD and LGAL.

Histological criteria to distinguish LGAL from marked lymphocytic-plasmacytic IBD include a relative absence of mixed lymphoid and granulocytic cells, which are replaced by monomorphous sheets of neoplastic lymphoid cells within the lamina propria that are sometimes distributed irregularly between villi in early neoplastic disease (Figure 17-7, A to C).[11,26,40,41] Other criteria include a lack of reactivity of enterocytes in the crypts and villi to the presence of neoplastic lymphoid cells,[40] effacement of the proprial-epithelial boundary, presence of epitheliotropism including aggregates of neoplastic lymphoid cells (microabscesses) (Figure 17-7, D),[9,26] the level of extension into the underlying submucosa, tunica muscularis, and serosa (Figure 17-7, E),[41] and the presence of neoplastic cellular infiltrates in mesenteric lymph nodes.[40-42] The irregular distribution of the lymphocytic infiltrates in early neoplastic lesions of LGAL is a key feature that differentiates it from lymphocytic-plasmacytic IBD. Heavily infiltrated villi with extensive epithelial invasion may be adjacent to villi with little or no infiltration (see Figure 17-7, A and B). In contrast, biopsies from patients with lymphocytic-plasmacytic IBD show a relatively uniform involvement of the villi in affected intestinal regions (Figures 17-7, F and 17-8).[11,43]

In addition to mimicking lymphocytic-plasmacytic IBD, LGAL may need to be differentiated from mast cell neoplasia because LGAL sometimes can be associated with an extensive paraneoplastic eosinophilic infiltrate.[11,12] In addition to the evaluation of sections stained by hematoxylin and eosin (HE), staining with toluidine blue and immunophenotyping should be performed when eosinophilic intestinal infiltrates are observed to

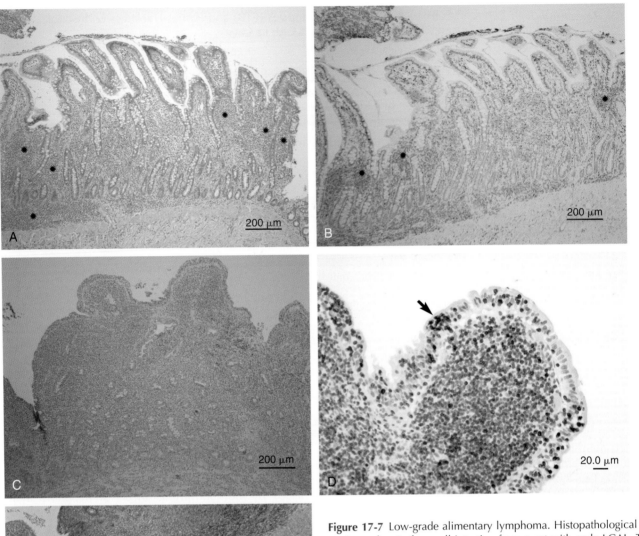

Figure 17-7 Low-grade alimentary lymphoma. Histopathological sections of part of a small intestine from a cat with early LGAL. The distribution of the neoplastic infiltrate is irregular and varies between and within villi. **A,** The infiltrate is denser in the lower parts of the villi at the left and right edges of the section *(asterisks)* (H&E stain). **B,** The neoplastic T-lymphocyte infiltrate primarily is affecting the base and center of the villi *(asterisks)* (anti-CD3 stain). **C,** The lamina propria of the mucosa and the submucosa are diffusely infiltrated with monomorphous sheets of small lymphocytes. There is severe villous blunting and distension, and the epithelial layer of villi is indistinct due to heavy infiltration with intraepithelial lymphocytes (H&E stain). **D,** The neoplastic lymphocytes are predominantly T cells. There is epitheliotropism with clustering of intraepithelial T lymphocytes *(arrow)* (anti-CD3-stain). **E,** Neoplastic infiltration can be seen between smooth muscle layers and the serosa *(arrows)* (H&E stain).

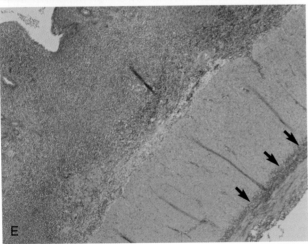

rule out intestinal mast cell neoplasia (see Chapter 67). In patients with lymphoma, eosinophil chemotaxis is thought to result from the production of interleukin-5 by neoplastic lymphocytes.[44] T-cell intestinal lymphoma with eosinophilic infiltrates also has been described in cats with high-grade disease and additionally in dogs and human beings.[45,46]

IMMUNOPHENOTYPING

Immunophenotyping is a useful adjunct to histological evaluation of HE-stained sections of gastrointestinal biopsies for the diagnosis of LGAL. Determination of immunophenotype can be accomplished by staining for T-cell markers, such as CD3, and B-cell markers, such as

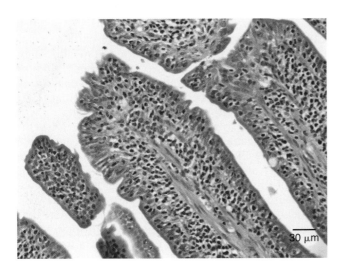

30 μm

Figure 17-8 Lymphocytic-plasmacytic inflammatory bowel disease. The lamina propria of the villi is heavily infiltrated with a mixture of small lymphocytes, plasma cells, and some eosinophils. The epithelial layer of the villi is uniformly arranged with occasional intraepithelial lymphocytes (H&E stain).

CD79a, CD45R, or BLA.36 (see Figures 17-7,*B* and 17-7,*D*). LGAL is widely considered to be a disorder of lymphocytes of the T-cell lineage.[9-11,26] A recent study documented T-cell immunophenotype in 30 of 33 cats with LGAL. The remaining three patients had B-cell lymphoma (n = 2) or non–T-, non–B-cell lymphoma (n = 1).[10] In another study of 32 cats diagnosed with alimentary lymphoma from HE-stained sections, immunohistochemical staining revealed that in five cats (15 per cent) the infiltrate was composed of a mixed population of small B- and T-lymphocytes and plasma cells, and these five cases were reclassified as IBD.[8] However, it should be noted that LGAL can not be diagnosed by identification of the T-cell phenotype alone because expansion of T-cell populations in intestinal mucosal–associated lymphoid tissue (MALT) also can occur in inflammatory intestinal disease in cats.[47]

CLONALITY TESTING

Determination of clonality of T-cell populations in the lymphocytic intestinal infiltrate by molecular techniques shows promise as an adjunct to histological and immunohistological phenotyping for diagnosing LGAL. Clonality testing was 89 per cent sensitive in the detection of T-cell lymphoma, based on clonal or oligoclonal T-cell populations that were considered to be neoplastic. Using PCR testing, 22 of 28 cats were found to have clonal rearrangements of the genes encoding the gamma variable region of the T-cell receptor, while three had oligoclonal rearrangements. In comparison, polyclonal rearrangements were detected in all three cats with normal intestinal histology and in all nine cats with lymphocytic-plasmacytic intestinal inflammation.[47]

RECOMMENDATIONS FOR BIOPSY

Histological evaluation of gastrointestinal FTB is more sensitive for the diagnosis of LGAL than histological evaluation of EB procured by gastroduodenoscopy.[30] In a study of 10 cats with LGAL, gastroduodenal EB specimens were compared with FTB from multiple gastrointestinal regions from the same cats. On evaluation of FTB, LGAL was detected in the jejunum and ileum of all 10 cats, in the duodenum in nine cats, and in the stomach of only four cats. On evaluation of EB, LGAL was diagnosed correctly in only three cats and suspected, but not diagnosed conclusively, in three cats, while it was diagnosed incorrectly as lymphocytic-plasmacytic IBD in another four cats. Difficulties in interpretation were encountered mostly with duodenal EB, and it was concluded that duodenal biopsies may be insufficient for accurate differentiation between IBD and LGAL.[30] Technical difficulties may have hampered the quality of EB specimens procured in this study because two cats had only partial duodenal assessment and duodenal biopsies were performed blindly in three cats with fewer samples taken. It has been shown that the quality of endoscopically obtained tissue samples has a profound effect on their sensitivity for identifying certain lesions.[48] One important factor affecting the quality of EB is the skill of the endoscopist and the number of tissue samples taken during endoscopy (see Table 17-3). A recent report showed that if six marginal- to adequate-quality duodenal or gastric biopsies were taken, as defined by presence of at least one villus and subvillous lamina propria, correct histological diagnosis was very likely to be achieved.[48] Optimal histological processing, including biopsy orientation and positioning, also is essential for samples to be considered adequate for interpretation.

Given the propensity of LGAL to invade the distal small intestine, it is likely that the sensitivity of the diagnosis of LGAL obtained through endoscopic biopsies could be improved if endoscopic studies were to routinely include ileal biopsies obtained by passage through the ileocecocolic valve. Further studies are required to compare the diagnostic utility of ileal biopsies collected by endoscopy or full-thickness biopsies for the diagnosis of LGAL in cats.

In summary, while EB are minimally invasive, a definitive diagnosis of LGAL requires significant expertise on the part of the endoscopist and the pathologist, as well as correct laboratory sample processing. FTB at celiotomy should be considered when these factors are not optimal. Laparoscopy is likely to increase in popularity because it serves as a minimally invasive alternative to celiotomy for the collection of FTB.

STAGING

Extraintestinal involvement in cats with LGAL is common, with more than 50 per cent of patients having disease outside the intestinal tract. Mesenteric lymph node involvement occurs in up to 60 per cent of cases, hepatic involvement in 30 per cent, and pancreatic or splenic involvement in fewer than 10 per cent of cases.[9,10,12,30] This may be an underestimate of the degree of systemic involvement because some studies have relied on EB to arrive at the diagnosis, and extragastrointestinal organs have not been biopsied routinely. Except for one study, which showed that histological evidence of liver involvement was not a negative prognostic factor for remission, there is no information on the influence of disease stage on prognosis.[12] When intestinal biopsies are collected during celiotomy or at laparoscopy, routine biopsy of other abdominal organs is recommended.

TREATMENT AND PROGNOSIS

CHEMOTHERAPY PROTOCOLS, REMISSION, AND SURVIVAL TIMES

Most cats with LGAL have an excellent response to treatment with oral slow-alkylating agents and prednisolone.[6,10,12] This probably is partly due to the low mitotic rate of the tumor. Induction chemotherapy protocols that have been utilized for the treatment of LGAL in cats are listed in Table 17-4. Treatment involves oral prednisolone and oral high-dose pulse chlorambucil therapy. Alternatively, the latter may be prescribed at a lower dosage q48h continuously. Compared with HGAL, cats with LGAL have longer remission and survival times. Histological grade therefore should be considered a prognostic factor for feline alimentary lymphoma. For HGAL, use of multiagent chemotherapy protocols that include doxorubicin is associated with a median survival time of 7 to 10 months.[2,3,18,49] In contrast, the median survival time for cats with LGAL who are treated with oral prednisolone and chlorambucil is 15 to 25 months (Table 17-5).[6,10,12] The presence of lethargy at the time of diagnosis was found to be a negative prognostic factor for remission in one report and for survival in another.[6,12] Clinical illness at diagnosis also has been shown to be a negative prognostic factor for survival in cats with HGAL.[1,17] Complete remission (CR), as defined by complete resolution of clinical signs for 30 days or more, occurred in 69 and 76 per cent of cats with LGAL in two separate studies.[6,12] In both studies, cats with a partial response were included in the no-response category because anything less than a CR was considered arbitrary due to insufficient data. As with HGAL, response to therapy was a prognostic factor for survival (see Table 17-5). In contrast, a recent report found a lower CR rate of 56 per cent, and no factors were significantly associated with survival times.[10] A key difference of this latter study and the other two studies was that a third response category of "partial response" (PR) was included, and was defined as a response of more than 50 per cent, but less than 100 per cent. In total, 95 per cent of the 39 cats for which treatment data were available in that study achieved either complete or partial remission, with median remission durations of 29 and 14 months, respectively. This would be considered a good outcome even in cats with a partial remission. Cats who achieve CR consistently have significantly longer survival times than do cats who do not achieve CR.

The dose of prednisolone should be reduced gradually once remission has been achieved in order to reduce side effects associated with long-term glucocorticoid use, such as diabetes mellitus and iatrogenic hyperadrenocorticism. Remission often can be maintained with a prednisolone dosage of 5 mg PO q24h or 2 to 3 mg/kg PO q48h.[10,12]

Cyclophosphamide (10 mg/kg PO q 3 to 4 weeks or 225 mg/m^2 PO q 3 weeks) in combination with prednisolone at induction doses can be used as a rescue protocol for cats who come out of clinical remission. In a small number of affected cats, reinduction was reported to be successful and the median survival time of 12 cats with successful reinduction using cyclophosphamide was 29 months.[6] (See Chapter 63 for a discussion of chemotherapy protocols for lymphoma.)

CHEMOTHERAPY—MONITORING AND ADVERSE EFFECTS

Oral chemotherapy usually is well tolerated and is associated with only low morbidity. Chlorambucil is a nitrogen mustard derivative that acts as a bifunctional alkylating agent. The most common adverse effects seen with chlorambucil are gastrointestinal toxicity and myelosuppression. Gastrointestinal signs usually are mild and self-limiting. Vomiting, diarrhea, and inappetence associated with treatment can be difficult to distinguish from clinical signs that are due to LGAL itself. Routine moni-

Table 17-4   Oral Induction Chemotherapy Protocols Used for the Treatment of LGAL

Protocol	Prednisolone	Chlorambucil
Fondacaro et al 1999[6]	10 mg/cat PO q24h	15 mg/m^2/24h PO for 4d q21d
Kiselow et al 2008[10]	5 mg/cat PO q12-24h	2 mg/cat PO q48h
Lingard et al 2009[12]	3 mg/kg PO q24h	15 mg/m^2/24h PO for 4d q21d

Table 17-5   Remission and Survival Data for Cats with LGAL

Author	N	Complete Remission (CR)	Median Survival Time (MST; Months)	MST[1] or Median Duration of Remission[2] for Cats Achieving CR (Months)
Fondacaro et al 1999[6]	29	69%	17	23[1]
Kiselow et al 2008[10]	39	56%	25	29[2]
Lingard et al 2009[12]	17	76%	15	19[1]

toring should include a CBC to assess the patient for neutropenia and thrombocytopenia.[12,50] After administration of high-dose pulse chlorambucil, a CBC should be performed prior to each 3-week chlorambucil treatment. A less common adverse effect of high-dose chlorambucil therapy is neurotoxicity. Seizures and myoclonus can occur in human beings and cats. These signs may be due to chloroacetaldehyde, a neurotoxic metabolite of chlorambucil.[12,50] The risk of neurotoxicity is reduced by ensuring a 24-hour interval between successive doses or by using low-dose chlorambucil q48h.

SUPPORTIVE TREATMENT

Because many cats with LGAL have low body condition scores and are inappetent or anorexic at presentation, provision of enteral nutrition is an important consideration. Esophagostomy or gastrostomy tubes should be placed routinely in these cats during general anesthesia for the intestinal biopsy procedure (see Chapter 12). When gastrointestinal ulceration is identified or suspected, treatment with proton-pump inhibitors (e.g., omeprazole) or H_2-antagonists (e.g., ranitidine or famotidine) and mucosal protectants (e.g., sucralfate) is indicated (Table 17-6). A further consideration is treatment of concurrent lymphocytic-plasmacytic IBD or dietary intolerance. Severe lymphocytic intestinal inflammation, secondary to food intolerance (for which the initial histological diagnosis from HE-stained intestinal biopsies was alimentary lymphoma), has been reported.[51,52] Dietary modification is important. The diet should

contain a novel protein component that should be single-source or hydrolyzed. The diet also should be gluten-free. The carbohydrate component also should be single-source and highly digestible (e.g., cooked rice). Commercial balanced diets that meet these criteria are available (see Chapter 8). Prebiotics, which constitute substrates used selectively by certain beneficial bacterial species, and probiotics, which are preparations of orally administered organisms that antagonize pathogenic bacteria and modulate the mucosal immune response, also may be of use (see Chapter 11). Administration of metronidazole may be beneficial for the treatment of small intestinal bacterial overgrowth, but also may have some immunomodulatory effects. Folate deficiency can be treated with oral folic acid supplementation. Cobalamin supplementation should be administered if the serum cobalamin concentration is subnormal. However, given the high incidence of hypocobalaminemia in cats with LGAL, routine cobalamin supplementation is warranted if the owner does not authorize measurement of serum cobalamin concentration.[10] Because cobalamin deficiency itself can result in inflammatory infiltration of the gastrointestinal mucosa and villous atrophy, response to chemotherapy may be suboptimal unless parenteral cobalamin supplementation is initiated (see Table 17-6). If serum cobalamin concentrations are high 1 month after the last monthly injection of cobalamin, supplementation can be discontinued. If serum cobalamin concentration is low or within the reference range, further supplementation is indicated. Serum cobalamin concentration also should be measured routinely in cats showing relapse of clinical signs.

Table 17-6 Supportive Therapies for Cats with LGAL

Strategy	Treatment
Enteral nutritional support	Esophagostomy or gastrostomy tube
Gastrointestinal ulceration	Omeprazole: 0.7-1.5 mg/kg PO q24h Sucralfate: 0.5-1 g PO q8h Ranitidine: 3.5 mg/kg PO q12h Famotidine: 0.5 mg/kg PO q12-24h

Treat concurrent IBD	Dietary modification
	  Protein: novel single-source or
	    hydrolyzed, gluten-free
	  Carbohydrate: single-source
	Prebiotics and probiotics
	Antibacterial therapy
	  Metronidazole: 10 mg/kg PO q12h,
	    or
	  Tylosin: 10 mg/kg PO q8h

Vitamin deficiencies	Folate deficiency
	  Folic acid: 1 mg/cat PO q24h
	Cobalamin (vitamin B_{12}) deficiency
	  Cobalamin: 250 µg/cat SQ q7d for
	    6 weeks, then q14d for 6 weeks,
	    then monthly
	  Adjust frequency by measurement
	    of serum concentrations

SUMMARY

LGAL is a chronic, indolent disease of middle-aged to older cats with clinical signs indistinguishable from those of other primary and secondary gastrointestinal diseases, including IBD. In the majority of affected cats, the disease is diffuse and involves more than one region of the gastrointestinal tract. The jejunum and ileum are the sites affected most frequently. Generalized intestinal thickening and mesenteric lymph node enlargement are detected commonly on physical examination and abdominal ultrasound. Focal intestinal masses also can occur. Although abdominal ultrasound may assist in the evaluation of these patients, histological examination is necessary to establish a definitive diagnosis of LGAL. In stark contrast to cats with intermediate- and high-grade disease, cats with LGAL generally show an excellent response to treatment with oral prednisolone and chlorambucil with durable remission times.

REFERENCES

1. Mahony OM, Moore AS, Cotter SM, et al: Alimentary lymphoma in cats: 28 cases (1988-1993), *J Am Vet Med Assoc* 207:1593, 1995.
2. Zwahlen CH, Lucroy MD, Kraegel SA, et al: Results of chemotherapy for cats with alimentary malignant lymphoma: 21 cases (1993-1997), *J Am Vet Med Assoc* 213:1144, 1998.

3. Rassnick KM, Mauldin GN, Moroff SD, et al: Prognostic value of argyrophilic nucleolar organizer region (AgNOR) staining in feline intestinal lymphoma, *J Vet Intern Med* 13:187, 1999.

4. Couto CG: Gastrointestinal neoplasia in dogs and cats. In Kirk RW, Bonagura JD, editors: *Current veterinary therapy XI*, Philadelphia, 1992, WB Saunders, p 595.

5. Gabor LJ, Canfield PJ, Malik R: Immunophenotypic and histological characterisation of 109 cases of feline lymphosarcoma, *Aust Vet J* 77:436, 1999.

6. Fondacaro JV, Richter KP, Carpenter JL, et al: Feline gastrointestinal lymphoma: 67 cases (1988-1996), *Eur J Comp Gastroenterol* 4:5, 1999.

7. Valli VE, Jacobs RM, Norris A, et al: The histologic classification of 602 cases of feline lymphoproliferative disease using the National Cancer Institute working formulation, *J Vet Diagn Invest* 12:295, 2000.

8. Waly NE, Gruffydd-Jones TJ, Stokes CR, et al: Immunohistochemical diagnosis of alimentary lymphomas and severe intestinal inflammation in cats, *J Comp Pathol* 133:253, 2005.

9. Carreras JK, Goldschmidt M, Lamb M, et al: Feline epitheliotropic intestinal malignant lymphoma: 10 cases (1997-2000), *J Vet Intern Med* 17:326, 2003.

10. Kiselow MA, Rassnick KM, McDonough SP, et al: Outcome of cats with low-grade lymphocytic lymphoma: 41 cases (1995-2005), *J Am Vet Med Assoc* 232:405, 2008.

11. Valli VE: Enteropathy-type T-cell lymphoma. In Valli VE, editor: *Veterinary comparative hematopathology*, Oxford, 2007, Blackwell Publishing, p 318.

12. Lingard AE, Beatty JA, Moore AS, et al: Low-grade alimentary lymphoma: clinicopathologic findings and response to treatment in 17 cases, *J Feline Med Surg* 2009 (in press).

13. Darbes J, Majzoub M, Breuer W, et al: Large granular lymphocyte leukemia/lymphoma in six cats, *Vet Pathol* 35:370, 1998.

14. Roccabianca P, Vernau W, Caniatti M, et al: Feline large granular lymphocyte (LGL) lymphoma with secondary leukemia: primary intestinal origin with predominance of a CD3/CD8aa phenotype, *Vet Pathol* 43:15, 2006.

15. Jackson ML, Wood SL, Misra V, et al: Immunohistochemical identification of B and T lymphocytes in formalin-fixed, paraffin-embedded feline lymphosarcomas: relation to feline leukemia virus status, tumor site, and patient age, *Can J Vet Res* 60:99, 1996.

16. Patterson-Kane JC, Kugler BP, Francis K: The possible prognostic significance of immunophenotype in feline alimentary lymphoma: a pilot study, *J Comp Pathol* 130:220, 2004.

17. Vail DM, Moore AS, Ogilvie GK, et al: Feline lymphoma (145 cases): proliferation indices, cluster of differentiation 3 immunoreactivity, and their association with prognosis in 90 cats, *J Vet Intern Med* 12:349, 1998.

18. Milner RJ, Peyton J, Cooke K, et al: Response rates and survival times for cats with lymphoma treated with the University of Wisconsin-Madison chemotherapy protocol: 38 cases (1996-2003), *J Am Vet Med Assoc* 227:1118, 2005.

19. Louwerens M, London CA, Pederson NC, et al: Feline lymphoma in the post-feline leukemia virus era, *J Vet Intern Med* 19:329, 2005.

20. Gabor LJ, Malik R, Canfield PJ: Clinical and anatomical features of lymphosarcoma in 118 cats, *Aust Vet J* 76:725, 1998.

21. Shelton GH, Grant CK, Cotter SM, et al: Feline immunodeficiency virus and feline leukemia virus infections and their relationships to lymphoid malignancies in cats: a retrospective study (1968-1988), *J Acquir Immune Defic Syndr* 3:623, 1990.

22. Torres AN, Mathiason CK, Hoover EA: Re-examination of feline leukemia virus: host relationships using real-time PCR, *Virology* 332:272, 2005.

23. Beatty JA, Lawrence CE, Callanan JJ, et al: Feline immunodeficiency virus (FIV)-associated lymphoma: a potential role for immune dysfunction in tumourigenesis, *Vet Immunol Immunopathol* 65:309, 1998.

24. Schafer M, Werner S: Cancer as an overhealing wound: an old hypothesis revisited, *Nat Rev Mol Cell Biol* 9:628, 2008.

25. Green PHR, Cellier C: Celiac disease, *N Engl J Med* 357:1736, 2007.

26. Valli VE, Jacobs RM, Parodi AL, et al: Tumors of lymphoid system. In *World Health Organization histological classification of hematopoietic tumors of domestic animals*, ed 2, Washington, DC, 2002, Armed Forces Institute of Pathology, p 25.

27. Krecic MR, Black SS: Epitheliotropic T-cell gastrointestinal tract lymphosarcoma with metastases to lung and skeletal muscle in a cat, *J Am Vet Med Assoc* 216:524, 2000.

28. Dubielzig RR, Everitt J, Shadduck JA, et al: Clinical and morphologic features of post-traumatic ocular sarcomas in cats, *Vet Pathol* 27:62, 1990.

29. McEntee MC, Page RL: Feline vaccine-associated sarcoma, *J Vet Intern Med* 15:176, 2001.

30. Evans SE, Bonczynski JJ, Broussard JD, et al: Comparison of endoscopic and full-thickness biopsy specimens for diagnosis of inflammatory bowel disease and alimentary tract lymphoma in cats, *J Am Vet Med Assoc* 229:1447, 2006.

31. Gookin J, Birkenheuer AJ, Breitschwerdt EB, et al: Single-tube nested PCR for detection of *Tritrichomonas foetus* in feline feces, *J Clin Microbiol* 40:4126, 2002.

32. Willard MD, Marks SL: Bacterial causes of enteritis and colitis. In August JR, editor: *Consultations in feline internal medicine*, vol 5, St Louis, 2006, Elsevier Saunders, p 39.

33. Ruaux CG: Laboratory tests for the diagnosis of intestinal disorders. In Steiner JM, editor: *Small animal gastroenterology*, Hannover, 2008, Schlütersche Verlagsbuchhandlung, p 50.

34. Goggin JM, Biller DS, Debey BM, et al: Ultrasonographic measurement of gastrointestinal wall thickness and the ultrasonographic appearance of the ileocolic region in healthy cats, *J Am Vet Med Assoc* 36:224, 2000.

35. Mattoon JS, Auld DM, Nyland TG: Abdominal ultrasound scanning techniques. In Nyland TG, Mattoon JS, editors: *Small animal diagnostic ultrasound*, ed 2, Philadelphia, 2002, WB Saunders, p 75.

36. Penninck DG, Moore AS, Tidwell AS, et al: Ultrasonography of alimentary lymphosarcoma in the cat, *Vet Radiol Ultrasound* 35:299, 1994.

37. Grooters AM, Biller DS, Ward H, et al: Ultrasonographic appearance of feline alimentary lymphoma, *Vet Radiol Ultrasound* 35:468, 1994.

38. Zwingenberger AL, Marks SL, Baker T, et al: Pattern recognition of thickened muscularis layer in diffuse feline small intestinal lymphoma and inflammatory bowel disease, *Proc Am Coll Vet Radiol* 22, 2007.

39. Day MJ, Bilzer T, Mansell J, et al: Histopathological standards for the diagnosis of gastrointestinal inflammation in endoscopic biopsy samples from the dog and cat: a report from the World Small Animal Veterinary Association Gastrointestinal Standardization Group, *J Comp Pathol* 138:S1, 2008.

40. Richter KP: Feline gastrointestinal lymphoma, *Vet Clin North Am Small Anim Pract* 33:1083, 2003.

41. Brown CC: Alimentary system. In Maxie MG, editor: *Jubb, Kennedy, and Palmer's pathology of domestic animals*, ed 5, vol 2, St Louis, 2007, Saunders Elsevier, p 124.

42. Ben-Ezra J: Small lymphocytic lymphoma. In Knowles D, Danile M, editors: *Neoplastic hematopathology*, Philadelphia, 2001, Lippincott Williams & Wilkins, p 773.

43. Valli VE: Enteropathy-type T-cell lymphoma. In Maxie MG, editor: *Jubb, Kennedy, and Palmer's pathology of domestic animals*, ed 5, vol 3, St. Louis, 2007, Saunders Elsevier, p 189.

44. Samoszuk M, Ramzi E, Cooper DL: Interleukin-5 mRNA in three T-cell lymphomas with eosinophils, *Am J Hematol* 42:402, 1993.

45. Barrs VR, Beatty JA, McCandlish IA, et al: Hypereosinophilic paraneoplastic syndrome in a cat with intestinal T cell lymphosarcoma, *J Small Anim Pract* 43:401, 2002.

46. Ozaki K, Yamagami T, Nomura K, et al: T-cell lymphoma with eosinophilic infiltration involving the intestinal tract in 11 dogs, *Vet Pathol* 43:339, 2006.

47. Moore PF, Woo JC, Vernau W, et al: Characterisation of feline T cell receptor gamma (TCRG) variable region genes for the molecular diagnosis of feline intestinal T cell lymphoma, *Vet Immunol Immunopathol* 106:167, 2005.

48. Willard MD, Mansell J, Fosgate GT, et al: Effect of sample quality on the sensitivity of endoscopic biopsy for detecting gastric and duodenal lesions in dogs and cats, *J Vet Intern Med* 22:1084, 2008.

49. Malik R, Gabor LJ, Foster SF, et al: Therapy for Australian cats with lymphosarcoma, *Aust Vet J* 79:808, 2001.

50. Benitah N, deLorimier LP, Gaspar M, et al: Chlorambucil-induced myoclonus in a cat with lymphoma, *J Am Anim Hosp Assoc* 39:283, 2003.

51. Wasmer ML, Willard MD, Helman RG, et al: Food intolerance mimicking alimentary lymphosarcoma, *J Am Anim Hosp Assoc* 31:463, 1995.

52. Ragaini L, Aste G, Cavicchioli L, et al: Inflammatory bowel disease mimicking alimentary lymphosarcoma in a cat, *Vet Res Commun* 27:791, 2003.

Andrea Valeria Scorza and Michael R. Lappin

The protozoans associated most frequently with gastrointestinal signs of disease in cats are the coccidians and the flagellates. More specifically, *Cryptosporidium* spp., *Isospora* spp., *Giardia* spp., and *Tritrichomonas foetus* are the most common protozoal organisms in cats and will be discussed in depth in this chapter. Although *Toxoplasma gondii* has an enteroepithelial cycle, gastrointestinal signs of disease are rare; *T. gondii* is associated more commonly with polysystemic diseases like fever and uveitis. Other coccidians with an enteric life cycle in cats include *Besnoitia* spp., *Sarcocystis* spp., and *Hammondia hammondi*; however, these organisms are rarely associated with gastrointestinal signs of disease. Finally, cats are infected occasionally by other protozoans, including *Balantidium coli*, *Blastocystis hominis*, *Entamoeba histolytica*, and *Enterocytozoon bieneusi*.

COCCIDIANS

CRYPTOSPORIDIUM SPP.

Etiology

In the past, most mammalian infections with *Cryptosporidium* spp. were attributed to *Cryptosporidium parvum*. However, recent genetic studies showed that most isolates from cats are *C. felis*.[1] In cats, sporulated oocysts (4 μm × 6 μm) are passed in the feces after completion of an enteric life cycle.

Epidemiology

Cryptosporidium spp.–infected cats have been documented worldwide (Table 18-1). However, the prevalence of *C. felis* varies based on the study population and on the diagnostic test used.[2-17] For example, in one study of 180

cats with diarrhea in the United States, the prevalence rates based on an immunofluorescent antibody assay and polymerase chain reaction (PCR) were 3 per cent and 29.4 per cent, respectively.[13] Therefore, while the true prevalence of *C. felis* is unknown, it is generally between 3 per cent and 20 per cent in cats with diarrhea. Also, in most of the studies, the prevalence tends to be higher in young cats and in shelter cats.

Pathogenesis

Little information is available concerning the pathogenesis of *C. felis* in cats. Thus, most information is extrapolated from what is known in human beings and mice after infection with *C. parvum*. *Cryptosporidium* spp. oocysts are sporulated when passed in feces. After excystation from oocysts, *Cryptosporidium* sporozoites attach to the intestinal epithelium between the cell membrane and the cell cytoplasm; this location may partially explain their resistance to chemotherapy.[18] The initial host-parasite interactions are complex and involve multiple parasite ligands and host receptors.[18] The intestinal epithelial cells serve as a physical barrier and produce a variety of cytokines and chemokines in response to the pathogen. *C. parvum* infection can induce mucosal infiltration with neutrophils, macrophages, and lymphocytes in the lamina propria underlying the epithelial cells, as well as intraepithelial infiltration with neutrophils and T lymphocytes. Proinflammatory cytokines are up-regulated during *C. parvum* infection.[18] Concurrently, antiinflammatory cytokines are produced and play a protective role in limiting the epithelial damage due to the infection.[18] Cellular immunity mediated by CD4+ and CD8+ α/β T cells is an important component for the resolution of *C. parvum* infection. Interferon-γ also appears to play an important role in innate immunity and in the cell-

200

Table 18-1 Prevalence of *Cryptosporidium* spp. in Cats

Number Tested	Country	Method	Prevalence (%)	Reference
162	Australia	Microscopy	1.2	2
10	France	Microscopy	0	3
300	Germany	Microscopy	1.3	4
13	Japan	Microscopy	38.5	5
608	Japan	Microscopy	3.8	6
57	Scotland	Microscopy	12.3	7
418	Australia	Microscopy	0	8
263	United States (New York)	Microscopy	3.8	9
206	United States (Colorado)	Microscopy	5.4	10
173	United States (North Carolina)	IFA	6.5	11
344	United States (California)	IFA	4.7	12
180	United States	IFA	3.3	13
145	United Kingdom	IFA	15.2	14
600	United States	Serology	8.3	15
258	Scotland	Serology (IgG)	74	16
135	Czech Republic	Serology	57	17
40	Australia	PCR	10	8
180	United States	PCR	29.4	13
145	United Kingdom	PCR	6.2	14

Modified from Lyndsay DS, Zajac AM: *Cryptosporidium* infections in cats and dogs, *Compend Contin Educ Pract Vet* 26:864, 2004.[4]

mediated response against *C. parvum*.[18] In otherwise healthy specific-pathogen–free cats, inoculation with *C. parvum* oocysts resulted in chronic infection, but minimal clinical signs of disease, even after the administration of glucocorticoids, suggesting that these organisms were minimally pathogenic in these healthy cats.[19]

Transmission

Cats are infected by *Cryptosporidium* spp. via the fecal-oral route by ingesting the oocysts in feces directly from mutual grooming, or indirectly from ingesting the oocysts in contaminated food or water. It also is possible that cats are infected by ingesting infected prey. *Cryptosporidium* spp. are extremely contagious because of the following characteristics: the oocysts are sporulated when passed in feces and thus are infectious immediately; a very low number of oocysts is enough to cause infection because autogenous reinfection occurs from the rupture of the thin-walled oocysts in the intestinal tract; and the oocysts are resistant to environmental stress and to most common disinfectants. *C. felis* oocysts generally are shed in the feces 3 to 6 days after infection.

Clinical Signs

Cats with *C. felis* infections can be infected clinically or subclinically, but most infections are subclinical. When clinical signs occur, cryptosporidiosis usually is characterized by small bowel diarrhea, anorexia, and weight loss. Most cats with *C. felis* infection and diarrhea have con-

current immunosuppression, preexisting disease in the intestinal tract, or coinfection with other infectious or noninfectious causes.[20-22] For example, coinfection with other protozoans, like *Giardia* spp. and *Tritrichomonas foetus*, may aggravate clinical signs of cryptosporidiosis in cats.[23-25] Noninfectious diseases associated with cryptosporidiosis in cats are lymphoma and inflammatory bowel disease.[20,26,27] Cats infected with *Cryptosporidium* spp. also can serve as subclinically infected carriers. The administration of glucocorticoids to some chronically infected, oocyst-negative cats, may induce repeated oocyst shedding.[19]

Diagnosis

C. felis oocysts are very small (4 μm × 6 μm) and are shed in low numbers by cats. Therefore results of fecal flotation generally are negative. Staining a thin fecal smear with modified Ziehl-Neelsen acid-fast stain (MZN) can be performed as an in-clinic test (Figure 18-1). A monoclonal antibody–based immunofluorescent antibody (IFA) assay (Merifluor *Cryptosporidium/Giardia*, Meridian Diagnostics, Cincinnati, OH) designed to detect *C. parvum* oocysts in human feces has been used in many feline studies and appears to detect *C. felis* oocysts. This assay has the advantage of detecting *Giardia* spp. cysts concurrently and thus can be used to identify parasites both by fluorescence and by morphology. However, this procedure requires a fluorescent microscope, and samples therefore must be sent to a reference laboratory. A recent study reported that IFA had a lower sensitivity than the MZN technique when a single fecal sample was tested.[28] The sensitivity of IFA and MZN were equal when two to four fecal samples were tested.[28]

Multiple commercially available enzyme-linked immunosorbent assays (ELISAs) designed to detect *C. parvum* antigen in human feces have been assessed for use with feline feces with variable results.[28,29] Our laboratory recently evaluated two lateral flow devices for the detection of *C. parvum* in human feces and found them to be inadequate for detection of *Cryptosporidium* spp. in feline feces.[29] This may relate to antigenic differences between *C. felis* and *C. parvum*. In another study, the ProSpecT Microplate Assay (Alexon Biomedical, Sunnyvale, CA) showed the highest sensitivity (71.4 per cent) and specificity (96.7 per cent) of a variety of commercial assays for the detection of *Cryptosporidium* when compared to IFA.[30]

Cryptosporidium spp. DNA can be amplified from feces by PCR testing, which is now commercially available at many diagnostic laboratories in the United States. The technique can be more sensitive than IFA.[2,19] However, currently there is no standardization between laboratories, and the level of quality control may vary widely between laboratories. The results of PCR also can be used for genotyping to determine whether the *Cryptosporidium* spp. detected is *C. parvum*, *C. felis*, or another *Cryptosporidium* species (Veterinary Diagnostic Laboratory, Colorado State University, Fort Collins, CO; http://www.dlab. colostate.edu). At this time, PCR is only recommended for assessment of cats with diarrhea because the clinical and zoonotic impact of oocyst-negative, but PCR-positive, healthy cats is unknown.

Treatment

It is impossible to determine whether *Cryptosporidium* spp. is causing diarrhea in a specific patient. However, when a cat with diarrhea is shown to be *Cryptosporidium* spp.–positive and there is no other obvious cause for the diarrhea, treatment may be indicated. More than 100 compounds have been evaluated for the treatment of cryptosporidiosis in human beings, cattle, and mice, and none control clinical signs of disease consistently or eliminate infection. There are few published reports of treated cryptosporidiosis in cats. Therefore the protocols described here can only be considered anecdotal (Table 18-2).

In one case report, administration of clindamycin hydrochloride to a cat with chronic cryptosporidiosis and lymphocytic duodenitis failed to resolve diarrhea or stop oocyst shedding.[20] However, after initiating tylosin therapy, the stool character normalized within 7 days and feces were negative for *Cryptosporidium* spp. oocysts over a period of 6 months. Also, the inflammatory changes in

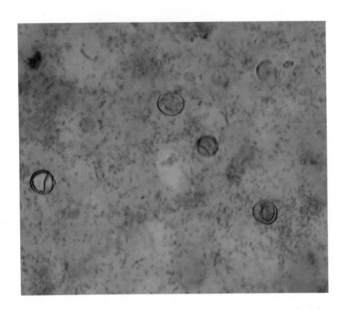

Figure 18-1 *Cryptosporidium* spp. oocysts (4-6 μm) stained with modified Ziehl-Neelsen acid-fast stain.

Table 18-2 Therapeutic Agents Commonly Used for the Treatment of Protozoal Infections in Cats

Drug	Dose	Route	Interval (Hours)	Minimum Duration (Days)	Organism
Azithromycin	10 mg/kg	PO	24	5-7	*Cryptosporidium* spp.
Febantel	56.5 mg/kg	PO	24	5	*Giardia duodenalis*
Fenbendazole	50 mg/kg	PO	24	5	*Giardia duodenalis*
Metronidazole	25 mg/kg	PO	12	7	*Giardia duodenalis*
Nitazoxanide	25 mg/kg	PO	12	7	*Giardia duodenalis*; *Cryptosporidium* spp.
Paromomycin	125-165 mg/kg	PO	12	5	*Giardia duodenalis*; *Cryptosporidium* spp.
Ponazuril	20-50 mg/kg	PO	24	1-2	*Isospora* spp.
Ronidazole	30 mg/kg	PO	24	14	*Tritrichomonas foetus*
Sulfadimethoxine	50-60 mg/kg then 25 mg/kg	PO	24	5	*Isospora* spp.
Tinidazole	30 mg/kg	PO	24	14	*Tritrichomonas foetus*
Tylosin	10-25 mg/kg	PO	12	14	*Cryptosporidium* spp.

the bowel resolved, and the cat was clinically normal over a 2-year period, which suggested a therapeutic response. We have treated other cats with presumed cryptosporidiosis with tylosin, and diarrhea has resolved in about 50 per cent of cases (Scorza and Lappin, unpublished observations, 2008). However, these observations are uncontrolled, and the signs in the affected cats may have resolved spontaneously without any treatment. However, it is likely that the antiinflammatory or antibacterial effects of tylosin play a role in the clinical response to the drug. Tylosin is not tolerated well by most cats because of its unpleasant taste and thus needs to be administered in capsules to many feline patients.

Recently, azithromycin has been shown to be effective for the management of cryptosporidiosis in some infected calves.[31] Azithromycin is well tolerated by cats and has been administered at 10 mg/kg PO q24h for a minimum of 10 days for the treatment of cryptosporidiosis with a variable response.

Paromomycin, an aminoglycoside for oral administration, was effective in clearing *Cryptosporidium* oocysts from the feces of a naturally infected cat with persistent diarrhea and in a group of experimentally inoculated cats.[32,33] However, the diagnostic tests used in the follow-up period in both studies may not have been adequately sensitive to detect cats who may have been in a carrier state. It is important to note that this drug should never be administered to cats with bloody diarrhea because it could be absorbed systemically. In one study of cats with *Tritrichomonas* infection treated with paromomycin, four out of 32 cats developed acute renal failure, and three of those four cats also became deaf.[34]

To date, nitazoxanide is the only drug approved by the U. S. Food and Drug Administration (FDA) for the treatment of diarrhea caused by *Cryptosporidium* in children and in adult human beings.[35] We are currently evaluating nitazoxanide for the treatment of a number of small-animal parasites. Some cats with *Cryptosporidium* spp. or *Giardia* spp. infections have shown resolution of diarrhea after the administration of nitazoxanide at a dosage of 25 mg/kg PO q12h for at least 5 days. However, the drug is a gastrointestinal irritant and commonly causes vomiting.

The optimal duration of therapy for feline cryptosporidiosis is unknown, and some cats treated with the protocols described in Table 18-2 may improve but may not resolve by the end of the suggested treatment period. In these cats, continued treatment may be indicated because a longer duration of therapy is sometimes needed to resolve the diarrhea. Cats with *Cryptosporidium* spp. and *Giardia* spp. coinfections seem to be more difficult to treat than cats infected with either organism alone. Some coinfected cats have required administration of paromomycin or nitazoxanide daily for more than 21 days to eliminate diarrhea.

Zoonotic Transmission

Most cats are infected with the cat-specific genotype *C. felis*.[1,14,36,37] Although *C. felis* DNA has been amplified from the feces of some human beings, molecular and epidemiological data suggest that the risk of zoonotic transmission of *Cryptosporidium* from companion animals to people is low.[38,39] However, care should be taken when handling the feces of cats with *Cryptosporidium* spp. infection and diarrhea.

Prevention

Cryptosporidium spp. are resistant to most common disinfectants, including commercial bleach. Formol saline (10 per cent solution) and ammonia (5 per cent) were effective in destroying the viability of the oocysts, but the required contact time was 18 hours. Exceptional sanitation and use of boiling water for the cleaning of water and food bowls should decrease the possibility of contamination within crowded environments. Housing cats indoors and feeding processed foods also may lessen the chances for exposure.

ISOSPORA (CYSTOISOSPORA) SPP.

Etiology

Isospora spp. that are capable of developing in intermediate hosts also are called *Cystoisospora* spp. Cats are infected commonly by *I. felis* and *I. rivolta*, which are obligate intracellular parasites with a direct life cycle or an indirect life cycle involving a paratenic host (frequently mice or other rodents). Unsporulated oocysts (*I. felis* = 27 to 31 μm × 38 to 51 μm; *I. rivolta* = 20 to 26 μm × 23 to 29 μm) are passed in feces after completion of an enteric life cycle in cats.

Epidemiology

While the prevalence of *I. felis* and *I. rivolta* infections vary depending on the study, it is thought that almost all cats will become infected with *Isospora* spp. in their lifetime. Enzootic infections occur frequently where cats are housed together or in close quarters like in shelters, pet stores, or catteries.

Pathogenesis

Infection occurs either through the ingestion of infective oocysts from the environment or when a cat eats a prey animal infected with the parasite. Oocysts are passed unsporulated in feces, and after exposure to warm temperature (20° C to 37° C) and humidity, sporulation occurs and two sporocysts are formed (Figure 18-2). Within each sporocyst are four infective sporozoites. After ingestion, sporozoites excyst in the intestinal lumen and undergo a series of asexual replications, followed by sexual replication, which leads to the formation of unsporulated oocysts that are shed in feces. Some sporozoites penetrate the intestinal wall and form unicellular cysts in the mesenteric lymph nodes or other extraintestinal tissues. These cysts may serve as a source of reinfection. Vomiting and diarrhea can occur and result from intestinal congestion, erosion of enterocytes, and atrophy of villi. These clinical signs occur mainly in kittens and young cats during the enteroepithelial cycle. *I. felis* generally is considered more pathogenic than *I. rivolta*.

Transmission

Isospora spp. are transmitted by ingestion of sporulated oocysts or by ingestion of infected transport hosts. The

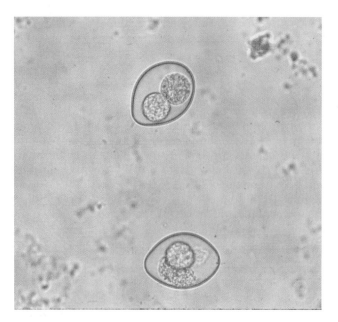

Figure 18-2 Sporulated *Isospora felis* oocysts (27-31 μm × 38-51 μm).

prepatent periods for *I. felis* and *I. rivolta* are between 7 to 10 days, and between 4 to 7 days or even more than 14 days, respectively.

Clinical Signs

Isospora spp. inhabit the small intestine of cats, and most infections cause no clinical signs of illness. Infection in kittens can be subclinical or cause clinical signs ranging from transient watery diarrhea to severe hemorrhagic diarrhea. Rarely, a heavily infected kitten may die. Kittens under condition of stress or immunosuppression, such as malnutrition and concurrent bacterial or viral infections, are most likely to become ill.

Diagnosis

Isospora spp. oocysts can be detected by fecal flotation and can be differentiated by the size of the oocysts. *Isospora felis* oocysts range in size from 27 to 31 μm by 38 to 51 μm, and *I. rivolta* oocysts range in size from 20 to 26 μm by 23 to 29 μm. Most cats with diarrhea from *Isospora* spp. infection are shedding large numbers of oocysts. However, several examinations may be required to document infection in some cats because shedding may be intermittent.

Treatment

It is questionable whether *Isospora* spp. infections cause chronic diarrhea in adult cats. If oocysts are found in feline patients with chronic diarrhea, the presence of another underlying disease should be considered. Sulfonamide-containing drugs have been used classically for treatment if clinical illness from *Isospora* spp. infection is suspected. However, these drugs are coccidiostatic, may be poorly tolerated by kittens, and have to be prescribed for long periods of time to be effective (see Table 18-2). Toltrazuril has been shown to be effective, but is currently not available in the United States.[40] Although no litera-

ture has been published on it, the related drug ponazuril is available for large animals and has been used safely for the treatment of *Isospora* spp. infection in kittens. Ponazuril (Marquis Paste, Bayer Animal Health) can be diluted at 1 g of paste to 3 mL of water, which gives a solution of 37.5 mg/mL. The drug is thought to be stable for several weeks after dilution. Ponazuril can be administered at 20 mg/kg PO q24h for 2 days, or at 50 mg/kg PO as a single dose. Both regimens appear to be safe and effective. Consideration should be given to treating cats who can be considered in-contact to the infected cat to attempt to prevent recurrent infection. Treatment of subclinically infected cats may lessen oocyst shedding and resultant environmental contamination. However, infection is not always cleared. In addition, the presence of a low-level infection can lead to premunition.

Prevention

Isospora spp. usually require several days in the environment to sporulate before they are infective, although under the right conditions, this time period can be as short as 6 to 8 hours. Therefore good litter box hygiene and prompt removal of feces can help to break the fecal-oral route of transmission in a multiple-cat environment. Utensils, runs, cages, and other implements should be disinfected by steam-cleaning or immersion in boiling water or by use of a 10 per cent ammonia solution. Cats should not be allowed to hunt. Insect control should be maintained because cockroaches and flies may serve as mechanical vectors of oocysts.

FLAGELLATES

GIARDIA SPP.

Etiology

Giardia duodenalis is a protozoan parasite with worldwide distribution that infects a variety of mammals. The *G. duodenalis* isolates from human beings and animals are indistinguishable morphologically. Molecular genetic studies have demonstrated that *G. duodenalis* is a species complex comprising seven assemblages (A to G). Some of the assemblages have been detected in animals and human beings, but some are host-specific. Cats can harbor the cat-specific assemblage F (Tables 18-3 and 18-4) and also occasionally the assemblages A and B, which represent the genotypes that have mainly been detected in human beings.[41-50] The organism exists in two stages, the motile trophozoite and the environmentally resistant cyst.

Epidemiology

Giardia spp. have been detected in feces from cats around the world (Tables 18-4 and 18-5). However, the prevalence of *Giardia* spp. varies, based on the study population and on the diagnostic test used.* Thus, although the true prevalence of *Giardia* spp. infections in cats is unknown, it is generally believed to be between 1 per

---

*References 9, 10, 12, 17, 42, 43, 51-61.

Table 18-3 Assemblages and Host Range of Isolates within the *Giardia duodenalis* Morphological Group

Assemblage	Host Range
A	Human beings, livestock, cats, dogs, beavers, guinea pigs, slow loris
B	Human beings, slow loris, chinchillas, dogs, beavers, rats, cats, siamang
C, D	Dogs
E	Cattle, sheep, pigs
F	Cats
G	Domestic rats

Modified from Thompson RCA: The zoonotic significance and molecular epidemiology of *Giardia* and Giardiasis, *Vet Parasitol* 126:15, 2004.[41]

Table 18-4 Genotypes of *Giardia duodenalis* Isolates from Cats

Number Tested	Country	Assemblage	Reference
21	Australia	9 A 2 B 2 C 7 D 1 E	42
14	Australia	Similar to dog genotype	43
3	Japan	F	44
1	Italy	F	45
1	Italy	A	46
19	Brazil	11 F 8 A	47
3	Colombia	F	48
9	United States	6 3B	49
17	United States	6A 11F	50

For assemblage host-range associations, see Table 18-3.

Table 18-5 Prevalence of *Giardia* spp. in Cats

Number Examined	Location	Method	Prevalence (%)	Reference
206	United States (Colorado)	Microscopy	2.4	10
263	United States (New York)	Microscopy	7.3	9
230	Chile	Microscopy	19.1	51
41	Canada	Microscopy	2.4	52
1355	United Kingdom	Microscopy	6	53
3167	Germany	Microscopy	10	54
81	Serbia	Microscopy	22	55
40	Australia	Microscopy	5	43
1063	Australia	Microscopy	2	56
131	Brazil	Microscopy	6.1	57
135	Czech Republic	Microscopy	1	17
305	The Netherlands	Microscopy	1	58
250	United States (Mississippi)	IFA	13.6	59
344	United States	IFA	9.8	12
4978	United States	Fecal ELISA	10.8	60
48	Italy	Fecal ELISA	4	61
48	United Kingdom	Fecal ELISA	15	53
135	Czech Republic	Serum	57	17
40	Australia	PCR	80	43

cent and 20 per cent in cats with diarrhea. Young, immunodeficient, and group-housed cats are thought to be more susceptible to infection and clinical disease.

Pathogenesis

Adherence of *Giardia* spp. trophozoites to the intestinal microvilli results in malabsorption by unknown mechanisms in some cats, which in turn can lead to small bowel diarrhea. Bacterial overgrowth syndrome may result from *Giardia* spp. infection, and clinical signs may be more severe in cats with other concurrent infections.

Transmission

In cats, trophozoites are found in the jejunum and ileum and can be passed in feces. However, because trophozoites rarely survive for a significant period outside the host, this stage is not considered infectious. *Giardia* spp. are transmitted among cats by ingestion of cysts that have been passed in the feces. After primary exposure, the prepatent period for *Giardia* spp. infections in cats ranges from 5 to 16 days. Shedding of *Giardia* cysts by cats may fluctuate from undetectable to concentrations of more than 1,000,000 cysts/g of feces.[62] Peaks of cyst shedding occur sporadically, and the duration between any two given peaks generally is between 2 and 7 days.[62] *Giardia* cysts can survive for weeks to months in the environment, and only a small number of cysts can cause infection.

Clinical Signs

Although most of the cats infected with *Giardia* spp. do not show clinical signs of disease, diarrhea occurs in some cats. The diarrhea is mucoid, pale, soft, and has a strong odor. Steatorrhea may be present as well. Mucus is common, and the stool sometimes contains traces of blood. Most infected cats are afebrile, do not vomit, and exhibit a normal serum total protein concentration and a normal complete blood count. Coinfections with *Giardia* and *Cryptosporidium* or *Tritrichomonas foetus* may result in more severe clinical illness that is more difficult to treat than *Giardia* infection alone.[23-25] Infection may be self-limited in 27 to 35 days or can be recurrent.

Diagnosis

A variety of different *Giardia* spp. tests have been evaluated for use in cats. There is no one test that can be performed on a single fecal sample that has 100 per cent sensitivity. Thus, a combination of diagnostic tests often is indicated. The American Association of Feline Practitioners recommends that all cats with diarrhea of 1 to 2 days in duration be evaluated by at least the combination of a direct fecal smear for trophozoites of *Giardia* spp. and a fecal flotation using a centrifugation technique.[63]

Liquid feces can be examined directly, or a small amount of mucus or feces can be mixed with saline on a microscope slide. With a coverslip placed, the sample then can be examined by light microscopy. At 100× magnification, trophozoites are recognized by their rapid motion, but their structural characteristics should be observed at 400×. The trophozoite is approximately 15 μm long and 8 μm wide, has a teardrop shape, and can be identified under light microscopy by the smiling

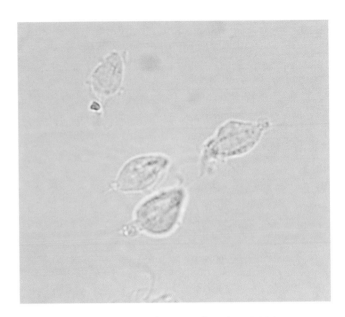

Figure 18-3 *Tritrichomonas foetus* trophozoites (10-26 μm × 3-5 μm) from culture.

face appearance. Because trophozoites may be associated with mucus, the only visible motility may be that of the flagella. *Giardia* trophozoites can be confused with trichomonads, in particular, *Tritrichomonas foetus*, because of their similar size (Figure 18-3). This organism can be differentiated from *Giardia* spp. by an undulating membrane, a rolling form of motility, the lack of a concave surface, and a single nucleus. The direct smear or wet mount examination should be performed on a fresh fecal sample. The application of Lugol's solution, methylene blue, or acid methyl green to the wet mount helps in the visualization of the internal structures of the trophozoites. Trophozoites are found rarely in solid feces. Thus, the direct smear or wet mount preparation is only indicated in cats with diarrhea.

Use of fecal concentration techniques, such as Sheather's sugar centrifugation or zinc sulfate centrifugation, are more sensitive than fecal cup flotation for detection of *Giardia* cysts and also can be used to evaluate for other parasitic infections. Cysts can be confused with yeast, but *Giardia* should be recognized easily because of its distinct structure. *Giardia* spp. of cats are approximately 12 μm long and 7 μm wide and contain internal structures like the nuclei and micronemes (Figure 18-4). Barium sulfate, several proprietary antidiarrheals, and enemas administered before the collection of the feces may interfere with the detection of the cysts. Cysts are shed intermittently, and therefore at least three samples should be examined over a period of about 1 week to exclude the possibility of a *Giardia* spp. infection.[64] Alternatively, additional diagnostic tests, such as a fecal antigen ELISA or IFA test, can be considered in an attempt to increase sensitivity. If the samples can not be examined immediately, they can be stored in the refrigerator for several days, but samples should not be frozen. Storage in the refrigerator prior to fecal flotation will lessen yeast overgrowth and also will block *T. gondii* oocyst sporulation if that agent is present.

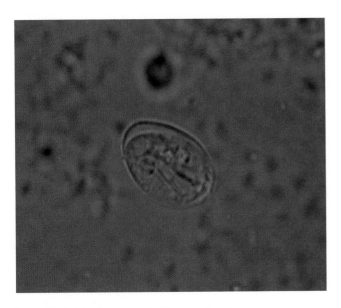

Figure 18-4 *Giardia* spp. cyst (12 μm × 7 μm).

If the feces contain much fat, formalin-ethyl acetate sedimentation is the best technique for detecting *Giardia* spp. cysts.

The monoclonal antibody-based immunofluorescent antibody assay mentioned earlier (Merifluor *Cryptosporidium/Giardia*, Meridian Diagnostics, Cincinnati, OH), which is used to detect *Cryptosporidium* spp. oocysts, also detects *Giardia* spp. cysts in feces. This assay was reported to be more sensitive and specific than zinc sulfate flotation, and was comparable to an antigen-detection technique when used on refrigerated feline fecal samples.[65] However, as noted previously, this assay can only be performed in diagnostic laboratories equipped with a fluorescence microscope.

A number of ELISAs are available for detection of *Giardia* spp. cysts in human feces, and one kit is labeled for use with dog and cat feces (SNAP*Giardia*, IDEXX Laboratories, Portland, ME).

Variable results have been seen with *Giardia* antigen tests when compared to other techniques. In one study, *Giardia* cysts were detected in 0 of 100 cats by microscopic examination (zinc chloride, sodium chloride flotation), and in 22 of 100 (22 per cent) of the cats in one commercially available fecal ELISA (ProSpecT *Giardia* Microplate Assay, Alexon Inc., Sunnyvale, CA), suggesting that the ELISA was more sensitive than the microscopic technique.[30] However, a different study found the same ELISA kit to be less sensitive than zinc sulfate flotation.[63] In a study performed in our laboratory, the agreement observed between several *Giardia* antigen tests and the IFA test ranged from 91.7 per cent to 100 per cent.[29] Recently, another study reported that the ProSpecT Microplate Assay had the highest sensitivity (91.2 per cent) and specificity (99.4 per cent) of any commercial assay for the detection of *Giardia* evaluated when compared to IFA.[28] In the same study, the SNAP *Giardia* antigen assay was as sensitive as fecal flotation and, when combined with fecal flotation, had a 97.8 per cent sensi-

tivity for *Giardia* spp.[28] At this time, fecal antigen tests are only recommended for assessment of cats with diarrhea because the clinical and zoonotic impact of an antigen-positive, cyst-negative healthy cat is unknown. In addition, it is currently unknown how long *Giardia* antigen assays remain positive after resolution of diarrhea. Therefore, if a veterinarian chooses to evaluate treated cats, only fecal flotation should be used for follow-up evaluation.

Several *Giardia* gene targets have been assessed in diagnostic PCR assays with varying results.[66,67] In addition, as for PCR assays for *Cryptosporidium* spp., there is no standardization between commercial laboratories providing these assays. It is unclear currently whether *Giardia* spp. PCR assays are more or less sensitive than other tests. However, the results of PCR can be used to determine whether the *Giardia* spp. detected was an assemblage that also infects people or a host-adapted assemblage (Veterinary Diagnostic Laboratory, Colorado State University, Fort Collins, CO 80523; http://www.dlab.colostate.edu/). At this time, PCR testing is only recommended for assessment of cats with diarrhea because the clinical and zoonotic impact of PCR-positive, cyst-negative healthy cats is unknown.

If the results of either a wet mount examination or fecal flotation are positive, the IFA, fecal antigen assay, or PCR is not needed, except to confirm results in questionable samples. These assays should be used as supplemental assays and should not replace fecal flotation and wet mount examination. Despite advances in immunological and molecular diagnostic assays, microscopic examination remains the gold standard for the laboratory diagnosis of cryptosporidiosis and giardiasis.[68]

Treatment

Cats with *Giardia* spp. infections and diarrhea generally are treated in an attempt to resolve diarrhea. When vomiting and small bowel diarrhea are the main clinical signs, highly digestible bland diets are indicated. If large bowel diarrhea is the principal clinical sign, high-fiber diets can be used instead (see Chapter 8). Use of probiotics also may improve clinical signs of disease[69,70] (see Chapter 11). However, although dietary manipulation often is used in cats with *Giardia* spp. infections, most veterinary clinicians also prescribe pharmaceuticals with anti-*Giardia* activity (see Table 18-2).

Metronidazole has been effective in eliminating *Giardia* cyst shedding in some naturally infected and experimentally infected cats.[71] Metronidazole also may help to correct secondary bacterial overgrowth and *Clostridium perfringens* overgrowth. Signs of toxicity, including gastrointestinal and central nervous system signs, have been associated with the administration of metronidazole to cats.[72] The neurological toxicity may develop following either chronic therapy or acute high doses.[72] There are two formulations of metronidazole available for oral administration. Metronidazole benzoate generally is well tolerated by cats.[71] Commercial products are available in some countries, and the drug is available for formulation in the United States. Metronidazole USP induces salivation and inappetence when administered orally to some cats.[73]

Fenbendazole is believed by many clinicians to be a good anti-*Giardia* drug, but to the authors' knowledge, it has only been evaluated in one study of cats (see Table 18-2). When fenbendazole was administered to cats infected concurrently with *Giardia* and *Cryptosporidium parvum,* cyst shedding was decreased in the treated cats when compared to controls, but only four of eight cats stopped shedding *Giardia* cysts.[23] Whether these results related to the presence of *Cryptosporidium* or to the strain of *Giardia* used is unknown. Fenbendazole should be considered for use when concurrent roundworm, hookworm, or *Taenia* infections are suspected. Albendazole can cause bone marrow suppression and should not be used in cats.[74] Febantel (Drontal Plus; febantel/pyrantel/praziquantel; Bayer Animal Health) is converted to fenbendazole and thus may also have anti-*Giardia* effects. When the drug was administered at 56.5 mg/kg PO for 5 days to six infected cats, there was a significant decrease in cyst shedding in the treated group when compared to controls, and four of the six treated cats stopped shedding *Giardia* cysts.[75]

The authors have administered paromomycin or nitazoxanide successfully to some cats with persistent diarrhea suspected to be due to *Giardia* spp. and *Cryptosporidium* spp. coinfection, using the protocols described for cryptosporidiosis. Other alternate drugs that have been used to treat *Giardia* infection in cats include tinidazole, ronidazole, and quinacrine. A *Giardia* vaccine was available in the United States for a short time and had been tried as an immunotherapy agent for the treatment of giardiasis in dogs and cats with variable results.[76,77] However, the feline product has now been discontinued.

Treatment failures are common in human beings and other animals with giardiasis. It is likely that no drug will be universally effective for the treatment of giardiasis in cats because different strains are likely to have different drug susceptibilities. In addition, there is no permanent immunity to *Giardia,* and cats can be reinfected within days of an apparently successful treatment. Therefore in clinical practice all options for treatment should be considered for the individual cat, and the drug and protocol may need to be varied. Some veterinarians recommend dual therapy with metronidazole and fenbendazole. Such dual therapy should be considered in chronic or recurrent cases of suspected *Giardia*-associated diarrhea and in concurrent disorders such as *Cryptosporidium* spp. infection, inflammatory bowel disease, bacterial overgrowth, exocrine pancreatic insufficiency, or immunodeficiency.

Prevention

A vaccine for *Giardia* spp. has been discontinued. Therefore the primary *Giardia* prevention strategies are to avoid exposure, stress, and coinfections. Housing cats indoors, providing only clean water, feeding processed foods, controlling potential transport hosts, providing strategic deworming, and providing a clean environment may lessen the risk for giardiasis. Once *Giardia* infection has been established in a group of cats, such as cats in shelters, multiple-cat households, or humane societies, it can be difficult to control recurrent infections. In these situations, the combination of the following strategies is used

to try to control the problem: (1) lessen environmental contamination by cleaning and disinfecting thoroughly with quaternary ammonium base compounds, (2) treat all cats, (3) clean cysts from coats of all cats, and (4) prevent reintroduction of infection by isolating cats with diarrhea. Cats can be bathed with regular pet shampoos and rinsed thoroughly. The perianal region can be cleaned with a quaternary ammonium base compound; however, these agents can be dermal irritants and should not be allowed to stay in contact with the skin for more than 3 to 5 minutes if used.[78]

Zoonotic Transmission

Giardia is the most common parasite infecting people worldwide. The majority of infections in human beings are acquired by drinking water or swallowing contaminated water while swimming in lakes or swimming pools. As discussed, cats are infected occasionally with the zoonotic assemblages A and B.[41-50] Although the detection of the same assemblages in human beings and cats is not conclusive evidence for zoonotic transmission, cats with diarrhea and *Giardia* cyst shedding in feces should be considered potential human health risks and should be treated with the primary goal to control diarrhea. If *Giardia* cysts are detected on a routine fecal flotation performed in a healthy cat, it should be discussed with the owner whether treatment should be attempted. Drug therapy is not 100 per cent safe or effective, and reinfection with *Giardia* is common. For example, in a recent study, 16 *Giardia* cyst–positive dogs with normal feces were treated with either fenbendazole or nitazoxanide.[79] Of the 16 dogs, eight had side effects related to the drug, and at the end of the 34-day study, five of the eight dogs were still infected.

TRITRICHOMONAS FOETUS

Etiology

Members of the order Trichomonadida are small and structurally complex flagellates that reproduce by binary fission and do not form cysts. In vertebrates, they are parasites of the gastrointestinal system, the reproductive system, and the upper portions of the respiratory tract. *Tritrichomonas foetus* infects the reproductive tract of both cows and bulls and can cause abortions. The organism also parasitizes the gastrointestinal system of cats. Genetic characterization of the internal transcribed spacer 1 region found differences between the bovine and feline isolates.[80] The trophozoite of *T. foetus* is 10 to 26 μm long and 3 to 5 μm wide, and has three anterior flagella (see Figure 18-3). Feline isolates of *T. foetus* remain in the reproductive tract of heifers but do not cause the same pathological changes as the bovine isolate.[80] Similarly, bovine isolates of *T. foetus* may not cause disease in cats as successfully as feline isolates.[80]

Epidemiology

Cats in crowded environments are infected more frequently, while infection of feral cats is uncommon. In an international cat show in the United States, 31 per cent of 117 cats owned by 89 different breeders were infected.[81]

In the United Kingdom, 16 of 111 (14.4 per cent) diarrhea samples were positive for *T. foetus* by PCR.[82] Both pure-breed and mixed-breed cats can be infected. Although *T. foetus*–associated diarrhea is common in kittens and young cats,[83] infection also is documented in adult cats with an age range from 3 months to 13 years.[81] Catteries with a recent history of refractory diarrhea, adult cats with *Isospora* spp. infections, and cats living in a facility with a small number of square feet per cat were more likely to be infected with *T. foetus*.[82,83]

Pathogenesis

Tritrichomonas foetus is an obligate parasite that depends on endogenous bacteria and host secretion for nutrients. In experimentally infected cats, *T. foetus* is restricted to the ileum, cecum, and colon. Fluctuations in the colonic microflora or other factors are necessary to produce the clinical signs of *T. foetus* infection. The organism can persist in cats without diarrhea, and diarrhea can become worse without an increased number of organisms.[25] An increased number of *T. foetus* and increased severity of diarrhea was associated with coinfection with *Cryptosporidium* spp.[25] It is unknown if immunosuppression predisposes to chronic infection with *T. foetus*. In one study, administration of prednisolone did not change the fecal consistency or the frequency of positive results on direct fecal exams.[25]

Clinical Signs

Clinical signs can be variable, ranging from asymptomatic infections to chronic intractable diarrhea. Clinical signs of disease often are intermittent and also often resolve with antimicrobial therapy, only to recur after therapy is discontinued. The diarrhea mainly is large bowel, with increased frequency of defecation and passage of semiformed to liquid, often malodorous, feces that sometimes are associated with fresh blood and mucus. When the diarrhea is severe, the anus becomes edematous and the cat can become incontinent. Although diarrhea may persist, most affected cats maintain a good health and body condition. In addition, *T. foetus* also has been detected in the uterine contents of a cat with endometritis/pyometra.[84]

Diagnosis

A direct smear should be performed on feces of all cats with large bowel diarrhea to evaluate for the presence of *T. foetus* trophozoites, using the technique described for *Giardia*. *T. foetus* is similar in size to *Giardia* but can be differentiated by the presence of an undulating membrane, rapid forward motion, the lack of a concave surface, and a single nucleus. A video clip demonstrating the classic motility can be seen at http://www.cvm.ncsu.edu/docs/personnel/gookin_jody.html. The sensitivity of a direct smear using samples from naturally infected cats was only 14 per cent in one study.[85] The sensitivity can be improved by analyzing multiple fecal smears. If *T. foetus* infection is still suspected after the initial diagnostic evaluation, culture can be performed using a commercially available culture system (In PouchTF, BioMed Diagnostics, Inc, White City, OR). The media utilized does not support the growth of *Giardia* spp. or *Pentatricho-monas hominis*, and positive test results likely correlate with infection by *T. foetus*.[85] Several PCR-based assays that are specific for *T. foetus* also are commercially available, and these assays are recommended for assessment of samples that were found negative by microscopy and fecal culture and for confirmation that microscopically observed or cultivated organisms are *T. foetus*.[86] PCR is specific for *T. foetus* and does not amplify *Giardia* or *P. hominis* DNA.[86] Recently, *P. hominis* DNA has been amplified from feces of cats coinfected with *T. foetus*, but whether this potentiates *T. foetus*–associated clinical disease currently is unknown.[87]

Treatment

Many treatment regimens have been attempted in cats with *T. foetus* infections with generally poor response.[88,89] In some cases, temporary improvement was noted with a variety of drugs, but relapse was invariable. Some of the apparent clinical improvement could be due to secondary effects of the drugs on the intestinal bacterial flora, although treatment also may prolong trophozoite shedding.[88,89]

Ronidazole has been the most effective drug used to date and currently is recommended at a dosage of 30 mg/kg PO q24h for 14 days.[90] Infection can relapse after treatment with ronidazole but can resolve after repeating the treatment regimen.[90] Higher doses of ronidazole can be associated with neurological signs.[91] Thus far, all reported cases of ronidazole-related neurotoxicity have been reversible, but irreversible neurotoxicity may occur.

Tinidazole administered at 30 mg/kg PO for 14 days suppressed *T. foetus* shedding to undetectable levels in two of four cats during a 33-week period posttreatment.[92] However, this drug currently is considered inferior to ronidazole because infections were not eliminated.

Zoonotic Transmission

Only a single case of an immunosuppressed human being infected with *T. foetus* has been reported. However, due to the poor host specificity of *T. foetus* and the close contact between cats and human beings, zoonotic transmission should be considered, and infected kittens with diarrhea should be handled with care.

Prevention

Kittens in crowded environments are more susceptible to infection due to stress or immunological immaturity. Therefore minimizing the stress and avoiding dense housing conditions likely would reduce the chances of exposure to *T. foetus*.

OTHER ENTERIC PROTOZOANS

AMEBIASIS

Entamoeba histolytica is a facultative parasitic amoeba that infects mainly human beings and nonhuman primates. Infection usually is acquired by ingestion of cysts from water or food that is contaminated with human feces. *E. histolytica* is a potentially invasive parasite, and dissemination of the amoeba throughout the body, especially the liver, lung, and the brain, via blood vessels and lymphatics occurs in some infected human beings. Experimental studies in cats suggest that invasion of other organs is rare in this species. *E. histolytica* was reported in a 3-year-old cat with bloody diarrhea and anorexia in Japan.[93] On necropsy examination, the cat showed marked thickening of the walls of the cecum and colon, and the mesenteric lymph nodes were significantly enlarged, similar to what is found in human patients infected with this protozoan. Information concerning the treatment of infected cats is not available. The potential for transmission from infected cats to people is unknown, but probably is unlikely.

BALANTIDIASIS

Balantidium coli is a ciliated protozoan that infects a wide variety of hosts. Infection in cats apparently is rare; the organism has only been reported in the feces of two of 100 healthy cats in Japan.[94] In people, infection rarely causes diarrhea and ulcerative lesions in the large intestine. Information concerning treatment of infected cats is not available. The potential for transmission from infected cats to people is unknown but probably is unlikely.

BLASTOCYSTOSIS

Blastocystis hominis is a protozoan parasite that inhabits the gastrointestinal tract of human beings and animals. *Blastocystis* spp. were found in 35 of 52 (67.3 per cent) fecal samples from cats in Australia.[95] The age of the infected cats ranged between 6 weeks and 7 years.[95] Some cats have a high number of organisms in the feces, but do not have any clinical signs of diarrhea. Information concerning treatment of infected cats is not available. A zoonotic potential has been suggested; however, *Blastocystis* spp. isolated from the feces of cats were smaller and irregular in shape compared to those found in human beings.[96]

MICROSPORIDIOSIS

Microsporidia are obligate intracellular spore-forming pathogens. Cats can harbor *Encephalitozoon cuniculi* and *Enterocytozoon bieneusi*.[48,97-100] *E. bieneusi* has been found in association with chronic diarrhea in human patients with acquired immunodeficiency syndrome. The prevalence of *E. bieneusi* in cats in Europe has been reported to be as high as 23 per cent, and a recent study reported a prevalence of 17 per cent in Colombia.[48,100] Genetic analysis of these isolates revealed that some of the genotypes found in cats also have been reported in human beings, suggesting that cats can be a potential source of infection for people.[48,100,101] Clinical signs in human beings consist of diarrhea, malabsorption, weight loss, rhinitis, and bronchitis. Whether similar syndromes occur in infected cats is unknown. An optimal therapy for *E. bieneusi* infection in human beings or cats is unknown.[102,103]

REFERENCES

1. Palmer CS, Traub RJ, Robertson ID, et al: Determining the zoonotic significance of *Giardia* and *Cryptosporidium* in Australian dogs and cats, *Vet Parasitol* 154:142, 2008.
2. Sargent KD, Morgan UM, Elliot A, et al: Morphological and genetic characterization of *Cryptosporidium* oocysts from domestic cats, *Vet Parasitol* 77:221, 1998.
3. Chermette R, Blondel S: Cryptosporidiose des carnivores domestiques, resultants preliminaries in France, *Bull Soc Franc Parasitol* 7:31, 1989.
4. Lyndsay DS, Zajac AM: *Cryptosporidium* infections in cats and dogs, *Compend Contin Educ Pract Vet* 26:864, 2004.
5. Iseki M: *Cryptosporidium felis* sp.n. (Protozoa: Eimririna) from the domestic cat, *Jap J Parasit* 5:285, 1979.
6. Arai H, Fukuda Y, Hara T, et al: Prevalence of *Cryptosporidium* infection among domestic cats in the Tokyo metropolitan district, *Jpn J Med Sci Biol* 43:7, 1990.
7. Nash AS, Mtambo MMA, Gibbs HA: *Cryptosporidium* infection in farm cats in the Glasgow area, *Vet Rec* 133:576, 1993.
8. McGlade TR, Robertson ID, Elliot AD, et al: Gastrointestinal parasites of domestic cats in Perth, Western Australia, *Vet Parasitol* 117:251, 2003.
9. Spain CV, Scarlett JM, Wade SE, et al: Prevalence of enteric zoonotic agents in cats less than 1 year old in Central New York State, *J Vet Intern Med* 15:33, 2001.
10. Hill S, Cheney J, Tatton-Allen GF, et al: Prevalence of enteric zoonoses in cats, *J Am Vet Med Assoc* 216:687, 2000.
11. Nutter FB, Dubey JP, Levine JF, et al: Seroprevalence of antibodies against *Bartonella henselae* and *Toxoplasma gondii* and fecal shedding of *Cryptosporidium* spp., *Giardia* spp., and *Toxocara cati* in feral and pet domestic cats, *J Am Vet Med Assoc* 225:1394, 2004.
12. Mekaru SR, Marks SL, Felley AJ, et al: Comparison of direct immunofluorescence, immunoassays, and fecal flotation for detection of *Cryptosporidium* spp. and *Giardia* spp. in naturally exposed cats in 4 northern California animal shelters, *J Vet Intern Med* 21:959, 2007.
13. Scorza V, Lappin MR: Detection of Cryptosporidium spp. by PCR in cats and dogs in the United States. Proceedings of the 23rd ACVIM Forum, Baltimore: (abstr), 2005.
14. Gunn-Moore DA, Scorza V, Wilmot A, et al: Prevalence of *Cryptosporidium* species in feces from cats in the United Kingdom. Proceedings of the 25th ACVIM Forum, Seattle: (abstr) 2007.
15. McReynolds C, Lappin MR, McReynolds LM, et al: Regional seroprevalence of *Cryptosporidium parvum* IgG specific antibodies of cats in the United States, *Vet Parasitol* 80:187, 1999.
16. Mtambo MMA, Nash AS, Wright SE, et al: Prevalence of specific *Cryptosporidium* IgG, IgM and IgA antibodies in cat sera using an indirect immunofluorescence antibody test, *Vet Parasitol* 60:37, 1995.
17. Svobodovà V, Konvalinova J, Svobodova M: Coprological and serological findings in dogs and cats with giardiosis and cryptosporidiosis, *Acta Vet Brno* 63:257, 1994.
18. Deng M, Rutherford MS, Abrahamsen MS: Host intestinal response to *Cryptosporidium parvum*, *Adv Drug Deliv Rev* 56:869, 2004.
19. Scorza AV, Brewer MM, Lappin MR: Polymerase chain reaction for the detection of *Cryptosporidium* spp. in cat feces, *J Parasitol* 89:423, 2003.
20. Lappin MR, Dowers K, Edsell D, et al: Cryptosporidiosis and inflammatory bowel disease, *Fel Pract* 25:10, 1997.
21. Goodwin MA, Barsanti JA: Intractable diarrhea associated with intestinal cryptosporidiosis in a domestic cat also infected with feline leukemia virus, *J Am Anim Hosp Assoc* 26:365, 1990.

22. Brizee-Buxton BL, Crystal MA: Coincident enteric crypto-sporidiosis (correspondence), *J Am Anim Hosp Assoc* 30:307, 1994.

23. Keith CL, Radecki SV, Lappin MR: Evaluation of fenbenda-zole for treatment of *Giardia* infection in cats concurrently infected with *Cryptosporidium parvum*, *Am J Vet Res* 64:1027, 2003.

24. Perez Trot G, Asanovic J, Petetta L: Resolucion de un caso complejo de diarrhea en una gata, *Rev Med Vet* 84:73, 2002.

25. Gookin JL, Levy MG, Law JM, et al: Experimental infection of cats with *Tritrichomonas foetus*, *Am J Vet Res* 62:1690, 2001.

26. Lent ST, Burkhardt JE, Bolka D: Coincident enteric crypto-sporidiosis and lymphosarcoma in a cat with diarrhea, *J Am Anim Hosp Assoc* 29:492, 1993.

27. Goodgame RW, Kimball K, Ou CN, et al: Intestinal function and injury in acquired immunodeficiency syndrome related-cryptosporidiosis, *Gastroenterology* 108:1075, 1995.

28. Marks SL, Hanson TE, Melli AC: Comparison of direct immunofluorescence modified acid fast staining, and enzyme immunoassay techniques for detection of *Crypto-sporidium* spp. in naturally exposed kittens, *J Am Vet Med Assoc* 225:1549, 2004.

29. Bachman D, Scorza AV, Brewer M, et al: Evaluation of chro-matographic immunoassays for the diagnosis of *Giardia* spp. and *Cryptosporidium* spp. of cats and dogs. Proceedings of the 25th ACVIM Forum, Seattle: (abstr), 2007.

30. Cirak VY, Bauer C: Comparison of conventional copro-scopical methods and commercially coproantigen ELISA kits for the detection of *Giardia* and *Cryptosporidium* infec-tions in dogs and cats, *Berl Münch Tierärztl Wochenschr* 117:410, 2004.

31. Elitok B, Elitok OM, Pulat H: Efficacy of azithromycin dihy-drate in treatment of cryptosporidiosis in naturally infected dairy calves, *J Vet Intern Med* 19:590, 2005.

32. McReynolds C, McReynolds LM, Brewer MM, et al: *Crypto-sporidium parvum* serum antibodies responses and oocyst shedding in experimentally inoculated cats. Unpublished data. Master's Defense, Colorado State University, 2001.

33. Barr SC, Jamrosz GF, Hornbuckle WE, et al: Use of paromo-mycin for treatment of cryptosporidiosis in a cat, *J Am Vet Med Assoc* 205:1742, 1994.

34. Gookin JL, Riviere JE, Gilger BC, et al: Acute renal failure in four cats treated with paromomycin, *J Am Vet Med Assoc* 215:1821, 1999.

35. Hemphill A, Mueller J, Esposito M: Nitazoxanide, a broad-spectrum thiazolide anti-infective agent for the treatment of gastrointestinal infections, *Expert Opin Pharmacother* 7:953, 2006.

36. Thomaz A, Meireles MV, Soares RM, et al: Molecular iden-tification of *Cryptosporidium* spp. from fecal samples of felines, canines and bovines in the state of São Paulo, Brazil, *Vet Parasitol* 150:291, 2007.

37. Huber F, da Silva S, Bomfim TC, et al: Genotypic character-ization and phylogenetic analysis of *Cryptosporidium* sp. from domestic animals in Brazil, *Vet Parasitol* 150:65, 2007.

38. Glaser CA, Safrin S, Reingold A, et al: Association between *Cryptosporidium* infection and animal exposure in HIV-infected individuals, *JAIDS* 17:79, 1998.

39. Brown RR, Elston TH, Evans L, et al: Feline zoonoses guide-lines from the American Association of Feline Practitioners, *Compend Contin Educ Pract Vet* 25:936, 2003.

40. Lloyd S: Activity of toltrazuril and diclazuril against *Isospora* species in kittens and puppies, *Vet Rec* 148:509, 2001.

41. Thompson RCA: The zoonotic significance and molecular epidemiology of *Giardia* and Giardiasis, *Vet Parasitol* 126:15, 2004.

42. Read CM, Monis PT, Thompson RCA: Discrimination of all genotypes of *Giardia duodenalis* at the glutamate dehy-drogenase locus using PCR-RFLP, *Infect Gen Evol* 4:125, 2004.

43. McGlade TR, Robertson ID, Elliot AD, et al: High prevalence of *Giardia* detected in cats by PCR, *Vet Parasitol* 110:197, 2003.

44. Itagaki T, Kinoshita S, Aoki M, et al: Genotyping of *Giardia intestinalis* from domestic and wild animals in Japan using the glutamate dehydrogenase gene sequencing, *Vet Parasitol* 133:283, 2005.

45. Lalle M, Pozio E, Capelli G, et al: Genetic heterogeneity at the β-giardin locus among human and animal isolates of *Giardia duodenalis* and identification of potentially zoonotic subgenotypes, *Int J Parasitol* 35:207, 2005.

46. Berrilli F, Di Cave D, De Liberato C, et al: Genotype char-acterization of *Giardia duodenalis* isolates from domestic and farm animals by SSU-rRNA gene sequencing, *Vet Para-sitol* 122:193, 2004.

47. Souza SLP, Genera SM, Richtzenhain LJ, et al: Molecular identification of *Giardia duodenalis* from humans, dogs, cats and cattle from the state of São Paulo, Brazil, by sequence analysis of fragments of glutamate dehydrogenase (gdh) coding gene, *Vet Parasitol* 149:258, 2007.

48. Santín M, Trout JM, Vecino JA, et al: *Cryptosporidium, Giardia* and *Enterocytozoon bieneusi* in cats from Bogota (Colombia) and genotyping of isolates, *Vet Parasitol* 141:334, 2006.

49. Van Keulen H, Macechko PT, Wade S, et al: Presence of human *Giardia* in domestic, farm and wild animals, and in environmental samples suggests a zoonotic potential for giardiasis, *Vet Parasitol* 108:97, 2002.

50. Vasilopulos RJ, Rickard LG, Mackin AJ, et al: Genotypic analysis of *Giardia duodenalis* in domestic cats, *J Vet Intern Med* 21:352, 2007.

51. Lopez JD, Abarca K, Paredes P, et al: Parasitos intestinales en caninos y felinos con cuadros digestivos en Santiago, Chile. Consideraciones en Salud Publica, *Rev Med Chile* 134:193, 2006.

52. Shukla R, Giraldo P, Kraliz A, et al: *Cryptosporidium* spp. and other zoonotic enteric parasites in a sample of domestic dogs and cats in the Niagara region of Ontario, *Can Vet J* 47:1179, 2006.

53. Tzannes S, Batchelor DJ, Graham PA, et al: Prevalence of *Cryptosporidium, Giardia* and *Isospora* species infections in pet cats with clinical signs of gastrointestinal disease, *J Feline Med Surg* 10:1, 2008.

54. Barutzki D, Shaper R: Endoparasites in dogs and cats in Germany 1999-2002, *Parasitol Res* (Suppl 3):S148, 2003.

55. Nikolic A, Dimitrijevic S, Djurkovic-Djakovic O, et al: Giar-diasis in dogs and kittens in the Belgrade Area, *Acta Vet (Belgr)* 52:43, 2002.

56. Palmer CS, Thompson RCA, Traub RJ, et al: National study of the gastrointestinal parasites of dogs and cats in Austra-lia, *Vet Parasitol* 151:181, 2008.

57. Barrientos Serra CM, Antunes Uchoa CM, Alonso Coimbra R: Parasitological study with fecal samples of stray and domiciliated cats *(Felis catus domesticus)* from the metro-politan area of Rio de Janeiro, Brazil, *Rev Soc Bras Med Trop* 36:331, 2003.

58. Robben SR, le Nobel WE, Döpfer D, et al: Infections with helminths and/or protozoa in cats in animal shelters in the Netherlands, *Tijdschr Diergeneeskd* 129:2, 2004 (abstract).

59. Vasilopulos RJ, Mackin AJ, Rickard LG, et al: Prevalence and factors associated with fecal shedding of *Giardia* spp. in domestic cats, *J Am Anim Hosp Assoc* 42:424, 2006.

60. Carlin EP, Bowman DD, Scarlett JM, et al: Prevalence of *Giardia* in symptomatic dogs and cats throughout the

United States as determined by the IDEXX SNAP *Giardia* test, *Vet Ther* 7:199, 2006.

61. Biancardi P, Papini R, Giuliani G, et al: Prevalence of *Giardia* antigen in stool samples from dogs and cats, *Revue Med Vet* 155:417, 2004.

62. Kirkpatrick CE, Farrell JP: Feline giardiasis: Observations on natural and induced infections, *Am J Vet Res* 45:2182, 1984.

63. Brown RR, Elston TH, Evans L, et al: Feline zoonoses guidelines from the American Association of Feline Practitioners, *Compend Contin Educ Pract Vet* 25:936, 2003.

64. Dryden MW, Payne PA, Smith V: Accurate diagnosis of *Giardia* spp. and proper fecal examination procedures, *Vet Ther* 7:4, 2006.

65. Lappin MR, Jensen WA, Taton-Allen G: Comparison of ZnSO$_4$ centrifugation, a fecal antigen assay, and an immunofluorescent antigen assay for diagnosis of giardiasis in cats, *J Vet Intern Med* 16:345, 2002 (abstract).

66. Barr SC, Bowman DD, Erb HN: Evaluation of two test procedures for diagnosis of giardiasis in dogs, *Am J Vet Res* 53:2028, 1992.

67. Cacciò SM, Ryan U: Molecular epidemiology of giardiasis, *Mol Biochem Parasitol* 160:75, 2008.

68. Chalmers RM: Advances in diagnosis—is microscopy still the benchmark? II International *Giardia* and *Cryptosporidium* Conference, Morelia, Michoacan, Mexico, 2007.

69. Chon SK, Kim NS: Evaluation of silymarin in the treatment of asymptomatic *Giardia* infections in dogs, *Parasitol Res* 97:445, 2005.

70. Benyacoub J, Perez PF, Rochat F, et al: *Enterococcus faecium* SF68 enhances the immune response to *Giardia intestinalis* in mice, *J Nutr* 135:1171, 2005.

71. Scorza AV, Lappin MR: Metronidazole for the treatment of feline giardiasis, *J Feline Med Surg* 6:157, 2004.

72. Caylor KB, Cassimatis MK: Metronidazole neurotoxicosis in two cats, *J Am Anim Hosp Assoc* 37:258, 2001.

73. Groman R: Metronidazole, *Compend Contin Educ Pract Vet* 22:1104, 2000.

74. Stokol T, Randolph JF, Nachbar S, et al: Development of bone marrow toxicosis after albendazole administration in a dog and cat, *J Am Vet Med Assoc* 210:1753, 1997.

75. Scorza AV, Radecki SV, Lappin MR: Efficacy of a combination of febantel, pyrantel, and praziquantel for the treatment of kittens experimentally infected with *Giardia* species, *J Feline Med Surg* 8:7, 2005.

76. Olson ME, Morck DW, Ceri H: The efficacy of a *Giardia lamblia* vaccine in kittens, *Can J Vet Res* 60:249, 1996.

77. Stein JE, Radecki S, Lappin MR: Efficacy of *Giardia* vaccination for treatment of giardiasis in cats, *J Am Vet Med Assoc* 222:1548, 2003.

78. Barr SC: Giardiasis. In Greene CE, editor: *Infectious diseases of the dog and cat*, ed 3, St Louis, 2006, Elsevier, p 736.

79. Lappin MR, Clarke M, Scorza AV: Treatment of healthy *Giardia* spp. positive dogs with fenbendazole or nitazoxanide. Proceedings of the 28th ACVIM Forum, San Antonio, TX: (abstr) 2008.

80. Stockdale HD, Lanaghan SC, Dykstra CC, et al: Molecular comparison of *Tritrichomonas foetus* from bovines and felines. Proceedings of the 53rd AAVP Annual Meeting, New Orleans, 2008.

81. Gookin JL, Stebbins ME, Hunt E, et al: Prevalence of and risk factors for feline *Tritrichomonas foetus* and *Giardia* infection, *J Clin Microbiol* 42:2707, 2004.

82. Gunn-Moore DA, McCann TM, Reed N, et al: Prevalence of *Tritrichomonas foetus* infection in cats with diarrhoea in the UK, *J Feline Med Surg* 9:214, 2007.

83. Gookin JL, Breitschwerdt EB, Levy MG, et al: Diarrhea associated with trichomonosis in cats, *J Am Vet Med Assoc* 215:1450, 1999.

84. Dahlgren SS, Gjerde B, Pettersen HY: First record of natural *Tritrichomonas foetus* infection of the feline uterus, *J Small Anim Pract* 48:654, 2007.

85. Gookin JL, Foster DM, Poore MF: Use of a commercially available culture system for diagnosis of *Tritrichomonas foetus* infection in cats, *J Am Vet Med Assoc* 222:1376, 2003.

86. Gookin JL, Birkenheuer AJ, Breitschwerdt EB, et al: Single-tube nested PCR for detection of Tritrichomonas foetus in feline feces, *J Clin Microbiol* 40:4126, 2002.

87. Gookin JL, Stauffer SH, Levy MG: Identification of *Pentatrichomonas hominis* in feline fecal samples by polymerase chain reaction assay, *Vet Parasitol* 145:11, 2007.

88. Foster DM, Gookin JL, Poore MF, et al: Outcome of cats with diarrhea and *Tritrichomonas foetus* infection, *J Am Vet Med Assoc* 225:888, 2004.

89. Mardell EJ, Sparkes AH: Chronic diarrhoea associated with *Tritrichomonas foetus* infection in a British cat, *Vet Rec* 158:765, 2006.

90. Gookin JL, Copple CN, Papich MG, et al: Efficacy of ronidazole for treatment of feline *Tritrichomonas foetus* infection, *J Vet Intern Med* 20:536, 2006.

91. Rosado TW, Specht A, Marks SL: Neurotoxicosis in 4 cats receiving ronidazole, *J Vet Intern Med* 21:328, 2007.

92. Gookin JL, Stauffer SH, Coccaro MR, et al: Efficacy of tinidazole for treatment of cats experimentally infected with *Tritrichomonas foetus*, *Am J Vet Res* 68:1085, 2007.

93. Shimada A, Muraki Y, Awakura T, et al: Necrotic colitis associated with *Entamoeba histolytica* infection in a cat, *J Comp Pathol* 106:195, 1992.

94. Nakauchi K: The prevalence of *Balantidium coli* infection in fifty-six mammalian species, *J Vet Med Sci* 61:63, 1999.

95. Duda A, Stenzel DJ, Boreham PFL: Detection of *Blastocystis* spp. in domestic dogs and cats, *Vet Parasitol* 76:9, 1998.

96. Greene CE: Blastocystosis. In Greene CE, editor: *Infectious diseases of the dog and cat*, ed 3, St Louis, 2006, Elsevier, p 744.

97. Dengjel B, Zahler M, Hermanns W, et al: Zoonotic potential of *Enterocytozoon bieneusi*, *J Clin Microbiol* 39:4495, 2001.

98. Lores B, del Aguila C, Arias C: *Enterocytozoon bieneusi* (microsporidia) in faecal samples from domestic animals from Galicia, Spain, *Mem Inst Oswaldo Cruz* 97:941, 2002.

99. Lobo ML, Xiao L, Cama V, et al: Genotypes of *Enterocytozoon bieneusi* in mammals in Portugal, *J Eukaryot Microbiol* 53(Suppl 1):S61, 2006.

100. Halánová M, Cisláková L, Valencáková A, et al: Serological screening of occurrence of antibodies to *Encephalitozoon cuniculi* in humans and animals in Eastern Slovakia, *Ann Agric Environ Med* 10:117, 2003.

101. Leelayoova S, Suputtamongkol Y, Subrungruang I, et al: Evidence supporting the zoonotic and non-zoonotic transmission of *Enterocytozoon bieneusi*, *Ann Trop Med Parasitol* 102:459, 2008.

102. Didier ES, Weiss LM: Microsporidiosis: current status, *Curr Opin Infect Dis* 19:485, 2006.

103. Didier ES, Maddry JA, Brindley PJ, et al: Therapeutic strategies for human microsporidia infections, *Expert Rev Anti Infect Ther* 3:419, 2005.

Mark E. Hitt

The terms *cholangitis, hepatitis,* and *cholangiohepatitis* are used to represent a group of disorders referred to as *feline inflammatory liver disease* (FILD). FILD is a broad term that refers to overlapping forms of disease processes. Liver disease is a relatively common problem in cats. The order of frequency for hepatopathies in cats seen in the author's specialty referral hospital is (1) acute neutrophilic cholangitis/cholangiohepatitis, (2) idiopathic hepatic lipidosis, (3) chronic forms of FILD, (4) neoplasia (particularly lymphoma), and (5) hepatocellular necrosis (e.g., toxic, drug-associated liver disease). This is similar to published reports, except that acute inflammatory disease is not the most common condition in these reports.[1]

Historically, terms to describe FILD have reflected concepts and descriptions based on such characteristics as duration of clinical signs (e.g., acute vs. chronic), suspected pathogenesis (e.g., infectious, idiopathic, or immunological), and histopathological description (e.g.,

location of inflammatory cells within the lobular and portal architecture, types of inflammatory cells present, extension through the limiting plate around portal triads, hepatocellular changes, presence and location of fibrosis, biliary epithelial and ductular changes, and/or vascular changes).[1-5] The most commonly cited names for forms of FILD over the past 2 decades include acute suppurative cholangitis/cholangiohepatitis, chronic nonsuppurative cholangiohepatitis, sclerosing-like cholangitis, lymphocytic cholangitis cholangiohepatitis complex (LCCC), cholangiohepatitis (CH) complex (with acute and chronic forms), progressive lymphocytic-plasmacytic cholangiohepatitis, and lymphocytic portal hepatitis (LPH).

The most recent terminology proposed to categorize FILD has been narrowed to five basic classifications (Box 19-1).[6] These definitions are still being refined based on ongoing discussions concerning the overlap in histological description and clinical presentation. Currently, it is

213

unclear whether there is a progression from one form of FILD to the next or a unique pathogenic pathway for each of these forms. The prevailing thought is that there is a relationship between the pathogenic pathways and these different forms of FILD.

Cats with FILD involving primarily the infiltration of neutrophils within and around the biliary ducts are considered to have the acute neutrophilic form (ANF) of cholangitis. Previous terminology would have used the term *suppurative cholangitis* for these cases. Ascension of bacteria through the bile ducts is thought to play a role in the pathogenesis of ANF.

If this inflammatory process progresses unchecked, additional infiltration with lymphocytes and plasma cells may occur along with the existing presence of the neutrophilic cellular components. This lymphocytic-plasmacytic infiltration, referred to as the chronic neutrophilic form (CNF) of cholangitis, can center on the bile ducts or be more extensive within the portal tracts.

According to the previous classification system, patients with minimal or absent neutrophilic infiltrations would have been described as having a nonsuppurative lymphocytic-plasmacytic cholangitis. If inflammatory cells extend beyond the limiting plate around portal tracts, the process is termed *cholangiohepatitis*. Injury to hepatocytes can occur due to the action of locally released inflammatory cytokines and a toxic microenvironment, direct hepatocellular injury due to inflammatory cells (cellular injury potentially may be reversible, but if necrosis has occurred it is nonreversible), and/or induction of hepatocellular apoptosis (i.e., a chain of events leading to programmed cell death of individual hepatocytes).

The third form of FILD, lymphocytic cholangitis (LC), involves pathological changes with a marked predominance of lymphocytes as inflammatory cells. This process is associated with a moderate to severe infiltration with small lymphocytes usually concentrated in portal areas but at times also in biliary ductules and the hepatic parenchyma. Small areas of lymphoid aggregates can be found on histopathological examination. A mixture of other inflammatory cells also may be seen in low numbers. This form also can be associated with biliary hyperplasia, distension of bile ductules, a mild degree of hepatocellular loss, and variable fibrosis. This form of cholangitis or cholangiohepatitis can be the result of an immune-mediated process as outlined in the next section.

The fourth form of FILD, lymphocytic portal hepatitis (LPH), is diagnosed clinically less often than the others. LPH occurs mostly in older cats, many of whom have no clinical suspicion for FILD. However, in one study 82 per cent of cats who underwent necropsy examination showed some degree of infiltration of the portal triads with small lymphocytes.[5] LPH is thought to be slowly progressive and associated with only minimal to modest changes in serum activities of hepatic enzymes. The etiology of LPH is not known, but it is suspected to be an extension of immune-mediated disease or a result of a nonspecific reactive response to extrahepatic disease. Patients with LPH tend to be diagnosed at an age greater than 10 years and have a comparatively good prognosis.

Finally, cholangitis associated with liver fluke infestation also is a variant of inflammatory liver disease in cats. This disease involves infestation by trematodes in the biliary system.[7-9] Several species of liver flukes can infect cats, the most common being *Platynosomum concinnum*. Cholangitis associated with liver flukes is considered separate from other forms of FILD because the etiology is known and often can be determined definitively.

ETIOLOGY AND PATHOGENESIS

Much remains to be clarified about the pathogenesis of FILD. Therefore the concepts proposed in this chapter should be considered hypotheses that likely will need to be refined and revised in the future as clinical experience and scientific information expand. As with many noninfectious inflammatory diseases, it is unclear if FILD is due to a single cause, such as an inflammatory response to a certain stimulus (e.g., infection, xenobiotics, or various toxins), inappropriate triggering of an immunological response, or loss of self tolerance, or if the disease is due to a combination of these factors or a progression through various stages involving these mechanisms. The hepatic parenchyma is exposed to portal blood returning from the intestines. This portal blood contains increased levels of bacterial waste products, small numbers of bacteria, endogenous and exogenous toxins, various xenobiotic compounds, and potential food-derived antigens or metabolites acting as potential haptens or neoantigens with the local immune system (e.g., gut-associated lymphoid tissues, [GALT]).

The liver plays an important role in the body's immune response. The defense mechanisms include innate immune cells (e.g., macrophages, natural killer T cells, and CD3+ T cells), hepatocellular metabolism (i.e., detoxification), biliary excretion of waste products (e.g., xenobiotics, enterotoxins, endotoxins, and others), the flushing action of bile flow, and elimination of microorganisms by endothelial cells and Kupffer cells. To defend against potentially toxic agents effectively and quickly, and to avoid launching a harmful systemic immune response against self, the liver needs to differentiate potential threats from nutrients. The ability for a differential recognition of pathogenic bacteria, normal flora, and self-related antigenic substances is critical to prevent an inappropriate activation of an inflammatory response in the biliary system.[10]

A complex theory concerning the pathogenesis of immune-mediated cholangiohepatitis has been described in the human medical literature. This theory involves many factors, including genetic and individual predispositions, the biosynthesis of a variety of soluble pathogen-recognition receptors (PRRs), previously generated toll-like receptors (TLR) that guide tolerance for the enteric flora, inappropriate loss of tolerance to enteric luminal antigens, development of biliary epithelial neo-antigens and subsequent activation of complement components, and chemotaxis of inflammatory cells.[11] Attention currently is focused on understanding how TLRs and germline-encoded PRRs activate the innate immune system and assist the process of differentiating pathogens from nonpathogens. The discovery of the toll-like receptors helped to identify the innate immune receptors responsible for tolerance towards the normal flora and self-antigens. It is interesting that TLRs seem only to be involved in the cytokine production and cellular activation of the immune system in response to microbes; they do not play a significant role in the adhesion and phagocytosis of microorganisms.[12] Activated immune cells can produce cytokines, which in turn will trigger inflammatory responses. Bacterial pathogens can be phagocytosed, digested, and processed for antigen recognition. The antigens can be presented to CD4+ T cells that release further cell signaling substances and cytokines.[13]

One of the primary theories concerning the pathogenesis of cholangitis in cats is that the disease process involves ascension of enteric bacteria into the bile ducts via the sphincter of Oddi, which serves as a valve between the duodenum on one side and the pancreatic duct and the common bile duct on the other. This in part may explain the relationship between pancreatitis, cholangitis, and inflammatory bowel disease that appears to exist in some cats. The liver's immune system plays an important role in controlling local innate immunity. The antigen-processing cells of the liver (e.g., Kupffer cells and dendritic cells), along with T cells of the GALT, are important in the development of immunological responses. Potentially aberrant immune responses directed against intestinal epithelial mucosal cells (as can result from failure of the mechanisms involving TLR and PRR) can lead to shared or similar antigenic recognition sites with the epithelial cells lining the biliary ducts, pancreatic ducts, and the intestinal mucosa.[13]

The interplay involving the misdirected immune response, the inflammatory reaction (e.g., mediated through cytokines and inflammatory cells), regenerative effects of hepatic tissue (e.g., through the action of hepatic growth factors, cytokines, and cellular signaling mechanisms), and progression to fibrosis is very complex. Progressive disease is associated with the development of fibrosis, sinusoidal capillarization, and alterations to structure and function of the lobular terminal hepatic venules. These latter changes also result in biliary hyperplasia or atrophy, cholestasis, and portal venous hypertension. The hepatocytes can be injured by activation of pathways that lead to apoptosis (premature programmed cell death). Some authors propose that unless there is an outright cause of hepatocellular necrosis (e.g., through primary hepatocellular injury), hepatocytes are only injured indirectly and that losses of hepatocytes result mostly from apoptosis. However, if the limiting plate is breached by inflammatory cells, further damage of hepatocytes is expected. This response to inflammation in the liver leads to a harmful microenvironment for hepatocytes via retention of bile acids, cell membrane injury, relative hypoxia, mitochondrial failure, and more shunting of blood to the terminal hepatic venules, which may in turn be compromised by fibrosis.[14,15] It has been postulated that CH begins to develop with a systemic infection or ascension of microorganisms via the biliary tree, followed by a response of the immune system that leads to inflammation. One hypothesis is that there is a progression from the acute neutrophilic form of the disease to the chronic neutrophilic form. This would be followed by a decreasing neutrophilic component and an increasing lymphocytic component, which would lead to the characteristic lesions of the lymphocytic form of FILD. The apparently less pathogenic form, LPH, might represent a less pronounced response of the liver to the everyday challenges of life because older cats commonly show some degree of LPH. Although this pathogenetic model is not documented in the literature, it is an interesting hypothesis to help explain the difficulty in understanding the overlaps seen between histopathological examination and clinical findings in the described forms of FILD.

There also is an ongoing effort to define small cell lymphoma involving the portal and biliary system because this condition can be confused easily with marked lymphocytic cholangitis. Determining the clonality of the involved lymphocytes may prove helpful in separating inflammation from lymphoma.

Many authors have suggested previously that bile is not normally sterile and that some degree of ascension of bacteria from the intestinal tract can occur even in normal cats.[16,17] However, there is contrasting evidence suggesting that bile within the gall bladder of normal cats usually is sterile when cultured for aerobic and anaerobic growth.[18] In one study, a group of feline and canine patients with hepatic inflammation was evaluated and seven of 30 (23.3 per cent) patients had positive bile cultures but only six of 103 (5.8 per cent) had positive hepatic cultures. *Escherichia coli*, *Enterococcus* spp., *Bacteroides* spp., *Streptococcus* spp., and *Clostridium* spp. were the most common isolates identified.[16] In another report, in six cats with cholangitis or cholecystitis, a similar pattern of bacterial cultures was identified, with *E. coli* being the predominant species. In addition, a *Streptococcus* organism and one *Salmonella enterica* serovar *typhimurium* also were cultured.[18] In this study, concurrent pathological changes involving the pancreas and intestines were found in three of the six patients. However, these data do not provide any proof whether bacteria are secondary or primary agents in the pathogenic sequence of events. More studies are needed to clarify the true role of bacteria in the pathogenesis of FILD. Newer methodologies such as fluorescent in situ hybridization (FISH) are being used to detect and localize the presence of specific bacterial deoxyribonucleic acid (DNA) sequences in hepatic specimens. Primary sclerosing cholangitis (PSC) is a severe, progressive liver disease of human beings. It is similar in histopathological appearance to more advanced cases of feline LPH, in which fibrosis is marked and cholestasis is severe. The etiology and pathogenesis of PSC in human beings remains unknown.[19] Also, as it does regarding LC and LPH in cats, controversy exists as to whether PSC in human beings should be considered an autoimmune disease.[20,21] A large number of autoantibodies have been identified in patients with PSC, suggesting that it is an autoimmune disease. However, the specificity of these antibodies generally is low, and the frequencies of the presence of these antibodies in affected patients vary greatly among different studies. In general, there appears to be a reversal of the common female gender predilection of many autoimmune disorders. It has been hypothesized that the presence of autoantibodies in patients with PSC may be the result of a nonspecific dysregulation of the immune system. It is interesting that the literature also points to the possible presence of specific antibody targets, including the biliary epithelium and neutrophilic granulocytes.[19] This relationship gives further support to the hypothesized pathogenic relationship among infections, the suppurative response, and the lymphocytic response directed against both the suppurative neutrophilic cells and the biliary epithelium. This hypothesis is similar to an older concept that infection-related haptens bind with innate cell membranes, leading to neoantigen formation as a mechanism for loss of self-tolerance and development of autoimmunity within the liver. Major histocompatibility complex Class II (MHC II) molecules normally are expressed by the epithelium of biliary ducts and Kupffer cells. In addition, there also are portal and bile duct intraepithelial lymphocytes (CD3+ or T lymphocytes). In one study involving immunohistochemical examination, cats who were diagnosed with progressive lymphocytic cholangitis showed increased numbers of CD3+ lymphocytes in the periportal and portal tissue.[17] There were fewer B cells forming aggregates or follicles within the most affected areas of lymphocytic infiltration. Low numbers of immunoglobulin A–positive plasma cells also were seen. It is interesting that both acute and chronic types of FILD had a similar composition of infiltrates. Expression of MHC class II was increased for the vascular endothelium and fibroblasts in areas of fibrosis, supporting the role of immunological stimulation.[14]

Chronic infections with organisms that are difficult to culture are suspected as one possible etiological cause for inflammatory liver disease in human beings and cats. Possible organisms being investigated in cats with cholangitis/cholangiohepatitis include common enteric bacteria, *Helicobacter* spp., and *Bartonella* spp.[22,23] Five *Bartonella* spp. have been shown to infect cats naturally (see Chapter 4 in the fifth volume of this series). However, in most instances, infections resolve spontaneously. In one study, DNA markers were used to look for the presence of *Helicobacter* sequences in hepatic tissue from cats with liver disease. DNA of *Helicobacter* spp. was found in hepatic tissue in two of 32 cats (6.3 per cent) with cholangiohepatitis and one of 16 cats (6.3 per cent) with noninflammatory liver disease.[22] These findings also suggest that *Helicobacter* spp. identified in the liver are distinct from those isolated normally from the stomach in cats. Although the low incidence of infection with *Helicobacter* spp. in cats with FILD would suggest that this organism is not a major cause of FILD, it represents an example warranting further research regarding infectious organisms and a possible and chronic stimulation of the immune system. *Bartonella henselae* (the main causative agent of cat scratch disease in human beings) is interesting as another example for the possible pathogenesis of inflammatory liver disease. Experimental studies have shown that *Bartonella* can cause chronic intraerythrocytic and vascular endothelial infections of multiple organs, including the liver.[23] It has been shown that the organism can persist in the host and cause lymphocytic hepatitis in healthy cats who were infected experimentally with *B. henselae* and/or *B. clarridgeiae* (coinfections).[24] In another study, *Helicobacter* spp. DNA was identified in the bile from four of 15 cats (27 per cent) with LPH and from eight of 51 cats (16 per cent) without LPH.[25] However, these results are not definitive proof of a cause-and-effect relationship; rather they provide a basis for further study of the role of infectious organisms such as *Helicobacter* and *Bartonella* spp. in the pathogenesis of chronic lymphocytic infiltration of the liver.

CLASSIFICATION

At this time, the classification of inflammatory liver disease in cats is based predominantly on histopathological criteria and focuses on the biliary tract (see Box 19-1). However, the patient's clinical history, clinicopathological data, and physical examination findings all play roles in determining the diagnosis because there is overlap among the histopathological patterns described above.

ACUTE NEUTROPHILIC FORM OF CHOLANGITIS/CHOLANGIOHEPATITIS

The ANF of cholangitis/cholangiohepatitis is thought to be the most common form of FILD. Associated mainly with a neutrophilic response, it is presumed to be a result of ascension of bacteria belonging to the normal intestinal microflora or of pathogenic bacteria via the common bile duct. Neutrophils, and occasionally bacteria, can be seen within the interepithelial areas of biliary walls and the lumen of bile ducts (Figure 19-1). If the disease is a first occurrence, there may be no fibrosis, marked distension of the bile ducts, or biliary epithelial hyperplasia. Often patients have been presented previously with a similar clinical episode. In these patients, fibrosis and biliary hyperplasia are more prominent. Because the distal portion of the common bile duct is shared with the pancreatic duct, there also is evidence of pancreatitis in some patients. The gall bladder and cystic duct can be affected, especially if bile sludge or other signs of cholestasis are present.

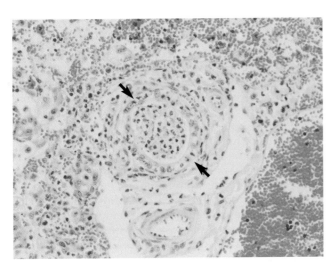

Figure 19-1 Acute neutrophilic cholangitis. This histopathological image shows neutrophils and cellular debris in the lumen of a bile duct *(between arrows)*. The neutrophilic infiltration also can be seen within the wall of the bile duct. (H&E stain.) (Courtesy Dr. John M. Cullen, North Carolina State University, Raleigh, NC.)

SIGNALMENT

In the author's experience, ANF occurs most commonly in younger cats, ranging from 1 to 9 years of age. There does not appear to be a breed or gender predisposition.

CLINICAL FINDINGS

The acute onset of clinical signs is the most obvious feature noted by a cat's owner. Abdominal pain, vomiting (either fluid in patients with an empty stomach or food that has been present in the stomach for several hours), diarrhea, and anorexia all are common presenting signs. Fever is a variable finding but supports the diagnosis of ANF when present. Dehydration is common. The author believes that many milder cases are never diagnosed definitively because owners often opt for symptomatic treatment with early use of antibiotics and supportive fluid therapy. However, a history of such an episode in the medical record can lead to a more focused diagnostic evaluation. Surgery may be advisable if a patient is not responding to treatment or shows worsening clinical signs or if there is the possibility of complete biliary obstruction or peritonitis.

DIAGNOSIS

An inflammatory leukogram, sometimes with a left shift, is more common with this form of FILD but does not occur in every patient. There is no consistent pattern of hepatic enzyme elevations. However, in the author's experience, serum alanine aminotransferase (ALT) and gamma-glutamyl transpeptidase (GGT) levels may increase earlier than levels of serum alkaline phosphatase (ALP) or serum bilirubin concentration. Rising serum bili-

rubin concentrations may be the only abnormal finding on a serum chemistry profile, which may be due to inspissations of bile admixed with purulent material and to edematous narrowing of the lumen of the biliary tree. Therefore a rising serum bilirubin concentration should lead to a concern for a potential secondary obstruction of bile flow and worsening of clinical signs if not treated. Often no dramatic increases of liver enzyme activities are observed initially if the cat is presented early enough in the course of the disease. A repeat serum chemistry profile is warranted 12 to 24 hours after initial presentation if the diagnosis still is unclear. Also, one of the main differential diagnoses in patients with this presentation is pancreatitis; therefore concurrent testing for pancreatitis (i.e., measurement of serum feline specific lipase immunoreactivity, SpecfPL) is warranted. An acute, severe presentation also warrants concurrent testing for systemic infections, including feline leukemia virus (FeLV), feline immunodeficiency virus (FIV) infections, feline infectious peritonitis (FIP), and toxoplasmosis.

IMAGING

As for any patient with significant signs of gastrointestinal disease, abdominal radiographs are indicated. These may be normal, but some patients can show evidence of hepatomegaly. Rarely evidence of radiopaque choleliths or emphysematous biliary ducts is identified. In chronic/recurring cases dystrophic mineralization of hepatic or pancreatic tissue can be present. Abdominal ultrasonographic assessment also is indicated, but in some cases the evaluation may not show overt abnormalities. However, abnormalities are found with enough frequency to justify routine use of this noninvasive procedure. Ultrasonographic findings can include distension of the common and cystic bile ducts; other, less common, findings include distension of intrahepatic bile ducts, evidence of luminal obstructive foci, thickening of the walls of the gall bladder, evidence of concurrent pancreatitis, and regional lymphadenomegaly. The finding of regional fluid adjacent to the hilar region of the liver (porta hepaticus) or around the gall bladder should prompt the clinician to consider fine-needle aspiration of the fluid or consider recommending exploratory surgery if the patient's condition is worsening. Although not common, regional bacterial peritonitis can occur in severe cases. Sequential monitoring of abdominal ultrasonography, along with serum chemistry analysis and complete blood count with white blood cell differential counts, is warranted if there is a lack of improvement.

OTHER DIAGNOSTIC TECHNIQUES

The use of fine-needle aspiration of the liver or adjacent peritoneal fluid can be helpful but has limitations. Because of the position of the normal liver within the costal arch, deeper targets (even with ultrasonographic guidance) may require an intercostal approach, which increases the risk of inadvertently hitting a major blood vessel or distended bile duct or obtaining a nondiagnostic sample. Cholecystocentesis (aspirating the gall bladder) can be accomplished relatively safely. The approach used may be direct or transhepatic (crossing liver tissue as a window to the gall bladder).[26-28] The aspirate can provide material for cytological examination and culture. The finding of septic bile, exudative peritoneal fluid, or hepatic cytological changes with an increased number of neutrophils (above the degree expected by comparison to peripheral blood) also supports the diagnosis. Histopathological evaluation of a liver biopsy is required for confirmation of the diagnosis. Hepatic tissue and bile should be submitted for culture (preferably for both aerobic and anaerobic culture). Techniques for liver biopsy include percutaneous needle-core biopsy (e.g., Tru-Cut as a cutting needle or Menghini as a suction needle) or, preferably, laparoscopic or surgical approaches that improve the sample quality. If a needle-core biopsy is used, the author prefers a 14-gauge disposable Tru-Cut–type needle. Specific requests for special stains should be made to assess the presence of bacteria, atypical organisms, and fibrosis. Immunophenotypical staining and assessment of clonality of lymphocytes can be requested if the diagnosis is more suggestive of the lymphocytic forms of cholangitis or cholangiohepatitis. The latter techniques, available through several pathology laboratories, help differentiate small cell lymphoma from lymphocytic cholangitis.

DIFFERENTIAL DIAGNOSES

The main differential diagnoses for ANF include acute gastritis, hairballs, acute food intolerance (change of diet), idiopathic hepatic lipidosis, hepatotoxicity, pancreatitis, toxoplasmosis, FIP, lymphoma, and inflammatory bowel disease. If clinical signs do not respond satisfactorily to antibiotics and supportive care, a full diagnostic evaluation is warranted.

TREATMENT

The initial treatment of ANF involves antibiotics and supportive care. The antibiotic selected to treat suspected ANF usually is an antimicrobial effective against a wide variety of common enteric bacteria. Treatment should be initiated quickly, although submission of collected specimens for culture is advised in case the patient fails to respond to the initial therapy. Intravenous or subcutaneous administration of antibiotics often is used initially because the patient is vomiting and anorexic. Intravenous ampicillin or a cephalosporin often is combined with a parenterally administered fluoroquinolone or aminoglycoside. Parenterally administered clindamycin or metronidazole also may be considered. Beta-lactamase–resistant antibiotics (e.g., ampicillin with sulbactam, ticarcillin, meropenem) also can be used if warranted.

Most patients begin to respond within 48 hours of initiating antibiotic therapy. If the patient is not improving, reassessment may be indicated, including repetition of some of the initial testing. Once vomiting has resolved, oral antibiotic treatment is initiated. Antibiotic therapy should be continued for a minimum of 2 to 4 weeks—longer if the patient has a known recurrent episode. It is essential to maintain hydration for adequate microvascular perfusion of the liver and to maintain normal electrolyte status. If the patient does not start to eat, partial parenteral nutrition should be considered (see Chapter 16 in the fifth volume of this series). If vomiting is controlled, nasoesophageal tubes are the easiest modality for liquid enteral nutrition. Few patients will tolerate an adequate volume and duration of oral syringe feeding, even if nausea has resolved. If surgery is required for any other reason, a jejunostomy tube can be placed. In a few institutions, endoscopic- or fluoroscopic-assisted placement of naso/gastro-jejunostomy tubes may be an alternative (see Chapter 12). Most cats with ANF begin to eat within a few days. Because biliary disease can be painful, an analgesic management plan should be implemented. Parenteral or transmucosal oral administration of buprenorphine is used most commonly in these patients. The author has used continuous rate infusions (CRI) of a combination of morphine, lidocaine, and ketamine (also known as MLK) when warranted for pain in these patients. Fentanyl patches also can be used, but this drug takes longer to reach appropriate blood levels and become effective. Often the patient is improving by this point. When the patient can tolerate oral medications, treatment with ursodeoxycholic acid (ursodiol, UDCA) should be initiated. The author uses 5 to 8 mg PO q24h initially until tolerance is established. The dose then is increased to 10 to 15 mg PO q24h. The author has avoided the use of UDCA when there is any suspicion of complete biliary obstruction. The primary goal of UDCA therapy is to increase bile flow. UDCA acts as a choleretic, making the bile less viscous. It also stabilizes cell membranes and is less toxic to the sinusoidal membranes than endogenous bile acids, the levels of which increase with cholestasis. UDCA also can increase survival of stressed or reversibly injured hepatocytes. It can be used long term with periodic monitoring of the patient's physical status and serum chemistry profile. Occasionally, the author has used a single dose of dexamethasone sodium phosphate (0.2 mg/kg IV) to help mitigate inflammation in patients who appear not to be improving in appetite and attitude despite other markers of clinical improvement. However, use of a corticosteroid in this situation carries obvious risks (e.g., immunosuppression, counter-regulatory to insulin, altering subsequent biopsy results). On the other hand, there are potential benefits from suppressing inflammation and reducing edema that may be narrowing the lumen of biliary ducts.[29]

Antiemetic medications often are needed in the first few days of the course of the disease. The use of metoclopramide as a constant rate infusion and/or the intramuscular injection of prochlorperazine (assuming that the patient is well hydrated) are the author's first choices. Other antiemetic drugs can be used (e.g., off-label use of dolasetron and/or maropitant) based on the attending veterinarian's experiences and comfort. The author commonly administers famotidine (0.5 mg/kg IV q12h) for several days after vomiting has resolved. In the author's opinion these patients have an altered gastric motility and hyperacidity that may increase the risks of reflux esophagitis and patient discomfort. However, there currently is no evidence to substantiate this hypothesis.

CHRONIC NEUTROPHILIC FORM OF CHOLANGITIS/CHOLANGIOHEPATITIS

As discussed previously, there is concern that ANF may progress to more chronic forms of FILD. The CNF may simply be the result of recurring ANF, repeated bacterial stimulation of the immune system, and developing degrees of inflammatory damage and fibrosis occurring in the portal triads. It is possible that the CNF serves as a bridge between ANF and the lymphocytic form of cholangitis. In past decades, CNF was described as nonsuppurative destructive cholangiohepatitis because neutrophils are a less prominent component of mixed inflammatory cells. Although the current nomenclature includes the term *neutrophilic,* there is mild to severe accumulation of plasma cells and lymphocytes in the portal regions, along with a variable number of neutrophils in the biliary tree. There is more significant injury to the portal triads, with necrosis and hyperplasia of biliary epithelium and often breaches in the limiting plate leading to hepatocellular damage. Fibrosis may be present, extending into the parenchyma of the lobule (Figure 19-2). Although rare in cats, histopathological findings may show some characteristics of cirrhosis.

SIGNALMENT

As with ANF, there is no particular breed or gender predilection for CNF. Affected cats tend to be middle-aged

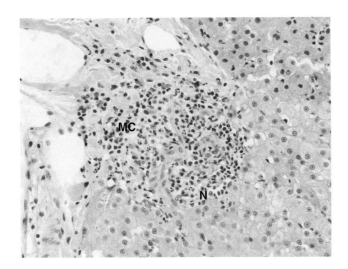

Figure 19-2 Chronic neutrophilic cholangitis. This histopathological image shows a mixed mononuclear cell infiltrate *(MC)* around a bile duct. Neutrophilic *(N)* infiltration of the wall and the lumen of the same bile duct also can be observed. Evidence of early fibrosis can be seen. (H&E stain.) (Courtesy Dr. John M. Cullen, North Carolina State University, Raleigh, NC.)

to older at presentation. The history can include prior episodes of confirmed or suspected hepatic or gastrointestinal upset that have never been diagnosed definitively.

CLINICAL FINDINGS

Clinical signs may have been intermittent over the past months or even years but with a tendency to worsen with each occurrence. Signs, which are often more vague than in patients with ANF, include vomiting, anorexia, soft stools, weight loss, and in some cases fever. The clinical history can vary in part because some of these patients have concurrent gastroenteritis (e.g., inflammatory bowel disease) and/or pancreatitis. Icterus is more common but may not be acute in its presentation, having developed slowly over a few days or even weeks in some cases. Patients can begin to appear unthrifty and have a low body condition score. In the author's experience clinical signs of hepatic encephalopathy (HE) are not common for patients with CNF, except for those with advanced disease.

DIAGNOSIS

Most cats with CNF have increased serum GGT and ALP levels and bilirubin concentration. Serum ALT activity ranges from normal to markedly increased. However, similar to patients with ANF, clinical chemistry abnormalities can be quite variable. If there is an acute superimposition of a new ascending bacterial infection, fever and leukocytosis can be present. Serum bile acid concentrations may be increased, but modest changes can be difficult to interpret due to concurrent hyperbilirubinemia. As with ANF, testing for pancreatitis is recommended. If surgery or laparoscopy is pursued, biopsies of the small intestine and stomach and examination of the pancreas should be performed, as well as liver biopsies and cultures of bile and liver tissue. It also is reasonable to repeat testing for FeLV and FIV in any cat with a chronic medical history. Although biopsies are valuable, the normal course is to treat with antibiotics and provide supportive and symptomatic care before deciding to perform a biopsy.

IMAGING

Abdominal radiography is valuable for the same reasons described for ANF. The liver may appear to have rounded margins and a normal or small size depending on the chronicity of the case. Ultrasound findings also can be similar to those in patients with ANF and have the same caveats. However, with increasing fibrosis and/or loss of hepatocellular mass, portobiliary markings within the hepatic parenchyma may take on a relative or true hyperechogenicity. In older patients, thoracic radiographs are warranted to check for metastasis of a possible neoplastic condition.

OTHER DIAGNOSTIC TECHNIQUES

Cytological examination of a fine-needle aspirate (FNA) is of lesser value in patients with CNF than in ANF. However, FNA can be used for cholecystocentesis. A liver aspiration also can be performed if more invasive and accurate techniques are declined by the client or precluded by the patient's status. The cytological description always has to be considered in context with the confidence in the sample collected and the clinical pathologist, the history of the patient, and the results of concurrent clinicopathological and imaging examinations. Correlation of cytological examination with biopsy results is controversial at best. (The reader is referred to Chapter 15 in the fourth volume of this series for a discussion of the use of fine-needle aspirates in the diagnosis of liver disease.)

Little advantage is likely to be gained from more advanced imaging modalities such as magnetic resonance imaging unless nodular changes or other abnormalities of other abdominal organs are a concern. Testing of prothrombin time (PT), partial thromboplastin time (PTT), and proteins invoked by vitamin K absence (PIVKA) should be considered if significant hepatic dysfunction is suspected or biopsies are to be pursued.[30] In patients with chronic liver disease the author also routinely performs a platelet count and an oral (buccal) mucosal bleeding time (OMBT) before collecting any biopsies.

DIFFERENTIAL DIAGNOSES

The main differential diagnoses for CNF include chronic gastritis, CNF with superimposed acute ascending biliary infection, idiopathic hepatic lipidosis if anorexia has been present for a sufficient length of time, chronic hepatotoxicity, chronic or recurrent pancreatitis, neoplasia (including lymphoma), FIP, inflammatory bowel disease (IBD), biliary obstruction, or a combination of these conditions. More aggressive diagnostic efforts (e.g., imaging and obtaining biopsies) often are considered more quickly when a longer history of CNF or a lack of improvement convinces the client of the need for action.

TREATMENT

The treatment of CNF initially involves the same considerations as described for ANF. The patient may be presented because of an acute crisis, recurrent episodes, or ongoing chronic signs. Treatment is most effective when based on biopsy results. Most cats with lymphocytic-plasmacytic inflammation will require long-term use of corticosteroids, given concurrently with antimicrobial therapy, to treat the inflammation and to reduce further fibrosis. A common dosage for prednisolone is 1 to 2 mg/kg PO q24h for the first 2 to 4 weeks, depending on the severity of signs. If parenteral administration is preferable, either prednisolone suspension (1 mg/kg SQ q24h) or dexamethasone sodium phosphate (0.25 mg/kg SQ or IV q24h for 2 to 3 days, then adjusting the dosage downwards) can be used. The long-term goal of treatment is to taper the patient's dose toward the lowest effective dosage of corticosteroids that reduces liver enzyme activities and that maintains the relative health of the patient. It is not uncommon to use prednisolone (0.5 to 1 mg/kg PO q48h) as a long-term treatment. Most cats tolerate corticosteroids well. However, diabetes mellitus may be unmasked in some patients due to the counter-regulatory effects of these drugs. Also, long-term corticosteroid use can have catabolic and immunosuppressive effects. If clinical signs and/or the liver enzyme activities do not improve, additional immunosuppressive medications are warranted because progression will occur without adequate treatment. Azathioprine has been described as an immunosuppressive treatment in cats for cholangitis and IBD. However, this drug has a fairly high rate of adverse drug reactions, including increases of liver enzyme activities and bone marrow suppression. Therefore use of azathioprine in cats is not recommended by the author.

Currently, the author's preference for added immunosuppression, if required, is chlorambucil, which is dosed initially at 0.25 mg/kg PO q72h. Monitoring of complete blood counts and serum chemistry profiles is necessary in cats treated with chlorambucil. Although this treatment usually is well tolerated, it can lead to bone marrow suppression at any point during its use in cats. Occasionally, a modest neutrophilic leukocytosis may be noted when chlorambucil is used at the above dosage. This may be the result of the disproportionately milder effects it has on T-helper cells than on T-suppressor lymphocytes. The dosage can be increased to q48h or decreased to q96h, depending on the patient's response. As mentioned previously, continued monitoring is necessary. Initially, a complete blood count is performed 10 days after starting chlorambucil. Then a complete blood count and serum chemistry profile are performed at 30 days. Thereafter, the author prefers to perform a complete blood count every 30 days and a serum chemistry profile and urinalysis every 90 days.

Hepatic encephalopathy occurs occasionally in cats with CNF. Lactulose enemas can be helpful in the treatment of acute hepatic encephalopathy. Lactulose also can be administered at a dosage of 0.5 to 1 mL/kg PO q8h. Diets restricted in protein, such as prescription diets or recipes designed for chronic kidney disease, often are useful. Management of hepatic encephalopathy also may include continued use of antibiotics to suppress anaerobic and aerobic intestinal microflora that generate ammonia and other toxic waste products. Because the enteric organisms of concern generally are not true pathogens, use of a relatively broad-spectrum antibiotic is recommended. The author prefers to use amoxicillin with clavulanic acid, amoxicillin, or fluoroquinolone antibiotics. Other authors recommend metronidazole or neomycin. It is controversial whether antibiotics can reduce enteric bacterial microflora long term. Treatment with ursodeoxycholic acid also is advised, following the same guidelines as discussed for ANF. If biopsies are performed, vitamin K_1 is administered SQ q24h on the day before and the day of the scheduled procedure.[30]

The clinical usefulness of nutritional supplements has not been proven but is thought helpful in providing an optimal environment for hepatocellular survival in situations of inflammation-related oxidative stress. Several nutritional supplements have been recommended for patients with chronic hepatopathies such as CNF. These include oral superoxide dismutase (Oxstrin, Nutramax Labs), omega-3 fatty acid supplements from marine fish oils, vitamin E, s-adenosylmethionine (SAMe), or silybin (derivative of milk thistle) prepared with phosphatidylcholine (Marin, Nutramax Laboratories). All of these may have beneficial effects, but large-scale, controlled studies that show positive effects of any of these nutraceuticals currently are lacking. For many of these nutraceuticals, the use of veterinary-labeled products is recommended instead of over-the-counter products. It should be emphasized to the client that long-term treatment and monitoring are needed for cats with CNF, even after clinical signs have resolved. Use of a gastrostomy tube for several weeks can provide calories and hydration that help the cat recover some of its body condition and facilitate administration of medications (see Chapter 12).

LYMPHOCYTIC CHOLANGITIS/ CHOLANGIOHEPATITIS

Lymphocytic cholangitis/cholangiohepatitis (LCC) is associated with an inflammatory infiltrate of the biliary system composed predominantly of small mature lymphocytes in the portal regions. Portal fibrosis and biliary hyperplasia are markers of its chronicity. LCC is thought to be a progressive disease and may or may not relate to the progression from CNF (Figure 19-3). The accumulation of lymphocytes usually is moderate to severe and often crosses into the adjacent hepatic parenchyma. The severity of lymphocytic infiltration suggests an immunological component, either primary or secondary. Fibrosis often is a more prominent finding in LCC. As the lobule loses hepatocytes and fibrosis progresses, the damage

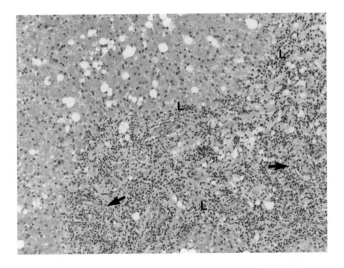

Figure 19-3 Lymphocytic cholangitis. Lymphocytic cholangitis is characterized by a diffuse infiltrate of small lymphocytes *(L)* surrounding the bile ducts and the presence of modest biliary hyperplasia *(arrows)*. (H&E stain.) (Courtesy Dr. John M. Cullen, North Carolina State University, Raleigh, NC.)

becomes more evident, as do changes of the bile ducts, evidenced by a tortuous hyperplastic appearance. This condition likely is slowly progressive. However, the author has seen patients in whom initial clinical signs were more consistent with an ascending biliary infection that has led to an acute presentation, and subsequent biopsy established the lymphocytic nature of the disease. As described previously, the pathogenesis of LCC is not defined; however, it is suspected to be associated with an autoimmune process, with a possible influence from antigens of bacterial origin.

SIGNALMENT

Lymphocytic cholangitis/cholangiohepatitis generally is seen in younger to mature cats, often less than 4 years of age. No gender predisposition has been noted. Persian cats are reported to be overrepresented.[29] This form of FILD may have a pathogenesis involving more of an autoimmune process.

CLINICAL FINDINGS

Most cats with LCC are presented for vague clinical signs (e.g., being a poor doer). They may have an intermittent history of vomiting and loss of appetite, a need to continually try novel diets, and a poor body condition score with gradual, long-term weight loss. Liver enzyme activities tend to be variable, with ALT activity being less severely increased in most cases. Serum ALP and GGT activities and serum bilirubin and bile acid concentrations often are increased. It is common to find a progressively increasing serum gamma globulin concentration on the serum chemistry profile. Fever and leukocytosis are not seen commonly. Ascites also is uncommon; if present, however, it is a poor prognostic indicator because it is evidence of portal hypertension. Abdominal fluid analysis should be pursued to increase the confidence in the diagnosis. Similarly, presence of hepatic encephalopathy should be considered as a significantly negative prognostic indicator.

DIAGNOSIS

The diagnosis of LCC depends to a great extent on a hepatic biopsy. Tests similar to those described for CNF and ANF are applicable for the diagnosis of this condition. Fine-needle aspiration of the liver may show increased numbers of small lymphocytes, but cytological examination is insufficient for a diagnosis of LCC.

IMAGING

Radiographic imaging of the liver often is normal in patients with LCC. However, there can be radiographic findings similar to those for other forms of FILD depending on concurrent disease and chronicity. Ultrasonographic findings generally are more prominent in this form of FILD, but they are far from pathognomonic. The portobiliary tracts often are prominent and hyperechoic. Some authors have described marked dilations and areas of stenosis of intrahepatic and/or extrahepatic bile ducts.[29]

OTHER DIAGNOSTIC TECHNIQUES

The options for additional diagnostic testing are few. Measurement of serum bile acid concentrations is indicated. If biopsies are collected, it is recommended to have immunohistochemical staining performed to help exclude lymphoma as a diagnosis. This has been shown for other tissues from cats with other inflammatory disorders.[31,32]

DIFFERENTIAL DIAGNOSES

The list of differential diagnoses is similar to that of other forms of FILD. With LCC, however, greater care needs to be taken, even with routine histopathological examination, to avoid incorrect differentiation of this disease from small cell lymphoma. The small intestine, stomach, pancreas, and regional lymph nodes should be biopsied during exploratory surgery, if possible, to identify concurrent diseases (see Chapter 17).

TREATMENT

The treatment for LCC is similar to that described for the chronic neutrophilic (with lymphocytic-plasmacytic components) form of FILD. However, corticosteroids alone often are inadequate for significant improvement and to stop the progression of this disease. Some form of combination immunosuppressive therapy—such as chlorambucil along with prednisolone, together with ursodeoxycholic acid—almost always is warranted. Cyclosporine may provide an alternative to chlorambucil, but clinical experience with this drug for the treatment of LCC is limited. Depending on the tolerance of the cat, the addition of nutraceuticals is recommended. However, there is little evidence at this point to support the clinical benefit of these medications in cats with LCC. It is common for the author to begin treatment with chlorambucil (0.25 mg/kg PO q48h), prednisolone (2 mg/kg PO q24h), and ursodeoxycholic acid (10 mg/kg PO q24h). Supplements then are added slowly over the course of several weeks to seek tolerance for both the total number of medications being administered and for each individual medication or supplement. Support of the pet's nutritional needs often is met with diets designed for cats with chronic kidney disease, which are moderately protein restricted but calorie dense. Placement of a gastrostomy tube to meet the caloric needs, maintain hydration, and administer medications may be helpful for many owners as well as for the patient during the first few weeks of therapy (see Chapter 12). Treatment is likely to be lifelong. The prognosis is variable; however, the cat may live for years if it tolerates treatments and the owner is faithful in monitoring the cat's status. Monitoring of the long-term use of chlorambucil is similar to the protocol described previously.

LYMPHOCYTIC PORTAL HEPATITIS

Lymphocytic portal hepatitis (LPH) is characterized by an infiltration of the portal triads with lymphocytes, a small number of neutrophils, and plasma cells. The bile ducts are affected much less in this form of FILD. The inflammatory component appears to be milder compared to that in the forms of FILD discussed previously. Lymphocytic portal hepatitis may represent a phenomenon related to aging or a reactive change rather than a true disease. There may be some mild fibrosis around biliary structures, but pseudolobule formation is not evident.

SIGNALMENT

LPH is common in older cats (generally 10 years of age or older). The pathogenesis of the disease is unknown.

CLINICAL FINDINGS

Most cats do not show overt clinical signs associated with LPH. There may be minimal to moderate increases in serum liver enzyme activities, but no specific pattern has been reported. Complete blood counts generally are unremarkable.

DIAGNOSIS

In the author's experience, LPH is found most commonly when a liver biopsy is requested during exploratory surgery for the collection of intestinal biopsies in patients with gastrointestinal signs or a suspicion of chronic pancreatitis.

IMAGING

Results of radiographic and ultrasonographic imaging generally are unremarkable or not specific for LPH. Because most cases occur in older cats, it is not uncommon to see subtle, nonspecific ultrasonographic changes in the liver that do not follow any particular pattern.

OTHER DIAGNOSTIC TECHNIQUES

Fine-needle aspiration and cytological examination generally are not rewarding.

DIFFERENTIAL DIAGNOSES

The list of differential diagnoses is similar to that of other forms of chronic FILD, presuming that increases of liver enzyme activities are observed.

TREATMENT

Unless there is concurrent evidence for a symptomatic hepatopathy, most cases are treated conservatively with ursodeoxycholic acid and/or nutritional supplements. The prognosis tends to be good with clinical signs of liver disease generally being minimal.

CHOLANGITIS ASSOCIATED WITH LIVER FLUKES

This form of FILD is due to an infestation of the biliary system by trematodes.[8-10] Several species of liver flukes are reported to infect cats. The fluke reported most commonly is *P. concinnum*. This fluke species, found in tropical and subtropical environments, is reported most commonly in the coastal regions of Florida, the Bahamas, the Caribbean islands, the states along the Gulf of Mexico, and Hawaii. Because many cats move with their owners around the country, the pet's history always should include geographical information. In the life cycle of the fluke, a land snail is the first intermediate host, followed by various lizards, toads, and geckos, which serve as second intermediate hosts.

SIGNALMENT

Young adult cats who hunt and eat second intermediate hosts are susceptible to infection with the flukes. The duration of fluke survival in cats when present in low numbers is unknown.

CLINICAL FINDINGS

Cats infected with large numbers of flukes may have signs of anorexia and lethargy. The flukes migrate to the bile ducts and, in some cases, to the pancreatic ducts. A modest eosinophilia often develops, peaking 4 to 5 months after infection. During the early stages of platynosomiasis, a transient but substantial increase in serum ALT activity is noted, as well as a significantly rising serum bilirubin concentration. When presented for veterinary care, the cats often show abdominal pain, similar to other forms of cholangitis with biliary obstruction. Cats may be presented for a chronic illness or may show an acute presentation. Clinical signs often are severe, with varying degrees of cholestasis, and also can include acute manifestations of secondary bacterial cholangiohepatitis. Vomiting, icterus, anorexia, fever, and abdominal tenderness are common signs in clinical cases.

DIAGNOSIS AND OTHER DIAGNOSTIC TECHNIQUES

Adult flukes and operculated eggs may be seen on histopathological examination of sections of liver biopsies. The flukes cause a marked inflammatory response, thickening and distension of the bile ducts, and subsequent biliary obstruction. Gross necropsy and histopathological findings include distension of the gall bladder and the bile ducts by very thick, viscous bile. Biliary hyperplasia and fibrosis of the ductal areas are common responses to chronic inflammation. Aspiration of bile and microscopic examination for operculated eggs can confirm the diagnosis. Fecal sedimentation examination also can be diagnostic. However, fecal flotation techniques usually are not helpful.

IMAGING

Ultrasonographic changes similar to those seen in cats with ANF, CNF, or LCC can be seen, along with evidence of biliary stasis or obstruction of extrahepatic or intrahepatic bile ducts.

DIFFERENTIAL DIAGNOSES

The clinical presentation of cats with cholangitis associated with liver flukes is similar to that of any of the above forms of FILD, and the differential diagnosis can be based on mechanisms that play a role in the pathogenesis of other forms of FILD (e.g., obstruction and cholestasis, secondary bacterial infection, inflammatory response, apparent fibrotic changes, and variable increases of serum clinical chemistry values).

TREATMENT

Treatment of liver flukes with praziquantel (30 mg/kg PO q24h for 5 to 10 days) is variably successful in cats. Surgical expression of the gall bladder and cannulation of the common bile duct may be helpful. The prognosis can be good, but surgery often is required even in cats with moderately severe disease.

SUMMARY

Feline inflammatory liver disease is a fairly common condition. The pathogenesis of FILD is complicated and not understood completely. The terminology for different forms of FILD continues to undergo revision. The interaction between pathologists, clinical pathologists, and clinicians is guiding the evolution of hypotheses for the pathogenetic mechanisms of these conditions. There are speculations that the different forms of FILD may be related and may even be a progression of one another to some extent. Similarities in treatment, overlapping laboratory values, and shared clinical signs add to the difficulty in separating these forms of FILD. Liver biopsies can clarify the diagnosis and help the clinician select the best treatment protocol.

REFERENCES

1. Gagne JM, Weiss DJ, Armstrong PJ: Histopathologic evaluation of feline inflammatory liver disease, *Vet Pathol* 33:521, 1996.
2. Day DG: Feline cholangiohepatitis complex, *Vet Clin North Am Small Anim Pract* 25:375, 1995.
3. Edwards M: Feline cholangiohepatitis, *Compend Contin Educ Pract Vet* 26:855, 2004.
4. Weiss DJ, Armstrong PJ, Gagne J: Inflammatory liver disease, *Semin Vet Med Surg (Small Anim)* 12:22, 1997.
5. Gagne JM, Armstrong PJ, Weiss DJ, et al: Clinical features of inflammatory liver disease in cats: 41 cases (1983-1993), *J Am Vet Med Assoc* 214:513, 1999.
6. van den Ingh TSGAM, Cullen JM, Twedt DC, et al: Morphological classification of biliary disorders of the canine and feline liver. In Rothuizen J, Bunch SE, Charles JA, et al, editors: *WSAVA standards for clinical and histopathological diagnosis of canine and feline liver diseases*, Edinburgh, 2006, Saunders/Elsevier, p 61.
7. Beilsa LM, Greiner EC: Liver flukes *(Platynosomum concinnum)* in cats, *J Am Anim Hosp Assoc* 21:269, 1985.
8. Hitt ME: Liver fluke infection in South Florida cats, *Feline Pract* 11:26, 1981.
9. Haney DR, Christriansen JS, Toll J: Severe cholestatic liver disease secondary to liver fluke (Platynosomum concinnum) infection in three cats, *J Am Anim Hosp Assoc* 42:234, 2006.
10. Allam R, Anders HJ: The role of innate immunity in autoimmune tissue injury, *Curr Opin Rheumatol* 20:538, 2008.
11. Gao B, Jeong W, Tian Z: Liver: An organ with predominant innate immunity, *Hepatology* 47:729, 2007.
12. Atkinson TJ: Toll-like receptors, transduction-effector pathways, and disease diversity: evidence of an immunobiological paradigm explaining all human illness? *Int Rev Immunol* 27:255, 2008.
13. Barrat FJ, Coffman RL: Development of TLR inhibitors for the treatment of autoimmune diseases, *Immunol Rev* 223:271, 2008.
14. Vergani D, Mieli-Vergani G: Aetiopathogenesis of autoimmune hepatitis, *World J Gastroenterol* 14:3306, 2008.
15. Shimizu Y: Liver in systemic disease, *World J Gastroenterol* 14:4111, 2008.
16. Wagner KA, Hartmann FA, Trepanier LA: Bacterial culture results from liver, gall bladder, or bile in 248 dogs and cats evaluated for hepatobiliary disease: 1998-2003, *J Vet Intern Med* 21:417, 2007.
17. Brain PH, Barrs VR, Martin P, et al: Feline cholecystitis and acute neutrophilic cholangitis: clinical findings, bacterial isolates and response to treatment in six cases, *J Feline Med Surg* 8:91, 2006.
18. Savary-Bataille K, Bunch SE, Spaulding KA, et al: Percutaneous ultrasound guided cholecystocentesis in healthy cats, *J Vet Intern Med* 17:298, 2004.
19. Silveira MG, Lindor KD: Primary sclerosing cholangitis, *Can J Gastroenterol* 22:689, 2008.
20. Hov JR, Boberg KM, Karlsen TH: Autoantibodies in primary sclerosing cholangitis, *World J Gastroenterol* 14:3781, 2008.
21. Day MJ: Immunohistochemical characterization of the lesions of feline progressive lymphocytic cholangitis/cholangiohepatitis, *J Comp Pathol* 119:135, 1998.
22. Greiter-Wilke A, Scanziani E, Soldati S, et al: Association of *Helicobacter* with cholangiohepatitis in cats, *J Vet Intern Med* 20:822, 2008.
23. Breitschwerdt EB: Feline Bartonellosis and cat scratch disease, *Vet Immunol Immunopathol* 123:167, 2008.
24. Kordick DL, Brown TT, Shin K, et al: Clinical and pathologic evaluation of chronic *Bartonella henselae* or *Bartonella clarridgeiae* infection in cats, *J Clin Microbiol* 37:1536, 1999.
25. Boomkens SY, Kusters JG, Hoffmann G, et al: Detection of Helicobacter pylori in bile of cats, *FEMS Immunol Med Microbiol* 42:307, 2004.
26. Herman BA, Brawer RS, Murtaugh RJ, et al: Therapeutic percutaneous ultrasound-guided cholecystocentesis in three dogs with extrahepatic biliary obstruction and pancreatitis, *J Am Vet Med Assoc* 227:1782, 2005.
27. Vörös K, Sterczer A, Manczur F, et al: Percutaneous ultrasound-guided cholecystocentesis in dogs, *Acta Vet Hung* 50:385, 2002.
28. Rivers BJ, Walter PA, Johnston GR, et al: Acalculous cholecystitis in four canine cases: ultrasonographic findings and use of ultrasonographic-guided, percutaneous cholecystocentesis in diagnosis, *J Am Anim Hosp Assoc* 33:207, 1997.
29. Twedt DC, Armstrong PJ: Feline inflammatory liver disease. In Bonagura JD, Twedt DC, editors: *Current veterinary therapy, vol 14*, St. Louis, 2009, Saunders/Elsevier, p 576.
30. Center SA, Warner K, Corbett J, et al: Proteins invoked by vitamin K absence and clotting times in clinically ill cats, *J Vet Intern Med* 14:292, 2000.
31. Waly NE, Gruffydd-Jones TJ, Stokeslow CR, et al: Immunohistochemical diagnosis of alimentary lymphomas and severe intestinal inflammation in cats, *J Comp Pathol* 133:253, 2005.
32. Weiss DJ: Differentiating benign and malignant causes of lymphocytosis in feline bone marrow, *J Vet Intern Med* 19:855, 2005.

CHAPTER

20 Exocrine Pancreatic Insufficiency

Jörg M. Steiner

Exocrine pancreatic insufficiency (EPI) is a condition caused by insufficient synthesis and secretion of pancreatic digestive enzymes from the exocrine portion of the pancreas. As such, EPI is a functional diagnosis, rather than an etiological or morphological diagnosis. This means that the condition has two components: (1) a decreased synthesis and secretion of pancreatic enzymes from that which is normal, and (2) an amount of digestive enzymes insufficient for normal digestion of the dietary components. For example, there are reports of German Shepherd Dogs who have a severely decreased serum trypsin-like immunoreactivity concentration and no identifiable pancreatic tissue during exploratory laparotomy, but with no clinical signs of EPI.[1] This is not surprising if one considers the physiology of digestion, which is a system characterized by great redundancy and exceptional functional reserve. For example, in cats dietary fat is digested by gastric and pancreatic lipase. The physiological importance of gastric lipase for fat digestion in cats is unknown, but it has been reported to be approximately 30 per cent in human beings and dogs.[2] Of course, 30 per cent is an average, and there may be a wide range between individuals. In addition, digestibility of fat does not have to reach 100 per cent to avoid clinical signs of loose stools. Therefore pancreatic lipase may play a less crucial role in some patients, and some cats may need little to no exocrine pancreatic function to maintain normal stool quality. However, in general, some exocrine pancreatic function will be required to ensure physiological digestion.

EPIDEMIOLOGY

Disorders of the exocrine pancreas, and especially EPI, traditionally have been thought to occur less frequently in cats than in dogs or human beings. However, several studies of postmortem examinations have shown that significant pathological lesions are quite common in feline pancreata, and EPI is now recognized quite frequently in cats.[3,4] Also, since the introduction of an assay (feline trypsin-like immunoreactivity [fTLI]) in 1995 for the diagnosis of feline EPI, the disease is now diagnosed much more frequently than before. For example, over a 10-year period (from the early 1980s to the early 1990s), of 180,648 cats entered into the Veterinary Medical Data Base (VMDB), located at that time at Purdue University, only 1027 cats (0.57 per cent) were recorded as diagnosed with disorders of the exocrine pancreas, and only 11 of those cats (0.006 per cent) were reported as being diagnosed with exocrine pancreatic insufficiency. In sharp contrast, over the last 5 years (2004 to 2008), the Gastrointestinal Laboratory at Texas A&M University assayed 84,523 serum samples for fTLI concentration and a total of 1342 samples had serum fTLI concentrations at or below 8.0 μg/L, which is diagnostic for feline EPI. Although these populations of cats are not the same, it is clear that the advent of this diagnostic test has led to a much more frequent diagnosis of EPI in cats.

Traditionally, EPI has been thought of as a condition of older cats. However, the age distribution of 882 cats with a serum fTLI concentration at or below 8.0 μg/L assayed over the last 5 years showed an even distribution of ages (Figure 20-1). Seven kittens were 6 months of age or younger, and 40 cats were 1 year of age or younger. Cats who were older than 12 years of age were represented less frequently, most likely due to a decreasing number of cats who are older than 12 years of age in the general feline population. A breed predilection has not been reported for feline EPI. The author recently has evaluated breed characteristics for a group of 610 cats with a serum fTLI concentration at or below 8.0 μg/L, for whom breed information was available (Figure 20-2). Although the data were not compared to the general cat population, there was no apparent overrepresentation of any particular breed.

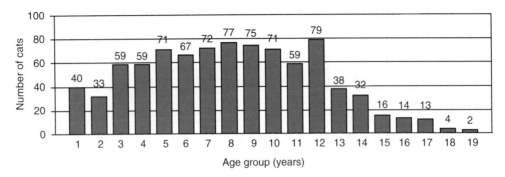

Figure 20-1 Age distribution of 881 cats diagnosed with EPI based on a serum fTLI concentration ≤8.0 μg/L. Each group represents cats belonging to an age group of 1 year each (e.g., age group 1: cats up to 1 year of age; age group 2: cats older than 1 year of age and up to 2 years of age). Seven kittens were up to 6 months of age, and 33 cats were more than 6 months of age and up to 1 year of age.

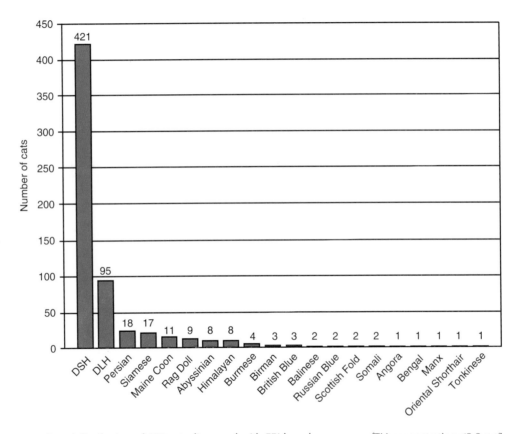

Figure 20-2 Breed distribution of 610 cats diagnosed with EPI based on a serum fTLI concentration ≤8.0 μg/L.

ETIOLOGY AND PATHOGENESIS

In theory, there are many potential causes of EPI, including pancreatic aplasia, pancreatic hypoplasia, pancreatic acinar atrophy (PAA), pressure atrophy due to pancreatic duct obstruction, and pancreatic destruction due to pancreatic inflammation. However, most of these theoretical causes of EPI have never been described in cats, and chronic pancreatitis is believed to be the most common cause of EPI in this species. Three cases of pancreatic acinar atrophy in cats have been mentioned in the literature, but none of these cases have been reported in detail.[5]

A few cases of EPI without preceding pancreatitis have been reported due to *Eurytrema procyonis* infestation.[6] These pancreatic flukes attach themselves to the wall of the pancreatic ducts and may cause mucosal proliferation, periductal fibrosis, and duct obstruction, without parenchymal inflammatory infiltration.[6] Adenocarcinomas of the exocrine pancreas or other neoplastic lesions in the area of the pancreatic duct or the duodenal papilla also can lead to obstruction of the pancreatic duct, followed by atrophy of acinar tissue; however, this also has never been reported in cats. Another rare cause of pancreatic duct obstruction may occur due to proximal duodenal resection, which occurs when the major duodenal papilla is damaged during surgery.[5] Finally, congenital pancreatic hypoplasia or aplasia has never been reported in cats.

The clinical syndrome of EPI does not require deficiency of all pancreatic digestive enzymes. For example, isolated pancreatic lipase deficiency has been reported as a rare cause of EPI in human beings and also has been reported recently in one dog.[7,8] However, isolated enzyme deficiency has not been reported previously in cats.

In human beings it has been shown that about 90 per cent of the functional reserve of the exocrine pancreas must be lost before clinical signs of EPI develop.[9] Digestive enzymes of pancreatic acinar origin play an integral role in assimilation of all major food components. A lack of pancreatic digestive enzymes will lead to maldigestion. However, there also are disturbances in the transport mechanisms for monosaccharides and disaccharides, amino acids, and fatty acids, leading to malabsorption. The exact reason for this malabsorption is not known, but it has been speculated that the exocrine pancreas secretes trophic factors that act on the intestinal mucosa and that the secretion of these trophic factors is decreased in patients with EPI. The large amount of nutrients remaining in the intestinal lumen usually leads to loose, voluminous stools and steatorrhea. At the same time, the lack of nutrient assimilation will cause weight loss and may lead to vitamin deficiencies in some patients. Serum cobalamin (vitamin B_{12}) concentrations are decreased in most cats with EPI.[10] Serum folate concentrations in cats with EPI are either decreased, indicating concurrent small intestinal disease, or within the normal range, which is in contrast to canine and human patients with EPI, who often show increased serum folate concentrations. A cat with EPI with secondary vitamin K–responsive coagulopathy has been reported.[11]

In cases of EPI caused by chronic pancreatitis, destruction of pancreatic tissue may not be limited to the acinar cells, and concurrent diabetes mellitus may be observed.[12,13] In fact, chronic pancreatitis has been recognized as an important cause of diabetes mellitus in human beings and dogs.[13,14] Diabetes mellitus also has been reported in cats with EPI.[12] Therefore cats with diabetes mellitus who have chronic loose stools should be evaluated for concurrent exocrine pancreatic disease. Also, because feline EPI in most cats is due to chronic pancreatitis, residual pancreatic inflammation may be present, and some cats may present with clinical signs that are compatible with both chronic pancreatitis and EPI.

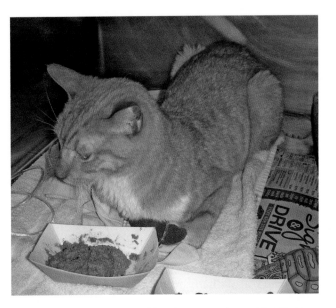

Figure 20-3 Theo, a 4-year-old male neutered cat with EPI. Note the thin appearance of the cat. (Courtesy Dr. Kenneth Jones, Jones Animal Hospital, Santa Monica, CA.)

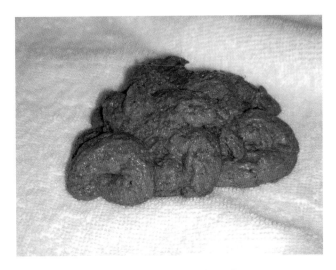

Figure 20-4 A large stool sample from Theo, the cat in Figure 20-3, with untreated EPI. Note the typical loose consistency and the light brown color. Also, the stool sample appears to contain a lot of undigested food particles. (Courtesy Dr. Kenneth Jones, Jones Animal Hospital, Santa Monica, CA.)

CLINICAL PICTURE AND DIAGNOSIS

Clinical signs reported most commonly in cats with EPI are weight loss, polyphagia, and loose stools (Figure 20-3).[12,15] Naturally, these clinical signs are nonspecific and also are seen in many cats with other disorders that are more common than EPI. Common causes of polyphagia in cats are hyperthyroidism, corticosteroid treatment, or diabetes mellitus. Common differential diagnoses for cats with weight loss are hyperthyroidism, dental and periodontal disease, chronic kidney disease (CKD), heart failure, neoplasia, and chronic intestinal disorders, such as inflammatory bowel disease. Finally, the most common disorders causing diarrhea are primary chronic intestinal disease or a variety of secondary disorders, such as hyperthyroidism, CKD, and liver failure.

The diarrhea is characterized by loose or semiformed voluminous stools, which may have a yellow to clay-colored appearance and may be quite malodorous (Figure 20-4). Some cats with EPI may develop watery diarrhea, but this is not common. The high fat content of the feces can lead to a greasy appearance of the haircoat, especially in the perianal and tail region. However, in a recent report of 20 cats with EPI, only one cat showed greasy soiling of the haircoat in the perineal region.[16]

Recently, severe D-lactic acidosis in a cat with clinical signs of episodic generalized weakness, ataxia, and lethargy was shown to be secondary to EPI.[17] The authors speculated that the D-lactic acidosis was due to massively increased bacterial fermentation in the intestinal lumen due to small intestinal bacterial overgrowth secondary to EPI.[17] The D-lactic acidosis and associated clinical signs resolved in this cat after enzyme supplementation.[17] (See Chapter 58 for a discussion on D-lactic acidosis and neurological signs.)

As mentioned previously, some cats with EPI have concurrent diabetes mellitus and may be presented with polydipsia and polyuria or even with acute complications of diabetic ketoacidosis. Also, patients may show residual signs of chronic pancreatitis, such as anorexia or abdominal discomfort. Similarly, many cats with chronic pancreatitis have concurrent inflammatory conditions of other abdominal organs, such as the intestines or the biliary system, and may show clinical signs associated with those inflammatory conditions (see Chapter 19).

Results of routine blood tests are within the normal range in most patients. Lymphopenia, lymphocytosis, neutrophilia, eosinophilia, and elevations of hepatic enzymes have been reported in a few affected cats.[5] It is unclear from the literature whether these laboratory abnormalities are rare changes associated with EPI or, more likely, are associated with concurrent conditions, such as diabetes mellitus, inflammatory bowel disease, or chronic cholangitis.

Abdominal radiographs or ultrasound also do not show any specific changes in most cats with EPI. In one report, two cats with EPI showed an inhomogeneous pancreatic parenchyma and pancreatic nodules, but this has not been reported elsewhere.[18] More common are radiographic and/or ultrasonographic changes due to concurrent conditions.

As mentioned above, EPI is a functional disease and thus requires a functional diagnosis. Several tests have been recommended to estimate exocrine pancreatic function in cats. The bentiromide absorption test (commonly known as PABA test), plasma turbidity, microscopic examination of feces for undigested fat, starch, or muscle fibers, and fecal proteolytic activity (FPA) all have been recommended for use in cats.[5,15,19-21] With the exception of FPA, all of these tests are unreliable and/or impractical in cats and are not recommended. Fecal proteolytic activity can be determined by a variety of methods. The simplest method uses a piece of unexposed radiographic film. A small stool sample is placed on the film, and one would expect a clear halo to develop around the fecal sample in healthy cats. Unfortunately, this method is unreliable and should not be performed. The azocasein or azoalbumin methods are more reliable. However, FPA is very labile, and false-positive results can occur due to inappropriate sample handling. At least three stool samples from consecutive days should be evaluated. Also, feces need to be frozen immediately and shipped on ice in order to prevent loss of FPA in the samples.[21] However, better diagnostic tests for feline EPI are now available,

and FPA should only be used for species for which more current tests are not available.

Immunoassays for the measurement of fTLI concentration have been developed and validated analytically.[10,22] Currently, there are only two assays for the measurement of serum fTLI available worldwide. The Gastrointestinal Laboratory at Texas A&M University offers a radioimmunoassay that uses purified feline cationic trypsin and a polyclonal rabbit antifeline cationic trypsin antiserum. This assay has been fully validated analytically.[23] The current reference range for serum fTLI measured at the Gastrointestinal Laboratory is 12 to 82 µg/L, with values of 8 µg/L or lower being diagnostic for EPI. There also is an enzyme-linked immunosorbent assay (ELISA) for the measurement of fTLI available exclusively in Europe. To the author's knowledge, the validation of this assay has not been described in the literature.

The assay for fTLI quantifies the amount of trypsin and related compounds in the serum. This is important because in healthy cats significant amounts of trypsin do not circulate in the blood stream. Instead, trypsinogen, the inactive zymogen of trypsin, circulates in the blood stream. Trypsinogen is synthesized by the pancreatic acinar cells and is stored in zymogen granules in the acinar cells. When the pancreas is stimulated to secrete digestive enzymes, zymogen granules are released into the pancreatic duct system by way of exocytosis. However, a small amount of zymogen granules are being released constantly into the vascular bed. The trypsinogen released can be measured in the serum with the fTLI assay. Theoretically, the assay also can detect some trypsin molecules that have been scavenged by proteinase inhibitors, such as α_1-proteinase inhibitor; however, this has not been studied specifically in cats and probably is of no clinical relevance for the diagnosis of feline EPI.

The fTLI assay has been used successfully to diagnose feline EPI for more than 10 years.[10,24] In one report clinical data from the first 20 cats with serum fTLI concentrations at or below 8 µg/L were evaluated; 17 of these 20 cats showed compelling evidence of EPI and the remaining three cats had supportive evidence of EPI.[16] All 20 cats in that study showed clinical signs compatible with EPI, and 17 cats showed a positive response to treatment. Two of the three cats who did not respond to therapy ultimately died, and a pancreatic biopsy strongly supported a diagnosis of EPI in both cases. The third cat who did not respond to therapy was vomiting and had decreased serum cobalamin and folate concentrations. Concurrent small intestinal disease or severe hypocobalaminemia may have impaired the therapeutic response to enzyme supplementation in this cat. On exploratory laparotomy, a small pancreas was noted by the surgeon, suggesting a diagnosis of EPI. However, a pancreatic biopsy was not collected. Two cats were 6 months old at the time of diagnosis. One cat showed poor growth and hair loss and responded to enzyme replacement therapy with weight gain and hair growth. The second cat was very thin and had a greasy haircoat. It also responded to enzyme replacement with weight gain. However, the cat was found dead 3 weeks after diagnosis and start of therapy, and a necropsy examination was not performed. Both cats responded with weight gain, but both still were immature at the time of diagnosis. Remission of some undiagnosed gastrointestinal disorder other than EPI may have led to growth and weight gain. It was strongly suspected that these three latter cats also had EPI, but evidence was not considered conclusive. Even if none of these three cats would have had EPI with false-positive test results, the specificity of serum fTLI concentration for EPI would still be 85 per cent. Therefore it was concluded that serum fTLI concentration is a specific test for EPI in cats.

Recently, it was shown that decreased renal function has a significant impact on serum fTLI concentrations and cats with renal failure may have falsely increased serum fTLI concentrations.[25] Therefore evaluation of serum fTLI concentrations in azotemic cats may obscure a diagnosis of feline EPI. However, no patient has been identified to date in whom a diagnosis of EPI was missed because of renal failure. The author would suggest reevaluating serum fTLI concentrations in azotemic cats who have a borderline fTLI concentration and in whom an alternative diagnosis for loose stools and weight loss can not be identified. In contrast to dogs, serum fTLI did not increase significantly after feeding of healthy cats.[26] However, this was not studied in cats with suspected EPI. Therefore the current recommendation is to withhold food whenever possible from cats for 12 hours before collecting a sample for measurement of serum fTLI concentration.

Most cats with EPI have severe serum hypocobalaminemia. In one study of 11 cats with EPI, serum cobalamin concentration was undetectable in 10 cats and subnormal in the remaining cat.[10] Because hypocobalaminemia can lead to various gastrointestinal and systemic effects and also can result in treatment failure in cats with EPI, the author recommends that serum cobalamin and folate concentrations should be measured in every cat suspected of having EPI.

MANAGEMENT

Most cats with EPI can be managed successfully by dietary supplementation with pancreatic enzymes. Dried extracts of bovine or porcine pancreas are available (e.g., Viokase or Pancrezyme); however, raw beef, pork, or game pancreas also can be given instead. If commercial products are used, powder is more effective than tablets or capsules, and enteric products should be avoided. Initially, one teaspoon per meal should be given. Because cats often do not like the taste of the pancreatic powder, it is best to mix the powder thoroughly with some canned food. If the cat refuses to consume the food with the powder, the enzymes can be mixed with fish oil and then stirred into the food. If raw pancreas is used, it should be chopped, portioned, and frozen in packages for single meals. Fresh-frozen pancreas can be kept frozen for several months without losing efficacy. Thirty to 60 grams of raw, chopped pancreas should be given per meal. Preincubation of the food with pancreatic enzymes or supplementation with bile salts is not necessary. Most cats respond quite rapidly to enzyme replacement therapy and show resolution of loose stools within 3 to 4 days.[24] When clinical signs have resolved, the amount of pancreatic enzymes given with each meal can be decreased gradually to the lowest effective dose, which may vary from patient to patient and also may vary between different batches of the pancreatic supplement.

Response to enzyme supplementation alone may not be satisfactory in many patients. This is not surprising if one considers that most cats with EPI have concurrent hypocobalaminemia. Cobalamin in cats can only be absorbed by specific carriers in the ileum if complexed with intrinsic factor. In contrast to its secretion in human beings, intrinsic factor is secreted almost exclusively by the exocrine pancreas in cats.[27] Also, cobalamin binds to R-protein in the stomach, which needs to be removed by pancreatic proteinases before cobalamin can bind to intrinsic factor. Finally, at least in dogs, EPI leads to a shift in the intestinal microbiota, which can lead to increased cobalamin utilization and cobalamin deficiency. The lack of intrinsic factor is believed to be the most crucial of these factors, and in one study of cats with EPI, serum cobalamin concentration was decreased in all 11 cats studied.[10] Hypocobalaminemia can lead to gastrointestinal lesions such as villous atrophy, intestinal inflammation, cobalamin malabsorption, and malabsorption of other nutrients.[28] It also can lead to systemic effects such as central and peripheral neuropathies and immunodeficiencies.[28] It is crucial therefore to measure serum cobalamin concentration in all cats suspected of having EPI and correct hypocobalaminemia in all cats with a decreased serum cobalamin concentration. Because cobalamin deficiency causes cobalamin malabsorption, oral supplementation is not effective in hypocobalaminemic cats. Also, multivitamin preparations do not contain sufficient amounts of cobalamin, and pure cobalamin is needed for therapy. In cats 150 to 250 µg is given subcutaneously based on body size. An injection is given once weekly for 6 weeks, followed by an injection every other week for 6 weeks, one more dose a month after that, and a recheck a month after the last dose. Some cats with EPI may require lifelong cobalamin supplementation.

The status of other vitamins has not been evaluated systematically in cats with EPI. In one study of dogs with EPI who had been treated with enzyme supplementation, total vitamin A, vitamin A components, and vitamin D concentrations were not different from healthy control dogs; however, serum vitamin E concentrations were lower than in healthy control dogs in two thirds of the dogs studied.[29] The decreased serum vitamin E concentration was not associated with any apparent negative impact on outcome in this study.[29] Because no data are available for cats and because no negative impact of decreased serum vitamin E concentrations has been shown for dogs with EPI, the author does not currently supplement cats with EPI with vitamin E or other fat-soluble vitamins. However, if the cat shows bleeding tendencies, a coagulation profile should be evaluated and, if indicated, the cat should be treated with vitamin K. To date only one cat with EPI and a vitamin K–responsive coagulopathy has been reported.[11]

Even patients who respond completely to enzyme therapy do not have a completely normalized fat absorption. This most likely is due to the fact that a portion of the pancreatic lipase of the supplement is being denatured irreversibly by the low pH in the stomach. This probably is the reason why some clinicians recommend feeding a low-fat diet to patients with EPI. However, decreasing the fat content of the diet also decreases the supply of fat-soluble vitamins and essential fatty acids, potentially leading to deficiencies of these essential nutrients. Therefore the author does not recommend decreasing the fat content in the diet routinely for cats with EPI. Several studies have evaluated the impact of diet on the treatment success in dogs with EPI, and none of these studies were able to show any impact of diet.[29-31] Because there are no studies available in cats, there are no specific dietary recommendations for cats with EPI. However, the author believes that it is prudent to avoid high-fiber diets because fiber may further hinder the digestion of fat.

Cats who fail to respond to therapy may benefit from treatment with an antacid. A proton pump inhibitor (e.g., omeprazole, 0.7 mg/kg PO q12h) would be expected to provide the most consistent gastric pH control.[32] This may decrease the degree of irreversible inhibition of exogenous pancreatic lipase in the stomach. However, it should be noted that antacid therapy has a negative effect on gastric lipase, so there may only be a minimal increase in fat absorption overall.

Some cats will not respond appropriately to enzyme supplementation and cobalamin administration. These cats may have concurrent small intestinal disease. This hypothesis is supported by the decreased serum folate concentrations observed in many cats with EPI. In one report of cats with EPI, six of 11 cats examined had decreased serum folate concentrations.[10] In addition, some cats with EPI may have secondary small intestinal bacterial overgrowth (SIBO), as has been noted in dogs with EPI.[33] Such patients may benefit from antibiotic therapy such as tylosin (25 mg/kg PO q12h) or metronidazole (15 to 25 mg/kg PO q12h). However, there is still a great deal of uncertainty about the normal intestinal microbiota and SIBO in cats.[34,35]

PROGNOSIS

Most cats with EPI have an irreversible loss of pancreatic acinar tissue and thus exocrine pancreatic function. Recovery is extremely rare and is poorly understood. However, with appropriate management and monitoring, these patients usually gain weight quickly (Figure 20-5), pass normal stools (Figure 20-6), and can go on to lead normal lives for a full lifespan.

SUMMARY

Exocrine pancreatic insufficiency is a syndrome caused by insufficient synthesis and secretion of pancreatic digestive enzymes by the exocrine portion of the pancreas resulting in insufficient delivery of these enzymes into the lumen of the small intestine. Clinical signs reported most commonly in cats are weight loss, loose and voluminous stools, steatorrhea, and in some cases

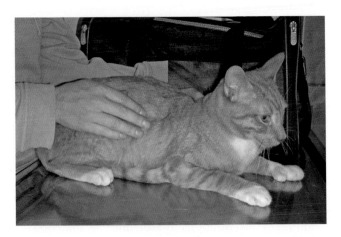

Figure 20-5 Theo, the cat in Figure 20-3, 2 months after starting pancreatic enzyme replacement therapy. He has gained almost 3 pounds during this time and is reported to be more active. (Courtesy Dr. Kenneth Jones, Jones Animal Hospital, Santa Monica, CA.)

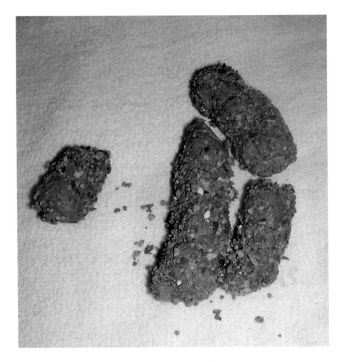

Figure 20-6 A stool sample from Theo, the cat in Figure 20-3, after treatment with pancreatic enzyme supplementation. The stool is now log shaped and has a normal dark brown color. (Courtesy Dr. Kenneth Jones, Jones Animal Hospital, Santa Monica, CA.)

greasy soiling of the haircoat. Serum fTLI concentration has been shown to be decreased in affected cats. Treatment of choice for cats with EPI consists of enzyme supplementation with either a powdered pancreatic extract or raw pancreas. Most cats with EPI also have severely decreased serum cobalamin concentrations and will require parenteral cobalamin supplementation.

REFERENCES

1. Wiberg ME, Westermarck E: Subclinical exocrine pancreatic insufficiency in dogs, *J Am Vet Med Assoc* 220:1183, 2002.
2. Carrière F, Laugier R, Barrowman JA, et al: Gastric and pancreatic lipase levels during a test meal in dogs, *Scand J Gastroenterol* 28:443, 1993.
3. Hänichen T, Minkus G: Retrospektive Studie zur Pathologie der Erkrankungen des exokrinen Pankreas bei Hund und Katze, *Tierärztliche Umschau* 45:363, 1990.
4. Spinaci M, Marcato P: Pancreatiti e altre patologie del pancreas esocrino nel gatto, *Obiettivi e Documenti Veterinari* 14:35, 1993.
5. Williams DA: Feline exocrine pancreatic insufficiency. In Kirk RW, Bonagura JD, editors: *Current veterinary therapy*, vol 12, Philadelphia, 1995, WB Saunders, p 732.
6. Fox JN, Mosley JG, Vogler GA, et al: Pancreatic function in domestic cats with pancreatic fluke infection, *J Am Vet Med Assoc* 178:58, 1981.
7. Xenoulis PG, Fradkin JM, Rapp SW, et al: Suspected isolated pancreatic lipase deficiency in a dog, *J Vet Intern Med* 21:1113, 2007.
8. Allenspach K, Suchodolski JS, McNeill FM, et al: Characterization of the bacterial microflora and innate immunity response in German Shepherd Dogs with antibiotic-responsive diarrhea, *J Vet Intern Med* 22:748 (abstract), 2008.
9. DiMagno EP, Go VLW, Summerskill WHJ: Relations between pancreatic enzyme outputs and malabsorption in severe pancreatic insufficiency, *N Engl J Med* 288:813, 1973.
10. Steiner JM, Williams DA: Validation of a radioimmunoassay for feline trypsin-like immunoreactivity (fTLI) and serum cobalamin and folate concentrations in cats with exocrine pancreatic insufficiency, *J Vet Intern Med* 9:193 (abstract), 1995.
11. Perry LA, Williams DA, Pidgeon G, et al: Exocrine pancreatic insufficiency with associated coagulopathy in a cat, *J Am Anim Hosp Assoc* 27:109, 1991.
12. Holzworth J, Coffin DL: Pancreatic insufficiency and diabetes mellitus in a cat, *Cornell Vet* 43:502, 1953.
13. Larsen S: Diabetes mellitus secondary to chronic pancreatitis, *Dan Med Bull* 40:153, 1993.
14. Fleeman LM, Rand JS, Steiner JM, et al: Chronic, subclinical, exocrine pancreatic disease is common in diabetic dogs, *J Vet Intern Med* 18:402 (abstract), 2004.
15. Dill-Macky E: Pancreatic diseases of cats, *Compend Contin Educ Pract Vet* 15:589, 1993.
16. Steiner JM, Williams DA: Serum feline trypsin-like immunoreactivity in cats with exocrine pancreatic insufficiency, *J Vet Intern Med* 14:627, 2000.
17. Packer RA, Cohn LA, Wohlstadter DR, et al: D-lactic acidosis secondary to exocrine pancreatic insufficiency in a cat, *J Vet Intern Med* 19:106, 2005.
18. Hecht S, Penninck DG, Mahony OM, et al: Relationship of pancreatic duct dilation to age and clinical findings in cats, *Vet Radiol Ultrasound* 47:287, 2006.
19. Pidgeon G: Exocrine pancreatic disease in the dog and cat. Part 2: Exocrine pancreatic insufficiency, *Canine Pract* 14:31, 1987.
20. Sherding RG, Stradley RP, Rogers WA, et al: Bentiromide:xylose test in healthy cats, *Am J Vet Res* 43:2272, 1982.
21. Williams DA, Reed SD: Comparison of methods for assay of fecal proteolytic activity, *Vet Clin Path* 19:20, 1990.
22. Steiner JM, Williams DA, Moeller EM, et al: Development and validation of an enzyme-linked immunosorbent assay (ELISA) for feline trypsin-like immunoreactivity (fTLI), *Am J Vet Res* 61:620, 2000.
23. Steiner JM: *Das Trypsin bei der Katze. Dr.med.vet. Thesis*, Germany, 1995, Universität München.
24. Browning T: Exocrine pancreatic insufficiency in a cat, *Aust Vet J* 76:104, 1998.
25. Steiner JM, Finco DR, Williams DA: Serum feline trypsin-like immunoreactivity (fTLI) in cats with experimentally induced chronic renal failure, *J Vet Intern Med* 16:385 (abstract), 2002.
26. Steiner JM, Williams DA: Feline exocrine pancreatic disorders, *Vet Clin North Am Small Anim Pract* 29:551, 1999.
27. Fyfe JC: Feline intrinsic factor (IF) is pancreatic in origin and mediates ileal cobalamin (CBL) absorption, *J Vet Intern Med* 7:133 (abstract), 1993.
28. Arvanitakis C: Functional and morphological abnormalities of the small intestinal mucosa in pernicious anemia—a prospective study, *Acta Hepato-Gastroenterol* 25:313, 1978.
29. Rutz GM, Steiner JM, Bauer JE, et al: Effects of exchange of dietary medium chain triglycerides for long-chain triglycerides on serum biochemical variables and subjectively assessed well-being of dogs with exocrine pancreatic insufficiency, *Am J Vet Res* 65:1293, 2004.
30. Batchelor DJ, Noble PJM, Taylor RH, et al: Prognostic factors in canine exocrine pancreatic insufficiency: Prolonged survival is likely if clinical remission is achieved, *J Vet Intern Med* 21:54, 2007.
31. Westermarck E, Wiberg M, Junttila J: Role of feeding in the treatment of dogs with pancreatic degenerative atrophy, *Acta Vet Scand* 31:325, 1990.
32. Bersenas AM, Mathews KA, Allen DG, et al: Effects of ranitidine, famotidine, pantoprazole, and omeprazole on intragastric pH in dogs, *Am J Vet Res* 66:425, 2005.
33. Williams DA, Batt RM, McLean L: Bacterial overgrowth in the duodenum of dogs with exocrine pancreatic insufficiency, *J Am Vet Med Assoc* 191:201, 1987.
34. Johnston KL: Small intestinal bacterial overgrowth, *Vet Clin North Am Small Anim Pract* 29:523, 1999.
35. Johnston KL, Lamport A, Batt RM: An unexpected bacterial flora in the proximal small intestine of normal cats, *Vet Rec* 132:362, 1993.

CHAPTER
21 Antiemetic Therapy

Karin Allenspach and Daniel L. Chan

Vomiting is defined as ejection of food and/or fluid from the stomach and/or the small intestine and is a common clinical sign in cats. It is important to remember that vomiting can result from various conditions of the gastrointestinal tract but also is seen in patients following intoxications, as well as in those with metabolic and endocrine disorders (e.g., uremia, hyperthyroidism), abdominal disorders (e.g., pancreatitis, peritonitis), and vestibular disorders (e.g., motion sickness). A thorough medical investigation to identify the underlying cause is indicated in any cat with signs of chronic vomiting. However, antiemetic treatment is initiated in many cases before the underlying cause can be identified. When using an antiemetic agent, it is useful to remember the pathophysiological mechanisms that are involved in vomiting to rationalize the use of specific antiemetic treatment regimens. The scientific evidence for the effectiveness of many antiemetic drugs that have been used for decades in feline medicine is mostly lacking. However, with the discovery of a new antiemetic drug class, the tachykinin inhibitors (i.e., neurokinin$_1$ inhibitors), new studies are emerging that will help us select specific antiemetic drugs in a more targeted fashion in the future.

PHYSIOLOGY OF EMESIS

The vomiting reflex consists of several neuronal pathways and centers. Activation of the neurons in the vomiting center within the reticular formation essentially occurs through two pathways. First, emetic substances such as toxins, medications, chemotherapeutic drugs, or uremic toxins reach the chemoreceptor trigger zone (CRTZ), which is located in the area postrema on the floor of the fourth ventricle. This area of the brain lies outside the blood-brain barrier and therefore can sense such stimuli

through the so-called humoral pathway. Triggering of neurons in the area postrema then leads to secondary activation of the vomiting center and the initiation of the vomiting reflex. The second pathway for activation of the vomiting center is through the so-called neuronal pathway. Specific receptors in the abdomen and the gastrointestinal tract are activated by inflammatory mediators and the stimulus travels via vagal and sympathetic afferent neurons directly to the vomiting center. Much in the same way, the vomiting center receives input from neurons from the vestibular apparatus and from cerebrocortical neurons.

It is crucial to remember these pathophysiological concepts when treating vomiting symptomatically because the efficacy of antiemetic agents depends on the presence of the respective neurotransmitters and their receptors in the brain. Specific receptors of neurotransmitters that have been detected in the brain of cats include dopamine (D_2-dopaminergic receptors), norepinephrine (α_2-adrenergic receptors), 5-hydroxytryptamine (5-HT-serotonergic receptors), acetylcholine (M_1-cholinergic receptors), histamine (H_1- and H_2-histaminergic receptors), and enkephalins (enkμ- and enkδ-enkephalinergic receptors).[1] Currently, there are no data available regarding the presence of neurokinin$_1$ receptors (NK$_1$-receptors) in the brain of cats. However, it is reasonable to assume that NK$_1$-receptors are present in cats because of the documented effectiveness of NK$_1$-inhibitors as antiemetic agents in that species (Figure 21-1).[2]

ANTIEMETIC AGENTS

Many antiemetic agents have been used traditionally in cats, and a summary of these agents along with their mechanism of action, recommended dosage, and side

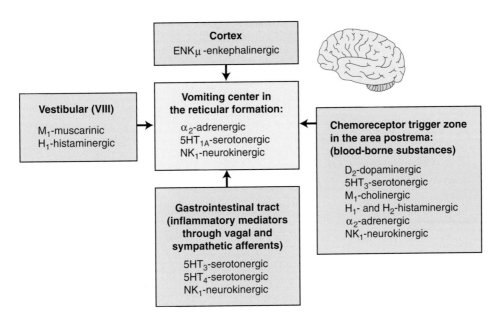

Figure 21-1 Activation of the vomiting center. The different pathways of activation of the vomiting center in the reticular formation: (1) the neural pathway, which consists of vagal and sympathetic afferents from the gastrointestinal tract and is stimulated by inflammatory mediators, (2) the humoral pathway, by which blood-borne substances activate the chemoreceptor trigger zone and subsequently the vomiting center, (3) vestibular stimuli, and (4) cortical stimuli. NK$_1$-receptors have not yet been identified for several regions of the brain in cats, and the areas displayed in this figure are based on studies in ferrets. However, because NK$_1$-inhibitors show effective control of vomiting in cats, these receptors also are assumed to be present in the brain of cats.

effects can be found in Table 21-1. However, it is important to remember that there are species-specific differences in the distribution of receptors in the brain, which may explain why some agents that have been shown to be effective in dogs are not effective in cats. A discussion of the various classes of antiemetics is provided to highlight the rationale for the use of these agents to treat vomiting in cats in different clinical situations.

α$_2$-ADRENERGIC ANTAGONISTS

Xylazine is the classic α$_2$-adrenergic agonist, which has potent emetic effects in cats but not in dogs. Many of the research models used to investigate the efficacy of antiemetic agents in cats are based on triggering vomiting by the administration of xylazine.[3-5] Antiemetic agents with good efficacy at the α$_2$-adrenergic receptors in the vomiting center include pure α$_2$-antagonists such as yohimbine, or mixed α$_1$/α$_2$-antagonists such as prochlorperazine and chlorpromazine.[3] The latter two are in the drug class of phenothiazines, which also have weak antagonistic effects on H$_1$- and H$_2$-receptors, M$_1$-cholinergic receptors, and D$_2$-dopaminergic receptors. Promethazine is another phenothiazine drug with antiemetic effects. There is evidence that NK$_1$-inhibitors can override the effect of xylazine on α$_2$-adrenergic receptors and provide good antiemetic efficacy.[5] Adverse effects possibly associated with drugs in this class include sedation and anticholinergic effects (e.g., dry mucous membranes).

D$_2$-DOPAMINERGIC ANTAGONISTS

Apomorphine is an emetic agent that acts specifically on D$_2$-dopaminergic receptors in the dog brain.[3] However, apomorphine is not a very effective emetic agent in cats, which is why it is believed that D$_2$-dopaminergic antagonists, such as metoclopramide, play a minor role as antiemetic agents in that species.[3,4] However, peripheral effects of D$_2$-dopaminergic antagonists in the gut, such as improved intestinal motility, may provide some antiemetic effects, but this has not been evaluated properly in cats. The exact action of metoclopramide in the gut is not known, but it appears that it sensitizes the upper gastrointestinal smooth muscle to the action of acetylcholine.[3] In cats, adverse reactions to metoclopramide include signs of frenzied behavior, disorientation, and constipation.

H$_1$- AND H$_2$-HISTAMINERGIC ANTAGONISTS

H$_1$- and H$_2$-histaminergic receptors have been demonstrated in the CRTZ in dogs and are believed to play a significant role in emesis in this species.[1] Antihistamines, such as dimenhydrinate and diphenhydramine, have been used widely to treat emesis, particularly related to motion sickness. The exact mechanism of action relating histamine receptor antagonism to an antiemetic effect is unknown, but these drugs appear to inhibit vestibular stimulation.[3] The presence of histamine receptors in the

Table 21-1 Antiemetic Agents Used in Cats

Drug	Mechanism of Action	Dosage	Side Effects
Chlorpromazine	Dopaminergic D_2 receptor antagonism	0.5 mg/kg IM q8h	Sedation, hypotension
Cimetidine	H_2 receptor antagonism	2.5-5 mg/kg IV q8h	Rarely: hepatotoxicity and nephrotoxicity
Cisapride	$5HT_4$ receptor agonism	0.1-0.5 mg/kg PO q8-12h	None reported in cats; GI signs possible
Dimenhydrinate	H_1 receptor antagonism	12.5 mg/kg PO q8h	CNS depression, xerostomia
Diphenhydramine	H_1 receptor antagonism	2-4 mg/kg PO, IM q8h	CNS depression, xerostomia
Dolasetron	$5HT_3$ receptor antagonism	0.6-10 mg/kg IV, PO q24h	Constipation
Famotidine	H_2 receptor antagonism	0.5 mg/kg IV, PO q12-24h	Possible hemolysis when administered chronically IV
Granisetron	$5HT_3$ receptor antagonism	0.1-0.5 mg/kg PO, IV q12-24h	None reported in cats
Maropitant	NK_1 receptor antagonism	0.5-1 mg/kg SQ q24h	Possible tremors
Meclizine	H_1 receptor antagonism	4 mg/kg PO q24h	Sedation, xerostomia, inappetence
Metoclopramide	Dopaminergic D_2 receptor antagonism	1-2 mg/kg/day as continuous rate infusion IV 0.2-0.5 mg/kg PO, SQ q8h	Frenzied behavior and disorientation; constipation
Mirtazapine	$5HT_3$ receptor antagonism, H_1 receptor antagonism	3-4 mg/cat PO q72h	Marked sedation, hypotension, vocalization, tachycardia, appetite stimulation
Ondansetron	$5HT_3$ receptor antagonism	0.1-1 mg/kg PO q12-24h	None reported in animals; constipation, extrapyramidal signs, arrhythmias, hypotension possible
Prochlorperazine	Mixed α_1/α_2 antagonism; dopaminergic D_2 receptor antagonism	0.1 mg/kg IM q6-12h	Sedation, hypotension
Promethazine	H_1 receptor antagonism	2 mg/kg PO or IM q24h	Sedation, xerostomia
Ranitidine	H_2 receptor antagonism	2 mg/kg/day continuous rate infusion; 2.5 mg/kg IV q8h	Rarely: cardiac arrhythmias and hypotension

CNS, Central nervous system; *GI,* gastrointestinal.

CRTZ has not yet been demonstrated in cats, and histamine receptor antagonists are not considered very effective in this species. Also, cats are believed to be relatively resistant to the emetic effects of histamine. Adverse reactions seen with antihistamines in general include central nervous system (CNS) depression, anticholinergic effects (e.g., dry mouth, urinary retention), and gastrointestinal disturbances (e.g., vomiting, diarrhea).

H_2-antagonists are a good choice perhaps as an antiemetic agent in uremic patients because they decrease gastrin secretion and in turn gastric acid production, which is believed to exacerbate uremic gastropathy associated with severe azotemia. Cimetidine, ranitidine, and famotidine all have been used based on this rationale. However, the treatment of gastric ulceration may require more effective inhibition of gastric acid secretion, which may only be achieved by use of proton-pump inhibitors, such as omeprazole. The efficacy of proton-pump inhibitors has not been evaluated in cats.

Piperazine antihistamines, such as meclizine, are believed to have a separate antiemetic effect in addition to their antihistaminergic effect; however, the mechanism of action is not completely understood.[6] It has been proposed that meclizine has central anticholinergic and CNS-depressant activity, particularly in the CRTZ, which may be responsible for its antiemetic effects. Adverse effects include sedation and, less frequently, anticholinergic effects (e.g., dry mucous membranes) and inappetence (especially in cats).

M_1-MUSCARINERGIC ANTAGONISTS

M_1-muscarinergic receptors and the neurotransmitter acetylcholine both have been demonstrated in the vestibular apparatus of cats.[1] Mixed M_1/M_2-receptor antagonists such as atropine and scopolamine, as well as pure M_1-receptor antagonists such as pirenzepine, have been used traditionally for the treatment of motion sickness in cats.[1] It is unclear, however, if the main action of these compounds is through muscarinic receptors alone or also through other pathways. This fact, as well as the side effects of sedation, xerostomia, and possible intestinal ileus, makes their use less preferable.[1]

5HT₃-SEROTONERGIC ANTAGONISTS

The central emetic effects of chemotherapeutic agents such as cisplatin are mediated through 5HT₃-serotonergic receptors in the CRTZ in cats.[1] Additionally, there are 5HT₃-receptors found peripherally on vagal nerve terminals.[1] It is unclear if the antiemetic effects of 5HT₃-antagonists are solely mediated centrally or if there are peripheral effects also. 5HT₃-selective antagonists such as ondansetron, dolasetron, and granisetron have been used widely for the treatment of chemotherapy-induced vomiting in cats and are believed to be very effective for this indication.[7,8] These agents also are reportedly effective when given preventively before administering the chemotherapeutic drug.[7,8] Advantages of some of these agents include infrequent dosing and the potential for parenteral administration.

A newer agent with some 5HT₃-serotonergic antagonistic effect is the tetracyclic antidepressant, mirtazapine. The antidepressant activity of mirtazapine appears to be mediated via antagonism of central presynaptic α_2 receptors, resulting in a net increase of norepinephrine, and this may contribute to its reported appetite-stimulating effects[6] (see Chapter 12). In addition, mirtazapine antagonizes several 5HT receptor subtypes and also histamine receptors (H₁). These effects are believed to be responsible for its antiemetic and antinauseant effects. The prominent sedative side effects of mirtazapine are related to its activity at H₁ receptors, while activity on peripheral α_1-adrenergic antagonism may explain the orthostatic hypotension associated with its use.[6] Other reported side effects include vocalization and tachycardia.[6] An important feature of mirtazapine metabolism is its dependence on glucuronidation for elimination. Because cats have limited capacity of glucuronidation, particularly when there is hepatic dysfunction, dosing intervals should be no more frequent than once every 72 hours.

5HT₄-SEROTONERGIC AGONISTS

Vagal efferent and myenteric neurons acting through 5HT₄-serotonergic receptors are responsible for the excitation and inhibition of the smooth muscles that are involved in the process of emesis. Cisapride is a very effective 5HT₄-agonist that has good antiemetic activity as well as having gastric, esophageal, and colonic prokinetic effects in cats.[9-11] Cisapride is a good choice as an antiemetic agent in patients with delayed gastric emptying. It also is useful for treatment of megacolon in cats. In these patients, cisapride is used primarily for its prokinetic effects on colonic smooth muscle cells and less for its antiemetic effects.[10] Availability of cisapride has become limited recently due to removal from the human market. However, cisapride for veterinary use is still available through many compounding pharmacies. Cisapride is known to interact with various cardiac drugs and can lead to serious arrhythmias in people, which is the reason why the drug was removed from the human market.

NEUROKININ₁-ANTAGONISTS (MAROPITANT)

Substance P is a neurotransmitter of the tachykinin family of neuroendocrine peptides that plays an important role in eliciting emesis. Substance P binds to neurokinin₁ receptors and has been detected in high concentrations in areas of the brain important for emesis, such as the nucleus tractus solitarius, the area postrema, and the dorsal motor nucleus of the vagus.[12] Although most of these data stem from studies in ferrets and human beings, it is likely that substance P also plays an important role in eliciting vomiting in cats (see Figure 21-1).[2] Many NK₁ receptor antagonists have become available for use in human medicine, and their wide application both as peripherally and centrally acting antiemetics has been a great success.

Recently, maropitant, a new NK₁ receptor antagonist, has been licensed for use in dogs and also has been used off-label widely in cats.[13] The recommended dosage for cats is 0.5 to 1 mg/kg SQ q24h, which is half the dosage recommended for dogs.[5] The safety and pharmacokinetics of this drug in cats have been reported recently.[5] The acute tolerance was tested in six cats at dosages of 1, 2.5, and 5 mg/kg for up to 15 days. No changes were identified in behavior, appetite, level of consciousness, physical examination, serum biochemistry profile, hematology, coagulation profile, and urinalysis. However, slight tremors during sleep were noted in one female cat after administration of dosages of 5 mg/kg SQ q24h.[5] In addition, reactions at the injection site were seen more often when doses above 1.5 mg/kg were administered SQ.[5] It is reasonable therefore to assume that the drug has a very good safety profile for use in cats. A pharmacokinetic study in cats indicated that maropitant has a serum half-life of 13 to 17 hours in this species, regardless of the route of administration. This study also suggested that the clearance was approximately four times slower than in dogs.[5] This information is clinically important because the antiemetic effects of maropitant can be expected to last up to 24 hours after administration to cats.

The efficacy of maropitant as an antiemetic agent has been tested in cats treated with xylazine, a potent α-adrenergic emetogenic drug in that species.[5] Maropitant administered at 1 mg/kg PO, SQ, or IV 2 hours prior to administration of xylazine reduced the number of emetic events significantly when compared to untreated cats.[5] The best effect with no emetic events in the treatment group was seen when maropitant was given IV. When maropitant was given orally 24 hours before administration of xylazine, the antiemetic effect was no longer statistically significant. However, a 66 per cent reduction in emetic events as compared to untreated cats was noted.

The efficacy of the drug also was tested for prevention of motion-induced emesis in cats.[5] To assess this effect, cats were placed in a motorized device resembling an amusement park Ferris wheel and rotated around a horizontal axis.[14] Seven of 32 (21.9 per cent) cats experienced nausea or vomiting in the wheel and were treated subsequently with maropitant 1 mg/kg SQ to assess its preventive antiemetic effect against motion sickness 4 hours before being placed in the wheel. Maropitant effectively reduced emetic events to zero, although the treated cats tended to retch more often than the untreated cats.[5]

In summary, initial data in cats have shown that maropitant is preventive as well as effective as a postevent antiemetic agent in xylazine-induced emesis in that species. In cats with motion sickness, there is evidence that it has good efficacy when used as a preventive treatment in susceptible patients. However, field studies investigating the efficacy of maropitant in various clinically relevant situations will be necessary to judge if it has a clinical antiemetic efficacy comparable to its effect in dogs. In the hands of the authors, maropitant has shown potent antiemetic efficacy in uremia-induced vomiting in cats.

RATIONAL CLINICAL USE OF ANTIEMETICS

CHEMOTHERAPY

Chemotherapy-induced nausea and vomiting is mediated through $5HT_3$-receptors in the CRTZ in cats.[1] This is in contrast to dogs and human beings, in whom chemotherapeutic drugs primarily cause inflammation in the gut, which then stimulates endocrine cells also in the gut to release mediators such as serotonin, substance P, and cholecystokinin. In turn, these mediators stimulate $5HT_3$-receptors on vagal afferent neurons, which then activate the vomiting center to elicit emesis.[1] This might be the reason why some chemotherapeutic agents have a different gastrointestinal toxicity in cats and dogs. The authors' clinical experience suggests that cyclophosphamide and gemcitabine are the chemotherapeutic drugs that elicit the most gastrointestinal toxicity in cats, followed by vincristine and doxorubicin. Chemotherapy-induced gastrointestinal toxicity in cats manifests itself as inappetence, nausea, vomiting, and/or diarrhea, usually beginning immediately after treatment and lasting until up to 5 days after treatment. Traditionally, metoclopramide has been used to treat and prevent chemotherapy-induced vomiting in cats. However, the more potent and directly effective $5HT_3$-antagonists ondansetron, dolasetron, and granisetron are much more effective.[7,8] Anecdotal evidence also suggests that maropitant, alone or in combination with ondansetron, is very effective in treating chemotherapy-induced emesis in cats. Also, a dose reduction of 20 per cent may be indicated if severe gastrointestinal toxicity occurs repeatedly after treatment with certain chemotherapeutic drugs.

INFLAMMATORY BOWEL DISEASE

Feline inflammatory bowel disease (IBD) is an important disease associated with clinical signs of vomiting, diarrhea, weight loss, and/or various degrees of inappetence. A clinical diagnosis is made on the basis of exclusion of all other known causes of such gastrointestinal signs, such as infectious agents (e.g., *Giardia*, feline leukemia virus, feline immunodeficiency virus), metabolic disease (e.g., hyperthyroidism), or gastrointestinal lymphoma. A complete diagnostic evaluation for cats with suspected IBD usually also includes histological evaluation of multiple intestinal biopsies. Cats with IBD show an infiltration of the gastrointestinal mucosa with lymphocytes and plasma cells, or with other types of inflammatory cells. Vomiting is seen frequently in cats with IBD, although it is rarely the only clinical sign. Because it is a sign of the underlying disease, an effort should be made to control vomiting and diarrhea by treating IBD.

There are no controlled clinical trials documenting the efficacy of various treatments in feline IBD. The traditional approach to the treatment relies on four components that can be used individually or most often combined: dietary modification, cobalamin supplementation, antibiotic therapy, and specific antiinflammatory and immunosuppressive drugs. Most specialists agree that dietary therapy is an important component of therapy, and up to one third of cats with IBD can be treated successfully with a dietary trial alone (see Chapters 8 and 22).[15] It is sometimes difficult to ensure that cats are fed a single diet exclusively, especially when they are outdoor cats. Prednisolone (given at a dosage of 1 to 3 mg/kg PO q12h) is the mainstay of antiinflammatory therapy in feline patients with IBD. Metronidazole (10 mg/kg PO q24h) also can be tried, although it tastes bitter and is often difficult to give over prolonged periods of time. If prednisolone fails to elicit a therapeutic response, chlorambucil can be added as a second-line treatment (1 to 2 mg/m² PO q48h). Cyclosporine has shown promise as a rescue treatment in dogs with IBD. However, anecdotal experience in cats suggests that it has less therapeutic efficacy in that species. If cyclosporine is used, it should be given for at least 4 weeks at dosages of 5 mg/kg PO q24h. It may be prudent to check serum concentrations of cyclosporine levels 1 to 2 hours after giving the drug to assess peak concentrations, which should be between 500 and 700 ng/mL. It also is important to remember that many cats with chronic gastrointestinal disease have low serum cobalamin concentrations, which may self-perpetuate any underlying gastrointestinal disease if left untreated.[16] It is imperative to correct this deficiency by parenteral supplementation (see Chapter 22). (The reader is referred to Chapter 13 in the fifth volume of this series for a complete discussion of the role of cobalamin in the diagnosis and treatment of chronic gastrointestinal disease.)

It is rare that vomiting due to IBD needs to be treated symptomatically in cats if the IBD is managed appropriately. If symptomatic antiemetic treatment is deemed necessary, maropitant could be a good choice, although there are no controlled studies available that prove efficacy in this setting.[5]

MOTION SICKNESS

Motion sickness is well-recognized in cats, although clinically it is a poorly described condition. Motion sickness in cats likely involves abnormalities of the vestibular system, the signals from which ultimately activate brainstem areas involved in emesis, including the nucleus tractus solitarius, the dorsal motor nucleus, and the area postrema. Motion sickness is a major inconvenience for pet owners, and most therapies are prescribed solely on description of clinical signs by the owner. Typically, this disorder is treated empirically with minimal medical investigation.

Cats affected with motion sickness are reported to display signs of nausea (e.g., hypersalivation) and discomfort that often lead to productive vomiting and is always associated with transport of the animal. Several antiemetic agents and tranquilizers are commonly prescribed off-label for the treatment of this disorder. Agents prescribed for motion sickness in cats include acepromazine, chlorpromazine, ondansetron, and metoclopramide. However, nonprescription drugs such as diphenhydramine, meclizine, and dimenhydrinate are used most commonly. The effectiveness of these agents is only reported anecdotally and known side effects associated with these agents include sedation, ataxia, and hypotension.

Although currently not licensed for use in cats, there are experimental data demonstrating effective treatment of motion sickness in cats with maropitant.[2,5] In one study, cats identified to be susceptible to motion-induced emesis were subjected to simulated motion and tested with maropitant versus placebo in a cross-over design.[5] Maropitant administered at 1 mg/kg SQ prevented motion-induced emesis effectively in all cats evaluated (n = 5) and reduced clinical signs indicative of nausea by at least 68 per cent compared to controls.[5]

UREMIA

Vomiting is a frequent finding in cats with uremia. The cause of vomiting is likely due to uremic toxins that, as of yet, have not been identified and are believed to act on the medullary emetic chemoreceptor trigger zone and also indirectly through uremic gastritis. Vomiting may exacerbate dehydration, the degree of azotemia, and electrolyte imbalances. Elevated serum gastrin concentrations due to decreased renal clearance may promote uremic gastropathy. Gastrin stimulates gastric acid secretion directly by stimulating receptors on parietal cells and by increasing histamine release, which in turn further promotes gastric acid secretion and gastric ulceration. Based on this rationale, H_2-antagonists such as cimetidine, ranitidine, or famotidine have been recommended for uremic cats who show nausea and/or vomiting. The efficacy of these agents on the frequency of vomiting has not been evaluated formally in cats. Gastric hyperacidity also is not identified universally in feline patients with uremia. Gastric ulceration with development of hematemesis may be treated with more potent gastric acid inhibitors, such as the proton-pump inhibitors (e.g., omeprazole).

Other considerations for vomiting in uremic cats could include the use of centrally acting antiemetic drugs. Metoclopramide infusions have been recommended previously in part due to their prokinetic effects on the stomach to promote gastric emptying, in addition to their centrally acting antiemetic effects. The use of the neurokinin$_1$-antagonist maropitant may be a more effective option for the treatment of vomiting associated with uremia. However, this has not been evaluated systematically to date.

PANCREATITIS

Pancreatitis can be associated with a variety of clinical signs in cats. While most cats with pancreatitis have nonspecific clinical signs, such as lethargy and anorexia, some cats can show vomiting.[17] It can be quite challenging to diagnose pancreatitis in cats. The incidence of vomiting associated with pancreatitis in cats is much lower than that in dogs. Even when present, the frequency and severity of vomiting often is less than that in dogs. It has been shown in human beings that early feeding is beneficial in patients with pancreatitis. In addition, unlike human beings, cats are at high risk for developing secondary hepatic lipidosis if they are not fed.[18] Therefore many authors recommend feeding cats with pancreatitis even when vomiting is present. Also, feline pancreatitis often is associated with concurrent disorders, such as IBD or hepatobiliary disease, and therefore vomiting may be related to these other conditions rather than to pancreatic inflammation alone.

Antiemetics can be used in feline patients who vomit but also can be used to decrease nausea and improve appetite. However, this is often ineffective. The α_2-adrenergic antagonists and $5HT_3$-antagonists have been suggested as effective antiemetics in cats with pancreatitis, but this has not been confirmed prospectively. Histamine- and bradykinin-induced increases in microvascular permeability are associated with the development of hemorrhagic necrosis in experimental models of feline pancreatitis. Based on this rationale, antihistamine receptor antagonists have been recommended for the treatment of naturally occurring feline pancreatitis, but efficacy has not been confirmed.[19] Agents that could cause hypotension (e.g., phenothiazines, antihistamines) may not be appropriate in cats with pancreatitis because hypoperfusion of the pancreas is believed to be a major component of this disease.

DELAYED GASTRIC EMPTYING

Abnormalities of gastric emptying or gastrointestinal motility in general are poorly described in cats. However, pooling or retention of fluid within the stomach due to delayed gastric emptying could result in alterations of the microbial gastrointestinal flora, as well as nausea and vomiting. Gastric stasis, or gastroparesis, is a functional disorder associated with delayed gastric emptying caused by abnormalities of myenteric neuronal or gastric smooth-muscle function. This disorder has been documented with inflammatory intestinal diseases and gastrointestinal injury in general. Gastroparesis also may occur secondary to hypokalemia, uremia, diabetes mellitus, various drugs (e.g., opioids, anticholinergics), pancreatitis, and peritonitis.

Documentation of gastroparesis generally is limited to subjective assessment of contrast radiography. Barium sulfate suspensions usually are used to evaluate gastric emptying of liquid-phase gastric contents. Barium-impregnated polyspheres may be more useful for evaluating gastrointestinal handling of solids, but this has not been well evaluated in cats (see Chapter 15). Measurement of gastric residual volumes (via aspiration of gastric feeding tubes) also may support the clinical suspicion of delayed gastric emptying. However, there are no established guidelines for acceptable residual volumes in cats. Anecdotally, it has been recommended that residual volumes greater than 50 per cent of the amount infused during the previous feeding, or accumulation of greater than twice the hourly infusion rate, should be considered excessive.[20]

Gastroparesis delays the implementation of nutritional support because vomiting often is used to justify withholding nutritional support. However, lack of enteral nutrition is known to lead to further gastrointestinal dysfunction, namely gastrointestinal atrophy, compromised intestinal mucosal barrier function, and an altered overall immune function. Gastroparesis also is known to be a predisposing factor of duodenogastric and gastroesophageal reflux, which have been associated with an increased risk of aspiration and nosocomial infections, although this has not been demonstrated in cats.

The use of prokinetic agents is the mainstay of therapy for gastroparesis. However, given the challenges of confirming the diagnosis, assessment of efficacy also is lacking. Agents used as prokinetic agents include $5HT_4$-serotonergic agonists and $5HT_3$-serotonergic antagonists (e.g., metoclopramide, cisapride), D_2-dopaminergic antagonists, α_2- and β_2-adrenergic antagonists (e.g., domperidone), acetylcholinesterase inhibitor and M_3-muscarinic agonists (e.g., ranitidine, nizatidine), and motilin receptor agonists (e.g., erythromycin).

In addition to its dopaminergic properties, metoclopramide also has $5HT_4$-receptor agonistic effects and $5HT_3$-receptor antagonistic effects. In animals, $5HT_4$-receptor agonism results in a prokinetic effect, whereas $5HT_3$ antagonism imparts a central antiemetic effect. Anecdotally, continuous rate infusion of metoclopramide appears to be superior as compared to intermittent subcutaneous or oral administration.

Cisapride is the best-known prokinetic agent, with its effects mediated by agonism of $5HT_4$-receptors of the enteric nervous system. Stimulation of these receptors results in acetylcholine release from postganglionic cholinergic neurons and smooth-muscle contraction. In addition to its $5HT_4$ effects, cisapride has antagonistic effects on $5HT_1$- and $5HT_3$-receptors, although the significance of these effects on gastrointestinal motility is questionable. Cisapride promotes gastrointestinal emptying and increases lower-esophageal sphincter tone. Additional effects include stimulation of jejunal and colonic motility. Unfortunately, cisapride has been associated with the development of serious cardiac arrhythmias in human patients, leading to its removal from the human market. However, no such side effects have been reported in cats, and cisapride continues to be used commonly in this species.

The close relationship between suspected gastrointestinal motility disorders and vomiting has led to the wide-spread use of H_2-antagonists (e.g., ranitidine and nizatidine) in affected patients. To date, no studies have evaluated the efficacy of this approach in cats. It is believed that the gastric prokinetic effects of ranitidine and nizatidine can be achieved with antisecretory doses. However, this has not been confirmed clinically.

Erythromycin is a macrolide antibiotic that increases gastrointestinal motility by acting on motilin receptors on smooth-muscle cells of the stomach. Erythromycin mimics the effects of motilin in the upper gastrointestinal tract. The prokinetic dose of erythromycin (1 mg/kg PO q12h) is much lower than the antimicrobial dose. Limited information is available about the efficacy of this treatment in cats.

REFERENCES

1. Beleslin DB: Neurotransmitter receptor subtypes related to vomiting. In Bianchi AL, editor: *Mechanisms and control of emesis*, Paris, 1992, Inserm, p 11.
2. Lucot JB, Obach RS, McLean S, et al: The effect of CO-99994 on the responses to provocative motion in the cat, *Brit J Pharmacol* 120:297, 1997.
3. King GL: Animal models in the study of vomiting, *Can J Physiol Pharmacol* 68:260, 1990.
4. Lang IM, Sarna SK: The role of adrenergic receptors in the initiation of vomiting and its gastrointestinal motor correlates in the dog, *J Pharmacol Exp Ther* 263:395, 1992.
5. Hickman MA, Cox SR, Mahabir S, et al: Safety, pharmacokinetics and use of the novel NK_1-receptor antagonist maropitant (Cerenia) for the prevention of emesis and motion sickness, *J Vet Pharmacol Ther* 31:220, 2008.
6. Plumb DC: *Plumb's veterinary drug handbook*, ed 6, Ames, Iowa, 2008, Blackwell.
7. Ogilvie GK: Dolasetron: A new option for nausea and vomiting, *J Am Anim Hosp Assoc* 36:481, 2000.
8. Rudd JA, Tse JYH, Wai MK: Cisplatin-induced emesis in the cat: effect of granisetron and dexamethasone, *Eur J Pharmacol* 391:145, 2000.
9. Washabau RL, Sammarco J: Effects of cisapride on feline colonic smooth muscle function, *Am J Vet Res* 57:541, 1996.
10. Hasler AH, Washabau RJ: Cisapride stimulates contraction of idiopathic megacolonic smooth muscle in cats, *J Vet Intern Med* 11:313, 1997.
11. Hall JA, Washabau RJ: Diagnosis and treatment of gastric motility disorders, *Vet Clin North Am Small Anim Pract* 29:377, 1999.
12. Hargreaves R: Imaging substance P receptors (NK_1) in the living human brain using positron emission tomography, *J Clin Psychiatry* 63(Suppl 11):18, 2002.
13. de la Puente-Redondo VA, Siedek EM, Benchaoui HA, et al: The anti-emetic efficacy of maropitant (Cerenia) in the treatment of ongoing emesis caused by a wide range of underlying clinical aetiologies in canine patients in Europe, *J Small Anim Pract* 48:93, 2007.
14. Crampton GH, Lucot JB: A stimulator for laboratory studies of motion sickness in cats, *Aviat Space Environ Med* 56:462, 1985.
15. Guilford WG, Jones BR, Markwell PJ, et al: Food sensitivity in cats with chronic idiopathic gastrointestinal problems, *J Vet Intern Med* 15:7, 2001.
16. Ruaux CG, Steiner JM, Williams DA: Early biochemical and clinical responses to cobalamin supplementation in cats with signs of gastrointestinal disease and severe hypocobalaminemia, *J Vet Intern Med* 19:155, 2005.

17. Hill RC, Van Winkle TJ: Acute necrotizing pancreatitis and acute suppurative pancreatitis in the cat. A retrospective study of 40 cases (1976-1989), *J Vet Intern Med* 7:25, 1993.

18. Akol KG, Washabau RJ, Saunders HM, et al: Acute pancreatitis in cats with hepatic lipidosis, *J Vet Intern Med* 7:205, 1993.

19. Whittemore JC, Campbell VL: Canine and feline pancreatitis, *Compend Contin Educ Pract Vet* 27:766, 2005.

20. Marks S: Enteral feeding devices: what's old, what's new. In *Proceedings of the WSAVA World Congress*, Vancouver, Canada, 2001, WSAVA, p 342.

CHAPTER

22 Therapeutic Approach to Cats with Chronic Diarrhea

Heidi S. Allen

Chronic diarrhea is defined as diarrhea that has persisted for at least 3 weeks. Intermittent chronic diarrhea is a term used to describe episodic diarrhea that has persisted for a period of time. The length of this period has not been defined specifically, because it depends on the frequency of the episodes that are being observed.

When determining therapeutic options for chronic diarrhea, it is important to know if the diarrhea is small or large bowel in origin (Table 22-1). Small bowel diarrhea is characterized by large quantities of loose to watery stool, which usually occurs one to two times a day (Figure 22-1). Large bowel diarrhea is characterized by small frequent bowel movements often with blood or mucus present (Figure 22-2). In some cases the diarrhea will have characteristics of both small and large bowel diarrhea (i.e., large quantities but some mucus or blood). The author uses the term *mixed bowel diarrhea* to describe this combination.

For appropriate management of chronic diarrhea in cats, it is crucial to first exclude endoparasite infections and treat accordingly. Also, for appropriate management of chronic diarrhea in cats, it is germane to exclude secondary causes of chronic diarrhea before a therapeutic trial is initiated.

This chapter discusses the various therapeutic approaches available for small and large bowel chronic diarrhea. Some treatment options also are discussed in more detail in other sections of this book and are thus referenced to those chapters.

ANTIPARASITIC AGENTS

A complete diagnostic evaluation for chronic diarrhea in a cat should always include a fecal smear and flotation. A *Giardia* fecal enzyme-linked immunosorbent assay (ELISA) test also may be beneficial. Even with negative results, it is essential to treat all patients with a broad-spectrum anthelminthic agent. The author uses praziquantel and pyrantel pamoate frequently in combination. One study evaluated the use of a combination of febantel, praziquantel, and pyrantel pamoate for the treatment of *Giardia* infection in cats. This combination therapy with febantel 56.5 mg/kg PO, pyrantel pamoate 11.3 mg/kg PO, and praziquantel 37.8 mg/kg PO for 5 days led to some success in treating giardiasis.[1] Also, the authors found that there were minimal complications, except for mild salivation after drug administration. Previous experiences with the same therapeutic protocol had shown transient neurotoxicity, which was not seen in this study.[1] Therefore this combination may be used as a broad-spectrum anthelminthic in cats.

Specific anthelminthics are recommended for different parasitic infections (Table 22-2). The anthelminthics used most commonly in cats include pyrantel pamoate, fenbendazole, and praziquantel. Pyrantel pamoate is effective against *Toxocara* (roundworms) and *Ancylostoma* (hookworms). Fenbendazole is effective for these nematodes, as well as *Strongyloides* (seen rarely in cats) and *Trichuris* (whipworms). Praziquantel is effective against

Table 22-1 Clinical Differentiation of Large Bowel and Small Bowel Diarrhea

Characteristic	Small Bowel Diarrhea	Large Bowel Diarrhea
Frequency of bowel movements	1 to 2 times a day	Multiple times a day
Amount with each bowel movement	Large amounts	Usually small amounts
Melena	Yes	No
Blood/mucus in stool	No	Yes
Tenesmus	No	Yes
Weight loss	±	Rarely
Vomiting	±	No

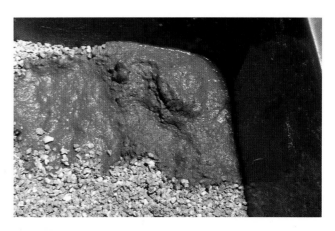

Figure 22-1 Small bowel diarrhea from a cat, which is characterized by a large quantity of liquid diarrhea.

Table 22-2 Anthelminthic Agents Used Commonly in Cats

Antiparasitic Agent	Usage	Dose	Side Effects
Pyrantel pamoate	*Toxocara cati* and *leonina*, *Ancylostoma tubaeforme*	5 mg/kg PO once, repeat in 2 weeks	Vomiting can occur rarely
Fenbendazole	*Toxocara cati* and *leonina*, *Ancylostoma tubaeforme*, *Trichuris serrata* and *campanula* *Strongyloides*	50 mg/kg PO q24h for 5 days	Vomiting can occur rarely
Praziquantel	*Dipylidium caninum*	5 mg/kg PO as fits into tablet size	Salivation, diarrhea
Metronidazole	*Giardia lamblia*	25 mg/kg PO q12h for 7 days	Anorexia, vomiting, salivation, tremors, seizures
Sulfadimethoxine	*Isospora felis* and *rivolta*	50 mg/kg PO once; then 25 mg/kg PO q24h for 14-20 days	Anorexia, leukopenia, anemia

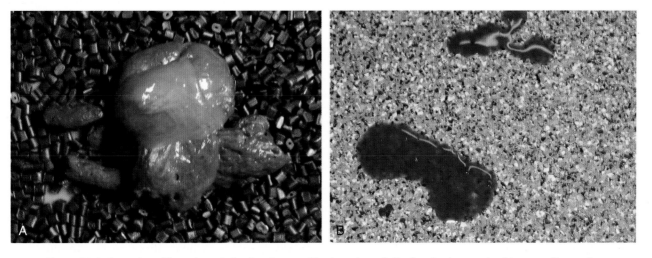

Figure 22-2 Examples of large bowel diarrhea in cats. The large bowel diarrhea is characterized by a small quantity of liquid stool with mucus (**A**) or blood (**B**).

Dipylidium caninum (tapeworms) and *Alaria* (the intestinal fluke). *Alaria* often is nonpathogenic and may not require therapy. It is important to note that the feline tapeworm, *D. caninum*, should be treated with praziquantel.

Protozoal infections that can cause chronic diarrhea in cats include *Giardia lamblia*, *Tritrichomonas foetus*, *Isospora felis* and *Isospora rivolta*, and *Cryptosporidium parvum* (see Chapter 18). A variety of protocols have been evaluated for the treatment of *Giardia* infections in cats. To date, metronidazole administered at 25 mg/kg PO q12h for 7 days has been shown to be most effective in eliminating *Giardia* cysts long term.[2] In one study none of the treated cats developed clinical signs of metronidazole toxicity at this dosage. However, it should be noted that this high dose was used only for 7 days.[2] Other therapies, such as fenbendazole and the combination treatment described in the preceding, have caused a decrease in the numbers of *Giardia* cysts, but not long-term resolution in all infected cats.[1,3] Also, *Giardia* vaccines have not shown efficacy in preventing giardiasis in cats.[4]

T. foetus is a protozoal organism causing infections that have been diagnosed with increasing frequency in cats over the last 10 years. The condition is self-limiting in many patients. However, it may take 9 months on average for resolution of clinical signs, and up to 2 years in some cats.[5] Currently ronidazole is considered the treatment of choice; however, neurotoxicity can develop and ronidazole should be used with caution. All cats with reported neurotoxicity after ronidazole treatment had reversible signs, but based on similar findings with metronidazole, irreversible signs may occur in some patients.[6,7]

C. parvum is another protozoal infection that occurs in cats. No therapeutic protocols have been shown to eliminate *Cryptosporidium* successfully and consistently, although the infection often can be self-limiting. *Isospora* spp. infections can be treated successfully with sulfadimethoxine (50 mg/kg PO q24h on day 1, then 25 mg/kg PO q24h for 14 days), although it is a self-limiting disease in most cases. (See Chapter 15 in the fifth volume of this series for further discussion about the diagnosis and treatment of these parasitic infections in young cats.)

NUTRITION

Nutrition is extremely important in the management of chronic diarrhea, and often is used alone or in conjunction with other therapies. This section briefly discusses nutritional options. Further information can be found in Chapter 8 of this volume.

Several dietary options are available for cats with chronic diarrhea, the first of which is a diet that is highly digestible and low in fat. These diets can be used in patients with small or large bowel diarrhea that are not the result of true food hypersensitivity. It is believed that unabsorbed fatty acids can lead to colonic water secretion, increased diarrhea, and water loss. However, fat is important as an energy source and high-fat diets are energy dense, which can be important for patients with chronic diarrhea. Therefore a moderate level of fat in the diet, approximately 15 to 22 per cent on a dry matter basis, is recommended for cats with small or large bowel chronic diarrhea.[8] However, cats with small bowel diarrhea may be able to tolerate higher dietary fat than dogs, and preliminary data suggest that low-carbohydrate, high-fat diets may be beneficial in some cats with chronic small bowel diarrhea.[8] Further studies are needed to validate these observations.

Several veterinary diets are highly digestible with low-fat content. Other options include boiled chicken, canned chicken in water, low fat deli meats, or baby foods, such as puréed chicken or turkey. Rice or corn can be used as a carbohydrate source, but it is often difficult to persuade cats to eat carbohydrates. If a homemade diet is to be used on a long-term basis, it is recommended that a nutritionist be consulted so that a balanced homemade diet is formulated for the patient (see Chapter 13).

Novel protein and hydrolyzed protein diets also can be used for cats with inflammatory bowel disease or food hypersensitivity. Novel protein diets have a single source of protein and a single source of carbohydrate, both of which should be new to the affected cat. This is important because all sources of carbohydrates contain a small amount of protein that can act as an allergen and cause food hypersensitivity. Hydrolyzed protein diets contain protein that has been broken down into small peptides that are less than 15,000 Daltons in size. It is important to note that the average size of the peptides in each of the diets may vary, and therefore the level of antigenicity also may vary between diets. Novel protein and hydrolyzed protein diets are used most commonly in cats with small bowel diarrhea, but they also can be used in cats with lymphocytic-plasmacytic colitis, which also may be caused by food hypersensitivity.[8] Several diets on the market contain novel or hydrolyzed proteins. It may take up to 6 to 8 weeks until a complete remission is achieved after initiating the diet; however, at a minimum, a partial response must be observed in the first 1 to 2 weeks of dietary therapy.

A diet trial with a novel or hydrolyzed protein diet may not lead to remission for several reasons. First, the patient may have an inherent allergy toward the protein source in the novel protein diet. Second, the peptides of the hydrolyzed protein diet may not be small enough to prevent an allergic reaction. Last, cats may have a hypersensitivity response to other components of these diets, including preservatives and supplements. A new diet may even worsen the diarrhea in some patients. Switching to another diet often is beneficial in these situations.

Fiber is beneficial in the treatment of chronic large bowel diarrhea and also can be beneficial in small bowel diarrhea in a small number of patients. There are two forms of fiber, soluble and insoluble. Soluble fiber forms a gel in solution, which helps to slow gastrointestinal transit time. Soluble fiber also increases bacterial fermentation in the colon, providing an additional source of nutrition for the colonocytes. Insoluble fiber does not form a gel in solution and is fermented to a lesser degree by bacteria. However, insoluble fiber adds bulk to the stool, helping to improve intestinal motility. Caution should be taken when administering insoluble fiber because of the possibility of turning the diarrhea into constipation. The addition of a soluble fiber (e.g., psyllium, ¼ to ½ tsp PO q12h) often is effective in cats with large bowel diarrhea (and sometimes small bowel diarrhea), and can be added to any of the diets described above. Psyllium is unflavored and is accepted readily by most cats because it does not change the flavor of the food. It is important to note that response to a particular diet usually is not predictable, and several diets often need to be evaluated in a feeding trial before the most effective diet for an individual patient is identified.

NUTRITIONAL SUPPLEMENTS

Fructo-oligosaccharides (FOS) are a form of soluble fiber that is specifically fermentable by *Bacteroides* and *Bifidobacterium* spp., allowing these bacteria to proliferate. These organisms have been shown to be beneficial for the health of colonocytes. Because FOS support the normal intestinal microflora, FOS are considered a prebiotic. In pigs, rabbits, and rats, FOS have been shown to lead to a decreased load of pathogenic bacteria, reduced mortality, and improved fecal quality.[9] In cats, studies have shown that FOS increase fecal *Lactobacillus* spp. numbers and decrease fecal *Escherichia coli* numbers.[10] However, more research is needed to demonstrate the beneficial effect of FOS in cats with chronic diarrhea.

Glutamine is an amino acid that serves as a preferred energy substrate for enterocytes. During the early stages of inflammation and damage, enterocytes can benefit from supplementation with oral glutamine solutions.[8] In later stages of the disease, supplementation with glutamine appears to be less beneficial.[8] The clinical benefit of glutamine in cats with chronic diarrhea has not been demonstrated and is questionable.

Probiotics are organisms in foods or supplements that have favorable effects on the gastrointestinal tract when taken orally. These beneficial bacteria help to decrease inflammation and normalize fatty acid production, which facilitate a reduction of water secretion into the intestinal lumen. Also, the deoxyribonucleic acid (DNA) of the probiotic species may have immunomodulatory effects.[11] Many probiotic products are on the market, including foods that contain probiotics. However, yogurt is not recommended for this purpose because the organisms present are often killed within the acid environment of the stomach. See Chapter 11 for a complete discussion about probiotics.

ANTIBIOTICS

Antibiotics may be the first line of treatment when pathogenic bacteria are suspected of causing chronic diarrhea. Diagnostic tests such as fecal cytology, fecal culture, and measurement of enterotoxin concentrations can be beneficial when trying to identify specific organisms (see Chapters 5 and 15 in the fifth volume of this series). A variety of antibiotics can be used, depending on the disease condition that is being treated. Table 22-3 lists antibiotics, and their indications, doses, and side effects.

Metronidazole and tylosin are excellent antimicrobial choices if a definitive diagnosis has not been made. Metronidazole has antibiotic properties against *Clostridium difficile* and *Clostridium perfringens*, and also has antiprotozoal activity against *Giardia*. In addition, metronidazole has antiinflammatory properties. The mechanism of action of the antiinflammatory properties are not understood completely; however, they may be related to an inhibition of cell-mediated immunity.[12] The recommended dosage for metronidazole is 10 to 15 mg/kg PO q12h. A lower dose of 7.5 mg/kg PO q12h or 15 mg/kg PO q24h can be used for antiinflammatory effect. Side effects include anorexia and neurological signs, such as head tremors and seizures. However, neurological side effects have not been reported at a dosage of 7.5 mg/kg PO q12h, even with long-term therapy. Metronidazole can be compounded into capsules, allowing more accurate dosing and preventing hypersalivation associated with the administration of pills and liquids.

Tylosin is bacteriostatic against gram-positive organisms at doses of 10 to 15 mg/kg PO q12h. Other susceptible organisms include *C. perfringens* and some gram-negative organisms, including *Campylobacter*, but not *Enterobacter* species. Tylosin is considered to be bactericidal at doses of 25 mg/kg PO q12h. Therefore tylosin can be used when one of these organisms is identified or when antibiotic-responsive diarrhea is suspected. As there

Table 22-3 Antibiotic Agents Used Commonly in Cats with Chronic Diarrhea

Antibiotic	Usage	Dose	Side Effects
Metronidazole	Antiinflammatory, antibiotic-responsive diarrhea, *Clostridium perfringens* and *difficile*	7.5 mg/kg PO q12h	Occasional GI side effects (usually anorexia)
		10-15 mg/kg PO q12h	Neurotoxicity at higher doses and long-term use
Tylosin	Antibiotic-responsive diarrhea, antiinflammatory, *Clostridium perfringens*, *Campylobacter* spp.	25 mg/kg PO q12h	Mild GI side effects
Erythromycin	*Campylobacter* spp., *Clostridium perfringens*	10-20 mg/kg PO q8h	GI side effects
Enrofloxacin	*Campylobacter* spp., *Salmonella* spp.	2.5-5 mg/kg PO q24h	Acute blindness at higher dosages; GI side effects
Amoxicillin	*Clostridium perfringens*	22 mg/kg PO q24h	GI side effects; possible anaphylactic reactions (rare)

is currently no diagnostic test for antibiotic-responsive diarrhea in cats, tylosin is used most commonly as a trial therapy in cats with chronic diarrhea who do not respond to dietary therapy alone.

Tylosin also has immunomodulatory effects, which may be responsible for decreasing intestinal inflammation.[13] Furthermore it appears that part of the beneficial effect of tylosin is a decrease in bacterial adherence to the intestinal mucosa, thereby reducing pathogenicity.[13] Further research is needed to determine the clinical efficacy of tylosin in cats with chronic diarrhea. The author uses tylosin most frequently in cats who have severely increased serum folate concentrations, but also in cats with well-controlled inflammatory bowel disease who develop an acute exacerbation of diarrhea. Rather than calculating the exact dose, 1/8 to 1/4 teaspoon (325 to 650 mg) can be given orally, which is significantly higher than the recommended dosage of 25 mg/kg; however, this dose is safe and is easier for the owner to administer. Also, 1/8 teaspoon fits conveniently into a gelatin capsule for owners who prefer to pill their cats. Otherwise, the tylosin can be sprinkled on the cat's food (preferably canned food). However, owners should be warned that tylosin may change the taste of the food adversely.

Several other antibiotics can be used for specific bacterial infections (see Table 22-3). *Campylobacter* spp. are sensitive to erythromycin, tylosin, and fluoroquinolones. The author uses erythromycin frequently, although it often causes gastrointestinal side effects. *C. difficile* is sensitive to metronidazole (10 to 15 mg/kg PO q12h), and *C. perfringens* is sensitive to amoxicillin, metronidazole, erythromycin, and tylosin. *Salmonella* spp. are sensitive to fluoroquinolones; however, it is important to note that *Salmonella* infection is a self-limiting disease. Because of the concern for development of antimicrobial resistance, salmonellosis should be treated with antibiotics only if the cat is bacteremic.

IMMUNOSUPPRESSANTS

Immunosuppressants are the cornerstone of therapy for inflammatory bowel disease in cats. However, these agents often are used without a definitive diagnosis. When the initial diagnostic evaluation has failed to reveal a definitive diagnosis and therapeutic trials have not led to resolution of clinical signs, immunosuppressant therapy may be appropriate if the owner can not afford further diagnostic tests or the patient is considered a poor candidate for additional evaluation. In these patients, it is important to ensure that the owner is aware that it may be more difficult to obtain a definitive diagnosis after immunosuppressant therapy is started. However, this only becomes a problem if the patient fails to respond to immunosuppressive therapy or if relapses occur.

Corticosteroids are the first therapeutic choice in most patients. Prednisone, or prednisolone preferably in cats, are corticosteroids with systemic activity, and a dose of 1 to 2 mg/kg PO q12h is effective in most cats with inflammatory bowel disease. Hepatic reduction of prednisone results in the formation of prednisolone, which is the active form. Some cats have decreased hepatic reduction

of prednisone and respond better to prednisolone. Therefore feline patients who have an unsatisfactory response to prednisone should be treated with prednisolone to determine if there is an improvement. The same dosage range is used for both drugs. Some clinicians prefer to treat cats with corticosteroids and an antimicrobial, such as metronidazole, concurrently, whereas others prefer monotherapy.

Budesonide exerts local corticosteroid activity in the intestinal tract. In human beings, budesonide is absorbed completely by the intestinal mucosa, but has a high first-pass effect in the liver.[14] Although budesonide works mainly on the intestinal mucosa, some systemic effects have been observed in human beings and dogs. Budesonide suppresses the pituitary-adrenocortical axis in normal dogs and dogs with inflammatory bowel disease, despite having minimal effect on serum ALP and ALT activities, serum glucose concentration, and urine specific gravity.[14,15] The author has seen a small number of patients who have developed heart failure or diabetes mellitus while on budesonide; however, these complications are extremely rare, and a cause-and-effect relationship has not been demonstrated for any species. Because budesonide is transported directly from the intestines to the liver, the drug bypasses the stomach and pancreas; therefore it is not recommended for cats with lymphoplasmacytic gastritis or concurrent pancreatitis. The dose of budesonide that is used most commonly in cats is 1 mg PO q24h. Budesonide must be compounded because capsules for human use are manufactured in a 3-mg size. The sustained release formula of budesonide must be used for compounding. Also, budesonide must be formulated into a capsule and not into a suspension because the liquid destroys the enteric coating of the active drug.

Chlorambucil (Leukeran) is a cell-cycle nonspecific alkylating immunosuppressive agent that inhibits primary and secondary immune responses, and diminishes antigen-trapping in lymph nodes.[12] Chlorambucil can be used if corticosteroids are not effective or are not tolerated by the cat. Minimal complications usually occur at the recommended dose of 2 mg PO q48h. A mild neutropenia or decreased appetite occasionally will develop; decreasing the dosage to 1 mg PO q48h or 2 mg PO q72h may resolve these side effects. Chlorambucil should be discontinued immediately if there are severe gastrointestinal side effects or bone marrow suppression (i.e., neutropenia, anemia, and/or thrombocytopenia). Lymphopenia is a common complication because chlorambucil kills antigen-reactive cells; however, this hematological side effect does not need to be addressed.

The author recommends initiating therapy with chlorambucil at a dose of 2 mg PO q48h. A complete blood count is checked after 10 to 14 days of therapy, then 3 to 4 weeks later, and every 4 to 6 weeks subsequently. As long as the patient is tolerating the chlorambucil satisfactorily at the second recheck, the author often will start decreasing the corticosteroid dose at that time. Owners must be advised to wear gloves when handling the chlorambucil.

Cyclosporine is an immunosuppressive agent that often is used for treatment of other diseases in cats, but there are no reports of its use for diseases of the gastrointestinal tract. (See Chapter 33 for a discussion of the use of cyclosporine in feline atopic disease.) Cyclosporine is used as a rescue agent for human patients with severe ulcerative colitis.[16] The drug has been used successfully in dogs with inflammatory bowel disease.[17] Further studies are required to determine whether cyclosporine also would be beneficial in cats with the same problem. Azathioprine is not recommended for use in cats because of its severe immunosuppressant properties in this species.

COBALAMIN

Cobalamin (vitamin B_{12}) is an important vitamin that is needed for several enzymatic reactions, two of which are extremely important from a medical standpoint. Methionine synthase facilitates the conversion of homocysteine to methionine. Methionine then is converted through several steps to L-methylmalonyl-CoA and methylmalonic acid. Methylmalonyl-CoA mutase is an enzyme that is required for the conversion of L-methylmalonyl-CoA to succinyl-CoA, which is involved in the tricarboxylic acid cycle (Figure 22-3).[18]

Cobalamin is absorbed in the ileum (see Figure 15-8). Cobalamin is released from dietary protein in the stomach through protein digestion. Cobalamin then binds to R-protein (haptocorrin) in the stomach. Once in the duodenum, pancreatic enzymes degrade the haptocorrin. Cobalamin then is bound to intrinsic factor, which is synthesized exclusively by the exocrine pancreas in cats. The cobalamin-intrinsic factor complexes bind to specific receptors in the ileum called cubilin. Cobalamin is absorbed by ileal enterocytes and then is transported into the blood stream. Cobalamin binds to transcobalamin 2 within the vascular space, allowing absorption of cobalamin by target cells.[19]

Cobalamin deficiency in human beings has been associated with megaloblastic anemia, decreased cognitive function, increased arteriosclerosis, and a risk of vascular thrombosis. In cats serum cobalamin levels can be used as a marker for gastrointestinal disease. However, cobalamin deficiency in itself is associated with weight loss and anorexia in cats with gastrointestinal disease.[20] Cats with gastrointestinal, hepatic, or pancreatic disease who also have hypocobalaminemia may have a poor response to other therapies if not supplemented.

For cats with chronic diarrhea and concurrent hypocobalaminemia, treatment should be initiated with pure cobalamin at a dose of 250 µg SQ q7d for 6 weeks. The frequency of administration then is decreased to q14d for 6 weeks. One more dose is given 1 month later. Serum cobalamin concentration should be rechecked 1 month after the last dose.[21] The reader is referred to Chapter 13 in the fifth volume of this series for a discussion of the role of cobalamin in the diagnosis and treatment of chronic gastrointestinal disease.

MISCELLANEOUS AGENTS

Activated charcoal and barium have been used successfully by some clinicians to treat cats with chronic diarrhea. In general, these agents have low toxicity but also low efficacy. The theory behind the mode of action of both agents is that they bind to bacterial toxins and soothe the inflamed intestinal mucosa. The author only uses barium in patients in whom there has been severe

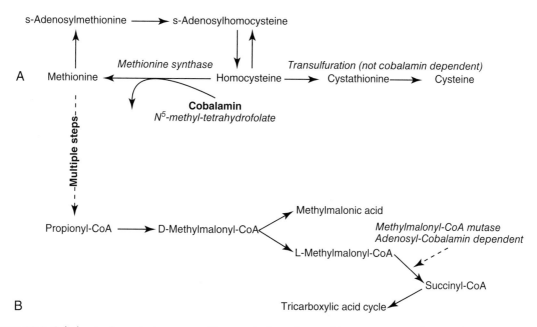

Figure 22-3 Cobalamin-dependent enzymes. The metabolic pathway of homocysteine to the tricarboxylic acid cycle. This pathway requires two cobalamin-dependent enzymes, methionine synthase and methylmalonyl-CoA mutase. (Reproduced with permission from Ruaux CG, Steiner JM, Williams DA: Early biochemical and clinical responses to cobalamin supplementation in cats with signs of gastrointestinal disease and severe hypocobalaminemia, *J Vet Intern Med* 19:155, 2005.)

Table 22-4 Uses, Dosage, and Side Effects for Nonantibiotic Therapeutic Agents Used for Chronic Diarrhea in Cats

Therapy	Uses	Dose	Side Effects
Prednisone or prednisolone	Inflammatory bowel disease	1-2 mg/kg PO q12h, then decreasing	Diabetes mellitus, gastrointestinal ulcerations, heart failure
Budesonide	Inflammatory bowel disease	1 mg PO q24h	Can lead to some systemic side effects
Leukeran	Inflammatory bowel disease	2 mg PO q48h	Anorexia, bone marrow suppression, lymphopenia
Cyclosporine	Possibly inflammatory bowel disease, colitis	Unknown at this time	Immunosuppression, anorexia, vomiting
Cobalamin	Hypocobalaminemia	250 μg SQ q7d for 6 weeks, then see text	None known
Barium	Gastrointestinal bleeding	5 mL PO q4h	Vomiting, aspiration, anorexia

gastrointestinal bleeding. A dose of 5 mL PO q4h is appropriate in such cases.

Bismuth has antienterotoxin, antibacterial, antisecretory, and antiinflammatory properties. Caution must be exercised when used in cats because many of the preparations containing bismuth also include salicylate compounds.

Opiate antidiarrheal drugs (e.g., Imodium) may help to control clinical signs by stimulating circular smooth muscle contraction and may also increase water absorption. However, opiates are not recommended for use in cats because they may lead to excitatory behavior.

SUMMARY

Many options are available for the treatment of chronic diarrhea in cats (see Tables 22-2 to 22-4). Therapeutic choices are based on a definitive diagnosis when available, or are part of the diagnostic evaluation itself. Noninvasive diagnostic tests, such as abdominal ultrasound, *Giardia* ELISA, *Clostridium* enterotoxin assays, serum concentrations of feline pancreatic lipase immunoreactivity, feline trypsin-like immunoreactivity, cobalamin and folate, fecal flotation, and fecal direct smear all may aid in obtaining a diagnosis. Often a definitive diagnosis cannot be made without more invasive diagnostic tests, such as intestinal biopsies. With a range of therapeutic options available, chronic diarrhea can be treated successfully in most affected cats.

REFERENCES

1. Scorza AV, Radecki SV, Lappin MR: Efficacy of a combination of febantel, pyrantel, and praziquantel for the treatment of kittens experimentally infected with *Giardia* species, *J Feline Med Surg* 8:7, 2006.
2. Scorza AV, Lappin MR: Metronidazole for the treatment of feline giardiasis, *J Feline Med Surg* 6:157, 2004.
3. Keith CL, Radecki SV, Lappin MR: Evaluation of fenbendazole for the treatment of *Giardia* infection in cats concurrently infected with *Cryptosporidium parvum*, *Am J Vet Res* 64:1027, 2003.
4. Stein JE, Radecki SV, Lappin MR: Efficacy of *Giardia* vaccination in the treatment of giardiasis in cats, *J Am Vet Med Assoc* 222:1548, 2003.
5. Foster DM, Gookin JL, Poore MF, et al: Outcome of cats with diarrhea and *Tritrichomonas foetus* infection, *J Am Vet Med Assoc* 225:888, 2004.
6. Gookin JL, Coople CN, Papich MG, et al: Efficacy of ronidazole for treatment of feline *Tritrichomonas foetus* infection, *J Vet Intern Med* 20:536, 2006.
7. Rosado TW, Specht A, Marks SL: Neurotoxicosis in 4 cats receiving ronidazole, *J Vet Intern Med* 21:328, 2007.
8. Davenport DJ, Remillard RL, Simpson KW, et al: Gastrointestinal and exocrine pancreatic disease. In Hand MS, Thatcher CD, Remillard RL, et al, editors: *Small animal clinical nutrition*, ed 4, Marceline, MO, 2000, Walsworth, p 725.
9. Gross KL, Wedekind KJ, Cowell CS, et al: Nutrients. In Hand MS, Thatcher CD, Remillard RL, et al, editors: *Small animal clinical nutrition*, ed 4, Marceline, MO, 2000, Walsworth, p 40.
10. Sparkes AH, Papasouliotis K, Sunvold G, et al: Effect of dietary supplementation with fructo-oligosaccharides on fecal flora of healthy cats, *Am J Vet Res* 59:436, 1998.
11. Watson JL, McKay DM: The immunophysiological impact of bacterial CpG DNA on the gut, *Clin Chim Acta* 364:1, 2006.
12. Plumb DC: *Plumb's veterinary drug handbook*, ed 6, Ames, IA, 2008, Blackwell.
13. Westermarck E, Skrzypczak T, Harmoinen J, et al: Tylosin-responsive chronic diarrhea in dogs, *J Vet Intern Med* 19:177, 2005.
14. Stroup ST, Behrend EN, Kemppainen RJ, et al: Effects of oral administration of controlled-ileal-release budesonide and assessment of pituitary-adrenocortical axis suppression in clinically normal dogs, *Am J Vet Res* 67:1173, 2006.
15. Tumulty JW, Broussard JD, Steiner JM: Clinical effects of short-term oral budesonide on the hypothalamic-pituitary-adrenal axis in dogs with inflammatory bowel disease, *J Am Anim Hosp Assoc* 40:120, 2004.
16. Swaminath A, Kornbluch A: Optimizing drug therapy in inflammatory bowel disease, *Curr Gastroenterol Rep* 9:513, 2007.
17. Allenspach K, Rufenacht S, Sauter S, et al: Pharmacokinetics and clinical efficacy of cyclosporine treatment of dogs with steroid refractory inflammatory bowel disease, *J Vet Intern Med* 20:239, 2006.

18. Ruaux CG, Steiner JM, Williams DA: Metabolism of amino acids in cats with severe cobalamin deficiency, *Am J Vet Res* 62:1852, 2001.

19. Simpson KW, Fyfe J, Cornetta A, et al: Subnormal concentrations of serum cobalamin (vitamin B12) in cats with gastrointestinal disease, *J Vet Intern Med* 15:26, 2001.

20. Ruaux CG, Steiner JM, Williams DA: Early biochemical and clinical responses to cobalamin supplementation in cats with signs of gastrointestinal disease and severe hypocobalaminemia, *J Vet Intern Med* 19:155, 2005.

21. Steiner JM: Diarrhea. In Ettinger SJ, Feldman EC, editors: *Textbook of veterinary internal medicine*, ed 6, St. Louis, Elsevier, 2005, p 137.

SECTION
IV

Endocrine and Metabolic Disease

Ellen N. Behrend, Section Editor

249

23 Answers to Commonly Asked Endocrine Diagnostic Questions

Robert J. Kemppainen

The following questions represent frequent enquiries received by our endocrine service regarding endocrine testing in cats. The questions center mainly on testing for adrenal and thyroid problems, because our laboratory provides assays evaluating function of these tissues. Questions regarding testing for reproductive problems are not covered. The questions and answers that follow may be considered, to a degree, to be lab-specific, because reference ranges and some interpretative advice vary among testing laboratories. Readers should understand that the endocrine testing field is evolving constantly, and options as to selection of the best test and how to interpret its results change over time. Therefore these answers are subject to change and it is always best to contact the laboratory to get the latest information.

GENERAL QUESTIONS

SHOULD I SUBMIT SERUM OR PLASMA SAMPLES FOR HORMONE ANALYSIS?

Testing laboratories vary in their recommendations for the type of sample for each assay. In our laboratory serum is preferred for thyroid hormone testing (total thyroxine [T$_4$] and free T$_4$). Samples for free T$_4$ measurement should be sent with refrigeration (i.e., frozen gel packs) if it is likely that transit to the lab will require more than 3 days. No cooling is needed for samples for total T$_4$. For cortisol measurement (e.g., dexamethasone suppression or adrenocorticotropic hormone [ACTH] stimulation testing), either serum or EDTA-plasma can be submitted. If serum is used, it is best to refrigerate samples during shipment. If EDTA-plasma is collected, samples do not require refrigeration if they are shipped to arrive within 2 days. We recommend serum for samples submitted for insulin measurement, whereas EDTA-plasma should be collected for endogenous ACTH determination.

QUESTIONS ABOUT ADRENAL FUNCTION TESTING

WHICH IS THE BEST TEST TO DIAGNOSE HYPERADRENOCORTICISM (CUSHING'S DISEASE) IN CATS?

We prefer the dexamethasone suppression test (over the ACTH stimulation test), using a dose of 0.1 mg/kg intravenously (IV) of dexamethasone. Note that this dose is equivalent to that used for high-dose dexamethasone testing in dogs. To perform the test, collect a presample of cortisol and then administer dexamethasone IV. Collect post-dexamethasone cortisol samples at 4 and 8 hours postinjection. Cats with spontaneous hyperadrenocorticism usually have post-dexamethasone cortisol concentrations (at 4 and/or at 8 hours) above 35 nmol/L (1.3 µg/dL).

Once the disease has been diagnosed differentiation of the pituitary-dependent form from a cortisol-secreting adrenocortical tumor is recommended. Tests that may be used for this purpose include high-dose dexamethasone suppression, following the same protocol given above except using 1 mg/kg of the drug. A post-dexamethasone cortisol concentration below 35 nmol/L and/or less than 50 per cent compared with the prevalue at 4 or 8 hours is consistent with pituitary-dependent disease. The failure to observe adequate suppression of cortisol concentrations can not be taken to confirm an adrenocortical tumor, and additional tests should be used in this instance. Other tests for differentiation include measurement of endogenous ACTH concentrations (high to high-normal in cats with pituitary-dependent disease, and low or not detectable in cats with functional adrenocortical tumors) and diagnostic imaging (ultrasound, radiography, computed tomography, and/or magnetic resonance imaging).

WHEN IS AN ACTH STIMULATION TEST OF USE IN CATS? HOW DO I PERFORM THE TEST?

The ACTH stimulation test can be used to diagnose spontaneous hyperadrenocorticism; however, the test is not as sensitive as the dexamethasone suppression test (in our experience) for this purpose (response to ACTH is normal in up to 50 per cent of cats with the disease).[1,2] The ACTH stimulation test is the method of choice to diagnose spontaneous hypoadrenocorticism (Addison's disease) and iatrogenic Cushing's disease, as well as to monitor therapy for hyperadrenocorticism if the cat is receiving a drug that inhibits adrenal cortisol secretion (e.g., mitotane, trilostane).

To perform the test, collect a presample of cortisol and administer Cortrosyn (Amphastar Pharmaceuticals, Inc, Rancho Cucamonga, CA; also known as cosyntropin or synthetic ACTH) at a dose of 0.125 µg per cat IV (this is equivalent to half of the ACTH in one vial). Collect a postsample cortisol 1 hour later. Intravenous injection is preferred; the adrenal response to Cortrosyn given intramuscularly (IM) is less and of shorter duration. In our laboratory normal resting (pre-ACTH) concentrations of cortisol in cats range from 10 to 110 nmol/L (0.4-4 µg/dL), and post-ACTH concentrations range from 210 to 330 nmol/L (7.6 to 12 µg/dL). If Cortrosyn is unavailable, compounded forms of ACTH could be considered for use; however, we have not evaluated their efficacy in cats. Compounded ACTH should be given IM and at least two post-ACTH cortisol samples should be submitted; the first at one hour, and the second at two hours after ACTH injection.

IS THERE VALUE IN MEASURING URINE CORTISOL:CREATININE RATIO IN CATS?

Yes. Determination of the urine cortisol:creatinine ratio can be a useful screening tool for spontaneous hyperadrenocorticism. A urine sample should be collected at home if feasible, to reduce possible stress-related effects associated with hospital collection. The finding of a normal ratio suggests that hyperadrenocorticism is unlikely. An elevated ratio means that hyperadrenocorticism is possible, and warrants a follow-up test such as dexamethasone suppression.

QUESTIONS ABOUT THYROID FUNCTION TESTING

DOES THE FINDING OF A NORMAL TOTAL T$_4$ LEVEL IN A HYPERTHYROID-SUSPECT CAT RULE OUT THE DISEASE?

No. The majority of, but certainly not all, cats with hyperthyroidism have total T$_4$ levels above the normal range. Cats with early or mild hyperthyroidism, or hyperthyroid cats affected concurrently by nonthyroidal disease (e.g., renal diseases, diabetes mellitus, systemic neoplasia, liver disease, chronic illness) may have total T$_4$ levels in the normal range. If hyperthyroidism is suspected in an older cat and the total T$_4$ concentration is in the upper part of the normal range (our normal range, 10 to 50 nmol/L [0.8 to 3.9 µg/dL]; upper normal, 25 to 50 nmol/L [1.9 to 3.9 µg/dL]), the disease should not be ruled out, particularly if a nodule is palpable in the neck. We recommend measuring free T$_4$ by equilibrium dialysis (see the following) in such cases.

WHAT IS THE VALUE OF MEASURING FREE T$_4$ LEVELS IN CATS?

This test is the one we recommend for hyperthyroid-suspect cats who have total T$_4$ levels in the upper normal range. The assay should be of the equilibrium dialysis type. Provided enough serum was collected, the test can be performed using the same sample submitted for total T$_4$. The majority of true hyperthyroid cats with total T$_4$ levels in the upper part of normal range will have elevated levels of free T$_4$ by dialysis. Free T$_4$ concentrations near the top of the normal range are suspicious for the disease and warrant retesting with total and free T$_4$ determinations in a few weeks or months; alternatively, these patients could be evaluated for hyperthyroidism using another test. Other endocrine tests used for this purpose include triiodothyronine (T$_3$) suppression and TRH stimulation.

It is important to note that it is NOT recommended to screen cats for hyperthyroidism by measuring free T$_4$ alone. The reason is that approximately 10 per cent of euthyroid cats with nonthyroidal disease have elevated free T$_4$ levels. What distinguishes these cats from being hyperthyroid is that they have low or low normal levels of total T_4, whereas total T_4 in hyperthyroid cats is high-normal or high.

DOES THE FINDING OF AN ELEVATED TOTAL T_4 IN A CAT MEAN THAT THE PATIENT IS HYPERTHYROID?

In our opinion the answer is yes. Aside from the possibility of sample submission error, laboratory error (it would be worth confirming the finding in young cats or cats not showing typical signs), or cats inadvertently receiving exogenous T_4, we know of no reason for a "false positive" total T_4 test result. We have not found, for example, that cats have T_4 autoantibodies, a phenomenon seen occasionally in dogs that is associated with falsely elevated total T_4 concentrations. Certainly the finding of an elevated total T_4 in an asymptomatic cat warrants a thorough physical examination and careful review of the patient's history. In addition, we would recommend periodic (every 3 to 4 months) retesting of total T_4 (and possibly free T_4) to evaluate trends in conjunction with noting any changes in the cat's condition, assuming the decision is made to not treat the cat for hyperthyroidism.

WHAT IS THE BEST WAY TO MONITOR METHIMAZOLE THERAPY?

Besides assessment of the clinical response, periodic measurement of total T_4 levels is highly recommended for monitoring purposes in all cats receiving methimazole. We do not see a reason to recommend use of the free T_4 assay for routine monitoring purposes. Total T_4 concentration is determined 2 to 3 weeks after starting methimazole, or after any dosage adjustments. For routine monitoring of cats on long-term therapy, measurement of total T_4 two to three times per year is recommended. The time of sample collection relative to methimazole administration (PO or topically) is not critical. Ideal total T_4 levels are in the lower half of the normal range (i.e., 10 to 25 nmol/L; 0.8 to 1.9 µg/dL). Depending on the clinical response, dosage adjustments can be made (up or down) to maintain total T_4 near this target range. Monitoring of the biochemical profile (especially liver enzymes and renal function) in conjunction with a complete blood count also is recommended every 2 to 3 weeks in the first 3 months of methimazole therapy, to monitor for renal failure and serious adverse effects (i.e., hepatopathy, thrombocytopenia, and agranulocytosis).

If iodinated contrast agents (e.g., ipodate or iopanoic acid) are used to manage hyperthyroidism, total T_3 concentrations should be determined for monitoring effectiveness, because these agents inhibit the conversion of T_4 to T_3.[3] Clinical signs also should be monitored, because some cats have ongoing clinical signs despite normalization of T_3 concentrations.

QUESTIONS ABOUT ACROMEGALY

I SUSPECT THAT THE INSULIN RESISTANCE IN THE DIABETIC CAT I AM TREATING MAY BE CAUSED BY ACROMEGALY. HOW DO I TEST FOR THIS PROBLEM?

Acromegaly in cats usually is caused by a growth hormone–secreting pituitary tumor. Virtually all affected cats have diabetes mellitus and are severely insulin-resistant. An interesting study reported that the incidence of acromegaly in diabetic cats may be significantly greater than thought previously.[4] There appears to be no single endocrine test at present that can diagnose the condition conclusively. Growth hormone measurement is becoming available in the United States, but some data suggest that measurement of this hormone is not diagnostic in all cases.[5] Probably the best endocrine test available presently is the measurement of insulin-like growth factor-1 (IGF-1) levels. Levels of IGF-1 usually are elevated in acromegalic cats.[6] False-positive results (elevated IGF-1 levels in cats not affected with acromegaly) have been reported, particularly in diabetic cats on long-term insulin therapy.[6] The finding of an elevated IGF-1 level in a diabetic cat with insulin resistance, in conjunction with signs consistent with the disease (e.g., being male or having weight gain, respiratory stridor, or enlargement of the head and feet) raise the suspicion of acromegaly to a high degree. Confirmation of the disease should be done using CT or MRI imaging of the pituitary gland (see Chapter 29).

REFERENCES

1. Peterson ME: Feline hyperadrenocorticism. In Mooney CT, Peterson ME, editors: *BSAVA manual of canine and feline endocrinology*, ed 3, Quedseley, Gloucester, UK, 2004, British Small Animal Veterinary Association, p 205.
2. Chiaramonte D, Greco DS: Feline adrenal disorders, *Clin Tech Small Anim Pract* 22:26, 2007.
3. Trepanier LA: Medical treatment of feline hyperthyroidism. In Bonagura JD, Twedt DC, editors: *Kirk's current veterinary therapy XIV*, St. Louis, 2009, Saunders, p 175.
4. Niessen SJM, Petrie G, Gaudiano M, et al: Feline acromegaly: an underdiagnosed endocrinopathy? *J Vet Intern Med* 21:899, 2007.
5. Reusch CE, Klet S, Casella M, et al: Measurements of growth hormone and insulin-like growth factor 1 in cats with diabetes mellitus, *Vet Rec* 158:195, 2006.
6. Berg RIM, Nelson RW, Feldman EC, et al: Serum insulin-like growth factor-1 concentration in cats with diabetes mellitus and acromegaly, *J Vet Intern Med* 21:892, 2007.

24 Primary Hyperaldosteronism

Kent R. Refsal and Andrea M. Harvey

Primary hyperaldosteronism (PHA) has been recognized as the leading cause of endocrine-mediated hypertension in human beings. Since Conn's first association of mineralocorticoid excess with an adrenocortical tumor,[1] hyperaldosteronism also has been attributed to primary idiopathic adrenal hyperplasia, defects in synthesis and metabolism of adrenal steroids, and rare instances of renin-secreting tumors. In the past decade, a series of case reports in cats has raised awareness of PHA as a cause of hypertension and hypokalemia, with the possibility of added complications of excesses of other adrenal steroids. The knowledge base from human medicine will be an invaluable asset as veterinarians improve the ability to diagnose and manage this disorder.

THE RENIN-ANGIOTENSIN-ALDOSTERONE SYSTEM AND CLASSIFICATION OF HYPERALDOSTERONISM

The renin-angiotensin-aldosterone system (RAAS) acts to maintain the volume of extracellular fluid, circulatory pressure, and electrolyte homeostasis through integrated effects of enzymes and hormones, chiefly on the vasculature and kidney (Figure 24-1), and continues to be a subject of review in the scientific literature.[2-4] The juxtaglomerular cells that line afferent arterioles of the renal glomeruli both synthesize prorenin and remove a segment of its N-terminus to form active renin, which is stored in

secretory granules. Both prorenin and renin are released from juxtaglomerular cells, the former in a tonic pattern and the latter in response to regulated pathways.[5] Active release of renin is stimulated predominantly by decreased renal perfusion detected by baroreceptors in the afferent arterioles. Other stimuli for renin release include a decrease in sodium content in glomerular filtrate, as detected by the macula densa cells of the proximal tubule, and sympathetic nerve stimulation via β-adrenergic receptors. In the circulation, renin acts on angiotensinogen, a protein synthesized in the liver, to cleave a decapeptide, angiotensin I, from the N-terminus. A peptidase, angiotensin-converting enzyme, removes two amino acids from the C terminal of angiotensin I to form angiotensin II, which has potent biological effects. The principal effects of angiotensin II arise from its binding to type 1 receptors to mediate vasoconstriction, promote renal tubular reabsorption of sodium, stimulate release of aldosterone from the adrenal cortex, and exert negative feedback on the release of renin.

Aldosterone is synthesized from cholesterol through a series of intermediary metabolites including progesterone, 11-deoxycorticosterone, and corticosterone (Figure 24-2) in the zona glomerulosa of the adrenal cortex. In addition to stimulus from angiotensin II, aldosterone is released in a direct response to hyperkalemia and to a lesser effect of adrenocorticotropic hormone (ACTH) from the anterior pituitary gland. After secretion into the circulation, aldosterone enters target tissues and exerts its effects through binding to mineralocorticoid receptors, which have affinity for, and are activated by, both cortisol and aldosterone. Mineralocorticoid-responsive tissues of epithelial origin (e.g., renal tubule, colon, sweat glands, and salivary glands) express the enzyme 11β-hydroxysteroid dehydrogenase type 2, which converts cortisol to cortisone, a steroid that does not bind to the mineralocorticoid receptor and enables access by aldosterone to the receptor. In the kidneys aldosterone acts on the distal collecting tubule and collecting ducts to stimulate activity of epithelial sodium channels, promoting sodium reabsorption with concurrent loss of potassium and hydrogen ions. Therefore, when stimulated, the classic cascade of events in the RAAS results in an increase of circulatory pressure via vasoconstriction and retention of sodium. Mineralocorticoid receptors in nonepithelial tissues have minimal 11β-hydroxysteroid dehydrogenase 2 activity and may be maintained in a tonic inactivated mode when occupied by cortisol.[6] The role of these receptors and aldosterone-mediated effects in inflammation and fibrosis occurring with cardiac, renal, and vascular disease, and metabolic syndrome is under active investigation.[6-9]

Hyperaldosteronism, or increased aldosterone secretion, can arise from a primary or secondary origin. PHA refers to excessive production from autonomous adrenal dysfunction. The ensuing effects of sodium retention and hypertension result in suppression of renin and angiotensin. Secondary hyperaldosteronism refers to increased aldosterone production in response to increased stimulation by the renin-angiotensin system. In most instances secondary hyperaldosteronism arises as a compensatory physiological response to counteract dehydration, hypotension, or sodium deficiency (reduced intake or increased loss). However, pathological manifestations of mineralocorticoid excess can arise from conditions of secondary hyperaldosteronism, notably from reduced renal perfusion secondary to renal disease or from rare instances of renin-secreting tumors.[10]

OVERVIEW OF PRIMARY HYPERALDOSTERONISM IN HUMAN BEINGS

ADRENAL ADENOMA AND IDIOPATHIC HYPERPLASIA

Three extensive reviews of these disorders have been published recently and serve as the main source of information for this discussion.[11-13] Adrenal adenoma and idiopathic hyperplasia account for more than 95 per cent of the diagnoses of human hyperaldosteronism, with idiopathic hyperplasia being more common than adrenal adenoma (60 per cent versus 35 per cent). Both conditions can occur with unilateral (most adenomas) or bilat-

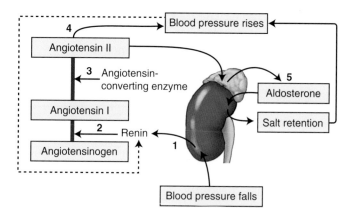

Figure 24-1 Sequence of physiological events in the renin-angiotensin-aldosterone system for regulation of blood pressure. (From *Am J Hypertens* 21:7, 2008, with permission.)

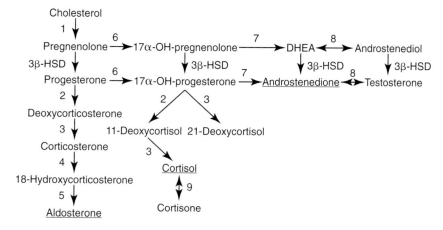

Figure 24-2 Illustration of the biosynthetic pathways and enzymes for mineralocorticoids, glucocorticoids, and androgens in the adrenal cortex. Enzymes involved (corresponding gene) are as follows: 1, cholesterol desmolase (*CYP11A*); 2, 21-hydroxylase (*CYP21*); 3, 11β-hydroxylase (*CYP11B1*); 4, 18-hydroxylase; 5, 18-oxidase; 6, 17β-hydroxylase (*CYP17*); 7, 17,20-lyase (*CYP17*); 8, 17β-hydroxysteroid dehydrogenase; 9, 11β-hydroxysteroid dehydrogenase. *3β-HSD*, 3β-Hydroxysteroid dehydrogenase/Δ5-Δ4-isomerase; *DHEA*, dehydroepiandrosterone. (From Sieber-Ruckstuhl NS, Boretti FS, Wenger M et al: Cortisol, aldosterone, cortisol precursor, androgen and endogenous ACTH concentrations in dogs with pituitary-dependent hyperadrenocorticism treated with trilostane. *Domest Anim Endocrinol* 31:63, 2006.)

eral (most hyperplasia) distribution. Risk factors to initiate screening for hyperaldosteronism include presence of refractory hypertension, unexplained hypokalemia, an adrenal mass, or a family history. Categorization of the lesion is based on histopathological examination of the adrenal cortex (hyperplasia versus microadenoma or macroadenoma). At the time of diagnosis more than 60 per cent of affected persons are normokalemic, with hypokalemia more likely to occur with adrenal adenomas.[13-15]

The steps for diagnostic evaluation are to document an inappropriate excess of aldosterone secretion, and then to determine whether it is from a unilateral or bilateral adrenal source. Localization of a unilateral lesion is of importance for the opportunity of resolving clinical signs with adrenalectomy. Bilateral conditions, whether caused by hyperplasia or adenoma, are best managed by mineralocorticoid receptor antagonists such as spironolactone or eplerenone. Thus a sequence of screening (or case finding) and confirmatory tests are performed, followed by procedures to distinguish unilateral from bilateral sources of aldosterone excess. These tests require preparatory measures by patients, do not always give conclusive results, and are not without risk of adverse reaction.

The aldosterone to renin ratio (ARR) is regarded as the most reliable screening test. Pretesting preparation includes an attempt to correct hypokalemia, an increase in sodium intake if on a restricted diet, and/or withdrawal of therapeutic agents that alter the ARR (e.g., mineralocorticoid receptor antagonists, potassium-sparing or -wasting diuretics, products containing licorice root) for at least 4 weeks.[13] False-positive ARR results most commonly are a result of very low renin activity, which may be attributable to performance capabilities of the renin activity assay, potassium or sodium loading, administration of other medications, or presence of concurrent diseases. Tests to confirm PHA assess the response to treatments designed to suppress circulating aldosterone concentrations. At present the tests considered most commonly are oral sodium loading, saline infusion, fludrocortisone administration with sodium supplementation, and the captopril challenge test,[13] but no confirmatory test is regarded as the "gold standard." An apparent increasing prevalence of PHA has raised controversy, with some authors suggesting an epidemic while others caution against overestimation of its occurrence.[12,16-20]

When screening and confirmatory tests support the existence of PHA, diagnostic measures are employed for localization. Often the initial test is a computed tomography (CT) scan of the adrenal glands to identify or exclude a large mass characteristic of an adrenocortical carcinoma. Limitations with CT include inconsistency in distinguishing small adenomas (<1 cm) from bilateral idiopathic hyperplasia or detection of an incidental nonfunctional neoplasm when there is bilateral hyperplasia. If the patient is a candidate for surgery, and CT results are not clearly indicative of an adrenal mass, adrenal venous sampling (AVS) is the procedure of choice. A catheter is inserted in a femoral vein and threaded into the caudal vena cava. Samples are collected from the inferior phrenic vein adjacent to the opening of the left adrenal vein and from the right adrenal vein. A "peripheral" sample is collected from the iliac vein. Aldosterone and cortisol concentrations are measured in all samples. Comparison of cortisol and aldosterone results in the three samples provides, first, an indication of the success of adrenal vein catheterization and, second, information on whether there is asymmetry of aldosterone concentrations in adrenal venous samples. If a patient is not a candidate for AVS or does not have access to a center performing the procedure, adrenal scintigraphy provides a means for localization of aldosterone production. Current protocols use ^{131}I-6β-iodomethyl-19-norcholesterol (NP-59) as the labeled agent. Patients are pretreated with dexamethasone and saturated potassium iodine to minimize uptake of NP-59 by adrenal cells for cortisol synthesis and to block thyroidal uptake of free ^{131}I. A summation of the diagnostic performance of scintigraphy across 11 studies showed an overall 82 per cent diagnostic sensitivity, 78 per cent specificity, and 82 per cent accuracy in identification of aldosterone-producing adenomas.[21] A limitation of this procedure is low uptake of labeled agent by small adrenal adenomas.

ADRENOCORTICAL CARCINOMA

Adrenocortical carcinomas account for less than 1 per cent of cases of PHA in human patients.[11] The diagnosis is based on screening and confirmatory tests as outlined, and on identification of an adrenal mass (usually >4 cm) on CT examination. Adrenal carcinomas also may exhibit variation in steroidogenic production, with clinical signs related to mineralocorticoid excess only, or mixed effects of glucocorticoid, mineralocorticoid, and/or sex steroid production.[22] Some carcinomas possess little or no 11β-hydroxylase activity, thus having minimal, if any, aldosterone secretion (see Figure 24-2). Signs of mineralocorticoid excess are caused by increased deoxycorticosterone production, leaving low or nondetectable circulating aldosterone concentrations, as has been reported in human beings and a dog.[22,23]

FAMILIAL CAUSES OF HYPERALDOSTERONISM

Familial hyperaldosteronism type I (glucocorticoid-remediable hyperaldosteronism) occurs in 0.5 to 1 per cent of cases of PHA. Affected persons usually are not hypokalemic but have a variable severity of hypertension. Suspicion for this disorder is raised by the presence of hypertension and cerebrovascular complications at a young age and a familial history of these occurrences. Initial confirmation of hyperaldosteronism is based on screening and confirmatory tests as described above. Findings of imaging studies and AVS testing are not unlike those of bilateral adrenal hyperplasia.[24] The etiology is a hybrid gene derived from the 5′ regulatory sequence of the 11β-hydroxylase gene (*CYP11B1*) with the 3′ coding sequence from the aldosterone synthetase gene (*CYP11B2*).[25-27] Therefore cells in the zona glomerulosa secrete aldosterone in response to ACTH rather than angiotensin II, and cells in the zona fasciculata produce hybrid steroids such as 18-hydroxycortisol or 18-oxo-cortisol. Measurement of 18-hydroxysteroids is the most definitive biochemical indicator in diagnosis.[24] Familial hyperaldosteronism type I has an autosomal dominant mode of inheritance and a genetic test is available.[26] Administration of dexamethasone results in decreases in glucocorticoid and mineralocorticoid concentrations, and blood pressure, serving as the basis for treatment of glucocorticoid-remediable hyperaldosteronism. Familial hyperaldosteronism type II (non–glucocorticoid-remedi-able hyperaldosteronism) refers to the familial occurrence of hyperaldosteronism owing to adrenocortical adenoma or hyperplasia. Genetic studies of families in Australia, Italy, and South America have identified a linkage of these causes of hyperaldosteronism with chromosome 7p22.[28]

Apparent mineralocorticoid excess is a rare disorder in which hypertension and hypokalemia are identified in young children. Plasma renin activity and circulating aldosterone concentrations are low. The etiology is a result of inactivating mutations of the gene encoding 11β-hydroxysteroid dehydrogenase type 2, which are inherited as an autosomal recessive trait. The mutations allow cortisol to gain access to the mineralocorticoid receptor.[29] The biochemical marker for this disorder is reduction of serum concentrations of cortisone and its metabolites in relation to cortisol. Nephrocalcinosis has been reported in association with apparent mineralocorticoid excess.[29,30] Restriction of dietary sodium is of benefit in controlling hypertension. Other therapeutic measures include administration of combinations of potassium supplementation, mineralocorticoid receptor antagonists, or hydrochlorothiazide.

FELINE PRIMARY HYPERALDOSTERONISM

BACKGROUND AND PATHOGENESIS

The first feline case of hyperaldosteronism related to an adrenocortical carcinoma was reported in 1983 involving a 17-year-old domestic shorthair cat presenting with hypokalemic polymyopathy.[31] Since 1999 PHA has been reported in 34 more cats. Adrenocortical adenoma or adenocarcinoma was identified in 23 cats.[32-41] Of these 23 cats, 13 were included in a single case series[36]; the series allowed a more detailed profile of this disease to be described. Interestingly, nine of the 13 cats were diagnosed at a single first opinion practice in the United Kingdom, raising the possibility that the condition might be more common than thought previously.

Unilateral adrenocortical neoplasia (adenoma or carcinoma) is the most commonly described cause of PHA in cats.[31-41] In contrast to human beings in whom adrenal carcinomas are very rare, unilateral adrenal adenomas and carcinomas appear to have approximately equal incidence in cats. Bilateral adrenal neoplasms also have been described in cats. Interestingly one patient initially had a left adrenal adenoma removed surgically, but by 2 years later the cat developed a right adrenal carcinoma.[33] Two cases of bilateral adrenal adenomas have been identified,

but for both cases the bilateral nature of adrenal disease was only discovered at postmortem examination, highlighting the necessity for careful evaluation of both adrenal glands.[36]

Aldosterone-producing adrenal neoplasms also have been recognized in conjunction with other endocrinopathies. Multiple endocrine neoplasia type 1 was reported in one cat with an aldosterone-producing adenoma and concurrent insulinoma and functional parathyroid adenoma.[38] One of the authors of this chapter (AH) has observed both hyperthyroidism and PHA in cats. Some adrenocortical tumors, especially carcinomas, may secrete glucocorticoids or sex steroids in addition to mineralocorticoids. Concurrent diabetes mellitus and primary hyperadrenocorticism have been reported.[32,37] To date there have not been detailed studies of steroid profiles in cats with PHA, but excessive co-secretion of glucocorticoid or progesterone may explain the occurrence of both hyperaldosteronism and diabetes mellitus.[37]

In 2005, a series of 11 cats were described as having nontumorous PHA, providing evidence for a feline counterpart of bilateral adrenal hyperplasia in human beings.[42] Most of these cats had laboratory evidence of mild renal disease. Three of the 11 cats with bilateral adrenal hyperplasia underwent necropsy with identification of bilateral nodular hyperplasia of the zona glomerulosa. Histopathological changes in the kidneys revealed hyaline arteriolar sclerosis, glomerular sclerosis, tubular atrophy, and interstitial fibrosis. Thus the causes of PHA (adrenal tumor or hyperplasia) that are most common in human beings also occur in cats.

FELINE PRIMARY HYPERALDOSTERONISM: ADRENAL ADENOMA AND CARCINOMA

SIGNALMENT

Feline PHA is a disease of middle-aged to older cats. Reported age of onset ranges from 5 to 20 years, with an average of 11 years. There does not appear to be any breed predispositions; most reported cases have been domestic shorthair cats, with one each of domestic longhair, Siamese, Burmese, and Burmilla. No gender predisposition exists; all reported cases have been neutered, with roughly equal proportions of female and male cats.

CLINICAL SIGNS RELATED TO MINERALOCORTICOID EXCESS

Most commonly the major presenting signs relate directly to increased aldosterone concentrations. The clinical presentation of cats can be divided broadly into two main groups: hypokalemic polymyopathy and acute onset blindness. The former is the most common presentation, with most reported cases presenting with various signs consistent with muscle dysfunction, including cervical ventroflexion (most common; Figure 24-3), hind limb weakness and ataxia, or, less commonly, limb stiffness, dysphagia, and collapse. In some cases the muscular features are mild and episodic, while in others they are

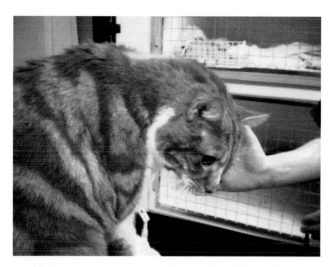

Figure 24-3 Cervical ventroflexion is a common manifestation of hypokalemic polymyopathy, a frequent presenting feature in cats with primary hyperaldosteronism, particularly those associated with adrenal neoplasia. (Courtesy Dr. Andrew Sparkes, Animal Health Trust, Newmarket, United Kingdom.)

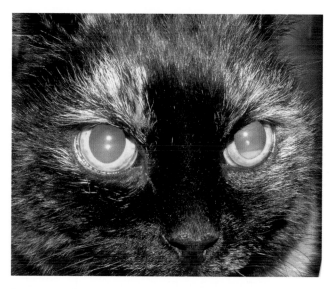

Figure 24-5 This image demonstrates more clearly the retinal detachment in a cat with systemic hypertension. (Courtesy Tim Knott, Rowe Veterinary Group, Bristol, United Kingdom.)

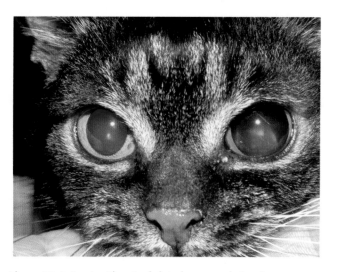

Figure 24-4 A cat with retinal detachment and vitreal hemorrhage, as a result of systemic hypertension. This is another clinical presentation of cats with primary hyperaldosteronism, and appears to be a more common presentation in cats with idiopathic hyperplasia than with adrenal neoplasia. (Courtesy Tim Knott, Rowe Veterinary Group, Bristol, United Kingdom.)

severe and acute in onset. One report described a cat presenting with respiratory distress, and the authors speculated that the respiratory failure was a manifestation of hypokalemic polymyopathy.[39] The cat was dehydrated upon admission and received intravenous fluids. With rehydration serum potassium became lower, presumably caused by dilution and because increased renal perfusion allowed more potassium loss. This response serves to illustrate that dehydration may mask the severity of hypokalemia or, perhaps, hypertension.

Intraocular hemorrhage or acute onset blindness resulting from retinal detachment (Figures 24-4 and 24-5) is the main presenting sign less commonly, occurring in

just two of the reported cases. In both patients, hypertension was severe (systolic blood pressure above 200 mm Hg), and no other clinical signs were reported. However, as stated, although not always the main presenting sign, subclinical hypertension is common.

Although not yet described specifically in association with hyperaldosteronism, hypertension also may result in central nervous edema, hemorrhage, or ischemia, which may contribute to neurological signs such as seizures, ataxia, and behavioral changes. Polyuria and polydipsia have been reported in about 15 per cent of cases, and may arise secondary to concurrent conditions such as hyperthyroidism; as a direct consequence of hypokalemia; or as a result of vasopressin resistance and increased osmotic threshold of vasopressin release, as has been documented in a canine case of PHA with polyuria and polydipsia.[43] Polyphagia also was reported in 10 per cent of cases, the cause of which was unknown; concurrent hypercortisolemia may be possible, although it has not been documented.

CLINICAL SIGNS RELATED TO OTHER STEROID EXCESS

The authors have encountered a few cats with aldosterone-secreting adrenocortical carcinomas who have had concurrent hyperprogesteronism. One of these cases is described briefly in Case Example 1. Clinical signs encountered by the authors are consistent with the clinical signs described in a reported case.[37] The signs of hyperprogesteronism usually predominate, resulting in very similar clinical signs to those encountered with hypercortisolemia, namely secondary diabetes mellitus, polyuria, polydipsia, polyphagia, poor coat condition, seborrhea, thin fragile skin, and a potbellied appearance. The glucocorticoid effect of elevated serum progesterone concentrations also may contribute to muscle weakness, which may be attributed initially to hypokalemic polymyopathy. Clinical signs of hypertension also may be present. Clinical signs of glucocorticoid and mineralocorticoid excess in two dogs were attributed to co-secretion of aldosterone and corticosterone by an adrenocortical tumor.[44,45] Measurement of corticosterone has not been described for assessment of adrenal tumors in cats.

CLINICAL SIGNS RELATED TO CONCOMITANT ILLNESS

Because cats affected with PHA are older, clinicians also must consider the possibility of concurrent diseases that may divert attention from hyperaldosteronism. Concomitant illness such as chronic kidney disease or hyperthyroidism may be assumed wrongly to be the cause of hypokalemia and/or hypertension (see Case Example 2). In general, hypertension associated with hyperthyroidism alone is mild; if severe hypertension is seen, the possibility of concurrent PHA should be considered. Left ventricular hypertrophy secondary to hypertension and/or concurrent disease such as hyperthyroidism may be present, resulting in typical clinical findings of cardiomyopathy such as a systolic heart murmur, tachycardia, gallop rhythm, or dysrhythmias (see Chapter 42). Development of congestive heart failure as a consequence of hypertension alone is rare. Cardiac disease associated solely with PHA has not been described in cats; however, the cardiac effects of elevated aldosterone are well recognized in human beings.[46]

CLINICOPATHOLOGICAL FEATURES

Hematology and Biochemistry

No specific hematological abnormalities of PHA have been identified. On a biochemical profile hypokalemia frequently is present; however, the degree is variable. Because hypokalemia is identified in cats for many other reasons (Box 24-1), a mild to moderate hypokalemia may be easily overlooked without consideration of hyperaldosteronism. Currently most reported cases of PHA are hypokalemic; however, this could, in part, reflect the fact that hypokalemia may be considered a prerequisite before evaluation for hyperaldosteronism is initiated. Persistence of hypokalemia despite supplementation with potassium is a common factor that prompts suspicion of hyperaldosteronism in cats. However, normokalemia does not exclude the possibility of PHA. Serum sodium concentrations usually are normal. Hypernatremia has been reported only in three feline patients with PHA and, in all cases, was mild.[32,33,36] The lack of significant hypernatremia may be explained by concurrent volume expansion secondary to sodium retention. Creatine kinase usually is elevated in cats with polymyopathy, with the degree of elevation also highly variable.

Blood urea nitrogen and creatinine may be elevated at the time of diagnosis, and progression of renal disease may be the cause of death in some cases. The presence of azotemia may hinder the diagnosis in some cases, because the presence of hypokalemia and/or hypertension may

---

Box 24-1 List of Differential Diagnoses for Hypokalemia and Hypertension in Cats

DIFFERENTIAL DIAGNOSES OF FELINE HYPOKALEMIA
Reduced Intake
Anorexia
IV fluids containing inadequate potassium
Increased Loss
Gastrointestinal loss
Vomiting
Diarrhea
Urinary loss
Renal disease
Diuretic administration
Postobstructive diuresis
Diabetic ketoacidosis
Primary hyperaldosteronism (PHA)
    Unilateral adenoma
    Unilateral carcinoma
        Aldosterone-secreting only
        Aldosterone- and progesterone-secreting
    Bilateral adenoma
    Bilateral adrenal hyperplasia
Hepatic insufficiency
Congestive heart failure
Intracellular Translocation
Metabolic alkalosis
Hyperthyroidism
Insulin therapy
Burmese hypokalemic polymyopathy

DIFFERENTIAL DIAGNOSES OF FELINE HYPERTENSION
Renal disease
Primary hyperaldosteronism (PHA)
    Unilateral adenoma
    Unilateral carcinoma
        Aldosterone-secreting only
        Aldosterone- and progesterone-secreting
    Bilateral adenoma
    Bilateral adrenal hyperplasia
Hyperthyroidism
Chronic anemia
?Diabetes mellitus
?Hyperadrenocorticism
?Obesity
?Liver disease

---

simply be considered a consequence of the renal disease itself. In human beings progressive renal disease is a recognized sequela to PHA.[46] Renal damage occurs because of a combination of elevated intraglomerular capillary pressure, inflammation, and fibrosis, which are a direct effect of angiotensin II and chronic hypokalemia.

Plasma Aldosterone Concentration

Baseline plasma aldosterone concentration (PAC) has been elevated with respect to laboratory reference values in all reported cases of feline PHA owing to adrenal neoplasia. However, there may be wide variation in PAC in normal cats (see Table 24-1 for examples). Therefore

Table 24-1 Baseline Concentrations of Aldosterone (ALDO) and Plasma Renin Activity (PRA) from Healthy Cats in Several Clinical Studies and in Cats with Primary Hyperaldosteronism

Cats Sampled in Study	Baseline Aldosterone	Reference
12 healthy pet cats, age range 1-12 years (median age, 3.5 years)	ALDO 11-1714 pmol/L range, median 388 pmol/L	Zimmer et al[66]
Healthy cats, 8>52 weeks 148 samples	ALDO 0-982 pmol/L range, mean ± SD, 160 ± 210 pmol/L	Yu and Morris[67]
10 healthy pet cats, 6 months-11 years	ALDO 69-291 pmol/L range, mean ± SD, 155 ± 67 pmol/L PRA 1.07-4.68 ng/mL/hr range, mean ± SD 2.82 ± 1.24 ng/mL/hr	Steele et al[64]
130 healthy pet cats, 4 months-14.5 years	ALDO 10-800 pmol/L range, median 235 pmol/L reference range, 110-540 pmol/L PRA 0.14-3.85 ng/mL/hr range,* median 0.94 ng/mL/hr,* reference range 0.28-2.96 ng/mL/hr*	Javadi et al[62]
24 cats with aldosterone-secreting adrenal tumors	ALDO 877-39,000 pmol/L range	Case reports[32-41]
11 cats with idiopathic primary hyperaldosteronism	ALDO 130-950 pmol/L range PRA 0.09-0.52 ng/mL/hr*	Javadi et al[42]

*PRA data reported in fmol/L/second, results in publication divided by 212.4 for conversion of units.

results must be assessed relative to clinical signs. There is no evidence for diagnostic benefit in performing an ACTH stimulation test for assessment of PHA. It has been the experience of the authors that the highest PAC occur with adrenocortical tumors, in which baseline aldosterone concentrations often are in excess of 1000 pmol/L (see Table 24-1).

Plasma Renin Activity

Distinguishing primary from secondary hyperaldosteronism requires assessment of activity of the renin-angiotensin system. The most commonly employed analysis has been the plasma renin activity (PRA) assay, based on in vitro generation of angiotensin I in a timed incubation. In human medicine accurate determination of a low PRA result may carry more weight to identify PHA than the PAC, hence the use of the ARR mentioned earlier in this chapter. In comparison with many other hormones, plasma concentrations of angiotensin I are very low, and immunoassay technology is strained to distinguish normal from suppressed concentrations. Plasma samples must be processed quickly and kept frozen until assay to minimize pre-assay renin activity. Another issue is related to in vitro activation of prorenin to renin, which could yield a falsely elevated PRA result. In human beings, so called cryoactivation of prorenin occurs between 25° C and freezing.[47] Cats are not susceptible to cryoactivation of prorenin.[48,49] Drugs (e.g., angiotensin-converting enzyme inhibitors and β-blockers), and dietary salt intake also may influence PRA. PRA results have been reported in five cases of feline PHA. Results were low in two cases[31,34] and normal in two others.[32] One cat had both a normal and low PRA result when measured on 2 consecutive days.[35] Therefore normal PRA values do not exclude the possibility of hyperaldosteronism caused by an

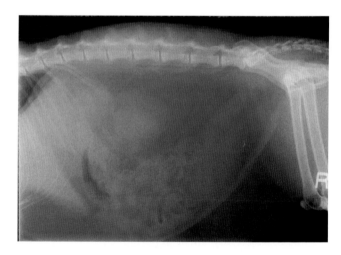

Figure 24-6 Lateral abdominal radiograph from a cat with primary hyperaldosteronism and hyperprogesteronemia, illustrating a large soft-tissue opacity cranial to the kidneys. This was suspected to be an adrenal adenocarcinoma. In human beings, and in our clinical experience with cats, the larger the adrenal mass, the more likely it is to be a carcinoma rather than an adenoma. In the reported cases of feline adrenal adenomas, a mass has not been visible radiographically.

adrenal tumor. Use of the ARR in the diagnosis of feline idiopathic hyperaldosteronism is discussed later.

Diagnostic Imaging

Adrenal masses are rarely visible radiographically, but if the mass is seen on radiographs, it is more likely to be an adrenocortical carcinoma than an adenoma (Figure 24-6). Pulmonary metastases can occur, albeit infrequently; therefore thoracic radiographs to screen for metastases should be performed prior to consideration of surgery (Figure 24-7). Currently ultrasonography is the best described imaging modality for detecting adrenal masses in dogs and cats. In all reported feline cases of PHA in which adrenal ultrasonography has been performed, unilateral adrenal enlargement with evidence of an adrenal mass has been identified, ranging from 10 to 35 mm in diameter (Figure 24-8). The contralateral adrenal gland may appear normal in appearance or may be unidentifiable. It is vital that the contralateral gland be assessed, because bilateral adenomas have been reported. Also the presence of a small or nondetectable contralateral adrenal gland would heighten concern for adrenal insufficiency in the intraoperative and postoperative periods after

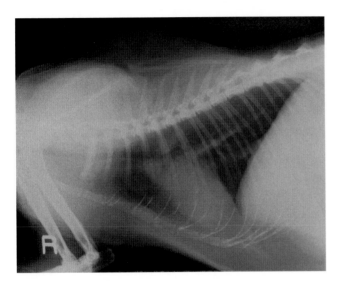

Figure 24-7 Lateral thoracic radiograph from a cat with an adrenocortical carcinoma. Two small soft-tissue opacity nodules can be seen in the second intercostal space, suggestive of pulmonary metastases. However, metastatic disease does not seem to be recognized commonly, and cats with adrenal carcinomas can have a good long-term prognosis following adrenalectomy.

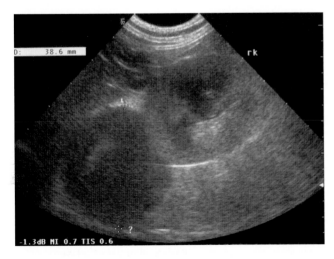

Figure 24-8 Ultrasound image demonstrating the typical hypoechoic appearance of an adrenal mass cranial to the right kidney. This was an adrenocortical carcinoma.

removal of the affected gland. Ultrasonography also should attempt to identify the presence and degree of invasion of the caudal vena cava by the tumor or related thrombus, and the presence of metastases to other organs.[32,40] A close association of the tumor with the caudal vena cava usually is evident; however, to date imaging has not been useful in preoperative assessment of the likely ease of surgical removal of adrenal masses.

Other imaging modalities, including magnetic resonance imaging (MRI), CT, and saphenous venography, have been reported in a small number of cases in an attempt to establish the extent of the adrenal mass before undertaking surgery. Results from MRI in one cat showed no evidence of extension into the caudal vena cava; however, the cat succumbed to fatal hemorrhage postoperatively.[36] Saphenous venography was used in one cat to demonstrate lack of invasion of the caudal vena cava by an adrenal tumor.[34] CT, the imaging modality of choice in human patients, has been used successfully in a cat and a dog, but further data are needed to define its diagnostic enhancement compared to ultrasound technology.[35,43] Radionuclide scintigraphy has not been reported in assessment of feline PHA.

DIAGNOSIS

Diagnostic algorithms are suggested (Figure 24-9), based on appropriate clinical signs and documentation of an elevated PAC. A related algorithm is based on initial identification of an adrenal mass.[50] However, implementation of any strategy currently is restricted by the difficulty in measuring PRA or lack of a defined mineralocorticoid suppression test in cats (see Figure 24-9, *B*). Because of the difficulty in measuring PRA, demonstration of the presence of adrenocortical neoplasia concurrently with a markedly elevated PAC is considered to be sufficient to make a diagnosis of aldosterone-secreting adrenocortical tumor in cats, especially in conjunction with persistent hypokalemia and hypertension.[36] However, it is possible that an incidental nonfunctional neoplasm can occur in conjunction with secondary hyperaldosteronism. As discussed previously, interpretation of PAC in the presence of azotemia can be problematic. Mean PAC values have been reported in cats with chronic kidney disease as 499 pmol/L and 2656 pmol/L.[51,52] Histopathological confirmation of the neoplasm together with resolution of clinical signs and PAC measurements postoperatively assist in confirming the diagnosis.

TREATMENT

Initial treatment of PHA is directed at controlling hypokalemia and/or hypertension. Potassium supplementation using potassium gluconate at doses of 2 to 6 mmol PO q12h has been used, and intravenous potassium chloride may be required in more severely hypokalemic cases. Amlodipine besylate (0.625 to 1.25 mg per cat PO q24h) is the initial treatment of choice for hypertension while test results are pending. Most hypertensive cats become normotensive with amlodipine treatment, but higher

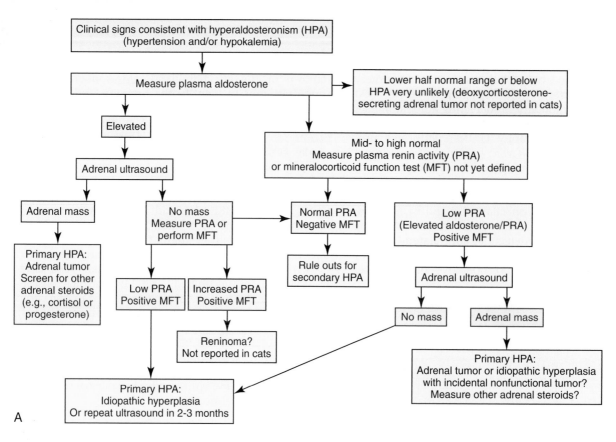

A

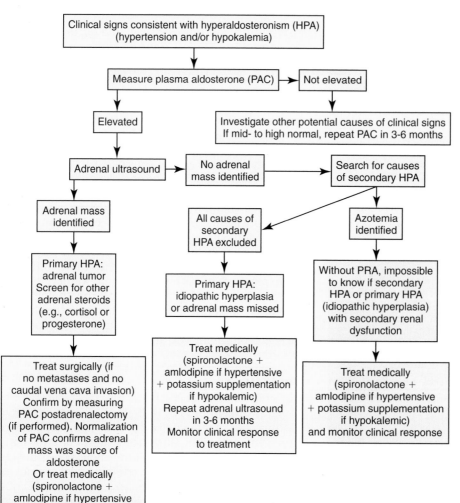

B

Figure 24-9 Proposed alternative algorithms for investigation for hyperaldosteronism in cats. **A,** Algorithm suggested when measurement of plasma renin activity (PRA) and mineralocorticoid function tests (MFT) are available. **B,** Algorithm suggested when measurement of plasma renin activity/mineralocorticoid function tests are not available.

doses sometimes are required. Hypertension can become refractory to treatment.

Spironolactone, a competitive aldosterone receptor antagonist, also is recommended (2 to 4 mg/kg PO q24h), assisting in the control of both hypokalemia and hypertension. Severe facial dermatitis has been reported recently in Maine Coon cats receiving spironolactone for management of hypertrophic cardiomyopathy.[53] Spironolactone has been associated with rare instances of cutaneous reactions and agranulocytosis in human beings.[54,55] It has lesser but significant affinity for progesterone and androgen receptors, and other adverse reactions of spironolactone in people include gynecomastia and menstrual irregularities.[56] Eplerenone has been developed as an alternative aldosterone receptor antagonist that has more selective affinity for mineralocorticoid receptors.[56,57] Eplerenone has been administered to dogs[58,59] in experimental studies, but the authors are not aware of its use in cats. Although medical treatment alone is unlikely to normalize potassium levels, control of clinical signs associated with myopathy usually is achieved.[35]

Adrenalectomy is a potentially curative treatment for unilateral adrenal masses (Figure 24-10). However, the procedure has been associated with high perioperative mortality; approximately 33 per cent of reported cases died intraoperatively or postoperatively, most commonly as a result of severe acute hemorrhage from the caudal vena cava. Patients should be stabilized medically prior to surgery and meticulous preoperative planning is required. A detailed description of perioperative and intraoperative management of an aldosterone-secreting adrenocortical carcinoma with attached caval thrombus has been reported recently.[40] Although clinicians must be vigilant, complications of postoperative adrenal insufficiency have not been associated with excision of aldosterone-secreting tumors in cats. Approximately 5 per cent of human patients develop postoperative hyperkalemia, requiring transient administration of fludrocortisone,[11]

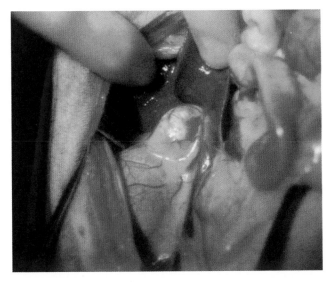

Figure 24-10 Intraoperative image showing the cream-colored right adrenal mass closely adherent to the kidney. (From Ganguly A: Primary aldosteronism, *N Engl J Med* 339:1828-1834, 1998.)

and one author (KR) is aware of similar occurrences in cats.

Cats with concurrent hyperprogesteronism or hypercortisolemia pose additional surgical risks, including wound dehiscence, sepsis, and thromboembolic disease. Effective medical management would necessitate suppression of progestin, glucocorticoid, and mineralocorticoid production, with the possibility of the additive effect of spironolactone. To date a protocol for such treatment has not been defined. One author (AH) has used trilostane in one cat with concurrent hyperaldosteronism and hyperprogesteronism. Treatment was only attempted for a short period of time when the clinical signs were quite advanced, and was not successful in suppressing progesterone concentrations. The cat continued to deteriorate and was euthanized (see Case Example 1). Use of aminoglutethimide also has been reported for preoperative stabilization but was of questionable benefit.[37]

PROGNOSIS

When medical management with combinations of potassium supplementation, amlodipine, and spironolactone is the chosen course of treatment, reported survival times in four of five treated cats ranged from 7 months to 984 days, with cats succumbing most commonly to chronic kidney disease or thromboembolic episode.[32,34,36] The survival time in one cat receiving medical treatment alone was limited to 50 days, attributed to noncompliance of the owners.[36] In some cases, hypertension becomes refractory to medical management. For patients who undergo adrenalectomy and survive the immediate perioperative and postoperative periods, the prognosis is good; eight of 17 adrenalectomized cats survived for at least 1 year, and two cats were alive 3.5 and 5 years postoperatively.[36] However, given the high perioperative mortality rate, the decision to undergo surgery should not be taken lightly. Interestingly the presence of an adrenal carcinoma does not appear to be associated with a poorer prognosis than an adrenal adenoma. Only one of three cats who were euthanized as a result of perioperative hemorrhage associated with surgery had an adrenal carcinoma; one cat with a carcinoma survived 1045 days following adrenalectomy. In contrast, the prognosis for human beings with adrenal carcinomas is much poorer than for those patients with adrenal adenomas.[60]

FELINE PRIMARY HYPERALDOSTERONISM: IDIOPATHIC HYPERPLASIA

CLINICAL FEATURES

In 2005 Javadi et al reported evidence of PHA in 11 cats who had pathological characteristics of the idiopathic or bilateral hyperplasia form recognized in human beings.[42] The cats included in the study were of similar signalment to those with adrenal neoplasia, being between 11 and 18 years of age and mostly of mixed breeds. The presenting complaints were similar to the previous reports of cats with hyperaldosteronism caused by adrenal neoplasia.

Only three of 11 cats in the report by Javadi et al presented with hypokalemic polymyopathy, and seven presented with retinal detachment or subretinal, intraretinal, and intravitreal hemorrhages associated with systemic hypertension. Overall, hypertension was more severe in Javadi et al's group of cats; all systolic blood pressures were above 185 mm Hg and were greater than 200 mm Hg in six cats. Ultrasonography and/or CT examination showed subtle abnormalities such as an increase in adrenal echogenicity or areas of calcification and thickening and/or rounding of one pole of one or both adrenal glands, but no evidence of adrenal neoplasia. Some cats had no adrenal changes.

CLINICOPATHOLOGICAL FEATURES

Clinicopathological features of cats with nontumorous or idiopathic hyperplasia generally were similar to those of cats with hyperaldosteronism associated with adrenal neoplasia. However, there are some subtle, but important, differences. Only six of 11 cats with the nontumorous form were hypokalemic (usually mild) at initial presentation. Mild azotemia also was common at initial presentation and tended to worsen over time in cats followed with serial sampling. Interestingly, there was not a corresponding increase in serum phosphate concentrations. Rather, serum phosphate concentrations were low-normal or low. Rats with experimentally induced hyperaldosteronism showed increased urinary calcium and magnesium excretion and a compensatory increase in parathyroid hormone, which could be a possible reason for the low phosphate concentrations.[61]

Mineralocorticoid function was assessed by comparison of baseline PAC, PRA, and ARR with those of a control population.[62] The 11 study cats had high-normal to increased PAC (see Table 24-1) and low-normal or decreased PRA. Elevation of the ARR was the evidence for inappropriate excess of aldosterone secretion.

One author of this chapter (AH) has directly encountered several cases similar to those reported by Javadi et al.[42] In the author's experience, these cats respond well in the short term to treatment with spironolactone with or without potassium supplementation. However, currently there is a lack of histopathological results and long-term follow-up available.

DIAGNOSTIC CHALLENGES FOR THE FUTURE

Given the challenge in diagnosing feline PHA, particularly the idiopathic form, it is highly possible that both forms of this condition are under-recognized in cats. Cats with renal disease and hypertension tend to have lower serum concentrations of potassium than those with normotensive renal disease.[63] In studies comparing diseased cats with normal controls, cats with renal disease and hypertension tended to have similar or higher PAC, whereas PRA could be low, normal, or elevated.[51,64] In another study, mean PAC results were similar among clinically normal cats, normotensive cats with renal disease, and cats with renal disease and hypertension, but

PRA was lowest in the latter group.[65] Therefore accessibility of PRA assays for veterinary diagnostic use would be of great value.

There also could be application of mineralocorticoid function tests, to follow the example from human medicine. An earlier study examined the effect of enalapril or benazepril on blood pressure, PAC, and PRA in cats with hypertension and chronic kidney disease and noted highly variable responses.[64] Some cats did respond with increases of PRA and decreases of both PAC and blood pressure, while others with very low initial PRA results showed no change in blood pressure, PRA, or PAC. In light of current knowledge, one may speculate that some of these latter cats had idiopathic PHA and could be identified by the lack of response to angiotensin-converting enzyme inhibitor administration. Measurement of urinary aldosterone-to-creatinine ratio in normal cats before and after suppression with increased dietary salt or fludrocortisone acetate has been reported recently,[41] and the same group is now investigating its use in assessment of feline hyperaldosteronism. Normal cats showed the most consistent decrease of the urinary aldosterone-to-creatinine ratio with administration of fludrocortisone acetate as compared with dietary salt supplementation, and one cat with an aldosterone-secreting adrenal carcinoma had an elevated ratio with no suppression. Advances in diagnosis and treatment will come in the wake of better characterization of the clinical and pathological spectrum of PHA in cats.

CASE EXAMPLE 1: ADRENOCORTICAL TUMOR

A 12-year-old neutered male domestic longhair cat presented with polyuria, polydipsia, weight gain, hind limb weakness, and poor coat condition (Figure 24-11). There had been a lack of hair regrowth after clipping for a wound repair 3 months previously (Figure 24-12). Additional findings on physical examination included thin

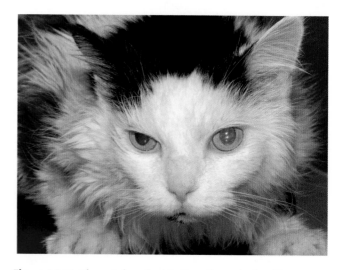

Figure 24-11 The cat described in Case Example 1, with hyperaldosteronism and hyperprogesteronism. Note the unkempt hair coat and crouched stance secondary to muscle weakness.

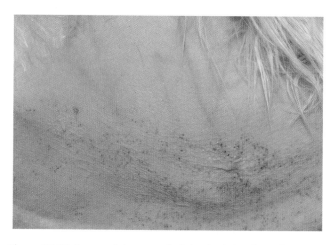

Figure 24-12 Image of the ventral abdominal skin from the cat in Figure 24-11, with hyperaldosteronism and hyperprogesteronism. Note the failure of hair regrowth and the thin skin with prominent subcutaneous blood vessels.

skin and a potbellied appearance. Evidence of mild hypertensive retinopathy was present, but the temperament of the cat precluded measurement of blood pressure. Laboratory investigations revealed hyperglycemia, elevated serum fructosamine concentration indicative of diabetes mellitus, and hypokalemia (2.5 mmol/L). Potassium supplementation, and amlodipine and insulin treatment, were initiated. Based on the clinical signs, hyperadrenocorticism was suspected. After achieving satisfactory control of the diabetes mellitus, the following investigations were performed:

Urine cortisol-to-creatinine ratio: 7.5 × 10^{-6} (reference 0.6 to 12.9 × 10^{-6}).

ACTH stimulation: Basal cortisol: 20 nmol/L, 1-hour post-ACTH cortisol: 335 nmol/L.

Low-dose dexamethasone suppression test: Basal cortisol: 37 nmol/L (reference 15 to 40 nmol/L), 3-hour post-dexamethasone cortisol: 42 nmol/L, 8-hour post-dexamethasone cortisol: 29 nmol/L (normal response post-dexamethasone <30 nmol/L). The results were deemed inconclusive for hyperadrenocorticism.

Abdominal radiographs showed a craniodorsal abdominal soft tissue mass (see Figure 24-6). Thoracic radiographs revealed possible pulmonary metastases (see Figure 24-7). Abdominal ultrasound revealed a 4-cm diameter irregular hypoechoic mass of the right adrenal gland (see Figure 24-8).

At this stage mild hypokalemia persisted (potassium 3.3 mmol/L, reference range 4 to 5 mmol/L) despite potassium supplementation, and the possibility of hyperaldosteronism was investigated. PAC was severely elevated at 2923 pmol/L (reference range 195 to 390 pmol/L). Treatment with spironolactone was initiated.

The cat continued to become progressively weaker and remained polyuric and polydipsic and mildly hypokalemic. The diabetes was well controlled. Progressive hypokalemic polymyopathy was considered to be the cause of the weakness. Hyperprogesteronism was considered because it can result in similar clinical signs as hypercortisolemia. A baseline progesterone concentration was

15.9 nmol/L (reference range <3 nmol/L). The addition of trilostane (30 mg PO q24h for 2 weeks, then 60 mg PO q24h for 4 weeks) did not suppress steroidogenesis. The cat's condition deteriorated and euthanasia was elected. Necropsy was not performed. The probable diagnosis: adrenal carcinoma with metastases, PHA, and hyperprogesteronism with secondary diabetes mellitus.

CASE EXAMPLE 2: IDIOPATHIC HYPERPLASIA

A 15-year-old spayed female domestic shorthair cat was presented following an episode of dyspnea and collapse. The cat also had a history of chronic cough. Physical examination revealed a grade 3 of 5 systolic heart murmur, wheezes on thoracic auscultation, and a small palpable goiter on the right side of her neck. Systolic blood pressure was 215 mm Hg (high definition oscillometry). Routine hematology was unremarkable. Serum biochemistry examination showed mildly elevated liver enzymes and a mild hypokalemia (3.5 mmol/L; reference range 4 to 5 mmol/L). Total serum thyroxine was elevated at 102 nmol/L (reference range 15 to 40 nmol/L). The hypertension was suspected to be a result of the hyperthyroidism. Treatment with methimazole (2.5 mg PO q12h) was initiated, resulting in normalization of laboratory parameters including serum potassium concentration. Reassessment of blood pressure on a few occasions over the following 2 months showed fluctuations between 150 and 220 mm Hg.

The cat was referred 2 months later owing to development of lethargy, twitching, hyphema, and blindness. Systolic blood pressure measurement (Doppler) revealed severe hypertension (270 mm Hg). Ophthalmic examination revealed complete retinal detachment in the left eye, and hypertensive retinopathy with retinal edema and small areas of retinal hemorrhage in the right eye. Otherwise examination was as described previously. The severity of hypertension was considered unusual as a result of hyperthyroidism alone, and therefore further diagnostic tests were undertaken to investigate the possibility of another underlying etiology. Immediate treatment with amlodipine besylate was initiated at 1.25 mg PO q24h, resulting in gradual reduction in systolic blood pressure to 180 mm Hg by the following day and a dramatic improvement in the cat's demeanor.

Routine hematological examination was unremarkable. Serum biochemistry examination revealed a mild azotemia (blood urea nitrogen 15 mmol/L, reference range 6.5 to 10.5 mmol/L; creatinine 171 μmol/L, reference range 133 to 165 μmol/L) and persistence of hypokalemia (3.9 mmol/L). Urine specific gravity was suboptimal at 1.020. Total serum thyroxine was 7 nmol/L (reference range 15 to 40 nmol/L). Thoracic radiographs showed a diffuse bronchial pattern suggestive of chronic lower airway disease. Abdominal radiographs were unremarkable. Echocardiography demonstrated mild left ventricular hypertrophy. Abdominal ultrasound showed no evidence of an adrenal mass, but mild bilateral enlargement of the adrenal glands. PAC was elevated (562 pmol/L; reference range 195 to 390 pmol/L). A PRA assay was not available.

Although secondary hyperaldosteronism associated with renal disease could not be excluded, the possibility of bilateral adrenal hyperplasia was considered. Treatment was continued with a reduced dose of methimazole and amlodipine, and the addition of spironolactone (12.5 mg PO q24h). At reassessment 10 days later, the cat had regained vision, the hypertensive retinopathy had resolved, systolic blood pressure was normal (150 mm Hg), serum thyroxine had normalized (32 nmol/L), and hypokalemia had resolved (4.1 mmol/L). Blood urea nitrogen remained mildly elevated but creatinine had normalized (171 μmol/L). Renal parameters, blood pressure, and serum potassium have since remained stable following each reassessment, now 6 months since presentation.

REFERENCES

1. Conn JW: Presidential address. Part I. Painting background. Part II. Primary aldosteronism, a new clinical syndrome, *J Lab Clin Med* 45:3, 1955.
2. Atlas SA: The renin-angiotensin aldosterone system: pathophysiological role and pharmacologic inhibition, *J Manag Care Pharm* 13(suppl S-b):S9, 2007.
3. Williams GH: Aldosterone biosynthesis, regulation, and classical mechanism of action, *Heart Fail Rev* 10:7, 2005.
4. Schweda F, Friis U, Wagner C, et al: Renin release, *Physiology* 22:310, 2007.
5. Toffelmire EB, Slater K, Corvol P, et al: Response of plasma prorenin and active renin to chronic and acute alterations of renin secretion in normal humans, *J Clin Invest* 83:679, 1989.
6. Yoshimoto T, Hirata Y: Aldosterone as a cardiovascular risk hormone, *Endocr J* 54:359, 2007.
7. Connell JMC, Davies E: The new biology of aldosterone, *J Endocrinol* 186:1, 2005.
8. Fuller PJ, Young MJ: Mechanisms of mineralocorticoid action, *Hypertension* 46:1227, 2005.
9. Rüster C, Wolf G: Renin-angiotensin-aldosterone system and progression of renal disease, *J Am Soc Nephrol* 17:2985, 2006.
10. Wong L, Hsu THS, Perlroth MG, et al: Reninoma: Case report and literature review, *J Hypertens* 26:368, 2008.
11. Young WF: Primary aldosteronism: renaissance of a syndrome, *Clin Endocrinol* 66:607, 2007.
12. Rossi GP, Pessina AC, Heagerty AM: Primary hyperaldosteronism: an update on screening, diagnosis and treatment, *J Hypertens* 26:613, 2008.
13. Funder JW, Carey RM, Fardella C, et al: Case detection, diagnosis, and treatment of patients with primary hyperaldosteronism: an Endocrine Society clinical practice guideline, *J Clin Endocrinol Metab* 93:3266, 2008.
14. Omura M, Sasano H, Saito J, et al: Clinical characteristics of aldosterone-producing microadenoma, macroadenoma, and idiopathic hyperaldosteronism in 93 patients with primary hyperaldosteronism, *Hypertens Res* 29:883, 2006.
15. Wu VC, Chueh SC, Chang HW, et al: Bilateral aldosterone-producing adenomas: differentiation from bilateral adrenal hyperplasia, *Q J Med* 101:13, 2008.
16. Kaplan NM: The current epidemic of primary aldosteronism: causes and consequences, *J Hypertens* 22:863, 2004.
17. Rossi GP, Bernini G, Caliumi C, et al: A prospective study of the prevalence of primary aldosteronism in 1,125 hypertensive patients, *J Am Coll Cardiol* 48:2293, 2006.
18. Calhoun DA: Is there an unrecognized epidemic of primary aldosteronism? Pro, *Hypertension* 50:447, 2007.
19. Kaplan NM: Is there an unrecognized epidemic of primary aldosteronism? Con, *Hypertension* 50:454, 2007.
20. Douma S, Petidis K, Doumas M: Prevalence of primary hyperaldosteronism in resistant hypertension: a retrospective observational study, *Lancet* 7:1921, 2008.
21. Simon DR, Palese MA: Noninvasive adrenal imaging in hyperaldosteronism, *Curr Urol Rep* 9:80, 2008.
22. Messer CK, Kirschenbaum A, New MI, et al: Concomitant secretion of glucocorticoid, androgens, and mineralocorticoid by an adrenal carcinoma: case report and review of literature, *Endocr Pract* 13:408, 2007.
23. Reine NJ, Hohenhaus AE, Peterson ME, et al: Deoxycorticosterone-secreting adrenocortical carcinoma in a dog, *J Vet Intern Med* 13:386, 1999.
24. Vonend O, Altenhenne C, Büchner NJ, et al: A German family with glucocorticoid-remediable aldosteronism, *Nephrol Dial Transplant* 22:1123, 2007.
25. Stowasser M, Gunasekera TG, Gordon RD: Familial varieties of primary aldosteronism, *Clin Exp Pharmacol Physiol* 28:1087, 2001.
26. Dluhy RG, Lifton RP: Glucocorticoid-remediable aldosteronism, *J Clin Endocrinol Metab* 84:4341, 1999.
27. McMahon GT, Dluhy RG: Glucocorticoid-remediable hyperaldosteronism, *Arq Bras Endocrinol Metab* 48:682, 2004.
28. Sukor N, Mulatero P, Gordon RD, et al: Further evidence for linkage of familiar hyperaldosteronism type II at chromosome 7p22 in Italian as well as Australian and South American families, *J Hypertens* 26:1577, 2008.
29. Nunez BS, Rogerson FM, Mune T, et al: Mutants of 11β-hydroxysteroid dehydrogenase (11-HSD2) with partial activity; improved correlations between genotype and biochemical phenotype in apparent mineralocorticoid excess, *Hypertension* 34:638, 1999.
30. Morineau G, Sulmont V, Salomon R, et al: Apparent mineralocorticoid excess: report of six new cases and extensive personal experience, *J Am Soc Nephrol* 17:3176, 2006.
31. Eger C, Robinson W, Huxtable C: Primary aldosteronism (Conn's syndrome) in a cat; a case report and review of comparative aspects, *J Small Anim Pract* 24:293, 1983.
32. Flood SM, Randolph JF, Gelzer AR, et al: Primary hyperaldosteronism in two cats, *J Am Anim Hosp Assoc* 35:411, 1999.
33. MacKay AD, Holt PE, Sparkes AH: Successful surgical treatment of a cat with primary aldosteronism, *J Feline Med Surg* 1:117, 1999.
34. Moore LE, Biller DS, Smith TA: Use of abdominal ultrasonography in the diagnosis of primary hyperaldosteronism in a cat, *J Am Vet Med Assoc* 217:213, 2000.
35. Rijnberk A, Voorhout G, Kooistra HS, et al: Hyperaldosteronism in a cat with metastasised adrenocortical tumour, *Vet Q* 23:38, 2001.
36. Ash RA, Harvey AM, Tasker S: Primary hyperaldosteronism in the cat: a series of 13 cases, *J Feline Med Surg* 7:173, 2005.
37. De Clue AE, Breshears LA, Pardo ID, et al: Hyperaldosteronism and hyperprogesteronism in a cat with an adrenal cortical carcinoma, *J Vet Intern Med* 19:355, 2005.
38. Reimer SB, Pelosi A, Frank JD, et al: Multiple endocrine neoplasia type 1 in a cat, *J Am Vet Med Assoc* 227:101, 2005.
39. Haldene S, Graves TK, Bateman S, et al: Profound hypokalaemia causing respiratory failure in a cat with hyperaldosteronism, *J Vet Emerg Crit Care* 12:202, 2007.
40. Rose SA, Kyles AE, Labella P, et al: Adrenalectomy and caval thrombectomy in a cat with primary hyperaldosteronism, *J Am Anim Hosp Assoc* 43:209, 2007.
41. Djajadiningrat-Laanen SC, Galac S, Cammelbeeck SE, et al: Urinary aldosterone to creatinine ratio in cats before and after suppression with salt or fludrocortisone acetate, *J Vet Intern Med* 22:1283, 2008.
42. Javadi S, Djajadiningrat-Laanen SC, Kooistra HS, et al: Primary hyperaldosteronism, a mediator of progressive renal disease in cats, *Domest Anim Endocrinol* 28:85, 2005.

43. Rijnberk A, Kooistra HS, van Vonderen IK, et al: Aldosteronoma in a dog with polyuria as the leading symptom, *Domes Anim Endocrinol* 20:227, 2001.

44. Behrend EN, Weigand CM, Whitley EM, et al: Corticosterone- and aldosterone-secreting adrenocortical tumor in a dog, *J Am Vet Med Assoc* 226:1662, 2005.

45. Machida T, Uchida E, Matsuda K, et al: Aldosterone-, corticosterone- and cortisol-secreting adrenocortical carcinoma in a dog: case report, *J Vet Med Sci* 70:317, 2008.

46. Rossi G, Sechi LA, Giacchetti G, et al: Primary aldosteronism: cardiovascular, renal and metabolic implications, *Trends Endocrinol Metab* 19:88, 2008.

47. Sealey JE, Gordon RD, Mantero F: Plasma renin and aldosterone measurements in low renin hypertensive states, *Trends Endocrinol Metab* 16:86, 2005.

48. Golin R, Morganti A, Busnardo I, et al: Cryoactivation fails to augment plasma renin activity in the cat, *Clin Exp Pharmacol Physiol* 9:665, 1982.

49. Glorioso N, Troffa C, Laragh JH, et al: The cat: an animal model for studies of inactive renin, *Am J Physiol* 252:E509, 1987.

50. Shiel R, Mooney C: Diagnosis and management of primary hyperaldosteronism in cats, *In Practice* 29:194, 2007.

51. Jensen J, Henik RA, Brownfield M: Plasma renin activity and angiotensin I and aldosterone concentrations in cats with hypertension associated with chronic renal disease, *Am J Vet Res* 58:535, 1997.

52. Mishina M, Watanabe T, Fujii K: Non-invasive blood pressure measurements in cats: clinical significance of hypertension associated with chronic renal failure, *J Vet Med Sci* 60:805, 1998.

53. MacDonald KA, Kittleson MD, Kass PH: Effect of spironolactone on diastolic function and left ventricular mass in Maine coon cats with familial hypertrophic cardiomyopathy, *J Vet Intern Med* 22:335, 2008.

54. Gupta AK, Knowles SR, Shear NH: Spironolactone-associated cutaneous effects: a case report and review of the literature, *Dermatology* 189:402, 1994.

55. Ibañez L, Vidal X, Ballarin E, et al: Population based drug-induced agranulocytosis, *Arch Intern Med* 165:869, 2005.

56. Garthwaite SM, McMahon EG: The evolution of aldosterone antagonists, *Mol Cell Endocrinol* 217:27, 2004.

57. Karagiannis A, Tziomalos K, Papageorgiou A: Spironolactone versus eplerenone for the treatment of idiopathic hyperaldosteronism, *Expert Opin Pharmacother* 9:509, 2008.

58. Cook CS, Zhang L, Fischer JS: Absorption and disposition of a selective aldosterone receptor antagonist, eplerenone, in the dog, *Pharm Res* 17:1426, 2000.

59. de Paula RB, da Silva AA, Hall JE: Aldosterone antagonism attenuates obesity-induced hypertension and glomerular hyperfiltration, *Hypertension* 43:41, 2004.

60. Wheeler MH, Harris DA: Diagnosis and management of primary aldosteronism, *World J Surg* 27:627, 2003.

61. Runyan AL, Chhokar VS, Sun Y, et al: Bone loss in rats with aldosteronism, *Am J Med Sci* 330:1, 2005.

62. Javadi S, Slingerland LI, van de Beek MG, et al: Plasma renin activity and plasma concentrations of aldosterone, cortisol, adrenocorticotropic hormone and alpha-melanocyte-stimulating hormone in healthy cats, *J Vet Intern Med* 18:625, 2004.

63. Syme HM, Barber PJ, Markwell PJ, et al: Prevalence of systolic hypertension in cats with chronic renal failure at initial evaluation, *J Am Vet Med Assoc* 220:1799, 2002.

64. Steele JL, Henik RA, Stepien RL: Effects of angiotensin-converting enzyme inhibition on plasma aldosterone concentration, plasma renin activity, and blood pressure in spontaneously hypertensive cats with chronic renal disease, *Vet Ther* 3:157, 2002.

65. Syme HM, Markwell PJ, Elliott J: Aldosterone and plasma renin activity in cats with hypertension and/or chronic renal failure, *J Vet Intern Med* 16:354, 2002(abstract).

66. Zimmer C, Hörauf A, Reusch C: Ultrasonographic examination of the adrenal gland and evaluation of the hypophyseal-adrenal axis in 20 cats, *J Small Anim Pract* 41:156, 2000.

67. Yu S, Morris JG: Plasma aldosterone concentration in cats, *Vet J* 155:63, 1998.

CHAPTER

25 Hyperthyroidism and the Kidneys

Thomas K. Graves

RENAL FUNCTION IN HYPERTHYROIDISM

Hyperthyroidism and chronic kidney disease are two of the most common disorders in feline medicine. Almost 30 per cent of cats over 15 years of age have chronic kidney disease,[1] and that estimate probably is conservative. Since the initial reports in 1979, hyperthyroidism has increased steadily in incidence, and it is widely considered the most common endocrine disorder diagnosed in cats over 8 years of age.[2] Although it is not surprising that two such common disorders as hyperthyroidism and chronic kidney disease can occur simultaneously in a given cat, it was not until the mid-1990s that investigators showed a clinically important interaction between the two diseases.[3-5]

At present it is well established that hyperthyroidism is associated with increased glomerular filtration rate (GFR) in cats, and that GFR declines after treatment of hyperthyroidism. Although the exact mechanism is unknown, it is likely that increased cardiac output and decreased peripheral vascular resistance associated with hyperthyroidism cause increased GFR by enhancing renal plasma flow.[6,7] In normal animals GFR remains constant across a wide range of mean arterial pressures, but this renal autoregulation apparently is lost in cats with hyperthyroidism. Similarly human patients with hyperthyroidism, and experimental animals treated with excess thyroid hormone, experience increased renal plasma flow and GFR.[8] It is not known if the thyrotoxic state is directly harmful to the kidneys, but renal insufficiency does not ensue after treatment of thyrotoxicosis in people or after withdrawal of thyroid hormone in experimental animals. On the other hand, many cats develop overt renal insufficiency after treatment of hyperthyroidism (Figure 25-1).

268

The reason is not established, but it may be that the increased GFR associated with hyperthyroidism can mask underlying renal insufficiency in a cat with both disorders. Upon reversal of the hyperthyroid state, renal blood flow and GFR decline, and renal insufficiency becomes more readily apparent. In one recent study 15 per cent of hyperthyroid cats developed overt renal insufficiency within 13 to 18 months of radioiodine therapy.[9] Other studies have shown posttreatment renal insufficiency in 17 to 38 per cent of hyperthyroid cats treated by a variety of methods.[3-5]

DIAGNOSIS OF HYPERTHYROIDISM IN CATS WITH KIDNEY DISEASE

Hyperthyroid cats with underlying kidney disease can present a diagnostic challenge. Multiple diseases can occur simultaneously in older cats, and nonthyroidal illness is thought to be one reason for the increasingly common finding of occult hyperthyroidism. The term *occult hyperthyroidism* refers to a condition in which clinical hyperthyroidism exists in the face of normal serum total thyroxine (TT_4) concentrations. Serum TT_4 concentrations are in the normal range in nearly 10 per cent of cats with hyperthyroidism overall, and in up to approximately 40 per cent of cats with mild hyperthyroidism.[10] Concurrent disease is a common finding in cats with occult hyperthyroidism; underlying kidney disease can falsely lower serum thyroid hormone concentrations, making a diagnosis of hyperthyroidism more difficult. In a large study of cats with nonthyroidal illness, serum TT_4 concentrations were below the normal range (less than 10 nmol/L) in almost 50 per cent of euthyroid cats with

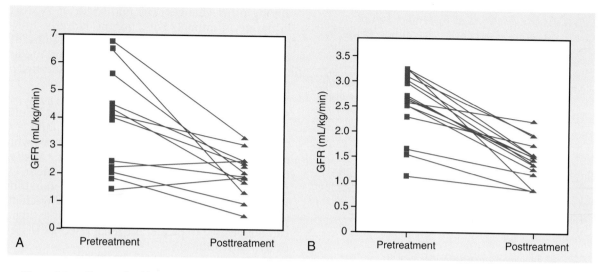

Figure 25-1 Glomerular filtration rate (GFR) was measured in cats before and 30 days after treatment of hyperthyroidism with methimazole (**A**) or thyroidectomy (**B**). GFR declined following treatment in 22 of 24 cats in the combined studies. The differences in the scale of GFR between **A** and **B** reflect different methods used for measurement. (Adapted from Graves TK, Olivier NB, Nachreiner RF, et al: Changes in renal function associated with treatment of hyperthyroidism in cats, *Am J Vet Res* 55:1745, 1994; and Becker TJ, Graves TK, Kruger JM, et al: Effects of methimazole on renal function in cats with hyperthyroidism, *J Am Anim Hosp Assoc* 36:215, 2000.)

kidney disease.[10] If the presence of kidney disease is associated with a marked reduction in serum TT_4 concentrations in euthyroid cats, it seems reasonable that serum TT_4 concentrations could be reduced in a cat with hyperthyroidism in addition to renal disease.

Measurement of serum concentrations of free thyroxine (FT_4) is thought to be a more sensitive test for feline hyperthyroidism than measurement of TT_4. Evaluation of FT_4 concentrations, however, may have unexpected pitfalls in cats with concurrent renal and thyroid diseases. In a recent report, serum FT_4 concentrations were high in 20 per cent of euthyroid cats with chronic kidney disease.[11] However, the cats all had TT_4 concentrations in the lower half of the normal range or lower. Based on that study and others, therefore, measurement of FT_4 is not recommended as a sole diagnostic test for hyperthyroidism in cats because of the high probability of arriving at a false-positive diagnosis.

The clinical finding of polyuria and polydipsia, a hallmark of chronic kidney disease in cats, also can be misleading in cats with hyperthyroidism. Polyuria and polydipsia occur commonly in feline hyperthyroidism, and could be caused by concurrent kidney disease or be unrelated to primary kidney disorders. The mechanism of polyuria and polydipsia in cats with hyperthyroidism is not known (see the following).

Just as kidney disease can obscure a diagnosis of hyperthyroidism, conversely, because thyroid hormone excess is associated with increased GFR, hyperthyroidism can cloud the diagnosis of chronic kidney disease in a cat. Treatment of cats with both diseases can be even more difficult, requiring frequent monitoring and careful manipulation of renal and thyroid functions to find the optimal balance for each individual patient.

CAN POSTTREATMENT RENAL INSUFFICIENCY BE PREDICTED?

Knowing which hyperthyroid cats are more likely to develop posttreatment renal insufficiency would be of great clinical value. Treatment of hyperthyroidism might be contraindicated in a cat with a high risk of developing renal insufficiency. In such cases a reversible form of treatment, such as antithyroid drug therapy, could have advantages over a more permanent treatment of hyperthyroidism with radioiodine therapy or surgical thyroidectomy.

Because GFR is increased in cats with hyperthyroidism, serum concentrations of creatinine are lower than they would be in the euthyroid state. For this reason serum creatinine concentration in a hyperthyroid cat can be even less useful an indicator of GFR than in a normal cat. Similarly blood urea nitrogen (BUN) concentration is a less useful indicator of GFR in a cat with hyperthyroidism. In hyperthyroidism BUN production is increased markedly because of excessive protein catabolism. Increased BUN/creatinine ratios have been reported in hyperthyroid people,[12] and also can be seen in many cats with hyperthyroidism. In our hospital we have observed elevations in the BUN/creatinine ratio not only in hyperthyroid cats compared with normal cats, but also in cats with occult hyperthyroidism when compared with normal cats (Table 25-1). BUN/creatinine ratio can not be used as a test for diagnosis of hyperthyroidism, but an elevated ratio could increase the clinical index of suspicion of the disease in a cat with a normal serum concentration of TT_4 (i.e., occult hyperthyroidism).

It is often stated that urine specific gravity (USG) can be used as an indirect indicator of renal sufficiency, and

Table 25-1 Concentrations of BUN and Serum Creatinine and BUN/Creatinine Ratios in Normal Cats vs. Cats with Occult Hyperthyroidism

	Normal Cats (n = 17)	Cats with Occult Hyperthyroidism (n = 7)
BUN (mg/dL)	21.2 ± 3.9*	28.3 ± 5.0*
Creatinine (mg/dL)	1.4 ± 0.1	1.2 ± 0.2
BUN/Creatinine	15.5 ± 2.7	23.6 ± 5.8*

Results are expressed as Mean ± SD.
*Denotes statistically significant difference.

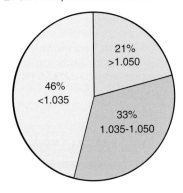

Pretreatment urine specific gravity in 24 cats with posttreatment renal failure

21% >1.050
33% 1.035-1.050
46% <1.035

Figure 25-2 Proportional representation of pretreatment urine specific gravity measurements in cats who developed renal insufficiency after treatment of hyperthyroidism. (Based on data reported in Aizawa T, Hiramatsu K, Ohtsuka H, et al: An elevation of BUN/creatinine ratio in patients with hyperthyroidism, *Horm Metab Res* 18:771, 1986.)

that cats with USG greater than 1.035 are less likely to suffer from renal insufficiency after treatment for hyperthyroidism.[2,13] Our studies of groups of cats that either did or did not develop renal insufficiency after treatment of hyperthyroidism, however, found that USG can not be used to predict the effect of treatment on renal function.[14] Figure 25-2 shows pretreatment USG data from cats experiencing renal insufficiency after treatment of hyperthyroidism. USG was greater than 1.035 in 54 per cent of the hyperthyroid cats who developed posttreatment renal insufficiency, and there was no statistically significant difference in USG between those cats who did and did not develop renal insufficiency.

It has been shown that USG is significantly lower in cats with hyperthyroidism compared with normal cats. The reason for this is unclear, but it might have little to do with the kidneys themselves. Certainly thyroid hormone has an effect on renal tubules, but those effects may not be clinically relevant. Renal tubular epithelial cells undergo hypertrophy in response to excess thyroid hormone, and many abnormalities in electrolyte and water metabolism exist in hyperthyroidism. Phosphate transport and sodium-potassium exchange are increased, among other changes. The end result of excess thyroid hormone in animals with normal kidneys, however, is normal urine. Although not clinically significant, some human patients with hyperthyroidism have mildly dilute urine, but it is caused by thyrotoxicosis-associated primary polydipsia.[8]

Measurement of GFR itself also is not a good predictor of the development of posttreatment renal insufficiency in feline hyperthyroidism. One study found a GFR of 2.25 mL/kg/min to be the cutoff point above which cats did not run the risk of renal insufficiency after radioiodine therapy.[5] However, very little agreement exists in measurement of GFR between the few laboratories that have published data on GFR in cats and between methods used, so an absolute GFR value based on a single study can not be used to predict the renal response to treatment of hyperthyroidism.

Lastly the N-acetyl-beta-D-glucosaminidase (NAG) index has been studied as a predictor of posttreatment renal insufficiency in hyperthyroid cats.[15] NAG is an enzyme found in proximal renal tubular epithelial cells, and it is proposed to be a marker for kidney disease in cats. However, the NAG index was found to be a poor predictor of posttreatment renal insufficiency.

ARE SOME TREATMENTS SAFER THAN OTHERS?

It is sometimes stated, based on anecdotal evidence at best, that methimazole therapy or radioiodine therapy is preferable to surgical thyroidectomy for treatment of feline hyperthyroidism because of a lower risk of posttreatment renal failure. It is thought that a slower return to euthyroidism observed in cats treated with radioiodine or antithyroid drugs might cause a more gradual and smaller decrease in GFR. Large studies comparing the effects of radioiodine, antithyroid drugs, and surgical thyroidectomy have not been reported, but one smaller study found no differences in posttreatment serum concentrations of creatinine, blood urea nitrogen, or TT_4 concentrations based on mode of treatment.[16] Figure 25-1 shows a comparison of changes in GFR between hyperthyroid cats treated with methimazole (see Figure 25-1, A) or thyroidectomy (see Figure 25-1, B). Although GFR was maintained posttreatment in some of the methimazole-treated cats versus all thyroidectomized cats experiencing a decrease in GFR, it is important to recognize that the two treatments were not examined together in the same study. Posttreatment renal insufficiency seems to be equally common regardless of the mode of treatment for hyperthyroidism.

METHIMAZOLE TRIALS

Because the development of posttreatment renal insufficiency is unpredictable based on laboratory testing, it is recommended that hyperthyroid cats undergo a therapeutic trial with methimazole, a reversible form of treatment of hyperthyroidism, prior to treatment with a more permanent therapy such as radioiodine or thyroidectomy. If a cat does not become azotemic or show clinical signs of renal failure when euthyroidism is achieved using methimazole, other treatments may be considered safe. It is important to note, however, that this hypothesis has not been studied, and it is possible that a given cat will still develop renal insufficiency after radio-iodine therapy or thyroidectomy, even if it was non-azotemic upon treatment with antithyroid drugs.

There are many different recommendations for how and when methimazole trials should be performed. Unfortunately there are few published data to guide these decisions. In some cats methimazole trials are impractical or not possible, as a result of adverse reactions to the drug or owner inability to administer oral medication. Transdermal methimazole may be a useful alternative for patients to whom owners are unable to give methimazole tablets by mouth. However, it should be noted that, with the exception of vomiting, side effects of methimazole are similar regardless of route of administration.[17]

Until recently it was difficult to determine the appropriate length of time for a methimazole trial, but a new study showed that the greatest decline in GFR occurs within the first month after treatment of hyperthyroidism, and that GFR remains relatively stable for the next 5 months.[18] Based on those results a 30-day methimazole trial would seem sufficient. A common mistake, however, is failure to recheck serum thyroid hormone concentrations during the methimazole trial. Because the serum half-life of TT_4 in cats is less than 8 hours, TT_4 concentration should be measured 1 week after starting a methimazole trial. If the TT_4 is not in the lower half of the reference range (i.e., the optimal level for hyperthyroidism control), the dose should be increased and the 30-day period should be started over. In addition, because of the possibility of life-threatening side effects of methimazole (e.g., hepatopathy, blood dyscrasia), it is never appropriate to wait 1 month before the initial reevaluation after starting methimazole therapy.

TREATMENT OF POSTTREATMENT RENAL INSUFFICIENCY

Despite efforts to predict posttreatment renal insufficiency in cats with hyperthyroidism, whether by methimazole trial or by other means, overt renal insufficiency can occur. In such cases the clinician is left with the decision of allowing a cat to remain relatively more thyrotoxic, in order to preserve renal blood flow and support GFR, or to tolerate a certain level of azotemia in order to prevent clinical signs and consequences of thyroid hormone excess. There is no established formula for management of these cases, and data to support recommendations for treatment of cats with renal insufficiency following treatment of hyperthyroidism are lacking.

In the author's practice hyperthyroid or previously hyperthyroid cats with renal failure are monitored carefully, and treatment is tailored to the individual cat. For example, if a cat is showing clinical signs of uremia (e.g., poor appetite, gastrointestinal signs, lethargy, dehydration), the decision might be made to maintain a higher-than-usual serum TT_4 concentration to achieve a better

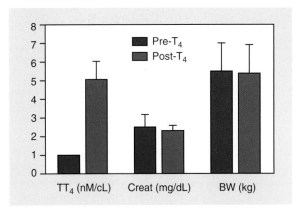

Figure 25-3 Serum concentrations of total thyroxine (TT_4) and creatinine (Creat), and body weight (BW) in five cats before (Pre-T_4) and after supplementation with thyroxine (Post-T_4) at 0.1 mg/cat PO q12h. All cats had renal azotemia following treatment with radioiodine, and thyroxine supplementation was given for 2 to 4 weeks between measurements.

quality of life for the patient. On the other hand, if clinical signs of thyrotoxicosis predominate (e.g., polyphagia, weight loss, hyperactivity), better control of hyperthyroidism might be preferred, even if a relatively higher level of azotemia is maintained. Experimental studies have shown that as thyroid hormone concentrations increase, GFR increases and serum creatinine concentration decreases. However, it has not been demonstrated convincingly that maintaining a relatively higher plane of hyperthyroidism will cause a decrease in serum creatinine concentration in a cat with renal failure following treatment for hyperthyroidism.

Figure 25-3 illustrates data from five cats with post–radioiodine renal insufficiency seen in the author's hospital. Supplementation with exogenous thyroxine resulted in the predicted increase in serum concentration of TT_4, but there was no observable change in creatinine concentrations or in body weight or clinical signs. Further work is needed to determine the proper strategy for managing these cases.

MANAGING HYPERTENSION

Controlling hypertension is an important aspect of management of cats with renal insufficiency following treatment of hyperthyroidism. Hypertension is harmful to the kidneys,[19] and control of hypertension and proteinuria is associated with longer survival in cats with renal disease (see Chapter 49). Drugs used to treat hypertension in cats fall into three categories: β-adrenergic antagonists, angiotensin-converting enzyme (ACE) inhibitors, and calcium-channel blockers (Table 25-2). While hypertension has been documented in cats with hyperthyroidism,[20,21] a cause-and-effect relationship has not been established. Hypertension is uncommon in people with hyperthyroidism; thyrotoxicosis is associated with decreased peripheral vascular resistance and blood pressure usually is normal. In some human patients with hyperthyroidism, marked tachycardia is thought to cause a summation

Table 25-2 Antihypertensive Drugs Used in Cats

Drug	Dosage	Notes
Amlodipine	0.625 mg/cat PO q24h	Calcium channel blocker Used for severe hypertension Decreases proteinuria Well tolerated in cats
Benazepril	0.5 mg/kg PO q12-24h	ACE inhibitor Not as effective as amlodipine Decreases proteinuria Delays progression of kidney disease Well tolerated in cats
Enalapril	0.5 mg/kg PO q12-24h	ACE inhibitor Not as effective as amlodipine No negative effects on kidneys Well tolerated in cats
Atenolol	3.125-6.25 mg/cat PO q12h	Selective β_1 antagonist Controls tachycardia Useful in hyperthyroidism Limited use for hypertension

of pressure in peripheral arteries with the pressure from systole, resulting in overall systolic hypertension.[22] Hypertension typically resolves in these patients upon treatment with β-blockers. Based on this, there is some rationale for the use of β-blockers in the treatment of hypertension in hyperthyroid cats. The calcium-channel blocker amlodipine, however, is probably the antihypertensive drug used most commonly in cats, with or without hyperthyroidism. Studies have shown a significant reduction in pathological proteinuria and slowed progression of kidney disease in hypertensive cats treated with amlodipine.[23]

In general, the ACE inhibitors enalapril and benazepril are less effective antihypertensive agents than amlodipine; however, there is considerable interest in their use in treating hypertension in cats with hyperthyroidism. Benazepril has beneficial effects on the kidneys.[24,25] Its administration slows the progression of glomerulosclerosis in cats, and its use is associated with decreased proteinuria in cats with chronic kidney disease. Therefore benazepril administration seems wise in cats with hyperthyroidism and renal failure, and the combination of an ACE inhibitor and a calcium-channel blocker sometimes is used in these patients. (See Chapter 49 for a further discussion on managing and monitoring hypertension.)

REFERENCES

1. Plantinga EA, Everts H, Kastelein AM, et al: Retrospective study of the survival of cats with acquired chronic renal insufficiency offered different commercial diets, *Vet Rec* 157: 185, 2005.
2. Mooney CT: Hyperthyroidism. In Ettinger SJ, Feldman ED, editors: *Textbook of veterinary internal medicine. Diseases of the dog and cat*, ed 6, St. Louis, 2005, Saunders, p 1544.
3. Graves TK, Olivier NB, Nachreiner RF, et al: Changes in renal function associated with treatment of hyperthyroidism in cats, *Am J Vet Res* 55:1745, 1994.
4. Becker TJ, Graves TK, Kruger JM, et al: Effects of methimazole on renal function in cats with hyperthyroidism, *J Am Anim Hosp Assoc* 36:215, 2000.
5. Adams WH, Daniel GB, Legendre AM, et al: Changes in renal function in cats following treatment of hyperthyroidism using 131I, *Vet Radiol Ultrasound* 38:231, 1997.
6. Bradley SE, Stephan F, Coelho JB, et al: The thyroid and the kidney, *Kidney Int* 6:346, 1974.
7. Klein I, Ojamaa K: Thyroid hormone and the cardiovascular system, *N Engl J Med* 344:501, 2001.
8. Moses AM, Scheinman SJ: The kidneys and electrolyte metabolism in thyrotoxicosis. In Braverman LE, Utiger RD, editors: *Werner and Ingbar's the thyroid: a fundamental and clinical text*, ed 7, Philadelphia, 1996, Lippincott-Raven, p 628.
9. Slater MR, Komkov A, Robinson LE, et al: Long-term follow-up of hyperthyroid cats treated with iodine-131, *Vet Radiol Ultrasound* 35:204, 1994.
10. Peterson ME, Melián C, Nichols R: Measurement of serum concentrations of free thyroxine, total thyroxine, and total triiodothyronine in cats with hyperthyroidism and cats with nonthyroidal disease, *J Am Vet Med Assoc* 218:529, 2001.
11. Wakeling J, Moore K, Elliott J, et al: Diagnosis of hyperthyroidism in cats with mild chronic kidney disease, *J Small Anim Pract* 49:287, 2008.
12. Aizawa T, Hiramatsu K, Ohtsuka H, et al: An elevation of BUN/creatinine ratio in patients with hyperthyroidism, *Horm Metab Res* 18:771, 1986.
13. Garrett LD: How to refer: the hyperthyroid cat, *NAVC Clinician's Brief* 4:79, 2006.
14. Riensche MR, Graves TK: An investigation of predictors of renal insufficiency following treatment of hyperthyroidism in cats, *J Feline Med Surg* 10:160, 2008.
15. Lapointe C, Bélanger MC, Dunn M, et al: N-acetyl-beta-D-glucosaminidase index as an early biomarker for chronic kidney disease in cats with hyperthyroidism, *J Vet Intern Med* 22:1103, 2008.
16. DiBartola SP, Broome MR, Stein BS, et al: Effect of treatment of hyperthyroidism on renal function in cats, *J Am Vet Med Assoc* 208:875, 1996.
17. Sartor LL, Trepanier LA, Kroll MM, et al: Efficacy and safety of transdermal methimazole in the treatment of cats with hyperthyroidism, *J Vet Intern Med* 18:651, 2004.
18. van Hoek I, Lefebvre HP, Kooistra HS, et al: Plasma clearance of exogenous creatinine, exo-iohexol, and endo-iohexol in hyperthyroid cats before and after treatment with radioiodine, *J Vet Intern Med* 22:879, 2008.
19. Brown S, Atkins C, Bagley R, et al: American College of Veterinary Internal Medicine. Guidelines for the identification, evaluation, and management of systemic hypertension in dogs and cats, *J Vet Intern Med* 21:542, 2007.
20. Kobayashi DL, Peterson ME, Graves TK, et al: Hypertension in cats with chronic renal failure or hyperthyroidism, *J Vet Intern Med* 4:58, 1990.
21. Maggio F, DeFrancesco TC, Atkins CE, et al: Ocular lesions associated with systemic hypertension in cats: 69 cases (1985-1998), *J Am Vet Med Assoc* 217:695, 2000.
22. Biondi B, Palmieri EA, Lombardi G, et al: Effects of thyroid hormone on cardiac function: the relative importance of

heart rate, loading conditions, and myocardial contractility in the regulation of cardiac performance in human hyperthyroidism, *J Clin Endocrinol Metab* 87:968, 2002.

23. Jepson RE, Elliott J, Brodbelt D, et al: Effect of control of systolic blood pressure on survival in cats with systemic hypertension, *J Vet Intern Med* 21:402, 2007.

24. Lefebvre HP, Brown SA, Chetboul V, et al: Angiotensin-converting enzyme inhibitors in veterinary medicine, *Curr Pharm Des* 13:1347, 2007.

25. Mizutani H, Koyama H, Watanabe T, et al: Evaluation of the clinical efficacy of benazepril in the treatment of chronic renal insufficiency in cats, *J Vet Intern Med* 20:1074, 2006.

26 Home Monitoring of Blood Glucose in Cats with Diabetes Mellitus

Claudia E. Reusch and Nadja S. Sieber-Ruckstuhl

Diabetes mellitus is a common endocrine disease in cats. A recent study reported an increase in hospital prevalence over 30 years from 0.08 per cent in 1970 to 1.2 per cent in 1999.[1] Currently it is assumed that approximately 80 per cent of these cats suffer from type 2–like diabetes, which is characterized by a combination of insulin resistance by peripheral tissues and liver and of β-cell failure. High blood glucose itself has negative effects on β-cell function and insulin sensitivity, a phenomenon called glucose toxicity. Immediate treatment may reverse these effects, at least in part, and the diabetes may go into remission. Remission usually occurs during the first 3 months of therapy; however, it may take 1 year or longer.[2] The possibility of diabetic remission is one of the reasons why close supervision and regular measurement of blood glucose is paramount. If remission occurs unnoticed and the administration of insulin is not discontinued, serious hypoglycemia may result.

The aim of therapy is to provide a good quality of life by eliminating clinical signs of diabetes (achieve remission, if possible), and by preventing complications such as hypoglycemia and ketoacidosis. Achieving normal blood glucose levels is not necessary, because most cats do well when the blood glucose concentration is maintained between 90 and 270 mg/dL.

Successful treatment requires that the owner be highly motivated and collaborate closely with the veterinarian, who should follow a precise protocol. Box 26-1 gives a brief overview of the protocol used in our hospital.

MONITORING IN THE HOSPITAL

Home monitoring (HM) of blood glucose by owners is an additional tool to improve long-term management of diabetes. However, it does not replace regular reevaluation by a veterinarian. The latter should include assessment of clinical signs and determination of serum fructosamine and blood glucose concentrations. The assessment of clinical signs by both owner and veterinarian is the most important parameter. A well-regulated cat has no or only very mild clinical signs of diabetes. In a cat with no clinical signs it is crucial to determine whether diabetic remission has occurred. In cats with persistent clinical signs, the cause must be identified and therapy optimized accordingly.

Fructosamine is the product of an irreversible reaction between glucose and the amino groups of various serum proteins, and its concentration reflects the mean blood glucose concentration of the preceding 1 to 2 weeks. Reference ranges differ slightly among laboratories but usually are around 200 to 360 μmol/L. In most cats with newly diagnosed diabetes, fructosamine levels are higher than 400 μmol/L and may be as high as 1500 μmol/L. Normal fructosamine levels may be seen in cats with a very recent onset of diabetes and in diabetic cats suffering from concurrent hyperthyroidism or hypoproteinemia.[3-5] Fructosamine concentrations increase when glycemic control worsens and decrease when glycemic control improves. Because even well-controlled cats are slightly

Box 26-1 Treatment and Management Protocol for Cats with Uncomplicated (Nonketotic) Diabetes Mellitus Used at the University of Zurich, Switzerland

AT THE TIME OF DIAGNOSIS
- Diagnosis (hyperglycemia, glucosuria, increased fructosamine) and evaluation for concurrent diseases (e.g., urinary tract infection [urine culture], hyperthyroidism [T$_4$], pancreatitis [abdominal ultrasonography, fPLI]).
- Cessation of diabetogenic drugs if possible.
- Start insulin therapy with intermediate-acting insulin (Caninsulin/Vetsulin or glargine, 1 to 2 U/cat q12h, depending on body weight and degree of metabolic derangement (i.e., severity of clinical signs, degree of hyperglycemia, and elevation of fructosamine).
- Hospitalization for 1 to 2 days.
- Measurement of blood glucose 3 to 4×/day (approximately every 4-6 hours); decrease insulin dose (by 25-50 per cent) if blood glucose drops by <90 mg/dL and reevaluation if dosage decrease was sufficient on the following day.
- Discharge after demonstration of injection techniques, with detailed written instructions; recommendation of high-protein, low-carbohydrate diet; weight loss if overweight. Possibility of home monitoring (HM) is mentioned.

RECHECK IN HOSPITAL 1 WEEK AFTER DIAGNOSIS
- History, body weight, physical examination.
- Blood glucose curve over 10 to 12 hours (insulin and food given at home, blood glucose measured every 1-2 hours). Fructosamine measurement.
- Adjustment of insulin dose if required (increments of 0.5-1 U/injection).
- HM and its advantages are discussed with the owner.

RECHECK IN HOSPITAL 3 WEEKS AFTER DIAGNOSIS
- History, body weight, physical examination, blood glucose curve, fructosamine measurement, dose adjustment (as after 1 week).

- Introduction to home monitoring of blood glucose if owner is interested.

HOME MONITORING OF BLOOD GLUCOSE BY THE OWNER
- Measurement of fasting capillary blood glucose 2×/week.
- Generation of 12-hour capillary blood glucose curve (measurement of glucose every 2 hours), 1×/month.

RECHECK IN HOSPITAL 6 TO 8 WEEKS AFTER DIAGNOSIS
- History, body weight, physical examination, blood glucose curve, fructosamine measurement, dose adjustment (as after 1 week).
- Reassessment of home monitoring techniques (if performed).
- Tests for underlying diseases if clinical suspicion (e.g., hypercortisolism, hypersomatotropism).

RECHECK IN HOSPITAL 10 TO 12 WEEKS AFTER DIAGNOSIS
- History, body weight, physical examination, blood glucose curve, fructosamine measurement, dose adjustment (as after 1 week).
- Reassessment of home monitoring techniques (if used).

FURTHER RECHECKS IN HOSPITAL EVERY 4 TO 6 MONTHS
- History, body weight, physical examination, blood glucose curve, fructosamine measurement, dose adjustment (as after 1 week).
- Reassessment of home monitoring techniques (if used).
- Urine culture once a year.

to moderately hyperglycemic throughout the day, fructosamine concentration usually will not decrease into the normal range. Accordingly a normal fructosamine concentration (particularly a fructosamine value in the lower half of the reference range) should raise concern about prolonged periods of hypoglycemia (e.g., insulin overdose, diabetic remission).

In general metabolic control is considered good when fructosamine levels are between 350 and 450 μmol/L, moderate when values are between 450 and 550 μmol/L, and poor when levels are higher than 550 to 600 μmol/L. In the latter case, fructosamine is not helpful in characterizing the problem because all of the possible reasons for poor regulation (e.g., insulin underdose, too short a duration of insulin effect, diseases causing insulin resistance, insulin absorption problems, Somogyi effect) have the same impact on fructosamine. In some cats fructosamine levels remain high, suggesting poor metabolic control, although clinical signs and blood

glucose levels are well-controlled. The reason for this discrepancy in most cats remains unknown. Therefore the assessment of clinical signs and blood glucose concentration are the most important criteria for treatment decisions.

Blood glucose curves (BGCs) are necessary to assess insulin efficacy, glucose nadir, duration of insulin effect, degree of blood glucose fluctuation, and the Somogyi effect. In general single glucose measurements are considered insufficient to assess metabolic control.

Evaluation of BGCs is of particular importance in the initial phases of diabetic regulation and in cats with persistence of clinical signs. For performance of an in-hospital BGC we prefer that owners give insulin and food at home, and then bring the cat to the hospital as soon as possible (within 2 hours). This approach eliminates the effect of lack of food intake on blood glucose levels if the cat refuses to eat in the clinic, at least in those cats who are only fed at the time of insulin administration. Only when technical difficulties are suspected are owners asked to bring the cat to the hospital before insulin administration and to carry out the entire injection procedure under supervision. Different approaches may be more appropriate depending on the circumstances; for instance, when the distance between the cat's home and the hospital is very long.

BGCs are generated by measuring the glucose concentration every 1 to 2 hours throughout the day until the next insulin dose is due. In our hospital, we avoid multiple venipunctures by collecting capillary blood from the ear using the same sampling technique and the same portable blood glucose meter (PBGM) as cat owners at home (see later).

Until recently BGCs were only created in the hospital because most owners are not skilled in collecting venous blood samples. However, there are several problems associated with serial blood glucose measurements in hospitalized cats. First, the procedure is time consuming and expensive; therefore in many patients it may not be carried out as often as indicated. Second, the concentration of blood glucose can be influenced markedly by stress or lack of food intake. Cats in particular are sensitive to stress caused by veterinary manipulation in an unfamiliar environment. Consequently the BGC may show a continual increase in glucose concentration or it may be elevated from the beginning. In the latter situation it is not possible to differentiate between stress-associated hyperglycemia, insulin underdose, and the many causes of insulin resistance. In cats who are brought to the hospital to generate a BGC before feeding or in cats who are used to nibbling food throughout the day, refusal to eat has a serious impact on blood glucose concentration. It is then difficult to decide whether lack of food intake or insulin overdose is the cause of low glucose concentrations.

SELF-MONITORING OF BLOOD GLUCOSE IN HUMAN BEINGS WITH DIABETES MELLITUS

In the late 1970s self-monitoring of blood glucose (SMBG) was introduced in human medicine.[6-8] For SMBG human patients obtain a drop of capillary blood, usually by pricking a fingertip, with the aid of a lancing device. The drop then is placed on a test strip, and the glucose concentration is measured using a PBGM. The sampling process is simple and has become relatively painless with the use of newer generations of lancing devices. The introduction of SMBG is regarded as the single most important advance in the management of diabetes since the discovery of insulin.[9] Today all diabetes treatment guidelines include SMBG as an integral part. Diabetic individuals (type 1 and 2) treated with insulin are advised to perform SMBG several times daily, and regular monitoring also is recommended in diabetics treated with oral hypoglycemic drugs or diet only.[10] More frequent SMBG is associated with better metabolic control, which in turn decreases the incidence and slows the progression of complications of long-standing diabetes.[9,11-13] SMBG has made it possible for patients to obtain immediate and precise feedback on their blood glucose concentration, allows them to understand the impact of food choices, physical activity, and concurrent illness, and gives them control of their disease.

Patients conducting SMBG need guidance and supervision because user technique is the major source of errors. All authorities recommend that each patient's monitoring technique be evaluated initially and at regular intervals thereafter. Patients also need to be taught how to use the data to adjust food intake, exercise, or drug therapy.

For human beings who find pricking a fingertip unpleasant, alternative site testing has been developed. Those sites where pricking may be less painful include the upper arm, forearm, base of the thumb, tip of the earlobe, and the thigh. Blood glucose levels obtained from alternative sites may differ slightly from those obtained from the fingertips.[14,15]

HOME MONITORING OF BLOOD GLUCOSE BY CAT OWNERS

BLOOD SAMPLING TECHNIQUES

Until a few years ago SMBG in diabetic pets was not thought to be feasible. However, several methods have been developed recently to obtain capillary blood by means of lancing devices manufactured for human patients. In 2000 two methods of capillary blood sampling from the ear were described.[16] One method, which used a conventional lancing device after prewarming the ear with a hair dryer, was applicable only to dogs. The other method, the "Vaculance method," was based on a new type of lancing device introduced at that time, the Microlet Vaculance (Bayer Diagnostics, Basel, Switzerland), and it was applied successfully in cats as well as in dogs (Figure 26-1). After lancing the skin the device creates a negative pressure, which enables the sampling of an adequate amount of blood in most instances. The details of the procedure for the Vaculance method are as follows. The tip of the ear is held between the thumb and index finger and the entire surface of the outer pinna is held flat using the remaining fingers of the same hand. With the other hand the lancing device is lightly placed on a nonhaired area of the inner pinna, such that an airtight seal is formed between the end cap of the device and the skin. When the plunger cap of the device is pressed, a lancet moves quickly back and forth one time. Pressure between the end cap and the skin is maintained while the plunger is slowly released. Because of the developing negative pressure, the skin of the ear begins to bulge into the end cap. The formation of a drop of blood is hastened by releasing the pressure exerted by the fingers on the outer surface of the pinna. When an adequate amount of blood appears on the skin, the plunger is pressed down to release the negative pressure and the lancing device is removed. Then the test strip of the PBGM is brought into contact with the blood drop and the required amount of blood is absorbed automatically (Figure 26-2).

The buccal mucosa has been described as another site for capillary blood sampling in dogs.[17] This site probably is not feasible in cats. Gums, lips, and footpads also have been mentioned as possible puncture sites,[18] but there are no studies that have investigated their suitability in cats. It is not known whether blood glucose levels vary with different sampling sites in cats, as is the case in human beings.

An alternative to capillary sampling is the collection of venous blood from the marginal ear vein. This tech-nique, called the marginal ear vein technique, has been used successfully in diabetic cats.[19,20] After localization of the marginal ear vein on the edge of the pinna, the vein is either punctured with a needle or a lancing device. Thompson et al[19] reported that a warm gauze sponge applied before puncture increased perfusion, and applica-tion of a thin film of petrolatum over the sampling site in long-haired cats allowed a drop of blood to form without dissipating into the fur. Van de Maele et al[20] prepared the puncture site in long-haired cats by shaving a small part of the pinna to improve visualization of the vein, and by placing a hard cylinder-shaped object, such as the empty roll from bandage material, behind the ear to provide stability. Afterwards pressure is applied to the punctured area to avoid excessive bleeding.

The Vaculance method has been used exclusively in our hospital and by our pet owners for almost 10 years, and therefore we do not have experience with the mar-ginal ear vein technique. The Vaculance method is easy to conduct, does not require warming of the ear or any other preparation of the puncture site, and generates a drop of blood within about 30 seconds. In contrast to the marginal ear vein technique, no bleeding is expected after capillary blood sampling and therefore no pressure is needed after the puncturing procedure.

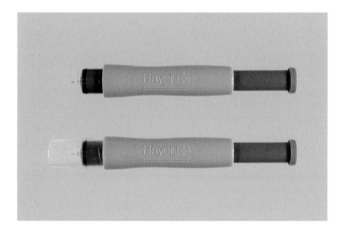

Figure 26-1 Lancing device Microlet Vaculance (Bayer Diagnostics).

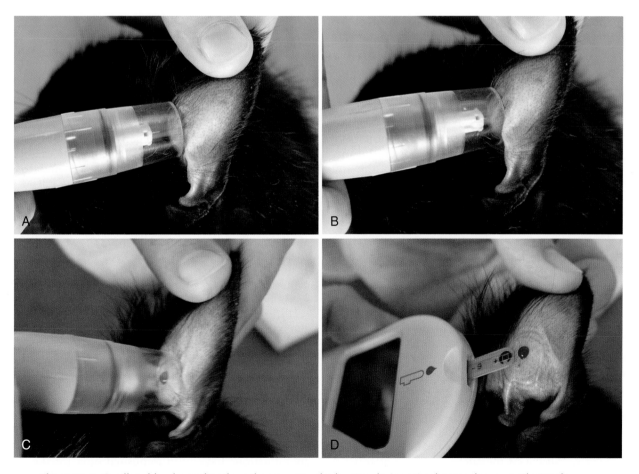

Figure 26-2 Capillary blood sampling from the ear using the lancing device Microlet Vaculance. **A,** Placing the lancing device on a nonhaired area of the pinna. **B,** Pressing the plunger cap of the device to move the lancet back and forth. **C,** Slowly releasing the plunger to develop a negative pressure between the end cap and the skin. **D,** Absorption of the blood drop by the test strip of the PBGM.

PORTABLE BLOOD GLUCOSE METER

The first PBGM was the Ames Reflectance Meter, patented in 1971 by the Ames Company. It was almost 20 cm long and required a very large drop of capillary blood, strips that had to be washed and wiped after blood application, and an electrical power outlet. The blood glucose concentration was indicated by the position of a needle on a graduated scale after 60 seconds.

Since then numerous models have been developed and marketed that are smaller, lighter, faster, and easier to handle. Today the average PBGM fits in the palm of a hand, is battery powered, requires a very small amount of blood, and provides rapid results on a display screen. Modern PBGMs have a memory capacity for the last series of test results, and some allow data to be transferred to a personal computer. Certain models require coding or calibration, a process used to match the PBGM with the test strips. Usually this is done by inserting a code strip or entering a code number into the meter each time a new box of test strips is opened. If this process is carried out incorrectly, the readings can be inaccurate. In some PBGMs a "no coding technology" is used, ensuring that the correct code is set automatically any time a new test strip is inserted. This reduces the risk of inaccurate blood glucose measurements and simplifies meter handling. Most new models function on the basis of electrochemical methods; for example, glucose-oxidase measurements are converted into electrical signals. PBGMs often are available at little or no cost; however, the price of the test strips can be substantial.

In human medicine, quality control of PBGMs is of ongoing concern. Factors that may affect the results of glucose measurements include variation in hematocrit, altitude, environmental temperature and humidity, hypotension, hypoxia, and triglyceride concentration.[21] The overall performance of a PBGM depends on the analytical accuracy of the unit, quality of the test strips, and proficiency of the user. The goal of the American Diabetes Association is that all measurements conducted with a PBGM be within 5 per cent of the laboratory value. However, this target is not met currently.[22]

In veterinary medicine the use of PBGMs has gained great popularity during recent years. They are not only an essential part of the HM procedure, but also are used frequently in veterinary hospitals for routine blood glucose measurements. However, it must be remembered that these devices have been designed for human beings, and most PBGMs currently available have not been validated for use in cats. However, a few studies have investigated the accuracy of PBGMs in cats.[16,19,23-25] In two studies PBGM measurements using capillary blood were compared with glucose measurements using venous blood and a reference method.[16,25]

In our own study[16] the PBGMs Glucometer Elite (Bayer Diagnostics) and Accu-Chek Simplicity (Roche Diagnostics, Inc., Indianapolis, IN) were evaluated. Using error grid analysis,[26] all PBGM measurements were in zones A and B, which is indicative of clinically acceptable results (Figure 26-3). The Glucometer Elite was considered the easiest to operate because it has no buttons to press and turns on automatically when the test strip is inserted; it

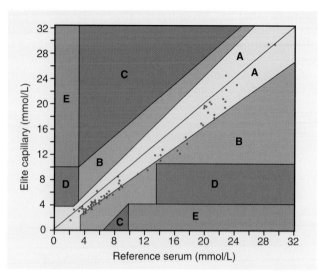

Figure 26-3 Error grid analysis for the Glucometer Elite using capillary blood. Values in zone A (clinically accurate) and zone B (benign estimate errors) are clinically acceptable. Values in zone C (unnecessary corrections), D (dangerous failure to detect) or E (erroneous treatment) are potentially dangerous and therefore not acceptable from a clinical point of view. For the Glucometer Elite all values were in zone A or B. Blood glucose values are given in mmol/L. Multiply by 18 to convert to mg/dL. (From Wess G, Reusch CE: Capillary blood sampling from the ear of dogs and cats and use of portable meters to measure glucose concentration, *J Small Anim Pract* 41:60, 2000, with permission.)

is the PBGM used in our hospital and by our pet owners. In contrast to other PBGMs, which underestimate or overestimate true blood glucose concentrations arbitrarily, the Glucometer Elite yielded underestimations consistently. In 2002 Bayer changed the brand name of their glucose monitor line, and the Glucometer Elite was renamed Ascensia Elite. Zeugswetter et al[25] compared capillary blood glucose values measured by the PBGM Free-Style Freedom (Abbott Laboratories, Abbott Park, IL) with venous blood glucose values measured by the reference method. The former were a mean of 32 mg/dL lower than the latter, and the error grid analysis showed that 96 per cent of the data measured with the PBGM were in zones A and B, and 2 per cent each were in zones C and E. Values in the latter zones are not acceptable from a clinical point of view.

Information about potential sources of error using PBGMs is scarce in veterinary medicine, and further studies are needed. To date it has only been shown that a low hematocrit results in a spurious increase in PBGM readings.[24]

Several companies are now marketing PBGMs for veterinary use and claim that they give more accurate results than PBGMs designed for human beings. Currently these devices include the GlucoPet or GlucoVet (ADM) and the AlphaTrak (Abbott Laboratories). However, independent investigations have been published only for the Alpha-Trak in dogs.[27] In that study six different PBGMs (including those designed for human and veterinary use) were evaluated using venous blood samples, and results were compared with those derived from the reference method.

The AlphaTrak was superior to all other PBGMs including the Ascensia Elite. According to preliminary studies in our hospital, this also may hold true for cats. Compared with the Ascensia Elite, the AlphaTrak is more demanding to operate; for example, it must be turned on manually and selection of a code number is required. However, these disadvantages probably are offset by the fact that the required blood volume is extremely small (0.3 µL) and the test time is very short (15 seconds). The measurement range of the AlphaTrak is 20 to 500 mg/dL.

In summary it is difficult to maintain a good general view of the accuracy of all available PBGMs because new devices are being developed constantly. PBGM readings usually differ to some extent from values measured by a reference method. However, these differences should be as small as possible to avoid treatment errors. Each new type of PBGM should be validated before it is used in cats.

INTRODUCTION OF CAPILLARY BLOOD GLUCOSE MEASUREMENT TO CAT OWNERS

Home monitoring of blood glucose concentration has been part of the routine protocol for long-term management of diabetic pets in our clinic since 1999. Owners are introduced to the technique in a stepwise fashion (see Box 26-1). The first step of the process takes place at the time of discharge after a definitive diagnosis of diabetes mellitus has been made. The owner receives detailed information on various aspects of diabetes mellitus, including dietary recommendations and insulin injection technique, and the concept of HM is introduced for the first time. This consultation takes approximately 45 minutes. The second step consists of reevaluation of the cat after 1 week. Owner observations are discussed, followed by a physical examination, fructosamine measurement, and generation of an in-clinic BGC. The insulin dose is adjusted, if necessary, in increments of 0.5 to 1 U/cat q12h. At the time of discharge the importance of the BGC in the control of the disease is emphasized. In addition, the advantages of HM are discussed, and the owner is informed that this procedure can be started after the next reevaluation.

The third step follows approximately 3 weeks after a diagnosis of diabetes has been made. Once again owner observations are assessed, a physical examination is performed, a BGC is generated, and the fructosamine concentration is determined. The owner then is given the opportunity to learn the technique of HM. This requires a minimum of 30 minutes and consists of repeated demonstrations of the use of the lancing device and the PBGM. The owner then practices the technique several times on his or her cat. The owner also is taught how to calibrate and check the accuracy of the PBGM (if this is required with the chosen PBGM) and record the blood glucose values on prepared forms (Figure 26-4). HM is not started before this time to allow the owner to become familiar with the disease and gain experience with the injection of insulin, which may pose a challenge in itself. Introduction of HM is delayed to a later date if the clinician has doubts that the owner is ready for the task. It is important that owners carry out the procedure on a regular basis to remain familiar with it, and that reassessments are done frequently.[28] Therefore the owners

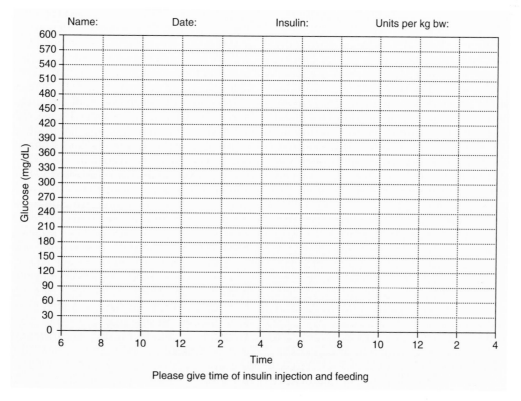

Figure 26-4 Form for cat owners to report blood glucose concentrations of a BGC.

are asked to measure fasting blood glucose concentrations at least twice per week and to generate a BGC (measurement of blood glucose every 2 hours for 12 hours) at least once per month. The former serves to detect morning hypoglycemia, in which case the owner is instructed to call the hospital. The BGCs generated by the owner are sent to the hospital by fax or e-mail, and appropriate changes in treatment are discussed over the phone. During the first few weeks of HM, periodic reassessment of the entire procedure in the hospital is advisable. Our protocol consists of having the owner measure the fasting blood glucose concentration, injecting the insulin, and feeding the cat at home. In the hospital, the owner takes another blood sample from the ear while a veterinarian watches the procedure. Possible technical problems can be discussed and remedied. During subsequent long-term management regular veterinary reevaluation of the diabetic cat is recommended (see Box 26-1), even if the owner is experienced with HM. Because HM has not been used widely in veterinary medicine, there are no studies to substantiate how often reevaluation should be scheduled. Currently we recommend that owners generate a BGC at least once per month and the patient be reassessed in the hospital approximately every 4 months (see Box 26-1).

PROBLEMS ENCOUNTERED IN HOME MONITORING

In a recent study owners of diabetic cats were asked to conduct one BGC per month over a 4-month period and to fill in a questionnaire covering all aspects of the procedure after each curve.[29,30] Twelve of 15 owners were able to determine blood glucose concentrations, whereas three could not because their cats were not cooperative.

Problems encountered initially included restraining the cat, producing negative pressure with the lancing device, generating a blood drop, absorption of the blood drop, and correct use of the test strips and the PBGM. At the end of the study problems occurred only occasionally and involved restraint of the cat, production of a blood drop, and generation of negative pressure using the lancing device. At the end of the study HM was considered straightforward by five owners, mostly straightforward by six, and difficult by one. Ten of the twelve owners conducted BG measurements on their own and two required help from another person.[30]

During instruction and demonstration of the HM procedure particular emphasis should be placed on those aspects of the procedure that cause the most problems. It is important that owners have ready access to veterinary support, if required. The majority of our clients call for advice at least once, especially after the start of HM. Some have specific questions regarding the procedure, while others just need reassurance that they are conducting the procedure correctly. Sometimes support via telephone is not sufficient and additional explanation or demonstration of the technique must be provided. By watching an owner carry out the procedure the clinician can identify and correct errors immediately. The prerequisite for good owner instruction is a knowledgeable veterinarian who is able to conduct the procedure correctly and is aware of all potential sources of error. Usually owners feel that their technique improves quickly, which leads to increased confidence in the test results. Many owners devise strategies for easier restraint of their cat and report that the cats tolerate blood collection better when placed in a favorite location, such as a windowsill or bed, or in a confined area such as a sink. The skin puncture does not seem to be painful, and the puncture sites are barely visible, even after numerous blood collections.[29,31]

INTERPRETATION OF BLOOD GLUCOSE CURVES GENERATED AT HOME AND COMPARISON OF HOME AND HOSPITAL BLOOD GLUCOSE CURVES

Our protocol for generation of a BGC at home is to have the owner measure the glucose concentration before the insulin injection and every 2 hours thereafter for 12 hours. More frequent measurements (hourly) should be suggested in cases with a suspected Somogyi effect. Owners certainly can be taught to interpret a BGC; however, we prefer that decisions regarding changes in the insulin dose be made by the veterinarian, and therefore BGCs be sent to the hospital. Interpretation of BGCs generated at home follows the same rules as BGCs generated in the hospital. Ideally the blood glucose concentration ranges from 220 to 270 mg/dL before the insulin injection and from 90 to 140 mg/dL at the time of maximal effect. The most important variables to assess are insulin efficacy, glucose nadir, and duration of effect. Insulin efficacy (i.e., the difference between the highest and the lowest glucose concentration) must be interpreted in light of the highest blood glucose concentration and the insulin dose. A small difference (e.g., 50 mg/dL) is acceptable when the highest blood glucose is less than approximately 200 mg/dL, but is not acceptable if the highest glucose level is greater than 300 mg/dL. An identical difference (e.g., 100 mg/dL) may indicate insulin efficacy in a cat receiving small amounts of insulin, but may point to insulin resistance if the insulin dose is high (>1.5 U/kg/injection). In the latter situation, technical problems and the counterregulatory phase of the Somogyi effect also must be considered.

The next variable to be assessed is the glucose nadir, which ranges ideally from 90 to 140 mg/dL. A lower nadir may occur in insulin overdose (including sudden improvement of insulin-resistant states), excessive overlap of insulin action, and lack of food intake. If the nadir is greater than 160 mg/dL, insulin underdose, the counterregulatory phase of the Somogyi effect, and technical problems involving the injection of insulin by the owner must be considered. In diabetic cats already receiving high doses of insulin (i.e., >1.5 U/kg/injection), concurrent diseases causing insulin resistance also are possible. Stressful situations causing an increase in the blood glucose concentration may occur not only in the hospital but also in the cat's environment at home. On several occasions we have seen nadirs that were somewhat lower (in the range of 60-80 mg/dL) than the recommended 90 to 140 mg/dL during HM. If the cats were well regulated and overdose of insulin was considered unlikely, insulin dose is not changed. We presume that blood glucose levels measured in a stress-free environment are generally lower than those measured in the hospital. Therefore the upper limit of 140 mg/dL of the recommended nadir range should not be exceeded when HM is used.

It is very important to identify the exact cause of glucose concentrations that are outside the target range, because treatment changes differ considerably depending on the underlying problem. Further corrective measures depend on the individual case and include careful questioning of the owner about the cat's food intake, concurrent disease, and stressful events (including potential problems with the generation of a blood drop). The owner may be asked to return to the hospital to practice insulin injection or blood sampling, or simply to generate another BGC to find out if the problem occurs repeatedly.

The duration of effect is defined as the time from insulin injection through the glucose nadir until the blood glucose concentration exceeds 220 to 270 mg/dL. If the duration is less than 8 to 10 hours, the cat usually has signs of diabetes, and if the duration is longer than 14 hours, the risk of hypoglycemia or the occurrence of the Somogyi effect increases with q12h dosing. Duration of action might improve with dietary manipulation. However, if this does not happen, a type of insulin with a different action profile is indicated. In the rare occasions when duration of action is longer than 14 hours, options such as reduction of dosage, q24h instead of q12h administration (in particular if duration of action is 20 to 24 hours), or a change to an insulin with shorter duration of action should be considered.

In human beings it is well known that blood glucose concentrations can vary markedly from day to day. These variations are associated primarily with differences in meal composition and size, different levels of physical activity, and emotional stress. However, even when these factors are kept constant, day-to-day variability in glucose concentration can persist. Causes for this include variable rate of insulin absorption, variation in length of insulin activity, and variation in insulin sensitivity and β-cell function. There also is a high degree of variability among BGCs of diabetic cats. Recently we compared BGCs generated at home with those generated in the hospital within the same week under the same conditions (i.e., same insulin dose, same blood sampling conditions).[30] In about 60 per cent of cases treatment decisions would have been the same, regardless of which of the two corresponding BGCs was used for evaluation; whereas in about 40 per cent of cases, the decisions would have differed. In a follow-up study BGCs generated on two consecutive days at home and on one day in the hospital within the same week were compared.[32] The insulin dose and amount and type of food were kept constant for all three BGCs. The differences between consecutive home curves also were relatively high and often not smaller than between home and clinic curves. Cats with good metabolic control tended to have more reproducible home curves than cats with moderate to poor metabolic control (Figure 26-5). One can conclude from these studies that single BGCs may not be reliable for treatment decisions, regardless of

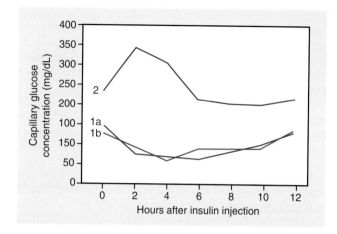

Figure 26-5 A case example in which the home BGCs matched very well. Two BGCs were generated at home on consecutive days (1a and 1b) and another BGC was generated in the hospital[2] during the same week in an 11-year-old castrated male domestic shorthair cat. The cat was considered to be well-regulated, clinical signs of diabetes had resolved, and fructosamine was 358 μmol/L. The two home curves look nearly identical and the glucose concentrations are within the target range. The blood glucose concentrations in the hospital were much higher and, particularly, the glucose nadir was above the target level. The higher glucose levels in the hospital were attributed to stress.

whether they are generated in the hospital or at home. However, one of the major advantages of HM is that it enables frequent generation of BGCs, which may be of particular importance in cats who are difficult to regulate. In those cats, more than one BGC can be generated at home before a change in treatment is initiated.

LONG-TERM COMPLIANCE WITH HOME MONITORING

In a recent study we investigated whether HM with all its challenges is feasible in the long-term and whether HM affects the frequency of reevaluation in the hospital.[33] Of 26 owners who had been taught the procedure, 65 per cent used HM on a regular basis. HM had been conducted for more than 1 year by 50 per cent of the owners, and one of them had used it for almost 4 years. This indicates that many owners are willing and able to conduct HM on a long-term basis. Thirty-five per cent of cat owners were not able to carry out HM because of technical difficulties or the fractious nature of the cat, and the majority of them gave up after the first few attempts. One cat was euthanized a few days after the start of HM (3 weeks after initiating insulin therapy) because the owner found coping with the disease too difficult. It is possible that the additional burden of HM was overwhelming and prompted the owner to have the cat euthanized. Therefore veterinarians must determine carefully whether and when an owner is prepared psychologically to start HM.

All cat owners who conducted HM successfully felt that it raised their self-confidence with regard to their ability to manage the disease in their cats. They were comfortable with the fact that if clinical changes developed they were able to measure blood glucose concentrations to determine whether hyperglycemia or hypoglycemia was a problem. Most cat owners complied with the HM protocol and generated a BGC every 2 to 4 weeks. Similar results were found in another study, which evaluated problems associated with HM and owners' perceptions.[20] All owners believed that HM helped in the glycemic control of their pet, and they appreciated their active participation in the management of the disease.[20]

Human diabetic patients quickly lose interest in self-monitoring of blood glucose if they are not taught how to interpret and act on test results, and if physicians do not review the test results during patient reevaluation. This probably applies to owners of diabetic pets as well. Therefore owners of diabetic cats who undertake HM should be informed of the optimal range of blood glucose concentration and the most frequently detected patterns of glucose response. However, owners also should be told to make adjustments in the insulin dose only after consultation with a veterinarian. Of the owners in the previously mentioned study,[33] 88 per cent complied with that recommendation and only 12 per cent changed their cat's dose of insulin without consultation. The frequency of in-hospital reevaluation of diabetic cats was not affected substantially by HM because the number of reevaluations did not differ significantly between cats managed with and without HM.

CONTINUOUS GLUCOSE MONITORING SYSTEMS

Continuous glucose monitoring systems (CGMS) have been introduced recently into veterinary medicine.[34] Studies using CGMS for HM of blood glucose have not been reported. However, the latest generation of devices that provide glucose levels in real time (e.g., Guardian Real Time System) may have great potential. The system uses a small electrode, which is inserted and fixed under the skin, to measure glucose levels in the interstitial fluid. The sensor is connected to a transmitter that sends glucose readings every 5 minutes in a wireless fashion to a monitor, which displays up to 288 readings per day. Currently the system still has some shortfalls: it requires calibration with a blood glucose measurement at least every 12 hours, the sensor can only be left in place for 72 hours, and it is expensive. However, with some further improvements, it is very likely that CGMS also will be used at home in the future.

CASE EXAMPLE 1

Uncomplicated diabetes mellitus was diagnosed in a 16-year-old, neutered male domestic shorthair cat, who weighed 6.6 kg and had polyphagia, weight loss, decreased activity, and increased blood glucose and fructosamine concentrations (glucose 486 mg/dL, reference range: 72 to 162 mg/dL; fructosamine 672 μmol/L, reference range: ≤340 μmol/L). The cat was started on 1 U insulin glargine

(Lantus) q12h and a high-protein, low-carbohydrate diet (Purina Veterinary Diets DM, canned) and sent home. Three weeks after the start of insulin treatment, the owner was introduced to HM and was advised to measure the fasting blood glucose concentration twice weekly, and to generate a 12-hour BGC once per month. Over the next few weeks the insulin dose was reduced to 0.5 U q12h. At a recheck 3 months after initiating insulin therapy, the owner reported that the cat had no clinical signs of diabetes. The fructosamine concentration was 454 μmol/L and the glucose levels measured in the hospital throughout the day were slightly below the target range (highest level 100 mg/dL, nadir 54 mg/dL). Serum biochemistry evaluation revealed increased blood urea nitrogen (BUN) and creatinine concentrations (BUN: 51 mg/dL, reference range: 20.7 to 35.3 mg/dL; creatinine 2.3 mg/dL, reference range: 1.08 to 1.79 mg/dL) and during further evaluation, a diagnosis of chronic kidney disease was made. A low-protein diet (Hill's Prescription Diet feline k/d) instead of a high-protein diet was recommended, and the insulin was left unchanged.

During the next 2 weeks the owner reported that the cat had increased thirst and decreased activity. Fasting glucose levels measured on several days at home were markedly elevated (504 mg/dL, 486 mg/dL, >594 mg/dL, 529 mg/dL), and a BGC generated at home confirmed that glycemic control had deteriorated (all glucose levels >300 mg/dL). The insulin dose was increased to 1 U q12h and the cat was reevaluated in the hospital 2 weeks later. At that time (4 months after insulin had been started), the cat still had polydipsia and decreased activity, the fructosamine level was 656 μmol/L, and the values of a BGC were clearly above the target range (highest value 331 mg/dL, nadir 264 mg/dL). The insulin was increased to 2 U q12h. Over the next month, clinical signs of diabetes persisted and two BGCs generated at home confirmed that glucose levels were still too high (highest values 466 mg/dL and 307 mg/dL, nadirs 369 mg/dL and 149 mg/dL). The insulin dose was increased in a stepwise fashion to 3 U q12h. Fourteen days after the last dose adjustment (5 months after starting insulin therapy), the owner called the hospital because of low glucose levels during a BGC generated at home (highest value 59 mg/dL, nadir 23 mg/dL) (Figure 26-6). The owner was advised to reduce the insulin dose by 50 per cent, watch the cat closely for signs of hypoglycemia and schedule a recheck in the hospital 1 week later. At the time of reevaluation, the cat was clinically normal, the fructosamine concentration had decreased to within the reference range (291 μmol/L) and a BGC revealed that glucose levels were still too low (highest value 54 mg/dL, nadir 29 mg/dL). The insulin dose was decreased to 0.5 U q12h, and the owner was advised to monitor the cat carefully and generate a BGC at home a few days later. The latter showed that glucose levels were no longer in the hypoglycemic range and that the highest glucose level was slightly lower than desired, but the nadir was within the target range (highest level 158 mg/dL, nadir 93 mg/dL). The insulin dose was not changed, and the owner was advised to monitor the cat frequently by HM (i.e., to generate a BGC at home every 2 to 3 weeks). Reevaluation of BUN (52 mg/dL) and creatinine (2.15 mg/dL) revealed that the

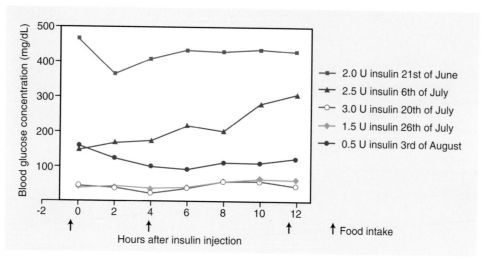

Figure 26-6 BGCs generated at home in case 1. The BGCs generated with 2 and 2.5 U insulin q12h revealed high glucose levels. Clinically, the cat still had signs of diabetes, and therefore the insulin dose was increased to 3 U q12h. Fourteen days after this dose adjustment, the BGC revealed levels in the hypoglycemic range. Although the insulin dose was decreased by 50 per cent, hypoglycemia persisted. Only after decreasing the insulin dose to 0.5 U q12h did the blood glucose concentrations normalize and the nadir of the BGC fall within the target range.

renal disease was stable, and feeding the low-protein diet was therefore continued. At the time of this writing, the cat was doing well receiving 0.5 U insulin q12h and the low-protein diet.

This case exemplifies the rapid change in insulin requirement that may occur during management of a diabetic patient. With HM dedicated owners can evaluate blood glucose concentration regularly and adjust the insulin dose after consulting a veterinarian. This increases the owner's compliance and self-confidence in the management of their cat's disease. In this case deterioration of glycemic control as well as hypoglycemia was recognized by HM, which allowed for prompt adjustment of the insulin dose. The increased insulin requirement after diet modification may have been caused by the different composition of the two diets. Hill's Prescription Diet feline k/d contains approximately 28 per cent protein and 30 to 40 per cent carbohydrate, whereas Purina Veterinary Diets DM contains approximately 51 per cent protein and eight per cent carbohydrate (expressed as per cent of the diet dry matter). High carbohydrate content predisposes cats to the development of higher postprandial blood glucose concentrations and worsens glycemic control. Another reason for deterioration of glycemic control may have been renal insufficiency. In cats with chronic kidney disease, insulin requirement can fluctuate unpredictably because of decreased renal clearance of insulin, decreased renal glucose production, and modified insulin sensitivity (insulin resistance).

CASE EXAMPLE 2

An 11-year-old spayed female domestic shorthair cat (3.8 kg) with polyuria/polydipsia, polyphagia, and decreased activity was diagnosed with uncomplicated diabetes mellitus (blood glucose 396 mg/dL, reference range: 72 to 162 mg/dL; fructosamine 447 μmol/L, reference range: ≤340 μmol/L). The cat was discharged on 1 U of an intermediate-acting insulin (Caninsulin/Vetsulin) q12h and a high-protein, low-carbohydrate diet (Hill's Science Plan, Feline Growth). After 1 week the owner was not yet confident of the injection technique, and therefore was advised to bring the cat to the hospital before feeding and insulin administration. Insulin was then injected under the supervision of a clinician, and the cat was hospitalized for the day to generate a BGC. There had been only a slight improvement in the clinical signs of diabetes, and the fructosamine concentration had not changed (454 μmol/L). The cat appeared to be extremely stressed in the hospital and refused to eat. Blood glucose levels fell from a fasting value of 529 mg/dL to a nadir of 61 mg/dL within 4 hours, which was attributed to lack of food intake. We decided to leave the insulin dose unchanged and to monitor the effect of the owner's improved injection technique. For future reevaluations, the owner was advised to give insulin and food at home before bringing the cat to the hospital, which is in accordance with our recommended protocol.

Three weeks after the start of insulin treatment the owner was introduced to HM and was advised to measure fasting blood glucose twice weekly and generate a 12-hour BGC once per month. Over the next 5 months the cat was evaluated regularly in the hospital and by HM and could be managed with insulin doses of 0.5 to 1 U q12h. Six months after initiating therapy the cat was hospitalized because the owner went on vacation. A BGC had been generated at home beforehand, revealing normal blood glucose levels. The lack of clinical signs of diabetes and a fructosamine concentration of 434 μmol/L indicated good glycemic control. A BGC also was generated during the cat's hospitalization. All of the glucose values were markedly elevated (>300 mg/dL) (Figure 26-7). The discrepancy between the values in the hospital and those

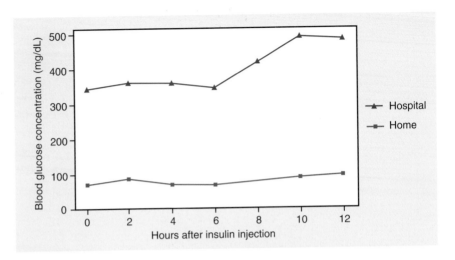

Figure 26-7 BGCs of case 2: an 11-year-old spayed female domestic shorthair cat, 3.8 kg. One BGC was generated at home, the other in the hospital three days later. At that time, the diabetes seemed well-controlled and the fructosamine concentration was 434 μmol/L. The discrepancies between the values in the hospital and at home were attributed to stress hyperglycemia.

at home was considered to reflect stress hyperglycemia, and the insulin dose was left unchanged. At reevaluations 1 and 2 months after that short period of hospitalization, the BGCs generated in the hospital differed substantially from those at home (glucose levels in the hospital were about three times as high as those at home). It was decided therefore to omit glucose measurement in the hospital and to base further monitoring on evaluation of clinical signs, fructosamine concentration, and glucose concentrations measured at home. The cat did well for 4 years, but then was diagnosed with pleural effusion and euthanized.

This case highlights two major problems associated with serial blood glucose measurements in hospitalized cats. First, there may be a severe drop in blood glucose levels if cats refuse to eat during hospitalization. Determining whether lack of food intake or insulin overdose is the reason for the decrease can be very difficult. Second, hospitalization and manipulation often stress cats immensely, which results in increased blood glucose levels; BGCs may show steadily increasing or consistently high glucose values throughout the day. Differentiation between stress hyperglycemia, insulin underdose, and insulin resistance is impossible. In both situations BGCs generated at home can be very helpful. However, treatment decisions also should be based on the assessment of clinical signs and fructosamine concentration.

REFERENCES

1. Prahl A, Guptill L, Glickman NW, et al: Time trends and risk factors for diabetes mellitus in cats presented to veterinary teaching hospitals, *J Feline Med Surg* 9:351, 2007.
2. Michiels L, Reusch CE, Boari A, et al: Treatment of 46 cats with porcine lente insulin—a prospective, multicentre study, *J Feline Med Surg* 10:439, 2008.
3. Reusch CE, Tomsa K: Serum fructosamine concentration in cats with overt hyperthyroidism, *J Am Vet Med Assoc* 215:1297, 1999.
4. Graham PA, Mooney CT, Murray M: Serum fructosamine concentrations in hyperthyroid cats, *Res Vet Sci* 67:171, 1999.
5. Reusch CE, Haberer B: Evaluation of fructosamine in dogs and cats with hypo- or hyperproteinaemia, azotaemia, hyperlipidaemia and hyperbilirubinaemia, *Vet Rec* 148:370, 2001.
6. Sönksen PH, Judd SL, Lowy C: Home monitoring of blood-glucose. Method for improving diabetic control, *Lancet* 1:729, 1978.
7. Walford S, Gale EAM, Allison SP, et al: Self-monitoring of blood glucose. Improvement of diabetic control, *Lancet* 1:732, 1978.
8. Skyler JS, Lasky IA, Skyler DL, et al: Home blood glucose monitoring as an aid in diabetes management, *Diabetes Care* 1:150, 1978.
9. Skyler JS: Self-monitoring of blood glucose. In DeFronzo RA, Ferrannini E, Keen H, et al, editors: *International textbook of diabetes mellitus*, ed 3, vol 2, Chichester, 2004, John Wiley & Sons Ltd, p 1671.
10. Bergenstal RM, Gavin JR: The role of self-monitoring of blood glucose in the care of people with diabetes: report of a global consensus conference, *Am J Med* 118(Suppl 9A):1S, 2005.
11. Schütt M, Kern W, Krause U, et al: Is the frequency of self-monitoring of blood glucose related to long-term metabolic control? Multicenter analysis including 24,500 patients from 191 centers in Germany and Austria, *Exp Clin Endocrinol Diabetes* 114:384, 2006.
12. Martin S, Schneider B, Heinemann L, et al: Self-monitoring of blood glucose in type 2 diabetes and long-term outcome: an epidemiological cohort study, *Diabetologia* 49:271, 2006.
13. Barnett AH, Krentz AJ, Strojek K, et al: The efficacy of self-monitoring of blood glucose in the management of patients with type 2 diabetes treated with a gliclazide modified release-based regimen, A multicentre, randomized, parallel-group, 6-month evaluation (DINAMIC 1 study). *Diabetes Obes Metab* 10:1239, 2008.
14. Fedele D, Corsi A, Noacco C, et al: Alternative site blood glucose testing: a multicenter study, *Diabetes Technol Ther* 5:983, 2003.
15. Toledo FG, Taylor A: Alternative site testing at the earlobe tip: reliability of glucose measurements and pain perception, *Diabetes Care* 27:616, 2004.
16. Wess G, Reusch C: Capillary blood sampling from the ear of dogs and cats and use of portable meters to measure glucose concentration, *J Small Anim Pract* 41:60, 2000.
17. Fleeman LM, Rand JS: Evaluation of day-to-day variability of serial blood glucose concentration curves in diabetic dogs, *J Am Vet Med Assoc* 222:317, 2003.
18. Mathes MA: Home monitoring of the diabetic pet, *Clin Tech Small Anim Pract* 17:86, 2002.
19. Thompson MD, Taylor SM, Adams VJ, et al: Comparison of glucose concentrations in blood samples obtained with a marginal ear vein nick technique versus from a peripheral

vein in healthy cats and cats with diabetes mellitus, *J Am Vet Med Assoc* 221:389, 2002.

20. Van de Maele I, Rogier N, Daminet S: Retrospective study of owners' perception on home monitoring of blood glucose in diabetic dogs and cats, *Can Vet J* 46:718, 2005.

21. Skyler JS, Cohen M: Self-monitoring of blood glucose. In Alberti KGMM, Zimmet P, DeFronzo RA, et al, editors: *International textbook of diabetes mellitus*, ed 2, Chichester, 1997, John Wiley & Sons Ltd, p 1031.

22. Boehme P, Floriot M, Sirveaux MA, et al: Evolution of analytical performance in portable glucose meters in the last decade, *Diabetes Care* 26:1170, 2003.

23. Link KR, Rand JS, Hendrikz JK: Evaluation of a simplified intravenous glucose tolerance test and a reflectance glucose meter for use in cats, *Vet Rec* 140:253, 1997.

24. Wess G, Reusch CE: Assessment of five portable blood glucose meters for use in cats, *Am J Vet Res* 61:1587, 2000.

25. Zeugswetter F, Benesch T, Pagitz M: Validierung des tragbaren Blutzuckermessgerätes FreeStyle Freedom bei Katzen, *Vet Med Austria/Wien Tierärztl Mschr* 94:143, 2007.

26. Clarke WL, Cox D, Gonder-Frederick LA, et al: Evaluating clinical accuracy of systems for self-monitoring of blood glucose, *Diabetes Care* 10:622, 1987.

27. Cohen T, Nelson R, Kass P, et al: Evaluation of six portable blood glucose meters in dogs, *J Vet Intern Med* 22:729, 2008 (abstract).

28. Reusch CE, Kley S, Casella M: Home monitoring of the diabetic cat, *J Feline Med Surg* 8:119, 2006.

29. Casella M, Wess G, Reusch CE: Measurement of capillary blood glucose concentrations by pet owners: a new tool in the management of diabetes mellitus, *J Am Anim Hosp Assoc* 38:239, 2002.

30. Casella M, Hässig M, Reusch CE: Home-monitoring of blood glucose in cats with diabetes mellitus: evaluation over a 4-month period, *J Feline Med Surg* 7:163, 2005.

31. Reusch CE, Wess G, Casella M: Home monitoring of blood glucose concentration in the management of diabetes mellitus, *Compend Contin Educ Pract Vet* 23:544, 2001.

32. Alt N, Kley S, Hässig M, et al: Day-to-day variability of blood glucose concentration curves generated at home in cats with diabetes mellitus, *J Am Vet Med Assoc* 230:1011, 2007.

33. Kley S, Casella M, Reusch CE: Evaluation of long-term home monitoring of blood glucose concentrations in cats with diabetes mellitus: 26 cases (1999-2002), *J Am Vet Med Assoc* 225:261, 2004.

34. Wiedmeyer CE, DeClue AE: Continuous glucose monitoring in dogs and cats, *J Vet Intern Med* 22:2, 2008.

27 Use of Long-Acting Insulin in the Treatment of Diabetes Mellitus

Jacqueline S. Rand

GOALS OF THERAPY

The principal goal for treatment of feline diabetes mellitus has changed over the last 5 years from ameliorating clinical signs to achieving euglycemia without the need for insulin therapy, commonly called diabetic remission. Remission or non–insulin dependence has enormous health and quality-of-life benefits for diabetic cats, and cost and lifestyle benefits for their owners. In cats who do not revert to non–insulin dependence the goals of therapy are to resolve clinical signs of polyuria, polydipsia, and weight loss while avoiding life-threatening hypoglycemia.

Because remission is so beneficial the treatment protocol selected should maximize the probability of remission. Recently new long-acting insulins for human use have become available, and data suggest their use in cats is associated with higher remission rates. To understand how and why they should be used to achieve remission, it is important to understand the pathogenesis of feline diabetes mellitus and the mechanisms associated with remission.

NON–INSULIN DEPENDENCE AND DIABETIC REMISSION

It is not clear whether cats in remission should be classed as diabetic (that is, non–insulin-dependent diabetics) or as truly being in diabetic remission. Only a very few cats in remission have undergone a glucose tolerance test, with some showing normal glucose tolerance and others showing abnormal glucose tolerance (Rand, unpublished data). It is likely that some previously diabetic cats are truly in diabetic remission, others have impaired glucose tolerance, and some should be considered non–insulin-dependent diabetics. For the purposes of this discussion they will be referred to as in remission, implying remission from insulin therapy rather than diabetic remission.

PATHOGENESIS OF FELINE DIABETES MELLITUS

To understand the potential for achieving remission it is important to understand the pathogenesis of diabetes mellitus in cats. Based on clinical and histological findings, in primary accession practice in the Western world the majority of cats have type 2 diabetes mellitus, characterized by a combination of impaired insulin secretion and insulin resistance.[1-4]

Five to 10 per cent of cats have diabetes classified as "other specific types of diabetes,"[2,5] which results from diseases that cause insulin resistance such as acromegaly or hyperadrenocorticism, or from conditions that destroy pancreatic beta cells such as neoplasia or pancreatitis.[6,7] The other specific types of diabetes constitute a much greater percentage of the diabetic population in referral practice, especially tertiary referral practice, where most referred diabetic cats are difficult to control and are atypical of the majority of diabetic cats seen in private practice.[2,5] Other specific types of diabetes also appear to be more prevalent in developing countries where obesity is rare. Achieving remission is only possible if there are functional beta cells remaining. Therefore cats with other specific types of diabetes mellitus that destroy beta cells, or cats with long-term poorly controlled diabetes mellitus that leads to chronic glucotoxic damage to beta cells, are unlikely to achieve remission, and the goals of therapy will be to control clinical signs.

TYPE 2 DIABETES MELLITUS

In human beings type 2 diabetes mellitus previously was called adult-onset diabetes; however, that name has been discarded because many new cases are in people less than 20 years of age.[8] It also was called non–insulin-dependent diabetes, but that name also is not recommended because many patients require insulin to achieve good glycemic control. Insulin resistance is a hallmark of type 2 diabetes. Diabetic cats on average are six times less sensitive to insulin than healthy cats, which is a similar magnitude of insulin resistance to human beings with type 2 diabetes.[9] In human beings insulin resistance predominantly is the result of the sum of the underlying insulin resistance (sensitivity), which is genetically determined, coupled with acquired insulin resistance, which is largely the result of obesity and physical inactivity. A range of insulin sensitivities are present in healthy, ideal-weight cats, and insulin sensitivity also is likely genetically determined in cats.[10] Cats with insulin sensitivities below the population median have three times the risk of developing impaired glucose tolerance with weight gain.[10] Weight gain of 44 per cent in cats over a period of 10 months decreased insulin sensitivity by half.[10] In human beings and dogs physical inactivity leads to insulin resistance independent of body weight, but whether this occurs in cats has not been investigated. Drugs, especially long-acting or repeated glucocorticoid administration, induce insulin resistance and are a frequent precipitator of clinical signs of diabetes in cats. Hyperglycemia also induces insulin resistance and is reversible with improved glycemic control.

Loss of beta cell function is another hallmark of type 2 diabetes. A major cause of beta cell loss in type 2 diabetes is thought to be apoptosis triggered by beta cell damage.[11] Beta cell damage is thought to be associated with chronic hyperfunction that occurs secondary to chronic insulin resistance. Other causes of loss of beta cells include pancreatitis and islet amyloid deposition.[2,5] Some loss of function is reversible, as occurs in the early stages of glucose toxicity. Loss of beta cells occurs in the later stages of glucose toxicity, resulting in irreversible loss of beta cell secretion. Logically the greater the loss of beta cells, the lower the probability for remission will be in an individual cat.

DIAGNOSIS OF DIABETES MELLITUS

In human beings type 2 diabetes is diagnosed when blood glucose is persistently above 126 mg/dL (7 mmol/L).[12] In cats diabetes usually is only diagnosed when blood glucose concentration is above the renal threshold, causing obligatory water loss and hence the signs of polyuria and polydipsia. This generally is associated with a blood glucose of 234 to 288 mg/dL (13 to 16 mmol/L) or above.[13] In cats no epidemiological studies have been performed to demonstrate the adverse health effects of persistent mild to moderate hyperglycemia, for example, between 144 and 252 mg/dL (8 and 14 mmol/L). In human patients the cutoff blood glucose concentration for diabetes mellitus has been lowered consistently over time as more information has become available on the adverse effects of mild hyperglycemia, including microvascular damage and retinopathy. Similar studies need to be performed in cats. It is likely that if cats were classified as diabetic with persistent fasting blood glucose concentrations of 180 mg/dL (10 mmol/L) or greater, most diabetic cats also would be non–insulin dependent and a much greater proportion could be controlled with weight loss and diet alone.

Measuring serum fructosamine is not a sensitive indicator of persistent hyperglycemia in cats. In healthy cats infused with glucose to maintain blood glucose concentrations at 306 mg/dL (17 mmol/L) for 6 weeks, serum fructosamine concentration was not consistently above the upper limit of the reference range.[14] Serum fructosamine assay is most useful in situations in which there is very poor clinical history and it is unknown whether hyperglycemia is associated with stress, or if it is truly persistent and associated with diabetes mellitus. However, this could be answered more simply, quickly, and less expensively by hospitalizing the cat and measuring blood glucose at least 3 hours later. Provided struggling does not occur with the second blood collection, blood glucose concentration should be in the normal range when measured 3 to 6 hours later, if hyperglycemia is caused by stress associated with the first blood collection. If blood glucose concentration is still mildly increased (180 to 252 mg/dL; 10 to 14 mmol/L), then measure it again the following morning to clarify the diagnosis. If blood glucose concentration is greater than 270 mg/dL (>15 mmol/L), institute therapy for diabetes immediately. If in doubt about the diagnosis, err on the side of diagnosing diabetes and institute appropriate treatment and monitoring of blood glucose concentration.

GLUCOSE TOXICITY

Glucose toxicity is an important phenomenon to understand because it relates to treatment goals, remission, and choice of insulin. Glucose toxicity describes the suppression of insulin secretion from beta cells secondary to prolonged hyperglycemia.[15,16] We have shown that insulin secretion in healthy cats is suppressed to concentrations found in insulin-dependent diabetic cats within three to seven days of blood glucose concentrations being maintained in the range of 540 mg/dL (30 mmol/L).[16] Glucose toxicity is dose-dependent, and less suppression occurs at lower glucose concentrations. Glucose toxicity is particularly important when superimposed on hyperfunctioning beta cells that are already compromised because of loss of beta cell mass from amyloid deposition or pancreatitis.[17] In this situation of hyperfunctioning beta cells, even low levels of hyperglycemia cause further rapid deterioration of beta cell function, worsening hyperglycemia, and eventually signs of overt diabetes mellitus.[17] Initially glucose toxicity causes reversible suppression of insulin secretion from beta cells, but later it causes irreversible loss of beta cells.

Achieving resolution of glucose toxicity is critically important to the goal of achieving diabetic remission. This is highlighted by data demonstrating that cats changed to a protocol to achieve excellent glycemic control within 6 months of diagnosis are much more likely to achieve non–insulin-dependent status than cats whose glucose concentrations are not strictly controlled until longer than 6 months after diagnosis.[4]

PREDICTORS OF DIABETIC REMISSION

In a study of 55 diabetic cats treated with glargine, only four variables were found to be associated with a higher probability of remission.[4] They were early implementation of intensive blood glucose control, prior glucocorticoid treatment, absence of signs of neuropathy, and lower maximal insulin dose. For cats who started intensive blood glucose control within 6 months of diagnosis of diabetes, the remission rate was 84 per cent. The remission rate decreased to 35 per cent for cats who were started on the same protocol more than 6 months after diagnosis; the difference was highly significant ($p = 0.0002$). Therefore it is critically important that excellent glycemic control be achieved sooner rather than later.

Cats treated with glucocorticoids in the 6 months prior to being diagnosed with diabetes were more likely ($p = 0.001$) to go into remission than cats without prior treatment with these drugs. The addition of marked insulin resistance secondary to glucocorticoid administration likely precipitates an acute onset of signs, which probably results in treatment being sought earlier, and hence earlier resolution of glucose toxicity than if the onset of signs had been slow and insidious.

Cats displaying a plantigrade stance at diagnosis or milder signs of peripheral neuropathy, such as a difficulty climbing stairs, were significantly less likely ($p = 0.02$) to go into remission. It is probable that cats with signs of neuropathy had uncontrolled hyperglycemia longer than cats without neuropathy, and hence greater loss of beta cells from the effects of prolonged glucose toxicity, and lower remission rates.

The mean maximum insulin dose required was lower in cats who became non–insulin-dependent during the study (0.43 IU/kg q12h) compared with cats who remained insulin-dependent (0.66 IU/kg q12h). Other factors examined that were not found to be predictors of remission were age at diagnosis, gender, weight at diagnosis, evidence of diabetic ketoacidosis at diagnosis, presence of chronic kidney disease or hyperthyroidism, and frequency of asymptomatic hypoglycemia. Obesity was not correlated negatively with remission.

INSULIN CHOICE

Because remission should be the initial major goal of therapy in newly diagnosed cats, the protocol selected must provide the cat the greatest probability of achieving this outcome. The intermediate-acting insulins such as neutral protamine Hagedorn (NPH) and Lente insulin have too short a duration of action to control blood glucose satisfactorily when given q12h. For porcine Lente insulin (Vetsulin, Caninsulin) given q12h, we have shown that typically for approximately 4 hours before each insulin dose there is minimal glucose lowering effect from the insulin, which translates to minimal insulin action for 8 hours out of every 24.[18] Although this duration of action is sufficient to control clinical signs in many cats, the marked hyperglycemia (>324 mg/dL; >18 mmol/L) twice daily continues to suppress and damage beta cells, leading to significantly lower remission rates compared with that achieved with longer-acting insulin.[3] NPH insulin tends to have a shorter duration of action than porcine Lente insulin, and is not recommended for use in cats. Although protamine zinc insulin (PZI) has a longer duration of action than Lente insulin, it appears to be associated with lower remission rates than the new long-acting insulin analogues glargine (Lantus, Aventis) and detemir (Levemir, Novo Nordisk).[3,19] In a small study of newly diagnosed diabetic cats, two of eight cats achieved remission with porcine Lente insulin, three of eight with PZI, and eight of eight with glargine.[3] Further evidence that glargine produces superior remission rates to Lente insulin is found in a recent study of 50 diabetic cats treated previously for a median of 16 weeks with other insulins, predominantly porcine Lente insulin, who failed to achieve remission. After changing to glargine and a protocol of intensive glucose monitoring, remission rates of 84 per cent were achieved if cats were started on the intensive protocol within 6 months of diagnosis.[4] In some countries veterinarians are required legally to use insulin registered for veterinary use as a first line of therapy. Because remission rates for cats are significantly lower if intensive glucose control is not instituted early, if diabetic remission does not occur within 4 to 8 weeks of using an insulin registered for veterinary use, it is recommended that the insulin be changed to glargine or detemir to facilitate remission.

Based on reported data the first choice of insulin in newly diagnosed diabetic cats is glargine. Early studies of limited numbers of cats indicate that there is little clinical difference between glargine and detemir.[19] Studies in healthy cats suggest that detemir has a longer duration of action than glargine and is perhaps the insulin of choice in cats.[20] Because there is substantially greater experience with the use of glargine in cats, and the pharmacokinetics and dynamics of glargine, but not detemir, have been reported in cats, glargine currently is the insulin of choice until more data are available. In the study of healthy cats detemir had a longer duration of action (median 800 minutes; range 525 to 915) than glargine (median 470 minutes; range 295 to 950 minutes) and less variation in duration of action between cats.[20] In human patients detemir also has been shown to be more consistent in its duration of action than glargine. Therefore, in cats in whom glargine appears to have too short a duration of action with q12h administration, detemir should be trialed. In countries where there is a legal obligation to first use a veterinary-use insulin, PZI would be the first-choice veterinary insulin if available, and porcine Lente insulin would be the second-choice veterinary insulin. It is recommended that if remission is not achieved within 4 to 8 weeks, the insulin be changed to glargine or detemir. It is likely that if excellent glycemic control can be achieved early and episodes of marked hyperglycemia avoided, the loss of beta cells associated with glucose toxicity is minimized and remission is facilitated.

MODE OF ACTION OF GLARGINE

Glargine is a synthetic insulin analogue and is produced using recombinant DNA technology utilizing *Escherichia coli*. The insulin molecule is modified by replacing asparagine at position 21 with glycine, and by adding two arginines at the terminal portion of the B chain. The glycine-arginine substitution is the basis for the name glargine. The modification shifts the isoelectric point, producing a molecule that is completely soluble at a pH of 4. However, in subcutaneous tissues with pH of 7.4 the acidic solution is neutralized, leading to the formation of microprecipitates.

Designed for q24h administration in human beings, glargine is marketed for people as a "peakless" insulin with respect to its glucose-lowering effect. The lack of peak is related to the glucose utilization rate of glargine, a parameter determined by the amount of intravenous glucose required to maintain a constant plasma glucose concentration after subcutaneous injection of insulin, and which indicates insulin activity. The blood glucose–lowering effect and duration in cats are similar to that in diabetic human beings.[21] However, there are definite peaks and nadirs in glucose and insulin concentrations associated with glargine use in diabetic and healthy cats.

Glargine has a very long duration of action, and after injection it forms hexameric microprecipitates in the subcutaneous tissue, which gradually break down. This slow release of glargine into the systemic circulation produces its sustained action. Because the formation of microprecipitates is dependent on the interaction of the acidic insulin (pH = 4) and the relatively neutral subcutaneous tissues (pH = 7), glargine should not be mixed or diluted before administration.

MODE OF ACTION OF DETEMIR

Detemir is a newer synthetic insulin analogue with a long duration of action that is produced using recombinant DNA technology in yeast *(Saccharomyces cerevisiae)*. The insulin molecule is modified by addition of an acylated fatty acid chain that enables reversible binding to plasma proteins, especially albumin, from where it is released slowly into plasma. The modification also prolongs self-association in the injection depot.[22] This leads not only to a prolonged absorption from subcutaneous tissue, but also to a buffering of the metabolic effect against variations in the blood flow rate at the injection site.[22]

STORAGE OF GLARGINE AND DETEMIR

Glargine is marketed for human use with a 28-day shelf-life at room temperature after opening. Glargine is somewhat fragile, but is chemically stable in solution for 6 months under refrigeration. Detemir is marketed with a 6-week shelf-life at room temperature after opening. The U.S. Food and Drug Administration (FDA) Microbiology Group has a policy of not recommending longer expiration periods on multiple-use injectable medication vials, even if a preservative is present, because of the risk of bacterial contamination. Glargine and detemir preparations contain the antimicrobial preservative metacresol, which is considered bacteriostatic, not bactericidal. The FDA believes that the vials may have a high probability of becoming contaminated with microbes by daily multiple punctures to withdraw medication past the arbitrary cutoff date. Neither Aventis nor NovoNordisk have submitted a microbiological study over 6-month or 12-month periods to show safety, and it is unlikely to be performed for economic reasons. For veterinary use we recommend that both insulins be kept refrigerated, although the antimicrobial agent may be more effective at room temperature. Owners of diabetic cats use refrigerated glargine or detemir routinely for up to 6 months without evidence of problems occurring. The insulin should be discarded immediately if any cloudiness or discoloration is noted.

DURATION OF ACTION AND ONCE- OR TWICE-DAILY ADMINISTRATION

In healthy cats administered glargine there was evidence of a carryover effect after 12 hours following q12h administration, and at 24 hours regardless of whether insulin was administered q24h or q12h.[21] Mean duration of action after a dose of 0.25 U/kg was at least 20 hours, but in some cats was as short as 14 hours. However, another study measuring glucose utilization rate in healthy cats found the median duration of glargine action was 8 hours but could be as short as 5 hours after administration of 0.5 U/kg. A pharmacodynamic study in diabetic cats needs to be performed to clarify the duration of action in diabetic cats.

Reducing the time on a daily basis that beta cells are exposed to marked hyperglycemia is thought to be important for recovery of beta cell function from the suppressive effects of glucose toxicity. In human beings and cats recovery of beta cell function is critical for subsequent diabetic remission.[16,23] Therefore it is likely that better glycemic control and reduced periods of hyperglycemia would be achieved in a greater proportion of diabetic cats if glargine is administered q12h rather than q24h. Clinical observations indeed suggest that remission rates in newly diagnosed diabetic cats are higher when glargine is administered q12h compared to q24h dosing.[3,4,24] Therefore it is recommended that glargine be dosed initially q12h, at least for the first 6 months, to facilitate recovery from glucose toxicity and remission.

HYPOGLYCEMIA

Biochemical hypoglycemia is detected frequently in glargine- and detemir-treated cats, but clinical hypoglycemia is rare. In a study of 55 cats treated with glargine using an intensive protocol designed to achieve euglycemia, asymptomatic or biochemical hypoglycemia was common, with 93 per cent of cats having a blood glucose concentration of greater than 40 to less than 50 mg/dL (>2.2 to <2.7 mmol/L) at some point in the study, as measured with a whole blood portable glucose meter calibrated for human blood.[4] Meters measuring glucose in whole blood typically read on average 18 to 36 mg/dL (1 to 2 mmol/L) lower than blood glucose measured by an automated serum chemistry analyzer or plasma equivalent meter. Glucose concentrations of greater than 20 to less than 30 mg/dL (>1.1 to <1.7 mmol/L) also were quite common, occurring at some point in 84 per cent of cats. However, there was only one mild episode of clinical hypoglycemia in 55 cats.[4]

Initial data collected by our group indicate that cats treated with Lente insulin have increased risk of clinical hypoglycemia compared to glargine.[3] In human type 1 and type 2 diabetics treated with glargine, the incidence of clinical hypoglycemia is reduced significantly compared with shorter-acting insulins such as NPH.[25,26]

SOMOGYI EFFECT

The Somogyi effect refers to marked hyperglycemia that follows a period of hypoglycemia. Numerous studies have shown that the Somogyi effect is uncommon in human diabetic patients. There are few studies in the veterinary literature documenting the Somogyi effect, although it is mentioned frequently in texts on feline diabetes. In a study of 55 diabetic cats treated with glargine, using a protocol designed for intensive glycemic control and monitored at home with an average of five blood glucose measurements per day, the Somogyi effect was docu-

mented rarely despite frequent occurrence of biochemical hypoglycemia.[27] A Somogyi effect being followed by insulin resistance, evidenced by the two subsequent insulin doses having almost no glucose-lowering effect, only occurred as four single events in four different cats. The Somogyi effect followed by insulin resistance appears to be more common with shorter-acting insulin such as Lente, which is associated with a rapid decrease in blood glucose concentration following insulin injection. This rapid and large decrease in blood glucose concentration, which triggers counter-regulation, is exacerbated because intermediate-acting insulin provides little insulin action for some hours prior to the next insulin injection, and subsequently there is marked hyperglycemia (e.g., >360 mg/dL; >20 mmol/L) at the time of the insulin injection. Further well-designed studies are required to document the relative incidence of the Somogyi effect with use of intermediate- versus long-acting insulins.

DIET

A restricted carbohydrate diet (<15 per cent of energy from carbohydrate) is critical for management of feline diabetic patients, and to achieve and maintain remission. Low carbohydrate diets reduce the demand on the beta cells to secrete insulin. Importantly, high carbohydrate diets result in significantly higher glucose concentrations for 3 to 18 hours after eating in cats fed q24h or q12h, and in concentrations that are continuously higher in cats fed *ad libitum*.[28] It is likely that in diabetic cats with no endogenous insulin, glucose concentrations rise even higher after eating high carbohydrate diets than in healthy cats. A restricted carbohydrate diet should be begun around the time of initiation of insulin therapy, and it is critical that the diet be continued during remission to minimize the demand on beta cells to secrete insulin. There are no data comparing postprandial glucose concentrations between diets ultra-low in carbohydrates (e.g., <8 per cent metabolizable energy) versus low carbohydrate diets (e.g., 8 per cent to 14 per cent metabolizable energy) to make evidence-based recommendations for the most appropriate level of carbohydrate restriction for diabetic cats.

Limited data on cats regarding feeding suggest that cats have a long postprandial period, and mean glucose concentrations are not different between cats that are meal-fed q24h or q12h and *ad libitum* fed cats.[28]

WEIGHT MANAGEMENT

In cats obesity decreases insulin sensitivity by 50 per cent, and requires more insulin to be secreted to maintain glucose concentrations in the normal range than for a lean body condition. Therefore it is critically important for cats to achieve an ideal body weight to have a greater probability of achieving and maintaining remission. Obese cats should be energy-restricted so they lose less than 2 per cent of body weight per week; for example, approximately 0.5 kg/month for an 8-kg cat. To minimize the demand on beta cells, feed a low carbohydrate diet

1#/month 17# cat

rather than a higher carbohydrate, low-fat, weight loss diet. See Chapter 19 in the fifth volume of this series for a discussion of the management of obesity.

MONITORING

Because of the long duration of insulin action and carryover effects seen in healthy cats, diabetic cats treated with glargine or detemir should have blood glucose measured just prior to insulin administration when using serial blood glucose monitoring to assess insulin dose. This is to ensure that cats with low preinsulin blood glucose concentrations are not overdosed. In most cats nadir glucose concentration does not occur consistently at the same time each day. In many cats nadir glucose concentration occurs around the time of the evening insulin injection.

Measuring water consumed at home reflects mean blood glucose concentration more accurately than does serum fructosamine concentration, and is an invaluable tool in providing additional clinical information on glycemic control.[29] Monitoring urine glucose concentration is more useful for adjusting insulin dose with glargine and detemir than intermediate-acting insulins; it is less useful for detecting remission because once cats are on the correct dose of glargine or detemir, they should only have negative or trace glucose concentrations present in urine. Measurement of water consumed and urine glucose concentration are useful in fractious cats in whom blood glucose concentration can not be measured without sedation or anesthesia. However, measurement of blood glucose concentration will provide more accurate information on which to base dose adjustments, and owners should be encouraged to perform home monitoring in fractious cats to maximize the probability for remission (see Chapter 26). In general, measurement of serum fructosamine concentration is of much less value than serial blood glucose measurements for dose adjustment, and is an imprecise measure of blood glucose concentration. Its greatest value is in cats for whom no clinical data are available or there is an inconsistency between blood glucose concentrations and the clinical data; for example, an owner who reports minimal clinical signs in a cat at home but blood glucose concentration measured in the veterinary clinic suggests poor control. Glargine and detemir are less potent insulins and seem to be less able to control hospital-induced hyperglycemia. Therefore, in cats in whom there is inconsistency between clinical signs and blood glucose concentration measured in the veterinary clinic, measurement of serum fructosamine concentration may be of use. However, home monitoring of blood glucose concentration would be more valuable.

DOSING

Two dosing protocols have been developed for use with glargine and work also with detemir and PZI (Tables 27-1 and 27-2). These protocols are designed for use with a glucometer made for human diabetic patients that measures glucose concentration in whole blood. Plasma glucose concentration measured using a plasma equivalent meter calibrated for human blood is on average 11 per cent higher.[30,31] It is important to note that the distribution of glucose between red blood cells and plasma is different in human beings, dogs, and cats. As a result, whole blood meters calibrated for human blood consistently read lower than the actual value measured in feline plasma. This translates to a value that on average is 20 to 40 per cent or 18 to 36 mg/dL (1 to 2 mmol/L) lower than the actual serum or plasma blood glucose concentration.[32,33] If a glucometer calibrated internally for feline use (e.g., AlphaTRAK, Abbott Laboratories, Abbott Park, IL) or a serum chemistry analyzer is used, add approximately 30 mg/dL (1.7 mmol/L) to the target glucose concentrations; for example, the protocol designed for home monitoring aims for a blood glucose concentration between 50 and 100 mg/dL (2.8 and 5.6 mmol/L) if measured with a whole blood meter calibrated for human use. If either a plasma-equivalent meter calibrated for feline blood or a chemistry analyzer is being used, aim for target glucose concentrations of approximately 80 to 130 mg/dL (4.4 to 7.2 mmol/L) (see Chapter 26).

Use syringes that allow measurement of very small insulin doses such as U100 0.3 mL syringes with half-unit increments. In newly diagnosed cats use an initial insulin dose of 0.25 to 0.5 U/kg of ideal body weight q12h, depending on blood glucose concentration (see Tables 27-1 and 27-2). In general, cats being treated with other types of insulin can be changed to the same dose of glargine or detemir, except if on a high dose of insulin. For cats on doses of four units or higher, caution is recommended until it is known how the cat will respond, and a lower dose should be tried initially. In the first three days of therapy monitor blood glucose concentrations carefully every 3 hours during the day, and decrease the insulin dose if the blood glucose concentration at any time is less than 50 mg/dL (2.8 mmol/L) measured with a whole blood glucose meter calibrated for human use, or less than 80 mg/dL (<4.4 mmol/L) with a plasma-equivalent meter calibrated for feline use or serum chemistry analyzer.

After the first 3 days of treatment there are two to three phases of treatment for diabetic cats. Initially there is a phase of increasing dose, followed by a phase of consistent dosing, and finally, for cats going into remission, a phase of decreasing dose. Even for cats who do not achieve remission, a phase of decreasing dose may be necessary once the insulin resistance associated with glucose toxicity resolves.

After the first three days after initiation of therapy, insulin dose is increased steadily every three to seven days until glucose concentrations for much of the day are consistently in the normal range or just above (see Tables 27-1 and 27-2). A common mistake that many veterinarians make when first using glargine or detemir is to stop insulin in the first weeks of insulin therapy when blood glucose concentration at the time of the next insulin injection is in the normal range or slightly above. There are three methods for dealing initially with low-normal blood glucose concentrations (50 to 100 mg/dL, 2.8 to 5.6 mmol/L with human meter; 65 to 120 mg/dL, 3.6 to 6.7 mmol/L with meter calibrated for feline blood) just

Table 27-1 Parameters for Changing Insulin Dosage When Using Insulin Glargine, Detemir, or PZI in Diabetic Cats and Monitoring Glucose Concentration Every 1 to 2 Weeks*

Parameter Used for Dosage Adjustment	Change in Dose
Begin with 0.5 U/kg if blood glucose ≥360 mg/dL (≥20 mmol/L) or 0.25 U/kg of ideal weight if blood glucose is lower; monitor response to therapy for first 3 days and decrease or increase dose as necessary. If no monitoring is occurring in the first week, begin with 1 U/cat q12h	
If preinsulin blood glucose concentration >216 mg/dL (>12 mmol/L) provided nadir is not in hypoglycemic range *or* If nadir blood glucose concentration >180 mg/dL (>10 mmol/L)	Increase by 0.25-1 U weekly
If preinsulin blood glucose concentration 180-216 mg/dL (≥10-≤12 mmol/L) *or* Nadir blood glucose concentration is 90-160 mg/dL (5-9 mmol/L)	Same dose
If preinsulin blood glucose concentration is 180 mg/dL (10 mmol/L). *or* If nadir glucose concentration is 54-72 mg/dL (3-4 mmol/L).	Use nadir glucose, water consumed, urine glucose, and next preinsulin blood glucose concentration to determine if insulin dose is decreased or maintained.
If preinsulin blood glucose concentration <180 mg/dL (<10 mmol/l) *or* If nadir blood glucose concentration <54 mg/dL (<3 mmol/l)	Reduce by 0.5-1 U *or* if total dose is 0.5-1 U q24h, stop insulin and check for diabetic remission
If clinical signs of hypoglycemia are observed	Reduce by 50%
IF BLOOD GLUCOSE MEASUREMENTS ARE NOT AVAILABLE:	
If water intake is ≤20 mL/kg on wet food or ≤60 mL/kg on dry food	Same dose
If water intake is >20 mL/kg on wet food or >60 mL/kg on dry food	Increase dose by 0.5-1 U
If urine glucose is >3+ (scale 0-4+)	Increase dose by 0.5-1 U
If urine glucose is negative	Decrease dose until 0.5-1 U q24h and then check for diabetic remission

*Doses are per injection.

Please note. Blood glucose concentrations were measured with a meter calibrated for human use that reads approximately 25-35 mg/dL (1.5-2 mmol/L) lower than actual blood glucose concentration or blood glucose measured with a meter calibrated for feline use. When using a meter calibrated for feline use or a serum chemistry analyzer, target glucose concentrations at the lower limit of the range should be adjusted accordingly by adding approximately 30 mg/dL (1.7 mmol/L) to the value listed in the protocol below. For example, a target value of >54 mg/dL (3 mmol/L) becomes >84 mg/dL (4.7 mmol/L) when using a serum chemistry analyzer or a meter calibrated for feline use.

Measure blood glucose concentrations at least once a week in the initial stages of stabilization to maximize the probability for remission.

Adapted from Rand JS, Marshall R: Diabetes mellitus in cats, *Vet Clin North Am Small Anim Pract* 35:211, 2005.

prior to the next insulin injection (see Table 27-2).[4] All of these methods are likely to lead to increased blood glucose concentrations. In most cats none of the three methods have been shown to work as well as consistent dosing. Fluctuations in blood glucose concentration are very common in the phase of increasing dose before glucose concentrations start to stabilize under consistent dosing.[4]

In the phase of increasing dose, many cats will react occasionally to an increased dose with increased glucose concentrations.[4] This occurs generally within the first 2 to 3 days after a dose increase and usually lasts for less than 24 hours. The dose should be held and the fluctuations ignored. If a glucose concentration is below normal (<50 mg/dL or <2.8 mmol/L human calibrated meter; <65 mg/dL or <3.6 mmol/L feline calibrated meter or serum chemistry analyzer) at any time, reduce the dose slightly.

The phase of stable dosing may last many months in some cats who eventually achieve remission, while in others it lasts only weeks. This phase also is the final phase for cats who remain insulin dependent. Periodic slight adjustments of the insulin dose are necessary in many cats. The average dose for cats who are stable on glargine or detemir treatment is 0.4 to 0.6 U/kg. Occasionally cats need high total doses of insulin (5 to 10 U/cat) to control blood glucose concentrations. Usually the dose can be reduced once control is achieved. Cats with acromegaly require large (>10 U/cat) and sometimes enormous doses (>50 U/cat) to control blood glucose concentration. Owners of cats with acromegaly should be encouraged to measure blood glucose concentration at home before each insulin injection, because growth hormone and blood glucose concentration can vary widely over time (see Chapter 29).

In the dose reducing phase, do not reduce the dose too quickly, because it will likely reduce the probability of remission by withdrawing insulin before beta cells have recovered from glucose toxicity. Phasing out of insulin is

Table 27-2 Parameters for Changing Insulin Dosage When Using Insulin Glargine (Lantus) or Detemir (Levemir) Together with Home Monitoring of Blood Glucose Concentrations in a Protocol Aimed at Achieving Intensive Blood Glucose Control

Parameter Used for Dosage Adjustment	Change in Dose
PHASE 1: INITIAL DOSE AND FIRST 3 DAYS ON GLARGINE OR DETEMIR	
Begin with 0.25 U/kg of ideal body weight q12h	
or	
If the cat received another insulin previously, increase or reduce the starting dose taking this information into account. Glargine has a lower potency than Lente insulin and PZI in most cats.	
Cats with a history of developing ketones who remain >300 mg/dL (>17 mmol/L) after 24 to 48 hours	Increase by 0.5 U
If blood glucose is <50 mg/dL (<2.8 mmol/L)	Reduce dose by 0.25 to 0.5 U depending on if cat is on low (<3 U/cat) or high (>3 U/cat) dose of insulin respectively
PHASE 2: INCREASING THE DOSE	
If nadir blood glucose concentration >300 mg/dL (>17 mmol/L)	Increase every 3 days by 0.5 U
If nadir blood glucose concentration 200 to 300 mg/dL (11-17 mmol/L)	Increase every 3 days by 0.25 to 0.5 U depending on if cat is on low or high dose of insulin respectively
If nadir blood glucose concentration <200 mg/dL but peak is >200 mg/dL (11 mmol/L)	Increase every 5 to 7 days by 0.25 to 0.5 U depending on if cat is on low or high dose of insulin respectively
If blood glucose is <50 mg/dL (<2.8 mmol/L)	Reduce dose by 0.25 to 0.5 U depending on if cat is on low or high dose of insulin respectively
If blood glucose at the time of the next insulin injection is 50 to 100 mg/dL (2.8-5.6 mmol/L)	Initially test which of the alternate methods is best suited to the individual cat: **a.** Feed cat and reduce the dose by 0.25 to 0.5 U depending on if cat is on low or high dose of insulin respectively **b.** Feed the cat, wait 1 to 2 hours and when the glucose concentration increases to >100 mg/dL give the normal dose. If the glucose concentration does not increase within 1 to 2 hours, reduce the dose by 0.25 U or 0.5 U (as above). **c.** Split the dose: feed cat, and give most of dose immediately and then give the remainder 1 to 2 hours later, when the glucose concentration has increased to >100 mg/dL. If all these methods lead to increased blood glucose concentrations, give the full dose if preinsulin blood glucose concentration is 50 to 100 mg/dL and observe closely for signs of hypoglycemia. In general for most cats, the best results in phase 2 occur when insulin dose is as consistent as possible, giving the full normal dose at the regular injection time.
PHASE 3: HOLDING THE DOSE. AIM TO KEEP BLOOD GLUCOSE CONCENTRATION WITHIN 50 TO 200 MG/DL (2.8-11 MMOL/L) THROUGHOUT THE DAY	
If blood glucose is <50 mg/dL (<2.8 mmol/L)	Reduce dose by 0.25 to 0.5 U depending on if cat is on low or high dose of insulin respectively
If nadir or peak blood glucose concentration >200 mg/dL (>11 mmol/L)	Increase dose by 0.25 to 0.5 U depending on if cat is on low or high dose of insulin and the degree of hyperglycemia
PHASE 4: REDUCING THE DOSE. PHASE OUT INSULIN SLOWLY BY 0.25 TO 0.5 U DEPENDING ON DOSE	
When the cat regularly (every day for at least 1 week) has its lowest blood glucose concentration in the normal range of a healthy cat, and stays under 100 mg/dL (<5.6 mmol/L) overall	Reduce dose by 0.25 to 0.5 U depending on if cat is on low or high dose of insulin respectively
If the nadir glucose concentration is 40 to <50 mg/dL (2.2 to <2.8 mmol/L) at least three times on separate days	Reduce dose by 0.25 to 0.5 U depending on if cat is on low or high dose of insulin respectively

Continued

Table 27-2   Parameters for Changing Insulin Dosage When Using Insulin Glargine (Lantus) or Detemir (Levemir) Together with Home Monitoring of Blood Glucose Concentrations in a Protocol Aimed at Achieving Intensive Blood Glucose Control—cont'd

Parameter Used for Dosage Adjustment	Change in Dose
If the cat drops below 40 mg/dL once (2.2 mmol/L)	Reduce dose immediately by 0.25 to 0.5 U depending on if cat is on low or high dose of insulin respectively
If peak blood glucose concentration >200 mg/dL (>11 mmol/L)	Immediately increase insulin dose to last effective dose

PHASE 5: REMISSION. EUGLYCEMIA FOR A MINIMUM OF 14 DAYS WITHOUT INSULIN

Adapted from Roomp K, Rand J: Intensive blood glucose control is safe and effective in diabetic cats using home monitoring and treatment with glargine, *J Feline Med Surg* 11(8):668-682, 2009.

Blood glucose should be measured at least three times daily with a glucometer. This has not been tested with veterinarian-measured blood glucose curves obtained once every 1-2 weeks, and Table 27-1 is recommended if intensive home monitoring is not being performed.

Please note. The blood glucose values were based on using portable glucose meters (Ascensia Contour, Bayer, Leverkusen, Germany; Accu-Chek Aviva, Roche Diagnostics, Basel, Switzerland) that use ≤0.6 μL of blood per test. These meters measure blood glucose concentration in whole blood and are calibrated for use with human blood. Values from meters calibrated for human blood that provide plasma-equivalent values are approximately 10 per cent higher than values from whole blood meters.

Please note. It is very important to note that blood glucose concentrations measured using a whole blood glucose meter calibrated for human blood may measure 30 to 40 per cent lower in the low end of the range than glucose concentrations measured using a serum chemistry analyzer or a plasma-equivalent meter calibrated for feline use. Therefore, if using a meter calibrated for feline use (e.g., AlphaTRAK, Abbott Laboratories, CA), target glucose concentrations at the lower limit of the range should be adjusted accordingly by adding approximately 30 mg/dL (1.7 mmol/L) to the value listed in the protocol. For example, instead of aiming for 50 to 100 mg/dL (2.8-5.6 mmol/L), aim for 80 to 130 mg/dL (4.4-7.2 mmol/L). Meters calibrated for feline use may read higher or lower than the actual value, in contrast to consistently lower readings for meters validated for human blood. See www.uq.edu.au/ccah for protocol using meters calibrated for feline use.

Please note. Mean median maximum dose in cats on detemir is about 30% less than for glargine (1.7 U/cat q12h; range, 0.5 to 4.0 U versus 2.5 U/cat q12h; range, 1.0 to 9.0 U q12h).

Dose increases are per injection per cat.

done slowly in a step-by-step manner (in 0.25 U or 0.5 U increments), depending on the overall dose being given. (Tables 27-1 and 27-2 show criteria for dose reductions.) At each newly reduced dose ensure the cat is still stable with blood glucose concentrations in the normal range for at least a week before reducing the dose further. If the blood glucose concentration does not remain in the normal range (50 to 100 mg/dL or 2.8 to 5.6 mmol/L with human meter; 80 to 130 mg/dL or 4.4 to 7.2 mmol/L with meter calibrated for feline blood) after a dose reduction during the day, increase the insulin dose immediately to the last effective dose. Sometimes, after a dose reduction blood glucose concentrations may remain in the normal range for 1 or 2 days, but the blood glucose concentrations then begin to increase again, and the dose needs to be increased. Once a cat is on a dose 0.25 to 0.5 U/cat q12h and blood glucose concentrations indicate the need for a further dose reduction, change to q24h dosing. Try to go from 0.25 U/cat to the smallest possible dose of insulin before stopping the insulin completely. For a few cats a small dose (e.g., 1 U) of insulin q48h is required when there is insufficient beta cell function to support euglycemia (remission), but daily dosing results in hypoglycemia.

DOSE VARIATIONS

In studies in healthy cats large individual variations occur in plasma insulin concentrations for a given calculated insulin dose, and are associated with large variations in blood glucose concentrations. The source of the variation is likely to be multifactorial, including differences in rates and percentage of absorption of insulin from the subcutaneous injection site, variation in insulin sensitivity between cats, and variation in the actual dose received per kg of metabolic weight.[21]

Similar variation in glucose responses also are reported in human[34-36] and dog studies.[37] Errors with insulin dosing are a potential source of variation in insulin and glucose concentrations. Many cats receiving q12h treatment receive less than 2 U at each injection. This very small volume of insulin makes dosage errors likely. It has been shown that pediatric nurses using 100 U 0.3 mL syringes were unable to dose any amount under 2 U accurately.[38] Glargine and detemir should not be mixed or diluted, so accurate dosing is difficult in most cats. These errors are likely to be minimized by use of insulin syringes designed for 100 U/mL insulin with 0.5 unit or smaller gradations.

HOME MONITORING

Some owners are willing to measure blood glucose concentrations at home (see Chapter 26). A study of 55 cats being monitored an average of five times daily at home showed that these owners were able to follow standard dosing rules and a protocol designed for intensive blood glucose control using glargine (see Table 27-2). With this protocol owners tested blood glucose concentration a minimum of three times each day. The protocol was designed for use with a glucometer made for human diabetic patients that measured whole blood (not plasma equivalent) and used a small volume (e.g., ≤0.6 µL) of blood per test. Owners using the protocol need to recognize the signs of hypoglycemia and must be able to take appropriate action and collaborate closely with their veterinarian.

MANAGEMENT OF CATS IN REMISSION

Once a cat is in remission, it is important to continue to feed a low or ultra-low carbohydrate diet. Glucocorticoid administration should be avoided if possible, because the addition of marked insulin resistance associated with long-acting or repeated glucocorticoid therapy can precipitate signs of overt diabetes. If glucocorticoids must be administered, concurrent low-dose glargine therapy, for example 0.5 to 1 U q24h, will help to maintain euglycemia. Glucose concentrations should be checked weekly for the first month for cats in remission, and ideally urine glucose should be measured most days. Measuring water intake also is a useful indicator to detect cats who are no longer in remission. If hyperglycemia occurs (e.g., >180 mg/dL or 10 mmol/L), insulin should be reinstituted immediately to prevent further damage to beta cells. A proportion of cats will achieve a second and, occasionally a third remission, if treated with insulin promptly once blood glucose concentration exceeds the normal range.

SUMMARY

In cats treatment with glargine is associated with a low risk of clinical hypoglycemia despite tighter glycemic control. Both glargine and detemir appear to result in a higher probability of remission in diabetic cats than Lente and PZI insulins, and they are the insulins of choice in newly diagnosed cats. They should be combined with low or ultra-low carbohydrate diets to minimize the demand on beta cells to produce insulin.

REFERENCES

1. Panciera DL, Thomas CB, Eicker SW, et al: Epizootiological patterns of diabetes mellitus in cats: 333 cases (1980-1986), *J Am Vet Med Assoc* 197:1504, 1990.
2. O'Brien TD, Hayden DW, Johnson KH, et al: High dose intravenous tolerance test and serum insulin and glucagon levels in diabetic and non-diabetic cats: relationships to insular amyloidosis, *Vet Pathol* 22:250, 1985.
3. Marshall R, Rand JR, Morton JM: Treatment of newly diagnosed diabetic cats with glargine insulin improves glycaemic control and results in higher probability of remission than protamine zinc and lente insulins, *J Fel Med Surg* 11:683, 2009.
4. Roomp K, Rand J: Intensive blood glucose control is safe and effective in diabetic cats using home monitoring and treatment with glargine, *J Fel Med Surg* 11:668, 2009.
5. Goossens MMC, Nelson RW, Feldman EC, et al: Response to treatment and survival in 104 cats with diabetes mellitus (1985-1995), *J Vet Intern Med* 12:1, 1998.
6. Nelson RW: Diabetes mellitus. In Ettinger EC, Feldman EC, editors: *Textbook of veterinary internal medicine*, ed 5, Philadelphia, 2000, Saunders, p 1438.
7. Rand JS, Marshall R: Diabetes mellitus in cats, *Vet Clin North Am Small Anim Pract* 35:211, 2005.
8. Dietz WH: Overweight and precursors of type 2 diabetes mellitus in children and adolescents, *J Pediatr* 138:453, 2001.
9. Feldhahn J, Rand JS, Martin GM: Insulin sensitivity in normal and diabetic cats, *J Feline Med Surg* 1:107, 1999.
10. Appleton DJ, Rand JS, Sunvold GD: Insulin sensitivity decreases with obesity, and lean cats with low insulin sensitivity are at greatest risk of glucose intolerance with weight gain, *J Feline Med Surg* 3:211, 2001.
11. Porte DJ: Beta-cells in type 2 diabetes mellitus, *Diabetes* 40:166, 1991.
12. The Expert Committee on the Diagnosis and Classification of Diabetes Mellitus: Report of the Expert Committee on the Diagnosis and Classification of Diabetes Mellitus, *Diabetes Care* 26(Suppl 1):S5, 2003.
13. Kruth SA, Cowgill LD: Renal glucose transport in the cat, Proceedings of the ACVIM Forum: 78, 1982 (Abstract).
14. Link KRJ, Rand JS: Changes in blood glucose concentration are associated with relatively rapid changes in circulating fructosamine concentrations in cats, *J Feline Med Surg* 10:583, 2008.
15. Unger RH, Grundy S: Hyperglycaemia as an inducer as well as a consequence of impaired islet cell function and insulin resistance: implications for the management of diabetes, *Diabetologia* 28:119, 1995.
16. Link KRJ: *Feline diabetes: diagnostics and experimental modelling* [doctoral thesis], 2001, The University of Queensland.
17. Imamura T, Koffler M, Helderman JH, et al: Severe diabetes induced in subtotally depancreatized dogs by sustained hyperglycemia, *Diabetes* 37:600, 1988.
18. Martin GJ, Rand JS: Control of diabetes mellitus in cats with porcine insulin zinc suspension, *Vet Rec* 161:88, 2007.
19. Roomp K, Rand JS: Evaluation of detemir in diabetic cats managed with a protocol for intensive blood glucose control, *J Vet Intern Med* 23:697, 2009.
20. Gilor C, Keel T, Attermeier KJ, et al: Hyperinsulinemic-euglycemic clamps using insulin detemir and insulin glargine in healthy cats, *J Vet Intern Med* 22:728, 2008 (abstract).
21. Marshall RD, Rand JS, Morton JM: Insulin glargine has a long duration of effect following administration either once daily or twice daily in divided doses in healthy cats, *J Feline Med Surg* 10:488, 2008.
22. Kurtzhals P: Engineering predictability and protraction in a basal insulin analogue: the pharmacology of insulin detemir, *Int J Obes Relat Metab Disord* 28(Suppl. 2):S23, 2004.
23. Robertson RP, Tanaka Y, Sacchi G, et al: Glucose toxicity of the β-cell: cellular and molecular mechanisms, In LeRoith D, Olefsky JM, Taylor SI, editors: *Diabetes mellitus*, New York, 2000, Lippincott Williams & Wilkins, p 125.
24. Weaver KE, Rozanski EA, Mahony OM, et al: Use of glargine and lente insulins in cats with diabetes mellitus, *J Vet Intern Med* 20:234, 2006.
25. Fonseca V, Bell DS, Berger S, et al: A comparison of bedtime insulin glargine with bedtime Neutral protamine Hagedorn in patients with type 2 diabetes: subgroup analysis of patients taking once-daily insulin in a multicenter, randomized, parallel group study, *Am J Med Sci* 328:274, 2004.
26. Fulcher GR, Gilbert RE, Yue DK: Glargine is superior to NPH for improving glycated hemoglobin and fasting blood glucose levels during intensive insulin therapy, *Int Med J* 35:536, 2005.
27. Roomp K, Rand JS: The Somogyi effect is rare in diabetic cats managed using glargine and a protocol aimed at tight glyce-

mic control, Proceedings of the *ACVIM Forum, San Antonio, TX (abstract) and in J Vet Intern Med* 22:790, 2008.

28. Farrow HA, Rand JS, Sunvold G: Diets high in protein are associated with lower postprandial glucose and insulin concentrations than diets high in either fat or carbohydrates in normal cats, *Proceedings of the 20*[th] *American College of Veterinary Internal Medicine Forum, May 2002 Texas, USA and in J Vet Intern Med* 16:360, 2008.

29. Martin GJ, Rand JS: Comparisons of different measurements for monitoring diabetic cats treated with porcine insulin zinc suspension, *Vet Rec* 161:52, 2007.

30. Steffes MW, Sacks DB: Measurement of circulating glucose concentrations: the time is now for consistency among methods and types of samples, *Clin Chem* 51:1569, 2005.

31. D'Orazio P, Burnett RW, Fogh-Andersen N, et al: Approved IFCC recommendation on reporting results for blood glucose (abbreviated). *Clin Chem* 51:1573, 2005.

32. Wess G, Reusch C: Assessment of five portable blood glucose meters for use in cats, *Am J Vet Res* 61:1587, 2000.

33. Reusch CE, Wess G, Casella M: Home monitoring of blood glucose concentration in the management of diabetes mellitus, *Compend Contin Educ Pract Vet* 23:544, 2001.

34. Bantle JP, Laine DC: Day-to-day variation in glycaemic control in type I and type II diabetes mellitus, *Diabetes Res* 8:147, 1988.

35. Bantle JP, Weber MS, Rao SMS, et al: Rotation of the anatomic regions used for insulin injections and day-to-day variability of plasma glucose in type I diabetic subjects, *JAMA* 263:1802, 1990.

36. Moberg E, Kollind M, Lins PE, et al: Day-to-day variation of insulin sensitivity in patients with type 1 diabetes: role of gender and menstrual cycle, *Diabet Med* 12:224, 1995.

37. Fleeman LM, Rand JS: Evaluation of day-to-day variability of serial blood glucose concentration curves in dogs, *J Am Vet Med Assoc* 222:317, 2003.

38. Casella SJ, Mongilio MK, Plotnick LP, et al: Accuracy and precision of low-dose insulin administration, *Pediatrics* 91:1155, 1993.

28 Diabetic Emergencies

Rebecka S. Hess

Uncomplicated diabetes mellitus is characterized by polyuria, polydipsia, polyphagia, and weight loss, and is diagnosed in clinically stable cats by documenting persistent hyperglycemia and glucosuria. Cats with uncomplicated diabetes can be treated as outpatients. Three diabetic emergencies that require intensive therapeutic intervention will be discussed here: diabetic ketoacidosis (DKA), the hyperosmolar hyperglycemic state (HHS), and insulin-induced hypoglycemia. All three states require intense emergency care and can be fatal, even when treated appropriately. While DKA and HHS are spontaneous complications of the diabetic state with complex pathophysiologies, insulin-induced hypoglycemia is an iatrogenic diabetic complication with a simple pathophysiology.

Traditionally DKA and HHS have been described as two extremes of diabetic complications, with DKA characterized by ketosis and acidosis and HHS characterized by severe hyperglycemia and dehydration.[1] In human beings DKA was believed to develop acutely, over a 24-hour period, in young patients with type 1 diabetes, whereas the HHS syndrome was thought to develop over a period of days to weeks in older patients with type 2 diabetes.[1] However, more recently, it has become apparent that about 40 per cent of human patients with DKA also have hyperosmolarity and that many individuals develop a diabetic complication that is a mixture of DKA and HHS.[1]

In cats very little has been reported regarding DKA or HHS; however, DKA appears to develop more commonly in diabetic cats than HHS and therefore will be discussed first.

DEFINITION AND PATHOPHYSIOLOGY OF DIABETIC KETOACIDOSIS

DKA is defined as a severe diabetic metabolic complication and clinical decompensation characterized by acidosis (venous pH <7.35) and ketonuria or ketosis. In the diabetic state glucose does not enter cells in sufficient amounts, and ketones are synthesized from fatty acids as a substitute form of cellular energy in order to meet metabolic demands. Ketone bodies are synthesized from acetyl-CoA, which is a product of mitochondrial β-oxidation of fatty acids. This adenosine triphosphate (ATP)–dependent catabolism is associated with breakdown of fatty acids two carbon fragments at a time, and results in formation of acetyl-CoA.

Synthesis of acetyl-CoA is facilitated by decreased insulin and increased glucagon concentrations. Insulin is an anabolic hormone, and its normal anabolic effects include conversion of glucose to glycogen and storage of amino acids as protein and of fatty acids in adipose tissue. On the other hand, the catabolic effects of glucagon include glycogenolysis, proteolysis, and lipolysis. Therefore low insulin and elevated glucagon concentrations contribute to decreased movement of fatty acids into adipose tissue and increased lipolysis, resulting in elevated acetyl-CoA concentration.

In nondiabetics acetyl-CoA and pyruvate enter the citric acid cycle to form ATP. However, in diabetics, glucose does not enter cells in adequate amounts and production of pyruvate by glycolysis is decreased. The activity of the citric acid cycle therefore is diminished, resulting in decreased utilization of acetyl-CoA. The net effect of increased lipolysis and acetyl-CoA production along with decreased utilization of acetyl-CoA in the citric acid cycle is an increase in the concentration of acetyl-CoA.[2]

The three ketone bodies synthesized from acetyl-CoA include β-hydroxybutyrate, acetoacetate, and acetone. Acetyl-CoA is converted to acetoacetate by two metabolic pathways, and acetoacetate then is metabolized to β-hydroxybutyrate or acetone. One of the pathways of acetoacetate synthesis involves condensation of two acetyl-CoA units and the other utilizes three units of acetyl-CoA. Ketone bodies are synthesized in the liver.[2]

Acetoacetate and β-hydroxybutyrate are anions of moderately strong acids. Therefore their accumulation results in ketotic acidosis. Metabolic acidosis and the electrolyte abnormalities that ensue are important determinants in the outcome of patients with DKA.[3]

One of the beliefs regarding the pathophysiology of DKA had been that patients who develop DKA have no or undetectable endogenous insulin concentration. While endogenous insulin concentration in cats with spontaneous DKA has not been reported, in one study five of seven dogs with DKA had detectable endogenous serum insulin concentrations, and two of these dogs had endogenous serum insulin concentrations within the normal range.[4] Similarly, a recent study described a group of seven cats with DKA who went on to develop diabetic remission lasting from 5 weeks to 24 months.[5] The ability to attain remission suggests that some cats with DKA have endogenous insulin secretory ability, allowing them to become independent of exogenous insulin therapy for various time periods. Therefore it is unlikely that zero or undetectable endogenous insulin concentration is a single important factor in the pathophysiology of DKA in cats.

A different factor that may be important in the pathophysiology of DKA is the presence of an elevated serum glucagon concentration, which could occur secondary to concurrent disease. While serum glucagon concentration in cats with spontaneous DKA has not been reported, a recent report of serum glucagon concentration in diabetic dogs found that a rise in glucagon concentration was significantly associated with an increase in ketone concentration.[6]

DEFINITION AND PATHOPHYSIOLOGY OF THE HYPEROSMOLAR HYPERGLYCEMIC STATE

HHS is defined as a severe diabetic metabolic complication and clinical decompensation characterized by profound hyperglycemia (≥600 mg/dL), hyperosmolarity (effective serum osmolality ≥320 mOsm/kg in cats or ≥330 mOsm/kg in human beings), and dehydration.[1,7] HHS also is defined by the absence of ketoacidosis.[1]

Osmolality is defined as the number of osmotically active particles per kilogram of water, and plasma osmolality can be estimated based on sodium, glucose, and blood urea nitrogen concentrations. However, urea can diffuse freely across cell membranes and does not contribute significantly to plasma osmolality. Therefore effective osmolality is calculated based on sodium and glucose concentrations alone, using one of several formulas including the following:

$$\text{Effective } P_{osm} \approx 2(\text{plasma}[Na^+]) + [\text{glucose}]/18$$

The pathophysiology of HHS is incompletely understood, but is believed to be similar to that of DKA in that increased glucagon concentration plays an important role in its development. Similar to DKA, insulin concentration is not zero in HHS.[1] It is not known why some diabetic individuals develop DKA whereas others develop HHS. The notion that HHS develops solely in older diabetic patients with type 2 diabetes mellitus has been refuted, because HHS has been reported in pediatric patients.[1,8] As in human beings, severely compromised diabetic cats exhibiting a mixture of the classic characteristics of DKA and HHS have been described.[8]

RISK FACTORS FOR DKA OR HHS

The mean age of cats with DKA is 9 years (range, 2 to 16 years),[9] whereas the mean age of cats with HHS is 12.6 ± 3.2 years.[7] Specific breed or gender has not been shown to increase the risk of DKA or HHS in cats.[7,9,10]

Concurrent disease is common in cats with DKA or HHS. It is possible that the presence of concurrent disease results in elevated serum glucagon concentrations, which increase the risk of DKA or HHS. Concurrent disease has been documented in about 90 per cent of cats with DKA. The most common concurrent diseases noted in cats with DKA are hepatic lipidosis, chronic kidney disease, acute pancreatitis, bacterial or viral infections, and neoplasia.[9] In a study that compared cats with HHS to those with DKA or uncomplicated diabetes, about 90 per cent of cats with HHS had a concurrent disorder.[7] Distribution of concurrent disease varied between disease states. Specifically, cats with HHS were significantly more likely to have chronic kidney disease or congestive heart failure as compared with cats with DKA or uncomplicated diabetes, and to have neoplasia or infections as compared with cats with uncomplicated diabetes (but not DKA).[7] Infections noted in the group of cats with HHS were upper respiratory or urinary tract infections, otitis, a necrotic toe, severe purulent dental lesions, and gastrointestinal parasites.[7] Acute pancreatitis was significantly more common in cats with DKA compared with cats with HHS or uncomplicated diabetes, and there was no significant difference in the rate of acute pancreatitis between cats with HHS and uncomplicated diabetes.[7] The rate of corticosteroid administration was not significantly different among the three groups of cats.[7]

Most cats with DKA are newly diagnosed diabetics.[9] However, about 70 per cent of cats with HHS were treated previously with insulin.[7] There is no apparent significant difference between duration of diabetes prior to diagnosis of HHS or DKA.[7,9]

The two most common risk factors for development of DKA or HHS in human beings are inadequate or inappropriate insulin therapy and infection.[1] Similarly 65 per cent of dogs with DKA are newly diagnosed diabetics who have not been treated previously with insulin, and 20 per cent have a urinary tract infection.

CLINICAL SIGNS AND PHYSICAL EXAMINATION FINDINGS IN CATS WITH DKA OR HHS

Clinical signs and physical examination findings may be attributed to chronic untreated diabetes, presence of concurrent disease, and the acute onset of DKA or HHS. The most common clinical signs of cats with DKA or HHS are polyuria and polydipsia, lethargy, inappetence or anorexia, vomiting, and weight loss.[7,9] Additional clinical signs reported in cats with HHS include ataxia or weakness, respiratory problems, inappropriate elimination, or neurological signs (e.g., circling, pacing, and unresponsiveness).[7]

Common abnormalities noted on physical examination of cats with DKA are a subjectively underweight body condition, dehydration, icterus, or hepatomegaly.[9] Common abnormalities noted on physical examination of cats with HHS are a subjectively overweight body condition, dehydration (noted in about 80 per cent of cats and classified as severe in about 50 per cent of cats with HHS), dental disease (noted in about 60 per cent of affected cats), respiratory compromise, and lower body temperature compared with cats with uncomplicated diabetes mellitus.

CLINICAL PATHOLOGY OF DKA OR HHS

Anemia and neutrophilia with a left shift are common features of feline DKA.[9] Cats with DKA also have significantly more red blood cell Heinz body formation compared with normal cats, and the degree of Heinz body formation is correlated with plasma β-hydroxybutyrate concentration.[11] In contrast, anemia is uncommon in cats with HHS and was observed in only three of 17 cats studied.[7] Four of 17 cats with HHS had Heinz body formation, and mature neutrophilia was noted in about 50 per cent of cats with HHS. [7]

Persistent hyperglycemia is apparent in all cats diagnosed with DKA or HHS, unless they have been treated with insulin.[7,9] As the definition of HHS implies, cats with HHS have a blood glucose concentration of 600 mg/dL or greater. However, it is possible for a cat to have a blood glucose concentration of 600 mg/dL or greater with diabetes mellitus that is not complicated by HHS or DKA. Elevations in alanine aminotransferase (ALT) activity and cholesterol concentration have been reported in about 80 per cent of cats with DKA, but they are not usually elevated in cats with HHS.[7,9,10] In comparison, aspartate aminotransferase (AST) activity was elevated in 11 of 11 cats with HHS.[7] Azotemia has been reported in approximately 50 per cent of cats with DKA and in about 90 per cent of cats with HHS.[7,9] Alkaline phosphatase (ALP) activity is normal in most cats with DKA or HHS, although it is elevated in almost all dogs with DKA.[2,7,9]

The pathophysiology of electrolyte abnormalities in cats with DKA and HHS differs between the two complications.[1,7,9] In DKA whole body potassium depletion usually is present, but may not be apparent at presentation. Cats with DKA often have a decreased potassium intake as a result of inappetence or anorexia, and increased loss through vomiting and osmotic diuresis. Hypokalemia may be exacerbated by binding of potassium to ketoacids. On the other hand, serum potassium concentration may be increased as excess hydrogen ions shift from the extracellular fluid into cells. Positively charged potassium ions then are shifted out of cells to compensate for the electric change associated with movement of positively-charged hydrogen ions into cells. Hyperglycemia and hypoinsulinemia also contribute to a shift of potassium

to the extracellular fluid. Initially a cat with DKA may even appear to have hyperkalemia because of decreased renal excretion, dehydration, and decreased insulin function. However, with rehydration, potassium ions are lost from the extracellular fluid and hypokalemia rapidly becomes apparent. Insulin therapy may worsen hypokalemia because insulin shifts potassium into cells. The most important clinical significance of hypokalemia in DKA is profound muscle weakness, which may result in ventroflexion of the neck and, in extreme cases, respiratory paralysis (see Chapter 59).

In HHS, acidosis is not the most important component of electrolyte movement. The most important factor in the pathophysiology of hypokalemia in HHS is severe osmotic diuresis. However, the other factors mentioned above such as anorexia, vomiting, binding of potassium to ketoacids, and insulin therapy also contribute to development of hypokalemia in HHS.

A study comparing serum potassium concentration of cats with DKA and HHS at the time of admission found that 36 cats with DKA had significantly lower potassium concentration (mean 3.1 ± 0.7 mmol/L) compared with 16 cats with HHS (mean 4.2 ± 0.9 mmol/L). In contrast, in human beings total body potassium depletion in HHS is thought to be more profound than in DKA.[1] However, severe dehydration in patients with HHS may mask total body potassium depletion at the time of initial examination more than in patients with DKA.[1] In 127 dogs with DKA, only 45 per cent of the patients were hypokalemic at the time of initial examination, but 84 per cent of dogs developed hypokalemia over the course of hospitalization.[3] Future studies comparing potassium concentration in rehydrated cats with DKA and HHS are needed in order to improve our understanding of potassium depletion in these patients.

In DKA hypophosphatemia develops when phosphate shifts from the intracellular to the extracellular space as a result of hyperglycemia, acidosis, and hypoinsulinemia. Osmotic diuresis or fluid therapy along with insulin therapy cause extracellular phosphate depletion leading to whole body phosphate depletion. In HHS the most important factor in the pathophysiology of hypophosphatemia is severe osmotic diuresis. Hypophosphatemia related to DKA has been associated with hemolysis in a cat and with seizures in a dog.[12] Additional clinical signs that may develop by reason of hypophosphatemia include weakness, myocardial depression, and arrhythmias. In human beings total body phosphate depletion in DKA is thought to be more profound than in HHS.[1]

Interestingly, while hypophosphatemia is recognized commonly in human patients with DKA and HHS and in dogs with DKA, hyperphosphatemia (rather than hypophosphatemia) actually is reported more commonly in cats with DKA and HHS.[1,3,7,9] The reason may be that studies in cats report serum phosphate concentration measured only at the time of admission when dehydration may mask hypophosphatemia. Furthermore, many cats with DKA and HHS have chronic kidney disease, which may contribute to increased phosphate concentration.

Decreased plasma ionized magnesium (iMg) concentration has been documented in four of five cats with

DKA, and may be caused by increased urinary magnesium excretion.[13] The clinical significance of hypomagnesemia in cats is unknown, but in human diabetics it includes insulin resistance, hypertension, hyperlipidemia, and increased platelet aggregation. Dogs with DKA usually do not have low iMg concentration at the time of initial examination.[3]

Serum sodium concentration can be high, normal, or low in patients with DKA or HHS. In human beings profound osmotic diuresis usually leads to a low serum sodium concentration at the time of initial examination. However, severe dehydration can mask sodium losses and may result in an initially normal or high serum sodium concentration. On the other hand, severe hyperglycemia can contribute to a pseudohyponatremia. Extracellular hyperglycemia results in fluid shifting from the intracellular to the extracellular space, causing dilution of the extracellular sodium (i.e., pseudohyponatremia). Various equations can be used to correct for pseudohyponatremia (e.g., the addition of 1.6 mEq to the measured serum sodium value for each 100 mg/dL glucose >100 mg/dL). For example, if the measured serum sodium concentration is 135 mEq/L and blood glucose concentration is 400 mg/dL, the corrected serum sodium concentration is 135 + (1.6 × 3) or 139.8 mEq/L.[1] Additionally, hyperlipidemia may interfere with sodium measurement and may contribute to a falsely decreased serum sodium concentration.

In one study of cats with HHS or DKA the median corrected sodium concentration of cats with HHS (159 mmol/L) was significantly greater than that (151 mmol/L) of cats with DKA.[7] In another study that compared cats with DKA to those with uncomplicated diabetes mellitus, 34 per cent of cats with DKA had hyponatremia in comparison to only 8 per cent with uncomplicated diabetes mellitus.[10] A third study found that 80 per cent of 42 cats with diabetic ketosis or diabetic ketoacidosis were hyponatremic.[9] In the two latter studies sodium concentration was not corrected for glucose. Hypochloremia also has been reported in human beings with DKA or HHS, and in cats and dogs with DKA.[1,3,7,9,10]

In patients with DKA and HHS, glucosuria usually is found on urinalysis, and proteinuria also may be apparent. In DKA, ketonuria may not be detected because the nitroprusside reagent in urine dipsticks reacts with acetoacetate but not with β-hydroxybutyrate, which is the dominant ketone body in DKA. Measurement of serum β-hydroxybutyrate concentration is more sensitive than measurement of urine ketones.[14] Urinary tract infections develop in about 13 per cent of diabetic cats.[15] The most common bacterial isolate is *Escherichia coli*.[15] In diabetic cats a urinalysis is a useful screening tool for a urinary tract infection, because most cats with a urinary tract infection have either white blood cells or bacteria identified in the urine sediment.[15] (See Chapter 48 in the fifth volume of this series for a discussion on bacterial urinary tract infections.)

Results of additional clinicopathological or imaging tests such as adrenal or thyroid axis testing, growth hormone and IGF-1 concentration, pancreatic lipase immunoreactivity, liver function tests, liver biopsy, abdominal ultrasound, thoracic radiographs, or brain magnetic resonance imaging depend on the presence of specific concurrent disorders.

DIFFERENTIAL DIAGNOSES

Differential diagnoses for the presence of ketosis include DKA, acute pancreatitis, starvation, intake of a low-carbohydrate diet, persistent hypoglycemia, persistent fever, or pregnancy. Differential diagnoses for a primary metabolic acidosis include DKA, renal failure, lactic acidosis, toxin exposure, severe tissue destruction, severe diarrhea, or chronic vomiting. Differential diagnoses for hyperosmolarity include HHS, dehydration, renal failure, and toxin exposure.

TREATMENT OF DKA OR HHS

The five components of treatment of DKA and HHS are correction of dehydration, electrolyte abnormalities, hyperglycemia, and acidosis, and treatment of any concurrent disorder. Administration and careful monitoring of intravenous (IV) fluid therapy is the most important component. No controlled studies in cats with DKA or HHS have examined the optimal fluid to be used for treatment. Therefore any commercially available isotonic crystalloid solution may be used. The use of 0.9 per cent saline has been advocated because of its relatively high sodium concentration[1]; however, its administration may be contraindicated in hyperosmolar diabetics in whom serum sodium concentration initially is high. Additionally, 0.9 per cent saline may contribute further to an acidosis owing to the high chloride concentration and its lack of a buffer. On the other hand, lactate (contained in lactated Ringer's solution) and acetate (contained in Plasma-Lyte and Normosol-R) are converted to bicarbonate and may contribute to treatment of acidosis. Another advantage of these buffer-containing crystalloids is that they contain potassium, which may blunt the acute decline in potassium concentration that can occur with initiation of fluid and insulin treatment. However, as long as a cat is monitored carefully, particularly in regard to hydration, mental status, and electrolyte concentrations, any of the above crystalloids can be used.

Because clinical trials regarding fluid therapy in cats with DKA and HHS have not been reported, it may be useful to turn to the American Diabetes Association (ADA) guidelines.[1] The ADA recommends treatment with 0.9 per cent saline for the first hour in patients with either DKA or HHS. After the first hour of fluid therapy DKA and HHS patients are treated with 0.45 per cent saline, if their corrected sodium concentration is high or normal, or with 0.9 per cent saline if their corrected sodium concentration is low. The rate of fluid administration depends on each patient's fluid losses, hemodynamic status, and cardiac function. In addition to rehydration, fluid therapy may contribute to a decrease in blood glucose concentration by improving renal perfusion and by decreasing the concentration of counter-regulatory hormones, most importantly glucagon.[16]

Box 28-1 Potassium Supplementation in Hypokalemic Cats	
Serum Potassium Concentration (mmol/L)	Potassium (mEq) Added to 250 mL Fluid Bag
1.6-2	20
2.1-2.5	15
2.6-3.0	10
3.1-3.5	7

*Not to exceed 0.5 mEq/kg/hour without electrocardiographic monitoring.

Table 28-1 Administration of IV Insulin in Cats with DKA or HHS*		
Blood Glucose Concentration (mg/dL)	Fluid Composition	Rate of Administration (mL/hr)
>250	0.9% NaCl	10
200-250	0.45% NaCl + 2.5% dextrose	7
150-200	0.45% NaCl + 2.5% dextrose	5
100-150	0.45% NaCl + 5% dextrose	5
<100	0.45% NaCl + 5% dextrose	Stop fluid administration

*2.2 U/kg of regular crystalline insulin added to 250 mL of 0.9% sodium chloride (NaCl) solution. The administration set must be flushed with 50 mL of the mixture prior to administration of the solution to the patient.

Correction and monitoring of electrolyte abnormalities is an extremely important component of therapy. Electrolyte supplementation must be monitored frequently (i.e., every 4 to 6 hours), because adjustment of supplementation rates may be required. A cat who is hyperkalemic at the time of initial examination may become hypokalemic shortly after fluid therapy has begun. Hypokalemia can be treated by administering potassium as an IV continuous rate infusion (CRI) at no more than 0.5 mEq/kg/hour (Box 28-1). If higher doses are required, continuous electrocardiographic monitoring should be performed simultaneously; and if a narrow T wave, prolonged QRS complex and PR interval, or depressed P wave amplitude are noted, potassium supplementation should be discontinued and serum potassium concentration measured. Hypophosphatemia (serum phosphate concentration <2.0 mg/dL) is corrected with an intravenous CRI of potassium phosphate (the solution contains 4.4 mEq/mL of potassium and 3 mM/mL of phosphate) at a rate of 0.03 to 0.12 mM phosphate/kg/hour. Administration of potassium must be taken into account when giving potassium phosphate for correction of hypophosphatemia.

A magnesium sulfate solution (containing 4 mEq/mL) given IV as a CRI of 1 mEq/kg/24h has been used successfully for correction of hypomagnesemia. Toxicity of erroneously administered IV magnesium has been reported in one diabetic cat and one dog with acute renal disease.[17] Signs of magnesium toxicity included vomiting, weakness, generalized flaccid muscle tone, mental dullness, bradycardia, respiratory depression, and hypotension.[17] Care must be taken to administer IV magnesium only to patients who have documented decreased iMg concentration.

As the hyperglycemia resolves, the sodium concentration is expected to appear higher secondary to the decrease in osmolality, and subsequent movement of free water from the intravascular space. If the hyponatremia and hypochloremia persist after 6 to 8 hours of fluid therapy, they should be corrected by administering 0.9 per cent saline or by increasing the rate of fluid administration if the cat is already receiving 0.9 per cent saline. Decisions regarding correction of sodium concentration should be based on the corrected sodium concentration.

Correction of hyperglycemia is performed by administering a rapidly acting insulin. At the author's institution, insulin administration is initiated after 6 hours of fluid therapy to allow for rehydration and initial correction of electrolyte abnormalities. Although several new rapidly acting insulin products have been introduced to the market and are being used successfully in the management of human patients with DKA, their clinical use in cats with DKA or HHS has not been investigated. Some human patients with mild DKA also are being treated with subcutaneous administration of rapidly acting insulins, such as lispro insulin, a practice driven by an attempt to decrease hospitalization expense; however, this strategy is not recommended currently in cats. At this time the use of regular insulin (Humulin R, Novolin R) is recommended for treatment of DKA or HHS in cats. Regular insulin is administered as an IV CRI (Table 28-1)[18] or intramuscularly (IM).[19] When IV regular insulin is administered as a CRI, blood glucose is measured every 2 hours. When insulin is administered IM, it is given every hour subsequent to measurement of blood glucose concentration. The initial dose for IM therapy is 0.2 U/kg regular insulin IM, followed by 0.1 U/kg regular insulin IM 1 hour later. Treatment with IM regular insulin is continued with 0.05 U/kg/hr, 0.1 U/kg/hr, or 0.2 U/kg/hr if blood glucose drops by more than 75 mg/dL/hr, between 50 to 75 mg/dL/hr, or by less than 50 mg/dL/hr, respectively.[19]

Acidosis usually is corrected with IV fluid administration and insulin therapy alone.[1,3,9,16] Giving bicarbonate for correction of acidosis in human patients with DKA is controversial because it has been shown to increase the risk for cerebral edema in children with DKA.[1,20] Possible additional risks associated with bicarbonate treatment in human beings with DKA include exacerbation of hypokalemia, increased hepatic ketone production, paradoxical cerebrospinal fluid acidosis, and worsening intracellular acidosis owing to increased carbon dioxide production.[16,21,22] The ADA recommends bicarbonate supplementation only in DKA patients in whom arterial pH remains less than 7.0 after 1 hour of fluid therapy.[1]

Bicarbonate treatment is not often given to most dogs and cats with DKA, yet acidosis typically resolves.[3,9] A recent retrospective study of 127 dogs with DKA reported that both the degree of acidosis and IV sodium bicarbonate administration were associated with a poor outcome.[3] It was not clear, however, if the poor outcome was because of the severe degree of acidosis that prompted such therapy or the bicarbonate therapy itself. Therefore bicarbonate administration should be done cautiously.

If bicarbonate therapy is deemed appropriate despite the potential risks, one treatment protocol is to administer IV over a 20-minute interval ½ to ⅓ of a dose as determined by the formula: sodium bicarbonate dose = [0.3 × body weight × negative base excess]. Treatment should be repeated hourly if needed after measurement of venous pH until venous pH is greater than 7.0. However, there are no studies to support this or any other specific bicarbonate treatment protocol in cats with DKA.

Presence of concurrent disease is believed to contribute to development of DKA and HHS. Therefore identifying any concomitant diseases and providing appropriate treatment is important. Treatment of concurrent disease may decrease glucagon secretion and contribute to improved diabetic regulation and resolution of DKA and HHS.

OUTCOME OF PATIENTS WITH DKA OR HHS

In one study of cats with DKA or ketosis without acidosis, most cats (70 per cent) survived to be discharged from the hospital.[9] Median hospitalization time for cats was 5 days, but up to 40 per cent of cats developed recurring episodes of DKA.[9]

In another study that compared cats with HHS to those with DKA, only six of 17 cats with HHS (35 per cent) survived to be discharged from the hospital.[7] Survival of cats with HHS was significantly lower than the survival of cats with DKA (31 of 37 cats, 84 per cent).[7] Of cats who survived to be discharged from the hospital, those patients with HHS had a shorter duration of hospitalization (median 3 days) compared with those with DKA (median 7 days).[7] The outcome of cats was not related to the presence of neurological signs or to serum glucose concentration, measured or corrected serum sodium concentration, or total and effective serum osmolality as measured at presentation.[7]

INSULIN OVERDOSE

Diabetic cats may receive an insulin overdose when there is a change in their insulin requirements or as a result of an error, which may happen at any time over the course of treatment. Insulin requirements may decrease because of resolution of a concurrent disorder or if the cat has transient diabetes and has gone into remission but continues to receive insulin (see Chapter 27).

An error in insulin administration may occur for a variety of reasons. One possible cause may be the use of a 40 U/mL insulin syringe for administration of a 100 U/mL insulin product. Care must be taken to ensure that owners of diabetic cats are educated in regard to the different insulin products and syringes, and that the proper insulin syringe is used.

An insulin overdose results in hypoglycemia, defined as a blood glucose concentration less than 65 mg/dL.[23] A recent review of medical records of 470 diabetic cats identified an insulin-induced hypoglycemic event in 17 per cent of these cats.[24] Diabetic cats are more likely to develop an insulin-induced hypoglycemic event compared with dogs, possibly because they are more likely to have transient diabetes mellitus.[23]

In one study cats who received an insulin overdose were predominantly neutered males with a median age of 12 years; however, this signalment is typical of diabetic cats in general.[23] Cats who had an insulin overdose had a greater median body weight (5.8 kg) compared with other diabetic cats (5.1 kg). Most cats who became hypoglycemic were receiving insulin doses greater than 6 U/injection, administered q24h or q12h.[23] The most common clinical signs associated with insulin overdose in cats were seizures, recumbency, anorexia, shaking, vomiting, ataxia, and dullness.[23]

Treatment consists of administration of dextrose, which usually is given intravenously, although in mild cases oral dextrose supplementation or feeding may be enough. Although median duration of hospitalization in 20 cats who had an insulin overdose was 20 hours, the duration of treatment varied, and lasted up to 10 days.[23] The dose of dextrose required to achieve euglycemia and the amount of time a cat needs to be on a glucose drip also can be unpredictable. In 14 cats, from 0.21 to 6.30 g/kg dextrose was needed to maintain euglycemia and the duration of dextrose supplementation ranged from 0.55 to 66 hours. In other words, hypoglycemia can recur even after a normal blood glucose concentration is attained and a dextrose drip may be required for up to approximately 3 days.[23] The administration of glucagon for treatment of insulin-induced hypoglycemia has been described anecdotally. In a report of 20 cats who had an insulin overdose, 90 per cent of cats survived to be discharged from the hospital after a median hospital stay of 20 hours.[23]

REFERENCES

1. Kitabachi AE, Umpierrez GE, Murphy MB: Hyperglycemic crises in adult patients with diabetes, *Diabetes Care* 29:2739, 2006.
2. Ganong WF: *Review of medical physiology*, ed 18, Stamford, 1997, Appleton & Lange.
3. Hume DZ, Drobatz KJ, Hess RS: Outcome of dogs with diabetic ketoacidosis: 127 dogs (1993-2003), *J Vet Intern Med* 20:547, 2006.
4. Parsons SE, Drobatz KJ, Lamb SV, et al: Endogenous serum insulin concentration in dogs with diabetic ketoacidosis, *J Vet Emer Crit* 12:147, 2002.
5. Sieber-Ruckstuhl NS, Kley S, Tschuor F, et al: Remission of diabetes mellitus in cats with diabetic ketoacidosis, *J Vet Intern Med* 22:1326, 2008.
6. Durocher LL, Hinchcliff KW, DiBartola SP, et al: Acid-base and hormonal abnormalities in dogs with naturally occurring diabetes mellitus, *J Am Vet Med Assoc* 232:1310, 2008.
7. Koenig A, Drobatz KJ, Beale AB, et al: Hyperglycemic, hyperosmolar syndrome in feline diabetics: 17 cases (1995-2001), *J Vet Emer Crit* 14:30, 2004.
8. Kershaw MJ, Newton T, Barrett TG, et al: Childhood diabetes presenting with hyperosmolar dehydration but without

ketoacidosis: a report of three cases, *Diabet Med* 22:645, 2005.

9. Bruskiewicz KA, Nelson RW, Feldman EC, et al: Diabetic ketosis and ketoacidosis in cats: 42 cases (1980-1995), *J Am Vet Med Assoc* 211:188, 1997.

10. Crenshaw KL, Peterson ME: Pretreatment clinical and laboratory evaluation of cats with diabetes mellitus: 104 cases (1992-1994), *J Am Vet Med Assoc* 209:943, 1996.

11. Christopher MM, Broussard JD, Peterson ME: Heinz body formation associated with ketoacidosis in diabetic cats, *J Am Vet Med Assoc* 9:24, 1995.

12. Willard MD, Zerbe CA, Schall WD, et al: Severe hypophosphatemia associated with diabetes mellitus in six dogs and one cat, *J Am Vet Med Assoc* 190:1007, 1987.

13. Norris CR, Nelson RW, Christopher MM: Serum total and ionized magnesium concentrations and urinary fractional excretion of magnesium in cats with diabetes mellitus and diabetic ketoacidosis, *J Am Vet Med Assoc* 215:1455, 1999.

14. Duarte R, Simoes DMN, Franchini ML, et al: Accuracy of serum beta-hydroxybutyrate measurements for the diagnosis of diabetic ketoacidosis in 116 dogs, *J Vet Intern Med* 16:411, 2002.

15. Bailiff NL, Nelson RW, Feldman EC, et al: Frequency and risk factors for urinary tract infection in cats with diabetes mellitus, *J Vet Intern Med* 20:850, 2006.

16. Glaser N, Kuppermann N: The evaluation and management of children with diabetic ketoacidosis in the emergency department, *Pediatr Emerg Care* 20:477, 2004.

17. Jackson CB, Drobatz KJ: Iatrogenic magnesium overdose: 2 case reports, *JVECC* 14:115, 2004.

18. Macintire DK: Treatment of diabetic ketoacidosis in dogs by continuous low-dose intravenous infusion of insulin, *J Am Vet Med Assoc* 202:1266, 1993.

19. Feldman EC, Nelson RW: Diabetic ketoacidosis. In Feldman EC, Nelson RW, editors: *Canine and feline endocrinology and reproduction*, Philadelphia, 2004, Saunders.

20. Glaser N, Barnett P, McCaslin I, et al: Risk factors for cerebral edema in children with diabetic ketoacidosis, *N Engl J Med* 344:264, 2001.

21. Chiasson JL, Aris-Jilwan N, Belanger R, et al: Diagnosis and treatment of diabetic ketoacidosis and the hyperglycemic hyperosmolar state, *CMAJ* 168:859, 2003.

22. Okuda Y, Adrogue HJ, Field JB: Counterproductive effects of sodium bicarbonate in diabetic ketoacidosis, *J Clin Endocrinol Metab* 81:314, 1996.

23. Whitley NT, Drobatz KJ, Panciera DL: Insulin overdose in dogs and cats: 28 cases (1986-1993), *J Am Vet Med Assoc* 211:326, 1997.

24. Chapman P, Cohen T, Hess R: Transient diabetes mellitus is an uncommon cause of hypoglycemic events in insulin treated diabetic cats, *J Vet Intern Med* 20:1522, 2006 (abstract).

29 Acromegaly

Stijn J.M. Niessen and David B. Church

ETIOLOGY

In contrast to the situation in dogs, in whom we encounter acromegaly mostly when induced by exogenous or endogenous progestogens, acromegaly in cats traditionally is thought to be caused by a functional somatotrophic adenoma in the pars distalis of the anterior pituitary gland, resulting in excessive growth hormone (GH) secretion[1] (Box 29-1). However, a recent report suggests that a proportion of acromegalic cats are suffering from somatotrophic hyperplasia rather than a specific adenoma[2] (Figure 29-1). Whether this represents a different group of acromegalics, or a rare subset of the same spectrum of disease, remains to be determined. Additionally, one case with a double pituitary adenoma causing both hyperadrenocorticism and acromegaly has been described.[3] Which processes initiate pituitary adenoma formation remain to be elucidated.

The expression of GH mRNA in mammary gland tissue, as seen in dogs, also can be found in cats and human beings, indicating that secretion of GH from mammary tissue also could occur in cats. Indeed, progestin-induced fibroadenomatous changes in the mammary glands of cats also are associated with locally enhanced GH expression. The mammary gene is identical to the pituitary-expressed gene and uses the same promoter for transcription. Nevertheless, feline cases of progestin-induced GH secretion from the mammary glands causing the clinical syndrome of acromegaly have yet to be described.[4,5]

EPIDEMIOLOGY

Acromegaly in cats previously was thought to be rare, with only approximately 30 cases reported in peer-reviewed literature before 2007.[6,7] Recent research has attempted to provide a more accurate insight into the possible true prevalence of this endocrinopathy. A large general screening study in the United Kingdom among diabetic cats with variable glycemic control (ranging from poor to adequate) who were not suspected initially to have acromegaly revealed that 59 out of 184 assessed subjects (i.e., 32 per cent of screened cats) had serum insulin-like growth factor 1 (IGF-1) concentrations strongly suggestive of the presence of acromegaly (Figure 29-2).[2] Of these 59 cats a subpopulation of 18 cats was assessed in more detail, leading to confirmation of the diagnosis in 94 per cent of assessed cases. Confirmation of acromegaly in such a high proportion of the subset suggests that the original estimation of prevalence in the 184 cats in the study, made on the basis of raised IGF-1 levels only, was likely to be an accurate approximation of the true prevalence in the greater diabetic population. Additionally, the data from this prospective British study were backed up by data from a retrospective North American study, which indicated that 26 per cent of diabetic cats met clinical criteria for the diagnosis of acromegaly.[8] The latter study did, however, include samples of diabetic cats that were submitted to the laboratory specifically for assessment for acromegaly, introducing a bias to the study. Overall, it remains a genuine possibility that we

304

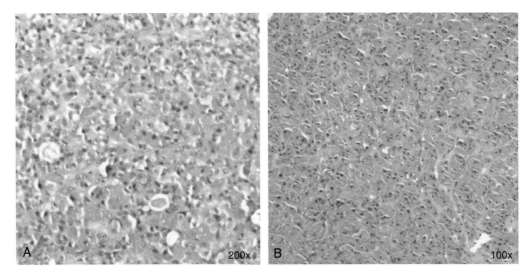

Figure 29-1 Microscopy images of histopathological examination (H&E stained, magnification indicated in right bottom corner) of normal **(A)** and hyperplastic **(B)** pars distalis of the anterior pituitary gland. Acidophilic cells (staining pink/red) predominate in the postmortem finding in a 9-year-old neutered male acromegalic domestic shorthair cat **(B),** whereas they are intermixed equally with basophilic cells in the normal pituitary gland **(A).**

Box 29-1 Brief Overview of Feline Acromegaly

1. Usually caused by pituitary adenoma
2. GH, IGF-1, and mass-induced effects
3. Diabetes mellitus, renal disease, cardiomyopathy, upper respiratory stridor, possible abdominal, facial, and limb conformational changes
4. In view of prevalence, "must have" differential diagnosis for insulin-resistant diabetes mellitus
5. Definite differential diagnosis for poorly controlled DM with weight gain
6. IGF-1 and fGH useful screening tool(s)
7. CT and/or MRI useful confirmation tool(s)
8. Adequate definitive treatment lacking; radiation therapy currently most advocated
9. Address neurological, cardiovascular, and renal complications

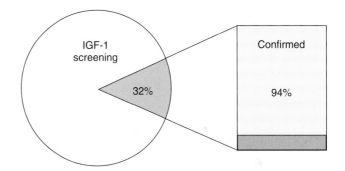

Figure 29-2 The results of a large prospective British screening study among diabetic cats.[2] Pie chart: 32 per cent of screened diabetics had an IGF-1 > 1000 ng/mL (purple segment), consistent with acromegaly. Bar chart: further evaluation of a subgroup of these 32 per cent (*n* = 18) confirmed acromegaly in 94 per cent (yellow segment) on the basis of intracranial CT, MRI, and/or postmortem findings.

are currently underdiagnosing acromegaly and revealing only the tip of the iceberg.[9]

In early reports acromegalic cats typically were middle-aged to older, neutered male mixed-breed cats with insulin-resistant diabetes mellitus.[1,6,10-14] Recent reports have confirmed this signalment, although insulin resistance was frequently but not consistently present at time of initial diagnosis. The authors found that of 59 cats with IGF-1 concentrations consistent with acromegaly, 52 were domestic shorthair cats, three domestic longhair, and four of unknown breed. Forty-seven were neutered males; six neutered females; five intact males; and one was of unknown gender. Their age ranged from 6 to 17 years (median, 11 years); body weight ranged from 3.5 to 9.2 kg (median, 5.8 kg), and median insulin dosage was 7 U per cat q12h (range, 1 to 35 U q12h), compared with 3 U per cat q12h in cats with IGF-1 concentrations below the acromegaly range.[2] However, because relatively few

cases have been documented to date, it seems prudent that clinicians remain open-minded with regard to this signalment.

PATHOGENESIS

Somatotrophic adenomas (and possibly somatotrophic hyperplasia) result in an increase in amplitude, duration, and frequency of the pulsatile release of GH, which in turn leads to elevated production of IGF-1, predominantly by the liver.[15] Affected cats suffer the catabolic and diabetogenic effects of GH, the anabolic effects of IGF-1, and, in some cases, the neurological consequences of an expanding intracranial neoplasm. A GH-induced postreceptor defect in insulin action at the level of target tissues is thought to explain why most reported cats with acromegaly have had concurrent insulin-resistant diabetes mellitus.* High IGF-1 concentrations induce excessive soft tissue growth, as evidenced by renal and myocardial pathology, hepatomegaly (although this is likely to be partly a result of hepatic lipid accumulation), adreno-megaly, and incidental thyroid enlargement, in addition to bone remodelling and thickening, resulting in arthropathy, broad facial features, and enlarged (so-called clubbed) paws.

In light of the change in renal size, renal disease is understood to be a possible complication in long-term untreated acromegalics. Abnormalities in renal histopathology reported in acromegalic cats include diffuse thickening of the glomerular basement membrane, thickening of Bowman's capsule, periglomerular fibrosis, and adipose and hydropic change with epithelial degeneration and regeneration of tubules.[2]

Pancreatic disease was reported previously by Gunn-Moore in two of 10 feline acromegalics,[6] and also was evident in two cats who underwent postmortem examination in the authors' study.[2] In the latter study the pancreas of one cat appeared grossly enlarged and firm and contained two cysts; on histopathological examination, diffuse hyperplasia with fibrous tissue, numerous interstitial lymphoid follicles, and marked vacuolation of the islet cells were noted. It remains to be determined if pancreatic disease is indeed more common in acromegalic diabetic cats, especially in view of the small number of cases in whom pancreatic pathology has been reported specifically and the potentially high prevalence of pancreatic disease in diabetic cats.[17]

Echocardiography in confirmed acromegalic cats has revealed variable changes ranging from no indication of structural abnormalities to atrial enlargement, generalized or focal interventricular septal thickening, and left ventricular free wall hypertrophy with thinning towards the apex. Diastolic dysfunction, systolic anterior motion of the mitral valve (SAM), mitral valve insufficiency, and increased left ventricular outflow velocity, as well as poor left atrial wall motion, spontaneous echo contrast, and a restrictive pattern of pulmonary venous flow all have been reported (Figure 29-3).[2] Overall myocardial changes seem common in acromegalic cats, and subsequent congestive heart failure can result. Kittleson et al reported increased GH concentrations among 31 cats with hypertrophic cardiomyopathy (HCM) when compared with 38 normal cats and 35 cats with cardiac disease of other cause. The serum GH concentrations in cats with HCM were less than those reported previously in cats with acromegaly. Pituitary tumors were not identified in eight of these cats with HCM on postmortem examination; however, presence or absence was not established for the remaining HCM cats.[18] These findings are supportive of a possible direct causal role of GH in the myocardial changes encountered in acromegaly.

Although hypertension has been regarded as common in acromegalic cats,[7,11] the largest and most recent study did not detect an increased prevalence of hypertension in acromegalics.[2] If indeed present in individual acromegalic cats, hypertension may result in (and, therefore,

---

*References 1, 2, 6, 8, 10, and 16.

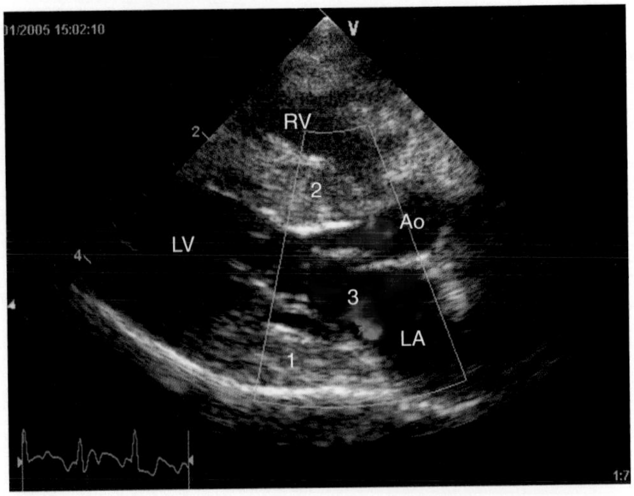

Figure 29-3 Right-sided parasternal echocardiogram (B-mode) with color-flow Doppler assessment of an acromegalic cat, showing thickening of the left ventricular free wall (1) and interventricular septum (2), as well as mitral valve regurgitation (3), likely induced by fGH and/or IGF-1 excess. *Ao,* Aorta; *LA,* left atrium; *LV,* left ventricle; *RV,* right ventricle.

cause a cat to be presented for) ocular hemorrhage, sudden blindness, or neurological abnormalities (see Chapter 49).

CLINICAL SIGNS

The soft-tissue and skeletal changes induced by IGF-1 have the potential to lead to a marked change in the overall or general appearance of an acromegalic cat. However, a recent study suggests the typical acromegalic phenotype is not particularly common.[2] Certainly the *absence* of a typical acromegalic appearance should not decrease a clinician's index of suspicion for the condition. Additionally, similar to the situation in human acromegaly, the feline disease has a gradual onset, often leading to late, or absence of, recognition of conformational changes by people in continuous contact with affected cats. Frequently comparison with pictures from past years is necessary to determine the difference in appearance and convince owners of these changes (Figure 29-4). Duration of the clinical signs (as perceived by the owners) in the cats seen by the authors indeed ranged broadly from 2 to 42 months (mean ± SD, 11.2 ± 11.4). In the authors' study the earliest clinical signs reported by the owners (Box 29-2) included those consistent with diabetes mellitus (i.e., polyuria/polydipsia [100 per cent of cats] and polyphagia [94 per cent]), but also weight gain (59 per cent). Some cats developed lameness (29 per cent), and some eventually displayed suspected or confirmed neurological signs, lethargy, impaired vision, circling, and vocalizing.[2] Initial weight loss followed by weight gain also has been reported.[1] Owners of the confirmed acromegalic cats in the authors' study had noted increased size of the paws in 12 per cent of cats, broader facial features in only one cat, and increased abdominal size in one cat. All cats were being treated with insulin at the

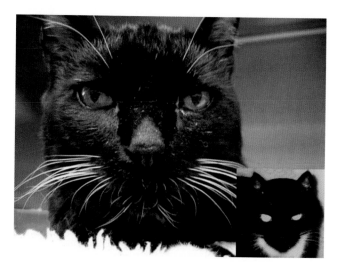

Figure 29-4 Broad facial features encountered in an acromegalic cat in 2005 *(main picture)* and compared with a picture of the same cat in 2000 *(inset)*. The owner had not noticed a clear difference in appearance until photographs were compared and differences were pointed out. (From Niessen SJ, Petrie G, Gaudiano F, et al: Feline acromegaly: an underdiagnosed endocrinopathy? *J Vet Intern Med* 21:899, 2007.)

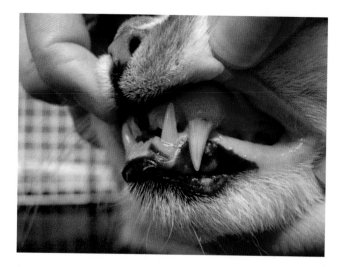

Figure 29-5 Prognathia inferior, as evidenced with a protrusion of the mandible, causing the distance between lower and upper canine teeth to increase. (From Niessen SJ, Petrie G, Gaudiano F, et al: Feline acromegaly: an underdiagnosed endocrinopathy? *J Vet Intern Med* 21:899, 2007.)

Box 29-2 Top 10 Clinical Signs of Feline Acromegaly
Polyuria
Polydipsia
Polyphagia (possibly extreme)
Weight gain (possibly initial weight loss)
Upper respiratory stridor
Broad facial features
Prognathia inferior
Abdominal enlargement/organomegaly
Clubbed paws
Neurological signs

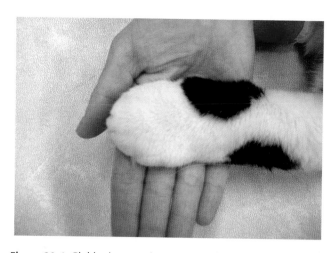

Figure 29-6 Clubbed paws of an acromegalic cat. (From Niessen SJ, Petrie G, Gaudiano F, et al: Feline acromegaly: an underdiagnosed endocrinopathy? *J Vet Intern Med* 21:899, 2007.)

time of diagnosis and all experienced difficulties in glycemic control, necessitating administration of increasing amounts of insulin before or after confirmation of the diagnosis of acromegaly. The median insulin dosage of the 17 confirmed acromegalic cats at time of initial examination in the study was 7 IU per cat q12h (range, 2 to 35 U q12h), higher than the 3 IU q12h for cats with IGF-1 below 1000 ng/mL.[2] Additional reported clinical signs include intermittent weakness (hypoglycemia) and behavioral changes.[1]

On physical examination of the 17 confirmed acromegalic cats, the authors noted enlarged liver and kidneys in 88 per cent, prognathia inferior (Figure 29-5) with increased distance between upper and lower canine teeth in 47 per cent, immature bilateral cataracts in 12 per cent, clubbed paws in 18 per cent (Figure 29-6), broad facial features in 82 per cent (see Figure 29-4), and systolic cardiac murmur in 24 per cent. They also noted gallop rhythm in one cat; respiratory stridor in 53 per cent; multiple limb lameness in 29 per cent; impaired vision, dilated pupils, reduced pupillary light reflex, reduced menace response, decreased facial sensation on the left and decreased postural reactions on the left, circling to the right, and vocalizing in one cat; decreased menace response bilaterally, confusion, and right-sided Horner's syndrome in another; and plantigrade stance of the hind limbs also in one patient. One cat experienced periods of open-mouth breathing and tachypnea when stressed which was attributable to congestive heart failure. Feldman and Nelson additionally reported the presence of a large tongue, increased interdental spacing, poor and unkempt hair coat, dullness, and increased soft tissue of the pharyngeal region in individual acromegalic cats.[1]

It is important to note that not all of these signs were present consistently in all cats seen by the authors in the most recent study. In fact, many cats were indistinguishable morphologically from nonacromegalic diabetic cats at the time of diagnosis, which could account for the possibility of current underdiagnosis of this endocrinopathy. Additionally, although polyphagia is a well-

Box 29-3 The Most Useful Diagnostic Tests When Acromegaly Is Suspected

Clinical image (insulin-resistant diabetes mellitus)
Hyperproteinemia, hyperglycemia, glycosuria, and/or
  possible other reported changes on serum
  biochemistry
fGH
IGF-1
CT with contrast enhancement
MRI with contrast enhancement

recognized consequence of diabetes mellitus, the degree of polyphagia seemed more extreme than in nonacromegalic diabetic cats.

DIAGNOSIS

Confirmation of acromegaly can be difficult because of the disorder's insidious onset, the cost of imaging procedures, and the frequent lack of a readily available feline growth hormone (fGH) assay.[1,19] As is the case in many diseases and specifically endocrinopathies, a combination of a suggestive clinical phenotype and indicative diagnostic aids is required to obtain an adequate level of confidence for a diagnosis of acromegaly (Box 29-3).

Acromegaly should be considered as a possible explanation for any animal with insulin-resistant diabetes mellitus. Other likely explanations include poor diabetes mellitus management through lack of owner compliance or inappropriate insulin storage and administration, leading to a false impression of the presence of insulin-resistant diabetes mellitus. For some guidelines to a possible approach when dealing with insulin-resistant diabetes mellitus, please refer to Figure 29-7.

Hyperadrenocorticism, and especially the pituitary-dependent form, deserves particular mention. Both acromegaly and hyperadrenocorticism are able to cause insulin resistance, can be associated with a pituitary tumor and adrenomegaly, and have a strong association with diabetes mellitus in cats. Consequently both diseases result in clinical signs related to poorly controlled diabetes mellitus; therefore differentiating between the two diseases can prove challenging. Both multifocal nodular hyperplasia of the adrenal cortices and generalized adrenomegaly have been reported in acromegalic cats,[10] and urine cortisol:creatinine ratios can be elevated in acromegalic cats as well.

When present the particular clinical signs of each disease (for acromegaly: broad facial features, clubbed paws, arthropathy, prognathia inferior; for hyperadrenocorticism: fragile skin, fur changes, bruising) may aid in the diagnostic process. It also is the authors' impression that acromegaly-induced insulin resistance can be more extreme in individual cases, compared with the resistance seen owing to hyperadrenocorticism, as evidenced by higher insulin requirements in acromegalic cats. Additionally, adrenocorticotropic hormone (ACTH) stimulation tests and low-dose dexamethasone suppression tests

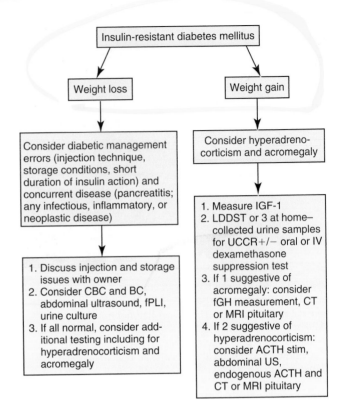

Figure 29-7 Diagram displaying a possible approach to insulin-resistant diabetic cats. *CBC,* Complete blood count; *BC,* biochemistry; *fPLI,* feline pancreatic lipase immunoreactivity; *LDDST,* low-dose dexamethasone suppression test; *UCCR,* urine cortisol to creatinine ratio; *ACTH stim,* adrenocorticotropic hormone stimulation test.

in general have proved useful in the discriminatory process.[1,2]

As in human beings hyperadrenocorticism and acromegaly can occur concurrently,[20] although there has been only one reported feline case: a cat with both pituitary-dependent hyperadrenocorticism and acromegaly caused by a "double" pituitary adenoma, consisting of histologically confirmed corticotroph and somatotroph adenomas separated by unaffected pituitary tissue.[3]

ROUTINE HEMATOLOGY, BIOCHEMISTRY, FRUCTOSAMINE, AND URINALYSIS

In view of the difficulty in attaining a diagnosis without costly diagnostic tests, the authors assessed the usefulness of routine hematology, serum biochemistry, and urinalysis in distinguishing between nonacromegalic and acromegalic diabetic cats.[21] Expectedly, hyperglycemia and glycosuria were present in both groups. Although fasting blood glucose concentrations showed a trend to be higher in acromegalic diabetic cats compared with nonacromegalic diabetics, the difference was not statistically significant (Figure 29-8). Similarly, serum fructosamine concentrations proved higher in acromegalic cats compared with nonacromegalic diabetics; however, overlapping values prevent this test from being a useful discriminating factor.

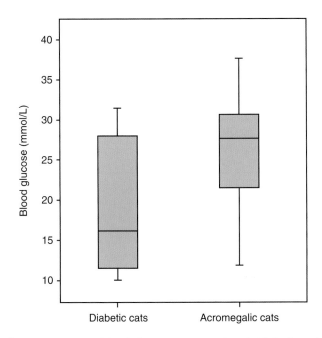

Figure 29-8 Fasting blood glucose concentrations in diabetic and acromegalic cats. No significant difference was found between the two groups, although acromegalic cats showed a trend toward higher fasting blood glucose concentrations.

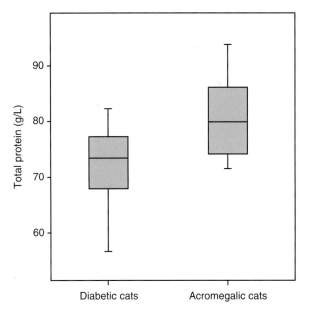

Figure 29-9 Total protein concentrations were significantly higher in acromegalic cats when compared with nonacromegalic diabetic cats.

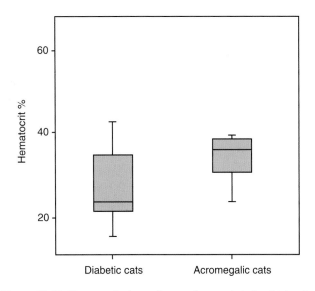

Figure 29-10 Hematocrit showed a trend towards being higher in acromegalic cats when compared with nonacromegalic diabetic cats; the difference, however, was not statistically significant.

Hyperproteinemia was the only factor truly overrepresented in the acromegalic group; hence its presence could suggest the need for further evaluation for acromegaly in an insulin-resistant diabetic cat (Figure 29-9). Indeed in Peterson et al's case series, nine of 14 acromegalic cats were hyperproteinemic.[10]

Previously hyperphosphatemia, possibly caused by GH-induced increased renal reabsorption; and erythrocytosis, possibly caused by an effect of GH or IGF-1 on bone marrow,[22] also have been suggested to be overrepresented in acromegalic cats[6,7,10] This could not be confirmed in the above mentioned authors' study, however, which was the only study using a diabetic control group to verify the findings. Additionally, hematocrit seemingly was higher in acromegalic cats, although statistical significance was not attained (Figure 29-10).

A range of other abnormalities have been associated anecdotally with feline acromegaly, including increased globulins, urea, creatinine, cholesterol, serum alanine aminotransferase (ALT), serum alkaline phosphatase (ALP), and calcium and decreased chloride. Many of these alterations can be expected in nonacromegalic diabetic cats and may simply represent the presence of unregulated diabetes and subclinical dehydration; indeed, these latter changes were not found to be overrepresented in acromegalics when compared with a nonacromegalic but diabetic control group. Azotemia was present in approximately 50 per cent of acromegalic cats in two reports published by Peterson et al[10] and Norman and Mooney.[11] Both authors suggested this may be attributable to GH- and/or IGF-1–induced nephropathy, diabetes mellitus, and/or possible hypertension. Interestingly, neither azotemia nor hypertension was demonstrable in the authors' described cases.[2]

INSULIN-LIKE GROWTH FACTOR 1

Because of the limited availability of a validated fGH assay, traditionally, serum total IGF-1 levels have been used as an aid in the diagnosis of feline acromegaly.[11] Compared with fGH, estimating serum IGF-1 levels has additional benefits because IGF-1 has nonpulsatile secretion and a relatively long half-life. However, increased IGF-1 concentrations have been reported in both acromegalic cats and nonacromegalic insulin-resistant diabetic cats, suggesting the possibility of false-positive results when using IGF-1 to diagnose acromegaly.[2,23,24] In addition, Norman and Mooney found normal IGF-1 concentrations at initial presentation in one cat later diagnosed with acromegaly (although increased serum IGF-1 concentration was documented eventually).[11]

Overall, however, IGF-1 estimation seems a valid initial screening tool. Berg et al found a sensitivity and specificity of 84 per cent (95 per cent confidence interval [CI] = 60.4 to 96.6 per cent) and 92 per cent (95 per cent CI = 81.3 to 97.2 per cent), respectively, and no significant correlation between serum IGF-1 concentration and duration of insulin treatment ($r = 0.23$, $p = 0.089$), insulin dosage ($r = 0.14$, $p = 0.30$), age ($r = 0.16$, $p = 0.12$), or pituitary volume ($r = 0.40$, $p = 011$). There was, however, some correlation between serum IGF-1 concentration and body weight ($r = 0.48$, $p < 0.0001$).[8]

FELINE GROWTH HORMONE

Evaluation of serum GH concentrations is not straightforward. First, GH secretion is influenced by many general factors such as sleep, food intake, gender, body mass, and stress. Second, the exact neuroendocrine control mechanisms of its release are still to be elucidated, and third, GH assays are not measuring a single substance; at least two major splice variants of GH exist in the circulation (20 and 22 kDa).[25]

Nevertheless, the duration, amplitude, and frequency of the pulsatile release of GH is increased in human beings with acromegaly,[15] and, despite some of its difficult characteristics, GH measurement can still be a valuable asset in the diagnosis of feline acromegaly. Single, random GH measurements have proved unreliable in confirming the diagnosis in human patients with occasional false negative results[25,26]; however, a high probability of acromegaly exists in people with single GH concentrations greater than 10 ng/mL.[26] This is in line with the situation in our feline patients with all published cases of feline acromegaly in whom GH estimation was performed having increased serum GH concentrations.* The authors therefore strongly recommend (whenever possible) using fGH estimation alongside IGF-1 determination. In the past, lack of availability of a suitable assay has proved prohibitive, although more recently, more centers are either offering or intending to offer this service.[19] A recent report indicated that fGH is relatively stable, allowing overnight transport of unseparated samples to be used reliably.[19] The mean (SD) basal fasting fGH level in 19 nonacromegalic, nondiabetic cats aged 2 to 16 years was 4.0 (1.4) ng/mL (range 1.9 to 6.3); 19 acromegalic cats had significantly higher fGH concentrations (range 8.5 to 33.2 ng/mL), with no overlap occurring between the two groups. However, in a second study eight out of 34 nonacromegalic diabetic cats had fGH concentrations that exceeded the upper limit of the reference interval of this particular assay (Table 29-1).[2] As only two of these eight cats had fGH concentrations that exceeded 10 ng/mL, a value of more than 10 ng/mL appears to be an acceptable cutoff level for determining acromegaly to be likely.[19] Specificity of this particular

*References 2, 10, 11, 19, 27-29.

Table 29-1 Endocrinological Data of Confirmed Acromegalic and Presumed Nonacromegalic Diabetic Cats

	Fructosamine (mM)	fGH (ng/mL)
Diabetics with IGF-1< 800	439; 219-790 (n = 34)	4.1; 2.2-16.7 (n = 34)
Confirmed acromegalics	553; 440-733 (n = 17)	16.1; 9.0-33.7 (n = 9)

Adapted from J Vet Intern Med, 2007, Blackwell-Synergy.[2]
fGH, Feline growth hormone; *IGF-1*, insulin-like growth factor 1;
n, number of samples.

assay proved to be 95 per cent and sensitivity 84 per cent at 10 ng/mL.

Glucose-induced GH suppression testing is undertaken commonly in human patients with suspected acromegaly, in an attempt to minimize the confounding effect of the pulsatile basal secretion of GH.[26] One report described the use of this test in an acromegalic cat[27]; another, however, found no suppression in four healthy cats,[30] and other investigators have suggested that this test is unlikely to be of benefit in cats.[11]

IMAGING: RADIOGRAPHY, ABDOMINAL ULTRASOUND, ECHOCARDIOGRAPHY, COMPUTED TOMOGRAPHY, AND MAGNETIC RESONANCE IMAGING

Radiographic abnormalities described in feline acromegalics include: increased oropharyngeal soft tissue; degenerative arthropathy with periarticular periosteal activation, osteophytes, soft-tissue swelling, and joint-space collapse; spinal spondylosis deformans; mandibular enlargement; hyperostosis of the calvarium; cardiomegaly and signs of congestive heart failure; hepatomegaly; and renomegaly.[1,10] Abdominal ultrasonography may be unremarkable or can reveal hepatomegaly, adrenomegaly, pancreatic changes, and/or renomegaly.[1] Echocardiographic changes similar to those found in HCM can be encountered and are described in the preceding.

Although several studies have reported computed tomography (CT) to be a useful tool in demonstrating a mass lesion of the pituitary gland in suspected acromegalic cats (Figure 29-11),[29,31,32] the sensitivity of contrast-enhanced CT studies to detect pituitary abnormalities in acromegalic cats has not been fully assessed. For example, Peterson et al reported one cat in whom a pituitary mass was not evident on CT imaging.[10] Moreover, two cats needed magnetic resonance imaging (MRI) after an unremarkable contrast-enhanced CT (Figure 29-12), and one cat proven to have acromegaly by pituitary histopathology had an unremarkable CT and MRI in a recent study.[2] Nevertheless, intracranial imaging with contrast enhancement clearly can be helpful in increasing the index of suspicion for acromegaly, although it obviously does not differentiate acromegaly from pituitary-dependent hyperadrenocorticism.

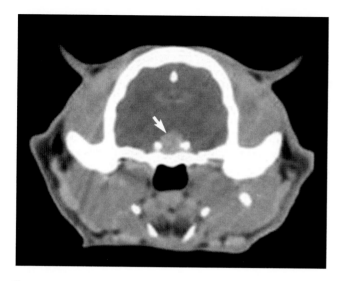

Figure 29-11 Transverse computed tomography view of the cranium of an acromegalic cat at the level of the pituitary gland, showing protrusion of a mass beyond the dorsal rim of the sella turcica (*white arrow, postcontrast enhancement*).

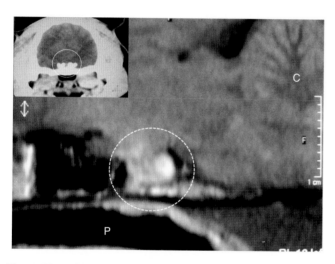

Figure 29-12 Main picture: Sagittal MRI image at the level of the pituitary gland of an acromegalic cat, showing irregular gadolinium uptake (*white circle*), suggesting a disturbed pituitary gland morphology. These subtle changes within the pituitary gland were missed with contrast-enhanced CT (*white circle, inset top left*). P, Pharynx; C, cerebellum.

BIOPSY AND POSTMORTEM EXAMINATION

Although acquiring a pituitary excisional biopsy is basic standard-of-care in human beings with acromegaly (usually using transsphenoidal endoscopy), it is a specialist procedure performed rarely on dogs, and even more seldom on cats. Hypophysectomy has been reported in one cat who had both acromegaly and hyperadrenocorticism and in seven cats with hyperadrenocorticism.[3,33] With the benefit of more advanced CT, MRI, and stereotactic software, hypophysectomy might become more feasible in our patients in the near future and would provide a means of definitive antemortem diagnosis. Unfortunately, postmortem examination currently remains the only route to histopathological confirmation of the disease. In addition, interpretation by a neuroendocrine pathologist and additional staining often are required.

TREATMENT

CONSERVATIVE TREATMENT

The most conservative treatment option involves solely treating the diabetes mellitus with insulin injections. However, obtaining glycemic control can prove to be a "utopia" and invariably problematic, requiring relatively high doses of insulin, with doses as high as 150 IU per cat reported. Using a combination of an intermediate or long-acting insulin with a short-acting insulin might prove helpful. However, most frequently the diabetes mellitus may be controlled only partially if at all and patients remain at risk for ketoacidosis.[11] Nevertheless, in the authors' experience high-dose insulin treatment can prove acceptable in individual patients and certainly should be attempted if more definitive treatment options are not plausible. Finding the appropriate dose is an empirical process, and increases are implemented until satisfactory clinical improvement is achieved. Because this approach does not address the underlying cause of the disease, the pituitary mass and GH- and IGF-1–induced consequences of the disease are left uncontrolled.

RADIOTHERAPY

An increasing body of evidence suggests that some form of radiotherapy, although far from ideal, currently is likely to be the optimal definitive treatment available to most veterinarians. The aims of radiation therapy for pituitary tumors are both to control the mass effect (i.e., the actual mass plus associated local edema) and to control the paraneoplastic effects, which in the case of acromegaly is especially the insulin resistance.[34] Table 29-2 provides an overview of the most frequently used radiation protocols and their reported success rates. Mayer et al found radiation therapy to be an effective primary treatment modality for cats presenting with neurological signs associated with a pituitary mass, and they were able to improve clinical signs associated with concurrent hyperadrenocorticism or acromegaly in cats with no neurological abnormalities.[35] The protocol included a total radiation dosage ranging from 45 to 54 Gray (Gy) administered Monday through Friday in 2.7 or 3.0 Gy fractions. Acute side effects were limited to epilation and mild otitis externa, whereas focal brain necrosis adjacent to regrowth of a pituitary carcinoma and a second tumor in the radiation field were reported as possible late effects. Median survival, regardless of cause of death of the eight cats subjected to this protocol, was 17.4 months (range: 8.4 to 63.1 months), with six cats alive at 1 year, and three cats alive at 2 years after treatment. Clinical signs caused by the concurrent endocrine disorder (seven cats with hyperadrenocorticism or acromegaly) began to improve within 1 to 5 months.

Table 29-2 Summary of Published Radiotherapy Results

Authors	Case Number	Radiotherapy Source	Dose	Protocol	Response	Survival
Peterson et al[10]	2	Cobalt-60	48 Gy	Not provided; over 4 weeks	1 CR, but relapsed at 6 months; 1 stable disease	Information not provided
Goossens et al[29]	3	Cobalt-60	48 Gy	12 fractions, 3/week	2 CR 1 PR	Alive 16 and 28 months Alive 16 months
Kaser-Hotz et al[36]	2	Electrons	38.5 Gy	11 fractions; 3/week	1 CR, died hypoglycemia	Dead 5 months
		Electrons and photons	42 Gy	12 fractions; 3/week	1 PR, unrelated death	Dead 8 months
Feldman and Nelson[1]	10	Lin Acc	45-48 Gy	15 fractions; 3 or 5/week	3 deaths—hypoglycemia 2 CR 2 CR then relapsed 1 PR	Dead within 3 months Alive >1 year Alive 1 and 3 years Alive 2 years
Brearley et al[34]	8	Lin Acc	38 Gy	5 fractions; 1/week	5 CR, 1 PR, 2 SD	Median survival: 72.3 wks Range: 16 to >181 wks (=16.6 months; 3.6-42 months)
Mayer et al[35]	8	Lin Acc	45-54 Gy	Divided into 2.7-3.0 Gy fractions, Monday through Friday	Neurological signs improved within 2 months in all five cats who presented with abnormal neurological signs. Clinical signs caused by a concurrent endocrine disorder began to improve within 1-5 months in the 7 cats with hyperadrenocorticism or acromegaly.	6 Alive >1 year; 3 alive >2 years

Adapted from Brearley et al, 2006[34] with the addition of recent studies.
CR, Complete response (i.e., off insulin); *Lin Acc,* linear accelerator; *PR,* partial response (i.e., reduced insulin); *SD,* stable disease.

Kaser-Hotz et al reported radiotherapy treatment of four cats with pituitary adenoma and one with pituitary carcinoma, based on CT or MRI.[36] Electrons were applied in four cats and electrons and photons in the fifth. Ten to 12 fractions of 3.5 to 4.0 Gy each were delivered on a Monday/Wednesday/Friday schedule. The mean total dose was 39 Gy with no severe acute side effects to treatment encountered. Follow-up CT examination was performed in four cats; the mass had disappeared in one cat and remained stable or slightly decreased in size in the other three patients. Survival was 5.5, 8, 15, 18, and 20.5 months, with two cats dying of causes unrelated to the tumor.

Goossens et al used cobalt-60 irradiation in three acromegalic cats, with none of the cats developing complications.[29] Each cat received a total dose of 48 Gy over 12 treatments. Insulin requirements decreased for all cats, although only temporarily in one cat, and two cats ceased to be diabetic. After treatment, decreases in insulin requirements correlated with decreases in plasma GH concentrations in the two cats in whom diabetes mellitus resolved. The correlation between decrease in insulin requirements and decreasing GH concentrations also was apparent in cases reported by the authors[19] and by Littler et al.[37] However, both latter reports also documented persistently elevated IGF-1 concentrations, which might suggest that radiotherapy may decrease GH concentration to a level such that diabetogenic effects are no longer evident but not to a level required to decrease IGF-1 secretion and its associated complications.[37] Indeed, Littler et al described a continued increase in the cat's size and appetite.[37]

In any endocrine abnormality caused by autonomous or excessive hormone secretion, the clinical signs are a result of an overall increase in target tissue exposure to the hormone in question. As the increased exposure relates more to uncontrolled hormone production than to the size of the endocrine tumor, inherently, radiotherapy is not an ideal therapeutic modality for hypersecreting endocrinopathies.

Additional disadvantages of radiotherapy as a treatment modality for any endocrine disorder include the need for multiple anesthetic episodes, hospitalization, cost, the unpredictable and variable response, and specifically the arbitrary timing of a possible response. The latter can lead to inadvertent overdosing with exogenous insulin in the postradiotherapy period if the onset of treatment response and concurrent decrease in insulin requirements are not noted in time.

MEDICAL THERAPY

In human beings somatostatin analogues (initially octreotide, followed by longer-acting lanreotide) have been used to treat patients in whom surgery and/or radiotherapy has failed, as well as a first-line therapy when other modalities are contraindicated or are unlikely to control GH and IGF-1 hypersecretion. Long-acting formulations, requiring once monthly injection only, have greatly improved the convenience and popularity of such analogues in human medicine. GH/IGF-I hypersecretion is controlled by these drugs in about 50 per cent of patients, with the remaining patients requiring additional different treatment. Pegvisomant, a GH-receptor antagonist, is effective in most of these remaining patients. Current research in human beings is focused on developing new somatostatin analogues with different somatostatin receptor selectivity and chimeric molecules that bind to both somatostatin and dopamine receptors, as well as gene therapy with the aim of increasing somatostatin sensitivity by increasing somatostatin receptor expression.[38,39]

Although somatostatin analogues have proved effective in many human patients, their efficacy in the limited number of feline acromegalics in whom they have been tried has been disappointing.[1,10,14] Hypothesized causes for the poor response include lack of somatostatin receptors or presence of mutated somatostatin receptors in feline pituitary adenomas, as well as incorrect dosing regimens. A longer-acting somatostatin analogue (lanreotide) is currently being tested in the authors' dedicated acromegaly clinic with promising preliminary results (marked decrease in insulin requirements) in individual, but not all, treated cats. Octreotide responsiveness has been shown recently on intravenous administration in individual acromegalic cats and was proposed as a qualifying test for such somatostatin treatment.[40] The usefulness of pegvisomant remains to be assessed in feline acromegaly. However, contrary to the situation with somatostatin, GH is poorly conserved across species, thus potentially limiting success with a human-specific GH-receptor antagonist.

Dopamine-agonist treatment with bromocriptine resulted in improved clinical signs and decreased serum GH concentrations in 70 per cent of human patients.[41] Bromocriptine treatment has not been evaluated robustly in acromegalic cats. Its use in canine hyperadrenocorticism resulted in unsatisfactory responses as well as unacceptable side effects (i.e., gastrointestinal signs, depression, and behavioral changes).[42] Use of L-deprenyl (Selegiline, a selective inhibitor of monoamine oxidase which inhibits breakdown of dopamine) has been assessed sporadically by the authors and its use has been reported in one acromegalic cat.[32] In the authors' experience and in the case report, L-deprenyl failed to reduce the need for high doses of insulin, nor did it reduce the clinical signs associated with the disease.

HYPOPHYSECTOMY

Although considered the treatment of choice in human patients with small pituitary adenomas, the only described experience with this treatment modality for feline acromegaly involved a single cat with a double pituitary adenoma suffering from concurrent hyperadrenocorticism and acromegaly.[3] In this individual cat insulin resistance resolved postoperatively, although the cat died unaccountably weeks after surgery. Slightly more information is available on hypophysectomy in cats with hyperadrenocorticism; microsurgical transsphenoidal hypophysectomy for the treatment of pituitary-dependent hyperadrenocorticism has been described in seven cats.[33] The procedure proved not without risk, with two cats dying within 4 weeks after surgery, although of apparently unrelated disease. In the remaining five cats the hyperadrenocorticism went into both clinical and biochemical remission. Hyperadrenocorticism recurred in one cat after 19 months, but no other therapy was given and the cat died at home 28 months after surgery. One cat died after 6 months because of undefined anemia, and another cat died after 8 months related to persistent nose and middle ear infection secondary to soft palate dehiscence after surgery. In the surviving two cats, the remission periods at the time of writing were 46 and 15 months. In the two cats with sufficient follow-up time, the concurrent diabetes mellitus disappeared at 4 weeks and 5 months after surgery.

CRYOTHERAPY

One cat with acromegaly was treated successfully by transsphenoidal cryosurgical ablation of the pituitary gland.[12] Sudden resolution of insulin-resistant diabetes mellitus 2 months postoperatively resulted in a hypoglycemic crisis caused by insulin overdose. The cat was treated, but lost its vision completely and suffered from additional neurological signs. Neurological deficits other than behavioral changes resolved over 3 months, but the cat remained blind for the next 9 months, at which time it was euthanized. Initially the blindness was attributed to acute cerebral necrosis; however, subsequently, the authors felt therapy with enrofloxacin was the most likely explanation for the retinal degeneration and permanent blindness, not radiation therapy or hypoglycemia.[43] A second case of acromegaly treated successfully with cryotherapy was published recently.[44] More cases need to be assessed in order to provide reliable recommendations with regard to this and other treatment modalities.

ADDITIONAL MANAGEMENT AND PROGNOSIS

In order to provide the best quality of life and longevity, acromegaly-associated concurrent diseases should be assessed and treated on an individual basis. Arthropathies might require analgesia, and congestive heart failure might require angiotensin-converting enzyme (ACE)-inhibitor and diuretic treatment. When using the latter, clinicians need to monitor carefully for electrolyte abnormalities, especially in view of concurrent aggravating diabetes-induced osmotic diuresis and possible concurrent nephropathy. Renal disease and hypertension will require additional attention using standard recommended therapy.

In general any cat on high-dose insulin treatment, but especially those having received radiation therapy, might suffer from hypoglycemic crises, which can prove fatal if not treated swiftly and appropriately. Client education and preparation is essential. In view of this possible complication, some authors suggest limiting insulin dose in acromegalic cats to a maximum of 15 IU per injection. Although this measure might prevent crises in a proportion of cats, the resultant excessive polydipsia, polyuria, and polyphagia might prove unbearable to both cat and owner without the use of higher insulin dosage administration. Home monitoring of urine glucose, or preferentially blood glucose, and close contact between attending clinician and owner can prove useful if not essential in the prevention or early detection of hypoglycemia (see Chapter 26).

If untreated with a definitive method (i.e., radiation therapy or hypophysectomy), most acromegalic cats eventually die or are euthanized as a result of the consequences of congestive heart failure, renal failure, hypoglycemia, respiratory distress, or pituitary mass–induced neurological signs. Survival times of both aggressively and conservatively treated cats vary enormously, with some cats not surviving more than a few weeks and others living for many years and dying from causes likely to be unrelated to acromegaly.

Further research is required to provide a better understanding of the clinical entity of feline acromegaly, especially as this appears to be a more common endocrinopathy than has been reported previously.

REFERENCES

1. Feldman EC, Nelson RW: Disorders of growth hormone. In Feldman EC, Nelson RW, editors: *Canine and feline endocrinology and reproduction*, ed 3, St. Louis, 2004, Saunders, p 69.
2. Niessen SJ, Petrie G, Gaudiano F, et al: Feline acromegaly: an underdiagnosed endocrinopathy? *J Vet Intern Med* 21:899, 2007.
3. Meij BP, Van der Vlugt-Meijer RH, Van den Ingh TS, et al: Somatotroph and corticotroph pituitary adenoma (double adenoma) in a cat with diabetes mellitus and hyperadrenocorticism, *J Comp Pathol* 130:209, 2004.
4. Mol JA, Van Garderen E, Selman PJ, et al: Growth hormone mRNA in mammary gland tumors of dogs and cats, *J Clin Invest* 95:2028, 1995.
5. Mol JA, Lantinga-van Leeuwen I, Van Garderen E, et al: Progestin-induced mammary growth hormone (GH) production, *Adv Exp Med Biol* 480:71, 2000.
6. Gunn-Moore D: Feline endocrinopathies, *Vet Clin North Am Small Anim Pract* 35:171, 2005.
7. Hurty CA, Flatland B: Feline acromegaly: a review of the syndrome, *J Am Anim Hosp Assoc* 41:292, 2005.
8. Berg RI, Nelson RW, Feldman EC, et al: Serum insulin-like growth factor-I concentration in cats with diabetes mellitus and acromegaly, *J Vet Intern Med* 21:892, 2007.
9. Peterson ME: Acromegaly in cats: are we only diagnosing the tip of the iceberg? *J Vet Intern Med* 21:889, 2007.
10. Peterson ME, Taylor RS, Greco DS, et al: Acromegaly in 14 cats, *J Vet Intern Med* 4:192, 1990.
11. Norman EJ, Mooney CT: Diagnosis and management of diabetes mellitus in five cats with somatotrophic abnormalities, *J Feline Med Surg* 2:183, 2000.
12. Abrams-Ogg ACG, Holmberg DL, Stewart WA, et al: Acromegaly in a cat: diagnosis by magnetic resonance imaging and treatment by cryohypophysectomy, *Can Vet J* 34:682, 1993.
13. Middleton DJ, Culvenor JA, Vasak E, et al: Growth hormone-producing pituitary adenoma, elevated serum somatomedin C concentration and diabetes mellitus in a cat, *Can Vet J* 26:169, 1985.
14. Morrison SA, Randolph J, Lothrop CD: Hypersomatotropism and insulin-resistant diabetes mellitus in a cat, *J Am Vet Med Assoc* 194:91, 1989.
15. Barkan AL, Stred SE, Reno K, et al: Increased growth hormone pulse frequency in acromegaly, *J Clin Endocrinol Metab* 69:1225, 1989.
16. Feldman EC, Nelson RW: Acromegaly and hyperadrenocorticism in cats: a clinical perspective, *J Feline Med Surg* 2:153, 2000.
17. Forcada Y, German AJ, Steiner JM, et al: Determination of fPLI concentrations in cats with diabetes mellitus, *J Feline Med Surg* 10:480, 2008.
18. Kittleson MD, Pion PD, DeLellis LA, et al: Increased serum growth hormone concentration in feline hypertrophic cardiomyopathy, *J Vet Intern Med* 6:320, 1992.
19. Niessen SJ, Khalid M, Petrie G, et al: Validation and application of an ovine radioimmunoassay for the diagnosis of feline acromegaly, *Vet Rec* 160:902, 2007.
20. Kageyama K, Nigawara T, Kamata Y, et al: A multihormonal pituitary adenoma with growth hormone and adrenocorticotropic hormone production, causing acromegaly and Cushing disease, *Am J Med Sci* 324:326, 2002.
21. Niessen SJ, Petrie G, Gaudiano F, et al: Routine clinical pathology findings in feline acromegaly. Proceedings of the BSAVA Congress, Birmingham, UK, 2007, p 482.
22. Casanueva FF: Physiology of growth hormone secretion and action, *Endocrinol Metab Clin North Am* 21:483, 1992.
23. Lewitt MS, Hazel SJ, Church DB, et al: Regulation of insulin-like growth factor-binding protein-3 ternary complex in feline diabetes mellitus, *J Endocrinol* 166:21, 2000.
24. Starkey SR, Tan K, Church DB: Investigation of serum IGF-I levels amongst diabetic and non-diabetic cats, *J Feline Med Surg* 6:149, 2004.
25. Butler J: Biochemical tests of growth hormone status in short children, *Ann Clin Biochem* 38:1, 2001.
26. Chang-DeMoranville J: Diagnosis and endocrine testing in acromegaly, *Endocrin Metab Clin* 21:649, 1992.
27. Eigenmann J, Wortman J, Haskins M: Elevated growth hormone levels and diabetes mellitus in a cat with acromegalic features, *J Am Anim Hosp Assoc* 20:747, 1984.
28. Lichtensteiger CA, Wortman JA, Eigenmann JE: Functional pituitary acidophil adenoma in a cat with diabetes mellitus and acromegalic features, *Vet Pathol* 23:518, 1986.
29. Goossens MM, Feldman EC, Nelson RW, et al: Cobalt 60 irradiation of pituitary gland tumors in three cats with acromegaly, *J Am Vet Med Assoc* 213:374, 1998.
30. Kokka N, Garcia JF, Morgan M, et al: Immunoassay of plasma growth hormone in cats following fasting and administration of insulin, arginine, 2-deoxyglucose and hypothalamic extract, *Endocrinology* 88:359, 1971.

31. Elliott DA, Feldman EC, Koblik PD, et al: Prevalence of pituitary tumors among diabetic cats with insulin resistance, *J Am Vet Med Assoc* 216:1765, 2000.
32. Abraham LA, Helmond SE, Mitten RW, et al: Treatment of an acromegalic cat with the dopamine agonist L-deprenyl, *Aust Vet J* 80:479, 2002.
33. Meij BP, Voorhout G, Van Den Ingh TS, et al: Transsphenoidal hypophysectomy for treatment of pituitary-dependent hyperadrenocorticism in 7 cats, *Vet Surg* 30:72, 2001.
34. Brearley MJ, Polton GA, Littler RM, et al: Coarse fractionated radiation therapy for pituitary tumors in cats: a retrospective study of 12 cases, *Vet Comp Oncol* 4:209, 2006.
35. Mayer MN, Greco DS, LaRue SM: Outcomes of pituitary tumor irradiation in cats, *J Vet Intern Med* 20:1151, 2006.
36. Kaser-Hotz B, Rohrer CR, Stankeova S, et al: Radiotherapy of pituitary tumors in five cats, *J Small Anim Pract* 43:303, 2002.
37. Littler RM, Polton GA, Brearley MJ: Resolution of diabetes mellitus but not acromegaly in a cat with a pituitary macroadenoma treated with hypofractionated radiation, *J Small Anim Pract* 47:392, 2006.
38. Chanson P: Emerging drugs for acromegaly, *Expert Opin Emerg Drugs* 13:273, 2008.
39. Acunzo J, Roche C, Thirion S, et al: Gene therapy of human somatotroph and lactotroph pituitary adenomas using an adenoviral virus expressing the somatostatin receptor type 2, *J Hum Gene Ther* 19:1107, 2008.
40. Slingerland LI, Voorhout G, Rijnberk A, et al: Growth hormone excess and the effect of octreotide in cats with diabetes mellitus, *Domest Anim Endocrinol* 35:352, 2008.
41. Thorner MO, Lee Vance M, Laws RE Jr, et al: The anterior pituitary. In Wilson JD, Foster DW, Kronenberg HM, et al, editors: *Williams textbook of endocrinology*, ed 9, Philadelphia, 1998, Saunders, p 249.
42. Drucker WD, Peterson ME: Advances in the diagnosis and management of canine Cushing's syndrome. Proceedings of the 31st Gaines Veterinary Symposium, Baton Rouge, LA, 1981, 17.
43. Abrams-Ogg A, Holmberg DL, Quinn RF, et al: Blindness now attributed to enrofloxacin therapy in a previously reported case of a cat with acromegaly treated by cryohypophysectomy, *Can Vet J* 43:53, 2002.
44. Blois SL, Holmberg DL: Cryohypophysectomy used in the treatment of a case of feline acromegaly, *J Small Anim Pract* 49:596, 2008.

SECTION
V

Dermatology

Karen A. Moriello, Section Editor

30 Anatomy of the Ear in Health and Disease

Paul B. Bloom

The pinna, the external ear canal (which is composed of a vertical ear canal and a horizontal ear canal), the middle ear, and the inner ear compose the organ called the ear. The ear is a remarkable organ. It adds beauty to animals, in addition to performing functions such as hearing and control of balance.

It is important to include an ear examination in any cat with skin disease, and to do a dermatological examination on any cat with ear disease. This is because diseases that affect the skin more often than not also affect the ear in some way.

The goal of this chapter is to describe the normal anatomy of the feline ear with an emphasis on identification of abnormalities that may enhance the clinician's ability to diagnose the cause of otitis in a cat.

EAR PINNA

The pinna, which is the first portion of the ear that is visible from a distance, is important to hearing because its anatomy is designed to capture sound waves. It also is involved with nonverbal communication between cats, and between cats and other animals, including human beings. Ear position, in association with facial expression and body position, can relay a number of feelings such as fear, anger, happiness, and curiosity.

Cats have pinnae that are more consistent in size and shape than in dogs. Most cats (except Scottish Folds) have erect pinnae unless a disease is present.

The pinna is triangular in appearance with the tip of the triangle distal (Figure 30-1). There is a concave surface that faces rostrolaterally and a convex surface that faces caudomedially. This shape is valuable in collecting sound and directing it toward the ear canal and eventually the tympanic membrane.

Both the concave and convex surfaces are covered by skin that is lightly haired compared with the cat's body. The concave surface is less haired than the convex surface. Sandwiched between these surfaces is the auricular cartilage. This cartilage is responsible for the shape of the pinna. When this cartilage is damaged, either through trauma or inflammation (e.g., auricular chondritis), the shape of the pinna will change (e.g., droop).

Because the epidermis, regardless of its location, is avascular, there are numerous small vessels located in the dermis to supply nutrients to the skin. When vessels rupture, the blood that escapes fills the space between the firm cartilage and the encasing epidermis, creating an aural hematoma. The exact cause of this occurrence is unclear. Historically it has been reported to be associated with otitis externa usually caused by ear mites; however, the author has seen more aural hematomas that are unassociated with concurrent ear infection. This may reflect the author's specialty practice.

The skin of the pinna is the same as other areas of the body, consisting of epidermis and dermis. The associated adnexal structures, hair follicles, and sebaceous and apocrine glands are present also.

Traveling more proximally, the auricular cartilage rolls to form a tube. This tube is a modified L-shaped structure; however, instead of the two parts of the L being unequal lengths, they are both approximately the same length—approximately 1 centimeter. Cats, in contrast to dogs, have a fairly constant length to their external ear canal.

The first step in an otic examination is to examine the pinna. This examination should be performed in a systematic manner in order not to miss an abnormality. Any alopecia, erythema, ulceration, crusting, scaling, or swelling present on the pinna should be noted, because these may be major clues of underlying disease. During the examination, note whether the lesions are primary or

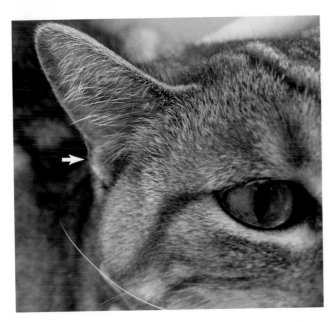

Figure 30-1 Cat pinna. Note the triangular appearance. Unlike dogs, the pinna of cats is almost uniform across breeds. The arrow points to the cutaneous marginal pouch.

secondary. Because certain primary lesions are associated with a limited number of diseases, identifying primary lesions is helpful in establishing a logical list of differential diagnoses. Primary lesions are changes in the skin caused directly by the disease process. Secondary lesions may evolve from primary lesions, or may be caused by scratching, trauma, infection, or the healing process. The distinction between a primary and secondary lesion is not always clear. Some lesions may be considered both a primary and secondary lesion depending on the disease process (e.g., alopecia).

PRIMARY LESIONS THAT MAY BE SEEN ON THE PINNA

Macule

A macule is a circumscribed flat area of the skin, less than one centimeter in diameter, which has a different color from the surrounding skin. Macules may be hyperpigmented, depigmented, or erythematous. When the skin is red it is called erythroderma. Erythroderma may be caused by erythema or purpura. Erythema occurs as the result of increased blood flow through the skin, or from dilatation and congestion of the cutaneous blood vessels. If pinnal erythema is present, an inflammatory process caused by infection (e.g., bacterial), neoplasia (e.g., squamous cell carcinoma), autoimmune disorder (e.g., vasculitis), hypersensitivities (e.g., atopy or cutaneous adverse food reaction), or a burn (radiation) should be considered as differential diagnoses. In addition, pinnal erythema may also be caused by exercise, fear, or excitement.

Erythroderma also may occur as a result of purpura. Purpura is hemorrhage in the skin. All forms of purpura involve microvascular disruption leading to extravasation of erythrocytes into the surrounding dermis. Descrip-

tion of purpura is modified depending on the size of the lesion. Petechiae are areas of hemorrhage one centimeter or less in diameter, whereas ecchymoses are purpuric lesions larger than one centimeter. The causes of purpura may be divided into two categories, intravascular and vascular. Intravascular causes are the result of platelet defects or coagulopathies; the most common vascular cause, excluding direct trauma, is vasculitis. Diascopy can be performed to differentiate erythema from purpura. To perform this procedure, a glass slide is pressed firmly on the area in question. The area under the slide then is evaluated to see if it has blanched. By applying pressure to the lesion, red blood cells that are present in the vessels are moved away from the lesional site. If erythroderma resolves while pressure is applied, the erythema is the result of inflammation. Purpuric lesions do not blanch with pressure. This is because the redness associated with purpura is caused by hemorrhage into the tissue rather than dilated or congested blood vessels that occur with erythema. Pressing on the tissue will not dramatically displace the red blood cells from the tissue.

Papule

A papule is a raised, circumscribed, firm elevation of skin less than one centimeter in diameter. This occurs because of cellular infiltration or edema in the epidermis or superficial dermis. When present on the pinna, etiological causes such as bacterial infections, fungal infection (e.g., dermatophyte), demodicosis, *Notoedres* infestation, fly bites (mosquito), and cutaneous drug reaction (systemic or topical) should be considered.

Plaque

A plaque is a coalescence of papules creating a raised portion of the skin larger than one centimeter in diameter. The same etiologies that induce papule formation cause plaques. Rarely ear tumors may present as plaques.

Pustule

A pustule is a circumscribed, elevated lesion that contains polymorphonuclear cells (neutrophils, eosinophils). It may be caused by infections (bacterial or fungal infection [e.g., dermatophyte]) or may be sterile such as in pemphigus foliaceus. Pemphigus foliaceus (PF) is the most common cause of pustules on the pinna of cats and cytological examination of these pustules often reveals acanthocytes compatible with PF (Figure 30-2). In fact, if pustules are seen on the pinna of a cat, the author considers PF to be the working diagnosis until histopathological examination proves otherwise. (See Chapter 29 in the fifth volume of this series for a complete discussion of pemphigus foliaceus.)

Alopecia

Alopecia is loss of hair (hypotrichosis is partial alopecia or thinning of hair). Alopecia occurs as a primary lesion in demodicosis, bacterial folliculitis, and dermatophytosis in cats. It also may occur in immune-mediated/autoimmune disease such as alopecia areata or pemphigus foliaceus. Congenital pinnal alopecia may occur in breeds such as the Sphynx or Abyssinian. Preauricular alopecia is normal in cats and is most obvious in darkly haired

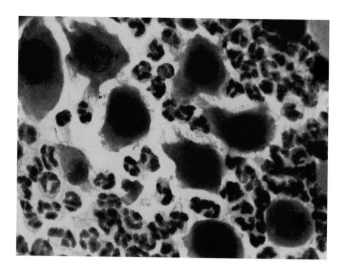

Figure 30-2 Impression smear of a pustule from a cat's ear. Note the rafts of deeply basophilic rounded epithelial cells. These are acantholytic cells, found commonly in pustules from animals with pemphigus foliaceus.

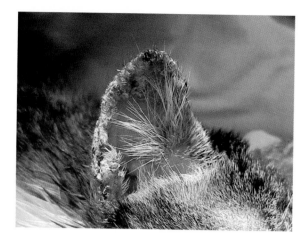

Figure 30-3 Severe crusting on the margin and concave surface of the pinna of a 7-month-old female cat with pemphigus foliaceus.

cats. These types of hair loss are noninflammatory. Alopecia also may be a secondary lesion. An example would be pruritus associated with a hypersensitivity reaction. If alopecia is present, the first step is to determine if it is posttraumatic alopecia. If it is posttraumatic, then atopy, flea allergy dermatitis, cutaneous adverse food reaction, dermatophytosis, and otitis externa would be possible etiological causes. Inflammatory alopecia is the most common cause of alopecia.

SECONDARY LESIONS THAT MAY BE SEEN ON THE PINNA

Scale

Scale is an accumulation of fragmented (desquamated) corneocytes from the stratum corneum. Scales per se are not abnormal; in fact, human beings shed approximately one billion cells each day.[1] Normally, scale fragments are so small that they are not visible to the naked eye. Abnormal scaling is an accumulation of these fragments so that they are visible without magnification. Any process that affects the degradation of the intercellular lipids or corneodesmosomes, or increases the proliferation of the basal keratinocytes, will create scale. Inflammation is a common cause of scale. Inflammatory cytokines that are produced when the epidermis is damaged include tumor necrosis factor-alpha (TNFα) and interleukin-6 (IL-6). Damaged epidermis also stimulates the production of lipid mediators. These inflammatory lipid mediators are produced by the metabolism of phospholipids in keratinocyte cell membranes into free arachidonic acid that is further metabolized into inflammatory eicosanoids, such as prostaglandins, thromboxanes, and leukotrienes. These cytokines and inflammatory eicosanoids stimulate epidermal proliferation in an effort to remove the noxious insult. However, this epidermal hyperproliferation also leads to defective differentiation of the keratinocytes. Inflammation that occurs with allergic skin

disease (atopy, cutaneous adverse food reaction), cheyletiellosis, *Otodectes* infestation, or dermatophytosis is a common cause of pinnal scaling. Pemphigus foliaceus, vasculitis, cutaneous T cell lymphoma, and cutaneous drug reaction (allergic or irritant) also may be accompanied by scaling.

Less common causes of pinnal scaling include nutritional and environmental causes (e.g., solar dermatitis). Deficiencies in a variety of vitamins, minerals, proteins, or essential fatty acids may cause scaling. Clinically these are very uncommon. In contrast to a true nutritional deficiency, scaling also may be associated with vitamin A–responsive or fatty acid–responsive dermatoses. In an arid environment there may be inadequate water content in the skin. With inadequate water content the enzymes necessary for separation of corneocytes (normal desquamation) will not occur, leading to scale.

Crusts

Crusts are the result of dry plasma or exudate on the skin. Cats frequently will have a lesion that is a combination of a papule and a crust known as a papulocrust. When crusts or papulocrusts are identified, dermatophytosis, autoimmune disease (PF, vasculitis, drug reaction), environmental allergen–induced atopic dermatitis, cutaneous adverse food reaction, flea allergy dermatitis, a bacterial skin infection (caused by an underlying hypersensitivity), *Notoedres cati* infestation, *Trombicula* (usually *Neotrombicula automnalis*) infestation, or a louse infestation (*Felicola subrostrata*) should be considered as possible causes (Figure 30-3).

On the caudal lateral surface of the proximal pinna is a small pouch, the cutaneous marginal pouch (see Figure 30-1). The purpose of this pouch is unknown; however, it is an easily accessible area for collecting skin biopsies of the pinna when needed (e.g., confirming PF, cutaneous small vessel vasculitis).

After examining the pinna visually, the external ear canals should be palpated for pain or firmness. Causes of firmness of the external ear canal include calcification of the cartilage of the external ear canal and thickening from fibrosis or edema.

EAR CANALS

The next step is an otoscopic examination, which involves examining the ear canals and tympanic membrane (Figure 30-4). To evaluate the ear canals and the tympanic membrane, the tip of the otoscope cone should be placed in the opening of the external vertical ear canal. In order to perform a proper otoscopic examination, it is important to understand the path that the vertical ear canal travels. Because the vertical canal travels ventrally and slightly rostrally, the otoscope cone initially should be directed vertically rather than horizontally, while gently pulling up on the pinna. There is a curve in the canal at the point where the vertical ear canal changes into the horizontal ear canal. This area is identified by a ridge of cartilage on the dorsal surface of the canal. This landmark is important to identify, because to gain entrance to the horizontal ear canal and visualize the tympanic membrane, the otoscope cone must be passed gently under this ridge. This is best accomplished by gently pulling on the pinna dorsally and laterally as the otoscope cone is advancing proximally in the ear canal.

The lining of the vertical and horizontal ear canal in cats contains very few to no visible hairs. The lining is a glistening pink and the dermal vessels should be visible on otoscopic examination. *The inability to visualize the dermal vessels is one of the first signs of inflammation in the ear canal.*

The most medial border of the horizontal ear canal ends at the tympanic membrane. As the auricular cartilage approaches the tympanic membrane, the annular cartilage replaces it. The annular cartilage ends just lateral to the tympanic membrane, and the osseous external

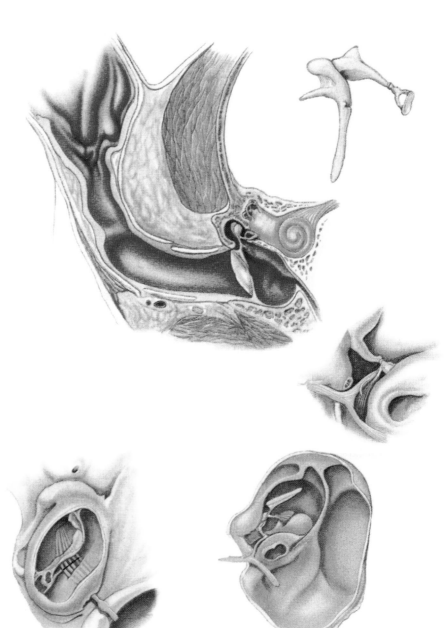

Figure 30-4 Schematic views of the feline middle and inner ear. (From Hudson LC, Hamilton WP: *Atlas of feline anatomy for veterinarians,* Philadelphia, 1983, Saunders.)

auditory meatus begins. This bony part of the external ear canal, which is an extension of the temporal bone, forms the most proximal part of the horizontal ear canal and terminates lateral to the tympanic membrane (see Figure 30-4). The temporal bones originate from the ventrolateral wall of the skull. Within the temporal bones are the sensory organs for hearing and balance (middle and inner ear). They also surround the proximal end of the external ear canal. This enclosure protects these important structures.

In contrast to our stereotypical skin, there are very few hairs in the ear canal of cats (unlike dogs, who may have copious amounts depending on breed). The external ear canal is lined by skin that, like skin on other parts of the body, contains hair follicles, and sebaceous and apocrine sweat glands. The sebaceous glands tend to secrete an oily substance, whereas the ceruminous glands (modified apocrine glands) secrete a milky white fluid that changes to a brown color when exposed to air. The combined product of these sweat glands is called cerumen. In human beings cerumen contains saturated and unsaturated long-chain fatty acids, cholesterol, cholesterol esters, wax esters, squalene, and triglycerides.[2]

Sweat glands (sebaceous and apocrine glands) secrete their contents into ducts by two different mechanisms. The first is known as holocrine secretion. In this process the secretion consists of the disintegrated cells of the gland. This is how sebaceous glands secrete their product. In contrast is apocrine secretion, in which just the apical portion of secretory cells is shed and incorporated into the secretion. This is the method by which ceruminous glands secrete their product.

Cerumen, along with trapped debris, normally is carried away from the tympanic membrane by the migration of the epithelial cells that line the ear canals. This movement of the epithelial cells is known as epithelial migration. Epithelial cells originate on the tympanic membrane and move from the tympanic membrane laterally to the opening of the vertical ear canal. This allows a "cleaning" mechanism to the ear canal. Defective epithelial migration may occur as the result of damage to the tympanic membrane from previous episodes of otitis externa, or from current inflammation (with or without a secondary bacterial or yeast infection) of the ear canal caused by allergies or previous *Otodectes* infestation. This defect leads to an accumulation of cerumen. The accumulation may appear as debris in the horizontal canal, or it may form into a large ball known as a ceruminolith. In the author's experience it is very common to see ceruminoliths in cats presented for neutering. When questioning the owners it is often reported that these cats have a history of previous *Otodectes* infestation. Once the ceruminolith is removed in these patients it does not recur. If it does recur, however, an additional underlying disease should be sought (e.g., environmental allergen-induced atopic dermatitis, cutaneous adverse food reaction).

There are different consistencies to the cerumen in human beings and dogs, varying from a very dry flaky appearance to the more typical moist form.[2] The type of cerumen that is present in human beings is a reflection of the macroenvironment, especially the humidity, and

also genetics. The author has not appreciated any pattern to the form that is present in dogs. Cats do not appear to have both forms, just the moist form.

Even though we focus frequently on cleaning ears to remove cerumen, it is important to understand that cerumen performs some very important functions. As mentioned previously, the purpose of cerumen is to protect the ear canals and the tympanic membrane by trapping and then mechanically removing resident bacteria and yeast and toxins produced by these organisms.[3] Cerumen also removes foreign material that may have entered the ear canal. The lipids and free fatty acids that are present in cerumen contribute to the barrier function of the epidermis of the ear canals. They perform this function by keeping the epidermis of the ear canals and the tympanic membrane moist. Also, by maintaining proper moisture, normal desquamation of the epidermis may occur.

Fatty acids present in cerumen are derived from the breakdown of sebaceous gland triglycerides. This hydrolysis occurs as the triglycerides are excreted onto the surface of the ear canal. The lipids that are present in cerumen have potent antibacterial activity. Recently two sebaceous gland–derived fatty acids (sapienic acid, C16:1D6, and lauric acid, C12:0) have been identified that are especially potent antimicrobial molecules.[4] The issue of whether cerumen has antimicrobial properties is undecided in human medicine.[5] What confuses the issue at this time is that in the presence of infection, cerumen, with its antimicrobial molecules, is produced in excess yet the infection continues.[6] This may be explained by studies suggesting that the lipid-rich cerumen is an ideal medium for proliferation of bacteria and fungi.[7,8] This apparent disconnect between the presence of excessive cerumen in cases of bacterial otitis externa and the antimicrobial properties of cerumen may be explained by differences in the components of the cerumen. When inflammation occurs in the ear canal, with or without a concurrent bacterial or yeast infection, the ceruminous glands will become hyperplastic and secretion from the glands will accumulate in the ear canals. In addition, the amount of sebaceous secretion decreases. Perhaps this difference in cerumen content has an impact on its antibacterial properties. Other investigators report that immunoglobulins, not cerumen, are responsible for protecting the external ear canal.[6] More research in this area will have to be performed before an answer is found.

As mentioned previously, the ability to visualize the dermal vessels of an inflamed ear canal is lost when performing an otoscopic examination. This may be caused by thickening of the epidermis and/or dermal edema. In addition, the epidermis of an inflamed ear canal will have a red appearance. Excessive waxy secretions and hyperplastic ceruminous glands may be present. These glands will create a "cobblestone" appearance to the lining of the ear canals. If inflammation continues, these glands will progress to form inflammatory polyps. These inflammatory polyps are not the same as the nasopharyngeal polyps that will be discussed later.

Treatment with a 10- to 21-day course of oral prednisolone and topical corticosteroids with or without antimicrobial agents, if appropriate, may reverse these hyperplastic and inflammatory changes, returning the ear canals to normal. In other situations they will only undergo partial regression, making the ear canal prone to infection owing to the inability of the natural ear-cleaning process to properly remove the cerumen and associated debris. In those cases an ear cleaning program should be established with appropriate owner education.

TYMPANIC MEMBRANE

The next structure to identify is the tympanic membrane (TM). The TM is part of the hearing mechanism. Vibrations (sound waves) detected by the TM are transmitted to the cochlea of the inner ear via the bones of the middle ear (malleus, incus, and stapes) and the oval (vestibular) window. The cochlea then converts this vibration into nerve impulses, which are transmitted to the auditory portion of brain via the eighth cranial nerve (auditory nerve).

The TM slants downward and inward obliquely so as to form an angle that ranges between 30 and 45 degrees with the floor of the horizontal canal.[9] The reason for this angle is not clear; however, in one study, the authors concluded that the "inclination of the eardrum allows a larger eardrum to fit inside a smaller ear canal diameter. This decreases the acoustic pressure in the ear canal needed to produce perceivable vibrations in the cochlea, while at the same time optimizing the amount of space used."[9] The authors calculated that by having the TM on an angle, a larger TM could be present in a given ear canal. However, because of the angle of the TM, debris and medication tend to accumulate at the junction of the ventral horizontal ear canal and the TM.

The TM is a concave semitransparent epithelial structure (Figure 30-5, *A*). The umbo is the most depressed part of the TM, and is formed where the tip of the manubrium of the malleus (one of the auditory ossicles) pulls the TM medially. The TM is divided into two parts. The smaller, dorsal opaque portion that is pink, loosely attached, and contains small blood vessels is the *pars flaccida*. This network of small blood vessels that extends across the TM is important in healing a damaged TM. The larger gray, semitransparent ventral portion is the *pars tensa*. The pars tensa is the major portion of the TM. In cats it is uncommon to appreciate and visualize the pars flaccida because of its much smaller size (Figure 30-5, *B*).

The TM has four layers. The outermost (lateral surface) is a continuum of the epithelium of the lining of the external ear canal. The next layer is the fibrous stratum that consists of two layers of collagen fibers. The innermost (medial) layer of the TM is lined by modified respiratory epithelium. This epithelium lacks goblet cells and cilia that are found in the respiratory tract.

The TM is thinner in the center and thicker at the periphery. This is because the fibrous layer of the pars tensa thickens laterally to form the tympanic annulus.

The normal barrier function of the TM is disrupted if it becomes inflamed. This leads to potential transmembrane migration of bacteria and absorption of otic medication that may cause otitis media (OM) and ototoxicity

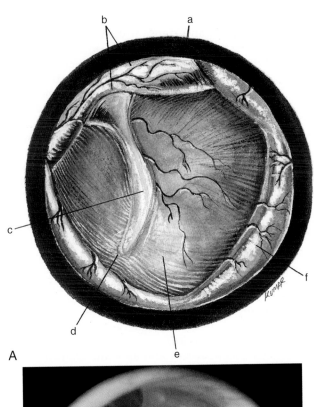

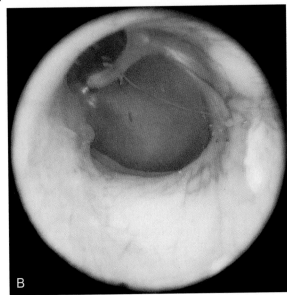

Figure 30-5 A, Tympanic membrane anatomy in the dog as observed through an otoscope. *a,* Rim of the otoscopic tube; *b,* flaccid part of the tympanic membrane; *c,* manubrium of malleus shining through the tympanic membrane; *d,* umbo of tympanic membrane; *e,* pars tensa of the tympanic membrane surrounding the manubrium; *f,* skin of the external acoustic meatus raised by the otoscope tube. **B,** Normal feline tympanic membrane. (**A,** Modified from DeLahunta A, Habel RE: *Applied veterinary anatomy,* Philadelphia, 1986, Saunders.)

respectively. Whether this actually occurs clinically is unclear. In contrast to acute inflammation, the epidermal layer of the TM becomes thickened with chronic inflammation, thereby decreasing these concerns.

When the TM is perforated it will heal by proliferation of the fibrous layer. This creates a thickened, opaque membrane in contrast to the normal translucent structure. It is impossible to differentiate a thickened TM associated with chronic inflammation because of otitis externa from a thickened TM resulting from previous (or current) OM without performing a myringotomy, surgical exploration (bullae osteotomy), or advanced imaging (computed tomography or magnetic resonance imaging).

Epithelial cell proliferation begins at the umbo and expands outward. It is important not to damage this area when performing a myringotomy (surgical incision into the TM), because this area contains the germinal epithelium where healing of a ruptured TM begins.

MIDDLE EAR (TYMPANIC CAVITY)

The middle ear is separated from the external ear canal by the TM. The middle ear (tympanic cavity [TC]) is an air-filled chamber that is lined by pseudostratified ciliated columnar epithelium containing goblet cells. This mucous membrane is continuous with that of the pharynx, through the Eustachian tube. There are mucus-producing goblet cells in the TC, but not in the external ear canal. If mucus is seen in the horizontal ear canal, it must have originated in the TC; therefore there must be a tear in the TM.

The TC in dogs is not sterile. A recent study of the TC of normal dogs revealed that aerobic bacteria were found in 25 of 30 TCs. *Staphylococci* or *Streptococcus* were isolated in 73 per cent of the TCs. The anaerobe *Clostridium perfringens* was found in 10 per cent of the TCs. Yeast organisms were not identified. These results supported the clinical impression that organisms in the TC are more consistent with organisms found in the nasopharynx than in the external ear canal. This is not surprising, because the mucous membrane of the TC is an extension of the nasopharyngeal epithelium. Whether the same microflora is present in cats is unknown at this time.

The TC contains three parts, described dorsally to ventrally: the attic or epitympanic recess, the tympanic cavity proper (TCP), and the tympanic bulla (TB) (Figure 30-6).

The attic is the smallest chamber and contains two of the three auditory ossicles, the head of the malleus, and the incus. The facial nerve canal is in this portion of the TC.

The middle portion of the TC (the TCP) lays adjacent to the TM. This portion of the TC contains the stapes (the third auditory ossicle) and part of the malleus (manubrium). The stapes is attached to the vestibular (oval) window. This window communicates directly with the inner ear. The manubrium of the malleus attaches to the fibrous layer of the pars tensa. In contrast to the dog, in whom the manubrium is C-shaped, the manubrium of the cat is much straighter. The outline of the manubrium of the malleus may be seen through the TM when the ear is examined.

The TB is the largest of the three compartments of the TC (Figure 30-7). It is in the ventromedial portion of the TC. In contrast to dogs, in whom a bony shelf partially separates the TCP from the TB, cats have a bony shelf that separates the two cavities completely (Figures 30-7, *D* and 30-8), except for a small defect in the shelf that is just lateral and caudal to the round window in the medial caudal portion of the TCP. Access to the TB from the TCP via myringotomy, which is important in the treatment of OM, is made especially difficult because of the limited opening (Figure 30-9).

The bony eminence (promontory) is on the medial wall of the TCP (Figure 30-10). This structure is directly across from the middorsal region of the TM on the medial wall of the TCP. On the medial side of the promontory is the cochlea of the inner ear. This promontory is visible occasionally through the TM. In contrast to dogs, in whom the sympathetic nerves cross near but not through the middle ear, these nerves cross through the TCP in cats, coursing across the promontory submucosally and making them susceptible to damage when performing a myringotomy or a middle ear lavage.

Also on the medial surface of the TCP are the eustachian tube (ET) and the vestibular (oval) and cochlear (round) windows (see Figure 30-10). The openings for the oval and the round windows are in the caudal portion of the TC, whereas the opening for the ET is in the rostral portion. The ET travels from the dorsal-lateral aspect of the pharynx and enters the rostral aspect of the TC. Typical of respiratory epithelium, the ET is lined with ciliated pseudostratified columnar epithelium that includes goblet cells. The ET normally is in a collapsed state; however, it will become inflated when pressure in the TC (medial surface of the TM) must be equalized with the pressure on the lateral surface of the TM.

The oval window is dorsal to the cochlear promontory (see Figure 30-10). The stapes covers the oval window. As mentioned previously, vibrations from the TM are transmitted from the malleus to the incus to the stapes. The stapes then transmits this vibration to the inner ear. The fluid (perilymph) in the inner ear converts mechanical energy (vibrations) to electrochemical energy (nervous impulse) that is transmitted to the auditory cortex in the temporal lobe of the cerebral cortex of the brain.

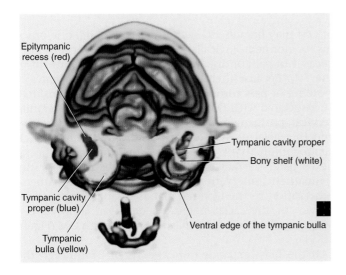

Epitympanic recess (red)

Tympanic cavity proper

Bony shelf (white)

Tympanic cavity proper (blue)

Ventral edge of the tympanic bulla

Tympanic bulla (yellow)

Figure 30-6 Schematic drawing of the three cavities of the feline tympanic bulla.

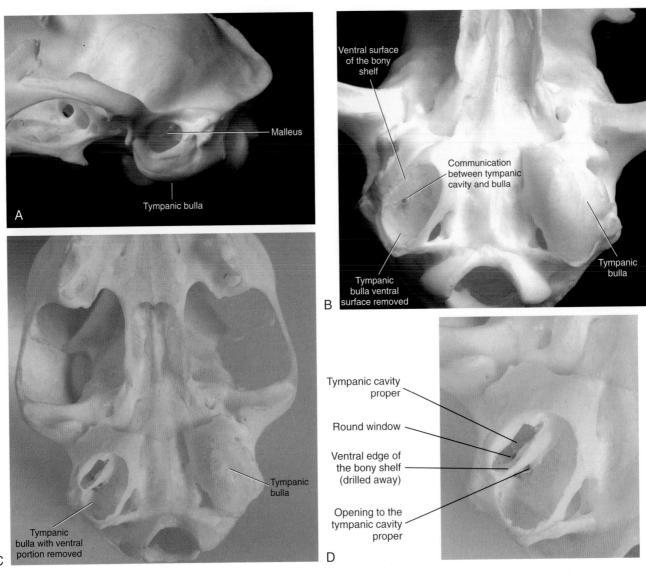

Figure 30-7 A, Lateral view of the feline skull showing the tympanic bulla and location of malleus. **B,** Ventral view of the feline skull showing the tympanic bulla. **C,** Ventral view of the feline skull showing a cut section of tympanic bulla. **D,** Close-up view of **A.**

At the caudal end of the promontory is the cochlear (round) window (see Figure 30-10). This window, which is covered by a mucous membrane, also communicates with the inner ear. The round window serves as a pressure valve, bulging outward as pressure rises in the inner ear.

Because we have discussed the external ear canal and the middle ear, it seems appropriate to apply this knowledge to a clinical example. It was discussed earlier that inflammatory changes in the ceruminous glands might lead to the development of an inflammatory polyp in the ear canal. This is not the same as a nasopharyngeal polyp. Nasopharyngeal polyp is an inflammatory lesion that originates from the TC or the ET rather than the external ear canal. With time this mass expands. If it expands into the inner ear, the cat will develop clinical signs of otitis interna (OI).

As the mass expands, the TM may rupture or become abnormal in appearance; for example, thickened, change in lucency (opaque), bulging, or discolored. Clinical signs

of OM may be present, such as head shaking, otic pruritus, or nonneurological head tilt (this may occur either because of pain or discomfort from fluid being present in the TC). Because there are nerves that are anatomically close to, or pass through the TC, neurological signs may be associated with OM. These nerves include the cranial cervical postganglionic sympathetic nerve (see below) and the facial nerve. Horner's syndrome (sympathetic), keratoconjunctivitis sicca (parasympathetic), and facial nerve paralysis may be present in cases of OM if the sympathetic innervation to the eye, the parasympathetic innervation to the lacrimal glands (branch of the facial nerve), or the facial nerve are damaged, respectively. Mechanical deafness also may be present with OM (Figure 30-11).

If the mass expands from the TC or ET through the TM into the external ear canal, the cat will have clinical signs associated with otitis externa such as head shaking, otic discharge, and otic pruritus. A mass will be visible in

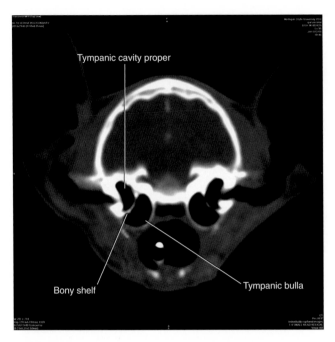

Figure 30-8 CT image of feline skull showing bony shelf in tympanic cavity.

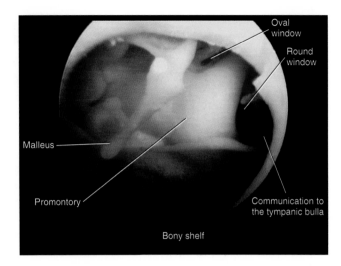

Figure 30-10 View of promontory and malleus.

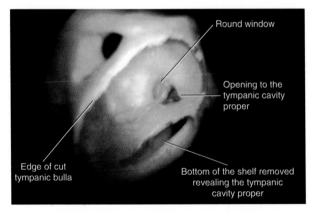

Figure 30-9 View of the round window and opening to the tympanic cavity.

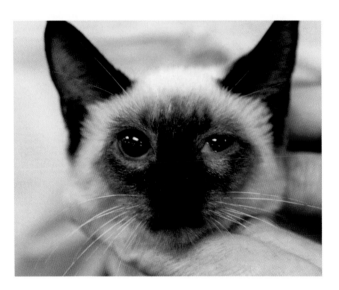

Figure 30-11 Left-sided Horner's syndrome in a 5-month-old female domestic shorthair cat with a large unilateral nasopharyngeal polyp (see Figure 30-13, **A** and **B**).

the horizontal ear canal when examined otoscopically (Figure 30-12).

Because of the anatomical relationship between the ET, the TC, and the nasopharynx, if the mass expands toward the nasopharynx the cat may have clinical signs that are associated with respiratory and or pharyngeal disease, such as dysphagia or signs of upper airway disease, such as nasal discharge, sneezing, or voice change. The cat also be may dyspneic or make a loud stertorous sound on inspiration (Figure 30-13).

Because the ET/TC and the external ear canals have different types of epithelium (epidermis vs. respiratory), an inflammatory polyp caused by ceruminous gland hyperplasia can be differentiated histologically from a nasopharyngeal polyp. Microscopic findings with naso-pharyngeal polyps include the presence of pseudostrati-fied ciliated columnar epithelium covering a core of fibrovascular connective tissue. Varying numbers of lym-

phocytes, plasma cells, and macrophages will be present. If the polyp is caused by ceruminous gland hyperplasia, the findings would include glandular hyperplasia associ-ated with epidermis, not respiratory epithelium.

FIBEROPTIC VIDEO ENHANCED OTOSCOPY VERSUS STANDARD OTOSCOPY

In contrast to standard otoscopy that only provides 10× magnification, fiberoptic video enhanced otoscopy (FOVEO) provides 25× magnification, allowing very detailed examination of the ear canal and the TM. Biopsy instruments can be inserted through the 2-mm working channel into the ear canal for collecting biopsies, remov-ing masses, performing myringotomies, or even laser therapy without obstructing the view, as would occur with a standard otoscope cone. Instrumentation needed for FOVEO includes a camera, an otoscope probe

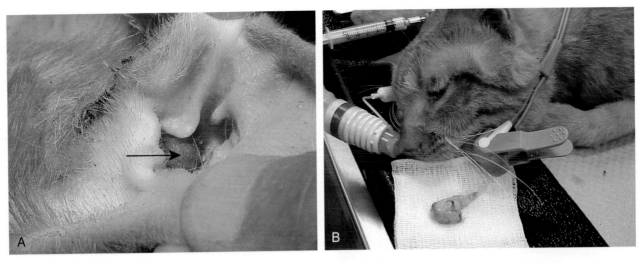

Figure 30-12 A, External ear canal polyp *(arrow)*, arising from the left middle ear cavity, in a 10-month-old neutered male domestic shorthair cat presented because of otorrhea and otic pain. **B,** The polyp removed by traction and avulsion from the patient in **A.** Bacterial otitis media was present.

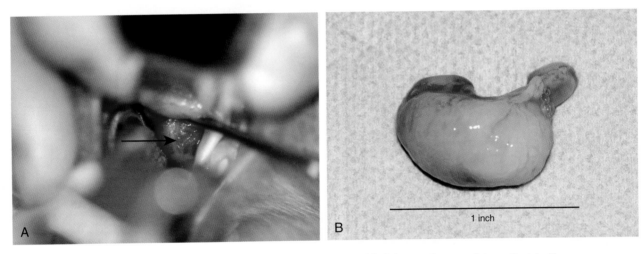

Figure 30-13 A, At induction of anesthesia, a large polyp *(arrow)* filled the oropharynx of the patient in Figure 30-11. Severe inspiratory dyspnea and stertor were the presenting complaints. **B,** The polyp from the same patient after removal by traction and avulsion.

containing magnifying rods and with a 2-mm working port, a fiber optic cable, and a powerful, focally intense 150 W halogen light source. The camera is connected to a video monitor, printer, and digital recorder that allow capture and documentation of normal or abnormal findings. These images then can be used to educate owners about ear disease. The reader is encouraged to read a more detailed explanation of otoscopy in a recently published article.[10]

EXAMINATION SUMMARY

The goal of this chapter was twofold: (1) to review the anatomy of the feline ear and (2) to describe a systematic examination process to aid in the diagnosis of feline otitis (Box 30-1). So that no abnormalities will be missed, the otic examination should be performed in a systematic manner beginning with the pinna. During the examina-

tion, record any findings such as pinnal alopecia, erythema, ulceration, crusting, scaling, or swelling. Next proceed to palpate the ear canals for pain, calcification, or thickening. Finally follow this by an otoscopic examination of the ear canals. To evaluate the ear canals and the TM, the tip of the cone of the otoscope should be placed in the opening of the external ear canal. The cone is advanced proximally by initially pulling straight up on the pinna. Because of the curve in the external ear canal, the ear canal must be straightened to see the horizontal canal and the TM. This is done by pulling the pinna laterally (outward). By stretching the pinna laterally into a straight line horizontally, the ear canal becomes straight. The otoscope is advanced into the horizontal ear canal as the canal is straightened. During the examination the presence, degree, and location of inflammation, ulceration, and proliferative changes should be noted (i.e., cobblestone hyperplasia) (Figure 30-14). The description of the size of both the vertical and horizontal canals along

Box 30-1 Differential Diagnoses of Ear Disease Based on Gross Examination Findings

EXTERNAL PINNA
- Swelling: aural hematoma, tumor, cellular infiltrate
- Abnormal droop: consider trauma, environmental factors, infiltrates
- Papules
  - Bacterial infections, dermatophytes, *Notoedres*, fly bites, cutaneous drug reactions (topical or systemic), eosinophilic infiltrates
- Plaque
  - Same causes as papules, rarely tumors
- Pustule
  - Bacterial, dermatophyte, PF (especially if on the inner pinna)
- Alopecia
  - Breed-related or normal (preauricular alopecia)
  - Feline demodicosis, bacterial folliculitis, dermatophytosis
  - Immune mediated: alopecia areata, later stages of PF
  - Congenital lesions
  - Secondary to pruritus (flea allergy, atopy, food allergy, drug reactions)
- Scale/Crusts
  - Any disease associated with pustules (e.g., PF)
  - Bacterial pyoderma, dermatophytosis, exfoliative dermatitis caused by *Malassezia*
  - Parasites: ear mites, *Cheyletiella*, *Notoedres*, *Trombicula*, lice

- Immune-mediated: PF, drug reactions, irritant reactions
- Solar damage
- Rare nutritionally-related or nutritionally-responsive (essential fatty acids, vitamin A)
- Excessive dryness in the environment
- Lack of grooming
- Secondary to inflammation from pruritus

EAR CANAL
- Lack of visualization of vessels: inflammation
- Increased cerumen: inflammation
- Cobblestone appearance: hyperplastic ceruminous glands caused by inflammation
- Obstruction: foreign body, ceruminolith, polyp, tumor

TYMPANIC MEMBRANE
- Intact and normally translucent?
- Ruptured: most likely cause is otitis media
- Discolored: abnormal consider otitis media, mass in ear canal
- Bulging?

PRESENCE OF HORNER'S SYNDROME
- Strongly consider OM

PRESENCE OF VESTIBULAR SIGNS
- Possible inner ear disease

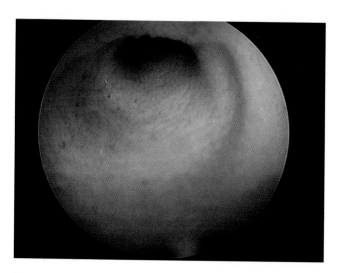

Figure 30-14 Cobblestone appearance of ear canal of cat with early ear disease. (Courtesy Dr. Karen Moriello, University of Wisconsin.)

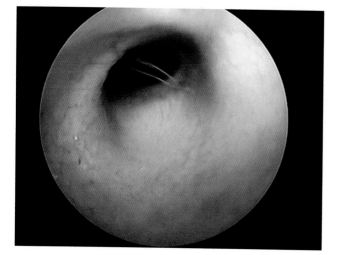

Figure 30-15 Note the small blood vessels in the wall of a healthy ear canal. (Courtesy Dr. Karen Moriello, University of Wisconsin.)

with the type, location, and quantity of debris or exudate also should be included in the medical record. Take note of the presence or absence of small blood vessels in the wall (Figure 30-15). The inability to see these vessels is one of the first signs of ear disease. Next, you should document if the TM is visible (Figure 30-16). If you are not able to do so, is it because of swelling, the presence of a ceruminolith, or is debris in the proximal horizontal

canal obstructing your view? Sometimes it is because the cat is in too much pain to allow deep examination of the ear canal. If you can visualize the TM, you should document if it is normal in appearance (see Figure 30-16). Changes noted may include discoloration or bulging.

It is important then to evaluate for concurrent middle or inner ear disease, because cats with chronic recurrent otitis externa may have concurrent OM. This process may

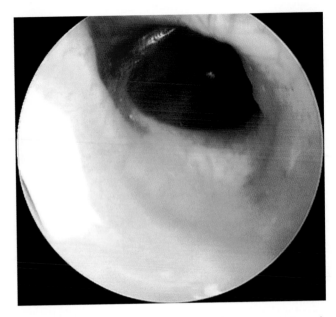

Figure 30-16 Normal feline tympanic membrane as seen through an otoscope. (Courtesy Dr. Karen Moriello, University of Wisconsin.)

require deep sedation or general anesthesia. Evidence of middle ear involvement includes a ruptured TM or an abnormal appearing TM (i.e., thickened, change in lucency [opaque], bulging, or discolored). Even though it has been stated that an intact TM does not exclude the presence of OM, it is important to follow that statement with "but the TM usually is *not* normal in appearance." Supporting this statement is a report in 1991 in which the authors diagnosed OM in 42 dogs via biopsy or necropsy examination of the middle ear.[11] The investigators reported that the TM was rarely torn in this group of dogs. (However, this was before FOVEO was available. It is possible that some of the dogs may have had tears in the TM that could not be appreciated without FOVEO.) The authors went on to state that the TM often was

thickened, supporting this author's opinion that the presence of OM with an intact normal TM is very rare.

During the examination, remember to look for evidence of Horner's syndrome, keratoconjunctivitis sicca (parasympathetic), or facial nerve paralysis that may be present. These clinical signs occur in cases of OM because of the close association of the respective nerves to the middle ear. Vestibular signs will be present only if OM extends to OI. Signs of OI include horizontal nystagmus, asymmetrical ataxia, and head tilt, circling, falling, or rolling toward the affected side.

REFERENCES

1. Milstone L: Epidermal desquamation, *J Derm Sci* 36:3, 2004.
2. Guest JF, Greener MJ, Robinson AC, et al: Impacted cerumen composition, production, epidemiology and management, *QJM* 97:8, 2004.
3. Gotthelf LN: Factors that predispose the ear to otitis externa. In Gotthelf LN, editor: *Small animal ear diseases: an illustrated guide*, Philadelphia, 2000, Saunders, p 46.
4. Drake DR, Brogden KA, Dawson DV, et al: Thematic review series: skin lipids. Antimicrobial lipids at the skin surface, *J Lipid Res* 49:4, 2007.
5. Campos A, Betancor L, Arias A, et al: Influence of human wet cerumen on the growth of common and pathogenic bacteria of the ear, *J Laryngol Otol* 114:925, 2000.
6. Sirigu P, Perra MT, Ferreli C, et al: Local immune response in the skin of the external auditory meatus: an immunohistochemical study, *Microsc Res Tech* 38:329, 1997.
7. Yassin A, Mostafa MA, Moawad MK: Cerumen and its microchemical analysis, *J Laryngol Otol* 80:933, 1966.
8. Stone M, Fulghum RS: Bactericidal activity of wet cerumen, *Ann Otol Rhinol Laryngol* 93:183, 1984.
9. Fay JP, Puria S, Steele CR: The discordant eardrum. Proceedings of the National Academy of Sciences. http://www.pnas.org.
10. Griffin CE: Otitis techniques to improve practice, *Clin Tech Small Anim Pract* 21:96, 2006.
11. Little CJ, Lane GJ, Pearson GR: Inflammatory middle ear disease of the dog: the pathology of otitis media, *Vet Rec* 128:293, 1991.

31 Diagnostic Imaging of the Ear

Lisa J. Forrest and Andrew Gendler

Imaging possibilities today for cats presenting with ear disease have increased beyond routine radiographs. Computed tomography (CT) and magnetic resonance imaging (MRI) provide cross-sectional images that are exceptionally useful when evaluating the complex anatomy of the skull. Most veterinary schools and many specialty practices have one or both of these imaging modalities, either in-house or readily available through human medical centers. It is important for the feline practitioner to understand how these imaging modalities work, and what the limitations, cost, and indications are of radiography, CT, and MRI.

IMAGING OPTIONS

Sophistication of imaging in veterinary medicine continues to increase, following the advancements seen in human medicine. The imaging possibilities for evaluating the feline ear include radiography, CT, and MRI. Each of these modalities works differently and has advantages and disadvantages with regard to cost, availability, limitations, and indications (Table 31-1).

RADIOGRAPHY

Conventional radiography remains the mainstay in private practice for evaluating the ear. This modality is available in all or most private practices, and equipment

cost and upkeep are reasonable. In addition, veterinarians have a high comfort level with evaluation of radiographs as compared with other modalities.

The radiographic image is the result of differential absorption of x-rays as the primary beam passes through the patient. Absorption and transmission of x-rays depends on the thickness, physical density, and effective atomic number of the patient being imaged. The x-ray photons that are not absorbed by the patient reach the radiographic film (transmitted) and determine the blackness and gray scale of the image.

Within radiography there are now two options for image capture. In all systems an x-ray tube is used to create the x-ray beam; the difference lies in the final display and generation of the image. The radiographic image can be captured with radiographic film that is developed either by hand-processing or an automatic processor. This is referred to as conventional film-screen radiography and is still used widely in veterinary practice. Digital radiography (DR) is beginning to replace conventional film-screen radiology in veterinary practice. Computed radiography (CR) is a form of DR. The x-ray beam interacts with the CR imaging plate and these imaging plates are processed by a plate reader, which creates a digital image on the computer. A computer image also is created with direct digital radiography (DDR), but there is no imaging plate to process. The DDR plate is incorporated into the radiographic table and sends the signal measured from the x-ray beam directly to a computer. With the increasing availability of digital radiography, computer manipulation and storage of radiographs are

Table 31-1 Feature Comparison of Imaging Modalities Used to Evaluate the Feline Ear

Modality	How It Works	Digital	Cost	Availability	Advantages	Limitations	Indications
Radiography	X-rays	±	$	+++	Superior spatial resolution	Superimposition of structures Limited gray scale	Simple otitis externa/media Screening technique
CT	X-rays	+	$$	++	Good contrast resolution	Cost Soft tissues better evaluated with MRI	Bony structures Middle and inner ear Radiotherapy computerized treatment planning
MRI	Magnetic field	+	$$$	+	Superior contrast resolution	Cost Geometric distortion Decreased accuracy of bone imaging	Middle and inner ear Evaluation of soft tissues

now possible. For more information on DR imaging, the reader is directed elsewhere.[1]

An important strength of radiography is the global information it can provide. In contrast, with cross-sectional imaging of CT and MRI, the anatomy is seen one "slice" at a time and the overall size and shape of organs must be reconstructed. Radiography is an excellent modality for bone imaging, which is what is evaluated in routine ear imaging (bullae, temporal bone). Radiography has high spatial resolution, which is the ability to discern small detail. The greatest disadvantage of radiography is the superimposition of overlying structures, which is at its greatest when imaging the skull. For example, it is not possible to image the brain with conventional radiography because of the overlying calvarium; the cross-sectional imaging modalities CT and MRI are more suitable for brain imaging. With conventional radiography it is not possible to discern whether the soft-tissue opacity within the bulla identified on radiographs is fluid or a mass because these two structures are the same opacity. However, CT and MRI can make that assessment more accurately, because these modalities have higher contrast resolution than radiography. Contrast resolution is the ability to discriminate between different tissues accurately and display these differences with varying shades of gray or brightness.[2] Although conventional radiography has limitations, it still has its place in imaging of the feline ear, for example, in the assessment of otitis media.

COMPUTED TOMOGRAPHY

CT images are computer-generated information obtained from x-ray detectors and are based on differences in x-ray absorption within the patient, which result from variances in physical density between tissues. In CT a thin x-ray beam emitted from an x-ray tube is directed at the patient as it rotates around the animal. X-ray detectors opposite the x-ray tube measure the transmitted radiation, which is relayed to the computer for reconstruction into the tomographic image (Figure 31-1).

CT offers distinct advantages over conventional radiography. The images are tomographic, in other words

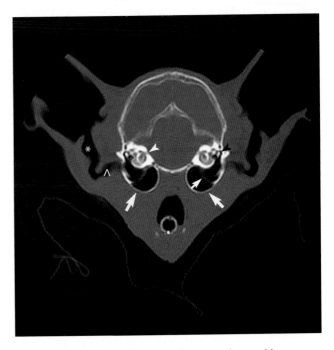

Figure 31-1 Transverse CT images (bone window and bone reconstruction algorithm) of the head of a normal cat at the level of the tympanic bullae. Air-filled vertical (*) and horizontal ear canals (^) are visible, and the thin-walled bony tympanic bullae *(white arrows)* delineate the middle ear. The bony septum *(short arrow)*, cochlea *(white arrowhead),* and auditory ossicles *(black arrowhead)* are well depicted.

"slices" of the patient. With tomographic images, superimposition of structures is not seen, which is a serious limitation of routine radiography. In CT imaging, contrast between structures is enhanced greatly because images are computer generated. There are only five radiographic opacities that we can identify on routine radiographs; and tissues, especially soft tissues, must be altered significantly in order to see a change. This is not true with CT images in which the range of tissue attenuation, or opacity, depiction is much greater (3000 to 4000 units), thereby increasing the accuracy of image interpretation.

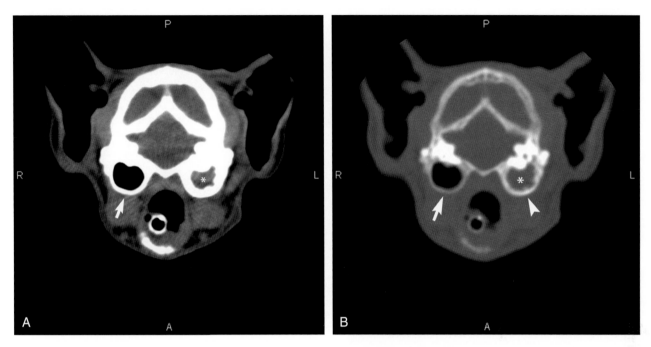

Figure 31-2 Transverse CT images of the tympanic bullae in a cat with left-sided otitis media. Note on the soft-tissue **(A)** and bone window **(B)** images the soft-tissue attenuating material in the left tympanic bulla (*). Only the bone window **(B)** depicts the bony thickening of the left bulla accurately *(arrowhead)*. Note the normal, air-filled, and thin-walled right tympanic bulla *(arrow)*.

CT technology can display a larger gray scale than radiography, enhancing contrast between structures. The human eye can not visualize, and monitors can not display, the full range of gray scale on one CT image; therefore images must be windowed. This allows viewing of images with both a soft-tissue and a bone window by adjusting the gray scale on the monitor, and is necessary to evaluate the tympanic bullae accurately (Figure 31-2).[3] Bone windows have window widths (WW) around 2000 Hounsfield units (HU) and window level (WL) of around 125 to 300, whereas a soft-tissue window will have a WW of 300 to 400 HU and a WL of 50 to 60 HU. A more in-depth discussion of CT image manipulation can be found elsewhere.[2]

Accurate detection of soft-tissue changes, delineation of tumors, and subtle bony lysis and proliferation are possible with the increased contrast afforded by CT. It has been shown that CT and radiographs have similar sensitivity for detection of otitis media.[4] Therefore radiography of tympanic bullae still remains a cost-effective screening tool for ear disease. Although CT is increasingly available for our veterinary patients, it is more costly than routine radiographs and may not have a primary role as a first-line screening technique, being reserved for more complicated cases of ear disease such as neoplasia (see Chapter 69).

MAGNETIC RESONANCE IMAGING

MRI is a tomographic imaging technique based on the properties of hydrogen atoms when placed in magnetic and radiofrequency fields. Hydrogen atoms are abundant in water and mammalian tissue, being highly prevalent in muscle and blood, and to a lesser extent in fat and bone. Because of this characteristic, MRI provides superior soft-tissue detail and is the imaging choice for the central nervous system. An in-depth discussion of the principles and equipment involved in image acquisition is beyond the scope of this chapter; additional information can be found elsewhere.[2]

Despite the superior soft-tissue detail obtained with MRI, there are instances when CT may be sufficient or a more desirable imaging modality. Because of the physical structure of bone, especially compact bone of the skull, the hydrogen atoms are not as movable and the bones of the skull appear black, an image void (Figure 31-3). Magnetic field inhomogeneity artifacts present with MRI can cause geometric distortion,[5] limiting the accuracy of measurements. This is not encountered in CT imaging. Therefore because structures are more geometrically precise with CT, this is the preferred modality for computerized radiotherapy treatment planning.

INDICATIONS FOR IMAGING CATS

Imaging should be used judiciously to answer a question and refine the differential diagnoses for cats presenting with clinical signs of ear disease. Imaging will help guide the clinician to the next diagnostic and/or therapeutic step when the following clinical signs are present:
- Ear exudate: suspect otitis
  - Radiography—bulla series
  - CT, if otitis not identified clearly on radiographs, or cat is unresponsive to appropriate therapy

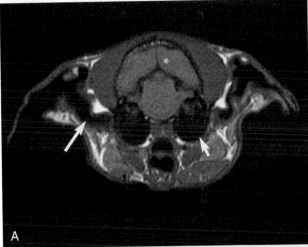
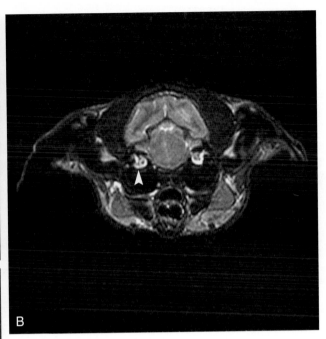
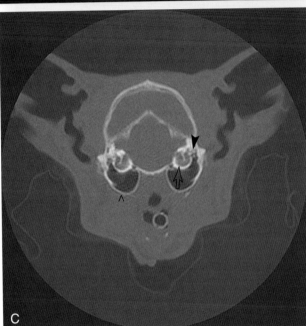

Figure 31-3 Transverse spin-echo T1-weighted (**A**) and T2-weighted (**B**) magnetic resonance images of the middle and inner ear in a normal cat. **C,** Transverse CT image at the same level is presented for comparison. **A,** T1-weighted magnetic resonance image has normal thin walls of the vertical ear canal *(long arrow)* and lining of the tympanic bulla *(short arrow)* that are isointense to the brain (*). **B,** T2-weighted magnetic resonance image, in which free fluid is bright white, provides excellent visualization of the endolymph within the labyrinth of the inner ear *(arrowhead)*. The tympanic bulla walls are black (on all sequences) because no magnetic resonance signal is detected from bone. **C,** CT gives excellent detail of the bony labyrinth of the inner ear, including the cochlea *(open arrow)*, bony ossicles *(black arrowhead)* and tympanic bulla *(^)*.

- Respiratory stridor, sneezing, nasal discharge in young cats: suspect nasopharyngeal polyp
  - Radiography—bulla series and lateral larynx radiograph
  - CT—more sensitive for polyp evaluation, also able to evaluate the nasal cavity
  - MRI—most sensitive with excellent contrast resolution
- Head tilt: central vs. peripheral vestibular disease
  - CT or MRI—best choice
  - Evaluate brain and bullae
  - Radiography—bulla series
  - Can start with screening radiographs. If bullae are normal, proceed to MRI to evaluate for brain lesion

GENERAL PROCEDURES FOR IMAGING CATS

Regardless of which imaging modality is chosen to evaluate cats with ear disease, immobilization is crucial to obtaining a diagnostic study. The patient must be heavily sedated or ideally under general anesthesia. Evaluation of the skull, particularly the auditory apparatus, requires comparison between the left and right sides. Additionally, as evaluators we are accustomed to viewing appropriately positioned images, which makes it easier to identify an abnormality when present. General anesthesia facilitates positioning of cats for a radiographic bulla series, making evaluation easier. When obtaining routine, screen-film radiographs of the feline auditory system, use the table-top technique; a grid is not needed because of the small size of the patient. Nonscreen film will provide superior detail, but requires a higher technique with longer exposures and can be used only when the patient is under anesthesia and secured with tape and foam wedges, with no personnel in the room during exposure. Single-emulsion film used in mammography also will produce high-detail radiographs with less exposure (technique) than needed for nonscreen film.

Radiographs of a bullae series include[6,7]:

- Lateral projection (Figure 31-4)
  - Use radiolucent material (foam, cotton) under mandible to obtain a true lateral view
  - Include cranial neck if nasopharyngeal polyps are suspected
- Lateral oblique projections (Figure 31-5)
  - Compare the left and right bullae
  - Cat is placed in right lateral recumbency without foam or cotton under chin
    - The left bulla will be highlighted
  - Cat is placed in left lateral recumbency without foam or cotton under chin
    - The right bulla will be highlighted
- DV projection (Figure 31-6)
  - Ensure that the mandible and maxilla are superimposed
  - Good view for evaluation of the external ear canals
- Rostroventral-caudodorsal oblique (open-mouth) projection centered on the bullae
  - Excellent view to evaluate bullae
  - Place cat in dorsal recumbency with neck flexed and nose pointed to x-ray tube, open mouth, and aim the x-ray beam at the back of the mouth.
- Rostro 10-degree ventro-caudodorsal oblique projection, alternative to the open mouth view (Figure 31-7).
  - Excellent, alternative view to evaluate the bullae
  - Place cat in dorsal recumbency with the hard palate at an angle of 10 degrees from vertical with the mouth closed. The primary beam is centered at the base of the mandibular body (see Figure 31-7, A).[7,8]

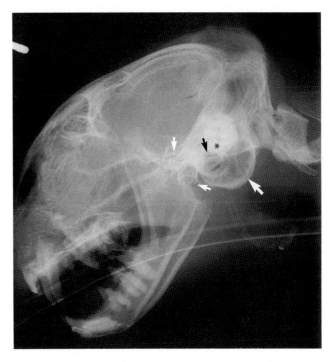

Figure 31-4 Lateral radiograph of the skull of a cat with an inflammatory polyp in the middle ear. Note the thickened bulla wall *(white arrow)* and increased soft-tissue opacity contained within it. It is impossible to determine which side the lesion is on from this view. The normal external acoustic meatus *(black arrow)* and petrous temporal bone (*) are visible. Both temporomandibular joints *(short white arrows)* can be seen owing to mild obliquity.

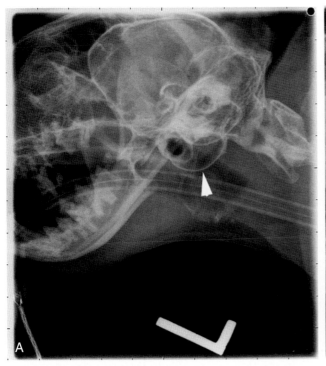

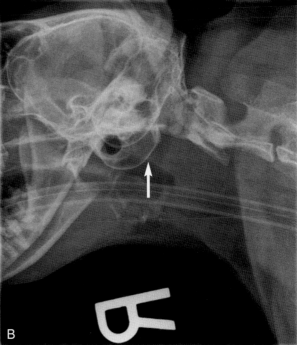

Figure 31-5 Left **(A)** and right **(B)** lateral oblique radiographs of the tympanic bullae in a normal cat. The left *(white arrowhead, **A**)* and the right *(white arrow, **B**)* bullae, positioned more ventrally, can be better visualized without superimposition of the opposite bulla or the petrous temporal bone.

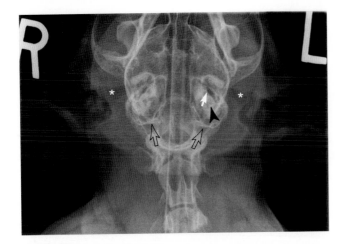

Figure 31-6 Dorsoventral radiograph of the external and middle ears in a normal cat. The external acoustic meatus *(arrow)* and petrous temporal bone *(arrowhead)* are superimposed with the tympanic bullae *(open arrows)*. Note the air-filled external ear canals approaching the middle ears (*).

COMPUTED TOMOGRAPHY AND MAGNETIC RESONANCE IMAGING

Precise skull positioning is equally important with CT and MRI. Precise positioning allows comparison of symmetry. Axial images should be obtained through the head to include the bullae, external ear canals, and nasopharyngeal region. CT imaging of the bony structures of the middle and inner ear is optimized by using a thin-slice collimation and increment or thick-section reformatting of the thinly collimated images.[9,10] It is important to view the images in both a soft-tissue and bone window on preadministration and postadministration of contrast medium. Iodinated contrast medium is injected intravenously to evaluate for inflammation and tumor extension. Tumors have an aberrant blood supply, which results in increased contrast enhancement as compared with normal tissues (Figure 31-8). Because MRI is true three-dimensional imaging, different imaging planes are obtained and include axial, dorsal, and sagittal planes. T1-weighted precontrast and postcontrast administration in the axial plane, and T1-weighted postcontrast administration in the dorsal and sagittal planes are obtained. T2-weighted precontrast images in the axial plane are obtained. The contrast medium that is used, gadolinium, is a paramagnetic substance that is best imaged with T1-weighted sequences.

IMAGE INTERPRETATION

Diseases of the ear that affect cats include inflammatory and noninflammatory conditions with otitis, inflammatory polyps, and neoplasia as the main differential diagnoses. Inflammatory diseases such as otitis and polyps will cause wall thickening of the tympanic bulla, which generally is smoothly marginated (Figure 31-9). Fluid accumulation in the bulla and inner ear can be seen alone

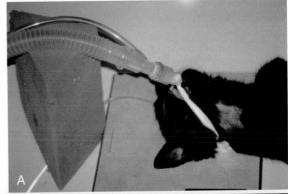

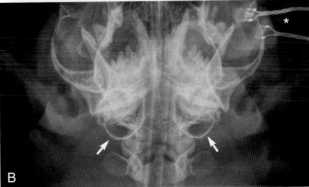

Figure 31-7 A, A normal cat is positioned in dorsal recumbency with its head extended 10 degrees from a line perpendicular to the tabletop to produce the rostro 10° ventro-caudodorsal oblique radiograph. **B,** Rostro 10° ventro-caudodorsal oblique radiograph of a normal cat with the left and right tympanic bullae *(arrows)* visible without superimposition of the mandible or occipital bone. Metallic wires from a pulse oximeter are attached to the left side of the tongue (*).

or with bony changes. Tumors of the ear canal are aggressive and cause bony lysis and irregular proliferation (Figure 31-10). Evaluation of radiographic and CT images use similar criteria because both imaging modalities use x-ray sources to obtain the image. Looking for symmetry between the right and left auditory apparatus is a good place to start the evaluation, and knowing normal radiographic anatomy of the bulla and adjacent bones is paramount to recognizing abnormalities (see Figures 31-5 to 31-8). Radiographs and CT images provide excellent bony detail. The clinician should evaluate the bullae for the following:

1. Tympanic bulla contour. The bulla is part of the temporal bone and is an air-filled enlargement extending medially from the air-filled external ear canal. The bullae are thin-walled, rounded bony structures with a smooth contour at the base of the skull.[9] The bullae are best seen on the lateral oblique and rostro 10-degree ventro-caudodorsal oblique projection (alternative to the open mouth view) radiographic views (see Figures 31-5 and 31-7) and on axial CT views in a bone window (see Figure 31-8).

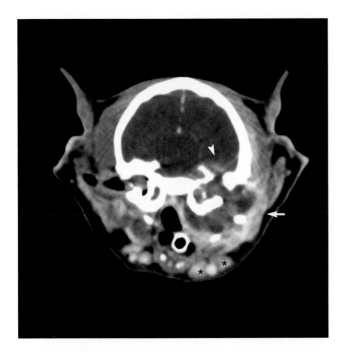

Figure 31-8 Transverse CT image (post IV contrast administration and soft-tissue window) at the level of the tympanic bullae of an 8-year-old, female-spayed domestic shorthair cat. There is an expansile soft-tissue mass *(arrow)* involving the left tympanic and the left horizontal ear canal. The mass is peripherally and heterogeneously contrast-enhancing, and there is osteolysis of the floor of the cranial vault, adjacent to the inner ear. Contrast enhancement is present in the ventral aspect of the left temporal lobe *(arrowhead)* consistent with mass extension into the cranial vault. Note the normal right ear canal and tympanic bulla for comparison. Contrast-enhanced mandibular lymph nodes *(black *)* around the linguofacial veins also are visible. The mass was diagnosed as a squamous cell carcinoma.

2. Bony proliferation or osteolysis of the bullae or surrounding bone (see Figures 31-9 and 31-10).
3. Presence of fluid/soft tissue opacity within the bulla. On radiographic views, one can not differentiate between fluid and soft tissue because both will have the same opacity. However, if there is contrast enhancement or an air-fluid interface within the bulla on CT images, then a determination of tissue and fluid can be made respectively (Figures 31-11 and 31-12).

Caution should be used when evaluating bulla wall thickness on CT images when fluid is present in the middle ear. A previous study[3] noted that the bony wall of a fluid-filled bulla appears thicker than an air-filled bulla. This volume-averaging artifact may result in a false diagnosis of bulla osteitis (chronic bone changes). When using CT to evaluate the middle ear, specificity can be improved with the smallest slice thickness possible.[9]

The normal bulla on magnetic resonance images, all sequences, is a signal void or black line. This is because the bulla contains air and is surrounded by cortical bone.[9] If fluid is present in the tympanic bulla, it appears as hyperintense (white) on T2-weighted images and isointense (same grey scale) to brain tissue on T1-weighted images, and it does not contrast enhance with gadolin-

ium (Figure 31-13). As with CT images, an air-fluid interface can be seen if present. Fluid within the inner ear can be seen on magnetic resonance images and will have the same signal intensity as described above.

COMMON FELINE EAR DISEASES

As discussed, feline ear disease is inflammatory (otitis, inflammatory polyp) or neoplastic.

OTITIS EXTERNA

A diagnosis of inflammation of the external ear canal generally is made on otic examination (see Chapter 30). Imaging can confirm the narrowing of the external ear canal or presence of cartilage mineralization (chronic disease), and allows evaluation of the middle ear and inner ear (CT and MRI).

OTITIS MEDIA

An imaging diagnosis of otitis media is based on thickening of the tympanic bulla, usually with the presence of soft tissue or fluid within the bullae. As stated previously, radiography is a sensitive imaging modality for otitis media (see Figure 31-9), but otitis media also can be seen with CT and MRI (see Figures 31-2 and 31-13).

OTITIS INTERNA

In order to make an imaging diagnosis of otitis interna, CT or MRI is necessary. The internal ear can not be distinguished on radiographs. Cross-sectional imaging is necessary to evaluate the inner ear. The inner ear is housed in the petrous part of the temporal bone and consists of the cochlea and semicircular canal; at the base of the inner ear, there are two exposed membranous surfaces, the oval and round windows.[9,11] Fluid normally is present in the inner ear, which dictates the appearance on CT and magnetic resonance images (see Figure 31-3). Otitis interna can result from extension of disease, such as neoplasia, that will cause bony destruction seen easily with CT imaging. With chronic otitis interna, the normal fluid of the inner ear is replaced with fibrous tissue, which changes the imaging results of MRI T2-weighted images; the normal hyperintense fluid signal of the inner ear (see Figure 31-3, *B*) shifts to an isointense to brain signal.[6,9,12] Because the inner ear connects to the central nervous system, extension of disease to the brain can occur, resulting in brain parenchymal changes and contrast enhancement on magnetic resonance images.[11,12,13]

BULLOUS EFFUSION IN CATS WITH SINONASAL DISEASE

Fluid in the middle ear has been noted in cats with sinonasal disease (Figure 31-14).[14] These cats did not exhibit

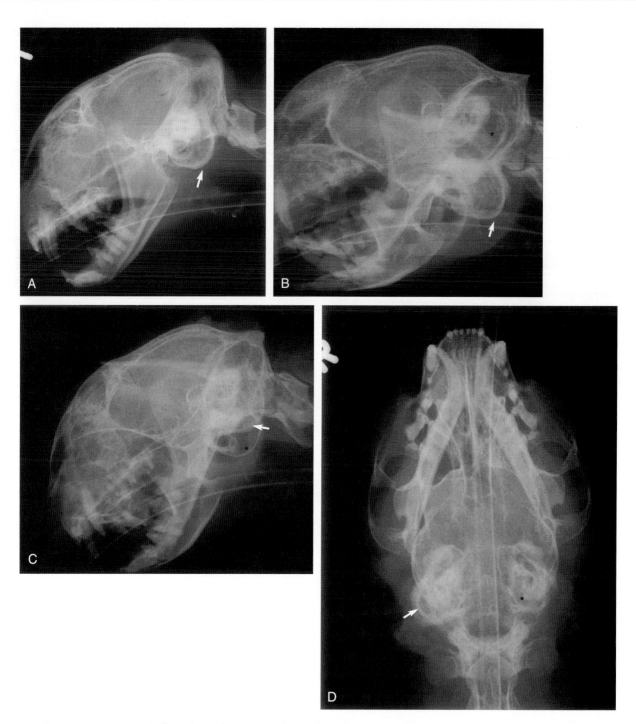

Figure 31-9 Tympanic bulla radiographic series including lateral view **(A),** right **(B)** and left **(C)** lateral oblique views, and ventrodorsal **(D)** view of a patient with a right-sided nasopharyngeal polyp and associated otitis media. The thickened bony wall and soft-tissue opacity contents of the right tympanic bulla (*arrow*) are easiest to detect on the right lateral oblique **(B)** and ventrodorsal **(D)** views. Compare these changes to the normal left tympanic bulla (*). The right lateral oblique view **(B)** in this patient is rotated enough that one can evaluate the left bulla adequately.

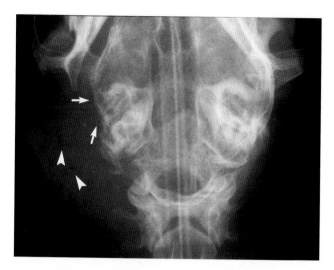

Figure 31-10 Dorsoventral radiographic projection of an aggressive soft-tissue mass lesion involving the left tympanic bulla. There is osteolysis *(arrows)* of the lateral aspect of the bony bulla and adjacent temporal bone associated with the large soft-tissue opacity. Small punctate gas opacities *(arrowheads)* are detected in the mass consistent with intralesional necrosis and/or prior needle aspiration.

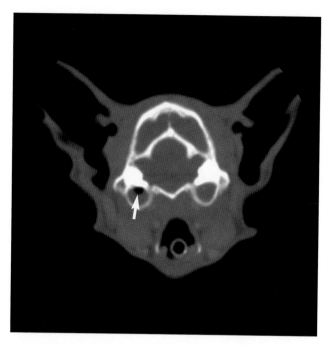

Figure 31-12 Transverse CT image (soft-tissue window) at the level of the tympanic bullae in a patient with chronic rhinitis and bilateral otitis media. Both tympanic bullae contain soft-tissue attenuating material. The concave meniscus and small volume of gas in the dorsal aspect of the right tympanic bulla *(arrow)* are consistent with fluid accumulation rather than a soft tissue mass. Based on the clinical and CT characteristics *(not pictured here)* of chronic rhinitis in this cat, auditory tube dysfunction was suspected as the cause for the fluid accumulation.

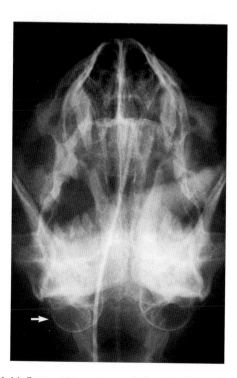

Figure 31-11 Rostro 10° ventro-caudodorsal radiographic projection of the tympanic bullae in a cat with right-sided otitis media. Note the increased soft-tissue opacity in the right bulla *(arrow)* compared to the left side. Both tympanic bullae have normal bone thickness.

clinical signs of middle ear disease, but had tomographic and clinical signs of rhinitis and/or sinusitis, including inflammatory, infectious, and neoplastic conditions. The working hypothesis is that auditory tube dysfunction may be responsible for development of fluid within the bullae.[14]

NASOPHARYNGEAL POLYPS

Nasopharyngeal polyps are benign masses that are thought to arise from the epithelial lining of the tympanic bulla, nasopharynx, or eustachian tube.[15-18] Polyps can be seen in cats of any age, and clinical signs depend on location of the polyp. Cats with polyps may present with stridor, nasal discharge, sneezing, dyspnea, voice change, vestibular signs, weight loss, and dysphagia (see Chapter 30).[18]

Nasopharyngeal polyps can be imaged with routine bullae radiographs and a straight lateral view that includes the cranial neck for complete evaluation of the nasopharynx (Figure 31-15). However, CT and MRI are more sensitive for evaluation of polyps.[9,15,16,18,19] Because of the cross-sectional nature of CT and MRI, it is easier to distinguish nasopharyngeal polyps in cats; CT provides better imaging of bone (Figure 31-16), whereas MRI is

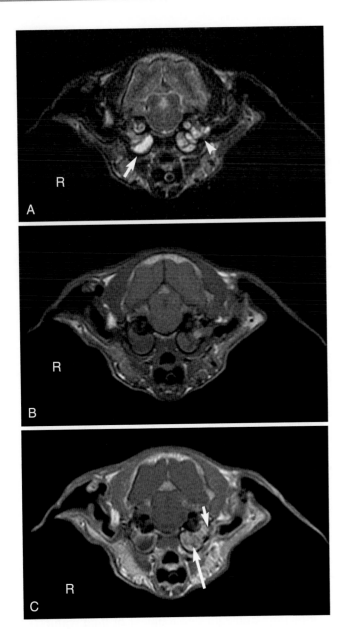

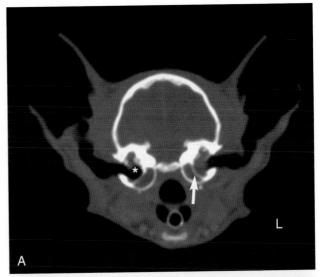

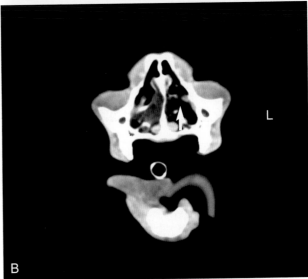

Figure 31-13 Transverse magnetic resonance images of the tympanic bullae in a cat with bilateral otitis media and regrowth of a nasopharyngeal polyp that was removed previously.
A, T2-weighted image has hyperintense medial compartments of both tympanic bullae, consistent with free fluid *(arrow)*. Both bony septa of the middle ears can be seen as a linear region of decreased signal adjacent to the free fluid. The lateral compartment of the right tympanic bulla and the horizontal ear canal have a heterogeneous hyperintensity suspected to be inflammatory changes with polyp regrowth *(arrowhead)*.
B, T1-weighted image with free fluid in the left tympanic bulla. Free fluid (hyperintense on T2 images) will appear isointense to grey matter on T1-weighted sequences. The medial compartment of the right tympanic bulla has more signal intensity than the left side, suggesting that this compartment contains thicker, more bound fluid such as an exudate, blood, or edematous tissue.
C, T1-weighted postcontrast image has a hyperintense mass lesion in the lateral aspect of the tympanic cavity and the horizontal ear canal *(short arrow)*. Irregular contrast enhancement also is detected in the peripheral aspects of the bulla *(long arrow)*. These changes are consistent with nasopharyngeal polyp regrowth, originating from the right tympanic bulla epithelium.

Figure 31-14 Bone window **(A)** transverse CT image of the tympanic bullae and a postcontrast soft-tissue window **(B)** transverse CT image at the level of the rostral maxillary turbinates in the same cat. Soft-tissue attenuating material fills both tympanic bullae, left worse than right **(A).** The meniscus interface with gas in the right ear canal (*) suggests the bulla is filled with fluid; however, lack of contrast enhancement would be conclusive in differentiating this material from a mass. Notice how well the bony septum *(arrow)* and the tympanic wall are delineated in this wide-window setting (WW-2500, WL-500). The tympanic wall can be misinterpreted as thickened in a narrow window setting or with thick slice acquisition. Diagnosis: bilateral otitis media. Maxillary turbinates in the rostral left nasal passage **(B)** are reduced in number *(arrow)*. There is mild, normal contrast enhancement of the remaining turbinates and the turbinates of the right nasal passage. Diagnosis: chronic rhinitis.

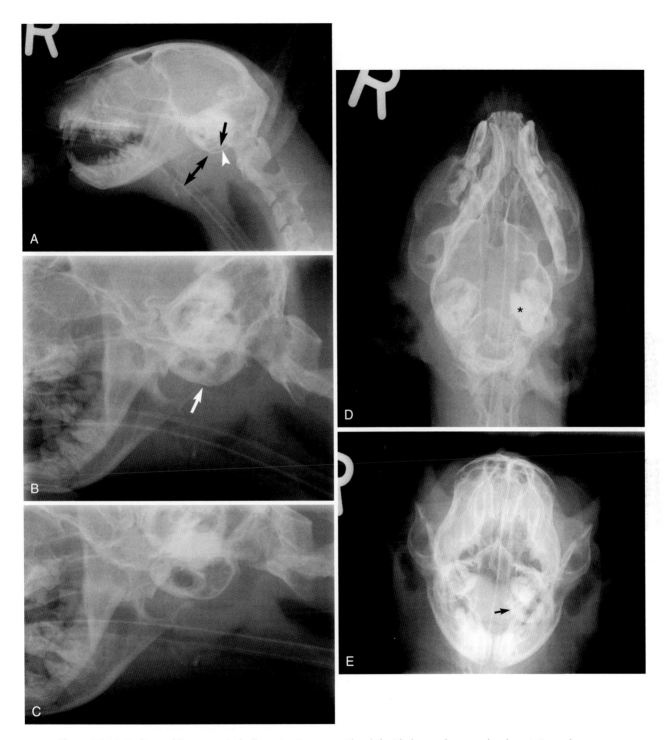

Figure 31-15 Radiographic tympanic bulla series in a cat with a left-sided nasopharyngeal polyp. **A,** Lateral radiograph has increased soft-tissue opacity and enlargement in the caudodorsal nasopharynx *(double-ended black arrow)*. Mild obliquity allows visualization of the tympanic bullae, one normal *(white arrowhead)* and the other thickened *(black arrow)*. **B,** Left lateral oblique view. The left tympanic bulla contains soft-tissue opacity and has a thickened bony wall *(white arrow)*. **C,** Right lateral oblique view. Normal right tympanic bulla. **D,** Dorsoventral view with the left petrous temporal bone (*) superimposed with the left tympanic bulla. Accurate localization of disease based on this view is suboptimal. **E,** Rostroventral-caudodorsal open mouth view. The left tympanic bulla contains soft-tissue opacity *(black arrow)* and a thickened bony wall.

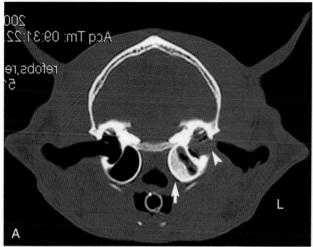

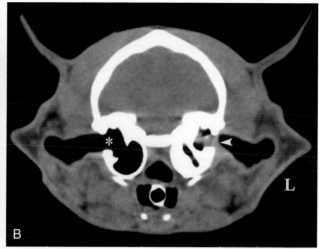

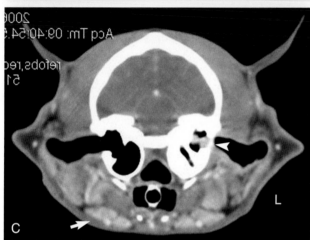

Figure 31-16 Transverse CT images of the tympanic bullae in a cat with a left-sided nasopharyngeal polyp, including bone reconstruction algorithm in a bone window **(A)**, precontrast **(B)**, and postcontrast **(C)** detail reconstruction images in a narrow soft-tissue window. The bony thickening of the left tympanic bulla *(long arrow)* is best appreciated in the bone algorithm and bone window image **(A)**. Soft tissue attenuating material is present in the lateral compartment of the left middle ear and the proximal left ear canal *(white arrowhead)* in all images **(A to C)**, and its homogeneous contrast enhancement *(white arrowhead, C)* is consistent with an inflammatory mass. Compare the left ear canal to the normal right ear canal (*).Contrast enhancement of the mandibular lymph nodes *(short white arrow)* is a normal finding.

optimal because of the superior soft-tissue imaging characteristics (Figures 31-13 and 31-17).

NEOPLASIA

Tumors of the feline ear are covered in detail in Chapter 69. Neoplastic masses present as aggressive disease on imaging, commonly resulting in bony lysis and expansile soft-tissue masses. Routine bullae radiographs (Figure 31-18) can identify bony lysis, but ideally CT is the best imaging modality when neoplasia is suspected (Figure 31-19). Soft-tissue and bony changes are more apparent on CT images than on radiographs. The aggressive behavior[20] and tumor extent, including tumor extension to the brain, can be determined easily with CT (see Figure 31-19). In addition to being the optimal cross-sectional imaging modality for bony changes, CT images are used for computerized radiotherapy treatment planning of these tumors. Often these tumors are treated with a combination of surgery and radiation therapy.[20]

SUMMARY

Imaging is an important part of evaluating the cat with ear disease. Routine bullae radiographs are good for screening cats with suspected ear disease and can diagnose otitis media easily. Cross-sectional imaging modalities (CT and MRI) are better for evaluating the skull, specifically the ears, because superimposition of bony structures is not a problem, thanks to the acquisition of "slices" of the patient with these methods. CT is best for evaluation of bony changes, which often are seen in cases of ear tumors and otitis media. CT also is the preferred imaging modality for computerized treatment planning because there is no image distortion and software programs recognize the x-ray attenuation of tissues imaged, resulting in more accurate portrayal of radiotherapy dose distribution within the patient tissues. MRI has superior soft-tissue detail and is the imaging modality of choice for nasopharyngeal polyps.

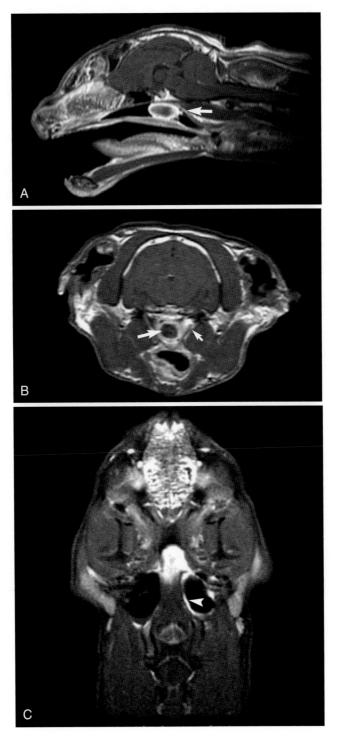

Figure 31-17 Multiplane T1-weighted postcontrast magnetic resonance images of a cat with a left sided nasopharyngeal polyp. **A,** On the sagittal plane image, an ovoid mass *(white arrow)* is present in the nasopharynx that is isointense to skeletal muscle and has marked peripheral contrast enhancement. **B,** The mass is seen on axial plane image *(long white arrow)* in the nasopharynx and a hyperintense stalk *(short white arrow)* extending up the left auditory tube is present. **C,** Dorsal plane image has hyperintensity of the lining of the left tympanic bulla *(white arrowhead),* consistent with the epithelial origin of the pedunculated nasopharyngeal polyp.

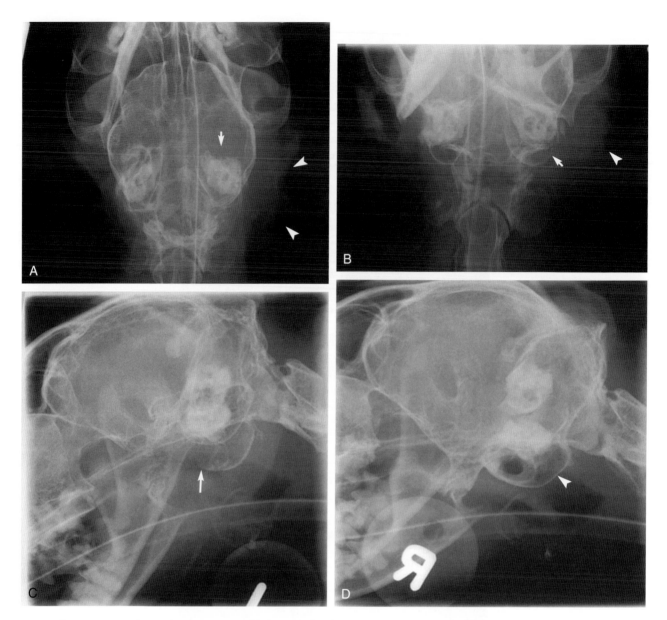

Figure 31-18 Radiographs of a 10-year-old domestic shorthair cat with a squamous cell carcinoma of the left ear, dorsoventral **(A),** rostro 10° ventro-caudodorsal oblique **(B)**, and lateral oblique **(C** and **D)** projections. In **A**, note the asymmetry of the bullae. The left bulla is less opaque *(white arrow)*. Also note the asymmetric soft-tissue swelling associated with the left ear *(white arrowheads)*. **B** highlights the bullae. Note the lysis of the left bulla *(white arrow)* and increased, asymmetric soft-tissue opaque thickening of the left ear region *(white arrowhead)*. **C** and **D** highlight the left and right bullae, respectively. In panel **C** note the lysis of the left tympanic bulla *(white arrow)* as compared with the unaffected right tympanic bulla in **D** *(white arrowhead)*. The radiographic evidence of bony lysis is indicative of an aggressive process, most consistent with neoplasia.

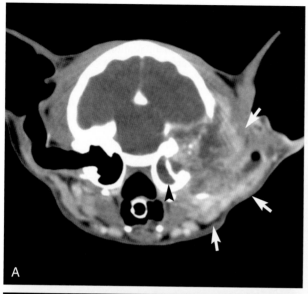

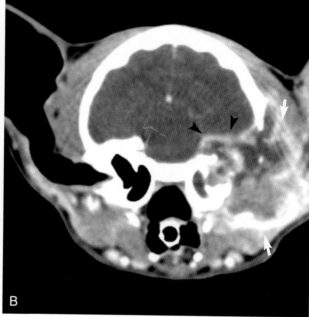

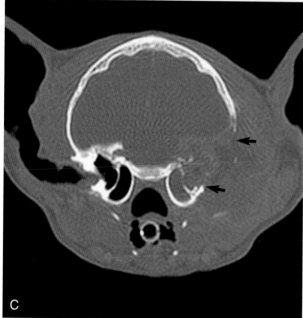

Figure 31-19 CT images of an 11-year-old, male castrated domestic shorthair cat with squamous cell carcinoma of the left ear. **A,** After administration of iodinated contrast medium using a soft-tissue display window. Note the heterogeneous contrast enhancement and thickening of the soft tissues of the left ear *(white arrows)* and the soft-tissue attenuating material in the left bulla *(black arrowhead)*. **B,** Postcontrast administration and soft-tissue display window. Note the large soft-tissue neoplasm with heterogeneous contrast enhancement *(white arrows)* and the meningeal enhancement *(black arrowheads)*; the latter indicates tumor extension into the brain. **C,** Computed tomographic image is displayed with a bone window, which enhances the bony lysis of the left calvarium and bulla *(black arrows)*.

REFERENCES

1. Armbrust LJ: Digital images and digital radiographic image capture. In Thrall DE, editor: *Textbook of veterinary diagnostic imaging*, ed 5, St. Louis, 2007, Saunders, p 22.
2. Tidwell AS: Principles of computed tomography and magnetic resonance imaging. In Thrall DE, editor: *Textbook of veterinary diagnostic imaging*, ed 5, St. Louis, 2007, Saunders.
3. Barthez PY, Koblik PD, Hornof WJ, et al: Apparent wall thickening in fluid filled versus air filled tympanic bulla in computed tomography, *Vet Radiol Ultrasound* 37:95, 1996.
4. Love NE, Kramer RW, Spodnick GJ: Radiographic and computed tomographic evaluation of otitis media in the dog, *Vet Radiol Ultrasound* 36:375, 1995.
5. Chen GTY, Pelizzari CA, Rietzel ERM: Imaging in radiotherapy. In Kahn FM, editor: *Treatment planning in radiation oncology*, Philadelphia, 2007, Lippincott Williams & Wilkins, p 10.
6. Bischoff MG, Kneller SK: Diagnostic imaging of the canine and feline ear, *Vet Clin North Am Small Anim Pract* 34:437, 2004.
7. Hammond GJ, Sullivan J, Weinrauch S: A comparison of the rostrocaudal open mouth and rostro 10-degrees ventrocaudodorsal oblique radiographic views for imaging fluid in the feline tympanic bulla, *Vet Radiol Ultrasound* 46:205, 2005.
8. Hofer P, Meisen N, Bartholdi S: Radiology corner: a new radiographic view of the feline tympanic bullae, *Vet Radiol Ultrasound* 36:14, 1995.
9. Garosi LS, Dennis R, Schwarz T: Review of diagnostic imaging of ear diseases in the dog and cat, *Vet Radiol Ultrasound* 44:137, 2003.
10. Porat-Mosenco Y, Schwarz T, Kass PH: Thick-section reformatting of thinly collimated computed tomography for reduction of skull-base-related artifacts in dogs and horses, *Vet Radiol Ultrasound* 45:131, 2004.

11. LeCouteur, RA, Vernau KM: Feline vestibular disorders. Part I: anatomy and clinical signs, *J Feline Med Surg* 1:71, 1999.

12. Garosi LS, Dennis R, Penderis J, et al: Results of magnetic resonance imaging in dogs with vestibular disorders: 85 cases (1996-1999), *J Am Vet Med Assoc* 218:385, 2001.

13. Klopp LS, Hathcock TJ, Sorjonen DC: Magnetic resonance imaging features of brain stem abscessation in two cats, *Vet Radiol Ultrasound* 41:300, 2000.

14. Detweiler DA, Johnson LR, Kass PH, et al: Computed tomographic evidence of bulla effusion in cats with sinonasal disease: 2001-2004, *J Vet Intern Med* 20:1080, 2006.

15. Kudnig ST: Nasopharyngeal polyps in cats, *Clin Tech Small Anim Pract* 17:174, 2002.

16. Stanton MLE: Feline nasopharyngeal and middle ear polyps. In Bojrab MJ, editor: *Disease mechanisms in small animal surgery*, Philadelphia, 1993, Lea & Febiger, p 128.

17. MacPhail CM: Atypical manifestations of feline inflammatory polyps in three cats, *J Feline Med Surg* 9:219, 2007.

18. Muilenburg RK, Fry TR: Feline nasopharyngeal polyps, *Vet Clin North Am Small Anim Pract* 32:839, 2002.

19. Seitz SE, Losonsky JM, Marrett SM, et al: Computed tomographic appearance of inflammatory polyps in three cats, *Vet Radiol Ultrasound* 37:99, 1996.

20. London CA, Dubilzeig RR, Vail DM, et al: Evaluation of dogs and cats with tumors of the ear canal: 145 cases (1978-1992), *J Am Vet Med Assoc* 208:1413, 1996.

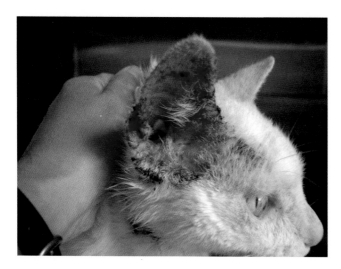

Figure 32-1 Cat with severe suppurative otitis externa and media caused by chronic ear mite infestation. Ear mites were found in the debris aspirated from the middle-ear lavage.

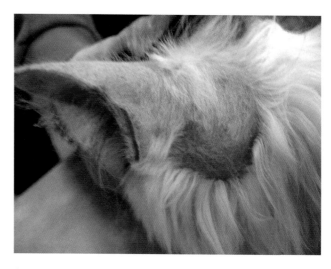

Figure 32-2 Cat with *Demodex gatoi* infestation presenting with severe otic pruritus. Mites were found on skin scrapings and on mineral oil microscopy.

environments are not treated as aggressively as they would have been if presented to a primary-care veterinarian. Cats with severe infestations often do not have their ears properly cleaned and medicated with an otic parasiticidal/corticosteroid medication; given the intense pruritus associated with ear mite infestations, otic corticosteroids are required for humane relief of pruritus. It is common for these organizations to use one application of a topical spot-on treatment (e.g., selamectin) in spite of the fact that studies have shown that at least two applications are needed (day 0 and day 30) (see Chapter 37).[12] Rarely do these cats receive a solid 30-day treatment protocol combined with regular flea control during their animal care days. Neither spot-on nor topical ear treatments will penetrate accumulated debris within the ears; ears still must be cleaned gently and debris must be removed for effective treatment. Mineral oil is a good choice for otic cleaning in these patients, because it is nonirritating and works to soften the debris in the ear canal for more effective removal.

Failure to repeat treatments will result directly in subclinical infestations within the population, otodectic whole-body mange, and treatment failures. Severe head and neck pruritus may be the result of a hypersensitivity reaction to small numbers of mites in subclinical infestations and/or repeat reinfestations from contact with exposed animals. Suppurative OE/OM usually is the result of many factors, including lack of removal of debris from the ears, overly aggressive removal of debris and damage to the otic epithelium, untreated pruritus with secondary self-trauma, and secondary infections. Aural hematomas are observed commonly in cats with ear mite infestations; the hematomas are secondary to the severe pruritus and head-shaking that result in repeated trauma to the pinnae. Deformed ear pinnae as a result of inappropriate treatment may predispose cats to recurrent yeast OE.

Veterinarians examining cats with OE/OM from shelters, animal rescue organizations, or pet stores should re-treat these patients for ear mites, and should ensure that these cats are receiving appropriate monthly flea control. In the authors' experience, these cats often have severe suppurative otitis and require systemic and topical antimicrobial treatment along with antipruritic therapy. If rod-shaped bacteria are present on the ear cytology, culture is recommended to ensure that *Pseudomonas* infection is not a complicating problem. General anesthesia and thorough ear cleaning almost always are beneficial; however, the authors often start medical therapy and have the cat return for ear cleaning 3 to 5 days later after the pain/pruritus has diminished. Middle-ear irrigation/bulla flushing often is indicated because ear mites can chew through the TM. This also may be the only way to remove concretions from the ear canal.

Cats with severe head and neck pruritus and/or otodectic mange will respond to a variety of treatments. The authors prefer whole-body application of fipronil *spray* every 2 weeks for three treatments, or twice weekly lime sulfur rinses for 2 to 4 weeks. Parenteral ivermectin (200 µg/kg SQ) can be used weekly or every other week; however, the authors always use a concurrent flea spray. These mites live very superficially on the skin and ivermectin alone has been inconsistently effective in the authors' experience with shelter cats.

OTIC DEMODICOSIS

Demodex cati (long and slender) and *Demodex gatoi* (short and fat) both can be found on mineral oil microscopy from the ears of cats with pruritic OE (Figure 32-2). The two most common presentations encountered by the authors are young cats with pruritic ears and older cats with pruritic ears. It also has been reported to be the cause of ceruminous otitis in cats.[12] In the latter case a concurrent systemic illness was either already diagnosed or diagnosed shortly thereafter. In young cats it is not uncommon to find concurrent *Otodectes* infestations and *Demodex* mites. In the authors' experience otic demodicosis has only been encountered in animals with clinical signs of ear disease. It has not been found in the ears of normal

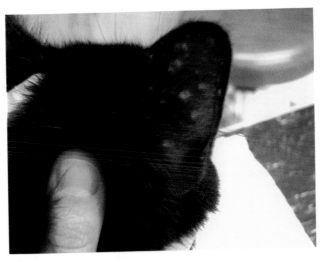

Figure 32-3 Cat with insect bite hypersensitivity. The bites on the ears started as pruritic crusts that developed into eosinophilic granuloma nodules.

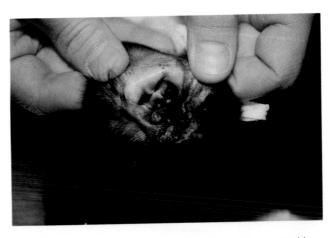

Figure 32-4 Atopic cat with obstructive otitis externa caused by fibrosis of the ear canal. The cat had a history of chronic pruritus and recurrent yeast otitis.

cats.[11] There are no products licensed for the treatment of feline otic demodicosis. Successful treatments include milbemycin 0.5 mg/kg PO q24h, or on a week-on/week-off basis, for 30 days; otic ivermectin; otic milbemycin; and otic preparations labeled for the treatment of ear mites in cats. Amitraz is not recommended for use in cats because it can be toxic. In young animals attention to general pediatric care usually will prevent recurrences. Otic demodicosis can be difficult to resolve in older cats if the underlying disease process (e.g., neoplasia, hyperthyroidism, diabetes mellitus) is not managed properly. Concurrent topical otic corticosteroids may be helpful in relieving the pruritus. The author has not encountered a case of feline otic demodicosis causing suppurative otitis.

INSECT BITE HYPERSENSITIVITY

Insect bite hypersensitivity usually involves the ears, face, and paws of cats. This is a seasonal disease that is more common in indoor/outdoor cats. Affected cats have pruritic crusts, papules, and erosions on their nose and outer ear pinnae (Figure 32-3). In some cases similar lesions may be seen at the junction of the haired skin and footpad. The diagnosis is based on history, clinical signs, and response to confinement. Glucocorticoids (methylprednisolone acetate 20 mg/cat SQ or IM every 1 to 2 months) can be administered during the insect season. Confinement indoors is the treatment of choice.

OBSTRUCTIVE OTITIS

The most common causes of obstructive otitis in cats are ear polyps, ear tumors, stenosis secondary to inflammation, ear deformity as a result of untreated aural hematomas, and ear debris concretions (Figures 32-4 to 32-6). The most common clinical signs associated with space-occupying obstructive lesions are chronic recurrent OE/OM, head shaking, and malodorous suppurative

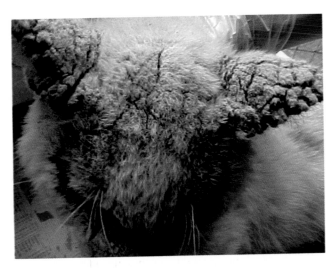

Figure 32-5 Cat with severe crusting and obstruction of the ear canals caused by *Notoedres* infestation.

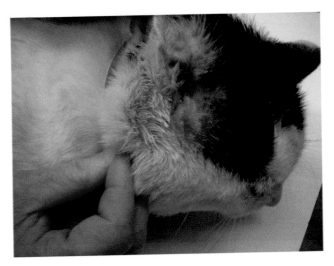

Figure 32-6 Cat with recurrent otitis because of a stenotic ear canal. The ear canal was palpably thickened on examination.

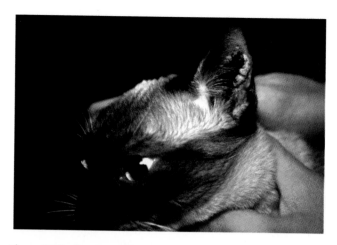

Figure 32-7 One-year-old Siamese cat with obstructive ear disease caused by a mast cell tumor.

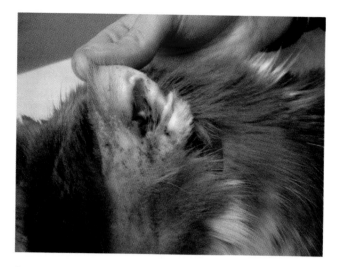

Figure 32-8 Typical presentation of a cat with allergic otitis. Frequently, yeast organisms can be found on skin cytology from the preauricular area.

discharge. These lesions tend to be unilateral; however, the author has seen several young cats present with bilateral OM caused by ear polyps. Mast cell tumors in young cats, particularly Siamese cats, can present as obstructive lesions (Figure 32-7). In the case of space-occupying lesions, resolution of the problem requires imaging of the ear canal to locate the obstruction so that it can be removed surgically. Because these cases tend to be chronic, affected cats usually have concurrent OM and need postoperative systemic and topical antimicrobial treatment based on culture and susceptibility testing. Irrigation of the ear canal and bulla also may be needed (see Otitis Media for details of procedure). These patients often have been treated previously with a variety of antibiotics, and subsequent antimicrobial therapy should be based on culture and sensitivity. It is important to remember to perform otic cytology, because this may help to guide initial antibiotic selection and identify concurrent yeast otitis that otherwise may not be diagnosed. Concurrent treatment of bacterial and yeast OM is common.

Stenosis of the external ear canal of cats is seen most commonly, but not exclusively, as a result of aural hematomas that have healed without surgical intervention. Intervention is needed if the obstruction is causing clinical discomfort and resulting in suppurative otitis. If the cat otherwise is not bothered by the problem, it is best left untreated. Prior to surgical intervention, a trial of medical treatment is indicated to determine if the ear stenosis still can be managed medically. If severe fibrosis is not present, the stenosis often can be relieved by either a trial of oral prednisolone (2 mg/kg PO q24h for 14d, then 1 mg/kg PO q24h for 14d), or methylprednisolone acetate 20 mg/cat SQ or IM every 2 weeks for two to three treatments. If this is successful, ear canal patency may be maintained with topical corticosteroids used at regular intervals (usually several times each week) for long-term maintenance.

ALLERGIC OTITIS

Allergic otitis in cats is a common complication of atopy and food allergy. The ideal treatment is appropriate man-

agement of the underlying allergic disease. Increasingly the authors are recognizing cats with seasonal atopic dermatitis in whom the predominant or most problematic clinical sign is facial and otic pruritus (Figure 32-8). Overall ear pathology tends to be minimal and owners usually report head-shaking and mild to moderate pruritus as the predominant clinical signs. Owners may complain about an increase in ceruminous discharge. Otic cytology often will reveal a concurrent yeast otitis; treatment of the yeast otitis may diminish but not fully eliminate the pruritus. These cats can be treated successfully with topical otic corticosteroids. The authors' favorite otic preparation is 1:1 combination of propylene glycol and injectable dexamethasone (2 to 4 mg/mL). Three to five drops are administered daily in each ear until the pruritus resolves, and then two to three times weekly or as needed. This product is easily formulated in a clinical practice and is nonirritating and inexpensive. One of the major advantages is that this formulation does not contain any antibiotics and/or antifungal agents. If only an antiinflammatory effect is needed, this compounded product is a good choice because it does not contain any unnecessary antimicrobials that could perpetuate the development of resistant organisms.

YEAST OTITIS

Recurrent chronic yeast otitis in cats is seen most commonly in patients with allergic ear disease caused by atopy or food allergy, mild obstructive ear disease, and commonly in cats with congenital hair coat abnormalities (i.e., Devon Rex, Sphynx). Because there are many species of *Malassezia*, morphology of the yeast organisms can vary considerably. One of the most common morphologies with which to be familiar is the "fat cocci" appearance of recently budded yeast. This form is very round and resembles a large coccal bacterium. Unless bacterial cocci are present in the microscopic field, it can be missed easily and mistaken for a bacterial organism. If a presumed staphylococcal infection has been treated and does not resolve, an ear culture specifically for yeast will help to differentiate between a resistant bacterial organism and a yeast infection.

Yeast organisms (*Malassezia* spp.) are common findings on otic cytology and there is considerable controversy as to "what number is significant?" As mentioned previously, the authors take a very practical approach to interpreting numbers of yeast on a slide. If yeast organisms are found on a cytological examination and the cat is asymptomatic, the authors do not treat the yeast infection. If, however, the cat is symptomatic, the authors treat the patient regardless of the number of yeast organisms per high-power field. One component of yeast otitis/dermatitis is a hypersensitivity reaction to byproducts of the organisms; therefore the number of yeasts may be less important than correlating clinical signs and cytological findings.

Because the authors' practice is composed primarily of referral cases, the most common treatment of choice is itraconazole 2 to 5 mg/kg PO q24h for 30 days, or q24h on a week-off/week-on protocol for 30 days. Fluconazole is being used increasingly as a treatment option because it is much less expensive than itraconazole. Ketoconazole is used commonly in dogs; however, cats do not tolerate this drug because of the increased potential for hepatotoxicity, and it is best avoided. Combination antifungal/antiinflammatory topical products may be very suitable and appropriate for mild cases or acute cases that are likely to be seen in a primary care facility.

Chronic recurrent yeast otitis may be caused by *Malassezia* OM. Definitive diagnosis may be made via diagnostic imaging and/or myringotomy with culture and cytology of exudate from the bulla. In the authors' experience, these cases require aggressive ear irrigation and systemic therapy for resolution. A careful reassessment of the case history should be made to determine if there is an underlying disease (e.g., allergies).

OTITIS MEDIA

OM in cats can be a sequela to an upper respiratory infection, it can occur as a complication of ear mite infestation or obstructive lesion such as a polyp, or it can be a primary disease in which organisms from the retropharynx ascend through the eustachian tube into the tympanic bulla. Many cats with OM have brown crumbly debris in the ears that looks very similar to ear mite infestations. The following is a summary of the authors' approach to medical management of OM in cats:

1. Administer general anesthesia and analgesics in preparation for sample collection and flushing of the bulla. Perform an otoscopic examination of the ear canal to determine whether or not the TM is ruptured (see Chapter 30).
2. If the TM is intact, a myringotomy should be performed in order to collect cytological and culture specimens. This can be done with a video-otoscope or with an operating head otoscope. Using an operating head otoscope, a sterile urethral catheter or 22-gauge, 6-inch spinal needle attached

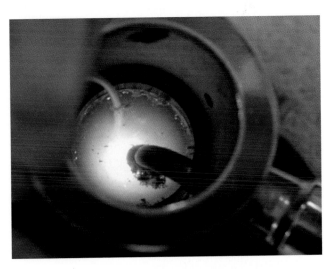

Figure 32-9 Middle-ear irrigation of a cat with chronic recurrent yeast infections. The debris seen in the fluid was dislodged from the middle ear cavity.

to a 3-mL syringe containing 1 mL of sterile saline is inserted through the TM; the fluid is flushed into the bulla and then aspirated back (Figure 32-9). This fluid can be used for both cytology and culture. Another technique that is equally useful uses a mini-tip culturette to perform both the stab incision and sample collection. The mini-tip culture swab is passed through a sterile ear cone attached to the operating head otoscope. It is used to puncture the TM and then is pushed into the bulla. The tip is rotated to collect specimens. This procedure is repeated to collect specimens for cytological examination. The needle, catheter, or swab is inserted through TM at the 5 and 7 o'clock positions. The caudoventral part of the TM is the largest and safest area to pass tubes and instruments, because it avoids the important vasculature and nerves, as well as the hearing apparatus (which is located craniodorsally).

If the TM can not be visualized, the ear canal should be cleaned and dried thoroughly using suction before collection of samples from the bulla. The authors recommend protection of the cat's face and eyes from ear cleaners and flushing fluid by gently wrapping the cat's head in a towel. If the TM is ruptured, samples can be collected from the bulla through the rent in the TM for both cytology and culture. Care must be taken not to contaminate the tips of the instruments with debris from the external ear canal. This can be accomplished by using a double catheter technique in which a large lumen catheter is used to shroud a small catheter within. Once the large catheter is safely in the bulla, the tip of the smaller catheter is pushed into the bulla to collect a sample. If liquid can not be aspirated, 1 mL of sterile saline is flushed into the bulla. The same shrouding technique can be performed using a sterile ear cone attached to operating otoscope. A sterile urinary catheter then is passed through the cone and used to collect a specimen by aspirating fluid. Again, if no fluid is obtained, 1 mL of sterile saline can be flushed into the bulla and aspirated.

3. Once samples have been collected, the bulla is flushed with copious amounts of warm sterile lavage fluid. Dilute povidone-iodine solution is used most commonly. Suction is used to remove the fluid. This process is continued until the fluid is clear. It is common for this process to dislodge large chunks of debris. A small amount of hemorrhage also is possible.

4. After flushing, the author instills enrofloxacin otic drops and dimethyl sulfoxide-fluocinolone otic solution into the bulla to decrease inflammation and to deliver a high concentration of antibiotics to the target area.

5. After the procedure, patients are treated with oral prednisone (1 to 2 mg/kg PO q24h for 2 weeks, and then the dose is tapered gradually over the next 2 weeks). Corticosteroids decrease inflammation, and decrease secretions and exudation in the bulla. If oral medication is difficult, alternatives include the use of injectable methylprednisolone acetate or intravenous dexamethasone (0.2 mg/kg) at the time of treatment and then once weekly.

6. Many cases of OM in cats are caused by *Malassezia* and/or a combined bacterial infection. Pending the results of culture and sensitivity, the authors often will prescribe marbofloxacin (3 to 5 mg/kg PO q24h) and itraconazole or fluconazole (3 to 5 mg/kg PO q24h).

7. Severe OM necessitating middle-ear irrigation and flushing of the bulla is best treated with concurrent topical antibiotics. One of the following antimicrobial agents is used most commonly: fluoroquinolones (ciprofloxacin, enrofloxacin, ofloxacin), ticarcillin, or ceftazidime (Box 32-2). It may be necessary to use a compounding pharmacy to make these otic solutions.

8. Pain medication will be needed in most cats after ear flushing for at least 5 to 7 days. Tramadol 1 to 4 mg/kg PO q8h is effective.

9. Long-term antibiotic therapy will be determined by the results of the cytology and culture. It is not uncommon for the cytological examination to reveal large numbers of yeast organisms, but negative results on yeast culture. Total treatment time varies, but owners should be expected to administer medication for at least 4 to 8 weeks.

10. Complications after flushing include head tilt, nystagmus, potential OI, and pain. Owners should be warned that small amounts of blood-tinged fluid may be seen in the ear canal after the procedure. This procedure is best done early in the day, and the patient released as late as possible in the day. Overnight hospitalization is ideal because it allows the cat to recover more fully and for the clinician to monitor the patient for adverse effects. Neurological side effects often are transient and are gone within 24 hours of flushing.

11. Cats with OM should be reexamined every 2 to 4 weeks during the treatment period.

Box 32-2   Safe Drugs to Use When the Tympanic Membrane Is Ruptured

ANTIBIOTICS
- Fluoroquinolones: ciprofloxacin, enrofloxacin, ofloxacin
- Aqueous penicillin G
- Carbenicillin
- Ticarcillin
- Ceftazidime
- Cefmenoxime

ANTIFUNGALS
- Clotrimazole
- Miconazole
- Nystatin
- Tolnaftate

ANTIINFLAMMATORY DRUGS
- Aqueous forms of dexamethasone and fluocinolone

CERUMENOLYTICS
- Most are not safe except for squalene

TRIS-BUFFERED EDTA

VESTIBULAR DISEASE AND OTITIS MEDIA/INTERNA

Space does not allow a detailed discussion of vestibular disease in cats; however, there are several important points to remember.
- Cats presenting with vestibular disease need a careful physical and neurological examination to determine if the vestibular signs result from peripheral or central causes.
- If clinical signs of OE/OM are present, it is likely that the vestibular signs are associated with the OM.
- OM can occur without obvious signs of otitis, making this determination difficult. Neurological examination and imaging usually are indicated in these situations. Diagnostic imaging is needed in cats with vestibular signs to confirm that there is no obstructive lesion (e.g., polyp) causing the signs and, hopefully, to confirm the presence of OM (see Chapter 31).

Patients with central vestibular disease (CVD) have a brainstem dysfunction.[6] In peripheral vestibular disease (PVD), cats have a rotary or horizontal nystagmus that does not change with the animal's head position. It may or may not be a constant finding in chronic cases, but sudden head movements usually can trigger the nystagmus and its direction is constant. The head tilt is always toward the side with the otitis; however, the fast phase of the nystagmus is away from the ear with the disease. Proprioception is normal in patients with PVD. In addition, PVD owing to OM/OI may be accompanied by ipsilateral facial nerve paresis and Horner's syndrome.

Patients with CVD can manifest any type of nystagmus, but vertical nystagmus is more common with CVD than with PVD. It has been reported that animals with

CVD have a nystagmus that changes in character or direction with a change in head position. Usually the nystagmus does not change, but if it does, then central disease is present. Abnormalities of cranial nerves other than VII and VIII are suggestive of CVD as is the presence of proprioceptive deficits. The most reliable abnormalities to look for in CVD are proprioceptive deficits and changes in mentation. Proprioceptive deficits can be difficult to assess in cats, even more so if they are ataxic.

The three major differential diagnoses for cats with peripheral vestibular disease are OI/OM, nasopharyngeal polyps, and idiopathic feline vestibular disease.[6] The latter condition is most common in the summer and fall, can affect cats of any age, and appears to be more common in cats who go outside. There is a sudden onset of ataxia, nystagmus, and head tilt consistent with a peripheral vestibular lesion. Facial paralysis, Horner's syndrome, and proprioceptive deficits are not features of this disease. OM/OI is a major differential diagnosis. Neurological signs typically improve spontaneously within about 2 weeks; this will not occur in cats with bacterial otitis. Some cats may have a mild persistent head tilt and ataxia. The cause is unknown; however, it has been suggested that this neurological problem may occur as a result of a virus or aberrant migration of *Cuterebra* larvae.

Otitis causes vestibular disease by one of two mechanisms.[6] Bacteria that infect the middle ear can produce toxins that inflame the labyrinth (OM), or bacteria may invade the labyrinth itself (OI). Bacterial OM/OI should be treated for at least 4 to 6 weeks with systemic antibiotics based on culture and sensitivity. Topical antibiotics are insufficient. Given that OM/OI can be difficult to diagnose via otoscopic examination and imaging, a treatment trial with antimicrobial drugs is recommended even if OM/OI can not be identified conclusively. Because of damage to the neuronal structures, there may be some residual head tilt, facial paralysis, or Horner's syndrome. (The reader is referred to Chapter 56 in the fifth volume of this series for a complete discussion on vestibular disorders.)

BENIGN PROLIFERATIVE CERUMINOUS CYSTS

This uncommon, nonneoplastic condition has an unknown etiology, but may be a sequela to OE. Affected cats often have multiple nodules or vesicles in the external ear canal and inner pinnae (Figure 32-10). The vesicles are small, measuring less than 2 mm on average. These lesions are deeply colored (dark blue, brown, or black) and may be mistaken for pigmented neoplasms. Biopsy of the lesions will confirm the diagnosis. The condition affects older cats primarily; however, it has been seen in young animals.[13] Surgical removal or laser ablation may be beneficial in symptomatic patients. Other treatments include lancing the cysts with a needle or blade, and using silver nitrate sticks as a chemical cautery. The cysts will dry and involute within several weeks. After several weeks the remaining cysts can be treated. Chemical ablation with trichloroacetic acid has been used successfully to treat these cysts when they occur around the eyelids. Cysts are débrided surgically

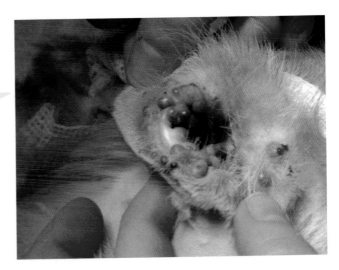

Figure 32-10 Benign proliferative ceruminous cysts in a cat.

and then treated topically with 20 per cent trichloroacetic acid.[14]

PROLIFERATIVE NECROTIZING OTITIS EXTERNA

Young kittens from 2 to 6 months of age are affected primarily by this visually distinctive condition. One case report, however, described the disorder in three young adult domestic shorthair cats between 3 and 5 years of age.[15] It is a rare condition with unknown etiology. The disorder is characterized by well-demarcated, erythematous plaques with annular or serpiginous borders. Thick keratinous debris also is present. Biopsy of the lesions will confirm the diagnosis. Lesions appear on the inner aspect of the pinnae, external ear canal, and sometimes the preauricular region on the face. Lesions develop rapidly and often progress to erosion and ulceration. The patient may or may not be pruritic. Often, secondary bacterial and yeast infections may be present. Lesions generally regress spontaneously by the time the cat is 12 to 24 months of age.[16] The disease may be more persistent in older cats. One study reported beneficial results when the cat was treated with tacrolimus ointment q24h.[15]

OTOTOXICITY CONCERNS

Aminoglycoside antibiotics (i.e., gentamicin, amikacin) have been shown to cause ototoxicity in particularly sensitive animals. The drug can reach very high concentrations in the ear leading to toxic side effects. In general, the development of ototoxicity depends on the duration of treatment, cumulative dose, average daily dose, peak and trough serum concentrations, concurrent use of diuretics, underlying disease status, and previous use of aminoglycoside antibiotics. The ototoxic effects generally are preceded by nephrotoxicity because the drug also is readily accumulated in kidney tissue. In dogs hearing loss is the most common presentation. Cats, however, generally show vestibular signs when ototoxicity occurs. Clinical signs may resolve eventually when the medication is withdrawn; however, the side effects are irreversible in some cases.[17]

Other drugs with the potential to cause ototoxicity include chlorhexidine, polymyxin B, ethacrynic acid, furosemide, salicylates, and cisplatin. The use of chlorhexidine as an ear cleaner is not recommended for this reason.[17]

REFERENCES

1. Hill RB, Lo A, Eden CA, et al: Survey of the prevalence, diagnosis, and treatment of dermatological conditions in small animals in general practice, *Vet Rec* 158:763, 2006.
2. August JR: Otitis externa: a disease of multifactorial etiology, *Vet Clin North Am Small Anim Pract* 18:731, 1988.
3. Detweiler DA, Johnson LR, Kass PH, et al: Computed tomographic evidence of bulla effusion in cats with sinonasal disease: 2001-2004, *J Vet Intern Med* 20:1080, 2006.
4. Gotthelf LN: Diagnosis and management of otitis media. In Gotthelf LN, editor: *Small animal ear diseases: an illustrated guide*, ed 2, St. Louis, 2005, Mosby, p 276.
5. Bensignor E: An approach to otitis externa and otitis media. In Foster A, Foil C, editors: *BSAVA manual of small animal dermatology*, ed 2, Gloucester, UK, 2003, British Small Animal Veterinary Association, p 104.
6. Axlund TW: Otitis interna and vestibular disease. In Gotthelf LN, editor: *Small animal ear diseases: an illustrated guide*, ed 2, St. Louis, 2005, Mosby, p 340.
7. Griffin CE: Otitis techniques to improve practice, *Clin Tech Small Anim Pract* 21:96, 2006.
8. Angus JC: Otic cytology in health and disease, *Vet Clin North Am Small Anim Pract* 34:411, 2004.
9. Murphy KM: A review of techniques for the investigation of otitis externa and otitis media, *Clin Tech Small Anim Pract* 16:235, 2001.
10. Nardoni S, Mancianti F, Rum A, et al: Isolation of *Malassezia* species from healthy cats and cats with otitis, *J Feline Med Surg* 7:141, 2005.
11. Sotiraki ST, Koutinas AF, Leontides SL, et al: Factors affecting the frequency of ear canal and face infestation by *Otodectes cynotis* in the cat, *Vet Parasitol* 96:309, 2001.
12. Guaguere E, Muller A, Degorce-Rubiales F: Feline demodicosis: a retrospective study of 12 cases, *Vet Derm* 15:34, 2004.
13. Gross TL, Ihrke PJ, Walder EJ, et al: Feline ceruminous cystomatosis. In *Skin diseases of the dog and cat: clinical and histopathologic diagnosis*, ed 2, Oxford, 2005, Blackwell Science, p 667.
14. Yang SH, Liu CH, Hsu CD, et al: Use of chemical ablation with trichloroacetic acid to treat eyelid apocrine hidrocystomas in a cat, *J Am Vet Med Assoc* 230:1170, 2007.
15. Mauldin EA, Ness TA, Goldschmidt MH: Proliferative and necrotizing otitis externa in four cats, *Vet Derm* 18:370, 2007.
16. Gross TL, Ihrke PJ, Walder EJ, et al: Proliferative necrotizing otitis of kittens. In *Skin diseases of the dog and cat: clinical and histopathologic diagnosis*, ed 2, Oxford, 2005, Blackwell Science, p 79.
17. Riviere JE, Spoo JW: Aminoglycoside antibiotics. In Adams HR, editor: *Veterinary pharmacology and therapeutics*, ed 8, Ames, 2001, Iowa State Press, p 841.

33 Rush and Conventional Immunotherapy

Ann M. Trimmer and Heide M. Newton

Feline atopic skin disease is very different from other diseases we treat and manage. No two patients or owners are the same. Each treatment plan must be customized to the individual patient. Additionally, atopy may be exceptionally debilitating but rarely is life-threatening. This fact may make it difficult to convince owners who do not have personal experience dealing with allergies that their cat needs treatment. Management of the pruritic patient requires the veterinarian to manage the owner successfully at the same time. Treating the pruritic cat is fraught with difficulty and challenge, but when successful, the reward for the patient, owner, and veterinarian is priceless. This chapter will delve into formulating an appropriate treatment plan for the atopic cat, along with comparing traditional allergen-specific immunotherapy (ASIT) and rush allergen-specific immunotherapy (RIT). RIT is best defined as the process of advancing an allergic patient to a maintenance dose of ASIT over a shorter period of time than that required for the traditional induction period.

DESIGNING THE TREATMENT PLAN

Once the diagnosis of atopic dermatitis has been made, a treatment plan can be created. To formulate this plan, the clinician must evaluate the patient, owner, and disease severity. When evaluating the patient, the clinician must consider factors such as other concurrent medical conditions, temperament at home and in the

hospital, environment (e.g., indoor only, outdoor only), and acceptance of medications. The veterinarian must evaluate the owner for similar factors, including concurrent medical illness (e.g., an owner with rheumatoid arthritis may not be able to administer allergy injections), previous compliance or lack thereof, attitude towards the patient, lifestyle, and potential financial constraints. Disease severity is considered separate from the patient, because this determines how quickly the patient may need relief. For example, in a cat with severe excoriations and alopecia secondary to intense pruritus, both an aggressive short-term and long-term plan for control may be necessary. In a cat with mild or more seasonal atopic dermatitis, a more conservative treatment plan may be adequate.

THERAPEUTIC OPTIONS

There are five generic categories of treatment options for atopic cats. These include ASIT, fatty acids, antihistamines, glucocorticoids, and other immunosuppressive medications (e.g., cyclosporine A).[1] Fatty acids, antihistamines, glucocorticoids, and other immunosuppressive medications focus on treating or modulating the inflammation triggered by the allergic reaction, whereas ASIT modulates the immune system to prevent the allergic reaction from developing. These categories are by no means exclusive nor are they the only potential treatment options. Instead, these categories are meant to be a starting point, and in the majority of patients either individually or in combination, these treatment options will provide relief for allergic cats. When creating the initial treatment plan, the veterinarian must take into account the benefits and disadvantages of each general category, and decide on a course of treatment in light of her or his observations about the patient, owner, and disease severity. For example, a cat with severe excoriations may benefit from the short-term use of oral glucocorticoids or antihistamines in combination with the initiation of immunotherapy. A noncompliant owner who may not administer allergy injections regularly may be best served by treating the patient with cyclosporine A in combination with rush induction of ASIT. On the other hand, ASIT may not be the best treatment choice in a feline patient with short seasonally recurrent disease. In the latter case a short course of antihistamines or oral glucocorticoids may be more appropriate. If this patient were to be treated with ASIT, the response to treatment could not be evaluated until the following year, but the owner would be required to administer allergy injections year round. Additionally, the expense of allergy testing and ASIT may be unwarranted for owners with financial constraints.

ALLERGEN-SPECIFIC IMMUNOTHERAPY

ASIT is the practice of administering gradually increasing quantities of an allergen extract to an allergic patient, the purpose of which is to reduce or eliminate the clinical signs associated with subsequent exposures to the causative allergen.[2] Although only well documented in human allergic patients and still considered a rare event, ASIT is the only therapeutic option for allergic diseases that may cure the patient through immunomodulation after years of therapy.[3] Multiple clinical studies have shown ASIT to be a safe and effective treatment for human beings and dogs with atopic dermatitis.[2,3] In contrast, fewer studies have been performed in feline atopic patients.[4] Those studies and anecdotal observations by veterinary dermatologists suggest that ASIT is an effective treatment option in atopic cats; however, its true success or failure rate is undocumented because no comprehensive studies have been completed.

MECHANISM OF ACTION

Atopic dermatitis in human beings and animals is characterized by the overproduction of allergen-specific immunoglobulin (Ig) E against normally innocuous environmental antigens. The inhalation of aeroallergens in sensitized human patients leads to Th2-biased immune deviation and subsequent production of cytokines that induce allergic disease.[5,6] In sensitized individuals allergen exposure induces cross-linking of FcERI receptor-bound IgE on effector cells. Once triggered this results in the immediate release of anaphylactic mediators and development of inflammation.

Although neither the underlying pathogenesis of atopic dermatitis nor the mechanism of action of ASIT in feline atopic patients has been fully elucidated, they are thought to be similar to that seen in human patients. Despite the fact that the use of ASIT in human beings began at the beginning of the twentieth century, the underlying mechanisms of ASIT are being elucidated to this day.[3,5-7] ASIT is postulated to normalize the dysregulated immune response that characterizes the allergic state. Both short- and long-term modulations of the immune system are initiated by ASIT, including alterations in the quantities and types of inflammatory cells, modifications in the secretion of inflammatory mediators, changes in the types and concentrations of allergen-specific immunoglobulins, and modulations of T-cell functions and cytokine production.[3,5-7]

Such modulations are exhibited classically in human patients undergoing venom immunotherapy. During the first few months of treatment, a decrease is noted in both mast cell and basophil activity for degranulation and systemic anaphylaxis. This alteration in activity is thought to result from the piecemeal release of anaphylactic mediators (histamine and leukotrienes) triggered by ASIT.[3] T regulatory (T reg) cells are a specific subclass of T lymphocytes that exhibit suppressive or regulatory functions. The generation of T reg cells and the suppression of allergen-specific Th1 and Th2 cells are noted in the early stages of ASIT.

T reg cells are generated within days of beginning ASIT, and contribute to the control of allergen-specific immune responses in five major ways. The first is the suppression of antigen-presenting cells; these cells support the development of Th1 and Th2 lymphocytes. Second, T reg cells suppress Th1 and Th2 cells directly. T reg cells also suppress allergen-specific IgE production along with mast cells, basophils, and eosinophils. Finally, T reg cells interact with local resident tissue cells and stimulate remodeling of these barriers. These actions eventually lead to a decrease in IgE/IgG4 ratios during ASIT. The levels of IgE allergen-specific antibodies decrease, and the levels of IgG4 blocking antibodies that prevent the cross-linking of the FcERI receptor increase over time (i.e., years). Therefore the entire desired effects of ASIT may take several years to achieve, making ASIT a long-term treatment option.[2,3,6,7]

BENEFITS VERSUS DRAWBACKS OF ALLERGEN-SPECIFIC IMMUNOTHERAPY

ASIT offers an effective and safe treatment option for cats. Reported success rates range from 60 to 78 per cent in feline atopic patients.[8,9] Additionally, the reported incidence of side effects in feline atopic patients undergoing ASIT is very low. A thorough literature search failed to reveal any documented cases of systemic reactions in feline patients undergoing traditional ASIT. Anecdotally, reported reactions in cats are rare and consist primarily of increased pruritus; however, anaphylaxis has been reported in a few cases. It has been reported anecdotally that one cat developed localized pruritus, vomiting, and diarrhea after an injection of 0.3 mL of approximately 20,000 PNU/mL. The cat was taken to an emergency clinic and responded well to treatment. Respiratory distress and gastrointestinal signs have been reported anecdotally in another cat within 3 hours of an injection. Anaphylaxis appears to be a rare event, although the complication must be considered a theoretical possibility.

The risk of an adverse reaction appears to increase in cats undergoing rush induction of ASIT. A pilot study investigating the use of a rush induction protocol reported the development of a localized injection site reaction in two of the four cats involved in the study. This study was conducted in feline patients with naturally occurring atopic dermatitis.[10] Separate studies evaluating the response of asthmatic cats sensitized to Bermuda grass allergen to more aggressive rush immunotherapy protocols have resulted in multiple systemic reactions during the induction.[5,11] These reactions will be discussed in greater detail later in this chapter.

The primary drawback to ASIT from a client's perspective appears to be the cost associated with initiating therapy. Allergy testing must be performed, and regardless of the method used, it can be cost-prohibitive for some owners. However, when one compares the costs of other therapeutic options and the monitoring required to maintain these therapies, ASIT typically is less expensive in the long term. The initial costs of ASIT may be substantial, but once maintenance therapy has been established, the costs are reasonable for most owners.

The primary drawback to ASIT for the veterinarian is the time commitment involved in ensuring successful completion of the ASIT protocol. Whether owners are administering the injections at home or bringing their cats to the hospital for their injections, the clinician or assistant/technician must follow up frequently with the client. In many patients a response to therapy is not seen for several months once therapy begins, and clients are tempted to stop prematurely before the treatment has had time to be effective. Additionally, some owners may notice adverse effects from the injections and fail to notify the clinician. Owners often believe that everything can be fixed quickly with minimal effort. A significant amount of hand holding is required to overcome this notion through the first few months of ASIT when no response to therapy is seen. Failure to follow through after beginning ASIT may lead to further frustration on the client's part and cause the clinician to lose a patient. Therefore the decision to offer ASIT as a therapeutic option to a client is not to be entered into without thorough evaluation of the client's and clinician's long-term commitment to follow through.

In areas where referral to a veterinary dermatologist is a feasible option, ASIT should be considered sooner rather than later. Patients who undergo ASIT in earlier stages of disease may respond better than those who have become chronic sufferers. Many clients become frustrated and fail to express their frustration to their attending veterinarian. Instead these clients choose to seek a second opinion, often from a different hospital. As tertiary care clinicians, the clients who are referred for our opinion before becoming frustrated tend to be happier and plan on returning to the same family veterinarian. Those clients who seek referral on their own frequently are frustrated and refuse to return to their previous veterinarians.

USE OF ALLERGEN-SPECIFIC IMMUNOTHERAPY IN FELINE ATOPY

Patient/Owner Selection

Feline dermatitis that responded to ASIT was first reported in 1982. Since then ASIT has been shown to be effective treatment for a wide variety of clinical syndromes associated with feline atopy. Pruritus, miliary dermatitis, noninflammatory alopecia, eosinophilic granuloma complex, otitis, pyoderma, and asthma all are commonly recognized clinical syndromes associated with feline atopy.[1] Management of each of these clinical syndromes is possible with ASIT.

One of the most common challenges when treating feline patients is administering medications. Even the most noncompliant cat often will accept injections without protest. ASIT is a safer treatment option than repeated repositol corticosteroid injections for cats who are difficult to medicate orally. Neither the duration of disease nor its severity are helpful in predicting which patients will improve with ASIT and which will fail to respond. Cats who are food motivated can be trained to associate the injections with an especially tasty treat, facilitating administration of the injections.

As noted, the temperament of the owner often is more important to the success of the treatment regimen than the temperament of the cat. Therefore consider the owner's previous efforts to comply with treatment instructions before choosing to begin ASIT therapy. If medications were sent home routinely and the owner failed to administer the complete course of treatment or return the cat for timely rechecks, ASIT may not be a good treatment option, especially if the chosen protocol requires owners to administer ASIT injections at home. Owners must be able to administer the injections, or their schedules must permit them to return to the hospital for timely administration of the injections. Monitoring the cat following an injection and for potential complications is essential for successful management. If an owner can not complete these tasks, ASIT will not control the cat's clinical signs successfully, leading to veterinarian and client frustration.

EXPLAINING ALLERGEN-SPECIFIC IMMUNOTHERAPY TO OWNERS

One of the most difficult tasks for the veterinarian is explaining to owners why ASIT would be a beneficial treatment option for their cat. The theory behind ASIT is complicated and difficult for most owners to understand; however, the following simple explanation can effectively convey the basis of ASIT and what the therapy can accomplish. The clinician can begin by explaining that the patient's allergy is an overreaction of the immune system to something in the environment that it perceives as harmful to itself. Whereas allergies in human beings lead to tearing and nasal congestion, allergies in cats lead to increases in grooming behaviors, licking, scratching, skin sores, and ear infections. Such a comparison helps to make an abstract concept more concrete. It also helps to explain that ASIT is a more specific therapeutic option that targets the cells in the body responsible for causing the clinical signs they are seeing, and induces tolerance to the offending allergens. Although evidence at this time remains anecdotal, rare, and controversial in feline atopic patients, it is important to emphasize that ASIT is the only therapeutic option that may "cure" their cat after years of therapy.[3] Cat owners often are concerned about shortening their pet's life expectancy with drugs. Emphasizing that ASIT is a much safer alternative to long-term medications may provide enough motivation for owners to choose ASIT for their cat.

Unrealistic client expectations often lead to premature discontinuation of ASIT. It must be made clear to clients that although ASIT therapy will take longer before the owner sees results, it represents a safer and more effective means of managing and possibly curing the cat's environmental allergies. Other therapies, such as injectable glucocorticoids, may work faster but potentially have more side effects. At the same time ASIT is not a cure-all. Sixty to 78 per cent of cats respond to ASIT; however, some of these cats still require additional medications on an intermittent or continual basis.[8,9] Some feline patients may improve with ASIT within a month, whereas others may show no improvement for 10 months or more. This variable timeline is frustrating, and there is no way to predict which cats will respond quickly. Clinicians should discuss these issues during the pretreatment conference and prepare clients for the possibility that their cat may require life-long therapy; at a minimum, they should expect that their cats will undergo ASIT therapy for at least 1 year.

CHOOSING ALLERGENS

Allergy testing is used solely to identify environmental allergens for treatment, and not to confirm a diagnosis of atopic dermatitis. Specific allergens should be identified for each individual patient based on a positive test score. Either intradermal skin testing (IDST) or serum allergy testing may be used to identify allergens. Although IDST is considered the gold standard by many dermatologists for canine and feline patients, IDST in the feline patient creates challenges.[9,12,13] Cats may have very subtle reactions, creating a higher incidence of false-negative reactions. In feline patients, IDST may be difficult to perform and interpret, and some dermatologists report that it has been associated with a higher incidence of anaphylaxis when compared with the procedure in dogs.[1] Additionally, cats must be sedated with minimal stress to permit IDST. Stress responses in cats may be so overwhelming that IDST will be completely negative. As a result, many veterinary dermatologists only perform serum allergy testing in cats, and use the results from these tests as a basis for ASIT. Several companies offer serum allergy testing; however, none of them have published studies that permit the clinician to evaluate their sensitivity and specificity in cats. Some companies offering serum allergy tests permit customization of the test itself (i.e., individual allergens may be added for testing,

in addition to the regional standard panel). This option should be considered strongly in situations in which the standard panel does not include tobacco extract and the owner smokes, or feather extract and the owner has a bird or numerous feather pillows.

A previous study comparing the results from serum allergy tests provided by one company with results from IDST in cats can not be interpreted globally because each company uses a different testing methodology.[14] In that study the authors concluded that serum allergy testing was not helpful diagnostically.[14] Neither serum nor intradermal allergy testing are diagnostic for atopy and should be used solely to select allergens for treatment. A retrospective study performed by Halliwell showed significant improvement in clinical signs in approximately 60 per cent of atopic cats that were treated with ASIT based on serum allergy testing.[8]

Regardless of the testing method used, only allergens with positive scores on either IDST or serum allergy testing should be included in the treatment mixture. Each testing method provides a guideline as to what constitutes a positive score. In general the higher the test score, the more likely that the allergen should be included in the mixture. The caveat to this statement is that reactions also must be interpreted in light of the season in which the patient is being tested. Generally scores to those allergens that are pollinating when the patient is tested are higher. Moreover the clinician should evaluate the patient's environment and history to ensure that the positive test scores on the allergy test correlate with this information. For example, if the cat's strongest positive reaction is to dog dander and the owner does not have a dog nor is the cat exposed to dogs through a kennel or grooming, the test results do not correlate well to the history and the patient should be reevaluated. Even strictly indoor cats may have strong seasonal pollen allergies. Allergens may be transferred into the home on the owner's clothing, on other animals, or even through the air conditioner or open windows. In areas that experience a true winter season where pollinating trees, weeds, and grasses die off, a cat with nonseasonal pruritus should have other positive test reactions such as house dust mites, molds, tobacco (if the owner smokes), or feathers.

BEGINNING ALLERGEN-SPECIFIC IMMUNOTHERAPY

Once the allergens have been selected and the allergen mixture has been compounded, the owner should schedule an appointment to come into the hospital so that the clinician or technician can discuss in detail the injection schedule and technique, and possible adverse effects. The clinician must evaluate each owner and decide whether to ask the owner to administer the injections at home or ask them to bring their cat to the hospital for the injections. Administering the injections at home may lead to better compliance, because bringing a cat into the hospital frequently for the injections leads to greater stress for patient and owner.

The first appointment is critical to the success of treatment and to the veterinarian-client relationship, because some owners will spend money for the allergy test and the treatment mixture and then fail to begin the injections because they do not understand the procedure or schedule. Given the proper guidance and treat incentives, the great majority of owners and cats comply with the injection schedule at home. Before starting the injections the owners can practice the treatment process at home to enhance the likelihood of success. Send home a capped syringe with the owners and tell them to practice daily for a week by putting the cat on their lap, a table, or counter top, and give the cat its favorite treat. Then touch the capped syringe to the back of the cat's neck and give it a follow-up treat, thereby training the cat to like or to accept the injections. Allowing the allergen solution to come to room temperature before administration will make the injection less objectionable for many cats.

Owners are instructed to monitor their cat for at least 2 hours after an injection. A written list of adverse effects to monitor is sent home with each owner but these also are discussed in detail in person. Although anaphylaxis is rare, owners are told that anxiousness, urticaria, vomiting, diarrhea, sudden collapse, or difficulty breathing all may represent an emergency requiring immediate treatment. A more common adverse effect is an increase in the level of pruritus. If this occurs, the owners are instructed to call before administering the next scheduled injection. Monitoring the injection site for localized swelling, warmth, or hair loss also is important.

Each of the companies that prepare allergy treatment mixtures proposes a slightly modified version of the injection schedule shown in Table 33-1. The schedule shows the administration of a gradually increasing amount of allergen over several weeks, followed by a gradual reduction in the frequency of injections while maintaining a constant volume. To ensure success, it is important that owners score their cat's level of pruritus before and after each injection throughout the treatment period. Pruritus may be scored on a scale of zero to 10, with 10 representing the cat's highest level of pruritus. This scoring system helps to monitor progress and provides a scale that owners can follow to see that, although the cat may still be pruritic, the level of pruritus has decreased in intensity. It also aids in adjusting treatment along the way. Owners also should track whether or not the cat received any additional medications, including topical agents, during this time.

The clients are contacted 7 to 10 days after initiating ASIT to make sure that they are not having problems administering the injections. Phone calls are made regularly during ASIT to ensure that the cat is not experiencing adverse reactions and that the owners are administering the injections correctly and on schedule. A follow-up examination usually is scheduled 6 to 8 weeks after the initiation of ASIT and every 4 months thereafter. It is helpful to have a consistent list of questions to ask owners each time they are contacted. Although the responses may vary, the questions remain constant, thereby permitting easier evaluation of the patient's progress. These are rough guidelines and each

patient and client will require different levels of monitoring during ASIT.

Table 33-1 Schedule for Allergen-Specific Immunotherapy

Day	Volume (mL)
VIAL #1	
1	0.1
3	0.2
5	0.3
7	0.4
9	0.6
11	0.8
13	1.0
VIAL #2	
15	0.1
17	0.2
19	0.3
21	0.4
23	0.5
25	0.5
5-DAY INTERVAL	
30	0.5
35	0.5
40	0.5
7-DAY INTERVAL	
47	0.5
54	0.5
61	0.5
68	0.5
10-DAY INTERVAL	
78	0.5
88	0.5
98	0.5
108	0.5
118	0.5

ADJUSTING ALLERGEN-SPECIFIC IMMUNOTHERAPY

Adjusting ASIT customizes treatment for each patient, often increasing the success of therapy. However, making adjustments to immunotherapy is frustrating for many clinicians. There is no strict set of guidelines to follow, and each patient may present a new set of challenges. Additionally, there is some disagreement about adjusting ASIT even among experts. Table 33-2 gives examples of common adjustments that may be made during ASIT.

Table 33-2 Adjustment Scenarios for Allergen-Specific Immunotherapy

Scenario	Adjustment	Reasoning
Injections every 10 days Cat is itchier 7 days after injection	Change injections to every 7 days Do not adjust volume	If itchier at day 7, then injections are not frequent enough so need to decrease time between injections
Injection every 14 days (0.5 mL) Cat is itchier after injection for 2 days	Do not adjust frequency Change volume to 0.4 mL	If itchier after injection then volume should be adjusted because the dose is too high
Injections every 7 days Itches after injection for 24 hours and begins itching again 5 days after injection	Change injections to every 5 days Change volume to 0.4 mL or less	Itchier after injection implies volume is too high, and itching before injection implies injections are too far apart
Injections every 14 days No itching noted	Change injection to every 21 days	If no reaction to the injections, then try to spread out injections to lessen burden on owner

DISCONTINUING ALLERGEN-SPECIFIC IMMUNOTHERAPY

There is no well-documented guideline as to when ASIT should be discontinued. This is true regardless of whether or not the patient is responding to treatment. Current recommendations are to encourage owners to administer ASIT for at least 1 year before discontinuing therapy. Improvement may be monitored by the dose and frequency required of additional medications and the pruritus scores that owners have assigned to their cat during the course of therapy. Thus one can compare the amount of medication or the number of ear infections or lesions that a patient had the previous year, even in cats who are not exhibiting marked improvement. Decreased dependence on medications and fewer ear or skin problems would indicate that there has been some response to ASIT.

When cats exhibit minimal to moderate amounts of improvement during the first year of ASIT, the clinician and owner must decide whether continuing ASIT will provide any ongoing therapeutic benefit. Many of these patients require lower dosages of other medications with significant side effects while they are undergoing ASIT. If the injections were well tolerated by cat and owner, then the recommendation would be to continue ASIT. ASIT should be discontinued for those patients who show minimal to moderate improvement on ASIT after 1 year, and when the cat or owner has difficulties with the injections.

ASIT should be discontinued, reevaluated, or modified for cats who show no response to ASIT after 1 year of treatment. Clinicians should reevaluate clinical signs and history prior to discontinuing therapy. If the owner had refused to perform a food trial previously, a lack of response to ASIT further supports the need for this diagnostic test; however, discontinuing ASIT before performing the food trial is not advisable. Clinicians also should consider repeating the allergy test or choosing an alternative method of testing if the cat fails to respond to ASIT. These guidelines are based on anecdotal reports and contradict what has been documented in human patients undergoing ASIT. Studies in human beings have shown that substantial levels of blocking antibodies can not be documented until year 2 or 3 of ASIT.[6] Therefore it is possible that the current guidelines for our feline patients erroneously recommend premature discontinuation of ASIT when an unsatisfactory response is seen after 1 year.

Atopic cats should receive year-round flea control to ensure that failure to respond to therapy is not because of another complicating allergy. Owners of predominantly indoor cats often balk at this recommendation, but every effort must be made to control complicating factors that could make it difficult to interpret response to therapy.

The frequency of injections should be decreased gradually over the subsequent year for patients who exhibit good to excellent initial response to ASIT after 6 months to 1 year. For example, if a cat's allergies are controlled and it is receiving an injection once every 3 weeks, the frequency of the injections should be reduced to once every 4 weeks for several months. If the cat's allergies are still controlled for 1 year without any clinical signs attributable to allergy or a need for other medications, the injections should be discontinued and the patient should be monitored for recurrence of clinical signs.

RUSH ALLERGEN-SPECIFIC IMMUNOTHERAPY

RIT is a technique for advancing an allergic patient to a maintenance dose of an extract over a shorter period of time than that required for the traditional induction period.[10] Typically this is an 8-hour period compared with the several days or weeks that comprise the induction phase of ASIT. An effective and safe protocol for RIT has been reported for dogs and human beings.[10,15] Additionally, RIT in dogs is associated with a higher success rate than conventional ASIT.

A pilot study evaluated the safety of a RIT protocol for four feline atopic patients.[10] Rush immunotherapy is an exciting alternative for feline patients, because successful completion of the prolonged induction period associated with traditional ASIT requires client and patient compliance. Clients may give up during the induction period because of frustration, and cats may object to the injections when they are more frequent. Although the true impact of missed injections on the overall success rate of ASIT is unknown, missed injections may increase the failure rate and the incidence of adverse reactions.

Although this study showed that RIT is a feasible alternative in cats, the true incidence of adverse reactions has not been established in atopic feline patients. Multiple RIT protocols have been evaluated in a colony of cats with experimentally induced asthma to Bermuda grass. These study protocols have evaluated immunotherapy with nonadjuvanted Bermuda grass allergen (doses 20 to 200 µg), and with extract adjuvanted with CpG oligodeoxynucleotides (immunostimulatory DNA sequences).[5,11] Rush immunotherapy with Bermuda grass alone resulted in multiple adverse reactions. Localized swelling was observed around the injection sites in all seven cats in the study.[5] In the previously mentioned study, two of four cats experienced a localized injection site reaction that was noted several days after RIT.[10] Additional adverse events noted in the seven asthmatic cats included an increase in respiratory rate greater than 30 per cent above baseline ($n = 4$), increased rectal temperature greater than 39.7 °C ($n = 3$), vomiting ($n = 3$), heart rate increased greater than 30 per cent above baseline ($n = 2$), agitation ($n = 2$), and systemic anaphylaxis ($n = 1$). These reactions occurred in spite of premedication with diphenhydramine. The cat who experienced systemic anaphylaxis received two intranodal injections of allergen. This protocol was adjusted based on this response.[5] In the subsequent cats only one injection was administered intranodally, whereas in the previous pilot study all injections were administered subcutaneously. A study conducted in canine atopic patients resulted in an increased rate of adverse reactions when the injections were administered intradermally.[10] These two studies suggest that increased exposure of allergen to antigen-presenting cells located in larger numbers in the dermis and lymph node may result in a higher reaction rate.[13]

The cellular responses noted with RIT in this colony of cats with experimentally induced asthma have been promising. Cats receiving RIT had reduced numbers of eosinophils in bronchoalveolar lavage fluid (BALF). Additionally, serum Bermuda grass allergen-specific IgG was higher in cats treated with RIT than in the control group at months 1 and 3. It is theorized that IgG molecules become blocking antibodies, thereby preventing IgE from triggering an allergic cascade. Surprisingly, no difference in allergen-specific IgE levels was noted between groups over time. Changes identified in this group of cats are similar to those noted in human patients undergoing ASIT.[3,5,11]

PERFORMING RUSH IMMUNOTHERAPY

Prior to performing RIT in an atopic cat, the patient should be premedicated with an antihistamine and potentially a glucocorticoid. An intravenous catheter should be placed to permit emergency venous access. Patients undergoing RIT must be monitored very closely. Vital signs should be collected every 30 minutes at a minimum. Deviations in heart and respiratory rates greater than 30 per cent of baseline should prompt a delay of subsequent injections until vital sign returns to normal. Severe adverse reactions that are indicative of anaphylaxis (for example, extreme agitation, vomiting,

diarrhea, or collapse) are stopping points for RIT and require immediate therapeutic intervention. Attempts should be made to spread out the injection sites, because this may lessen the localized reactions noted previously. Once the final injection of the protocol has been administered, monitoring should continue for at least 2 hours in the hospital.[5,10] When RIT has been completed, the patient advances to the maintenance phase of ASIT in which an injection is administered once weekly.

The use of RIT holds great promise for feline patients by accelerating the response rate to therapy and by relieving the burden on the owner to administer injections reliably during the induction period of traditional ASIT. The previously mentioned studies have shown that RIT can not be performed without full disclosure of the potential risks, including death, to the owner. Rush immunotherapy should not be entered into lightly, and the patient must be monitored closely to ensure that all reactions are noted and addressed before becoming life-threatening.

CONCURRENT USE OF MEDICATIONS

The use of concurrent medications during the induction and maintenance phases of ASIT is controversial. There are no published data on the effect of concurrent medications on the success of ASIT in cats or dogs. Many patients are uncomfortable during the initial months of ASIT and require concurrent medications to maintain a good quality of life. In these cases the clinician may attempt to taper the medications required each month to assess the effects of ASIT on the patient. Concurrent medications may include antihistamines, glucocorticoids, or cyclosporine A, and each is discussed in greater detail in the following. It also is important to emphasize the need for treatment of secondary bacterial and yeast infections.

In human patients undergoing ASIT the concurrent administration of H_1 antihistamines resulted in an accelerated response to treatment. Administering an H_1 antihistamine is thought to result in the up-regulation of H_2 receptors, which have regulatory and suppressive effects. These effects are thought to result in enhanced peripheral T-cell tolerance and possible active suppression of the inflammatory or immune responses.[7] These are the desired immunomodulations stimulated by ASIT.

ANTIHISTAMINES

Antihistamines are H_1 receptor antagonists. Histamine released from activated mast cells binds endothelial cell H_1 receptors, resulting in edema, erythema, and inflammation. Blockade of H_1 receptors by antihistamines prevents the pruritus created by those effects of histamine.

Several antihistamines are recommended frequently for pruritic cats, including cetirizine, chlorpheniramine, clemastine, cyproheptadine, diphenhydramine, and hydroxyzine. Few studies of the efficacy, pharmacokinetics, or safety of antihistamines in cats have been performed; however, many feline patients benefit with no or few perceived adverse effects. Because patient response varies, several different antihistamines should be evaluated, each for a period of seven to 21 days. In the authors' experience, cetirizine and chlorpheniramine have been the most effective antihistamines for our feline patients.

Cetirizine often is recommended as effective, and recently has become available over the counter (Cetirizine hydrochloride, Zyrtec). Anecdotal dosing recommendations range from 5 to 10 mg/cat PO q12-24h. However, a recent pharmacokinetic study showed that a dose of 5 mg/cat (approximately 1 mg/kg) PO was well tolerated, and maintained plasma concentrations higher than those considered effective in human beings for 24 hours.[16] This study suggests that 5 mg PO q24h may be the appropriate dose for cetirizine in cats. No published studies were discovered regarding the efficacy of cetirizine for pruritus.

Chlorpheniramine dosed at 2 mg/cat PO q12h was reported to eliminate pruritus in 19 of 26 cats without significant side effects.[17] Another clinical trial showed that six of 11 cats who failed to respond to chlorpheniramine or a fatty acid supplement alone had an excellent response to the combination without adverse effects.[18] Therefore it has been suggested that the combination of an antihistamine and fatty acid supplement may produce superior antipruritic effects than either agent alone.

Clemastine was shown to be useful in controlling pruritus in five of 10 atopic cats at a dose of 0.67 mg/cat PO q12h.[19] Likewise, cyproheptadine, which has both antihistaminic and antiserotonergic activities, showed antipruritic effects in nine of 20 cats at 2 mg/cat PO q12h; however, eight of these nine cats also experienced adverse effects including polyphagia and behavior changes.[20] No published data were discovered regarding the use of diphenhydramine or hydroxyzine in cats, although these are recommended commonly in textbooks at the doses shown below (Table 33-3).

GLUCOCORTICOIDS

Systemic glucocorticoids are a commonly prescribed and generally effective therapy for managing feline pruritus. The authors prefer oral glucocorticoids to injectable treatment because of the increased flexibility in controlling the dose and resulting side effects. Although cats often are considered to have a high tolerance for glucocorticoids compared with dogs, serious and well-recognized adverse effects can occur, such as weight gain and diabetes mellitus. Therefore we prefer to exhaust all other medical options before turning to long-term glucocorticoids as a mainstay treatment for feline atopic dermatitis.

Oral glucocorticoids used in cats include dexamethasone, methylprednisolone, prednisolone, prednisone, and triamcinolone. Prednisolone is sometimes preferred over prednisone because there is some concern about the efficiency of feline hepatic conversion of prednisone to prednisolone, but no scientific documentation of this concern has been discovered. Oral regimens are determined by the needs of the patient, but consist of initial daily doses for several days following by progressive tapering of the dose and interval. For example, prednisolone might be given at 2.2 mg/kg PO q24h for 5 to 7 days, then tapered to q48h for another 7 to 10 days, and then decreased to 2.2 mg/kg PO twice weekly or 1.1 mg/kg PO q48h depending on clinical response. The specific dosing schedule is a product of the patient's response to treatment (improvement of pruritus), signs of adverse effects, and the veterinarian's clinical judgment. The goal is to use the lowest dose and longest dosing interval effective to control the clinical sign of pruritus. Close monitoring is recommended, including periodic serum blood chemistry panels and urinalyses, for any cat remaining on long-term oral glucocorticoid therapy. Combination therapy of an oral glucocorticoid and an oral antihistamine may have a steroid-sparing effect.

The most commonly employed injectable glucocorticoid treatment in cats is repositol methylprednisolone acetate (Depo-Medrol, Pfizer) given SQ or IM. Injections typically are dosed at 5 mg/kg or 20 mg/cat, and should be given no more frequently than every 8 to 12 weeks. Glucocorticoid injections often are the preferred treatment in cats who are difficult to medicate orally; however, injectable therapy is more likely than controlled oral treatment to create significant adverse effects. One study showed that a single injection of 5 mg/kg repositol methylprednisolone causes plasma volume expansion secondary to glucocorticoid-mediated hyperglycemia.[21] That study concluded that methylprednisolone administration may predispose cats with cardiovascular disorders and impaired compensatory mechanisms to congestive heart failure. Another report, derived from different data collected from the same cats, showed significant serum biochemical changes in some cats, with individual variability.[22] Iatrogenic hyperadrenocorticism has been

Table 33-3 Antihistamines

Antihistamine	Common Dose	Reported Adverse Effects
Cetirizine HCl	5 mg/cat PO q24h	None reported
Chlorpheniramine maleate	2-4 mg/cat PO q12h	Drowsiness
Clemastine fumarate	0.68 mg/cat PO q12h	Diarrhea, lethargy
Cyproheptadine HCl	2-8 mg/cat PO q12h	Polyphagia, sedation, behavioral changes, vomiting
Diphenhydramine HCl	0.5 mg/kg PO q12h	Hyperexcitability
Hydroxyzine HCl	5-10 mg/cat PO q12h	Depression, behavioral changes

reported in a cat who received 20 mg methylprednisolone subcutaneously weekly for 4 weeks.[23] In another case report, a cat who had received 8 mg (3.3 mg/kg) triamcinolone acetonide subcutaneously three times over a 4-month period was shown to have dermatological changes consistent with iatrogenic Cushing's syndrome as well as a steroid hepatopathy.[24]

CYCLOSPORINE

Cyclosporine is a calcineurin inhibitor that prevents the allergic immune response by blocking T-cell activation, cytokine production, and mast cell and eosinophil degranulation. It is licensed for use in dogs with canine atopic dermatitis and has been shown to be effective in controlling pruritus, but it is not licensed for use in cats. Nevertheless, cyclosporine is used frequently in cats with good results. Cyclosporine has two formulations—modified and unmodified. Only the modified form should be used because of increased absorption.

Cyclosporine is administered to atopic cats at a dose of 5 mg/kg PO q24h for 4 weeks. If the cat is responding well at the end of that time, the dose is decreased to q48h and tapered further to twice weekly based on clinical response. The authors recommend baseline laboratory evaluation including complete blood count, serum chemistry profile, serological tests for feline immunodeficiency virus and feline leukemia virus, and serum titers for *Toxoplasma gondii* prior to starting treatment. Complete blood counts and serum chemistry profiles should be repeated no less often than every 6 months during cyclosporine therapy. Many patients receive great clinical benefit from the medication, and it is particularly useful when corticosteroid avoidance is preferred.

Few studies have been published evaluating the efficacy of cyclosporine in atopic cats; however, the existing reports demonstrate that cyclosporine can be beneficial in reducing pruritus in allergic cats.[25,26] In a double-blind, randomized, prednisolone-controlled study, there was no significant difference in the reduction of pruritus or improvement of lesions between cats treated with cyclosporine 5 mg/kg PO q24h for 28 days, and those treated with prednisolone 1 mg/kg PO q24h.[27] Adverse effects generally are mild and include vomiting and diarrhea; however, fatal systemic toxoplasmosis has been reported in cats receiving cyclosporine.[28,29]

The effects of cyclosporine with concurrent ASIT are unknown. It has been suggested that cyclosporine may support or interfere with the suspected mechanisms of successful immunotherapy.[30]

REFERENCES

1. Bettenay SV: Feline atopy. In Bonagura J, editor: *Kirk's current veterinary therapy XIII*, Philadelphia, 2000, Saunders, p 564.
2. Olivery T, editor: ACVD task force on canine atopic dermatitis, *Vet Immunol Immunopathol* 81:143, 2001.
3. Crameri R: Allergy diagnosis, allergen repertoires and their implications for allergen specific immunotherapy, *Immunol Allergy Clin North Am* 26:179, 2006.
4. Trimmer AM: Feline immunotherapy, *Clin Tech Small Anim Pract* 21:157, 2006.
5. Reinero CR, Byerly JR, Berghaus RD, et al: Rush immunotherapy in an experimental model of feline allergic asthma, *Vet Immunol Immunopathol* 110:141, 2006.
6. Verhagen J, Blaser K, Akidis CA, et al: Mechanisms of allergen-specific immunotherapy: T-regulatory cells and more, *Immunol Allergy Clin North Am* 26:207, 2006.
7. Jutel M, Blaser K, Akidis CA: Histamine receptors in immune regulation and allergen specific immunotherapy, *Immunol Allergy Clin North Am* 26:245, 2006.
8. Halliwell REW: Efficacy of hyposensitization in feline allergic diseases based upon results of in vitro testing for allergen-specific immunoglobulin E, *J Am Anim Hosp Assoc* 33:282, 1997.
9. Reedy LN: Results of allergy testing and hyposensitization in selected feline skin diseases, *J Am Anim Hosp Assoc* 18:618, 1982.
10. Trimmer AM, Griffin CG, Boord MJ, et al: Rush allergen specific immunotherapy protocol in feline atopic dermatitis: a pilot study, *Vet Derm* 16:324, 2005.
11. Reinero CR, Cohn LA, Delgado C, et al: Adjuvanted rush immunotherapy using CpG oligodeoxynucleotides in experimental feline allergic asthma, *Vet Immunol Immunopathol* 121:241, 2008.
12. Schleifer SG, Willemse T: Evaluation of skin test reactivity to environmental allergens in healthy cats and cats with atopic dermatitis, *Am J Vet Res* 64:773, 2003.
13. Novak N: Targeting dendritic cells in allergen immunotherapy, *Immunol Allergy Clin North Am* 26:307, 2006.
14. Foster AP, O'Dair H: Allergy testing for skin disease in the cat: in vivo vs in vitro tests, *Vet Derm* 4:111, 1993.
15. Bettenay SV, Mueller RS: Evaluation of the safety of an abbreviated course of injections of allergen extracts (rush immunotherapy) for the treatment of dogs with atopic dermatitis, *Am J Vet Res* 62:307, 2001.
16. Papich MG, Schooley EK, Reinero CR: Pharmacokinetics of cetirizine in healthy cats, *Am J Vet Res* 69:670, 2008.
17. Miller WH Jr, Scott DW: Efficacy of chlorpheniramine maleate for management of pruritus in cats, *J Am Vet Med Assoc* 197:67, 1990.
18. Scott DW, Miller WH: The combination of antihistamine (chlorpheniramine) and an omega-3/omega-6 fatty acid-containing product for the management of pruritic cats: results of an open clinical trial, *N Z Vet J* 43:29, 1995.
19. Miller WH Jr, Scott DW: Clemastine fumarate as an antipruritic agent in pruritic cats: results of an open clinical trial, *Can Vet J* 35:502, 1994.
20. Scott DW, Rothstein E, Beningo KE, et al: Observations on the use of cyproheptadine hydrochloride as an antipruritic agent in allergic cats, *Can Vet J* 39:634, 1998.
21. Ployngam T, Tobias AH, Smith SA, et al: Hemodynamic effects of methylprednisolone acetate administration in cats, *Am J Vet Res* 67:587, 2006.
22. Sharkey LC, Ployngam T, Tobias AH, et al: Effects of a single injection of methylprednisolone acetate on serum biochemical parameters in 11 cats, *Vet Clin Pathol* 36:184, 2007.
23. Ferasin L: Iatrogenic hyperadrenocorticism in a cat following a short therapeutic course of methylprednisolone acetate, *J Feline Med Surg* 3:87, 2001.
24. Schaer M, Ginn PE: Iatrogenic Cushing's syndrome and steroid hepatopathy in a cat, *J Am Anim Hosp Assoc* 35:48, 1999.
25. Noli C, Scarampella F: Prospective open pilot study on the use of cyclosporin for feline allergic skin disease, *J Small Anim Pract* 47:434, 2006.

26. Vercelli A, Raviri G, Cornegliani L: The use of oral cyclosporin to treat feline dermatoses: a retrospective analysis of 23 cases, *Vet Dermatol* 17:201, 2006.

27. Wisselink MA, Willemse T: The efficacy of cyclosporine A in cats with presumed atopic dermatitis: a double blind, randomised prednisolone-controlled study, *Vet J* 180:55, 2009.

28. Barrs VR, Martin P, Beatty JA: Antemortem diagnosis and treatment of toxoplasmosis in two cats on cyclosporin therapy, *Aust Vet J* 84:30, 2006.

29. Last RD, Suzuki Y, Manning T, et al: A case of fatal systemic toxoplasmosis in a cat being treated with cyclosporin A for feline atopy, *Vet Dermatol* 15:194, 2006.

30. Robson DC, Burton GG: Cyclosporin: applications in small animal dermatology, *Vet Dermatol* 14:1, 2003.

34 Methicillin-Resistant Staphylococci

Daniel O. Morris

ETIOLOGY OF STAPHYLOCOCCAL INFECTIONS

Bacteria of the genus *Staphylococcus* are gram positive, facultatively anaerobic cocci that exist as part of the normal cutaneous and mucosal microflora of mammals and birds. Many staphylococcal species also are opportunistic pathogens capable of causing serious infections of the skin and other body tissues and cavities.[1,2] When cutaneous or systemic disease disrupts the skin's surface defense mechanisms, skin infection (pyoderma) or otitis externa may result from these same staphylococcal species. Invasive infections involving the genitourinary tract, respiratory tract, joints, and body cavities also may result either from ascension along epithelial tracts, introduction via penetrating wounds, or hematogenous spread.

Although the coagulase-negative staphylococci are receiving renewed attention with regard to their medical importance,[3,4] it is the coagulase-positive species that have long been considered to be the important pathogens in veterinary medicine. Although both groups have been isolated from healthy feline skin and from cats with skin lesions, reports of pathogenic coagulase-negative staphylococci in cats remain rare.[5]

The coagulase-positive species that normally colonize the skin of the domestic cat are *Staphylococcus intermedius* and *Staphylococcus aureus*, although there is disagreement in the veterinary literature regarding which is dominant, and this factor may vary by geographical region.[6-9] *S. aureus* also is the primary species colonizing human skin, and some investigators have suggested that feline carriage of *S. aureus* is reflective of human-to-cat transmission.

S. intermedius was first recognized as a species distinct from *S. aureus* in the mid-1980s, and the phylogenetic structure and nomenclature of *S. intermedius* has changed again as a result of advances in molecular characterization.[10,11] The *S. intermedius* group (SIG) is now comprised of three genetically demonstrable species: *S. intermedius*, *S. pseudintermedius*, and *S. delphinii*, each of which occupy distinct ecological niches.[10] The primary canine pathogen is now known to be *S. pseudintermedius*, and this is likely to be the case for cats as well. However, for discussion purposes the author uses the nomenclature common to the feline literature, keeping in mind that most reports on *S. intermedius* prior to late 2007 are likely to refer in actuality to *S. pseudintermedius*.

Finally, *Staphylococcus hyicus* and *Staphylococcus schleiferi* also have been isolated from the skin of healthy cats and from cats with skin lesions.[5] *S. schleiferi* is a coagulase-variable species, with both coagulase-positive and negative subspecies. *S. schleiferi* subsp. *coagulans* is thought to be the primary subspecies occurring in dogs, in whom it causes infections that are commonly associated with prior antibiotic use.[12,13] In human beings it is the coagulase-negative variant (*S. schleiferi* subsp. *schleiferi*) that has been shown to be most commonly pathogenic, causing postsurgical skin and soft-tissue infections.[14] Isolation of either subspecies of *S. schleiferi* from cats remains exceedingly rare[5] and will not be considered further in this text. However, principles discussed for other staphylococcal species apply to *S. schleiferi* as well.

ETIOLOGY OF METHICILLIN RESISTANCE

Since the inception of antibiotic use in the practice of modern medicine, staphylococci have evolved in response to the presence of antimicrobial drugs in their environments. Currently all staphylococcal species that infect human beings and domestic animals exhibit some degree of antimicrobial resistance.[15,16] Even nonpathogenic staphylococci harbor drug resistance factors that can be transferred to pathogenic species. In human medicine, methicillin resistance (MR) in *S. aureus* has contributed to the scope of multiple drug resistance (MDR) since the early 1960s, whereas MR in staphylococci of feline origin has been recognized as a serious and widespread problem only within the past decade.

Methicillin and oxacillin are members of a class of antibacterial agents known as the semisynthetic penicillinase-resistant penicillins (SSPRP). Because of its superior stability in vitro, oxacillin is now used by most microbiology laboratories as the surrogate for testing the susceptibility of bacteria to this entire class of antibiotics.[16] Even so, the term *methicillin resistant* has persisted in the common vernacular and in most scientific publications. The SSPRP class was developed to circumvent staphylococcal resistance to the first generation penicillins, which is mediated by bacterial production of penicillinase enzymes. Although the SSPRP class is unaffected by penicillinases, it is susceptible to an acquired penicillinbinding protein (PBP), known as PBP2a or PBP2'. This staphylococcal PBP is encoded by the *mec*A gene, which confers an intrinsic resistance to all beta-lactam antibiotics and their derivatives (including all classes and generations of penicillins and cephalosporins).[17] Methicillin-resistant staphylococcal strains may express coresistance to any combination of other drug classes, including aminoglycosides, fluoroquinolones, macrolides, tetracyclines, fucidic acid, and mupirocin, in which case they are referred to as MDR. However, the mechanism of resistance is distinct for each of these antimicrobial classes (i.e., owing to mechanisms other than PBP).

EPIDEMIOLOGY

METHICILLIN-RESISTANT *STAPHYLOCOCCUS AUREUS* (MRSA)

Since the early 1960s the incidence of MR has escalated within human hospital strains of *S. aureus*, and hospital-acquired methicillin-resistant *S. aureus* (HA-MRSA) now has become the most prevalent pathogen causing nosocomial infections of people throughout the world.[18] More recently MRSA strains that cause skin and soft tissue infections in people with no known nosocomial risk factors have arisen de novo within the community.[18,19] The proliferation of these community-acquired (CA-MRSA) strains has been global, and although variations exist according to geographic area and ethnic populations, at least half of the persons colonized with MRSA in the United States now carry CA-MRSA strains.[20]

The population biology of MRSA has been studied extensively, and it has been determined that several international epidemic clones exist, resulting from the horizontal transmission of the *mec*A gene, which encodes methicillin resistance.[20] The *mec*A gene is a small part of a much larger genetic element that is integrated precisely into the *S. aureus* chromosome. This staphylococcal chromosome cassette *mec* (SCC*mec*) varies in size but always

contains the *mec*A gene. Five prototypic forms of SCC*mec* (I-V) have now been defined, and although the same types often are associated with divergent clonal lineages, particular clones have been shown to be associated with single SCC*mec* elements.[21] SCC*mec* types I, II, and III typically are associated with HA-MRSA strains, whereas SCC*mec* types IV and V typically are identified in CA-MRSA cases.[22] Recently CA-MRSA strains have been displacing the "traditional" nosocomial strains within some hospitals, and HA-MRSA strains have migrated into community settings.[18] Therefore the term *health-care associated* (HCA)–MRSA may be used to describe hospital strains that have spread into the community and caused subsequent community-onset infections. These may be mistaken for "true" CA-MRSA based on patient demographics and inadequate molecular and epidemiological data.[23]

Although the prevalence of nasal colonization by MRSA in the U.S. population has been estimated most recently to be 1.5 per cent,[23a] the proportion of *S. aureus* infections that are methicillin resistant has been reported to be as high as 72 per cent among local community-onset cases.[20] Risk factors associated with transmission of CA-MRSA include crowded living conditions and shared bathing facilities (e.g., military ships, prisons, day cares, sports teams, residential facilities). Risk factors for HA-MRSA transmission include immunosuppressive conditions, invasive medical instrumentation, surgery, and hospitalization. These epidemiological definitions do not appear to be globally applicable to animal MRSA cases (see the following).

Although rates of human MRSA infection have been monitored closely for several decades, the prevalence of MRSA infections in domestic animals is difficult to estimate. A retrospective analysis of pets presented to the author's institution during the 24-month period of January 1, 2003 through December 30, 2004, showed that MRSA infection occurred with equal prevalence (one case per 1000 admissions) in dogs and cats.[24] Overall the proportion of feline *S. aureus* infection isolates exhibiting MR was 28 per cent. However, it should be noted that the prevalence of resistance reported in this study is likely to be higher than in more general patient populations, as a result of referral bias and case selection bias (for bacterial culture) by specialist clinicians.

METHICILLIN-RESISTANT *S. INTERMEDIUS* (MRSI)/*S. PSEUDINTERMEDIUS* (MRSP)

In recent years, MRSI has emerged as a clinically important pathogen that causes treatment-resistant infections of dogs and cats.[24,25] Like MRSA strains, phenotypic resistance of *S. intermedius* isolates to methicillin has been shown to be mediated by penicillin-binding protein 2a, which is encoded by a *mec*A gene.[26] Also, as observed with HA-MRSA strains (see the following), most MRSI isolates coexpress resistance to other classes of antimicrobials, such as the fluoroquinolones, macrolides, tetracyclines, and aminoglycosides.[24,25] For the first-generation fluoroquinolones in particular, the disparity in resistance between MRSI and methicillin-susceptible *S. intermedius*

(MSSI) is striking, where only 55 to 57 per cent of MRSI isolates were susceptible to enrofloxacin and marbofloxacin respectively, whereas 98.5 per cent of MSSI isolates maintained susceptibility to both.[24]

Because human MRSA isolates have a clonal population structure and global dissemination has occurred, it has been hypothesized that MRSI isolates also would be highly clonal. A recent study of the population genetic structure of *S. intermedius* isolates by multilocus sequence typing showed that all previously identified MRSI were actually of the *S. pseudintermedius* phylotype, and were highly clonal.[10] These isolates had been obtained from several countries, including the United States, Canada, Japan, United Kingdom, and several other European Union nations. Additionally, sequencing of the *mec*A gene revealed a high degree of homology (95 to 100 per cent) with the *mec*A gene of *S. aureus*, suggesting horizontal transfer of the gene. The structure of the MR-*S. pseudintermedius* phylogenetic tree suggests that the *mec*A gene has been received by this staphylococcal species on multiple occasions on several different continents.[10]

PATHOGENESIS

In human beings most CA-MRSA strains have maintained antimicrobial susceptibility profiles comparable to methicillin-sensitive *S. aureus* (MSSA), with the obvious exception of resistance to beta lactams. However, HA-MRSA strains commonly express resistance to several other classes of antimicrobial agents, which likely has resulted from selective pressure exerted by antimicrobial use in health care facilities.[18,26] The broad antimicrobial resistance patterns inherent to HA-MRSA contribute significantly to the morbidity and mortality associated with human nosocomial MRSA infection. Meta-analyses of *S. aureus* bacteremia and surgical site infections in people have demonstrated that methicillin resistance is associated independently with increased length of hospital stay, hospital charges, and mortality, compared with MSSA infections.[27] Although CA-MRSA strains generally exhibit less multidrug resistance than health care–associated (HA-MRSA) strains, some CA-MRSA strains express virulence factors, such as necrolytic toxins and super antigen production, that HA-MRSA do not.[22] These virulence factors increase their pathogenicity in otherwise healthy persons, and may produce characteristic clinical signs, such as cutaneous abscesses and necrotizing hemorrhagic pneumonia.

An association between MRSA infection, subcutaneous abscesses, and lymphadenitis has been reported in a series of feline surgical biopsy specimens.[28] Ozaki and colleagues reported a histological pattern that included central abscesses with colonies of bacterial cocci, surrounded by collagenous granulation tissue and prominent eosinophilic inflammation. In 15 of 17 cases tested, gram-positive cocci were positive for PBP2′ using an immunohistochemical technique. A retrospective study by the author and colleagues hypothesized that MRSA infection would affect a different population of cats, produce more severe clinical signs, and carry a less favorable prognosis than MSSA infection.[29] However, the results did not indicate a discernible difference in signalment, clinical signs, or outcomes between the two groups, despite all isolates being SCC*mec* Type II (HA-MRSA) strains. The authors also documented three cases with lymph node pathology similar to that reported by Ozaki, but all three were associated with culture-confirmed MSSA infections, suggesting that this inflammatory pattern may represent an unusual response to *S. aureus* in general, rather than a specific response to MRSA. Caution is advised in interpreting these data because of the relatively low number of MRSA cases and lack of complete records for several animals.

TRANSMISSION

In recent years individual case reports and small case series have been published that suggest that transmission of MRSA from human beings to pet animals (zooanthroponosis) has occurred.[30] More rarely, reports have suggested that MRSA-infected or colonized animals have passed the organism back to people (reciprocal zooanthroponosis). For example, a cluster outbreak of MRSA cases in a nursing home was linked to a colonized cat who served as the facility mascot.[31] Other than nontargeted and limited targeted surveillance of veterinary hospital personnel and animals, no published data regarding the prevalence of MRSA colonization within the general population of dogs and cats are available. Weese and colleagues reported recently that in households in which an MRSA-infected or colonized pet resided, at least one person in each household was positive for subclinical colonization. All MRSA isolated were Canadian epidemic MRSA strain 2, a strain type that has "escaped" from hospital settings and is now the predominant community-onset strain in Canada (known in the United States as strain USA 100).[32]

Among the household contacts of human patients with MRSA infection, a frequency of colonization of 14.5 per cent has been demonstrated.[33] Close contacts, defined as a spouse, parent, child, or caregiver, were at a 7.5-fold greater risk of carriage versus casual contacts (other individuals such as roommates, siblings, and friends). The person-pet relationship often will meet the criterion of close contact. Still, a study designed to assess the role of subclinical MRSA carriage in pets belonging to people with active infection has not been published, making it impossible to know how often colonized pets might be a "weak link" in control of recurrent/cyclical MRSA infections within human household members.

In regard to veterinary health care workers, prevalence studies have been conducted in small regional surveys.[34] Isolates of MRSA strains from pets and veterinary personnel often have been indistinguishable, suggesting some mode of cross-transmission (although directionality of transmission is entirely speculative). This has been true for both horses and small animals. In a veterinary teaching hospital the prevalence of MR staphylococcal colonization of feline and canine outpatients recently ranged from 13 to 19 per cent.[5,35] However, risk factors for colonization of pets and people have not been assessed systematically.

At the 2005 American College of Veterinary Internal Medicine Forum in Baltimore, 417 attendees consented to nasal swabbing for targeted MRSA surveillance.[34] Of these, 27 (6.5 per cent) were MRSA-positive, including 15 of the 96 (15.6 per cent) persons in large animal practice; 12 of the 271 (4.4 per cent) persons in small animal practice; and none of the 50 persons in industry or research. The strains isolated were dominated by two distinct clones. Large animal practitioners harbored a strain (known as USA 500) that is uncommon in people other than horse owners and people who work with horses. However, small animal practitioners harbored strain USA 100. In this study there was lower overall risk for small animal practitioners, although they were still colonized at a rate exceeding that estimated for the general population of the United States.[34]

Although the zoonotic potential of the SIG is not understood completely, *S. intermedius* generally is not considered to be a human pathogen. However, it has been reported to cause severe infections of human beings occasionally,[36,37] and evidence suggests that people may commonly harbor *S. intermedius* strains identical to those that infect their pets.[38] Additionally, MDR strains of *S. intermedius* have been isolated from owners of dogs presenting with deep pyoderma.[39] Perhaps of more concern than direct zoonosis of MRSI is the potential for horizontal transmission of the *mecA* gene from MRSI to susceptible strains of other *Staphylococcus* species. In such a case domestic pets could serve as reservoirs for dissemination of methicillin resistance. Longitudinal population-based cohort studies will be required to define the frequency of transmission and potential risk factors for cross-colonization and infection more accurately.

CLINICAL SIGNS

The clinical signs of feline MRSA or MRSI infection may include any of the possible pathogenic effects of staphylococcal infection. Because staphylococcal infection may occur in any organ or tissue, signs may span a very wide range. In the author's dermatology practice the most common presentations of feline staphylococcal infection are otitis externa, facial acne, and surface pyoderma superimposed upon eosinophilic plaques and indolent lip ulcers. In a retrospective study conducted at the author's institution, the majority of *S. aureus* infections were of deep soft tissues, fluids, and body cavities, whereas *S. intermedius* infections were predominantly of the skin and external ear canals. The overwhelming majority of both MRSA and MRSI isolates were MDR, exhibiting resistance to at least three classes of antibiotics in addition to oxacillin.[24]

DIAGNOSIS

The Clinical Laboratories Standards Institute (CLSI) is the organization in the United States that instructs clinical laboratories on standard procedures and reporting protocols. The CLSI classifies antimicrobial agents into four groups, A to D.[40] Compounds in Groups A to C may be reported routinely or selectively as determined by the laboratory, in consultation with veterinarians. Selective reporting should help to improve the clinical relevance of reports and rational antimicrobial use by practitioners, so as to minimize the selection of multidrug-resistant strains by overuse of broad-spectrum agents. Selective reporting is controversial among veterinarians, as is the use of some drugs (e.g., linezolid for MRSA or MRSI), because these drugs have major implications for successful treatment of life-threatening staphylococcal infections of human beings.

The minimum inhibitory concentration (MIC) is the lowest concentration of an antimicrobial that inhibits bacterial growth in vitro. This does not always equate to clinical effect, because of potential issues with drug absorption and distribution to tissues in individual patients. The CLSI publishes MIC breakpoints for reporting by microbiology laboratories, for all appropriate microbe-drug combinations.[40] Again, selective reporting may limit the repertoire of drugs listed on reports for clinicians. For example, many laboratories will not report linezolid susceptibility for staphylococci of veterinary origin.

Broth microdilution plates include a range of antibiotic concentrations in accordance with CLSI breakpoints. When growth occurs in all wells, the MIC is reported as greater than the highest concentration in the plate (e.g., for *S. aureus*, oxacillin >2 μg/dL), and these isolates are resistant to the drug. When no growth occurs in any of the wells, the MIC is reported as *less than or equal to* the lowest concentration in the plate (e.g., for *S. aureus*, oxacillin <0.25 μg/dL) and these isolates are susceptible to the drug. An absolute value is shown when the MIC falls within the range of drug concentrations in the plate (e.g., for *S. aureus*, oxacillin = 1 μg/dL). These isolates may be either resistant or susceptible depending on the MIC, so an interpretation is always given.

Many laboratories continue to use the disc diffusion (Kirby Bauer) method for bacterial susceptibility testing. This method gives a qualitative approximation of an antibiotic's effect by measuring how well it inhibits bacterial growth on solid culture media. The zone of growth inhibition is measured in millimeters and the zone size is interpreted and reported as susceptible, intermediate, or resistant (as derived from standardized regression curves) based on CLSI guidelines. The method used for susceptibility testing is less important than the laboratory's adherence to standardized protocols, and the disc diffusion method is entirely acceptable in a clinical setting although many researchers and clinicians prefer MICs. Regardless, clinicians should communicate with the laboratory manager to ensure that CLSI guidelines have been adopted into the laboratory's standard operating procedures, and to determine which packaging and shipping protocols the laboratory prefers for different types of specimens (e.g., fluids, tissues, swabs). Veterinary microbiology laboratories generally will be more familiar with the animal pathogens that are not common in human beings (e.g., *S. intermedius* and *S. schleiferi*), although medical microbiology laboratories can serve veterinary clientele well in most cases. Again, communication with laboratory personnel is essential.

TREATMENT

Despite the reported escalation of MR in staphylococci of veterinary origin, the majority of staphylococcal strains residing on cats continue to be susceptible to most classes of antibiotics, including the beta-lactams.[5] Therefore empirical therapy of first-time skin and soft-tissue infections with "cat friendly" drugs, such as amoxicillin-clavulanic acid, first-generation cephalosporins, and clindamycin, continues to constitute acceptable practice. However, when clinical suspicion of antimicrobial resistance arises because of initial treatment failure, samples for culture and susceptibility testing should be collected as early in the therapeutic process as possible. This is especially important because even ineffective antimicrobial therapy may continue to select for multiresistant strains. In particular, sequential empirical therapies should no longer be considered the standard for recurrent urinary tract infections, recurrent pyoderma, and non-healing wounds.

Antimicrobial susceptibility to other (non–beta-lactam) drugs is nearly impossible to predict in MR staphylococcal isolates. Clindamycin and the fluoroquinolones are rarely wise choices in cats because of the high prevalence of resistance in MRSA and MRSI strains.[24,25] In fact, there is evidence that the use of fluoroquinolones may provoke enhanced resistance to methicillin in *S. aureus* isolates, suggesting that early diagnosis can be essential to a positive chemotherapeutic outcome.[41] Conversely, potentiated sulfa drugs continue to be effective against the majority of MRSA and MRSI strains,[24,25] and these drugs have a high margin of safety in cats. Therefore the author will often initiate therapy with trimethoprim-sulfadiazine while culture results are pending.

The most problematic therapeutic decisions come when an isolate is resistant to all drug classes discussed in the preceding. Fortunately even MDR strains of MRSA and MRSI have maintained a high prevalence of susceptibility to chloramphenicol and amikacin, although each of these drugs presents its own challenges owing to cumbersome dosing regimens and/or concerning toxicity profiles. The author strongly recommends that clinicians consult a veterinary pharmacology resource for dosing protocols, pharmacotoxicology information, and potential interactions with coadministered drugs before prescribing oral chloramphenicol or amikacin (subcutaneously) for cats.

Topical amikacin is often effective for otic infections, whereas polymyxin-B is effective for *S. intermedius* only (*S. aureus* is inherently resistant to polymyxin-B). In the United States commercial otic products containing these ingredients are not available, so they must be compounded.[42] For localized pyoderma, such as facial acne and eosinophilic lesions with surface infection, fusidic acid (not available in the United States) and 2 per cent mupirocin (Bactroban, GlaxoSmithKline and generics) are reasonable choices, although resistance has arisen in some MRSA strains. For more regional or generalized pyoderma, benzoyl peroxide (author's preference) or chlorhexidine shampoos can be quite helpful, but topical antimicrobials generally are incapable of clearing deep pyodermas, such as abscesses and wound infections, when used for monotherapy.

Finally, vancomycin (intravenous) and linezolid (orally) continue to be mainstays for therapy of multiresistant MRSA infections of human beings, many of which may be disfiguring or life-threatening. As such their use in animals is highly controversial. Because vancomycin requires intravenous administration and is a potent nephrotoxin, its use in cats would rarely be pursued. Linezolid may be administered orally and therefore is an attractive option to some clinicians. Although the astronomical cost of the drug and lack of pharmacodynamic data in pets should help to minimize its use in cats, such use has been reported anecdotally. However, the ethical considerations of using the "last resort" drug for human therapy begs a lengthy (and likely emotional) discussion among veterinarians and the healthcare community at large. The author's institution currently enforces a policy prohibiting use of linezolid in animal patients.

An interesting frontier for future studies is the use of strain-specific bacteriophage therapy.[43] Bacteriophages (phages) are viruses that infect and lyse bacteria; they have no pathogenic effect on mammalian or plant cells. Phages are ubiquitous in the environment, such that human beings and animals are exposed to them routinely at high levels through food and water without adverse effect. Some phages are approved by the U.S. Food and Drug Administration (FDA) for use as food additives. These phages specifically target bacterial species that may cause contamination of human foods (e.g., *Listeria* spp. in the production of retail meats and cheeses).[44] Phages are classified by the FDA as GRAS (Generally Recognized as Safe) for human consumption. Although phages are not approved for use as alternatives to antibiotics for the treatment of human bacterial infections, they have been used extensively for this purpose in Russia and eastern European countries, where significant safety data have accrued. A clinical trial to assess the ability of anti-MRSA phages to clear subclinical colonization of dogs and cats is in the planning stage.

MANAGEMENT

In the case of MDR bacteria, management refers not only to treatment of the infected patient, but also to reduction of risk for transmission within hospital/clinic settings and the community (including the home environment). Risk reduction, in the ideal scenario, would involve identification and isolation of all infected *and colonized* individuals (via surveillance cultures), and use of contact or barrier nursing precautions in handling both patient groups. In regard to nosocomial transmission, the subclinical colonization of healthcare workers can be a weak link, because of the obvious risk of transmission to immunocompromised patients. However, contamination of clothing (including gloves and gowns), medical equipment, and the environment all have been clearly implicated in transmission between patients as well. This appears to be true also in veterinary hospitals. A report of nosocomial transmission in a small animal intensive care unit has illustrated the utility of patient screening and barrier precautions in small animal care settings, once an index case has been identified.[45] These measures were successful in arresting the outbreak, but might be impractical in many general practice settings.

Decolonization of nasal carriers has been a major challenge in human medicine for several decades. Regimens generally involve the use of nasal mupirocin coupled with antiseptic baths, because other body sites also may be colonized. Attempts at decolonization generally are performed in healthcare workers only in the context of nosocomial outbreaks. Family members of persons (especially pediatric patients) with recurrent MRSA infection occurring within the home also may undergo decolonization therapy. In healthcare workers, recolonization occurs in 17 to 48 per cent within 4 weeks to 6 months.[46] The rise in mupirocin resistance among MRSA strains and the need for environmental decontamination within the home also are factors that may confound success. Regardless, veterinary healthcare workers who are concerned about their personal status and potential nosocomial transmission to their animal patients should seek advice from a physician specializing in infectious disease medicine.

Potential regimens for decolonization/suppression of MRSA in pets have not been explored in an organized manner, and before such attempts can be advocated, longitudinal studies of the duration of pet colonization are warranted. Because dogs are not ideal hosts for *S. aureus* colonization,[35] it could be that longitudinal persistence in that species routinely will be short term, and this seems to be supported by anecdotal reports.[47] The potential situation for cats is even less clear, because up to 50 per cent of cats may harbor *S. aureus* naturally (within some geographic areas),[5] and MRSA nasal colonization in a kitten was documented to persist for 9 months.[45] In extreme circumstances systemic therapy[48,49] or topical (nasal) therapy[50] of colonized pets has been declared successful in breaking cyclical recurrence in human patients, although these pets were not cultured at sites other than the nares to prove global bodily clearance. Studies of MR staphylococcal carriage sites in dogs and cats suggest that nasal therapy alone is likely to be futile, because there were no differences in carriage between nares, oral cavity, anus, groin, and hair/skin of the cranium.[5,35] Regardless, it is the author's strongly held opinion that systemic antibiotics for colonized pets should be discouraged in favor of barrier precautions or isolation from other susceptible pets and people in the household.

For pet owners, as well as attending veterinary staff, barrier precautions should include covering of wounds and avoidance of contact with exudates; use of protective disposable gloves; scrupulous hand hygiene procedures after each patient contact (including glove changes); daily washing of food and water dishes and laundering of pet bedding; and complete restriction of the pet from beds and furniture. Immunocompromised persons, and those with a personal history of MRSA infection, should not be involved in wound care or grooming of a pet harboring MRSA or MRSI infection. The British Small Animal Veterinary Association has posted very helpful guidelines on the World Wide Web.[51]

In human hospitals where MRSA prevalence exceeds 5 to 10 per cent, surveillance cultures and patient isolation/cohort nursing can be expected to be cost effective. Such measures actually are highly cost effective compared with universal gowning/gloving as the primary control mechanism.[46] Because of the comparative rarity of nosocomial MRSA and MRSI transmission in veterinary hospitals, such continuous surveillance measures are very unlikely to be cost effective, and will remain research tools until more concrete data can be collected. In the meantime practices should be targeted toward reducing transmission of MDR bacteria between veterinary staff and animals by excellent hand hygiene, barrier precautions, and (when possible) cohort nursing practices within veterinary care facilities.

REFERENCES

1. Patel A: Bacterial pyoderma. In August JR, editor: *Consultations in feline internal medicine*, vol 5, St. Louis, 2006, Saunders, p 251.
2. Kloos WE, Musselwhite MS: Distribution and persistence of *Staphylococcus* and *Micrococcus* species and other aerobic bacteria on human skin, *Appl Microbiol* 30:381, 1975.
3. Huebner J, Goldmann DA: Coagulase-negative staphylococci: role as pathogens, *Annu Rev Med* 50:223, 1999.
4. Patel A, Lloyd DH, Howell SA, et al: Investigation into the potential pathogenicity of *Staphylococcus felis* in a cat, *Vet Rec* 150:668, 2002.
5. Abraham JL, Morris DO, Griffeth GC, et al: Surveillance of healthy cats and cats with inflammatory skin disease for colonization of the skin by methicillin-resistant coagulase-positive staphylococci and *Staphylococcus schleiferi* ssp. *schleiferi*, *Vet Dermatol* 18:252, 2007.
6. Lilenbaum W, Nunes ELC, Azeredo MAI: Prevalence and antimicrobial susceptibility of staphylococci isolated from the skin surface of clinically normal cats, *Lett Appl Microbiol* 27:224, 1998.
7. Lilenbaum W, Esteves AL, Souza GN: Prevalence and antimicrobial susceptibility of staphylococci isolated from saliva of clinically normal cats, *Lett Appl Microbiol* 28:448, 1999.
8. Patel A, Lloyd DH, Lamport AI: Antimicrobial resistance of feline staphylococci in south-eastern England, *Vet Dermatol* 10:257, 1999.
9. Igimi S, Atobe H, Tohya Y, et al: Characterization of the most frequently encountered *Staphylococcus* sp. in cats, *Vet Microbiol* 39:255, 1994.
10. Bannoehr J, Ben Zakour NL, Waller AS, et al: Population genetic structure of the *Staphylococcus intermedius* group: insights into *agr* diversification and emergence of methicillin-resistant strains, *J Bacteriol* 189:8685, 2007.
11. Sasaki T, Kikuchi K, Tanaka Y, et al: Reclassification of phenotypically identified *Staphylococcus intermedius* strains, *J Clin Microbiol* 45:2770, 2007.
12. Frank LA, Kania SA, Hnilica KA, et al: Isolation of *Staphylococcus schleiferi* from dogs with pyoderma, *J Am Vet Med Assoc* 222:451, 2003.
13. May ER, Hnilica KA, Frank LA, et al: Isolation of *Staphylococcus schleiferi* from healthy dogs and dogs with otitis, pyoderma, or both, *J Am Vet Med Assoc* 227:928, 2005.
14. Hernández JL, Calvo J, Sota R, et al: Clinical and microbiological characteristics of 28 patients with *Staphylococcus schleiferi* infection, *Eur J Clin Microbiol Infect Dis* 20:153, 2001.
15. Werckenthin C, Cardoso M, Martel JL, et al: Antimicrobial resistance in staphylococci from animals with particular

reference to bovine *S. aureus*, porcine *S. hyicus*, and canine *S. intermedius*, *Vet Res* 32:341, 2001.

16. Chambers HF: Methicillin resistance in *Staphylococci*: molecular and biochemical basis and clinical implications, *Clin Microbiol Rev* 10:781, 1997.

17. Berger-Bachi B, Rohrer S: Factors influencing methicillin resistance in staphylococci, *Arch Microbiol* 178:165, 2002.

18. Diederen BMW, Kluytmans JAJAW: The emergence of infections with community-associated methicillin resistant *Staphylococcus aureus*, *J Infect* 52:157, 2006.

19. King MD, Humphrey BJ, Wang YF, et al: Emergence of community-acquired methicillin-resistant *Staphylococcus aureus* USA 300 clone as the predominant cause of skin and soft-tissue infections, *Ann Intern Med* 144:309, 2006.

20. Graham PL, Lin SX, Larson EL: A U.S. population-based survey of *Staphylococcus aureus* colonization, *Ann Intern Med* 144:318, 2006.

21. McDougal LA, Steward CD, Killgore GE, et al: Pulsed-field gel electrophoresis typing of oxacillin-resistant *Staphylococcus aureus* isolates from the United States: establishing a national database, *J Clin Microbiol* 41:5113, 2003.

22. Fey PD, Said-Salim B, Rupp ME, et al: Comparative molecular analysis of community- or hospital-acquired methicillin-resistant *Staphylococcus aureus*, *Antimicrob Agents Chemother* 47:196, 2003.

23. Del Giudice P, Blanc V, Durupt F, et al: Emergence of two populations of methicillin-resistant *Staphylococcus aureus* with distinct epidemiological, clinical, and biological features, isolated from patients with community-acquired skin infections, *Br J Dermatol* 154:118, 2006.

23a. Gorwitz RJ, Kruszon-Moran D, McAllister SK, et al: Changes in the prevalence of nasal colonization with *Staphylococcus aureus* in the United States, 2001-2004, *J Infect Dis* 197:1226, 2008.

24. Morris DO, Rook KA, Shofer FS, et al: Screening of *Staphylococcus aureus*, *S. intermedius*, and *S. schleiferi* isolates obtained from small companion animals for antimicrobial resistance: a retrospective review of 749 isolates (2003-2004), *Vet Dermatol* 17:332, 2006.

25. Jones RD, Kania SA, Rohrbach BW, et al: Prevalence of oxacillin- and multidrug-resistant staphylococci in clinical samples from dogs: 1,772 samples (2001-2005), *J Am Vet Med Assoc* 230:221, 2007.

26. Bemis DA, Jones RD, Hiatt LE, et al: Comparison of tests to detect oxacillin resistance in *Staphylococcus intermedius*, *Staphylococcus schleiferi*, and *Staphylococcus aureus* isolates from canine hosts, *J Clin Microbiol* 44:3374, 2006.

27. Cosgrove SE, Qi Y, Kaye KS, et al: The impact of methicillin resistance in *Staphylococcus aureus* bacteremia on patient outcomes: mortality, length of stay, and hospital charges, *Infect Control Hosp Epidemiol* 26:166, 2005.

28. Ozaki K, Yamagami T, Nomura K, et al: Abscess-forming inflammatory granulation tissue with Gram-positive cocci and prominent eosinophilic infiltration in cats: possible infection of methicillin-resistant *Staphylococcus*, *Vet Pathol* 40:283, 2003.

29. Morris DO, Mauldin EA, O'Shea K, et al: Clinical, microbiological, and molecular characterization of methicillin-resistant *Staphylococcus aureus* infections of cats, *Am J Vet Res* 67:1421, 2006.

30. Weese JS: Methicillin-resistant *Staphylococcus aureus*: an emerging pathogen in small animals, *J Am Anim Hosp Assoc* 41:150, 2005.

31. Scott GM, Thomson R, Malone-Lee J, et al: Cross-infection between animals and man: possible feline transmission of *Staphylococcus aureus* infection in humans? *J Hosp Infect* 12:29, 1998.

32. Weese JS, Dick H, Willey BM, et al: Suspected transmission of methicillin-resistant *Staphylococcus aureus* between domestic pets and humans in veterinary clinics and in the household, *Vet Microbiol* 115:148, 2006.

33. Calfee DP, Durbin LJ, Germanson TP, et al: Spread of methicillin-resistant *Staphylococcus aureus* (MRSA) amongst household contacts of individuals with nosocomially acquired MRSA, *Infect Control Hosp Epidemiol* 24:422, 2003.

34. Hanselman BA, Kruth SA, Rousseau J, et al: Methicillin-resistant *Staphylococcus aureus* colonization in veterinary personnel, *Emerg Infect Dis* 12:1933, 2006.

35. Griffeth GC, Morris DO, Abraham JL, et al: Screening for skin carriage of methicillin-resistant coagulase-positive staphylococci and *Staphylococcus schleiferi* in dogs with healthy and inflamed skin, *Vet Dermatol* 19:142, 2008.

36. Mahoudeau I, Delabranche X, Prevost G, et al: Frequency of isolation of *Staphylococcus intermedius* from humans, *J Clin Microbiol* 35:2153, 1997.

37. Pottumarthy S, Schapiro JM, Prentice JL, et al: Clinical isolates of *Staphylococcus intermedius* masquerading as methicillin-resistant *Staphylococcus aureus*, *J Clin Microbiol* 42:5881, 2004.

38. Goodacre R, Harvey R, Howell SA, et al: An epidemiological study of *Staphylococcus intermedius* strains from dogs, their owners and veterinary surgeons, *J Analyt App Pyrolysis* 44:49, 1997.

39. Guardabassi L, Loeber ME, Jacobson A: Transmission of multiple antimicrobial-resistant *Staphylococcus intermedius* between dogs affected by deep pyoderma and their owners, *Vet Microbiol* 98:23, 2004.

40. Clinical Laboratory Standards Institute: *Performance standards for antimicrobial disk and dilution susceptibility tests for bacteria isolated from animals: informational supplement. Document M31-S1*, Wayne, PA, 2004, National Committee for Clinical Laboratory Standards.

41. Venezia RA, Domaracki BE, Evans AM, et al: Selection of high-level oxacillin resistance in heteroresistant *Staphylococcus aureus* by fluoroquinolone exposure, *J Antimicrob Chemother* 48:375, 2001.

42. Morris DO: Medical therapy of otitis externa and otitis media, *Vet Clin North Am Small Anim Pract* 34:541, 2004.

43. Hanlon GW: Bacteriophages: an appraisal of their role in the treatment of bacterial infections, *Int J Antimicrob Agents* 30:118, 2007.

44. Daniells S: *FDA approves viruses as food additive for meat.* http://www.foodnavigator-usa.com/news/ng.asp?id=70066-intralytix-bacteriophages-listeria-fda. 2006.

45. Weese JS, Dick H, Faires M, et al: Cluster of methicillin-resistant *Staphylococcus aureus* colonization in a small animal intensive care unit, *J Am Vet Med Assoc* 231:1361, 2007.

46. Muto CA, Jernigan JA, Ostrowsky BE: SHEA guidelines for preventing nosocomial transmission of multi-drug resistant strains of *Staphylococcus aureus* and *Enterococcus*, *Infect Control Hosp Epidemiol* 24:362, 2003.

47. Weese JS: Personal communication, February 2008.

48. Sing A, Tuschak C, Hormansdorfer S: Methicillin-resistant *Staphylococcus aureus* in a family and its pet cat, *N Engl J Med* 358:1200, 2008.

49. van Duijkeren E, Wolfhagen MJ, Box AT, et al: Human-to-dog transmission of methicillin-resistant *Staphylococcus aureus*, *Emerg Infect Dis* 10:2235, 2004.

50. Manian FA: Asymptomatic nasal carriage of mupirocin-resistant, methicillin-resistant *Staphylococcus aureus* (MRSA) in a pet dog associated with MRSA infection in household contacts, *Clin Infect Dis* 36:e26, 2003.

51. The British Small Animal Veterinary Association: *MRSA in animals—epidemiology and infection.* http://www.mrsainanimals.com/BSAVA.html. 2006

35 Acne

Edward Jazic

Acne is a common skin disease or reaction pattern of cats. The aim of this chapter is to describe the clinical and histopathological features of acne as well as to provide current therapeutic and management treatment strategies.

ETIOLOGY AND PATHOGENESIS

Acne is a disorder of follicular keratinization and is a well-recognized skin disease pattern in the cat.[1,2] The etiopathogenesis of acne is not understood. Unproven causal factors have included changes in the hair growth cycle, poor grooming habits, stress, underlying seborrheic predisposition, abnormal sebum production, immuno-suppression, and the effect of chronic viral infections.[1,3] In human beings acne is a multifactorial disease of the pilosebaceous unit (sebaceous glands, hair follicles), and factors such as the alterations in the pattern of follicular keratinization, excessive sebum production, and hormonal imbalances are believed to play important roles. In contrast to human beings, acne is not confined to adolescence in cats.[1,2,4] No breed predilections have been noted. There may be a gender predilection for neutered males.[2]

CLINICAL SIGNS

Mild, early cases of acne are characterized by the presence of comedones, scattered areas of dark crusts or keratinous debris, and mild alopecia (Figure 35-1). These lesions are located most commonly along the chin region, the lower lip, and occasionally the upper lip. At this stage most cats are asymptomatic. Some cats will remain in this comedonal stage and not progress to develop other signs. Other cats progressively begin to develop erythema, papules, pustules, alopecia, variable swelling, and pruritus (Figures 35-2 and 35-3). In more severe and chronic cases painful firm nodules will develop in conjunction with diffuse edema, thickening, fistulation, and eventual scarring (Figures 35-4 and 35-5).[1,2,4] Regional lymphadenopathy also may be prominent. Some cats can have so much pain that lethargy and anorexia ensue.

DIAGNOSIS

The diagnosis of "chin acne" is a clinical diagnosis. In the majority of cases of acne, the clinical diagnosis is straightforward and is based on the presence of classical lesions (comedones, keratinous debris, alopecia, papules) on the chin and lips. The major challenge faced by the clinician is to determine whether there is an underlying treatable cause.

Skin scrapings should be performed to rule out demodicosis. This may require sedation, depending on the degree of pain in the affected area. Cytological examination of the superficial skin and exudates should be performed to look for complicating bacterial and/or *Malassezia* infections. In cats with comedones, contents of the comedones should be examined cytologically; yeast organisms and/or demodectic mites may be found.[1,2] These parasites can be primary or contributing causes. In addition, appropriate specimens should be collected for a fungal culture to rule out dermatophytosis. If furunculosis is present, cytological examination of exudates and tissue culture is indicated to identify primary and secondary bacterial or fungal infections. The most commonly isolated bacteria from acne lesions in cats are coagulase-positive staphylococci and alpha-hemolytic streptococci.[2,3] Other organisms isolated less commonly include *Micrococcus* sp., *Pasteurella multocida*, and beta-hemolytic streptococci.[2,3] In human beings, *Propionibacterium acnes* is the principal organism involved with inflammatory acne lesions.

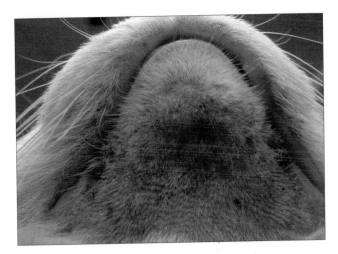

Figure 35-1 The hair has been clipped to provide better visualization of the mild erythema, comedones, and dark keratinous debris.

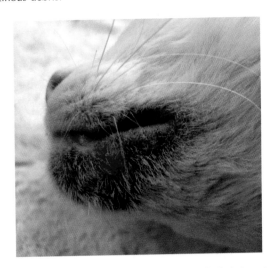

Figure 35-2 Extensive comedone formation with dark keratinous debris, alopecia, erythema, and swelling. Note the lesions extend to the upper lip region.

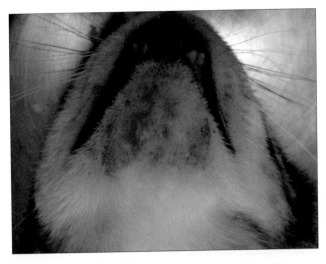

Figure 35-3 The chin has been clipped to provide better visualization of the erythema, papules, keratinous debris, comedones, and exudate.

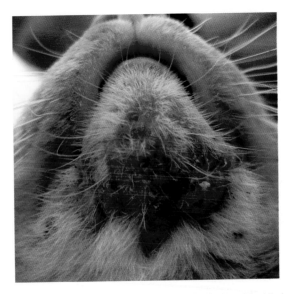

Figure 35-4 Severe chin furunculosis and edema with dried crusts, papules, erythema, alopecia, and comedones.

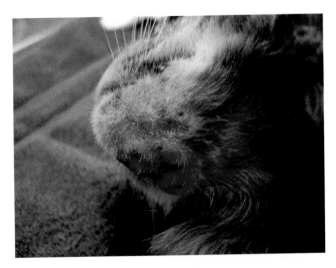

Figure 35-5 The chin has been clipped to provide better visualization of the numerous erythematous, draining furuncles, and proliferative scar tissue.

Although the diagnosis of chin acne is relatively easy, identification of the underlying trigger may be more challenging. A thorough history and physical examination should be performed to look for an underlying cause. Often chin acne is a clinical sign of a whole-body skin disease. Some cats with underlying allergic skin disease (atopy, food hypersensitivity) will have the chin and perioral region involved as part of their pruritic distribution.[1,2] An eosinophilic granuloma should be considered as a differential diagnosis for pronounced chin swelling; in these cats the chin is hard (Figure 35-6).[1] Cats with chin edema also may have mastocytoma (Figure 35-7) (see Chapter 67). Chronic, refractory lesions should be biopsied and submitted for histopathological examination to determine the underlying cause (see the following section).

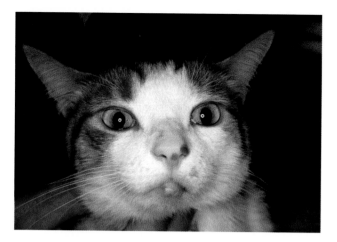

Figure 35-6 Cat with eosinophilic chin granuloma.

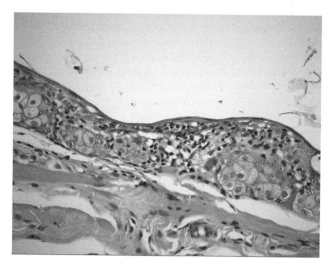

Figure 35-8 Skin biopsy from cat with chin acne. This section shows the extensive lymphoplasmacytic periductal inflammation.

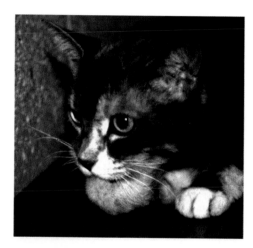

Figure 35-7 Cat with chin edema caused by mastocytoma.

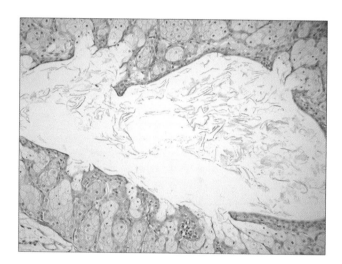

Figure 35-9 Skin biopsy from cat with chin acne. This section shows marked sebaceous gland dilatation with mild lymphoplasmacytic periductal inflammation.

Outbreaks of acne in multiple-cat households have been reported and an infectious etiology has been suspected.[2,4,5] In these cases differential diagnoses to consider include *Demodex gatoi*, dermatophytosis, viral infections (feline herpesvirus, feline calicivirus), and primary irritant contact dermatitis. A recent study demonstrated feline calicivirus antigen, via immunohistochemical staining from a cat with chronic acne, in a household of multiple cats with acne.[2]

HISTOPATHOLOGICAL FEATURES

Skin biopsy procedures will require sedation and infiltration of local anesthesia because these areas are so painful. It is important to sample representative lesions for the best chance of getting a diagnostic specimen. Disposable skin biopsy punches (6 mm) are recommended.

Discrete comedones represent ideal punch biopsy specimens. With early lesions the most common histopathological findings include lymphoplasmacytic periductal inflammation (Figure 35-8), sebaceous gland duct dilatation (Figure 35-9), and follicular keratosis with plugging and dilatation (Figures 35-10 and 35-11).[2] Superficial hair follicles are distended with keratin to form comedones in patients in whom the cause is a follicular keratinization disorder. Attached sebaceous ducts commonly become distended with sebum. The epidermis may demonstrate mild acanthosis and spongiosis with some crusting. More advanced cases will demonstrate folliculitis (Figures 35-12 and 35-13), furunculosis, pyogranulomatous sebaceous adenitis and dermatitis, and epitrichial gland occlusion and dilatation (Figure 35-14).[2,4] Staphylococcal organisms, as well as *Malassezia* spp. organisms, may be found in surface crusts and comedones. Cats with evidence of folliculitis and furunculosis commonly have secondary bacterial infections. With severe furunculosis, dermatophytosis may be a causative or complicating factor; special stains such as Gomori's methenamine silver or periodic acid–Schiff can be used to aid in identification of the organisms. Special stains also may be needed for the identification of mast cell tumors/mastocytosis (see Chapter 67).

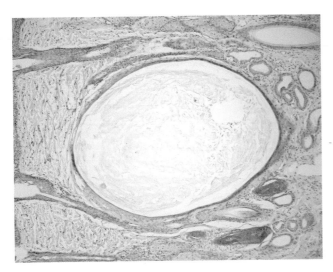

Figure 35-10 Skin biopsy showing small comedone formation.

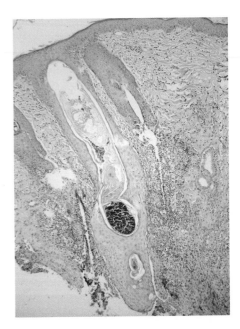

Figure 35-12 Cross section of skin showing large comedone formation and suppurative folliculitis/furunculosis.

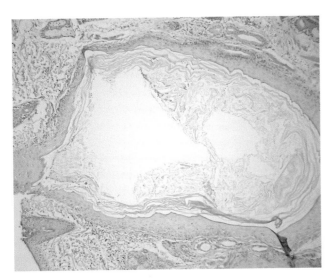

Figure 35-11 Skin biopsy showing large comedone formation. Note the surrounding inflammation.

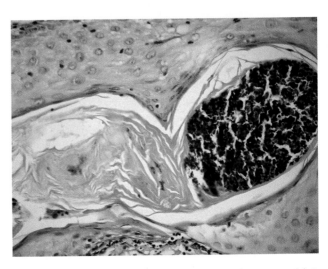

Figure 35-13 Closer view of Figure 35-10. Note keratinous debris and extensive suppurative folliculitis.

TREATMENT

The lesion severity of acne determines the need, type, and intensity of the treatment that will be required to manage each case successfully. Asymptomatic cats in the comedonal stage typically require topical treatments, or observation alone in some cases. The progression to papules, furuncles, edema, and draining tracts requires both topical and systemic treatment modalities. The ultimate goal of acne management is to disrupt, dislodge, and resolve comedone formation, and to treat any secondary or complicating infections.

TOPICAL ANTISEBORRHEIC DRUGS

The ease and efficacy of topical therapy can be improved significantly by initially clipping the hair in the affected area. The severity of skin lesions often is masked by the hair coat (Figure 35-15). Sedation may be needed. Warm water compresses are indicated prior to the administration of any topical treatments, especially when furuncles and draining tracts are present. By soaking the lesions, comedones are softened and drainage is promoted. Manual expression of the comedones, pustules, and furuncles is strongly discouraged, because this can enhance the inflammatory response and exacerbate the lesions.

A wide array of topical medications are available that have keratoplastic, comedolytic, and follicular flushing properties. Keratoplastic agents attempt to normalize the keratinization and epithelialization abnormalities that are present in disorders such as acne. Antiseborrheic agents are available as gel, lotion, shampoo, and cleansing pad formulations. The following products are applied

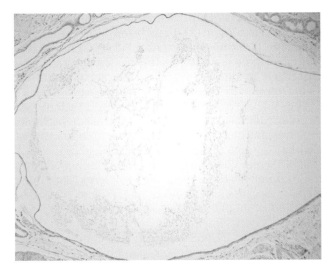

Figure 35-14 Severe epitrichial gland dilatation.

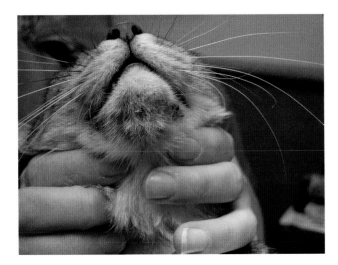

Figure 35-15 Chin acne obscured by hair coat. Compare with Figure 35-1.

q24h for seven to 10 days, and then administered two to three times weekly for maintenance if needed.

Benzoyl peroxide is a potent, broad-spectrum antibacterial agent that has follicular flushing, antipruritic, degreasing, keratolytic, and keratoplastic properties.[1] It is the most well-recognized topical therapy for human and feline acne patients. It is available in a 2.5 per cent gel formulation as well as a variety of 2.5 or 3 per cent shampoos (Pyoben, OxyDex, SulfOxyDex, Benzoyl-Plus). Benzoyl peroxide can be irritating in some cats. Irritant reactions can include erythema, excessive dryness, and pruritus. It also can bleach hair and clothing.

Salicylic acid inhibits comedogenesis by promoting the desquamation of follicular epithelium. It is available at a concentration of 0.5 to 2 per cent in a variety of over-the-counter lotions, creams, and pads. Salicylic acid is well-tolerated and less irritating than benzoyl peroxide. Commonly used acne cleansing pads include Stri-Dex, Fostex, and Clearasil. These pads contain variable amounts of salicylic acid, benzoyl peroxide, sulfur, and aloe vera. Sulfur has keratoplastic, keratolytic, follicular flushing (mild), antibacterial, antifungal, and antiparasitic properties.[1] *Sulfur* and *salicylic acid* exhibit synergistic activity; as such, all sulfur-containing shampoos typically will contain salicylic acid. Commonly used shampoos include Sebalyt, Sebolux, and Seba-Hex.

Topical retinoids should be considered for patients in whom the comedogenic process can not be disrupted or resolved. These drugs function by slowing down the desquamation process. In cases of human acne, topical retinoids are the most effective comedolytic agents available. Commonly used products include tretinoin (Retin A, 0.01 to 0.05 per cent cream or lotion), adapalene (Differin, 0.1 per cent gel or solution), and tazarotene (Tazorac, 0.05 to 0.1 per cent gel). The most common side effects of topical retinoid treatment include skin irritation and the potential for initial worsening of acne. Because oral retinoids are potent teratogens, topical retinoids are not recommended for use in pregnant queens and queens used for breeding purposes.

TOPICAL ANTIMICROBIALS

Topical antimicrobials should be considered when papules, furuncles, and draining tracts are present. Mupirocin (pseudomonic acid) is produced from *Pseudomonas fluorescens* and is not chemically related to any other antibiotic.[6] It acts by inhibiting isoleucyl tRNA synthetase competitively, resulting in the failure of isoleucine incorporation into growing polypeptide chains. Mupirocin shows activity mainly against gram-positive bacteria (*Staphylococcus, Streptococcus*), whereas most gram-negative bacteria are highly resistant to the drug. Currently it can be obtained in a 2 per cent ointment. It is well tolerated by the vast majority of cats, and has shown excellent clinical efficacy in acne patients complicated with secondary bacterial infections.[3] However, it should be noted that mupirocin is supplied in a water-soluble ointment base of propylene glycol. The prolonged use of large amounts of topical mupirocin can induce toxicity if ingested, especially in cats with impaired renal function.

Fusidic acid is an antimicrobial steroidal substance produced originally by strains of *Fusidium coccineum*.[6] The most susceptible organisms to fusidic acid are *Staphylococcus* spp. and *Streptococcus* spp. It is almost completely inactive against gram-negative organisms. Fusidic acid interferes with protein synthesis by inhibiting a factor involved in the translocation of polypeptide units and elongation. Fucidin is available in a 2 per cent ointment formulation. Some formulations of Fucidin contain hydrocortisone or betamethasone. These steroid-containing products are not recommended, because topical glucocorticoids can induce comedone formation.

Additional topical antimicrobial lotions or ointments containing clindamycin (BenzaClin, 5 per cent benzoyl peroxide and 1 per cent clindamycin), tetracycline (Topicycline, 2.2 per cent solution), or erythromycin (Benzamycin, 5 per cent benzoyl peroxide and 3 per cent erythromycin), also have been reported to be effective.[5]

Through its antibacterial and antiinflammatory properties, 0.75 per cent metronidazole gel (MetroGel) also may be useful. Triple antibiotic preparations containing neomycin, polymyxin B, or bacitracin are not recommended by the author. Neomycin has more potential for allergic sensitization than most other topical drugs. Bacitracin and polymyxin B are inactivated rapidly by purulent exudates, do not penetrate well, and often can result in treatment failures.

TOPICAL ANTIFUNGALS

For acne complicated by *Malassezia* overgrowth, commonly used topical drugs include but are not limited to miconazole (Conofite lotion or spray, 1 per cent miconazole nitrate), chlorhexidine (Chlorhexiderm Shampoo, 2 to 4 per cent chlorhexidine), ketoconazole (KetoChlor Shampoo, 1 per cent ketoconazole and 2 per cent chlorhexidine), and Malaseb Pledgets or Wipes (miconazole nitrate, 2 per cent and chlorhexidine gluconate, 2 per cent).

SYSTEMIC THERAPEUTIC OPTIONS

In most circumstances, the presence of furuncles and draining tracts is indicative of extensive bacterial folliculitis and furunculosis, and systemic antimicrobial therapy is required. Solid empirical choices include amoxicillin-clavulanic acid (12.5 to 25 mg/kg PO q12h), cefpodoxime (5 mg/kg PO q24h), clindamycin (6 to 11 mg/kg PO q12h), cefadroxil (20 mg/kg PO q12h), and cephalexin (15 to 20 mg/kg PO q12h). Fluoroquinolones such as marbofloxacin (2.5 to 5.5 mg/kg PO q24h) or orbifloxacin (2.5 to 7.5 mg/kg PO q24h)) should be reserved for gram-negative infections or for infections confirmed with sensitivity testing. Treatment should be continued for a minimum of 4 to 8 weeks.

For patients with extensive *Malassezia* dermatitis, oral itraconazole (5 to 10 mg/kg PO q24h) or fluconazole (5 to 10 mg/kg PO q24h) should be administered for 3 weeks.

Cats with recurrent acne may benefit from fatty acid supplementation.[5] Fatty acids can reduce inflammation and normalize keratinization.

Some cats who exhibit severe edema and furunculosis will benefit significantly from a 10- to 14-day tapering course of prednisolone (1 to 2 mg/kg PO q24h). This treatment also may reduce scar tissue formation. Bacterial and fungal infections should be ruled out prior to administering corticosteroids.

The use of synthetic retinoids should be considered for cats who are not tolerant of topical management or who are refractory to therapy in general. The major benefit of retinoids in the management of the follicular keratinization disorder that occurs with acne is their ability to regulate proliferation, growth, and differentiation of epithelial tissues. In addition, all retinoids have antiinflammatory and immunomodulatory effects. Retinoids affect humoral and cellular immunity, cellular adhesion and communication, proteases, and prostaglandins.[7] Some cats have responded to the administration of isotretinoin (Accu-

tane, 2 mg/kg PO q24h).[5] Isotretinoin should be administered for a minimum of 60 days before assessing response to therapy. If improvement is noted, daily administration typically can be reduced to q48-72h. The most common side effects in cats include periocular crusting and erythema, conjunctivitis, diarrhea, vomiting, and anorexia.[8,9] In dogs side effects and laboratory changes include keratoconjunctivitis sicca, hypertriglyceridemia, hypercholesterolemia, and increased levels of alanine aminotransferase, aspartate aminotransferase, and alkaline phosphatase.[8,9] Periodic serum chemistry panels and Schirmer tear tests are recommended for cats on long-term isotretinoin therapy. Because all retinoids are potent teratogens, isotretinoin should not be administered to pregnant queens or queens intended for breeding purposes.

Cyclosporine (Neoral, Atopica) has immunomodulatory and antiproliferative effects (see Chapter 33). It functions by inhibiting calcineurin-mediated cytokine regulation. Cyclosporine blocks IL-2 transcription and T cell responsiveness to IL-2, resulting in impaired T-helper and T-cytotoxic lymphocyte function. In human beings acne has been implicated as a side effect of cyclosporine. For now cyclosporine can be recommended only at a dosage of 5 mg/kg PO q24h for chin dermatitis resulting from atopic dermatitis or eosinophilic granuloma formation. To the author's knowledge no studies have been conducted utilizing cyclosporine as a treatment for acne in cats.

Interferons are a family of regulatory proteins that have immunomodulatory functions against viral and bacterial infections, among many other effects (see Chapter 36). Anecdotal reports of improvement with low-dose alpha interferon (30 IU PO q24h on a week-on/week-off treatment schedule) suggest that a viral etiology might be present in some cases. Other alternatives include weekly dosing of omega interferon (Virbagen Omega) at 1 MU/kg weekly SQ for at least three treatments.

PROGNOSIS

The prognosis for acne is good; however, lifelong therapy is needed in the majority of cases. There usually is some underlying disease (e.g., atopy, food allergy) or an inherent disorder of keratinization in cats with acne. Maintenance topical medications are required in most affected cats to minimize comedogenesis and prevent secondary bacterial folliculitis and furunculosis.

REFERENCES

1. Scott DW, Miller WH, Griffin CE: Keratinization defects. In *Small animal dermatology*, ed 6, Philadelphia, 2001, Saunders, p 1042.
2. Jazic E, Coyner K, Loeffler D: An evaluation of the clinical, cytological, infectious and histopathological features of feline acne, *Vet Dermatol* 17:134, 2006.
3. White SD, Bourdeau PB, Blumstein P, et al: Feline acne and results of treatment with mupirocin in an open clinical trial: 25 cases (1994-96), *Vet Dermatol* 8:157, 1997.
4. Gross TL, Ihrke PJ, Walder EJ, et al: *Skin diseases of the dog and cat: clinical and histopathologic diagnosis*, ed 2, Oxford, 2005, Blackwell Science, p 437.

5. Rosenkrantz WS: The pathogenesis, diagnosis, and management of feline acne, *Vet Med* 86:504, 1991.
6. Werner AH, Russell AD: Mupirocin, fusidic acid and bacitracin: activity, action and clinical uses of three topical antibiotics, *Vet Dermatol* 10:225, 1999.
7. Peck GL, DiGiovanna JJ: The retinoids. In Freedberg IM, et al, editors: *Fitzpatrick's dermatology in general medicine*, ed 5, New York, 1999, McGraw-Hill, p 2810.
8. Kwochka KW: Retinoids and vitamin A therapy. In Griffin CE, et al, editors: *Current veterinary dermatology*, St. Louis, 1993, Mosby-Year Book, p 203.
9. Power HT, Ihrke PJ: Synthetic retinoids in veterinary dermatology, *Vet Clin North Am Small Anim Pract* 20:1525, 1990.

36 Use of Interferon Omega for Skin Diseases

Meret E. Ricklin Gutzwiller

REVIEW OF COMPOUND

INTERFERONS IN GENERAL

Interferons (IFNs) are naturally produced glycoproteins first discovered in 1957. They are divided into two groups: type I, also called viral IFNs, and type II or immune IFNs. Type I IFNs include IFN-α and IFN-ω (also called IFN-alphaII1), both synthesized predominantly by leukocytes, and IFN-β, synthesized by most cell types but particularly by fibroblasts. All three bind to the IFN I-receptor. Type II IFN has only one member, the IFN-γ, which is synthesized mainly by T-lymphocytes and natural killer-cells (NK-cells) in response to antigenic or mitogenic stimuli.[1] The goal of this chapter is to familiarize the reader with mechanistic and clinical uses of feline IFN omega (IFN-ω) in veterinary dermatology.

RECOMBINANT FELINE INTERFERON-OMEGA

Recombinant feline IFN-ω (rFeIFN) has a 170 amino acid (AA) sequence with a molecular weight of 25 kDa and is N-glycosylated. Its sequence shows a 60 per cent homology with human IFN-α and human IFN-ω, and a 35 per cent homology with human IFN-β. It belongs to the type I IFN group according to its specific AA sequence at the N-terminus, and its subclass is IFN-ω. The commercially available formulation (rFeIFN) is produced industrially by silk worm larvae (Bombyx mori) that have been infected with a recombinant baculovirus vector containing FeIFN cDNA.[2]

The purified rFeIFN-omega is acid-stable for more than 50 days at 4° C, and in vitro studies have shown that it has dose-dependent antiviral activities against feline herpesvirus, feline coronavirus, feline calicivirus (FCV), feline panleukopenia virus, and antitumor activities against a wide range of tumor cell lines of cats and dogs.[1,3,4]

PHARMACOKINETICS

Elimination after intravenous administration is biphasic and rapid. In the first or distribution phase, the half-life is 5 minutes. In the second or metabolic phase, the half-life is 31 minutes. rFeIFN is distributed mainly into kidneys and liver and is metabolized quickly in these two organs. The highest concentration of inactivated rFeIFN in urine can be measured within 15 minutes postadministration. rFeIFN does not cross the blood-brain barrier. The highest concentrations are found in kidney, liver, and thyroid tissue, and the lowest concentrations in muscle and adipose tissue.[2]

After subcutaneous administration of 5 million units (MU)/kg of rFeIFN, serum concentrations increase gradually and a maximum concentration (C_{max}) of 577 U/mL occurs at 1.47 hours postadministration. Thereafter concentrations decrease slowly and are nondetectable after 24 hours. The elimination half-life is 1.72 hours.[5] Even though serum levels are very short-lived, rFeIFN induces the activity of 2'-5' oligoadenylate synthetase (OAS) in leukocytes in the peripheral blood and keeps the level elevated for 3 days.[6] At least four isoenzymes of OAS are described in human beings. They are activated by double-stranded ribonucleic acid (RNA) and catalyze the formation of adenosine monophosphate (AMP) oligomers linked by a 2'-5' diester bond. These oligomers then activate an RNAse, which is responsible for degradation of RNA at specific sequences, thus providing a system for the control of virus replication and gene expression.[7]

ADVERSE EFFECTS AND TOXICITY

Potential transient adverse effects postadministration include mild apathy, decreased appetite, sinus tachycardia, mild transient leukopenia, thrombocytopenia, and anemia. To date there are no studies on the long-term effects of rFeIFN. Its safety has not been determined in kittens less than 9 weeks of age, puppies younger than 1 month of age, and pregnant animals.[5]

Intravenous administration of 20 MU/kg rFeIFN to cats provoked a sinus tachycardia, mild apathy, mild increase of respiratory rate and body temperature; the latter two parameters were still within normal range.[8]

COMMERCIAL PREPARATION

rFeIFN is available commercially as Virbagen Omega (Virbac Santé Animale S.A., Carros, France) as a lyophilized powder plus solvent in 5 × 1 MU, 2 × 5 MU, or 10 × 1 MU per vial with a shelf life of 2 years when stored at 4° C. The product does not contain any preservatives and should be used immediately after reconstitution. The compound is stable for approximately 3 weeks at 4° C. Reconstituted Virbagen Omega can be frozen at –20° C and is stable for at least 6 months. Freeze-thaw cycles, however, should be avoided.

Virbagen Omega is licensed for use in the treatment of cats with feline leukemia virus (FeLV) and/or feline immunodeficiency virus (FIV) infection and for the treatment of parvovirus infections in dogs in the European Union, Switzerland, Argentina, Brazil, New Zealand, Australia, and Mexico. The drug currently is not licensed in the United States; however, there are ongoing discussions for licensing in the United States, Canada, and South Africa.

MECHANISM OF ACTION

Type I IFNs have multiple antiviral, antiproliferative, and immunomodulatory activities and exhibit autocrine as well as paracrine activities (Box 36-1).[1] The IFN response is very fast and limits virus spreading, thereby buying time for the generation of an acquired immune response to the invading virus. IFNs exert their actions through cell surface receptors.

IFNs use the Janus kinase Jak/STAT (signal transducers and activators of transcription) pathway. The main induction event is the redistribution from the cytoplasm to the nucleus of the transcription factor NF-κB that plays a role in the transcriptional induction of many immunomodulatory genes, including other cytokines, MHC-I, and cell adhesion molecules that normally are expressed at low levels or are quiescent.

The IFN I receptor is composed of two major subunits, IFNAR1 (IFN-a receptor 1), associated with tyrosine kinase Tyk2, and IFNAR2 associated with Jak1. IFNAR 1 and 2 associate when IFN I binding occurs, thereby facilitating the transphosphorylation and activation of the two kinases, and creating a new docking site for STAT2 that is then phosphorylated and recruits itself STAT1, which also becomes phosphorylated. The phosphorylated STAT1/STAT2 heterodimers dissociate from the receptor and translocate to the nucleus where they associate with deoxyribonucleic (DNA)-binding protein p48 to form a heterotrimeric complex, ISGF3 (IFN-stimulated gene factor 3), which binds the ISRE (IFN-stimulated response element) of IFN I–responsive genes (Figure 36-1).

Box 36-1 The Activities of IFN Type I

ANTIPROLIFERATIVE ACTIVITIES OF IFN I
- Growth-suppressive effects contributed by PKR and RNase L.
- Negative regulation of the cell cycle by the up-regulation of p21, a tumor suppressor gene.
- Repression of the cell cycle by down-regulating the p202 IFN-I inducible, mitogenic gene product.
- Down-regulation of c-myc transcription.
- Induction of apoptosis by activated PKR, 2′-5′ oligoadenylate synthetase system and by inducing both Fas and Fas-ligand.

ANTIVIRAL RESPONSE
Double-Stranded RNA-Dependent Protein Kinase R (PKR)
- Activated PKR has a number of important cell-regulatory activities because it:
  - Phosphorylates the alpha subunit of the eukaryotic translation initiation factor eIF2 and prevents viral protein synthesis.
  - Mediates signal transduction in response to ds-RNA and other ligands.

- Aids in clearance of viral infections by mediating apoptosis in a direct and indirect manner.

2′-5′ Oligoadenylate Synthetase System
- Leads to inhibition of protein synthesis by catalyzing cleavage of preferentially viral mRNA by activating L-RNAse and also by ribosomal inactivation leading to a translational inhibition.

Mx Proteins
- These are highly conserved GTPases that interfere with virus replication, probably by inhibiting the trafficking or activity of virus polymerases.

IMMUNOMODULATORY FUNCTIONS
Interferons Enhance
- The expression of MHC-I proteins and thereby promote CD8+ T cell responses
- The cytotoxicity of NK-cells by up-regulating the levels of perforins

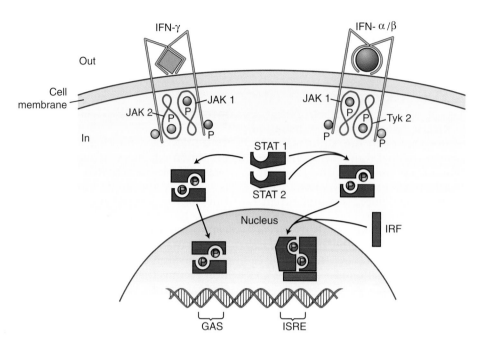

Figure 36-1 Schematic of IFN signaling by the Jak-STAT pathway: The signaling process is initiated by binding of the IFN ligand to its specific receptor, thereby activating Jak and Stat transcription factors by phosphorylation. In IFN I Tyk-2 and Jak-kinases are activated, which leads to phosphorylation and activation of Stat-1 and -2 proteins with subsequent translocation along with the IRF to the nucleus. The complex of these three proteins, called IFN-stimulated gene factor 3 (ISGF-3), activates the transcription of IFN-I-inducible genes through the ISRE. With IFN-γ, Jak-1 and -2 are activated, which leads to phosphorylation and homodimerization of STAT-1 and subsequent translocation to the nucleus where it activates the transcription of IFN-γ inducible genes through the gamma-interferon activated sequence (GAS) enhancer element. (Adapted from *Interferons in small animal medicine*, Suffolk, 2007, Virbac Ltd., p 7 figure 1, by Severin Gutzwiller.)

IFN-γ induces a phosphorylation of only STAT1 and therefore another DNA-binding element GAF (gamma-IFN activating factor, which is a STAT1 dimer) is created. GAF binds to DNA sequence GAS (gamma-IFN activated sequence).

The primary step usually is inhibition of viral replication, induction of the protein kinase PKR, 2′,3′-oligoadenylate synthetase, and RNAse L. All three of these induce apoptosis; RNA-specific adenosine deaminase ADAR1 and protein MxGTPase induce iNOS (inducible nitric oxide synthetase), repression of the cell cycle by the p202 IFN-I inducible gene product, downregulation of c-myc transcription, and increase of MHC-I and -II molecules, all of which play an important role in immune responses to infections.[7]

Mainly by influencing Th1 type cytokine and chemokine induction and by regulating cytokine and chemokine receptor gene expression, IFN type I induces a Th1 type response and an adaptive CD8+ T-cell response that is likely to be efficacious against both chronic viral infections and neoplastic diseases that affect cats.[9]

ANTIVIRAL ACTIVITY

This action is mainly dependent on two enzymes activated by double-stranded RNA; the OAS and the protein kinase p68 (PKR) that are both induced by IFNs. OAS leads to inhibition of protein synthesis on the one hand by catalyzing the cleavage of preferentially viral mRNA through activation of an L-RNAse, and on the other hand by inactivation of ribosomes leading to a translational inhibition. Among other activities, PKR interferes with viral protein synthesis by inactivating the eukaryotic translation initiation factor (eIF2) that then impairs viral protein synthesis. PKR also mediates programmed cell death (apoptosis) and therefore aids in viral clearance.

ANTIPROLIFERATIVE ACTIVITY

Proliferation is reduced by induction of apoptosis through PKR and also L-RNAse as explained previously, as well as through Fas and Fas-Ligand. IFNs inhibit the cell cycle by up-regulating p21, a tumor suppressor, down-regulating p202, an IFN-inducible mitogenic gene product, and by down-regulating transcription of the protooncogene c-myc.

IMMUNOMODULATORY ACTIVITY

IFNs type I induce MHC-I protein expression and therefore promote a CD8+ T-cell response. They also increase the activity of NK-cells with their cytolytic activity. By inhibiting integrins that are important for cell migration of inflammatory cells, IFNs inhibit the access of the immune cells to the inflammatory site.[7]

Mainly by influencing Th1 type cytokine and chemokine induction and by regulating cytokine and chemokine receptor gene expression, IFN type I induces a Th1 type response and an adaptive CD8+ T-cell response that is likely to be efficacious against both chronic viral infections and neoplastic diseases that affect cats.[9]

USE IN SKIN DISEASES

rFeIFN is a relatively new compound and the commercial product has been available for only a short time. Descriptions of the use of rFeIFN are limited to a small number of well-controlled studies, case reports, personal communications, and information provided by the manufacturer. Increased use will clarify treatment efficacy and schedules.

VIRAL SKIN DISEASES

Feline Herpesvirus Infections

Feline herpesvirus dermatitis is an uncommon, predominantly facial skin disease caused by feline herpesvirus type I (FHV-I). This virus is a double-stranded DNA virus that replicates in the nucleus of the host cells, producing intranuclear inclusion bodies. It is one of the major causes of upper respiratory tract disease. Transmission occurs through close contact and transfer of body fluids.

Feline herpesvirus dermatitis is a rare disease seen most commonly in cats with latent herpesvirus infections. A history of ocular disease and upper respiratory tract infections is not always present. Skin lesions can be triggered by stress and immunosuppression.[10] The primary sites of replication are epithelial tissues. The virus invades epithelial cells, causing a cytopathogenic effect when it replicates and breaks out of the cell. This results in surface epithelial erosions and inflammation. Secondary bacterial infections worsen the inflammatory response. α-Herpesviridae, by definition, develop neuronal latency. Reactivation of the virus may occur periodically with the virus transported anterograde via the axon from the nerve cell body to the original site of peripheral infection.[11]

Clinically, cats present with an erosive or ulcerative, vesicular and crusting dermatitis with variable erythema, swelling, and exudation on the nasal planum or haired skin of the face (Figure 36-2). In rare cases it can be associated with ulcerative stomatitis. Regional lymphadenopathy may be present, and lesions may be painful or pruritic. Some cats also may have systemic signs such as depression, sneezing, pyrexia, inappetence, anorexia, and serous nasal discharge.

The major differential diagnoses include mosquito bite hypersensitivity, food allergy, squamous cell carcinoma, mast cell tumor, and dermatophytosis. Definitive diagnosis requires ruling out other causes of facial dermatitis, and a skin biopsy. Histological findings include severe eosinophil-rich necrosis and epidermal ulceration, with extension of the necrosis into hair follicles and underlying dermis and intranuclear inclusion bodies in the epithelium and adnexal epithelia. The intranuclear inclusions

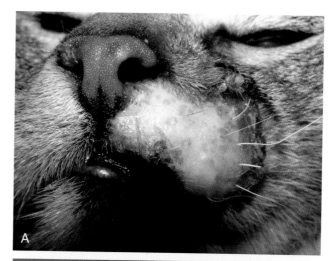

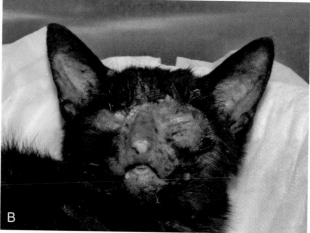

Figure 36-2 A, Face of a cat with herpes dermatitis. Notice the plaque-like lesion on the muzzle with alopecia, erosions, and crusts, and a small erosive lesion on the right ala of the nose. **B,** Severe erosive and exudate facial dermatitis caused by feline herpesvirus I in a 6-month-old female domestic shorthair cat.

are lightly basophilic and amphophilic, and have a smudged or homogeneous appearance with margination of nuclear chromatin (Figure 36-3). If intranuclear inclusions are overlooked or absent on histological examination of skin biopsy specimens, confusion with eosinophilic dermatoses can occur.[12] Polymerase chain reaction testing is very sensitive, but needs to be interpreted carefully because it does not discriminate between viable, cultivable virions and immature, immunologically inactivated or noncultivable viruses or DNA-fragments.[13] Serology is not useful because a high titer can not be differentiated from a vaccine titer.

The following 24-day protocol using rFeIFN has been used successfully to treat this disease.[12] On day 0, 1.5 MU/kg is injected perilesionally. On day 2 and day 10, 0.75 MU/kg is injected perilesionally and 0.75 MU/kg is administered SQ. The drug protocol used on day 2 and 10 is repeated on days 20, 22, and 24. Sedation is needed for perilesional injections. Antibiotics and analgesics also may be needed. Immunosuppressive drugs should be avoided. The expected result is resolution of the lesions with slight scarring.[12]

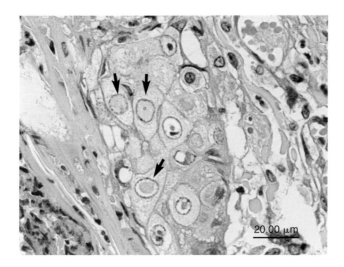

Figure 36-3 Skin biopsy from a cat with herpes dermatitis. Note the intranuclear eosinophilic inclusion bodies with margination of the nuclear chromatin.

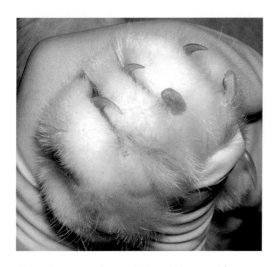

Figure 36-4 Cutaneous horns: FIV-positive cat with a cutaneous horn on the footpad. (Courtesy Ekatarina Kunetsova, Moscow.)

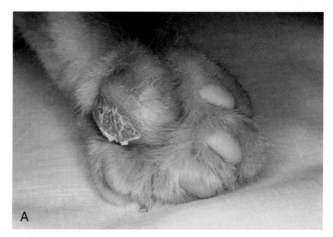

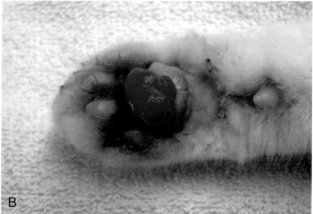

Figure 36-5 A, Feline plasma cell pododermatitis. The surface of the swollen and discolored central pad of the paw of a cat shows white, scaly, silvery, crosshatched appearance with stria. The small digital foot pads are normal. **B,** Feline plasma cell pododermatitis. The lesions shown in this cat were acute and proliferative. Diagnosis was confirmed by biopsy.

Retroviral Infection

FeLV is an oncogenic immunosuppressive retrovirus. It commonly affects the skin by its cytosuppressive actions. Skin lesions associated with FeLV are characterized by chronic or recurrent gingivitis or pyoderma, poor wound healing, seborrhea, exfoliative dermatitis, generalized pruritus, and cutaneous horns (Figure 36-4).[14] Histological findings of skin biopsies may show syncytial-type giant cell formation in the epidermis and outer root sheath of the hair follicles. FIV infections often occur concurrently with FeLV and skin lesions may overlap. Cats with FIV infections may present with signs of plasma cell stomatitis and plasma cell pododermatitis. FeLV and FIV infections can not be differentiated based on clinical signs alone. The following treatment is recommended. In addition to appropriate supportive or symptomatic therapy, administer three 5-day courses of feline omega IFN. On days 0, 1, 2, 3, and 4, give 1 MU/kg rFeIFN SQ. Repeat this 5-day course in 2 weeks, and again 2 months

from day 0 if RBC values are stable or improving.[15] Improvement in clinical signs and laboratory values are prognostic indicators that the cat may be a good responder.

Plasma Cell Pododermatitis

This is an uncommon skin disease in cats. The etiology is unknown but the marked plasmacellular infiltrate, the consistent hypergammaglobulinemia, and the response to immunomodulating and/or immunosuppressive therapy suggest an immune-mediated etiology. The association with FeLV or FIV infection is controversial.[14]

The clinical lesions are highly characteristic, with soft, spongy swelling and variable ulceration usually affecting multiple paw pads. The swelling is uniform; therefore the normal symmetry of the pad usually is not disturbed. Central larger pads are involved most consistently. The appearance of the surface of the pad varies, and may be deeply purple in color. Central ulcerations may be present. In older lesions, there may be a white, scaly, silvery, crosshatched appearance with stria (Figure 36-5). Owners may report lameness in some affected cats. In a minority of cases, there maybe concurrent plasma cell stomatitis, immune-mediated glomerulonephritis, or renal amyloidosis.[14]

Diagnosis is based on history, clinical signs, and skin biopsy. Histological sections show acanthosis with variable erosions, ulceration, and exudation. The dermis and adipose tissue are infiltrated by plasma cells that obscure the normal dermal architecture.[16] Spontaneous remission or periodic recurrence may be observed. Treatment is reported with equal success using doxycycline, corticosteroids, or surgical excision.[17,18] Treatment with rFeINF may be beneficial because of the suspected immune-mediated etiology and possible association with FeLV/FIV.

Cats with plasma cell pododermatitis have been treated with rFeIFN as follows.[19] On week 1, using a total of 5 MU/cat, 1 MU was injected into each affected paw and 1 MU was injected SQ on the lateral thorax. On weeks 2 and 3, 5 MU/cat was injected SQ. Doxycycline (5 mg/kg PO q24h) may be used concurrently.

Pox Virus

Pox lesions in cats are induced by orthopox virus. Rodents are the reservoir of infection and it is presumed that affected cats contract the disease via hunting. The disease is more common in cats living in rural environments who are allowed outdoors and in the fall when rodents are most active.

Early lesions present as a small ulcer or area of abscessation or cellulitis, usually on the face or a distal part of a limb. After 7 to 10 days, multiple nodular lesions develop following viral replication in the regional lymph node and a leukocyte-associated viremia. Typically, lesions are focal, raised, and erythematous. Initially they are vesicular, rapidly crusting, and variably pruritic. Lesions generally resolve after 4 to 6 weeks in otherwise healthy cats unless infected with FIV or secondary bacterial infections.

Definitive diagnosis may be made by virus isolation, serology, or skin biopsy. Histologically lesions are characterized by severe ulceration, serocellular crusting, and ballooning degeneration of keratinocytes. There usually are numerous, large, intracytoplasmic, brightly eosinophilic inclusions of variable size.[16] (The reader is directed to Chapter 30 of the fifth volume in this series for more information about this disease.)

There is no specific treatment except for supportive symptomatic therapy. Immunosuppressive treatment must be avoided. As in other viral infections, IFN therapy can be beneficial. rFeIFN was used to treat cats with feline pox by administering 1 MU/kg q48h starting on day 0, 2, and 4. Half the dose was administered perilesionally and the remainder SQ.[20] Antimicrobial therapy also may be needed, if secondary colonization of lesions with bacteria is present.

Acne

Acne is discussed in detail in Chapter 35. Briefly, it is a reaction pattern and the underlying etiology is multifactorial. Clinically cats may present with any combination of comedones, alopecia, crusts, papules, and erythema (Figure 36-6). Pruritus is variable. Histological findings include any combination of lymphoplasmacytic periductal inflammation, sebaceous gland duct dilatation, fol-

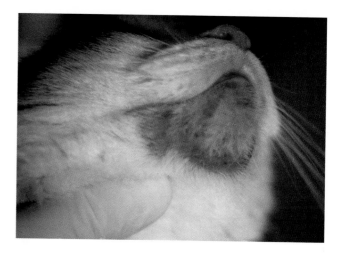

Figure 36-6 Chin of a cat with acne. Note the comedones, erythema, alopecia, and swelling of the chin. (Courtesy Clinical Dermatology Unit, University of Bern.)

licular keratosis with plugging and dilatation, epitrichial gland occlusion and dilatation, folliculitis, pyogranulomatous sebaceous adenitis, and furunculosis.[21] In addition to topical treatment and systemic antibiotics, rFeIFN has been used to treat acne. It was administered once weekly for 3 weeks at a dose of 1 MU/kg SQ.[22]

Chronic Gingivostomatitis

Gingivostomatitis is a disease that is becoming increasingly common in cats. The etiology often is unknown; however, various infectious agents have been implicated in the development of the disease including FCV, FIV, and FeLV. Anaerobic bacteria in dental plaque also play an important role as well as dental and periodontal diseases.[23] Cats typically present with any combination of halitosis, ptyalism, dysphagia, pawing at the mouth, poor grooming, weight loss, or apathy.

Examination of the oral mucosa commonly reveals severe inflammation, often with ulceration of the gingival and oral mucosa.[23] Close inspection reveals proliferation and/or ulcerative erythematous inflammation of the pharynx; gingival, buccal, or palatal mucosa; fauces; or tongue (Figure 36-7). Two sites are commonly affected: the glossopalatine mucosa (palatoglossitis) and the buccal mucosa overlying the premolar/molar arches (buccostomatitis).[24] As mentioned, the pathophysiological basis of the disease is not fully understood; however, an inadequate immune response to a chronic oral antigenic stimulation is suspected as part of the etiology.

Histological examination of tissues shows two distinct inflammatory patterns.[23] The first is a lichenoid dermalepidermal infiltration of predominantly plasma cells and smaller numbers of neutrophils, lymphocytes, and macrophages, suggestive of an immune reaction or "overreactive" patient. The other, less common histological presentation is a leukocytic exocytosis suggesting an immunocompromised patient.

In addition to good dental hygiene, antibiotics for a sufficient length of time, appropriate analgesics, and good nutrition, the addition of rFeINF has been shown to be beneficial with cessation of viral shedding.[24]

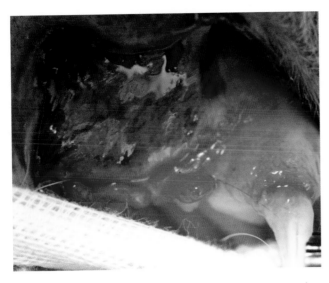

Figure 36-7 Oral cavity of a cat with gingivostomatitis. Note the severe buccostomatitis. (Courtesy Philippe Roux, University of Bern.)

Mild cases were treated with perilesional injections (1 MU/kg) into the submucosa on days 0, 15, and 30. This series of injections can be repeated in 2 months from day 0, depending on the cat's response to treatment. In moderate to severe cases the protocol described above was used concurrently with 1 to 2 MU/kg SQ q48h for five treatments.[25] An alternative treatment schedule is to administer 1 MU/kg SQ q48h for five treatments, and then administer 10,000 U in 2 mL NaCl PO q24h for 2 months and then q48h for the third month.[24]

Fibrosarcoma

Fibrosarcomas are common in cats and comprise 40 per cent of feline skin tumors. The scope of this chapter does not allow for a detailed discussion and review of the tumor biology. Briefly, this is a common skin tumor of cats that is locally invasive with a high rate of recurrence and potential for metastasis. The pathogenesis of some of these tumors is associated with vaccination; however, because vaccines with and without adjuvant have resulted in sarcoma development, the role of adjuvants in tumorigenesis is not clear.[26] Extensive surgery with 3-cm margins is the treatment of choice.[27] Recurrence rates decrease with additional preoperative radiation therapy in patients with clean margins postoperatively.[28] In an open, non–placebo-controlled study, rFeIFN was used preoperatively and postoperatively in cats with fibrosarcomas. All treatments used a dose of 1 MU/kg. During week 1 the cats received one dose injected into the tumor for 3 days. During week 2 a fourth treatment dose was injected into the tumor. Doses five and six were injected subcutaneously at the postexcision site 2 consecutive days after excision. During the next 3 weeks cats received two doses per week subcutaneously at the treatment site for a total of 12 doses over the treatment period. In this study the recurrence rate was 45 per cent. Because this was not a controlled study, it was not possible to determine if the treatment had a significant effect on the rate of recurrence. Previous studies have reported recurrence rates of 20 per cent to 70 per cent.[29]

REFERENCES

1. Goodbourn S, Didock L, Randall RE: Interferons: cell signaling, immune modulation, antiviral responses and virus countermeasures, *J Gen Virol* 81:2341, 2000.
2. Ueda Y, Sakurai T, Yanai A: Homogeneous production of feline interferon in silkworm by replacing single amino acid code in signal peptide region in recombinant baculovirus and characterization of the product, *J Vet Med Sci* 55:251, 1993.
3. Truyen U, Blewaska S, Schultheiss U: Antiviral potency of interferon-omega (IFNω) against selected canine and feline viruses, *Der Praktische Tierarzt* 83:862, 2002.
4. Siebeck N, Hurley DJ, Garcia M, et al: Inhibitory effects of recombinant feline omega interferon on the replication of feline herpesvirus I in vitro. Proceedings of the International Veterinary Ophthalmology Meeting, Munich, 130, 2004.
5. Virbac Animal Health: Virbagen Omega, the veterinary interferon. http://www.virbagenomega.com
6. Ueda Y, Sakurai T, Kasama K, et al: Pharmacokinetic properties of recombinant feline interferon and its stimulatory effect on 2',5'-oligoadenylate synthetase activity in the cat, *J Vet Med Sci* 55:1, 1993.
7. Samuel CE: Antiviral actions of interferons, *Clin Microbiol Rev* 14:778, 2001.
8. EMEA, Committee for Veterinary Medicinal Products: Interferon-omega Scientific Discussion. European Agency for the Evaluation of Medicinal Products, London. http://www.emea.europa.eu/vetdocs/PDFs/EPAR/virbagenomega/10850len6.pdf/, May 1, 2009.
9. Baldwin S, Powell TD, Sellins KS, et al: The biological effects of five feline IFN-α subtypes, *Vet Immunol Immunopathol* 99:153, 2004.
10. Hargis AM, Ginn PE, Mansell J, et al: Ulcerative facial and nasal dermatitis and stomatitis in cats associated with feline herpesvirus 1, *Vet Dermatol* 10:267, 1999.
11. Stiles J: Feline herpesvirus, *Clin Tech Small Anim Pract* 18:178, 2003.
12. Ricklin Gutzwiller ME, Brachelente C, Taglinger K, et al: Feline herpes dermatitis treated with interferon omega, *Vet Dermatol* 18:50, 2007.
13. Maggs DJ, Clarke HE: Relative sensitivity of polymerase chain reaction assays used for detection of feline herpesvirus and commercial vaccines, *Am J Vet Res* 66:1550, 2005.
14. Scott DW, Miller WH, Griffin CE: *Muller and Kirk's small animal dermatology*, ed 6, Philadelphia, 2001, Saunders.
15. De Mari K, Maynard L, Sanquer A, et al: Therapeutic effects of recombinant feline interferon-ω on feline leukemia virus (FeLV)-infected and FeLV/feline immunodeficiency virus (FIV)-coinfected symptomatic cats, *J Vet Intern Med* 18:477, 2004.
16. Gross TL, Ihrke PJ, Walder EJ, et al: *Skin diseases of the dog and cat: clinical and histopathologic diagnosis*, ed 2, Oxford, 2005, Blackwell Publishing.
17. Scarampella F, Ordeix L: Doxycycline therapy in 10 cases of feline plasma cell pododermatitis: clinical, haematological and serological evaluations, *Vet Dermatol* 15(S1):27, 2004.
18. Dias Pereira P, Faustino AMR: Feline plasma cell pododermatitis: a study of 8 cases, *Vet Dermatol* 14:333, 2003.
19. Florant E: Essay préliminaire de traitement de la pododermatite plamacytaire feline par l'Interferon Oméga. Proceedings of AFVAC, Bordeau, 2006.
20. Nagele A: Successful treatment of feline cowpox infection in two kittens, *Virbac Tiergesundheit* 20:2007.

21. Jazic E, Coyner KS, Loeffler DG, et al: An evaluation of the clinical, cytological, infectious and histopathological features of feline acne, *Vet Dermatol* 17:134, 2006.

22. Florant E: A severe case of feline acne treated with Omega Interferon, *Informations dermatologiques vétérinaires* 10:2004.

23. Lyon KF: Gingivostomatitis, *Vet Clin North Am Small Anim Pract* 25:891, 2005.

24. Southerden P, Gorrel C: Treatment of a case of refractory feline chronic gingivostomatitis with feline recombinant interferon omega, *J Small Anim Pract* 48:104, 2007.

25. Mihaljevic SY: First clinical experiences with omega-Interferon in the treatment of chronic gingivitis-stomatitis-oropharyngitis of cats, *Der Praktische Tierarzt* 84:350, 2003.

26. Hendrick MJ: Feline vaccine-associated sarcomas: current studies on pathogenesis, *J Am Vet Med Assoc* 213:1425, 1998.

27. Macy DW, Couto CG: Prevention and treatment of injection-site sarcomas, *J Feline Med Surg* 3:169, 2001.

28. Kobayashi T, Hauck ML, Dodge R: Preoperative radiotherapy for vaccine associated sarcoma in 92 cats, *Vet Radiol Ultrasound* 43:473, 2002.

29. Hampel V, Schwarz B, Kempf C, et al: Adjuvant immunotherapy of feline fibrosarcoma with recombinant feline interferon-ω, *J Vet Intern Med* 21:1340, 2007.

CHAPTER

37 How to Treat Common Parasites Safely

Marcia Schwassman and Dawn Logas

Great advances in feline ectoparasite control have been made in the past decade. In particular the development of many new flea control products has made killing fleas without harming their host cat easier than ever before. These new products have both great efficacy and safety. Some of these new flea control products also are effective against other ectoparasites including ticks, mites, and lice.

FLEAS

The cat flea, *Ctenocephalides felis felis*, is the most important ectoparasite of domestic cats. In addition to causing flea-allergy dermatitis, fleas are the intermediate host for a tapeworm *(Dipylidium caninum)*, and can serve as vectors for some rickettsial organisms, as well as *Bartonella henselae*. Severe flea infestations can lead to anemia in affected cats, as well as annoyance for the human members of the household.

A basic understanding of the life cycle of the cat flea is essential to developing an effective flea control program. Adult cat fleas spend their entire life on their host. Female fleas will mate as soon as 8 hours after initiating feeding and will begin laying eggs as soon as 24 hours after initiating feeding. Female fleas are prolific egg layers, capable of laying 40 to 50 eggs daily. Eggs and flea feces fall off the host cat into the environment, with the greatest concentration of eggs found in areas where the pet sleeps or rests. Eggs usually hatch within 2 to 10 days. The larvae feed on adult flea feces, nonviable eggs, and other larvae

as they progress through three larval stages. Flea larvae prefer higher ambient temperatures and relative humidity and can be ready to pupate in 8 days when reared at 32° C and 75 per cent relative humidity. The majority of flea larvae inside the home develop at the base of carpets. In the outside environment, flea larvae develop best in warm, moist areas (e.g., in leaf litter or mulch under trees and shrubs). Once the larvae are ready to pupate, they spin a cocoon. The cocoon surface is sticky and environmental debris will adhere to its surface. The preemergent adult inside the cocoon can emerge in as few as 5 days, or given favorable conditions, can remain dormant for 200 days if no host is available. Heat and mechanical pressure that indicate the presence of a host stimulate adult emergence from the cocoon. The newly emerged adult flea jumps onto a mammalian host and the cycle starts again.

It is important to note that the cat flea has broad host specificity and also will readily accept dogs, ferrets, rabbits, opossums, and raccoons as hosts.[1] Under ideal conditions the entire flea life cycle can be completed in as little as 14 days, or can be delayed by 6 months. It also is important to note that adult fleas represent only 5 per cent of the entire flea population, whereas the immature life cycle stages (eggs, larvae, and pupae) represent the vast majority (95 per cent) of the population.

The concept of integrated pest management is advocated as the most effective way to eliminate existing flea populations quickly as well as prevent reinfestations. Integrated pest management involves the routine use of flea adulticides on the pet to eliminate the most visible part of the flea infestation, as well as control of egg and larval populations in the environment. Both on-pet and premise products are available to control immature stages of the flea life cycle. The preemergent adult fleas within their protective cocoons are the stage most resistant to destruction by any means. Integrated pest management also should provide the added benefit of delaying the development of resistance to the newer insecticides that are so valuable to us. The convenience and outstanding effectiveness of the newer insecticides may tempt the clinician into forgoing good client education and the principles of integrated pest management, but we must avoid this trap if we wish to preserve the effectiveness of these new insecticides (Table 37-1).

In addition to knowledge of flea biology, proper client education concerning the new flea control products also is important. Misconceptions regarding these newer flea control products are common. Many pet owners think that these products repel adult fleas, and therefore assume fleas have become resistant to a product if they see any fleas on their pet during the month after application of the product. In reality they are not seeing resistant fleas, but rather newly hatched adults that have developed from already existing immature stages in the environment. Complete eradication of the entire flea population takes time. Current extensive monitoring efforts have not detected any field collected strains of fleas resistant to imidacloprid,[2] although the KS1 laboratory strain of fleas has demonstrated some reduced susceptibility to various insecticides, including imidacloprid and fipronil.[3,4] Only one isolate of fleas collected in 1998 from Florida has shown some reduced susceptibility to fipronil.[4]

Flea control programs also must take into account whether or not the patient is flea allergic. Control of flea populations is desirable to prevent flea-induced anemia and transmission of parasites and infectious diseases; however, complete eradication of fleas from a cat's environment may be necessary if a cat is extremely flea allergic. Products that stop flea feeding quickly and/or kill adult fleas quickly will be the most beneficial. The amount

Table 37-1 Summary of Commonly Used Flea Control Products in Cats

Drug	Class	Mode of Action	Application	Target Parasites	Age of Use
Imidacloprid (Advantage) Primarily an adulticide Larvicidal activity	Neonicotinoid	Acts as agonist at polysynaptic nicotinic acetylcholine receptors; results in paralysis and death of adult fleas	Spot-on that spreads over the skin by translocation and is not absorbed systemically; must be applied to skin not hair coat	Fleas	Labeled for use in cats 8 weeks of age or older
Imidacloprid with moxidectin (Advantage multi)	Neonicotinoid and avermectin	Moxidectin is an avermectin and causes paralysis	Spot-on	Fleas, heartworm prevention, ear mites, hookworms, and roundworms	Labeled for use in cats 9 weeks of age or older
Fipronil (Frontline) Also available with methoprene (Frontline Plus) Adulticide	Phenylpyrazole	Binds at GABA-gated chloride channel causing excessive neuronal stimulation, paralysis, and death of adult fleas	Spray or spot-on Spreads over skin by translocation via the surface lipids on the skin, and is stored in sebaceous glands where it is constantly resecreted onto the hair and skin Not absorbed systemically Must be applied to skin	Fleas and ticks	Labeled for use in cats 8 weeks of age or older, and is safe in breeding, pregnant, and lactating cats
Selamectin (Revolution) Adulticide but has ovicidal and larvicidal activity	Semisynthetic avermectin	Binds to receptors on glutamate-gated (and possibly GABA) chloride channels leading to flaccid paralysis and death	Topical spot-on Absorbed through skin into the blood and then is redistributed to sebaceous glands	Fleas, heartworm prevention, control of ear mite infestations, control of hookworms and roundworms	Labeled for use in cats 6 weeks of age or older, and is safe for breeding, pregnant, and lactating cats

Continued

Table 37-1 Summary of Commonly Used Flea Control Products in Cats—cont'd

Drug	Class	Mode of Action	Application	Target Parasites	Age of Use
Nitenpyram (Capstar) Adulticide	Systemically active neonicotinoid	See imidacloprid	Orally administered	Adult fleas	Labeled as safe for cats 4 weeks of age or older weighing at least 2 pounds Safe in breeding, pregnant, or lactating cats Can be used with imidacloprid, fipronil, pyrethrins, lufenuron
Metaflumizone (Promeris)	Semicarbazone	Works by blocking voltage-dependent sodium channels leading to blocking of nerve impulses causing paralysis and death	Spot-on Spreads over skin in 24 to 48 hours Minimal systemic absorption	Fleas	Labeled as safe for use in cats 8 weeks of age or older
Dinotefuran (Vectra)	Neonicotinoid	See imidacloprid	Spot-on formulation combined with insect growth regulator pyriproxifen Spreads over body and adheres to skin and hair, absorbed on contact with fleas	Fleas	Labeled for use in cats 8 weeks of age or older
Pyrethrins and pyrethroids	Pyrethrin and synthetic pyrethroids	Affect voltage-dependent sodium channels of neurons and cause paralysis	Sprays and sponge-ons	Adult fleas, ticks, lice, *Cheyletiella*, ear mites, fur mites	Read label of each product Pyrethroids, especially >2%, can be extremely toxic to cats

of effort required will vary, given the degree of hypersensitivity of each individual patient, as well as differences in local environment.

INSECTICIDES/ADULTICIDES

Imidacloprid

Imidacloprid (Advantage) was the first newer generation insecticide released for control of fleas in 1996. It is a topical spot-on that spreads over the skin by translocation and is not absorbed systemically. It is a neonicotinoid (chloronicotinyl nitroguanidine) that acts as an agonist on the postsynaptic nicotinic acetylcholine receptors. By keeping the receptor channels open, it causes constant neuronal stimulation and therefore paralysis

and death of adult fleas. Imidacloprid has a very high margin of safety as a result of the affinity of the compound for insect acetylcholine receptors over mammalian acetylcholine receptors. Imidacloprid is absorbed through the flea intersegmental membranes and does not require ingestion by the flea to be effective.[5]

Imidacloprid kills adult fleas rapidly, with 100 per cent efficacy achieved within 12 to 24 hours after application.[6] Efficacy decreases slightly by 28 days after application, with 90 to 96 per cent of newly applied fleas killed in 24 hours.[7] One earlier study showed that imidacloprid's efficacy decreased to below 100 per cent by approximately 3 weeks after application, and that some viable eggs were produced after this time period.[3] Therefore initial application of imidacloprid every 3 weeks may be beneficial for the very flea-allergic cat. Imidacloprid also has good larvicidal activity,[8] although the principles of integrated pest management would discourage the use of a single chemical as both an adulticide and a larvicide. Imidacloprid is labeled for use in cats 8 weeks of age and older, and can be administered as often as once a week. The label recommends following veterinary advice for use on debilitated, aged, pregnant, or lactating cats.

Proper application of these topical parasiticidal products is essential for optimal effectiveness. The product must be applied to the skin, not the haircoat, to ensure adequate dispersal over the entire body. The product must be applied at the base of the skull. If the product is applied further down the neck incorrectly, the cat may be able to remove much of the product by grooming itself. The authors have seen a few localized reactions consisting of erythema, alopecia, papules, and crusts at the site of application, as well as a few cats who exhibit generalized pruritus following application of the product. Should any adverse reaction be seen, thorough bathing with a degreasing shampoo should remove most of the product. It is unknown if the reactions are to the imidacloprid itself or to the vehicle in the product.

Imidacloprid is available by itself (Advantage) or in combination with moxidectin (Advantage multi). Moxidectin is an avermectin that acts at the γ-aminobutyric acid (GABA) and glutamate-gated chloride channels, causing paralysis of parasites. In addition to controlling fleas, Advantage multi also prevents heartworm disease caused by *Dirofilaria immitis*, ear mite *(Otodectes cynotis)* infestations, and controls intestinal hookworms *(Ancylostoma tubaeforme)* and roundworms *(Toxocara cati)*. Advantage multi is labeled for use in cats 9 weeks of age and older as a once-monthly spot-on. Advantage multi for dogs is labeled for use against lice and *Sarcoptes scabiei*, so it would be expected to have activity against the cat louse *(Felicola subrostratus)* as well as *Notoedres cati*.

Fipronil

Fipronil (Frontline) was introduced shortly after imidacloprid in 1996. It is a phenylpyrazole insecticide with activity against adult fleas and ticks. It binds at the GABA-gated chloride channel, causing excessive neuronal stimulation, paralysis, and death of adult fleas. Some evidence suggests it is the glutamate-gated chloride channels that are affected rather than the GABA-gated chloride channels. Fipronil's high affinity for insect receptors over mammalian receptors is responsible for its safety in animals. Fipronil kills insects by contact or by ingestion.[9] It is available as a spray (Frontline spray), as a spot-on formulation (Frontline Top Spot), and in combination with the insect growth regulator methoprene as the spot-on formulation Frontline Plus.

Fipronil spreads over the skin by translocation via the surface lipids on the skin and is stored in the sebaceous glands from where it is constantly resecreted onto the skin and hair. It is not absorbed systemically. Because of its dependence on the skin surface lipid layer, many dermatologists recommend that fipronil be applied 24 to 48 hours before or after bathing, because bathing can disrupt the surface lipid layer. Fipronil reaches 100 per cent flea kill by 24 hours after application; however, like imidacloprid, efficacy decreased to below 100 per cent by 3 to 4

weeks after application, allowing some viable egg production.[3] Viable egg production is prevented by the methoprene in Frontline Plus. These data indicate that some extremely flea-allergic cats may not have adequate flea control with fipronil alone for the full 4 weeks. Unfortunately fipronil is an EPA-registered product, and clinicians are advised that it is a violation of federal law to deviate from the label instructions stating the product should not be reapplied before 30 days. The authors are aware of cases in which fipronil has been used more frequently (e.g., every 3 weeks) without any adverse effects. Clinical trials have demonstrated the effectiveness of fipronil in reducing the clinical signs of flea-allergy dermatitis in cats.[10] It is labeled for use in cats 8 weeks and older, and is safe for use in breeding, pregnant, and lactating cats.

Proper application of the product to the skin and not the haircoat at the base of the skull is important for adequate dispersal of the product. Some cats may develop inflammation at the site of application, and the authors have seen a few cats who developed generalized pruritus following application of the spot-on formulation of fipronil. Should any adverse reaction occur, thorough bathing with a degreasing shampoo should remove the majority of the product. As with imidacloprid it is not known if the reaction is to the fipronil itself or to its vehicle. Frontline for dogs also is labeled for use against *Sarcoptes scabiei* and chewing lice, and appears to have activity against *N. cati*, cat lice, and *O. cynotis*.

Selamectin

Selamectin (Revolution) was introduced in 1999. It is a semisynthetic avermectin derived from a bioengineered strain of *Streptomyces avermitilis*. Selamectin binds to receptors on glutamate-gated (and possibly GABA-gated) chloride channels, leading to flaccid paralysis and death of parasites. Selamectin's greater affinity for insect chloride channel receptors accounts for its safety in animals. Selamectin is a topical spot-on formulation that is absorbed through the skin into the blood and then is redistributed to the sebaceous glands. Selamectin achieves 100 per cent flea kill by 24 hours after application[6]; however, by 28 days after application, flea kill has decreased to less than 100 per cent.[6,11] Selamectin also has ovicidal and larvicidal activity, but as with imidacloprid, principles of integrated pest management would discourage use of a single product as an adulticide and larvicide. Selamectin has been shown to decrease clinical signs in flea-allergic cats when applied monthly.[12] Although some reports demonstrated slower flea kill by selamectin compared with other flea adulticides, selamectin was shown to decrease flea feeding more than imidacloprid or fipronil.[13]

In cats selamectin is labeled for the control of flea infestations, prevention of heartworm disease caused by *D. immitis*, control of ear mite *(O. cynotis)* infestations, and control of the intestinal parasites *A. tubaeforme* and *T. cati*. Selamectin can be used in cats 6 weeks of age and older. It also is safe for breeding, pregnant, and lactating cats. Adverse events are infrequent. As with all topical spot-on flea control products, local irritant reactions at the site of application have been reported. Rare instances of vomiting, loose stool, anorexia, lethargy, tachypnea, and muscle tremors also have been reported. Selamectin has been reported to be effective against *Cheyletiella* spp. when used once monthly for 3 months,[14] and for *Notoedres cati* when used every 2 weeks for three applications.[15]

Nitenpyram

Nitenpyram (Capstar) is a systemically active neonicotinoid insecticide approved in 2000 for killing adult fleas on dogs and cats. It binds to insect nicotinic acetylcholine receptors in postsynaptic nerve membranes and blocks transmission of nerve impulses, thereby causing paralysis and death of adult fleas. It is given orally and begins killing fleas within 30 minutes after administration,[16] and can achieve 100 per cent flea kill by 3 hours after administration.[17] Effective flea kill is maintained for 48 hours after administration (100 per cent at 24 hours and 98.6 per cent at 48 hours).[18] Not only does nitenpyram kill adult fleas quickly, it also causes a rapid decrease in feeding.[13] For both of these reasons, nitenpyram also causes a dramatic decrease in egg production.[18] The product is extremely safe and is labeled for use in cats 4 weeks and older, weighing at least 2 pounds. Nitenpyram is safe for use in pregnant and nursing cats, and can be safely given together with imidacloprid, fipronil, pyrethrins, and lufenuron.[16] Tablets can be given daily with or without food. Some flea-infested cats may show increased pruritus (as evidenced by scratching, licking, twitching) for several hours after administration of nitenpyram. This effect is caused by the altered movement of fleas affected by nitenpyram.[18,19]

Metaflumizone

Metaflumizone (Promeris), released in 2008, was the first semicarbazone insecticide approved for flea control in the United States. Metaflumizone acts by blocking voltage-dependent sodium channels, thereby blocking propagation of nerve impulses along axons. This results in paralysis and death of fleas. Metaflumizone is available as a spot-on formulation that spreads over the skin by 24 to 48 hours after application.[20] Systemic absorption is minimal.[20] Flea reduction of 74 to 98 per cent is reported by 24 hours after application, and greater than 90 per cent reduction in flea counts is maintained for up to 7 weeks in some studies.[6,21] Other studies indicate less complete control of adult fleas at 5 to 6 weeks after application; therefore monthly product application would seem prudent.[6] Flea egg production is essentially zero for more than 30 days.[22] Metaflumizone is labeled for use in cats 8 weeks of age and older. It has a high margin of safety. Application of up to five times the recommended dose to 8-week-old kittens produced no adverse effects. The authors have no clinical experience with this product because of its recent release at the time this text was written.

Dinotefuran

Dinotefuran (Vectra) is the latest of the neonicotinoid insecticides to be released in the United States for flea control. It is available in a spot-on formulation in combination with the insect growth regulator pyriproxifen. Dinotefuran is absorbed on contact with the flea. It binds to a unique site on the insect acetylcholine receptor and causes paralysis and death of adult fleas. Dinotefuran spreads over the body and adheres to the skin and hair. Dinotefuran kills adult fleas quickly with up to 99 per cent flea reduction by 6 hours after application, and up to 100 per cent flea reduction by 12 hours after application. By day 30 after application flea infestation had decreased by 93.3 per cent; therefore some extremely flea-allergic cats may benefit from more frequent application (e.g., every 3 weeks) (Figures 37-1 to 37-3). Egg production also was greatly decreased for the month following application of Vectra and none of the few eggs produced hatched. Dinotefuran is labeled for use in cats older than 8 weeks of age.[23]

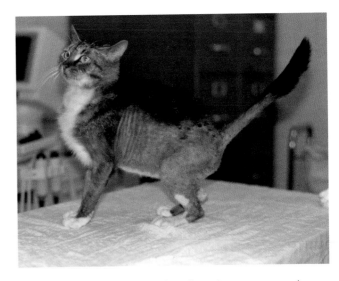

Figure 37-1 Flea-allergic cat. Flea allergy in cats can vary in severity from mild to severe. Note the extensive hair loss on the trunk of the patient.

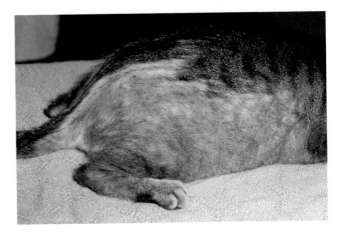

Figure 37-2 Closer view of cat in Figure 37-1. Hair loss is symmetrical and flea-allergy dermatitis can mimic other pruritic skin diseases of cats (e.g., atopy).

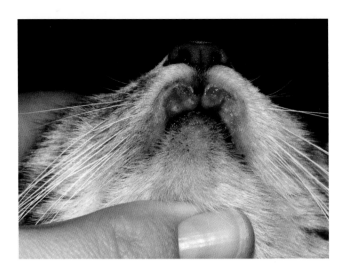

Figure 37-3 Flea-allergic cat. In this picture the major lesion is a bilaterally symmetrical lip ulcer or "rodent ulcer." Similar lesions can be seen with atopy or food allergy; however, flea-allergy dermatitis should be ruled out early in the diagnostic process.

Pyrethrins and Pyrethroids

Pyrethrins and their synthetic cousins the pyrethroids have good activity against adult fleas. They affect the voltage-dependent sodium channels of neurons and cause paralysis and death of parasites. In addition to killing adult fleas, they also are effective against ticks, lice, *Cheyletiella* spp., ear mites *(O. cynotis),* and the cat fur mite *(Lynxacarus radovsky).*[24] Most cats tolerate up to 0.1 per cent solutions well; however, the higher concentrations of two per cent or more found in some dog and equine products are extremely toxic to cats and must be avoided. The disadvantages of pyrethrin/permethrin-based products for flea control are short duration of activity and formulation of products. Most of these products are manufactured as sprays or dips, neither of which is particularly easy to apply to cats.

INSECT GROWTH REGULATORS

Methoprene and Pyriproxifen

Methoprene (Precor) and pyriproxifen (Nylar) are juvenile hormone analogues that arrest the development of flea larvae. The larvae die instead of progressing through their normal developmental stages. These insect growth regulators have extremely low mammalian toxicity, so they are ideal for both on-pet and environmental use. Methoprene is degraded by ultraviolet (UV) light, so outdoor use is not recommended. It is available for indoor environmental use, as well as in several on-pet products. Methoprene and pyriproxifen spread by translocation, so collars or spot-on formulations are effective. Methoprene remains effective in the environment for 1 to 2 months or longer after application. Pyriproxifen is more UV light–stable, making it suitable for both indoor and outdoor use. It remains effective in the environment for 2 to 4 months after application, depending on environmental

conditions. Pyriproxifen is available as an environmental spray as well as in on-pet products.

INSECT DEVELOPMENT INHIBITORS

Lufenuron

Lufenuron (Program) is a benzoylphenyl urea that inhibits chitin biosynthesis. It has both ovicidal and larvicidal activity against fleas. Lufenuron concentrates in the fat from where it is slowly released into the bloodstream. It is available in tablet, liquid, and 6-month injectable formulation for use in cats 6 weeks of age and older. The tablet and liquid forms should be given with a meal to ensure complete absorption. Lufenuron is extremely safe for cats because mammals have no chitin. No adverse effects in kittens were noted when the tablet or liquid formulations were administered to nursing cats. The safety of the injectable formulation has not been established in reproducing cats. Some cats may experience discomfort with the injection, and a few local reactions were seen at the injection site.

ENVIRONMENTAL FLEA CONTROL

The need for aggressive environmental flea control has decreased greatly since the introduction of highly effective adulticides, especially when used in combination with insect growth regulators or lufenuron. For indoor cats faced with a mild flea infestation, initial use of a flea adulticide combined with on-pet use of methoprene, pyriproxifen, or lufenuron should eliminate the problem relatively quickly. However, if the infestation is heavy, additional environmental control measures may be needed to speed control of the infestation.

Indoor Flea Control

Vacuuming removes a large percentage of flea eggs and larvae from carpets; therefore regular vacuuming of infested areas is recommended. Spraying the indoor environment with methoprene or pyriproxifen also will kill a large percentage of the immature flea stages.

Sodium Polyborates

Sodium polyborate powders kill flea larvae and eggs by desiccation and are particularly effective in carpeted areas. Professional application is recommended and usually comes with a 1-year guarantee provided the carpet is not steam cleaned during that period.

Outdoor Flea Control

Flea larvae develop best in warm, humid areas; therefore removal of leaf litter and mulch from shaded areas may be helpful in heavy infestations. Pet access to damp, dark areas such as under foundations, decks, and porches should be prohibited. Keeping out free-roaming pet animals (e.g., dogs, cats) as well as urban wildlife (e.g., raccoons, opossums) can decrease continued contamination of the area with new flea eggs. The application of pyriproxifen outdoors to areas favorable for flea larval

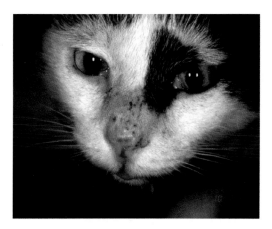

Figure 37-4 Cat with insect bite hypersensitivity. Note the symmetrical lesions on the face and nose. Insect bite hypersensitivity should be a differential diagnosis in cats with facial dermatitis.

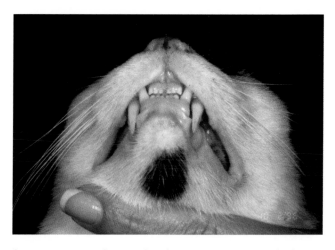

Figure 37-5 Cat with insect bite hypersensitivity. Note the lesions on the lips and chin.

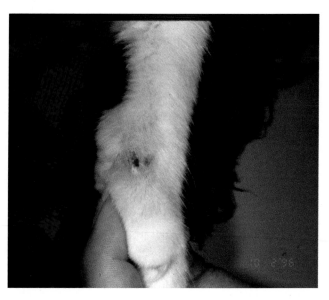

Figure 37-6 Cat with insect bite hypersensitivity. Note the lesions at the base of the nail bed. Insect bite hypersensitivity lesions are common at the junction of skin and thinly haired areas.

development can decrease the environmental flea burden greatly.

Steinernema carpocapsae

Biological control using the beneficial nematode *Steinernema carpocapsae* also can eliminate much of the environmental flea burden. These nematodes kill flea larvae and pupae. The nematodes survive best in outdoor areas that are well shaded and that have much organic material on the ground. These nematodes may need to be applied monthly and are killed by extreme heat and cold. The nematodes are formulated as a powder that is mixed with water and sprayed on the yard. It is important to remember that these nematodes are living organisms, so their use with other pesticides is incompatible. Spraying flea adulticides in the environment usually is not necessary unless the infestation is particularly heavy. Because the newly hatched adult fleas are seeking a mammalian host, it makes more sense to apply the adulticides to the host and use products that stop the development of the immature stages of the flea in the environment.

MOSQUITO AND *CULICOIDES* HYPERSENSITIVITY

Classic mosquito bite hypersensitivity reactions in cats were documented by Mason and Evans in 1991.[25] Lesions involve the nasal planum and bridge of the nose most commonly, and can consist of papules, nodules, edema, erosions, crusts, alopecia, depigmentation, and scarring (Figure 37-4). Lesions also may be seen on the ear pinnae, footpads, chin, paws, and lips (Figures 37-5 and 37-6). Pruritus is variable. Diagnosis is confirmed by skin biopsy, lack of response to flea control, and positive reaction to intradermal injection of mosquito extract. Resolution of clinical signs when the cat is confined to the inside of the house or to a screened-in area free of mosquitoes provides further confirmation of the diagnosis and is the preferred method of treatment.

Few descriptions of hypersensitivity reactions in cats to the bites from *Culicoides* spp. biting gnats ("no-see-ums") exist in the literature,[26] although *Culicoides* hypersensitivity is well-documented in horses. In cats clinical signs can include pruritus, papules, nodules, crusts, excoriations, erythema, and alopecia of the head and ear pinnae, and less often, body and limbs. Diagnosis is confirmed by lack of response to flea control, positive reaction to intradermal testing with *Culicoides* spp. antigen, and resolution of clinical signs when the cat is kept strictly indoors. Access to screened porches also must be prohibited because regular screening is not a barrier to *Culicoides* spp.

If the cat with mosquito or *Culicoides* bite hypersensitivity can not be confined indoors, insect repellents must be used as much as possible. Products containing 0.1 per cent permethrin have some repellent activity against mosquitoes and *Culicoides* spp.; however, they must be applied frequently and usually are only partially effective. The higher concentrations of permethrins required for good mosquito and *Culicoides* spp. repellency are toxic to cats so they can not be used. Avon Skin so Soft bath oil is supposed to have repellent activity against *Culicoides* spp., so it can be tried in place of permethrins. Repellent products containing diethyltoluamide (DEET) are not recommended because they can be toxic to cats. Resolution of clinical signs of mosquito or *Culicoides* spp. hypersensitivity is extremely difficult if cats can not be made strictly indoor pets.

TICKS

Other than pyrethroid products, which are not particularly effective at safe concentrations, fipronil is the only product labeled for use against ticks on cats. Selamectin is labeled for use against ticks in dogs so it may have some effectiveness in cats also. Advantix and Vectra 3D both contain levels of permethrin toxic to cats; therefore owners with dogs and cats in the household must take care to apply the correct product to the correct species.

DEMODICOSIS

Feline demodicosis is caused by two different species of mites, *Demodex cati* and *Demodex gatoi*. (See Chapter 27 in the fifth volume of this series for a detailed discussion of demodicosis in cats.)

DEMODEX GATOI

This demodectic mite with the short, blunted abdomen causes a contagious, often severely pruritic dermatitis in cats. *D. gatoi* can be difficult to demonstrate, sometimes necessitating the use of response to therapy as a diagnostic test. Weekly dipping with a two per cent lime sulfur solution is the most effective treatment for *D. gatoi*. A series of six dips is recommended and clinical improvement should be seen after three dips. Lime sulfur is a very safe compound for topical use. Adverse reactions are rare and typically consist of erythema, excessive dryness, and increased pruritus.

Despite the demonstrated efficacy and safety of lime sulfur, clients may be reluctant to use the product because of its unpleasant odor. Ivermectin dosed at 300 µg/kg PO q24h or q48h for a minimum of 6 weeks also is effective. Clients must be advised that this constitutes off-label use of the drug and toxic reactions (neurological) are possible. For this reason the authors recommend using test doses of 50 µg/kg, 100 µg/kg, then 200 µg/kg PO before giving the full dose. Some textbooks list amitraz as a recommended treatment for feline demodicosis; however, because of concerns about toxic reactions, the authors prefer not to use this product. All in-contact cats should be treated because *D. gatoi* is contagious.[27]

DEMODEX CATI

D. cati can cause generalized dermatitis and ceruminous otitis. This follicular mite is similar in appearance to the demodectic mite of dogs, and also is often seen secondary to immunosuppression. Feline leukemia virus infection,

feline immunodeficiency virus infection, diabetes mellitus, and neoplasia all have been seen in association with *Demodex cati* infestation. Resolution of the underlying disease process by itself may result in elimination of the mites, or specific miticidal therapy may be needed. Ivermectin and lime sulfur at the same doses used to treat *D. gatoi* usually are effective. If ivermectin is not a viable option, off-label use of amitraz at 0.0125 to 0.025 per cent applied every 5 days for 4 to 6 weeks usually is effective.[28] Cats should be treated until two sets of skin scrapes for mites are negative.

EAR MITES *(OTODECTES CYNOTIS)*

Many products currently are available for the treatment of ear mites in cats. Topical otic preparations containing thiabendazole (Tresaderm), ivermectin (Acarexx) or milbemycin (Milbemite) all have good efficacy against ear mites. Selamectin once monthly is labeled for control of ear mites, and provides the additional benefit of killing ear mites that have left the ear canal to also infest the skin on the head and neck. Studies have shown that two applications (day 0 and day 30) are required for eradication of the mites.[29] More frequent application (i.e., every 2 weeks) of selamectin is considered by some clinicians to be more efficacious. Moxidectin (Advantage multi) applied once monthly also is labeled for control of *O. cynotis* in cats. With the wide availability of effective, label-approved products for treatment of ear mites, the off-label use of ivermectin is discouraged.

FELINE SCABIES *(NOTOEDRES CATI)*

Various topical products are effective against *N. cati* (Figure 37-7). Once weekly dips with a 2 per cent lime sulfur solution for 4 to 6 weeks are recommended. Selamectin is effective against *N. cati* although it is not labeled for this use. Three applications at 2-week intervals are recommended.[15,24] Ivermectin dosed at 200 to 400 µg/kg PO or SQ q7-14d for 4 to 6 weeks also is effective; however,

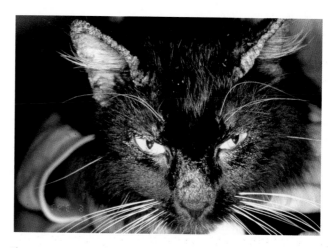

Figure 37-7 Cat with *Notoedres* infestation. Note the facial distribution of lesions and the thick crusting on the ears. This is an intensely pruritic disease and mites are found easily.

this is off-label use and idiosyncratic toxic reactions to ivermectin can be seen in cats.[15]

CHEYLETIELLOSIS

Cheyletiella spp. infestations in cats are caused most often by *Cheyletiella blakei*. Treatment options include pyrethrins, permethrin, and lime sulfur dips.[24] Selamectin applied once monthly for 3 months was effective at eliminating *Cheyletiella* spp. from cats.[14] Ivermectin dosed at 200 to 300 µg/kg PO q7-14d for 6 to 8 weeks also is effective.[15]

CAT FUR MITE *(LYNXACARUS RADOVSKY)*

Cat fur mite infestations are reported sporadically. This parasite is more common in some geographic areas than others. A single dose of ivermectin at 300 µg/kg PO has been reported to be effective.[15] Lime sulfur dips also are thought to be effective in the treatment of fur mite infestations.[30]

PEDICULOSIS

Felicola subrostratus is the biting louse of cats. Ivermectin dosed at 200 µg/kg SQ or selamectin applied one time at the label dose are effective against *Felicola subrostratus*.[15] Lime sulfur dips, fipronil, pyrethrins, and synthetic pyrethroids also should be effective.[30]

REFERENCES

1. Dryden MW, Broce AB, Cawthra J, et al: Urban wildlife as reservoirs of cat fleas, *Ctenocephalides felis*. Am Assoc Vet. Parasitol 40th Annual Meeting, Pittsburgh: 65, 1995 (Abstr).
2. Blagburn BL, Dryden MW, Payne PA, et al: New insights into flea resistance, *Compend Contin Educ Pract Vet* 30(Suppl):4, 2008.
3. Dryden MW: Laboratory evaluations of topical flea control products: Proceedings British Veterinary Dermatology Study Group: 14, 1998.
4. Payne PA, Dryden MW, Smith V, et al: Effect of 0.29% w/w fipronil spray on adult flea mortality and egg production of three different cat flea, *Ctenocephalides felis* (Bouche), strains infesting cats, *Vet Parasitol* 102:331, 2001.
5. Melhorn H, Hansen O, Mencke N: Comparative study on the effects of three insecticides (fipronil, imidacloprid, selamectin) on developmental stages of the cat flea (*Ctenocephalides felis* Bouche 1835): a light and electron microscopic analysis of in vivo and in vitro experiments, *Parasitol Res* 87:198, 2001.
6. Schnieder T, Wolken S, Mencke N: Comparative speed of efficacy of imidacloprid against *Ctenocephalides felis* in experimentally infested cats, *Compend Contin Educ Pract Vet* 30(Suppl):18, 2008.
7. Jacobs DE, Hutchinson MJ, Krieger KJ: Duration of activity of imidacloprid, a novel adulticide for flea control against *Ctenocephalides felis* in cats, *Vet Rec* 140:259, 1997.
8. Jacobs DE, Hutchinson MJ, Ewald-Hamm D: Inhibition of immature *Ctenocephalides felis felis* (Siphonaptera: Pulicidae) development in the immediate environment of cats treated with imidacloprid, *J Med Entomol* 37:228, 2000.
9. National Pesticide Telecommunications Network: Fipronil, EPA. http://ace.orst.edu/info/nptn/factsheets/fipronil.htm. 1998.
10. Medleau L, Hnilica KA, Lower K, et al: Effect of topical application of fipronil in cats with flea allergic dermatitis, *J Am Vet Med Assoc* 221:254, 2002.
11. McTier TL, Shanks DJ, Jernigan AD, et al: Evaluation of the effects of selamectin against adult and immature stages of fleas (*Ctenocephalides felis felis*) on dogs and cats, *Vet Parasitol* 91:201, 2000.
12. Dickin SK, McTier TL, Murphy MG, et al: Efficacy of selamectin in the treatment and control of clinical signs of flea allergy dermatitis in dogs and cats experimentally infested with fleas, *J Am Vet Med Assoc* 223:639, 2003.
13. McCoy C, Broce AB, Dryden MW: Flea blood feeding patterns in cats treated with oral nitenpyram and the topical insecticides imidacloprid, fipronil and selamectin, *Vet Parasitol* 156:293, 2008.
14. Chailleux N, Paradis M: Efficacy of selamectin in the treatment of naturally acquired cheyletiellosis in cats, *Can Vet J* 43:767, 2002.
15. Burrows A: Avermectins in dermatology. In Bonagura JD, Twedt DC, editors: *Kirk's current veterinary therapy XIV*, St. Louis, 2009, Mosby, p 390.
16. Novartis Animal Health NADA 141-175 Capstar® (Nitenpyram).
17. Schenker R, Tinembart O, Humbert-Droz E, et al: Comparative speed of kill between nitenpyram, fipronil, imidacloprid, selamectin and cythioate against adult *Ctenocephalides felis* (Bouche) on cats and dogs, *Vet Parasitol* 112:249, 2003.
18. Rust MK, Waggoner MM, Hinkle NC, et al: Efficacy and longevity of nitenpyram against adult cat fleas (Siphonaptera: Pulicidae), *J Med Entomol* 40:678, 2003.
19. Mahoney R, Tinembart O, Schenker R: Flea-related itching in cats and dogs after treatment with nitenpyram, *Compend Contin Educ Pract Vet* 23(Suppl):20, 2001.
20. DeLay RL, Lacoste E, Delprat S, et al: Pharmacokinetics of metaflumizone in the plasma and hair of cats following topical application, *Vet Parasitol* 150:258, 2007.
21. Holzmer S, Hair JA, Dryden MW, et al: Efficacy of a novel formulation of metaflumizone for the control of fleas (*Ctenocephalides felis*) on cats, *Vet Parasitol* 150:219, 2007.
22. Dryden MW, Payne P, Lowe A, et al: Efficacy of a topically applied formulation of metaflumizone on cats against the adult cat flea, flea egg production and hatch, and adult flea emergence, *Vet Parasitol* 150:263, 2007.
23. Vectra technical monograph, Summit VetPharm, www.summitvetpharm.com.
24. Kennis R: Parasiticides in dermatology. In Campbell K, editor: *Small animal dermatology secrets*, Philadelphia, 2004, Hanley and Belfus, p 65.
25. Mason KV, Evans AG: Mosquito bite-caused eosinophilic dermatitis in cats, *J Am Vet Med Assoc* 198:2086, 1991.
26. Moriello K: Eosinophilic dermatoses. In Foster A, Foil C, editors: *BSAVA manual of small animal dermatology*, ed 2, Gloucester, 2003, British Small Animal Veterinary Association, p 233.
27. Beale KA, Morris DO: Feline demodicosis. In Bonagura JD, Twedt DC, editors: *Kirk's current veterinary therapy XIV*, St. Louis, 2009, Mosby, p 438.
28. Craig M: Demodicosis. In Foster A, Foil C, editors: *BSAVA manual of small animal dermatology*, ed 2, Gloucester, 2003, British Small Animal Veterinary Association, p 153.
29. Blot C, Kodjo A, Reynaud MC, et al: Efficacy of selamectin administered topically in the treatment of feline otoacariasis, *Vet Parasitol* 112:241, 2003.
30. Scott DW, Miller WH, Griffin CE: *Small animal dermatology*, ed 6, Philadelphia, 2001, Saunders, p 423.

Cardiology and Respiratory Disorders

Matthew W. Miller, Section Editor

38 Cardiac Blood Tests

Mark A. Oyama

The assessment of feline cardiac function relies traditionally on electrocardiography, radiography, and echocardiography. These diagnostic modalities are relatively time-consuming, expensive, and in the case of echocardiography, may be of limited availability. Blood-based cardiac testing is an emerging field offering important advantages over traditional diagnostic tests, including lower financial cost and wide availability. The clinical utility of blood-based testing relies on the specificity and sensitivity of the assay to detect underlying heart disease and provide information regarding disease severity, response to treatment, and prognosis. Sensitivity refers to the ability of a test to detect affected individuals, whereas specificity refers to the ability to detect individuals not affected by the condition in question. A clinical test that yields a yes or no (binary) result represents a conflicting balance between sensitivity and specificity. That is, gains in sensitivity typically are offset by losses of specificity and vice versa. Tests that yield continuous (e.g., numerical) results can provide additional information regarding severity of the disease (i.e., higher assay values signify more severe disease), allow risk stratification and prognostication, as well as the ability to guide therapy.

Cardiac blood testing is widely accepted in human medicine. In fact, blood-based detection of cardiac "biomarkers" represents the diagnostic standard for detection of acute myocardial infarction and congestive heart failure.[1,2] A biomarker is defined as a substance elaborated by a specific tissue, detected in circulation, released in proportion to a particular disease process that provides information regarding presence and severity of disease, and is relatively stable and easy to detect by routine clinical laboratory methods. Detection of biomarkers for disease of organs other than the heart is both familiar and routine. For example, bilirubin is a commonly used biomarker to detect hepatic disease. In cats B-type natriuretic peptide (BNP), atrial natriuretic peptide (ANP), and cardiac troponin have demonstrated the greatest potential as cardiac biomarkers.

NATRIURETIC PEPTIDES

ANP and BNP, released from the myocardium primarily in response to elevated wall stress, elicit vasodilation, diuresis, and natriuresis. In this respect the biological activity of ANP and BNP counters that of the renin-angiotensin-aldosterone system, which also is activated in cats with heart disease and heart failure. Production of ANP occurs primarily within the atrial myocardium, whereas in cats with heart disease, both the atrial and ventricular myocardium secrete BNP.[3-5] Both hormones are produced initially as prohormones, and upon secretion are cleaved subsequently by serum proteases to form the active hormone (C-terminal ANP and C-terminal BNP), as well as an inactive N-terminal portion (NT-proANP and NT-proBNP). Detection of the circulating N-terminal fragments is facilitated by their longer half-life and greater stability as compared with the C-terminal molecules. Thus the commercially available feline ANP and BNP tests detect the N-terminal molecules specifically.

In human beings ANP and BNP assays are used to (1) detect asymptomatic disease in high-risk populations, (2) assess severity of disease, (3) confirm or exclude a diagnosis of heart failure in emergent patients, (4) provide prognosis, and (5) guide treatment through use of sequential measurements.[2,6,7]

DETECTION OF UNDERLYING HEART DISEASE

Circulating concentrations of C-ANP and C-BNP are elevated in cats with heart disease,[8] and plasma C-ANP concentrations correlate strongly with left atrial pressure in cats.[9] NT-proANP and NT-proBNP are similarly elevated in affected cats.[10] Median (95% CI) concentration of NT-proANP in healthy control cats, cats with heart disease without heart failure, and cats with heart disease and heart failure was 682 (530 to 834) pmol/L, 1176 (810 to 1543) pmol/L, and 1865 (1499 to 2231) pmol/L, respectively.[10] Using a cutoff value of 960 pmol/L, NT-proANP assay possessed a sensitivity of 84 per cent and specificity of 82 per cent in distinguishing healthy controls from cats with heart disease or heart failure. Overall, NT-pro-ANP assay classified 83 per cent of the 78 cats correctly in the study. In the same study[10] median (95% CI) concentration of NT-proBNP in healthy control cats, cats with heart disease without heart failure, and cats with heart disease and heart failure was 34 (11 to 56) pmol/L, 184 (111 to 257) pmol/L, and 525 (437 to 612) pmol/L, respectively. Using a cutoff value of 49 pmol/L, NT-proBNP assay possessed 100 per cent sensitivity and 89 per cent specificity, and 96 per cent of all cats were classified correctly. Thus every cat with heart disease or heart failure ($n = 50$) was detected by NT-proBNP assay. The detection of heart disease in cats using NT-proBNP assay is further supported by a study of 80 healthy control cats and 86 cats with asymptomatic heart disease.[11] In this population an NT-proBNP cutoff value of 40 pmol/L yielded 90 per cent sensitivity and 85 per cent specificity for detecting cats with asymptomatic heart disease. These results indicate that detection of asymptomatic or occult cardiomyopathy is possible using natriuretic peptide assay, and in particular NT-proBNP assay. Cats with preclinical cardiomyopathy are a particularly important subpopulation, because by definition they demonstrate no clinical signs referable to their underlying disease. Cats with preclinical disease frequently escape detection until overt sequelae (i.e., pulmonary edema, pleural effusion, systemic thromboembolism) develop, at which time prognosis is very poor.

In general, screening tests are most useful when the assay in use is highly sensitive and is applied to a high-risk population with a relatively high prevalence of disease.[12] In a feline population this may include breeds at high risk (e.g., Maine Coon), older cats, or cats with heart murmurs or gallop rhythms. This combination of high sensitivity and relatively high prevalence maximizes the predictive power of the test by reducing the number of false-positive and false-negative results.

ASSESSMENT OF DISEASE SEVERITY

In cats with cardiomyopathy, circulating NT-proANP and NT-proBNP concentrations correlate with traditional indices of disease severity, such as vertebral heart size, left ventricular wall thickness, and left atrial size.[10,13] These results agree with findings in human beings with hypertrophic cardiomyopathy (HCM).[14,15] It should be noted, however, that the precise clinical utility of circulating BNP concentrations for quantification of disease severity in any *individual* patient is still a subject of great debate.[16,17] Importantly NT-proBNP may not detect very early and mild disease (i.e., a false-negative result). More studies in this specific population are needed. The importance of detecting very early disease can be viewed in different ways. On the one hand, a false-negative result would allow a cat with mild disease to remain undetected, and this may negatively impact breeding decisions made for animals young enough to still be bred. In this regard identification and screening for specific causative genetic mutations remains the gold standard (see Chapter 39). On the other hand, proponents of cardiac blood testing argue that the impact of a false-negative result on any individual animal outside of breeding considerations is relatively low, such that very mild disease is not typically associated with clinical signs, nor are there proven medical interventions that alter the course of disease at this early stage. Thus no practical intervention other than rechecking disease at a later date is typically performed in cats with very mild disease. Based on previous studies indicating a high degree of sensitivity and specificity in cats with moderate to severe disease,[10,11,13] one could reasonably expect that serial NT-proBNP assay in these cats could be used to detect progressive disease.

DETECTING HEART FAILURE IN THE CAT WITH RESPIRATORY SIGNS

In cats with respiratory signs BNP assay helps to differentiate causes of dyspnea. In a study of 137 cats who presented with respiratory signs, plasma NT-proBNP higher than 265 pmol/L yielded a sensitivity of 91 per cent and specificity of 85 per cent in detecting those cats with heart failure ($n = 84$) versus those with primary respiratory diseases such as asthma, pneumonia, or neoplasia ($n = 53$).[13] Similarly, Connolly et al[10] reported that NT-proBNP higher than 220 pmol/L possessed 94 per cent sensitivity and 88 per cent specificity, whereas NT-proANP higher than 986 pmol/L possessed 94 per cent sensitivity and 80 per cent specificity, in 41 cats with respiratory disease and 33 cats with heart failure. Finally Wess et al[18] reported that NT-proBNP higher than 277 pmol/L achieved 95 per cent sensitivity and 85 per cent specificity in 21 cats with respiratory disease and 20 cats with heart failure. Thus the cumulative results of these studies suggest that NT-proANP, and in particular, NT-proBNP, are useful as part of the diagnostic evaluation of cats who present with respiratory signs. Those cats with elevated NT-proBNP concentrations likely suffer from congestive heart failure, whereas those with lower values are more likely to have primary respiratory disease. The value of such testing is especially pertinent to patients who are not stable enough for routine diagnostic tests (e.g., thoracic radiography, echocardiography, transtracheal wash). The development of rapid pet-side assays is needed to fulfill the potential of these tests maximally for use in the emergent patient.

PROGNOSTIC VALUE AND GUIDE TO TREATMENT

Little data regarding the use of cardiac biomarkers as guides to therapy or prognostic indicators are available in cats. In human beings, however, BNP measurement has proven to be useful in risk stratification and as a predictor of survival. In one study[19] of 48,629 hospitalizations in people with heart failure, BNP possessed a strong linear relationship to in-hospital mortality. Patients with the highest BNP concentrations were 2.2 times more likely to die than those with the lowest values. Importantly, this study included a large number ($n = 18,164$) of people with heart failure but preserved systolic function, which is similar to the most common forms of feline cardiomyopathy (i.e., hypertrophic and restrictive cardiomyopathy). In a study of human patients with hypertrophic cardiomyopathy, Magga et al[20] reported that BNP concentration correlated with the degree of pathologic myocardial remodeling, and this may help to explain the correlation between elevated BNP and decreased survival.

In cats prediction of either survival or risk of morbid events such as congestive heart failure or thromboembolism is particularly difficult. It is generally believed, however, that both the severity of left ventricular hypertrophy and the degree of atrial enlargement is predictive of outcome in cats with heart disease.[21] Therefore biomarkers that are released in response to atrial and ventricular stretch such as NT-proBNP may have prognostic value. Treatment of feline heart disease generally is guided by clinical signs and echocardiographic findings. In human patients with HCM, progressively elevated BNP concentration is associated with clinical deterioration,[22] and BNP-directed treatment may improve outcome. In one study[23] therapy designed specifically to decrease BNP concentration to less than 100 ng/L resulted in a 50 per cent reduction of death from heart failure or rehospitalization versus control.

CARDIAC TROPONINS

Contraction of the cardiac muscle is initiated by release of intracellular calcium ions and the subsequent cross bridging of actin and myosin filaments. The cardiac troponin complex, which acts in conjunction with the actin filament, is a critical regulator of this process. The troponin complex is formed by three distinct units, cardiac troponins I (cTnI), T (cTnT), and C. During the initiation of contraction, cardiac troponin-C binds intracellular calcium and relieves the inhibitory effect of cTnI on the actin and myosin, thus allowing cross bridging to begin. Subsequent disassociation of calcium from troponin-C effectively ends contraction and allows the muscle to relax.

In cases of cardiac injury, the troponin subunits detach from the actin filament, leak into the interstitial space, and gain entry into the general circulation. The cTnI and cTnT isoforms present in cardiac muscle are distinct from those in skeletal muscle, and detection of either cardiac isoform in plasma or serum is a highly specific and sensitive indicator of cardiac injury. Although the exact kinetics of troponin release from feline myocardium are relatively unknown, the characteristics of cardiac troponin release appear similar in most mammalian species.[24,25] In human beings the release kinetics of cardiac troponin are biphasic with rapid leakage of small amounts of cytosolic troponin followed by greater and more sustained release of bound troponin, resulting in detection of rising troponin levels within 4 hours of injury and peaking between 12 and 48 hours. Elevated concentrations can persist after acute myocardial infarction for as long as 2 weeks.[26]

Due to a high degree of homology between human and veterinary species,[27] detection of feline cardiac troponin can be accomplished using immunoassays designed for detection of human troponin. The majority of studies performed in cats utilize assays that test specifically for cTnI. Although results between different commercial immunoassay machines are not likely to be directly comparable, the concentration of circulating cTnI in healthy cats should be uniformly low. Most healthy cats possess cTnI concentrations below any particular assay's detection limit (typically <0.03 to 0.05 ng/mL).[28] The particular sample type that is used (i.e., plasma, serum, or whole blood) depends on each manufacturer's assay. It is important to note that elevated cardiac troponin is indicative of myocardial cell damage, but is not specific for any particular etiology. Thus a variety of causes have been associated with increased cTnI in cats, including cardiomyopathy,[29,30] blunt myocardial trauma,[31] hyperthyroidism,[32] and renal disease.[33]

In human beings, troponin testing is used primarily for the diagnosis of acute myocardial infarction secondary to atherosclerotic disease. In cats, this particular cause of myocardial infarction is rare; however, small infarctions secondary to coronary artery and myocardial hypertrophy are a prominent feature of feline cardiomyopathy.[34,35] Acute infarction in cats would result in a biphasic release of troponin similar to that seen in human beings. This release pattern is in contrast to cases of chronic cardiac disease in which chronic low-level myocardial injury produces mild but persistently elevated troponin concentrations.[36] In human patients with chronic heart disease, elevated troponin is associated with increased mortality and hospitalization.[37,38] In cats with moderate to severe HCM, cTnI is elevated and is correlated to ventricular wall thickness as well as the presence or absence of congestive heart failure.[29,30] Therefore higher elevations of cTnI are thought to signify greater myocardial injury, and it is tempting to speculate whether cTnI values correlate with survival. In human beings persistently elevated troponin levels predict worse outcome, whereas treatment producing a decrease in troponin is associated with a corresponding decrease in mortality.[39-41] These data suggest that cTnI has prognostic value and potentially could be used to guide treatment.

Due to its specificity for cardiac muscle, cTnI assay can assist in the differentiation of cardiac and noncardiac causes of dyspnea in cats.[29,42] In cats with respiratory distress, the median plasma cTnI concentration in cats with congestive heart failure was 10-fold higher than in cats with primary respiratory disease such as asthma. Plasma cTnI concentration higher than 1.43 ng/mL was 100 per cent specific (but only 58 per cent sensitive) for identifying cats with congestive heart failure.[42] Thus detecting a very elevated cTnI will reliably signal heart failure; however, because of the relatively low sensitivity, use of this cutoff point also will generate many false-negatives. The use of cardiac blood tests in combination, such as performing both NT-proBNP and cTnI assay, may help to improve sensitivity and specificity, but specific clinical studies are lacking (Figure 38-1).

	NT-proBNP	Cardiac troponin
Diagnose heart disease	+++	++
Assess disease severity	++	++
Differentiate cardiac vs. noncardiac dyspnea	+++	+
Guide treatment	?	?
Prognosis	?	?

Figure 38-1 Author's evaluation of the current utility of NT-proBNP and cardiac troponin testing for various indications in cats. +++, Data available, good utility; ++, data available, moderate utility; +, data available, limited utility; ?, no data available.

cTnI is elevated in cases of blunt myocardial trauma,[31] hyperthyroidism,[32] and renal disease.[33] In the case of trauma and hyperthyroidism, the underlying myocardial cell injury producing these elevations is thought to be limited. Thus cTnI levels presumably would return to normal once the primary condition is remedied. In a study of hyperthyroid cats,[32] elevated cTnI values tended to return to normal after successful radioactive iodine treatment. Cardiac troponin is cleared from circulation by the reticuloendothelial system as well as by renal excretion. In a small study involving 14 cats with azotemia, cTnI was elevated in eight of 14 cats (57 per cent),[33] and these findings are consistent with human patients with chronic kidney disease in whom troponin is elevated in approximately 50 per cent of cases.

LIMITATIONS OF CARDIAC BLOOD TESTING

Many unknowns exist regarding the clinical application of natriuretic peptide and cardiac troponin testing in cats. To date studies investigating the diagnostic potential of these assays have been promising, but many important limitations remain. As with any diagnostic assay, the results of cardiac blood tests should be interpreted in conjunction with the patient signalment, history, physical examination findings, and other diagnostic test results. In this regard cardiac blood tests should augment, not replace, conventional diagnostic tests such as electrocardiography, radiography, and echocardiography. In many instances blood-based testing may help to increase confidence in pursuing further diagnostic tests; however, the information obtained by natriuretic peptide or troponin assay is not a substitute for further evaluation. Proper sample collection, handling, and shipping are particularly important for feline NT-proBNP assay, and strict adherence to the manufacturer's instructions is required to obtain accurate results.

For both NT-proBNP and cardiac troponin, little is known about the assay's ability to guide therapy and improve outcome. Ideally, improved cardiac function could be detected by serial cardiac blood tests, much in the same way that improved renal function is detected by serial declines in serum creatinine values. In human

beings BNP-guided therapy leads to improved outcome in patients with heart failure,[23] but these types of studies in veterinary species are lacking. In cases of renal disease, both NT-proBNP and cardiac troponin may be falsely elevated, and results must be interpreted cautiously. This limitation is particularly germane to an older population of cats in whom concurrent renal and cardiac disease is common.

In summary, feline cardiac blood tests represent a rapidly developing field from which several indications appear reasonable. Cats with preclinical (occult) cardiomyopathy can be detected with an acceptable degree of sensitivity and specificity. Initial blood testing in cats with suspected disease may help to determine which patients should undergo further diagnostic tests such as electrocardiography, radiography, or echocardiography. Blood testing can help to determine the etiology of respiratory signs in cats with an acceptable degree of sensitivity and specificity, and use of blood testing may permit more specific and timely treatment. In cats with heart disease, the natriuretic peptides and cardiac troponin are correlated with severity of underlying morphological and functional changes. Further studies are needed to determine if this relationship can predict risk of death or morbid events and if cardiac blood tests can be used to help tailor individualized treatments aimed at minimizing the severity of, or preventing, the occurrence of these outcomes.

REFERENCES

1. Wu AH, Apple FS, Gibler WB, et al: National Academy of Clinical Biochemistry Standards of Laboratory Practice: recommendations for the use of cardiac markers in coronary artery diseases, *Clin Chem* 45:1104, 1999.
2. Arnold JM, Howlett JG, Dorian P, et al: Canadian Cardiovascular Society Consensus Conference recommendations on heart failure update 2007: prevention, management during intercurrent illness or acute decompensation, and use of biomarkers, *Can J Cardiol* 23:21, 2007.
3. Mifune H, Suzuki S, Noda Y, et al: Fine structure of atrial natriuretic peptide (ANP)-granules in the atrial cardiocytes in the hamster, guinea pig, rabbit, cat and dog, *Jikken Dobutsu* 41:321, 1992.
4. Biondo AW, Liu ZL, Wiedmeyer CE, et al: Genomic sequence and cardiac expression of atrial natriuretic peptide in cats, *Am J Vet Res* 63:236, 2002.
5. Biondo AW, Ehrhart EJ, Sisson DD, et al: Immunohistochemistry of atrial and brain natriuretic peptides in control cats and cats with hypertrophic cardiomyopathy, *Vet Pathol* 40:501, 2003.
6. Heart Failure Society of America: HFSA 2006 Comprehensive Heart Failure Practice Guideline, *J Card Fail* 12:e1, 2006.
7. Tang WH, Francis GS, Morrow DA, et al: National Academy of Clinical Biochemistry Laboratory Medicine practice guidelines: clinical utilization of cardiac biomarker testing in heart failure, *Circulation* 116:e99, 2007.
8. Sisson DD, Oyama MA, Solter PF: Plasma levels of ANP, BNP, epinephrine, norepinephrine, serum aldosterone, and plasma renin activity in healthy cats and cats with myocardial disease, *J Vet Intern Med* 17:438, 2003 (abstract).
9. Hori Y, Yamano S, Iwanaga K, et al: Evaluation of plasma C-terminal atrial natriuretic peptide in healthy cats and cats with heart disease, *J Vet Intern Med* 22:135, 2008.

10. Connolly DJ, Magalhaes RJ, Syme HM, et al: Circulating natriuretic peptides in cats with heart disease, *J Vet Intern Med* 22:96, 2008.

11. Fox PR, Oyama MA, MacDonald KA, et al: Assessment of NTproBNP concentration in asymptomatic cats with cardiomyopathy, *J Vet Intern Med* 22:759, 2008 (abstract).

12. Nakamura M, Tanaka F, Sato K, et al: B-type natriuretic peptide testing for structural heart disease screening: a general population-based study, *J Card Fail* 11:705, 2005.

13. Fox PR, Oyama MA, Reynolds CA, et al: Utility of plasma N-terminal pro-brain natriuretic peptide (NT-pro BNP) to distinguish between congestive heart failure and non-cardiac causes of acute dyspnea in cats, *J Vet Cardiol* 2009; in press.

14. Kaski JP, Tome-Esteban MT, Mead-Regan SJ, et al: B-type natriuretic peptide predicts disease severity in children with hypertrophic cardiomyopathy, *Heart* 94:1478, 2008.

15. Panou FK, Kotseroglou VK, Lakoumentas JA, et al: Significance of brain natriuretic peptide in the evaluation of symptoms and the degree of left ventricular diastolic dysfunction in patients with hypertrophic cardiomyopathy, *Hellenic J Cardiol* 47:344, 2006.

16. Binder J, Ommen SR, Chen HH, et al: Usefulness of brain natriuretic peptide levels in the clinical evaluation of patients with hypertrophic cardiomyopathy, *Am J Cardiol* 100:712, 2007.

17. Arteaga E, Araujo AQ, Buck P, et al: Plasma amino-terminal pro-B-type natriuretic peptide quantification in hypertrophic cardiomyopathy, *Am Heart J* 150:1228, 2005.

18. Wess G, Daisenberger P, Hirschberger J: The utility of NT-proBNP to differentiate cardiac and respiratory causes of dyspnea in cats, *J Vet Intern Med* 22:707, 2008 (abstract).

19. Fonarow GC, Peacock WF, Phillips CO, et al: Admission B-type natriuretic peptide levels and in-hospital mortality in acute decompensated heart failure, *J Am Coll Cardiol* 49:1943, 2007.

20. Magga J, Sipola P, Vuolteenaho O, et al: Significance of plasma levels of N-terminal Pro-B-type natriuretic peptide on left ventricular remodeling in non-obstructive hypertrophic cardiomyopathy attributable to the Asp175Asn mutation in the alpha-tropomyosin gene, *Am J Cardiol* 101:1185, 2008.

21. Fox PR, Liu SK, Maron BJ: Echocardiographic assessment of spontaneously occurring feline hypertrophic cardiomyopathy. An animal model of human disease, *Circulation* 92:2645, 1995.

22. Pieroni M, Bellocci F, Sanna T, et al: Increased brain natriuretic peptide secretion is a marker of disease progression in non-obstructive hypertrophic cardiomyopathy, *J Card Fail* 13:380, 2007.

23. Jourdain P, Jondeau G, Funck F, et al: Plasma brain natriuretic peptide-guided therapy to improve outcome in heart failure: the STARS-BNP Multicenter Study, *J Am Coll Cardiol* 49:1733, 2007.

24. Cummins B, Cummins P: Cardiac specific troponin-I release in canine experimental myocardial infarction: development of a sensitive enzyme-linked immunoassay, *J Mol Cell Cardiol* 19:999, 1987.

25. O'Brien PJ, Smith DE, Knechtel TJ, et al: Cardiac troponin I is a sensitive, specific biomarker of cardiac injury in laboratory animals, *Lab Anim* 40:153, 2006.

26. Mair J, Thome-Kromer B, Wagner I, et al: Concentration time courses of troponin and myosin subunits after acute myocardial infarction, *Coron Artery Dis* 5:865, 1994.

27. Rishniw M, Barr SC, Simpson KW, et al: Cloning and sequencing of the canine and feline cardiac troponin I genes, *Am J Vet Res* 65:53, 2004.

28. Adin DB, Milner RJ, Berger KD, et al: Cardiac troponin I concentrations in normal dogs and cats using a bedside analyzer, *J Vet Cardiol* 7:27, 2005.

29. Connolly DJ, Cannata J, Boswood A, et al: Cardiac troponin I in cats with hypertrophic cardiomyopathy, *J Feline Med Surg* 5:209, 2003.

30. Herndon WE, Kittleson MD, Sanderson K, et al: Cardiac troponin I in feline hypertrophic cardiomyopathy, *J Vet Intern Med* 16:558, 2002.

31. Kirbach B, Schober KE, Oechtering G: Diagnosis of myocardial cell injuries in cats with blunt thoracic trauma using circulating biochemical markers, *Tieraerztl Prax* 28:30, 2000.

32. Connolly DJ, Guitian J, Boswood A, et al: Serum troponin I levels in hyperthyroid cats before and after treatment with radioactive iodine, *J Feline Med Surg* 7:289, 2005.

33. Porciello F, Rishniw M, Herndon WE, et al: Cardiac troponin I is elevated in dogs and cats with azotaemic renal failure and in dogs with non-cardiac systemic disease, *Aust Vet J* 86:390, 2008.

34. Kittleson MD, Meurs KM, Munro MJ, et al: Familial hypertrophic cardiomyopathy in Maine coon cats: an animal model of human disease, *Circulation* 99:3172, 1999.

35. Cesta MF, Baty CJ, Keene BW, et al: Pathology of end-stage remodeling in a family of cats with hypertrophic cardiomyopathy, *Vet Pathol* 42:458, 2005.

36. Healey JS, Davies RF, Smith SJ, et al: Prognostic use of cardiac troponin T and troponin I in patients with heart failure, *Can J Cardiol* 19:383, 2003.

37. Metra M, Nodari S, Parrinello G, et al: The role of plasma biomarkers in acute heart failure. Serial changes and independent prognostic value of NT-proBNP and cardiac troponin-T, *Eur J Heart Fail* 9:776, 2007.

38. Horwich TB, Patel J, MacLellan WR, et al: Cardiac troponin I is associated with impaired hemodynamics, progressive left ventricular dysfunction, and increased mortality rates in advanced heart failure, *Circulation* 108:833, 2003.

39. Mueller C: Risk stratification in acute decompensated heart failure: the role of cardiac troponin, *Nat Clin Pract Cardiovasc Med* 5:680, 2008.

40. Peacock WF, De Marco T, Fonarow GC, et al: Cardiac troponin and outcome in acute heart failure, *N Engl J Med* 358:2117, 2008.

41. La Vecchia L, Mezzena G, Zanolla L, et al: Cardiac troponin I as a diagnostic and prognostic marker in severe heart failure, *J Heart Lung Transplant* 19:644, 2000.

42. Herndon WE, Rishniw M, Schrope D, et al: Assessment of plasma cardiac troponin I concentration as a means to differentiate cardiac and non-cardiac causes of dyspnea in cats, *J Am Vet Med Assoc* 233:1261, 2008.

39 Genetic Screening of Familial Hypertrophic Cardiomyopathy

Kathryn M. Meurs

Hypertrophic cardiomyopathy is the most common form of heart disease in cats.[1] It is an adult-onset myocardial disease known to be inherited in the Maine Coon and Ragdoll breeds, and causative genetic mutations now have been identified in both of these breeds.[2,3] A number of small families of cats with several affected members have been observed in a few additional breeds including the Norwegian Forest cat, British and American Shorthair, Sphynx, Siberian, and Bengal. This may suggest that hypertrophic cardiomyopathy also is an inherited disease in these breeds, although conclusive genetic studies have not been performed to date. Given the familial nature of hypertrophic cardiomyopathy in the Ragdoll and Maine Coon breeds, as well as the significant clinical consequences of the disease, cat breeders have expressed increased interest in genetic testing. Additionally, pet owners often are curious to know more about the underlying cause of their cat's disease. Although this chapter will emphasize the current state of genetic testing for hypertrophic cardiomyopathy in Maine Coon and Ragdoll cats, a useful and frequently updated Web site for veterinarians and cat breeders interested in future developments in familial feline hypertrophic cardiomyopathy as well as other feline inherited diseases is maintained by the Feline Advisory Board.[4]

406

ETIOLOGY

MAINE COON HYPERTROPHIC CARDIOMYOPATHY

A familial form of hypertrophic cardiomyopathy in the Maine Coon cat was reported by Dr. Mark Kittleson at the University of California, Davis, in 1999.[5] Breeding studies demonstrated that it was an autosomal dominant trait. Autosomal dominant traits should have the following criteria: males and females generally are affected equally, every affected individual should have at least one affected parent, and the trait generally is observed in every generation (Figure 39-1). Affected animals may carry the genetic mutation on one or both copies of the gene. If the mutation is on both copies of the gene (one inherited from each parent), they are called homozygous for the mutation and will pass one copy of the mutation to all of their offspring. They are defined as heterozygous if they have one gene with the mutation and one normal gene. Heterozygous cats have a 50 per cent chance of passing on the genetic mutation to their offspring. This does not mean that 50 per cent of a litter of kittens will have the mutation, but rather that each kitten has a 50 per cent chance of having the mutation. The litter may

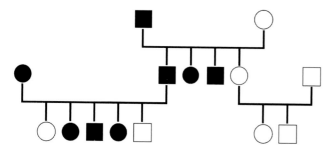

Figure 39-1 Example of a family of cats with an autosomal dominant mode of inheritance of hypertrophic cardiomyopathy. Male cats are depicted as a square, females as a circle. Affected cats are indicated by solid black symbols and unaffected cats are indicated by solid white symbols. Autosomal dominant traits should have equal (or almost equal) numbers of affected males and females, every affected individual should have at least one affected parent, and the trait generally is observed in every generation.

actually have from zero to 100 per cent of kittens born with the mutation.

An additional important, but poorly understood, aspect of the inheritance of hypertrophic cardiomyopathy in the Maine Coon cat is that hypertrophic cardiomyopathy appears to be inherited with incomplete penetrance. This means that cats who have the mutation will have different degrees of disease severity depending on the "penetrance" of the trait in that animal. Even within the same litter, two siblings may have the same mutation; however, one sibling may show a more severe form than the other, and some cats may never actually show a clinical form of the disease.

In the Maine Coon cat a genetic mutation has been identified in the myosin binding protein C (MYBPC3) gene.[2] Myosin binding protein C is a cardiac sarcomeric protein involved in cardiac contraction. It is the second most commonly mutated gene responsible for the human form of the disease.[6] In the Maine Coon cat the mutation is a single base pair change from a guanine to a cytosine in the 31st codon of the gene. The mutation changes the highly conserved amino acid that is produced from alanine to proline, a large amino acid with a ring. Additionally, the alteration of the amino acid is predicted to change the structure of myosin binding protein C in this region, and alters the ability of the cardiac protein to interact with other contractile proteins.

Homozygous (two copies of the mutated gene) Maine Coon cats are thought to typically, but not always, develop a more severe form of hypertrophic cardiomyopathy and may show clinical signs before 4 years of age.[2] Heterozygous (one copy of the mutated gene) cats may develop the disease at a later age and have milder signs. As mentioned a small percentage of cats with the mutation may never show clinical signs of the disease, as a result of incomplete penetrance. Genetic modifiers that affect the expression and penetrance of the disease are likely, but have yet to be determined.

The Maine Coon mutation appears to be quite breed-specific. It is unlikely to be associated with hypertrophic

cardiomyopathy in other breeds of cats unless they are closely related to the Maine Coon breed.

RAGDOLL CARDIOMYOPATHY

A substitution mutation also has been identified in the myosin binding protein C gene in the Ragdoll cat.[3] The Ragdoll mutation, however, is different from that in the Maine Coon cat and appears to be breed-specific to the Ragdoll. In the Ragdoll cat the mutation is a cytosine to thymine substitution in the 820th codon, and the amino acid produced in affected cats is tryptophan rather than the arginine that is observed in normal cats. It is extremely unlikely that the Maine Coon and Ragdoll mutations were inherited from a common ancestor, because the mutations are different and are located in such different regions of the gene. It is more likely that these are two novel mutations that developed independently. Although the mode of inheritance of this mutation in the Ragdoll cat has not been identified through breeding studies, it is most likely an autosomal dominant trait as well.

In the Ragdoll, homozygous cats appear to be very severely affected with the development of heart failure and thromboembolic episodes, often before 2 years of age. Heterozygous cats appear to have a much more mild form of the disease that may include only mild papillary muscle hypertrophy.

MUTATION SCREENING

Genetic testing is now available to test a cat for either mutation by submitting a deoxyribonucleic acid (DNA) sample to a reputable screening laboratory. Good quality DNA samples can be obtained either from a blood sample submitted in an ethylenediaminetetraacetic acid (EDTA) tube, or by brushing the oral gums of the cat with a special buccal swab, although many laboratories will even accept samples submitted on a cotton swab. Buccal swabbing is particularly helpful for testing young kittens from whom it may be difficult to obtain a blood sample. Additionally, an owner can perform the buccal swabbing at home without stressing a difficult adult cat and mail the swabs directly to the screening laboratory.

Once the sample is provided to the laboratory it can be analyzed in a number of ways. The gold standard for testing is to perform DNA sequencing for actual visualization of the mutation (Figure 39-2). Less reliable assays are available, but often have not been validated.

The test results should verify that the cat is negative, heterozygous, or homozygous for the mutation. Cats who test negative do not have the mutation. This does not mean that they can not ever develop hypertrophic cardiomyopathy; it simply means that they will not develop the form of the disease caused by that specific genetic mutation. Although the mutations described have been shown to be the cause of hypertrophic cardiomyopathy in many Maine Coon and Ragdoll cats, there are some cats who are positive on echocardiographic examination for hypertrophic cardiomyopathy who do not have the

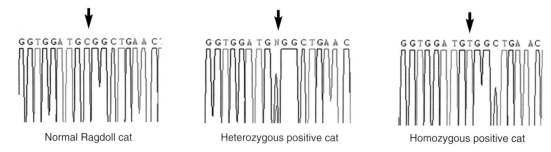

Figure 39-2 DNA sequencing of the Ragdoll hypertrophic cardiomyopathy mutation allows visualization of the mutation for accurate diagnosis. The arrow denotes the base pair of interest. The normal Ragdoll has a C (cytosine), the heterozygous cat has an N meaning that both a C (cytosine) and a T (thymine, the abnormal base) are observed, and the homozygous cat only has a T (thymine, the abnormal base).

specific mutations. Cats who test as positive heterozygous or positive homozygous have an increased risk of developing disease as discussed in the preceding under each breed.

EPIDEMIOLOGY

It is difficult to estimate the prevalence of these mutations within the Maine Coon and Ragdoll populations because testing for the mutations is limited to those cats whose owners choose to screen them. Therefore evaluation of results from screening laboratories will have some bias.

Test results of submissions to Washington State University for the Maine Coon and Ragdoll are provided here as baseline information for the clinician; however, the inherent bias of the population should be considered.[7] Over an approximately 1-year period starting in December of 2005, 3100 Maine Coon submissions were evaluated.[8] Thirty-five per cent (1089) of the samples were positive for the mutation. Only 9 per cent (101 submissions) were homozygous for the mutation.[8] Positive submissions were submitted from 21 countries.

Over a 1-year period starting in June 2007, 1800 Ragdoll samples were submitted to the same laboratory for evaluation. Twenty-eight per cent (500 submissions) were positive for the mutation; however, only 8 per cent (40) were homozygous. Positive submissions were received from the United States, Japan, Australia, Canada, Portugal, France, Belgium, Germany, and the Netherlands.

BREEDING RECOMMENDATIONS

Due to the apparently high prevalence of the mutation in both breeds, it would seem to be unwise to recommend that all cats with the mutation be removed from the breeding programs because this could result in dramatically altering the genetic makeup of these breeds. Additionally, it should be emphasized that not all cats who have the mutation, particularly if they are heterozygous, will develop a clinical form of the disease. Our current recommendations for both breeds are to not use cats who are homozygous for the mutation for breeding purposes because they will certainly pass on the mutation to all of

their offspring and they have the highest risk of developing the disease. Heterozygous cats should be evaluated carefully. Cats who have many strong positive breed attributes and are disease-negative at time of breeding could be bred to a mutation-negative cat. Their lack of clinical disease may suggest that they have a less penetrant form of the disease or that they just do not show evidence yet of this adult-onset clinical disease. Therefore these cats should only be used if they are exceptional for the breed and they should be evaluated clinically for the disease every year. If they develop the clinical disease, they should be kept in the breeding program no longer. The offspring of the mating of a positive heterozygous and a negative should be screened for the mutation, and if possible, a mutation-negative kitten with the desirable traits of its parents should be selected to replace the mutation-positive parent in the breeding colony. Over a few generations this will decrease the prevalence of the disease mutation in the population, hopefully without greatly altering the genetic makeup of the breed too significantly. Finally, disease-negative but mutation-positive cats should be evaluated annually for presence of disease.

OTHER CAUSES OF HYPERTROPHIC CARDIOMYOPATHY IN THE MAINE COON AND RAGDOLL

Not all Maine Coon cats or Ragdoll cats with hypertrophic cardiomyopathy have one of the identified mutations. The cause of the disease in these individual cases is unknown at this time. In human beings there are more than 400 genetic mutations that lead to the development of hypertrophic cardiomyopathy; therefore it is likely that cats may have many genetic causes (and nongenetic causes) as well.[6]

HYPERTROPHIC CARDIOMYOPATHY IN OTHER BREEDS OF CATS

There appear to be examples of familial hypertrophic cardiomyopathy in other breeds of cats including the British Shorthair, Bengal, Norwegian Forest Cat, and Sphynx among others, although extensive breeding studies have not been done. There is no evidence that any of these breeds share the same mutations as Maine Coon or Ragdoll cats, and screening these breeds with the two genetic tests is not likely to be useful. There may be some benefit to screening breeds of cats who have a known familial relationship to the Maine Coon or Ragdoll if they have hypertrophic cardiomyopathy.

REFERENCES

1. Kittleson MD: Feline myocardial disease. In Ettinger SJ, Feldman EC, editors: *Textbook of veterinary internal medicine*, ed 6, St. Louis, 2005, Saunders, p 1082.
2. Meurs KM, Sanchez X, David RM, et al: Identification of a missense mutation in the cardiac myosin binding protein C gene in a family of Maine Coon cats with hypertrophic cardiomyopathy, *Hum Mol Genet* 14:3587, 2005.
3. Meurs KM, Norgard MM, Ederer MM, et al: A substitution mutation in the myosin binding protein C gene in Ragdoll cats, *Genomics* 90:261, 2007.
4. Feline Advisory Bureau. FAB Inherited disease registry. http://www.fabcats.org/breeders/inherited_disorders/index.php, 2008.
5. Kittleson MD, Meurs KM, Munro MJ, et al: Familial hypertrophic cardiomyopathy in Maine Coon cats: an animal model of human disease, *Circulation* 24:3172, 1999.
6. Keren A, Syrris P, McKenna WJ: Hypertrophic cardiomyopathy: the genetic determinants of clinical disease expression, *Nat Clin Pract Cardiovasc Med* 5:158, 2008.
7. Hypertrophic cardiomyopathy genetic mutation testing service for cats. http://www.vetmed.wsu.edu/deptsVCGL/felineTests.aspx, 2008.
8. Fries R, Heaney AM, Meurs KM: Prevalence of the myosin binding protein C in Maine Coon cats, *J Vet Intern Med* 22:893, 2008.

40 Diastolic Dysfunction in Feline Cardiomyopathies

Jean-Paul Petrie

Cardiomyopathies are a significant cause of morbidity and mortality in the feline population. Cardiomyopathy refers to a group of diseases in which the predominant feature is a structural and functional impairment of the heart muscle. These diseases are distinctive because they are not associated with pericardial, hypertensive, congenital, valvular, ischemic, or metabolic causes. Improvements in diagnostic techniques have increased the awareness of primary cardiomyopathy in the feline population and allowed for a more accurate description of the changes in the structure and function of the heart muscle.[1-8] Classification of cardiomyopathies has been difficult because of the overlapping nature of many cases that do not fit into one of the major groups. Both morphological and structural classifications are attempted based on information obtained from the two-dimensional, M-mode, and Doppler echocardiograms. The major morphological classifications include hypertrophic, restrictive, dilated, and right ventricular cardiomyopathy.[9] Despite the popularity of the morphological descriptions in clinical practice, an attempt to identify the underlying physiological consequences should be made. Morphological myocardial changes result in alterations of systolic function, diastolic function, or both (Figure 40-1). An understanding of the physiological implications of the disease ultimately will allow for more focused therapy. Publications continue to emerge on diastolic dysfunction in normal cats and in cats with heart disease.

Diastolic dysfunction is the primary functional disturbance in hypertrophic and restrictive cardiomyopathies.[10,11] Physical examination, electrocardiography (ECG), and thoracic radiographs are unreliable in the diagnosis of diastolic dysfunction. Accurate assessment of diastolic function previously required the use of more invasive testing, including measurements of cardiac pressures, rate of left ventricular relaxation, and left ventricular compliance.[12,13] Doppler echocardiography is a noninvasive emerging method in feline cardiology to allow earlier and more accurate estimation of diastolic function.[14-19] Quantification of diastolic dysfunction will provide us with a baseline to be able to assess therapeutic efficacy in future clinical trials. Ideally, therapy would target a specific physiological process and the response to therapy measured quantitatively through long-term follow-up echocardiographic data.[20,21]

Assessment of hemodynamic properties requires basic understanding of cardiac physiology, including diastolic properties and left ventricular filling patterns. This chapter serves as an introduction to the concept of diastology by discussing the definition, physiology, diagnostic testing, diseases, and potential therapeutic options. A detailed description of feline cardiomyopathies, including clinical presentation, diagnosis, and therapy, can be found in Chapters 33 and 34 of the fifth volume of this series.

DEFINITION

Diastolic dysfunction is defined as the inability to fill the left ventricle to a normal end-diastolic volume without an abnormal increase in left ventricular end-diastolic or mean left atrial pressure. A failure to increase left ven-

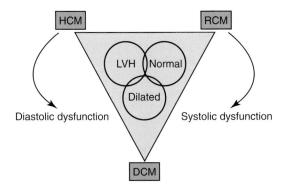

Figure 40-1 Historical classification of feline cardiomyopathies is based on morphological changes. In cats these morphological classifications tend to overlap with features of each classification present. An attempt to understand and identify the two major physiological consequences is recommended: diastolic and systolic dysfunction. *HCM,* Hypertrophic cardiomyopathy; *RCM,* restrictive cardiomyopathy; *DCM,* dilated cardiomyopathy.

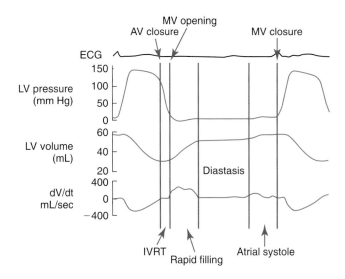

Figure 40-2 Diastole can be broken down into four distinct phases beginning with the closure of the aortic valve including (1) isovolumic relaxation time (IVRT), (2) early diastolic filling (rapid filling), (3) diastasis, and (4) atrial systole.[4]

tricular end-diastolic volume resulting in an elevated filling pressure leads to reduced exercise capacity and signs of pulmonary congestion.[22-24]

PHYSIOLOGY

Diastole is the period of the cardiac cycle defined as beginning with closure of the aortic valve and ending with closure of the mitral valve. Ventricular relaxation begins at approximately the time of peak ventricular pressure and is manifested as a reduction in left ventricular pressure. Diastole is divided into four phases: (1) isovolumic relaxation (IVR), (2) early diastolic filling, (3) diastasis (mid-diastole), and (4) atrial contraction (Figure 40-2). The first phase, IVR, begins when the left ventricular pressure falls below the aortic pressure, resulting in cessation of forward aortic flow and closure of the aortic valve. During this phase the left ventricular volume remains constant as left ventricular pressure continues to decline. Geometrical changes to the left ventricle continue during this period. The isovolumic phase ends when the left ventricular pressure falls below left atrial pressure, the mitral valve opens, and ventricular filling begins. During the second phase, early diastolic filling, blood enters the left ventricle from the left atrium down a pressure gradient generated by continued ventricular relaxation. Although the act of relaxation is an active process, blood fills the ventricle passively along its gradient. Negative pressure can be generated during relaxation in the left ventricle, creating a "sucking" effect. Under normal conditions this phase represents the most rapid period of ventricular filling. Because of a reduction in ventricular relaxation, ventricular filling, and atrial emptying, the atrioventricular pressure gradient decreases. When left ventricular and atrial pressure equilibrate, ventricular filling stops. The third phase, diastasis, is the phase in diastole when atrial and ventricular pressures are in equilibrium and little or no filling occurs. Flow from the pulmonary veins may continue to contribute slightly to ventricular filling. The duration of this period is affected

by heart rate and can be abolished at higher heart rates. The final phase, atrial contraction, often is defined as the late filling phase. In normal conditions atrial contraction results in a second phase of ventricular filling. During this phase under normal conditions, almost all of the blood flows forward into the left ventricle and little into the pulmonary veins. Left atrial contraction contributes approximately 10 to 30 per cent of the total ventricular filling volume and is affected by many arrhythmias and disease.[23]

DETERMINANTS OF DIASTOLIC FUNCTION

Determinants of left ventricular diastolic performance are affected by systolic performance, heart rate, and cardiac conduction. Two major diastolic properties are left ventricular relaxation and left ventricular compliance (Figure 40-3). In early diastole the rate of ventricular filling is related to the pressure difference between the left atrium and left ventricle when the mitral valve opens. This pressure gradient is mostly determined by the left atrial pressure and the rate of active decline in the left ventricular pressure (ventricular relaxation). Left ventricular relaxation is an active process that requires energy expenditure within the myocardial cells. The active process of relaxation is mostly completed by mid-diastole (diastasis). During the later portion of diastole, the passive properties of the myocardium predominate (myocardial compliance). The transmitral gradient (TMG), which determines the left ventricular filling pattern, is influenced by many factors including both left ventricular relaxation and compliance.[24] Faster left ventricular relaxation results in a larger early TMG, more filling in early diastole, and less filling in late diastole. Slower left ventricular relaxation results in a lower early TMG and proportionally less early diastolic filling compared with late diastolic filling. For the same rate of left ventricular relax-

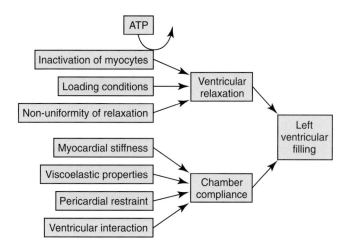

Figure 40-3 The two significant diastolic properties that influence left ventricular filling are ventricular relaxation and chamber compliance. Several factors affect these properties, resulting in diastolic dysfunction.

ation, decreased left ventricular compliance and increased left atrial pressure have the opposite effect on the TMG and can offset a slower rate of relaxation. Changes in rates of left ventricular relaxation and left atrial pressure are a continuum resulting in many different filling patterns for given situations. Therefore the same filling pattern may occur with different combinations of increased left atrial pressure and left ventricular relaxation.[24]

PATHOGENESIS OF DIASTOLIC DYSFUNCTION

HYPERTROPHIC OBSTRUCTIVE/ NONOBSTRUCTIVE CARDIOMYOPATHY

Hypertrophic cardiomyopathy is a disease characterized by abnormal concentric or asymmetric left ventricular hypertrophy.[2] Secondary causes of hypertrophy including acromegaly, hypertension, aortic stenosis, and hyperthyroidism should be excluded prior to making the definitive diagnosis. The left ventricle is nondilated with a broad variation in phenotypic changes. The entire left ventricle can be hypertrophied or it may be isolated to a particular wall segment. The hypertrophy can be mild to severe. No single pattern is "classic" or characteristic for the disease. Systolic anterior mitral valve motion (SAM) resulting in a dynamic left ventricular outflow tract obstruction is commonly associated with interventricular septal hypertrophy. The mitral valve is displaced anteriorly during systole, resulting in a pressure gradient midway through systole across the left ventricular outflow tract and a corresponding posteriorly directed mitral regurgitation. The left ventricle typically is hyperdynamic owing to the increased muscle mass.

The primary physiological consequences of ventricular hypertrophy are an elevated left ventricular end-diastolic pressure with a normal or reduced left ventricular end-diastolic volume. These changes result from a stiff and noncompliant ventricle along with alterations in early diastolic filling or ventricular relaxation. Compliance is affected as a result of the increased muscle mass, increased amount of myocardial fibrosis, and disorganization of the ventricular myocytes (see Chapter 43). The presence of a dynamic outflow tract obstruction secondary to SAM results in increased left ventricular systolic pressures, myocardial wall stress, and impedes left ventricular ejection. The left atrium dilates in response to the elevated left ventricular filling pressure, leading eventually to elevated pulmonary venous pressures and congestive heart failure.[25,26]

RESTRICTIVE CARDIOMYOPATHY

Restrictive cardiomyopathy has been used to morphologically describe nonhypertrophied ventricles with normal systolic function. A presumptive diagnosis of restrictive cardiomyopathy is made based on morphology, but further verification of diastolic function is essential to making a more accurate diagnosis. Left ventricular chamber dimensions usually are normal or mildly reduced, systolic function is normal, and wall thickness is normal to mildly increased. Regional areas of ventricular thinning and scarring may represent myocardial atrophy or infarction. Focal or diffuse areas of hyperechoic and thickened endocardium or wall segments are associated with excessive scarring and fibrous tissue. Fibrous bands of tissue may be seen adjacent to myocardial walls, bridging areas of myocardial thinning, or in some cases bridging the septum, papillary muscles, and free wall obliterating the left ventricular apex (see Chapter 43).[4]

The physiological consequences of restrictive cardiomyopathy are alterations in the diastolic filling properties of the left ventricle. Changes in ventricular relaxation and chamber compliance are the primary alterations. Elevation in left ventricular end-diastolic pressure with normal or mildly elevated end-systolic volumes result in progressive increases in left atrial pressure. Characteristic mitral inflow velocity profiles have been used to imply restrictive ventricular filling. Several Doppler echocardiographic variables can be used together to determine the extent of diastolic functional impairment.[27]

DILATED CARDIOMYOPATHY

Dilated cardiomyopathy is a myocardial disease associated with a reduction in systolic function. Dilated cardiomyopathy refers to the classic description seen as dilation of all four cardiac chambers with global wall thinning and a marked reduction in fractional shortening or ejection fraction. The left ventricular end-diastolic and systolic volumes are increased. Regional areas of hypokinesis often are associated with wall thinning and regional scarring.

Reduction in left ventricular systolic function leads to elevation in end-diastolic pressures caused by reduced systolic emptying and increased residual end-systolic volumes. A reduction in cardiac output leads to clinical signs of pulmonary congestion, pleural and abdominal effusions, and in some cases cardiogenic shock.[28]

ASSESSMENT OF DIASTOLIC FUNCTION

Two-dimensional echocardiography identifies, characterizes, and quantifies diseases that result in diastolic dysfunction. The two-dimensional and M-mode images also are evaluated for the presence of systolic function. Certain disease entities are associated almost exclusively with diastolic dysfunction and can be diagnosed using two-dimensional echocardiography. For example, the combination of left ventricular hypertrophy, normal systolic function, left atrial enlargement, and absence of valve insufficiency is strong evidence for the presence of diastolic dysfunction and elevated filling pressure. The supplemental Doppler imaging is used to confirm and quantify the degree of diastolic dysfunction. There are numerous echocardiographic techniques for evaluating left ventricular diastolic function. These methods are being validated and investigated in a variety of feline myocardial diseases. The mitral inflow, isovolumic relaxation time, pulmonary venous flow, and tissue Doppler imaging of the mitral annulus have had the most clinical utility. Additional diastolic techniques need to be further defined and validated.

ISOVOLUMIC RELAXATION TIME

Isovolumic relaxation time (IVRT) represents the time during left ventricular relaxation between closure of the aortic valve and opening of the mitral valve. The IVRT can be readily measured by spectral Doppler echocardiography (Figure 40-4). Simultaneous mitral inflow and aortic outflow tract velocity signals are obtained. The aortic closure and mitral opening interval can be determined.[23,24] Normal IVRT has been reported as 71 ± 17 ms in normal anesthetized cats, and 46.2 ± 7.6 ms in conscious cats.[29,30] When compared with invasive measures of diastolic function, IVRT was well correlated and a good

indicator of diastolic function in anesthetized cats.[29] IVRT is prolonged in early diastolic dysfunction (relaxation) and shortened with restrictive cardiomyopathy, because the markedly elevated left atrial pressures result in early opening of the mitral valve. In cats with hypertrophic cardiomyopathy, IVRT was shown to be prolonged.[31,32] As with many other Doppler indices of diastolic function, IVRT has been shown to be correlated with age in cats. In a study comparing different age ranges of conscious cats, there was a progressive increase in the IVRT with age.[30]

TRANSMITRAL FLOW

Blood flow through the mitral valve is proportional to the atrioventricular pressure gradient (Figure 40-5). The typical pulsed wave Doppler measurement of transvalvular flow is characterized by two phases. The early phase, or E wave, represents flow during the rapid filling phase. The second phase, or A wave, represents transmitral flow

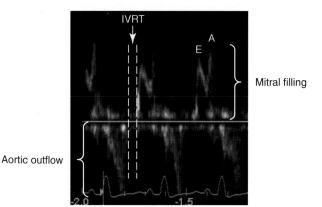

Figure 40-4 Isovolumic relaxation time (IVRT) is represented as the time from closure of the aortic valve to opening of the mitral valve. Aortic outflow is shown below the baseline and mitral filling is noted above the baseline. The time between the two velocities represented by the dashed lines is the IVRT.

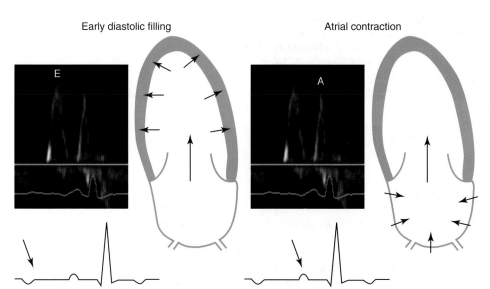

Figure 40-5 The development and timing of the mitral filling velocity tracings is represented in this figure. The early mitral filling (E) begins with opening of the mitral valve and is timed on the ECG just following the T wave. The atrial systolic component (A) is left ventricular filling during atrial contraction and is timed on the ECG just following the P wave.

associated with atrial contraction. The E and A waves are two well-defined peaks that have a measurable upslope and downslope (Figure 40-6). At higher heart rates the period of diastasis decreases and the peaks may become fused and indistinguishable. This can be a problem in many cats because of the inherent faster heart rates in this species. The author has had some success in pressing the nasal planum firmly for 20 to 30 seconds to result in a reduction in heart rates and separation of the waves (Figure 40-7). Although the values of these velocities are affected by a variety of hemodynamic and physiological factors, certain patterns of mitral filling have been associated with varying degrees of diastolic dysfunction (Figure 40-8). Thus three distinct clinical patterns of abnormal transmitral flow have been described: impaired relaxation, pseudonormal, and restrictive. Impaired relaxation is characterized by a prolonged E wave deceleration time and a reduced peak E and an increased peak A wave velocity. A delay in relaxation results in a reduction in the early transmitral filling gradient. A second transmitral filling pattern is restrictive and is characterized by a shortened deceleration time, increased E wave, and a diminished A wave. Increased early filling occurs with rapid equilibration of the atrioventricular pressures. Subsequently there is a reduced atrial contribution to filling caused by a relatively nondistensible left ventricle. A third pattern termed pseudonormal has characteristics of normal transmitral filling velocities. This results from a balancing of abnormal relaxation and reduced ventricular compliance (restrictive forces). This pattern is an intermediate form representing a transition from abnormal relaxation to restrictive physiology. The pseudonormal pattern shows nearly equal E and A wave velocities with a normal or shortened deceleration time.[24] Mitral filling patterns are influenced by age, heart rate and rhythm, loading condition, systolic function, atrial function, and respirations.[23,24] Normal mitral filling variables are listed for both anesthetized and conscious cats in Table 40-1. Aging in dogs and human beings has shown a corresponding change in the mitral filling profile, with the peak late diastolic flow velocity exceeding the peak early passive filling velocity, resulting in an E:A ratio of less

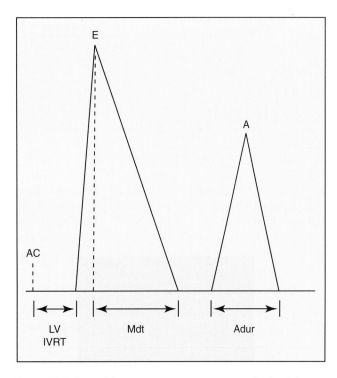

Figure 40-6 Several important measurements are obtained from the mitral filling tracings including isovolumic relaxation time (IVRT), early filling velocity (E), late filling velocity associated with atrial contraction (A), early filling velocity deceleration from the peak of the E wave to baseline (Mdt), and the duration of the A wave (Adur). AC represents closure of the aortic valve.

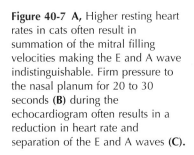

Figure 40-7 A, Higher resting heart rates in cats often result in summation of the mitral filling velocities making the E and A wave indistinguishable. Firm pressure to the nasal planum for 20 to 30 seconds **(B)** during the echocardiogram often results in a reduction in heart rate and separation of the E and A waves **(C).**

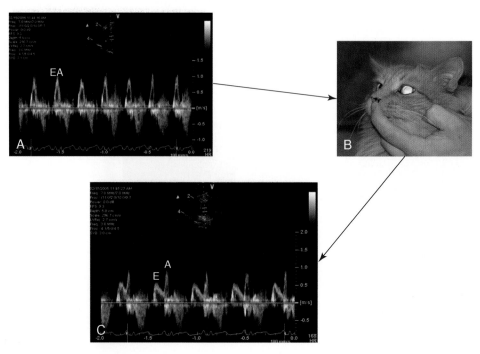

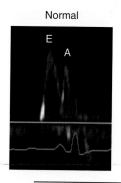
Normal

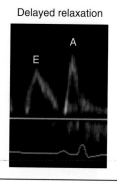
Delayed relaxation

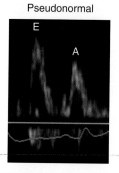
Pseudonormal

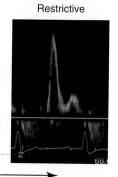
Restrictive

Figure 40-8 Mitral filling velocities have been shown to represent gradual progression of diastolic dysfunction from mild (delayed relaxation) to severe (restrictive). *E* represents early diastolic filling and *A* represents late diastolic filling.

Table 40-1 Normal Mitral Filling Values in Anesthetized and Conscious Cats		
Variable	**Anesthetized**[25]	**Conscious**[26]
Mitral E (m/s)	0.67 ± 0.14	0.70 ± 0.14
Mitral A (m/s)	0.33 ± 0.11	0.65 ± 0.14
E deceleration time (ms)	66 ± 13	NA
E:A	2.27 ± 1.0	1.12 ± 0.22

than one.[33,34] In healthy conscious cats, the peak early diastolic velocity (E) is weakly associated with age. There was no important change in the peak late diastolic velocity (A) and the ratio of early to late diastolic velocities (E:A).[30] In cats with hypertrophic cardiomyopathy there was a significantly reduced early E wave velocity, prolongation of E wave deceleration, and increased A wave velocity.[32]

TISSUE DOPPLER IMAGING

Tissue Doppler imaging (TDI) allows for quantitative measurement of myocardial velocity rather than blood flow during the cardiac cycle. TDI is used for the assessment of both global and regional cardiac function. This method has been described in normal cats and in cats with cardiomyopathy.[15,16,29,31,35] An apical left-sided image is obtained and a spectral Doppler tracing is obtained from a sample volume placed at the annulus of the mitral valve (Figure 40-9). The trace obtained is a mirror image of that acquired during mitral filling (Figure 40-10). The typical pattern will demonstrate a single systolic velocity and two diastolic velocities. The two diastolic velocities represent early and late diastolic motion. This method appears to be relatively insensitive to the effects of preload, and therefore will help differentiate normal versus pseudonormal mitral filling patterns. If an early relaxation abnormality is present, mitral annulus motion during late diastole is increased. Mitral annulus velocity is markedly reduced with restrictive cardiomyopathy. Normal values for TDI are listed in Table 40-2. The location of the sample volume is an important consideration when comparing values. A difference has been shown between the lateral and mitral annulus for cats.[16] A reduction in the peak diastolic velocity (E') was seen in cats

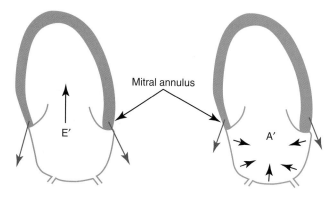

Figure 40-9 Movement of the mitral valve annulus *(green arrows)* opposite the flow of blood into the left ventricle during diastole. This downward motion in this plane occurs as the heart elongates. The initial movement is in early diastole during rapid filling (E') and a second movement is during atrial contraction (A').

Table 40-2 Normal Tissue Doppler Imaging Values Obtained from the Mitral Annulus in Conscious Cats[16]		
	Septal Annulus	**Lateral Annulus**
E' (cm/s)	6.42 ± 1.83	8.39 ± 2.58
A' (cm/s)	6.57 ± 2.4	6.2 ± 2.43
E':A'	1.02 ± 0.25	1.47 ± 0.59

with hypertrophic and unclassified cardiomyopathy compared with normal cats.[16,31,36] Familial hypertrophic cardiomyopathy in Maine Coon cats has been associated with an abnormal myosin binding protein C gene (see Chapter 39). TDI showed a reduction in peak mitral annular velocity (E') in cats with the genetic mutation and no hypertrophy, suggesting a potential identifier of abnormal diastolic function in those cats who have not yet developed hypertrophy.[35] Normal TDI values have been published previously in Maine Coon cats.[37]

PULMONARY VEIN FLOW

Doppler flow recorded in the pulmonary venous system has provided useful information regarding the

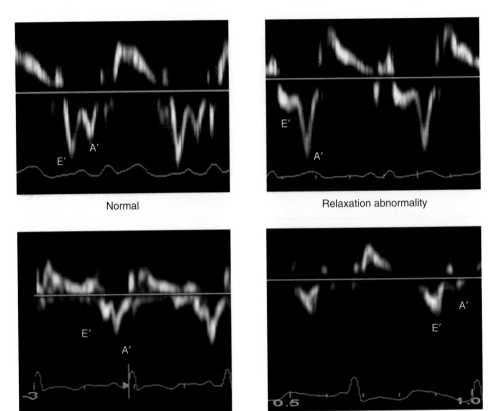

Figure 40-10 Tissue Doppler images of the mitral valve annulus showing different degrees of diastolic dysfunction from normal to restrictive.

Normal

Relaxation abnormality

Pseudonormal

Restrictive

physiology of left ventricular filling and diastolic function.[23] The sample volume is placed in the pulmonary vein near the entrance into the left atrium. The pattern is determined predominantly by transmitral flow and left atrial function. The pattern consists of two forward waves and one reverse wave (Figure 40-11). The first forward wave occurs during systole (S) and coincides with left atrial relaxation immediately after atrial contraction. The second wave occurs during diastole (D) and coincides with the early transmitral flow and ventricular filling. Pulmonary venous blood flows through the left atrium, which acts as a conduit from the pulmonary veins to the filling left ventricle. Reverse flow is a small brief velocity signal below the baseline during atrial contraction and is commonly referred to as the atrial reversal (AR) wave. Early diastolic dysfunction results in a reduction in the D wave and a shift of the flow to the systolic phase, S wave. Restrictive physiology results in a reduction in systolic flow, a marked elevation in the diastolic filling phase (D wave) with an abrupt cessation, and a variable AR wave depending on the properties of the left atrium. If atrial contractile properties are preserved, an increased AR wave amplitude results because of reflux of blood flow into the pulmonary veins as resistance to forward emptying is elevated during atrial contraction. Pulmonary venous flows are influenced by age, loading conditions, and mitral regurgitation.[24] Normal values have been published in anesthetized and conscious cats.[29,30] Normal values are listed in Box 40-1. This technique remains to be validated in cats with cardiomyopathy.

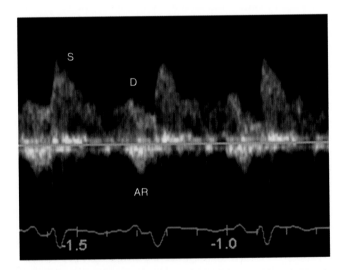

Figure 40-11 Normal pulmonary venous flow in a cat. The first flow wave is the systolic flow (S) as the blood enters the left atrium during ventricular contraction and a closed mitral valve. The second phase is the diastolic flow (D) as blood enters the pulmonary veins during ventricular filling and an open mitral valve. The third flow phase is the atrial reversal (AR) as blood flows forward into the left ventricle and backward up the pulmonary vein during atrial contraction.

Box 40-1 Normal Pulmonary Venous Flow Values in Conscious Cats[30]

Variable	Value
Peak systolic velocity (S) (m/s)	0.48 ± 0.14
Peak diastolic velocity (D) (m/s)	0.47 ± 0.10
Peak retrograde velocity (AR) (m/s)	0.23 ± 0.06

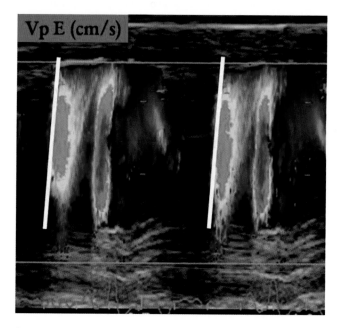

Figure 40-12 Example of color M-mode flow propagation in a normal cat. The *white line* represents the slope of the early flow propagation (Vp E) and recorded in cm/s.

COLOR M-MODE FLOW VELOCITY PROPAGATION

Color M-mode Doppler allows for the assessment of velocities both temporally and spatially over a line. An M-mode is obtained with the line through the long axis of the left ventricle, mitral valve, and left atrium with the color Doppler mode activated. The color aliasing velocity is reduced and an isovelocity (aliasing) line is recorded from the early diastolic signal. The slope of this velocity propagation (Vp) line is calculated (Figure 40-12). The slope of this line is reduced with different degrees of diastolic dysfunction. In anesthetized cats Vp was shown to be well-correlated with invasive measures of diastolic function.[29] Because of the technical challenges of this technique in conscious cats with higher heart rates, its clinical value remains unknown.

No single measurement of diastolic function is reliable. A combination of the above Doppler methods, in addition to two-dimensional and M-mode echocardiography, provides an assessment of diastolic function (Figure 40-13). The information obtained helps understanding of the physiological alteration and provides a baseline to follow the progression of disease. These methods are being validated continually in normal cats,

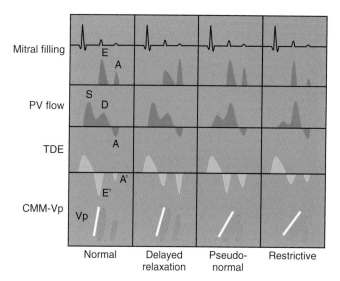

Figure 40-13 This figure summarizes the results of the different diagnostic techniques described for various progressive states of diastolic dysfunction. It is important to recognize that no single measurement of diastolic function is reliable. A combination of these Doppler methods, in addition to two-dimensional and M-mode echocardiography, provides an assessment of diastolic function for each individual patient.

different age groups, and various myocardial disease states.

THERAPY

The primary cause of diastolic heart failure in human beings is systemic hypertension. Therapeutic trials in human patients have focused on the chronic long-term management of systemic hypertension as a primary therapy for diastolic heart failure.[38] Nonhypertensive diastolic heart failure is less studied. The cornerstone of therapy is the regulation of ventricular filling pressure by diuretics in a range that prevents dyspnea and allows for adequate cardiac output. Additional therapeutic agents used commonly in cats with diastolic disease include beta-blockers, calcium channel blockers, angiotensin-converting enzyme (ACE) inhibitors, and aldosterone blocking agents (e.g., spironolactone).

Beta-blockers are used to improve diastolic function by a reduction in heart rate and prolongation of left ventricular filling. Beta-blockers have been shown to have a more beneficial effect on the dynamic left ventricular gradient seen in hypertrophic obstructive cardiomyopathy.[39] In patients with more advanced diastolic dysfunction, the effective filling volume is reduced and further reduction in heart rate may lead to a drop in cardiac output and clinical decompensation.[38] Careful titration of beta-blockers in these patients is critical.

Calcium channel blockers have negative chronotropic effects and some negative inotropic effects. Verapamil has been studied in human patients with diastolic failure and exerts its effects primarily through a reduction in systemic blood pressure.[40] Diltiazem has minimal effect on peripheral vasculature and has been shown to improve ventricular relaxation.[41] The reduction in heart rate allows more time for ventricular filling and for a reduction in myocardial oxygen consumption. Diltiazem is not as effective as beta-blockers in reducing dynamic outflow tract gradients.[39]

Activation of the renin-angiotensin-aldosterone systems (RAAS) is increased in cats with hypertrophic cardiomyopathy and in cats with congestive heart failure.[42] Activation of the RAAS results in aldosterone-mediated salt and water retention, vasoconstriction, and sympathetic nervous system activation. In addition, angiotensin II and aldosterone stimulate myocyte hypertrophy and fibrosis.[43,44] The effects of the ACE inhibitor ramipril were evaluated in Maine Coon cats with hypertrophic cardiomyopathy and no congestive heart failure.[42] Treatment with ramipril did not result in any change in left ventricular mass, diastolic function, myocardial fibrosis, or plasma brain natriuretic peptide within a 1-year period. Spironolactone, an aldosterone antagonist, also was evaluated in Maine Coon cats with hypertrophic cardiomyopathy to evaluate its effect on diastolic function and left ventricular mass.[45] There was no improvement in diastolic function parameters or left ventricular mass over a 4-month treatment period.

The evaluation of different pharmacological interventions on diastolic function is needed in cats with cardiomyopathic disease. The further development of diagnostic testing to better evaluate diastolic dysfunction is ongoing. Currently, therapy is empirical based on theoretical and anecdotal information. Long- and short-term studies are required to provide needed justification for therapy in these patients with moderate risk of congestive heart failure and thromboembolic disease. Current therapies used for the management of cardiomyopathic disease should be studied and evaluated using the parameters of diastolic function listed above. A better understanding of the mechanisms and physiological consequences of disease will help us to identify future therapeutic directions.

REFERENCES

1. Atkins CE, Gallo AM, Kurzman ID, et al: Risk factors, clinical signs, and survival in cats with a clinical diagnosis of idiopathic hypertrophic cardiomyopathy: 74 cases (1985-1989), *J Am Vet Med Assoc* 201:613, 1992.
2. Fox PR, Liu S, Maron BJ: Echocardiographic assessment of spontaneously occurring feline hypertrophic cardiomyopathy, *Circulation* 92:2645, 1995.
3. Fox PR, Maron BJ, Basso C, et al: Spontaneously occurring arrhythmogenic right ventricular cardiomyopathy in the domestic cat: a new animal model similar to the human disease, *Circulation* 102:1863, 2000.
4. Fox PR: Endomyocardial fibrosis and restrictive cardiomyopathy: pathologic and clinical features, *J Vet Cardiol* 6:25, 2004.
5. Kittleson MD, Meurs KM, Munro MJ, et al: Familial hypertrophic cardiomyopathy in Maine Coon cats: an animal model of human disease, *Circulation* 99:3172, 1999.
6. Liu SK, Maron BJ, Tilley LP: Feline hypertrophic cardiomyopathy: gross anatomic and quantitative histologic features, *Am J Pathol* 102:388, 1981.
7. Pion PD, Kittleson MD, Rogers QR, et al: Myocardial failure in cats associated with low plasma taurine: a reversible cardiomyopathy, *Science* 237:764, 1987.
8. Rush JE, Freeman LM, Fenollosa N, et al: Population and survival characteristics of cats with hypertrophic cardiomyopathy: 260 cases (1990-1999), *J Am Vet Med Assoc* 220:202, 2002.
9. Richardson P, McKenna W, Bristow M, et al: Report of the 1995 World Health Organization and International Society and Federation of Cardiology Task Force on the Definition and Classification of Cardiomyopathies (see comments), *Circulation* 93:841, 1996.
10. Bonow RO: Left ventricular diastolic function in hypertrophic cardiomyopathy, *Herz* 16:13, 1991.
11. Child JS, Perloff JK: The restrictive cardiomyopathies, *Cardiol Clin* 6:289, 1988.
12. Grossman W, McLaurin LP, Ellis L: Alterations in left ventricular relaxation and diastolic compliance in congestive cardiomyopathy, *Am J Cardiol* 81:180, 1998.
13. Mandinov L, Eberli FR, Seiler C, et al: Diastolic heart failure, *Cardiovasc Res* 45:813, 2000.
14. Bright JM, Herrtage ME, Schneider JF: Pulsed Doppler assessment of left ventricular diastolic function in normal and cardiomyopathic cats, *J Am Anim Hosp Assoc* 35:285, 1999.
15. Sampedrano CC, Chetboul V, Gouni V, et al: Systolic and diastolic myocardial dysfunction in cats with hypertrophic cardiomyopathy or systemic hypertension, *J Vet Intern Med* 20:1106, 2006.
16. Koffas H, Dukes-McEwan J, Corcoran BM, et al: Pulsed tissue Doppler imaging in normal cats and cats with hypertrophic cardiomyopathy, *J Vet Intern Med* 20:65, 2006.
17. Bright JM, Golden AL: Use of relaxation half-time as an index of ventricular relaxation in clinically normal cats and cats with hypertrophic cardiomyopathy, *Am J Vet Res* 51:1352, 1990.
18. Gavaghan BJ, Kittleson MD, Fisher KJ, et al: Quantification of left ventricular diastolic wall motion by Doppler tissue imaging in healthy cats and cats with cardiomyopathy, *Am J Vet Res* 60:1478, 1999.
19. Chetboul V, Sampedrano CC, Gouni V, et al: Two-dimensional color tissue Doppler imaging detects myocardial dysfunction before occurrence of hypertrophy in a young Maine Coon cat, *Vet Radiol Ultrasound* 47:295, 2006.
20. Temporelli PL, Corra U, Imparato A, et al: Reversible restrictive left ventricular diastolic filling with optimized oral therapy predicts a more favorable prognosis in patients with chronic heart failure, *J Am Coll Cardiol* 31:1591, 1998.
21. Capomolla S, Pinna GD, Febo O, et al: Echo-Doppler mitral flow monitoring: an operative tool to evaluate day-to-day tolerance to and effectiveness of beta-adrenergic blocking agent therapy in patients with chronic heart failure, *J Am Coll Cardiol* 38:1675, 2001.
22. Givertz MM, Colucci WS, Braunwald E: Clinical aspects of heart failure; pulmonary edema, high output heart failure. In Zipes DP, Libby P, Bonow RO, et al, editors: *Braunwald's heart disease: a textbook of cardiovascular medicine*, Philadelphia, 2005, Saunders, p 541.
23. Nishimura RA, Tajik AJ: Evaluation of diastolic filling of left ventricle in health and disease: Doppler echocardiography is the clinician's Rosetta stone, *J Am Coll Cardiol* 30:8, 1997.
24. Appleton CP, Firstenberg MS, Garcia MJ: The echo-Doppler evaluation of left ventricular diastolic function. A current perspective, *Cardiol Clin* 18:513, 2000.
25. Geske JB, Sorajja P, Nishimura RA, et al: Evaluation of left ventricular filling pressures by Doppler echocardiography in patients with hypertrophic cardiomyopathy. Correlation with direct left atrial pressure measurement at cardiac catheterization, *Circulation* 116:2702, 2007.

26. Nishimura RA, Holmes DR: Clinical practice: hypertrophic obstructive cardiomyopathy, *N Engl J Med* 350:1320, 2004.

27. Kushwaha SS, Fallon JT, Fuster V: Restrictive cardiomyopathy, *N Engl J Med* 336:267, 1997.

28. Fans R, Coats AJ, Henein MY: Echocardiography derived variables predict outcome in patients with nonischemic dilated cardiomyopathy with or without a restrictive filling pattern, *Am Heart J* 144:343, 2002.

29. Schober KE, Fuentes VL, Bonagura JD: Comparison between invasive hemodynamic measurements and noninvasive assessment of left ventricular diastolic function by use of Doppler echocardiography in healthy anesthetized cats, *Am J Vet Res* 64:93, 2003.

30. Disatian S, Bright JM, Boon J: Association of age and heart rate with pulsed-wave Doppler measurements in healthy, nonsedated cats, *J Vet Intern Med* 22:351, 2008.

31. Gavaghan BJ, Kittleson MD, Fisher KJ, et al: Quantification of left ventricular diastolic wall motion by Doppler tissue imaging in healthy cats and cats with cardiomyopathy, *Am J Vet Res* 60:1478, 1999.

32. Bright JM, Herrtage ME, Schneider JF: Pulsed Doppler assessment of left ventricular diastolic function in normal and cardiomyopathic cats, *J Am Anim Hosp Assoc* 35:285, 1999.

33. Mantero A, Gentile F, Gualtierotti C, et al: Left ventricular diastolic parameters in 288 normal subjects from 20-80 years old, *Eur Heart J* 16:94, 1995.

34. Schober KE, Fuentes VL: Effects of age, body weight, and heart rate on transmitral and pulmonary venous flow in clinically normal dogs, *Am J Vet Res* 62:1447, 2001.

35. MacDonald KA, Kittleson MD, Kass PH, et al: Tissue Doppler imaging in Maine Coon cats with a mutation of myosin binding protein C with or without hypertrophy, *J Vet Intern Med* 21:232, 2007.

36. MacDonald KA, Kittleson MD, Garcia-Nolen T, et al: Tissue Doppler imaging and gradient echo cardiac magnetic resonance imaging in normal cats and cats with hypertrophic cardiomyopathy, *J Vet Intern Med* 20:627, 2006.

37. Chetboul V, Sampedrano CC, Tissier R, et al: Reference range values of regional left ventricular myocardial velocities and time intervals assessed by tissue Doppler imaging in young nonsedated Maine Coon cats, *Am J Vet Res* 66:1936, 2005.

38. Lester SJ, Tajik AJ, Nishimura RA, et al: Unlocking the mysteries of diastolic function. Deciphering the Rosetta stone 10 years later, *J Am Coll Cardiol* 51:679, 2008.

39. Wey AC, Kittleson MD: Comparison of the efficacy of intravenous diltiazem and esmolol to reduce left ventricular outflow tract velocity and heart rate in cats with hypertrophic obstructive cardiomyopathy, *J Vet Intern Med* 14:335, 2000.

40. Staro JF, Zaret BL, Schulman DS, et al: Usefulness of verapamil for congestive heart failure associated with abnormal left ventricular diastolic filling and normal left ventricular systolic performance, *Am J Cardiol* 66:981, 1990.

41. Betocchi S, Piscione F, Losi AM, et al: Effects of diltiazem on left ventricular systolic and diastolic function in hypertrophic cardiomyopathy, *Am J Cardiol* 78:451, 1996.

42. MacDonald KA, Kittleson MD, Larson RF, et al: The effect of ramipril on left ventricular mass, myocardial fibrosis, diastolic function, and plasma neurohormones in Maine Coon cats with familial hypertrophic cardiomyopathy without heart failure, *J Vet Intern Med* 20:1093, 2006.

43. Tan LB, Jalil JE, Pick R, et al: Cardiac myocyte necrosis induced by angiotensin II, *Circ Res* 69:1185, 1991.

44. Pitt B, Zannad F, Remme WJ, et al: The effect of spironolactone on morbidity and mortality in patients with severe heart failure, *N Engl J Med* 341:709, 1999.

45. MacDonald KA, Kittleson MD, Kass PH: Effect of spironolactone on diastolic function and left ventricular mass in Maine Coon cats with familial hypertrophic cardiomyopathy, *J Vet Intern Med* 22:335, 2008.

41 Congenital Heart Disease

Risa M. Roland

Cardiac congenital abnormalities account for less than 3 per cent of all cardiac abnormalities seen in cats. Definitive diagnosis of most congenital abnormalities can be accomplished with a combination of historical findings, physical examination findings, thoracic radiographs, echocardiography, and electrocardiography (ECG). The more common feline cardiac congenital abnormalities, including mitral and tricuspid valve dysplasia, patent ductus arteriosus, aortic stenosis, pulmonic stenosis, ventricular septal defect, atrial septal defect, tetralogy of Fallot, endocardial fibroelastosis, and peritoneopericardial diaphragmatic hernia, have been summarized previously.[1] This chapter will provide updated information on the more common feline cardiac congenital abnormalities and an expanded discussion of the less common congenital abnormalities.

MITRAL VALVE DYSPLASIA

Mitral valve dysplasia (MVD), in the most general sense, is a developmental anatomical abnormality of the mitral valve apparatus. This may include malformations of the valve leaflets, valve annulus, chordae tendineae, papillary muscles, or a combination thereof (Figure 41-1). The abnormality results most commonly in mitral regurgitation, but stenosis of the mitral valve has been reported.[2] Additionally, dynamic left ventricular outflow tract obstruction and mitral regurgitation may occur as a result of systolic anterior motion (SAM) of the mitral valve associated with mitral valve malformation. If the outflow tract obstruction is severe, left ventricular concentric hypertrophy may occur. This may be difficult to distinguish from primary hypertrophic cardiomyopathy with secondary systolic anterior motion of the mitral valve (hypertrophic obstructive cardiomyopathy). Cats with

significant outflow tract obstructions and mitral regurgitation secondary to SAM of the mitral valve can present with clinical signs of syncope, exercise intolerance, and left-sided congestive heart failure (lethargy, respiratory difficulty) as kittens or young adult patients. Physical examination reveals a left apical sternal systolic murmur of mitral regurgitation, a left basilar systolic ejection murmur, or both. Two-dimensional echocardiography reveals SAM of the mitral valve (Figure 41-2) in addition to the other anatomical abnormalities consistent with MVD. If SAM of the mitral valve is present, the transaortic velocities are increased commensurate with the degree of obstruction and the spectral Doppler envelope may assume a dagger shape commensurate with the degree of obstruction (Figure 41-3). Beta-blocker therapy may help to alleviate the left ventricular outflow tract obstruction and may promote resolution of attendant hypertrophy.

Cats with mitral stenosis may present with lethargy, exercise intolerance, and signs of left-sided congestive heart failure. Physical examination findings may reveal a left apical diastolic murmur, although this is exceptionally difficult to appreciate in most cats because of the high heart rate. In cases of isolated mitral stenosis, there will be discordance between the severity of the enlargement of the left atrium and the left ventricle, the degree of left atrial enlargement being significantly greater than that of the left ventricle because of diastolic obstruction of blood flow from the left atrium to the left ventricle. Two-dimensional echocardiography reveals valve leaflets with a decreased diastolic excursion. Color and spectral Doppler echocardiography reveal high velocity, disturbed transmitral flow with a prolonged pressure half-time.[3] Definitive treatment of a stenotic valve involves cardiopulmonary bypass and has not been reported in the veterinary literature. Balloon dilation of a stenotic mitral valve is another interventional option. Severe mitral

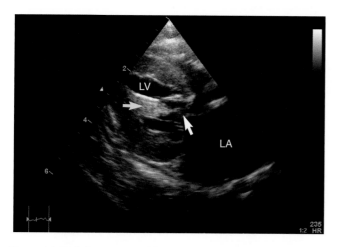

Figure 41-1 Right parasternal long axis view in a cat with mitral valve dysplasia. Note the bright, thickened single left ventricular papillary muscle *(yellow arrow)*. In addition, there is an elongated, thickened anterior mitral valve leaflet that attaches directly to this papillary muscle *(white arrow)*. The left atrium is severely enlarged. *LA,* Left atrium; *LV,* left ventricle.

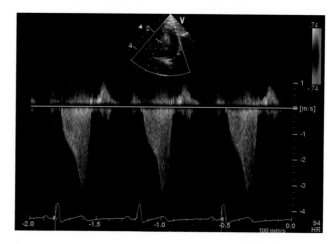

Figure 41-3 Spectral Doppler analysis depicting the velocity across left ventricular outflow tract in a cat with mitral valve dysplasia. Note the dagger-shaped appearance of the Doppler envelope suggesting a dynamic obstruction to blood flow. The velocity across the outflow tract is increased (3.4 m/s; 46 mm Hg), indicating a mild left ventricular outflow tract obstruction.

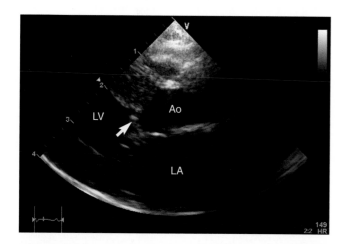

Figure 41-2 Right parasternal long axis view (systolic frame) in a cat with mitral valve dysplasia. Note the systolic anterior motion of the mitral valve *(white arrow)* and the left atrial enlargement. *LA,* Left atrium; *LV,* left ventricle; *Ao,* aorta.

regurgitation may develop following dilation, making this a less desirable treatment choice. Therefore medical management of left-sided congestive heart failure secondary to mitral stenosis is utilized and includes the use of diuretics and angiotensin-converting enzyme inhibitors. Potent vasodilators must be used with caution, if at all, because the obstructed left ventricular inflow may predispose to severe systemic hypotension. Isolated mitral valve stenosis puts patients at high risk for thromboembolism; therefore therapy with clopidogrel and aspirin is warranted.

TRICUSPID VALVE DYSPLASIA

Tricuspid valve dysplasia (TVD) is characterized by an anatomical abnormality of the tricuspid valve apparatus, which may include the valve leaflets, valve annulus, chordae tendineae, papillary muscles, or a combination of these structures. Most commonly lesions associated with TVD lead to a regurgitant jet and signs of right ventricular and right atrial eccentric hypertrophy, although tricuspid stenosis has been reported.[4] The stenosis may be present in addition to tricuspid regurgitation. Many cats who present with tricuspid valve stenosis are asymptomatic, and cats with mild lesions may remain asymptomatic through adulthood or develop signs of congestive heart failure during adulthood. Signs of heart failure, including lethargy, dyspnea, weight loss, anorexia, and abdominal distension, may be present in young cats with significant lesions.[5] Physical examination findings in cats with tricuspid stenosis reveal a right-sided parasternal diastolic murmur (in addition to a systolic murmur if regurgitation of the valve is present). With tricuspid stenosis there is significantly greater enlargement of the right atrium than the right ventricle because of impaired diastolic filling of the right ventricle. The valve leaflets have a decreased excursion in diastole, and color and spectral Doppler echocardiography reveal turbulent blood flow in the right ventricle just distal to the tricuspid valve. As with MVD, definitive treatment of the abnormal valve apparatus involves cardiopulmonary bypass and valve replacement. Because of their small size and cost of the procedure, this often is not a viable option for cats. Balloon dilation of a stenotic tricuspid valve is a possibility, because the residual tricuspid regurgitation is not as hemodynamically significant as that associated with the original stenosis. However, this procedure has not been reported to date, to the best of the author's knowledge. Therefore medical management of right-sided congestive heart failure is instituted and includes the use of diuretics and angiotensin-converting enzyme inhibitors, with or without vasodilator therapy.

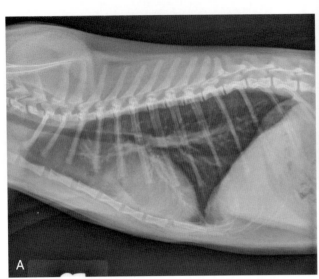
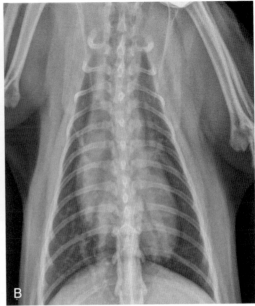

Figure 41-4 A, Lateral radiograph from a cat with a left-to-right shunting PDA documenting elongation of the cardiac silhouette consistent with left ventricular enlargement. Notice the prominent pulmonary vasculature and mild increase in pulmonary interstitial markings consistent with pulmonary overcirculation and incipient heart failure. **B,** Ventrodorsal view showing evidence of left ventricular enlargement and pulmonary overcirculation.

PATENT DUCTUS ARTERIOSUS

Failure of a patent ductus arteriosus (PDA) to close after birth results in a shunting of blood from the descending aorta to the pulmonary artery, resulting in a volume load placed on the pulmonary vasculature and left heart. Although the murmur of PDA in dogs is classically continuous, the high heart rate in cats sometimes makes appreciation of the diastolic component challenging in this species. Thoracic radiography documents variable degrees of left heart enlargement and pulmonary overcirculation commensurate with volumetric shunting (Figure 41-4). Echocardiography is used to confirm the diagnosis by documenting the presence of continuous disturbed flow within the main pulmonary artery (Figure 41-5). Surgical ligation is the more common definitive treatment; however, transvenous coil embolization has been reported in cats, representing an additional method of definitive treatment.[6]

Figure 41-5 Left cranial parasternal short axis view in a cat with a patent ductus arteriosus (PDA). Note the funnel-shaped PDA is observed easily in this echocardiographic view. *Ao,* Aorta; *MPA,* main pulmonary artery; *PDA,* patent ductus arteriosus.

PULMONIC STENOSIS

Lesions of pulmonic stenosis can be primarily valvular, supravalvular, or subvalvular in location, resulting in right ventricular concentric hypertrophy secondary to the pressure load induced by the stenosis. In addition to fixed anatomical obstruction, a dynamic component often is present. Definitive diagnosis is confirmed with echocardiography. Common features of moderate to severe pulmonic stenosis include accelerated transpulmonary flow velocity, global right ventricular hypertrophy, and flattening of the interventricular septum (Figure

41-6). Beta blockade may help to alleviate any dynamic component, but relief of the anatomical obstruction requires either surgical repair or an interventional catheterization procedure. Balloon valvuloplasty has been reported in cats with favorable outcomes.[7] In addition, balloon valvuloplasty has been performed successfully in cats who have infundibular stenosis (the muscular portion of the right ventricular outflow tract extending between the right ventricle and the pulmonary valve).[8]

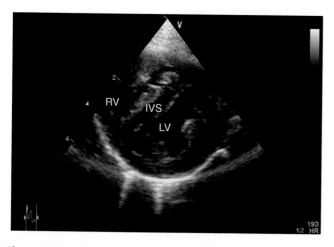

Figure 41-6 Right parasternal short axis view in a cat with severe pulmonic stenosis. There is severe right ventricular enlargement present and flattening of the interventricular septum secondary to the elevated right ventricular pressure. *RV,* Right ventricle; *LV,* left ventricle; *IVS,* interventricular septum.

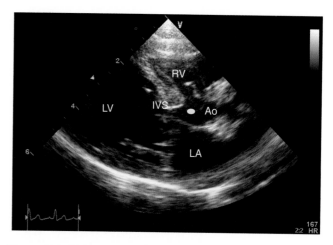

Figure 41-7 Right parasternal long axis inflow-outflow view in a cat with a ventricular septal defect. Note the defect directly above the interventricular septum *(yellow spot).* This represents the ventricular septal defect. *LA,* Left atrium; *LV,* left ventricle; *Ao,* aorta; *RV,* right ventricle.

VENTRICULAR SEPTAL DEFECT

Ventricular septal defect (VSD) is a common congenital abnormality in cats. The diagnosis and management have been well described. In some cases of VSDs, the defect may become partially or completely covered by adherence of tricuspid valve tissue to the defect or by proliferation of fibrous tissue around the margins of the defect.[9] The result is a membrane of tissue that blocks the flow of blood across the VSD. Because the left ventricular pressure is higher than that in the right ventricle, the membrane usually bulges toward the right ventricle in systole, resulting in a membranous ventricular septal aneurysm (MVSA).[9] Two-dimensional echocardiography is used in patients with VSDs to assess the size of the lesion as well as to determine if an MVSA is present (Figures 41-7 and 41-8).

PERITONEOPERICARDIAL DIAPHRAGMATIC HERNIA

Peritoneopericardial diaphragmatic hernia (PPDH) is a relatively common feline congenital abnormality. A high incidence has been reported in male Persian cats.[10] In cats a diagnosis of PPDH typically is first suspected based on thoracic radiographic evaluation and confirmed with echocardiography (Figure 41-9). Lateral thoracic radiographs may demonstrate a dorsal peritoneopericardial mesothelial remnant, a radiopacity located between the caudodorsal border of the heart and diaphragm and ventral to or superimposed over the caudal vena cava.[11] This finding may be useful in diagnosing the lesion. There is controversy with regard to the need to repair these lesions, especially in older asymptomatic cats in whom the diagnosis is incidental.

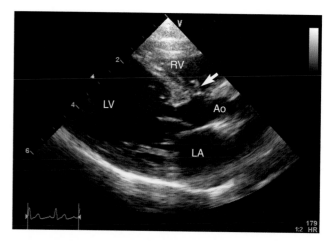

Figure 41-8 Right parasternal long axis inflow-outflow view in a cat with a membranous ventricular septal aneurysm. Note the fibrous tissue present directly above the interventricular septum and adjacent to the septal leaflet of the tricuspid valve *(arrow).* This represents a membranous ventricular septal aneurysm, which prevents blood flow across a ventricular septal defect.

ATRIOVENTRICULAR CANAL DEFECTS OR ATRIOVENTRICULAR SEPTAL DEFECTS

Atrioventricular (AV) canal defects result from a failure of the endocardial cushions to fuse in utero. The endocardial cushions are an integral part of the formation of the interatrial and interventricular septum as well as the AV valve leaflets. This defect has been described as a hereditary lesion in a family of Persian cats.[12] In addition, abnormalities of the tricuspid valve have been observed in some cats with a common AV canal.[5] AV canal defects may be partial or complete, and the distinction is made

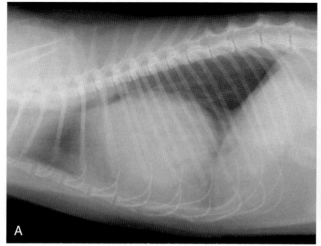

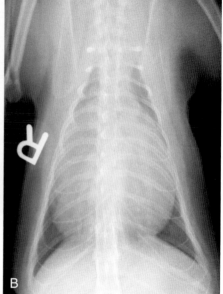

Figure 41-9 A and **B,** Lateral and ventrodorsal radiographs from a cat with PPDH. Notice the lack of separation between the diaphragm and the markedly enlarged pericardial silhouette.

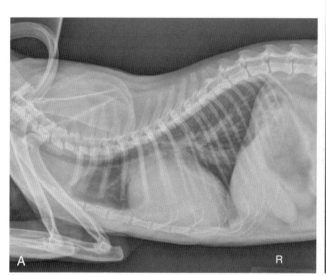

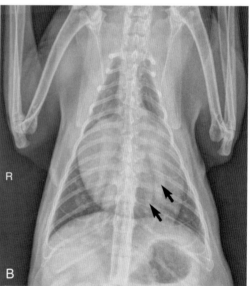

Figure 41-10 A, Right lateral thoracic radiograph of a cat with a partial atrioventricular canal. Note the severe generalized cardiomegaly as well as the dilated caudal vena cava and the pulmonary overcirculation. **B,** The dorsoventral thoracic radiograph from the same cat demonstrates severe generalized cardiomegaly as well as pulmonary artery and pulmonary venous distension *(arrows).*

based on the extent of the defect. With a complete AV canal, the AV septum is absent. The AV septum normally is located between the left ventricular outflow tract and the right atrium.[13] If the septum is absent, there is a common AV orifice and a five leaflet valve often is present that bridges the heart. Frequently the papillary muscles are oriented abnormally. With a complete AV canal, there is complete communication between all four chambers resulting from an atrial septal defect, a ventricular septal defect, and valvular regurgitation across the five leaflet valve. If the valve leaflets have a connection to the interatrial septum or the interventricular septum, a partial AV canal is present.

The presence of an AV canal results in severe volume overload of the right and left heart. Affected cats can present with stunted growth as well as a left sternal systolic heart murmur secondary to regurgitation of the AV valves. If heart failure is present, respiratory difficulty or abdominal effusion may be present. The ECG commonly reveals conduction abnormalities, especially bundle branch blocks, and the heart is markedly enlarged on thoracic radiographs (Figure 41-10).[13] Pulmonary edema or pleural effusion also may be present if heart failure has developed. Echocardiography reveals dilation of all four chambers with lack of an interventricular and interatrial septum if the cushion defect is complete (Figure 41-11).

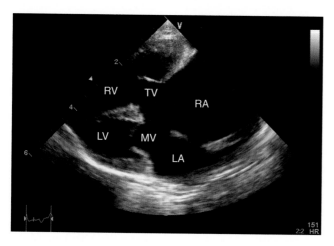

Figure 41-11 Right parasternal short axis view of a cat with a partial atrioventricular canal. Note the absence of a complete interatrial septum and the attachment of the mitral valve leaflet to the interventricular septum. There is severe right atrial and right ventricular enlargement present. *RA*, Right atrium; *LA*, left atrium; *RV*, right ventricle; *LV*, left ventricle; *TV*, tricuspid valve; *MV*, mitral valve.

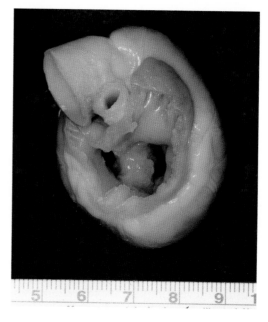

Figure 41-12 Dorsal view of a postmortem specimen from a cat with an atrioventricular canal defect. The dorsal portion of the atria has been removed to reveal the lack of a developed atrial septum and malformation of a common atrioventricular valve.

Incomplete cushion defects will have evidence of an intact atrial septum with a defect in the interventricular septum, or an intact interventricular septum with a defect in the interatrial septum (Figure 41-12). If the defect is severe, cats generally succumb to the disease secondary to left heart failure. If the defect is not severe, cats may be asymptomatic until adulthood or never develop clinical signs of disease. Medical management is aimed at controlling signs of congestive heart failure with diuretics, angiotensin-converting enzyme inhibitors, and vasodilators. Clopidogrel and aspirin also may be administered to prevent aortic thromboembolism.

SUPRAVALVULAR MITRAL STENOSIS AND COR TRIATRIATUM SINISTER

Supravalvular mitral stenosis (SMS) refers to a fibrous membrane present above the mitral valve leaflets. It is very rare in cats and often is present with other signs of dysplasia of the mitral valve apparatus.[14] Cor triatriatum sinister is a rare congenital abnormality characterized by an accessory atrial chamber separated from the actual atrial chamber by a fibromuscular membrane. These malformations may be difficult, if not impossible, to differentiate clinically without surgical exploration. In SMS the left auricle is proximal (relative to pulmonary venous blood flow) to the dividing membrane; however, in cor triatriatum sinister, the left auricle is distal to the dividing membrane relative to pulmonary venous blood flow. Both malformations result in the left atrium being partitioned into two distinct chambers and are similar pathophysiologically. The additional atrial chamber collects pulmonary venous drainage.[10,15,16] The membrane has either a single variable-sized hole or multiple perforations that allow blood flow to the left atrium. Cor triatriatum

sinister is thought to result from lack of incorporation of the common pulmonary vein into the left atrium, whereas SMS is a form of MVD.[12,16] Clinical signs associated with either condition are related to the severity of the obstruction of blood flow across the membrane. The obstruction to left atrial filling results in pulmonary edema or pulmonary hypertension.[17] Clinical signs in affected cats consist of small stature, lethargy, and dyspnea. Physical examination may or may not reveal a murmur. The respiratory rate may be increased secondary to left-sided congestive heart failure. Thoracic radiographs reveal an enlarged left atrium and pulmonary edema or signs of pulmonary hypertension including right atrial and right ventricular enlargement and dilated, tortuous pulmonary arteries. The accessory membrane that creates the secondary left atrial chamber can be appreciated on two-dimensional echocardiography as well as left atrial enlargement. Color and spectral Doppler echocardiography can be used to visualize the high velocity turbulent blood flow across the accessory atrium and determine the severity of the obstruction. Surgical correction of the defect is the definitive treatment.[18] If surgery is not elected, medical management of left-sided congestive heart failure can be instituted, including the use of diuretics, angiotensin-converting enzyme inhibitors, and vasodilators. Clopidogrel and aspirin also may be administered in an effort to prevent aortic thromboembolism. Sildenafil may be administered in an attempt to decrease the clinical signs associated with pulmonary hypertension; however, this treatment carries the risk of profound systemic hypotension because of the fixed nature of the obstruction.

DOUBLE-OUTLET RIGHT VENTRICLE

The malformation of double-outlet right ventricle (DORV) results in both great vessels originating from the right ventricle. Usually a large VSD accompanies this defect, providing outflow from the left heart to the systemic circulation.[19] Pulmonary overcirculation occurs and can lead to left-sided congestive heart failure unless there is concurrent pulmonic stenosis present or pulmonary hypertension develops.[10] Clinical signs include lethargy, weakness, and respiratory difficulty if left-sided congestive heart failure develops. Physical examination may reveal a systolic murmur and a widely split second heart sound. Cyanosis is present commonly.[19] The ECG and thoracic radiographs may reveal right atrial and right ventricular enlargement. Echocardiography typically documents substantial right ventricular hypertrophy and the presence of a large VSD. Agitated saline contrast studies usually reveal important bidirectional shunting. Complete characterization of the anatomy of the great vessels is challenging; however, identification of two discrete great vessels helps to differentiate this lesion from a truncus arteriosus (see below). Surgical repair has been reported in one cat, but the procedure is technically challenging and expensive.[20] This is a complex lesion and is associated with a very poor prognosis.

DOUBLE-CHAMBERED RIGHT VENTRICLE

Double-chambered right ventricle (DCRV) results from anomalous muscle bundles extending from the interventricular septum to the right ventricular free wall, or from hypertrophy of the crista supraventricularis and right ventricular free wall.[21,22] Anomalous muscle bundles may arise secondary to incomplete absorption of the embryonic myocardium.[22] The muscle bundles or hypertrophy divide the right ventricle into a proximal (relative to blood flow) high pressure chamber and a distal normal pressure chamber.[21] Physical examination reveals a systolic murmur present on the left or right side and normal femoral pulses.[21,22] Pulmonary auscultation is normal unless there is right-sided congestive heart failure, in which case dull lung sounds may be present secondary to pleural effusion. The ECG reveals right heart enlargement patterns as well as a right axis shift; however, important rhythm disturbances are uncommon. Thoracic radiographs reveal right heart and caudal vena cava enlargement with small pulmonary vasculature. Abnormalities seen commonly with two-dimensional echocardiography include a discrete band of tissue traversing the right ventricle from the interventricular septum to the right ventricular free wall. Proximal to this band, there is marked right ventricular concentric hypertrophy and dilatation, whereas distal to this band the infundibulum is commonly dilated. Right atrial enlargement also may be present. The left heart appears underfilled and there may be regional flattening of the interventricular septum and paradoxical septal motion caused by the high pressure in the proximal right ventricular chamber.[22] Mild to moderate regurgitation of the tricuspid valve may be

observed.[21] SAM of the mitral valve may be present secondary to abnormal left ventricular loading conditions and interventricular septal hypertrophy.[22]

The prognosis for cats with DCRV is variable. Cats may live into adulthood with no signs of congestive heart failure or may not develop congestive heart failure until late in life. On the other hand, severely affected cats may be profoundly compromised in the first year. Balloon valvuloplasty of the defect has been reported; however, the outcome was not favorable long term, most likely because of the anatomy of the fibromuscular band that is not sufficiently compliant to alleviate the obstruction after ballooning.[21,22] Partial ventriculectomy using an incised patch graft technique under total venous inflow occlusion has been reported and may provide an option for cats with severe disease.[21] Treatment with beta blockers to decrease any dynamic component to the obstruction may be helpful in cats for whom surgical correction is not an option. If signs of right heart failure develop, medical management (diuretics, angiotensin-converting enzyme inhibitors) can be employed, but typically is of minimal clinical benefit.

RIGHT-TO-LEFT SHUNTING (REVERSE) PATENT DUCTUS ARTERIOSUS

PDA defects that ultimately reverse (rPDA) and shunt right to left usually are very large defects. The shunting of blood from the left to right across a very large PDA could result in peracute death owing to massive volume overload and left-sided congestive heart failure. Presumably this does not occur because the pulmonary vascular resistance does not decrease significantly after birth, thereby limiting volumetric shunting.[23] This persistent elevation in pulmonary artery pressure (pulmonary hypertension), coupled with the large shunt, leads to progressive increases in pulmonary artery pressure and ultimately right to left shunting across the ductus.[23,24] Cats with rPDA present with signs of respiratory difficulty, lethargy, and weakness, especially in the hind limbs, and cyanosis in the caudal extremities with pink cranial mucous membranes (differential cyanosis). Signs of respiratory difficulty may occur, especially with exercise. Physical examination reveals no murmur and a split second heart sound secondary to the presence of pulmonary hypertension. Additionally, the right apical precordial impulse may be accentuated because of right heart enlargement. The hematocrit frequently is increased in excess of 65 per cent.

Electrocardiographic criteria for right atrial and right ventricular enlargement often are present. Thoracic radiographs reveal a ductal aneurysm (dilation of the descending aorta in the area where the ductus arteriosus originates) on the dorsoventral view as well as right heart enlargement. The main pulmonary artery appears dilated and the pulmonary vasculature may be undercirculated. Two-dimensional echocardiography reveals right ventricular concentric hypertrophy as well as a dilated pulmonary artery. A large conduit, consistent with a PDA, may be visualized between the aorta and pulmonary artery. Color and spectral Doppler echocardiography may reveal right-to-left shunting laminar blood flow across the ductus. Pulmonary hypertension can be documented and quantified by measuring pulmonic and tricuspid insufficiency velocities. Confirmation of the rPDA can be determined by contrast studies using agitated saline. First, a study of the heart must be performed to exclude a right-to-left intracardiac shunt. An additional study then is performed and the abdominal aorta is imaged to determine if microbubbles are present after injection. If microbubbles are present in the abdominal aorta and an intracardiac shunt has been excluded, an rPDA is presumed to be present. Treatment of rPDA involves periodic phlebotomy in an attempt to decrease the hematocrit to about 60 to 65 per cent, and avoidance of strenuous exercise. Sildenafil may be administered in an attempt to decrease the clinical signs associated with pulmonary hypertension and to minimize right-to-left shunting. Surgical ligation or interventional closure of a rPDA is contraindicated.

TRUNCUS ARTERIOSUS

Truncus arteriosus occurs when there is no partitioning between the aorta and pulmonary artery resulting in a large single vessel that allows flow from the ventricles to the pulmonary, systemic, and coronary circulations.[25] It occurs when there is failure of the spiral septum to form embryologically, such that the conal septum and the truncal septum fail to separate.[10,12,25] A large VSD also is invariably present. Because of the large VSD and the single outflow tract, blood in the ventricles mixes, with clinical signs dependent on the ratio of pulmonary to systemic blood flow.[10] In early stages of life, left heart failure develops as a result of volume overload and it is presumed that most kittens succumb to the disease at this point. If the kitten survives, over time the increased pulmonary blood flow leads to pulmonary hypertension, and clinical signs of cyanotic heart disease occur, including cyanosis, exercise intolerance, and respiratory difficulty. Affected cats may be polycythemic. Physical examination may reveal a heart murmur and cyanosis, but these findings are not pathognomonic for this defect. Echocardiography reveals a VSD with one large great vessel originating above it. An agitated saline contrast study reveals admixture of blood from both ventricles into the single large great vessel. Medical management is aimed at controlling polycythemia. Sildenafil may be administered in an effort to decrease the clinical signs associated with concurrent pulmonary hypertension. The prognosis is guarded and most cats may succumb to the disease early in life; however, cats surviving into adulthood have been reported.[26]

PULMONARY ARTERY STENOSIS

This congenital defect involves stenosis of the main or branched pulmonary arteries with variable degrees of main pulmonary artery dilation proximal to the stenotic lesion.[27] The right heart may develop concentric hypertrophy secondary to the obstruction across the pulmonary arteries. Most cats are asymptomatic on presentation and present for evaluation of a murmur. Clinical signs of the disease are exercise intolerance and respiratory difficulty especially with exercise. Physical examination reveals a basilar systolic murmur, with or without a diastolic murmur, that may be present on the left or right side of the thorax.[27] Electrocardiographic examination and thoracic radiographs may reveal signs of right heart enlargement. Two-dimensional echocardiography reveals the stenosis in the pulmonary arteries as well as pulmonary artery dilation proximal to the stenosis. Right ventricular enlargement, with or without right atrial enlargement, also may be seen. Color and spectral Doppler echocardiography documents turbulent blood flow across the stenosis as well as the velocity of blood flow across the stenosis. Most affected cats survive into adulthood with no clinical signs; however, some patients develop signs of lethargy or exertional dyspnea.[27] The use of interventional procedures including balloon dilation or stenting of these peripheral lesions, although performed commonly in human beings, has not been reported in cats.

REFERENCES

1. Brown WA: Congenital heart disease. In August JR, editor: *Consultations in feline internal medicine*, vol 3, Philadelphia, 1997, Saunders, p 263.
2. Matsuu A, Kanda T, Sugiyama A, et al: Mitral stenosis with bacterial myocarditis in a cat, *J Vet Med Sci* 69:1171, 2007.
3. Bonagura JD: Feline echocardiography, *J Feline Med Surg* 2:147, 2000.
4. Lord PF, Liu SK, Carmichael JA: Congenital tricuspid stenosis with right ventricular hypoplasia in a cat, *J Am Vet Med Assoc* 153:300, 1968.
5. Liu SK, Tilley LP: Dysplasia of the tricuspid valve in the dog and cat, *J Am Vet Med Assoc* 169:623, 1976.
6. Schneider M, Hildebrandt N: Transvenous embolization of the patent ductus arteriosus with detachable coils in 2 cats, *J Vet Intern Med* 17:349, 2003.
7. Johnson MS, Martin M: Balloon valvuloplasty in a cat with pulmonic stenosis, *J Vet Intern Med* 17:928, 2003.
8. Schrope DP: Primary pulmonic infundibular stenosis in 12 cats: natural history and the effects of balloon valvuloplasty, *J Vet Cardiol* 10:33, 2008.
9. Thomas WP: Echocardiographic diagnosis of congenital membranous ventricular septal aneurysm in the dog and cat, *J Am Anim Hosp Assoc* 41:215, 2005.
10. Bonagura JD, Lehmkuhl LB: Congenital heart disease. In Fox PR, Sisson D, Moïse NS, editors: *Textbook of canine and feline cardiology*, Philadelphia, 1999, Saunders, p 471.
11. Berry CR, Koblik PD, Ticer JW: Dorsal peritoneopericardial mesothelial remnant as an aid to diagnosis of feline congenital peritoneopericardial diaphragmatic hernia, *Vet Radiol Ultrasound* 31:239, 1990.
12. Kogure K, Miyagawa S, Ando M, et al: AV canal defect in a feline species. In Nora JJ, Takao A, editors: *Congenital heart disease: causes and processes*, Mt. Kisco, NY, 1984, Futura, p 69.
13. Kittleson MD: Other congenital cardiovascular abnormalities. In Kittleson MD, Kienle RD editors: *Small animal cardiovascular medicine*, St. Louis, 1998, Mosby, p 282.
14. Stamoulis ME, Fox PR: Mitral valve stenosis in three cats, *J Small Anim Pract* 34:452, 1993.

15. Fine DM, Tobias AH, Jacob KA: Supravalvular mitral stenosis in a cat, *J Am Anim Hosp Assoc* 38:403, 2002.

16. Koie H, Sato T, Nakagawa H, et al: Cor triatriatum sinister in a cat, *J Small Anim Pract* 41:128, 2000.

17. Heaney AM, Bulmer BJ: Cor triatriatum sinister and persistent left cranial vena cava in a kitten, *J Vet Intern Med* 18:895, 2004.

18. Wander KW, Monnet E, Orton EC: Surgical correction of cor triatriatum sinister in a kitten, *J Am Anim Hosp Assoc* 34:383, 1998.

19. Jeraj K, Ogburn PN, Jessen CA, et al: Double outlet right ventricle in a cat, *J Am Vet Med Assoc* 173:1356, 1978.

20. Northway RB: Use of an aortic homograft for surgical correction of a double-outlet right ventricle in a kitten, *Vet Med Small Anim Clin* 74:191, 1979.

21. Koffas H, Fuentes VL, Boswood A, et al: Double chambered right ventricle in 9 cats, *J Vet Intern Med* 21:76, 2007.

22. MacLean HN, Abbott JA, Pyle RL: Balloon dilation of double-chambered right ventricle in a cat, *J Vet Intern Med* 16:478, 2002.

23. Kittleson MD: Patent ductus arteriosus. In Kittleson MD, Kienle RD, editors: *Small animal cardiovascular medicine*, St. Louis, 1998, Mosby, p 218.

24. Connolly DJ, Lamb CR, Boswood A: Right-to-left shunting patent ductus arteriosus with pulmonary hypertension in a cat, *J Small Anim Pract* 44:184, 2003.

25. Chuzel T, Bublot I, Couturier L, et al: Persistent truncus arteriosus in a cat, *J Vet Cardiol* 9:43, 2007.

26. Nicolle AP, Tessier-Vetzel D, Begon E, et al: Persistent truncus arteriosus in a 6-year-old cat, *J Vet Med A Physiol Pathol Clin Med* 52:350, 2005.

27. Schrope DP, Kelch WJ: Clinical and echocardiographic findings of pulmonary artery stenosis in seven cats, *J Vet Cardiol* 9:83, 2007.

42 Rhythm Disturbances: Recognition and Therapy

Matthew W. Miller

Arrhythmias are commonly associated with both primary cardiac and extracardiac disease in cats.[1,2] Arrhythmias are associated most frequently with primary myocardial disease, by far the most common form of adult-onset feline heart disease, but also may complicate severe congenital cardiac malformations. The most common extracardiac diseases complicated by arrhythmias include hyperthyroidism, systemic hypertension, and severe electrolyte derangements, such as hyperkalemia (Figure 42-1), associated most frequently with urinary tract obstruction.[3,4]

Although specific comparative studies of dogs and cats have not been reported, it is generally accepted that the frequency of clinically important arrhythmias is lower in cats.[5] Nonetheless, arrhythmias are detected regularly during evaluation of cats with suspected heart disease. Despite the fact that some arrhythmias require no specific intervention, others cause important, potentially life-threatening hemodynamic compromise, making the ability to recognize and manage these rhythm disturbances imperative for optimal patient management. Goals of cardiac rhythm management should include abolishing and preventing recurrence of the rhythm derangement when possible, minimizing the hemodynamic impact of any arrhythmia that can not be terminated, and avoiding therapy-associated morbidity.[6] Several antiarrhythmic drugs are used clinically in cats;

however, specific studies comparing the utility of individual agents generally are lacking (Table 42-1).

IDENTIFICATION OF RHYTHM DISTURBANCES

Careful physical examination is the best screening test for detection of rhythm disturbances in cats. Clinical signs associated with important rhythm disturbances, including exercise intolerance and worsening heart failure, are challenging to recognize in cats. Even more dramatic clinical manifestations, including syncope, can be missed as a result of the frequently reclusive behavior displayed by some cats with important heart disease. Arrhythmias are detected commonly in combination with other physical examination abnormalities, including jugular venous distension, abnormal lung sounds, cardiac murmurs, or a gallop rhythm. Detection of any of these abnormalities on physical examination should prompt the clinician to pay particular attention to cardiac rhythm. Careful auscultation with simultaneous femoral pulse palpation usually will allow the observant examiner to detect a persistent or frequently occurring paroxysmal rhythm disturbance. Femoral pulse deficits are alterations in the perceived regularity of the cardiac rhythm; in the presence of other findings consistent with cardiac disease,

Table 42-1 Antiarrhythmic Drugs Used in Cats

Drug	Class	Dose (per cat)	Dose (mg/kg)
Dilacor XR (diltiazem)	Calcium channel blocker	30 mg PO q12-24h	4-6 mg/kg PO q12-24h
Atenolol	Beta-blocker	5-25 mg PO q12-24h	1-5 mg/kg PO q12-24h
Sotalol	Class III antiarrhythmic	10 mg PO q12h	1-3 mg/kg PO q12h
Lidocaine	Class I antiarrhythmic	1 mg IV bolus PRN up to a total of 5 mg, given slowly over 5 min	0.25-0.1 mg/kg IV given slowly over 3-5 minutes followed by a 10-40 μg/kg/min CRI
Procainamide	Class I antiarrhythmic	NA	2-5 mg/kg PO q8-12h

CRI, Constant rate infusion; *IV,* intravenous; *NA,* not applicable; *PO,* By mouth; *PRN,* as needed.

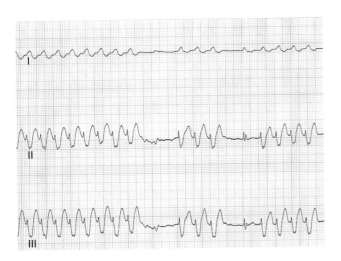

Figure 42-1 Three-lead (I, II, III) electrocardiogram demonstrating a paroxysmal wide complex tachycardia in a cat with hyperkalemia (8.6 mEq/L) caused by urethral obstruction. Paper speed 25 mm/sec, 1 cm = 1 mV calibration.

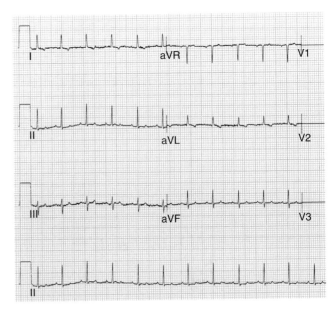

Figure 42-2 Six-lead electrocardiogram documenting normal sinus rhythm with a heart rate of approximately 150 bpm. Notice that the small amplitude upright P waves in lead II are consistently followed by a primarily upright QRS complex and a subsequent T wave. Additionally, the R-R interval varies less than 10 per cent. Paper speed 25 mm/sec, 1 cm = 1 mV amplitude calibration.

these alterations warrant recording of an electrocardiogram (ECG).

Diagnostic ECGs by convention are recorded with the cat in right lateral recumbency. Chemical restraint rarely is necessary and may alter the diagnostic recording most notably by influencing heart rate and the proarrhythmic effects of some frequently employed agents such as ketamine and medetomidine. The improvement in the recording quality rarely outweighs the risk associated with chemical restraint and should be avoided. In patients who have respiratory embarrassment, recording the ECG in sternal recumbency or with the patient standing may provide a diagnostic recording while minimizing patient stress. When a rhythm disturbance is persistent, it may be characterized adequately with a short recording. With paroxysmal arrhythmias, longer duration recordings are required and 24-hour ambulatory (Holter) monitoring may be required to fully describe the arrhythmia. Optimal determination of response to antiarrhythmic drugs and characterization of arrhythmias ideally is accomplished with serial Holter examinations. Unfortunately, this is an underutilized technique in cats. Excellent review papers describe the technique for recording resting ECGs and Holter monitoring in cats.[7-9]

SINUS RHYTHM AND SINUS TACHYCARDIA

In normal healthy cats, normal sinus rhythm (NSR) is the most common underlying cardiac rhythm. NSR is defined electrocardiographically as having regularly spaced (<10 per cent P-P variation) P waves, and for every P wave there is an associated QRS complex followed by a T wave. The heart rate in cats with NSR typically is between 140 and 200 beats per minute (bpm) (Figure 42-2). Once these same morphological criteria are met, but the rate exceeds 200 bpm, a rhythm diagnosis of sinus tachycardia (arguably a normal rhythm in cats) is more appropriate (Figure 42-3).

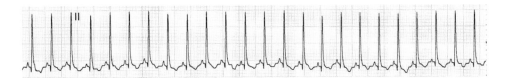

Figure 42-3 Lead II electrocardiogram documenting sinus tachycardia in a cat. Notice the consistent P-QRS-T relationship despite the elevated heart rate (240 bpm). The increased R-wave amplitude (1.6 mV) is suggestive of left ventricular enlargement. Paper speed 25 mm/sec, 1 cm = 1 mV amplitude calibration.

THERAPY

Sinus tachycardia should be viewed as an indicator of high sympathetic tone typically requiring no directed therapy. When associated with primary cardiac disease and heart failure, optimizing cardiac output and eliminating congestion usually are sufficient interventions. Sinus arrhythmia, and to a lesser extent sinus bradycardia, are caused most commonly by high vagal tone, the cause of which needs to be identified and eliminated if possible. Medications that are administered chronically to elevate heart rate, including the methylxanthine bronchodilators and propantheline, frequently are associated with unacceptable adverse side effects and are not used routinely.[10]

SUPRAVENTRICULAR TACHYARRHYTHMIAS

Supraventricular tachyarrhythmias originate by definition at or above the bundle branches and therefore include arrhythmias of both atrial and junctional origin. The QRS morphology typically is normal because the ventricular depolarization occurs along the normal conduction pathways. However, abrupt variations in rate, tachycardia, and primary cardiac disease can cause interventricular conduction abnormalities or aberrancy, resulting in a wide and morphologically bizarre QRS complex despite a supraventricular origin.

ATRIAL PREMATURE OR SUPRAVENTRICULAR PREMATURE COMPLEXES

Atrial premature complexes are associated most commonly with atrial enlargement secondary to primary cardiac disease but may be caused by a variety of extracardiac diseases, including hyperthyroidism. Atrial premature complexes occur by definition earlier than the next anticipated sinus impulse, have demonstrable atrial activity (P), and the QRS complex is morphologically similar if not identical to that associated with a normal sinus origin impulse (Figure 42-6). Frequently, the more generic term of *supraventricular premature complexes* is used to encompass an atrial, nodal, or junctional origin. Although isolated commonly, atrial premature complexes also can occur in couplets and triplets. If four or more atrial premature complexes occur sequentially, they are classified as paroxysmal atrial or supraventricular tachycardia.

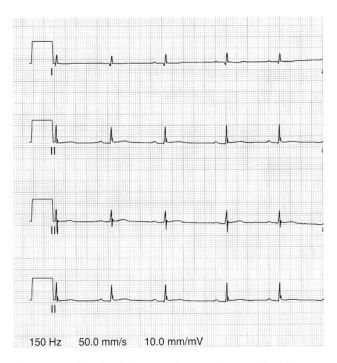

150 Hz   50.0 mm/s   10.0 mm/mV

Figure 42-4 Three-lead electrocardiogram documenting sinus bradycardia in a cat with head trauma secondary to being struck by a car. Notice the consistent P-QRS-T relationship and lack of R-R variability (<10 per cent). The calculated instantaneous heart rate is approximately 120 bpm. Paper speed 50 mm/sec, 1 cm = 1 mV amplitude calibration.

SINUS BRADYCARDIA AND SINUS ARRHYTHMIA

Heart rates less than 140 bpm in which the previously described P-QRS-T relationships are maintained is consistent with a diagnosis of sinus bradycardia (Figure 42-4). Sinus arrhythmia is an abnormal rhythm in cats. It is defined electrocardiographically by a gradual variation in P-P intervals that exceeds 10 per cent, which is often associated with respiration. The P-QRS-T relationships for sinus bradycardia are the same as described in the previous section. This rhythm abnormality is associated most commonly with disease that causes substantial increases in vagal tone, including intracranial disease, elevated intraocular pressure, and important primary respiratory diseases (Figure 42-5).

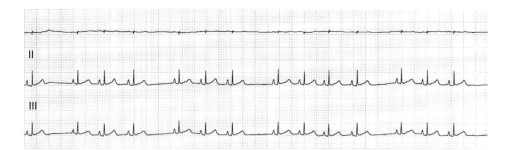

Figure 42-5 Three-lead (I, II, III) electrocardiogram demonstrating sinus arrhythmia in a cat with asthma. Notice the gradual predictable rhythmic variation in heart rate. A consistent P-QRS-T relationship is maintained. The heart rate is low at 120 bpm. Paper speed 25 mm/sec, 1 cm = 1 mV amplitude calibration.

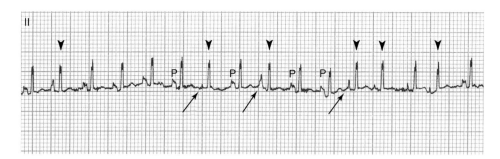

Figure 42-6 Lead II electrocardiogram from a cat with mitral valve dysplasia, mitral regurgitation, and substantial left atrial dilation. The underlying cardiac rhythm is sinus with a heart rate of 180 bpm. Notice the frequent atrial premature complexes *(APC)*. Although the QRS morphology of the APC is identical to that of the sinus impulses, the APC P-wave morphology *(arrows)* is substantially different to that of the P-wave morphology *(P)* of the normal sinus beats. Paper speed 25 mm/sec, 1 cm = 1 mV amplitude calibration.

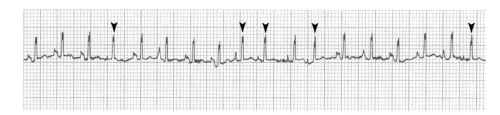

Figure 42-7 Lead II electrocardiogram from a cat with hypertrophic cardiomyopathy. Notice the rapid (300 bpm) rate, regular R-R interval, and narrow QRS morphology consistent with a supraventricular origin tachycardia. Paper speed 25 mm/sec, 2 cm = 1 mV amplitude calibration.

PAROXYSMAL ATRIAL OR SUPRAVENTRICULAR TACHYCARDIA

Paroxysmal atrial or supraventricular tachycardia is defined as the sequential occurrence of four or more supraventricular premature complexes. This arrhythmia usually is indicative of primary cardiac disease and substantial atrial enlargement. These arrhythmias can be sustained or can occur in short bursts with abrupt onset and spontaneous termination. Instantaneous rates in excess of 270 bpm are common and sometimes approach 400 bpm (Figure 42-7).

ATRIAL FIBRILLATION

Cats must have substantial atrial enlargement to have the critical mass of atrial tissue required to sustain atrial fibrillation; therefore, almost without exception, the presence of this arrhythmia implies the presence of clinically important cardiac disease, most commonly myocardial disease. It is defined electrocardiographically as a rapid, irregular, frequently chaotic rhythm with no demonstrable P waves in any lead. Fluctuations in atrioventricular (AV) nodal and interventricular conduction often result in variable QRS morphology, further complicating the diagnosis. The ventricular rate may vary from 170 to 260 bpm (Figure 42-8). Because important myocardial disease and atrial enlargement are present so often, additional arrhythmias, most notably isolated ventricular premature complexes, are seen commonly with atrial fibrillation (Figure 42-9).

THERAPY

Specific antiarrhythmic therapy rarely is required with isolated and infrequent supraventricular premature complexes. Even short periods of paroxysmal supraventricular tachycardia may be well tolerated. The hemodynamic impact of these arrhythmias is influenced substantially by the severity of the associated underlying cardiac disease. Frequently, successful management of congestive heart failure (CHF) is sufficient to alleviate clinical signs and to make specific antiarrhythmic therapy unnecessary.

Atrial fibrillation and paroxysmal or sustained high-rate supraventricular tachycardia require intervention to mitigate the adverse hemodynamic impact with which they are associated. The goal of therapy in this group of arrhythmias is to either eliminate the arrhythmias with restoration of sinus rhythm or to simply control ventricular response rate.[11,12] Although digoxin is featured prominently in the literature for therapy of most supraventricular tachyarrhythmias, including atrial fibrillation, the author rarely uses digoxin in cats because of an unacceptable incidence of clinically important adverse side effects. No firm data exist comparing the efficacy of different antiarrhythmic drugs in the management of supraventricular tachycardia, including atrial fibrillation in cats. Although the goal of therapy is to abolish the arrhythmia and restore sinus rhythm, this is often idealistic. In the case of atrial fibrillation, control of ventricular response rate below 150 to 160 bpm is a more reasonable therapeutic goal. The author prefers using sotalol or atenolol in patients who are not demonstrating evidence of CHF or recent arterial thrombosis. Therapy with diltiazem is preferred for this subset of patients. Once clinical signs of CHF or arterial thrombosis have resolved, therapy with sotalol or atenolol can be initiated. The clinical conundrum often is that resolution of CHF can not be achieved without adequate rhythm management.

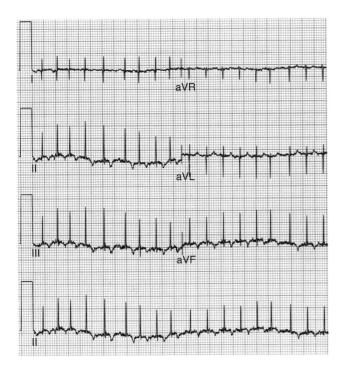

Figure 42-8 Six-lead (I, II, III, aVR, aVL, aVF) electrocardiogram from a cat with severe hypertrophic cardiomyopathy and congestive heart failure. The cardiac rhythm is irregularly irregular and rapid (220 bpm) despite therapy with diltiazem. There is no demonstrable P-wave activity in any lead that is consistent with a diagnosis of atrial fibrillation. Paper speed 25 mm/sec, 1 cm = 1 mV amplitude calibration.

ABNORMALITIES OF ATRIOVENTRICULAR NODAL CONDUCTION

Normally, the only electrical communication between the atria and ventricles is through the AV node. The sinus impulse is slowed at this location, giving time for the ventricles to fill before depolarization of the ventricles through the bundle of His, the bundle branches, and subsequently the Purkinje fibers. In addition to optimizing the timing between atrial emptying and ventricular contraction, the AV node serves to protect against the dramatic ventricular rate responses associated with supraventricular tachyarrhythmias. Abnormalities of AV nodal conduction can be broken down simply into those associated with prolongation of AV nodal conduction

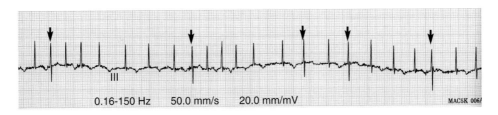

Figure 42-9 Lead III rhythm strip from a cat with restrictive cardiomyopathy. The underlying cardiac rhythm is atrial fibrillation as evidenced by the rapid (280 bpm) irregularly irregular R-R interval and lack of demonstrable P waves. Additionally, notice the occasional isolated monomorphic ventricular premature complexes (arrows). Paper speed 50 mm/sec, 2 cm = 1 mV amplitude calibration.

(first-degree AV block), intermittent complete block (second-degree AV block), and persistent complete block (third-degree AV block).

FIRST-DEGREE ATRIOVENTRICULAR BLOCK

In first-degree AV block, all P waves are conducted across the AV node and result in an associated QRS-T complex. The conduction across the AV node, however, is slowed, as evidenced by a prolonged P-R interval typically in excess of 90 msec. This arrhythmia results in no overt clinical signs and requires no specific therapy; however, it is documented commonly in association with myocardial failure. Conditions that result in elevated vagal tone (increased intraocular or intracranial pressure), or administration of medications (narcotic drugs, beta-blockers, calcium channel blockers, and digitalis glycosides) that slow AV nodal conduction directly or indirectly, may result in this conduction abnormality.

SECOND-DEGREE ATRIOVENTRICULAR BLOCK

Second-degree AV block is defined as the failure of one or more P waves to be conducted to the ventricles and cause a resultant QRS-T complex. The P-R interval in the conducted complexes may be normal or prolonged. Although the conditions that cause first-degree AV block potentially can result in second-degree AV block, most cats with second-degree AV block have demonstrable evidence of primary myocardial disease.

THIRD-DEGREE (COMPLETE) ATRIOVENTRICULAR BLOCK

In third-degree, or complete, AV block, there is absolute interruption of AV nodal conduction. An independent pacemaker drives the atria and ventricles, and the ventricular (escape) rate is markedly slower than the atrial rate (Figure 42-10). The morphology of the escape QRS complex is variable, depending on its origin. A variable QRS morphology is suggestive of an unstable escape mechanism, making management of the arrhythmia more urgent. Third-degree AV block almost always is associated with primary organic heart disease. Clinical signs may include weakness and lethargy, worsening heart failure, and syncope. Syncopal events associated

with complete AV block may be misinterpreted as seizure activity.[13,14]

THERAPY

AV block induced by chronic oral drug administration, including beta-blockers, calcium channel blockers, and digitalis glycosides, usually responds to discontinuation or dosage reduction of the causative medication. If the bradyarrhythmia is associated with sedation or anesthesia, discontinuation of inhaled anesthetic agents, narcotic reversal, or administration of a parasympatholytic agent (atropine sulfate 0.02 to 0.04 mg/kg; glycopyrrolate 0.005 to 0.01 mg/kg) may be sufficient. If cardiac output is impacted substantially and the arrhythmia is not alleviated by these measures, temporary rate support may be achieved by intravenous (IV) administration of a sympathomimetic agent (isoproterenol 0.02 to 0.04 μg/kg/min or dopamine 2 to 5 μg/kg/min).[15] These interventions rarely augment AV nodal conduction, providing support instead by driving the ventricular escape rate.

Where available, temporary transvenous pacing is an effective way to control ventricular response rate provisionally in patients with high-grade second- or third-degree AV block as a bridge to final therapy. Definitive long-term management of cats with symptomatic high-grade second- or third-degree AV block requires implantation of a permanent cardiac pacemaker.[16] Because of the relatively rapid escape rates, often greater than 100 bpm, seen commonly in cats with complete heart block, many patients are asymptomatic or display only mild clinical signs and therefore require no definitive therapy.

VENTRICULAR PREEXCITATION

Ventricular preexcitation occurs when a conduction pathway connects the atrium to the ventricles directly, thereby bypassing the AV node. This allows activation of a portion of the ventricle earlier than would be expected relative to conduction of the atrial impulse across the AV node, and several different forms of preexcitation have been reported in cats.[17,18] Premature stimulation of a portion of the ventricle alone does not result in clinical signs. In fact, this conduction disturbance almost certainly is markedly underdiagnosed. Clinical signs, when present, may include lethargy, weakness, or even

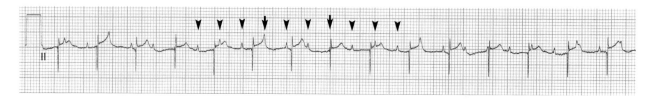

Figure 42-10 Lead II rhythm strip from a cat with chronic kidney disease and systemic arterial hypertension. Notice how the P waves (*arrowheads*) with a rate of 240 bpm are unrelated to the QRS complexes occurring at a heart rate of 120 bpm. The P waves occasionally are superimposed on the QRS or the T wave (*arrows*). Paper speed 25 mm/sec, 1 cm = 1 mV amplitude calibration.

collapse and are caused by paroxysmal or sustained tachycardia.

Although several forms of preexcitation occur, there are common electrocardiographic features of this conduction abnormality. The PR interval often is shortened and may be less than 40 msec. In some instances, the P wave is partially inscribed in the initial portion of the QRS complex, making the PR segment essentially absent. The QRS appearance depends on several factors, including type of preexcitation, the relative conduction velocities of the bypass tract, and the normal conduction pathways, as well as the direction of conduction across the bypass tract (antegrade or retrograde). In some cats, the morphology of the QRS complex can appear normal, whereas in others it may be splintered and wider than normal. If a reentrant conduction loop is established, paroxysmal or sustained tachyarrhythmias may be noted. Rapid sustained tachycardia with a wide splintered QRS complex secondary to preexcitation poses a diagnostic challenge because it appears similar to sustained ventricular tachycardia (Figure 42-11).

THERAPY

Preexcitation without clinical signs typically is not treated. If clinical signs are noted, they usually are due to the associated severe reentrant tachyarrhythmias and resultant reductions in cardiac output. Vagal maneuvers (application of vigorous ocular and ideally carotid sinus pressure) should be attempted and may terminate or slow the arrhythmia by altering conduction through the AV node. If this intervention is ineffective, cautious administration of IV diltiazem (0.1 to 0.25 mg/kg IV slowly) or esmolol (200 to 500 µg/kg IV slowly) may be effective. The administration of drugs that alter the conduction of the accessory pathway preferentially, such as procainamide or quinidine, has been advocated in dogs and human beings; however, reports of their use in cats are lacking. Definitive therapy of patients nonresponsive to medical management requires surgical or catheter-based ablation, and to the author's knowledge, the use of these procedures has not been reported in cats.[19]

VENTRICULAR ARRHYTHMIAS

Ventricular arrhythmias are some of the most common rhythm disturbances documented in cats. By definition, they originate distal to the AV node and can originate in the specialized conduction fibers or ventricular myocardium. Because the ventricular conduction does not occur along the normal intraventricular conduction pathways, the QRS complexes inscribed by most ventricular premature complexes and paroxysmal or sustained ventricular tachycardias are wide and bizarre when compared to the QRS morphology of a normal sinus impulse. Ventricular arrhythmias are the most common feline arrhythmias. They are seen commonly in older cats with no overt evidence of heart disease or heart failure. They also are associated commonly with all forms of primary myocardial disease, hyperthyroidism, and severe congenital

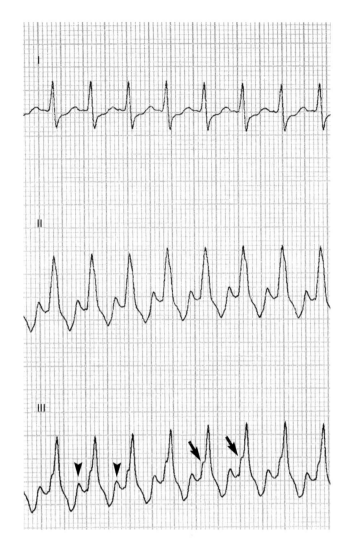

Figure 42-11 Three-lead (I, II, III) electrocardiogram from a cat with an intermittent arrhythmia. P waves *(arrowheads)* can be seen buried in the preceding T wave. The P-R interval is short, and a notch *(arrows)* can be seen in the upstroke of the QRS indicative of preexcitation of a portion of the ventricle. Paper speed 25 mm/sec, 1 cm = 1 mV amplitude calibration.

malformations.[20] Primary myocardial disease and CHF increase the likelihood of ventricular arrhythmias, whereas the development of ventricular arrhythmias may cause CHF in a cat with previously well-compensated heart disease.[5]

VENTRICULAR PREMATURE COMPLEXES

Ventricular premature complexes (VPCs) by definition occur earlier than the next anticipated sinus impulse. They have no demonstrable associated atrial activity and the QRS complex is morphologically dissimilar, frequently both wide and bizarre, when compared with that of a normal sinus origin impulse (Figure 42-12). The T wave is almost always large, having the opposite polarity of the main deflection of the QRS complex and blending frequently into the QRS complex. Fusion beats, complexes caused by simultaneous depolarization of the ventricles by a VPC, and a sinus beat sometimes are seen and confirm the presence of VPCs. Although usually isolated, VPCs also can occur in couplets and triplets. Although generally considered more important when multiform or frequent in nature, no studies have confirmed this supposition. If four or more VPCs occur sequentially, they are classified as paroxysmal ventricular tachycardia.

PAROXYSMAL AND SUSTAINED VENTRICULAR TACHYCARDIA

Paroxysmal ventricular tachycardia is defined as the sequential occurrence of four or more VPCs interspersed with spontaneous reversion to sinus rhythm, whereas sustained ventricular tachycardia is persistent, not resolving without intervention. These arrhythmias usually are indicative of primary cardiac disease, most notably primary myocardial disease. Instantaneous rates greater than 250 bpm are common but rarely exceed 300 bpm (Figure 42-13). The term *idioventricular tachycardia* is used

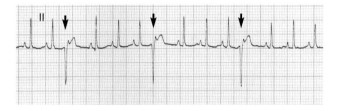

Figure 42-12 Lead II electrocardiogram from a cat with thyrotoxic heart disease. The predominant cardiac rhythm is sinus (180 bpm) with occasional isolated monomorphic ventricular premature complexes. Notice how dramatically different the morphology of the VPC is relative to the QRS of the normal sinus complex. Additionally, the associated T wave is large and in opposite polarity to major deflection of the VPC. Paper speed 25 mm/sec, 1 cm = 1 mV amplitude calibration.

for patients in whom the rate of the ventricular arrhythmia is only slightly greater than and often competing with the underlying sinus rate (Figure 42-14). Idioventricular tachycardia frequently is well tolerated and often does not require specific antiarrhythmic therapy but responds to supportive management of an underlying noncardiac condition.

THERAPY

There are few data to support administration of specific antiarrhythmic drugs for therapy of asymptomatic ventricular arrhythmias. Pursuing a diagnosis of and managing a metabolic cause for the arrhythmia or optimizing therapy for heart failure are more appropriate strategies. It has been suggested that even when asymptomatic, ventricular arrhythmias should be treated if deemed to be unstable. Criteria proposed include the presence of multifocal VPCs, R-on-T phenomenon in which the R wave of the VPC falls in the T wave of the preceding impulse, or sustained ventricular tachycardia (Figure 42-15). It is important to realize that supportive literature for this suggestion is lacking and that administration of ventricular antiarrhythmic drugs carries the possibility of worsening the arrhythmia (proarrhythmia). Therapy should be instituted in patients in whom the arrhythmia results in hemodynamic compromise (i.e., hypotension, weakness, syncope, CHF, and shock) and instability. Resolution of signs of CHF may be impossible without adequate rhythm management; however, elimination of all VPCs typically is not possible or necessary. Optimal antiarrhythmic therapy should be based on serial Holter monitoring, although this may be impractical in some patients.

In situations in which the arrhythmia is life-threatening, requiring immediate intervention, therapy with lidocaine is the author's therapy of choice (initial dose of 0.25 to 1 mg/kg IV over 5 minutes [up to a total of 4 mg/kg]

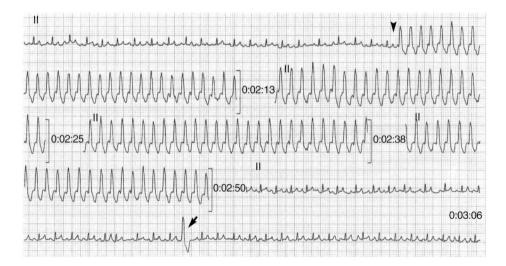

Figure 42-13 Lead II electrocardiogram. The initial rhythm is sinus with a heart rate of 160 bpm, followed by a long episode of ventricular tachycardia *(arrowhead)* that reverts spontaneously to sinus rhythm with a single ventricular premature complex *(arrow)*. Paper speed 25 mm/sec, 1 cm = 1 mV amplitude calibration. (Courtesy Dr. J-P Petrie.)

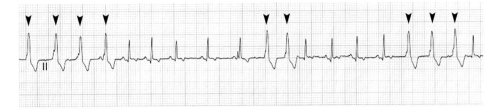

Figure 42-14 Lead III rhythm strip from a cat with unclassified cardiomyopathy and systolic dysfunction. The underlying cardiac rhythm is sinus. There are frequent monomorphic ventricular premature complexes *(arrowheads)* that occur at a rate very similar to that of the sinus mechanism. This results in the rhythm alternating between normal sinus rhythm and an accelerated idioventricular rhythm. Paper speed 50 mm/sec, 2 cm = 1 mV amplitude calibration.

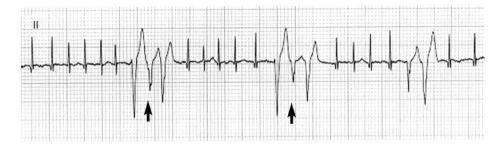

Figure 42-15 Lead II electrocardiogram from a cat with mitral valve endocarditis and congestive heart failure. The underlying cardiac rhythm is atrial fibrillation with a ventricular response rate of 240 bpm. Notice the closely coupled (R-on-T) bursts of ventricular premature complexes *(arrows)*. Paper speed 25 mm/sec, 1 cm = 1 mV amplitude calibration.

followed by a 20 to 40 µg/kg/min constant rate infusion [CRI]). If the arrhythmia is unresponsive to this initial therapy, esmolol (50 to 500 µg/kg IV bolus, or 50 to 200 µg/kg/hour CRI) may be added or used as monotherapy. Chronic maintenance therapy is achieved most commonly using sotalol (0.5 to 2.0 mg/kg PO q12h) or less frequently atenolol (1 to 5 mg/kg PO q12h). Infrequently, procainamide (3 to 5 mg/kg PO q8-12h) is added when monotherapy is ineffective and arrhythmia suppression is deemed necessary.[21]

REFERENCES

1. Côté E, Harpster NK: Feline cardiac arrhythmias. In Bonagura JD, Twedt DC, editors: *Current veterinary therapy XIV*, St Louis, 2009, Saunders Elsevier, p 731.
2. Harpster NK: The cardiovascular system. In Holzworth J, editor: *Diseases of the cat: medicine and surgery*, Philadelphia, 1987, WB Saunders, p 837.
3. Norman BC, Côté E, Barrett KA: Wide-complex tachycardia associated with severe hyperkalemia in three cats, *J Feline Med Surg* 8:372, 2006.
4. Peterson ME, Keene BW, Ferguson DC, et al: Electrocardiographic findings in 45 cats with hyperthyroidism, *J Am Vet Med Assoc* 180:934, 1982.
5. Fox PR, Harpster NK: Diagnosis and management of feline arrhythmias. In Fox PR, Sisson DD, Moise NS, editors: *Textbook of canine and feline cardiology*, ed 2, Philadelphia, 1999, Saunders, p 386.
6. Tilley LP: *Essentials of canine and feline electrocardiography*, ed 3, Philadelphia, 1992, Lea & Febiger.
7. Sisson DD, Ettinger SJ: The physical examination. In Fox PR, Sisson DD, Moïse NS, editors: *Textbook of canine and feline cardiology*, ed 2, Philadelphia, 1999, Saunders, p 386.
8. Petrie JP: Practical application of Holter monitoring in dogs and cats, *Clin Tech Small Anim Pract* 20:173, 2005.
9. Ware WA: Twenty four hour ambulatory electrocardiography in normal cats, *J Vet Intern Med* 13:175, 1999.
10. Gelzer AR, Kraus MS: Management of atrial fibrillation, *Vet Clin Small Anim Pract* 34:1127, 2004.
11. Côté E, Harpster NK, Laste NJ, et al: Atrial fibrillation in cats: 50 cases (1979-2002), *J Am Vet Med Assoc* 15:256, 2004.
12. Crijins HJ: Rate versus rhythm control in patients with atrial fibrillation: what the trials really say, *Drugs* 12:1651, 2005.
13. Penning VA, Connolly DJ, Gajanayake I, et al: Seizure-like episodes in three cats with intermittent high grade atrioventricular dysfunction, *J Vet Intern Med* 23:200, 2009.
14. Côté E, Ettinger SJ: Electrocardiography and cardiac arrhythmias. In Ettinger SJ, Feldman EC, editors: *Textbook of veterinary internal medicine*, ed 6, St Louis, 2005, Elsevier, p 1040.
15. Petrie JP: Permanent transvenous cardiac pacing, *Clin Tech Small Anim Pract* 20:164, 2005.
16. Kellum HB, Stepien RL: Third-degree atrioventricular block in 21 cats (1997-2004), *J Vet Intern Med* 20:97, 2006.
17. Hill BL, Tilley LP: Ventricular pre-excitation in seven dogs and nine cats, *J Am Vet Med Assoc* 187:1026, 1985.
18. Ogburn PN: Ventricular pre-excitation (Wolff-Parkinson-White syndrome) in a cat, *J Am Anim Hosp Assoc* 13:171, 1977.
19. Wright KN: When where and how to perform cardiac radiofrequency catheter ablation, *J Vet Cardiol* 8:95, 2006.
20. Côté E, Jaeger R: Ventricular tachyarrhythmias in 106 cats: associated structural cardiac disorders, *J Vet Intern Med* 22:1444, 2008.
21. Fox PR: Right ventricular cardiomyopathy in cats. In Bonagura JD, Twedt DC, editors: *Current veterinary therapy XIV*, St Louis, 2009, Saunders Elsevier, p 815.

CHAPTER
43 Pathology of Primary Myocardial Disease

Philip R. Fox

THE ROLE OF CARDIOVASCULAR PATHOLOGY IN PRACTICE

Necropsy plays a vital role in medical and scientific discovery.[1-4] Indeed, necropsy permits recognition of disease patterns, facilitates understanding of pathophysiology, validates technical processes (imaging, serological tests), and helps to assess therapeutic efficacy and toxicities. It also is a method to detect diagnostic errors, and to provide knowledge that can be applied to future cases. Collectively these activities advance medical diagnosis and patient care.

Gross or histopathological lesions can be detected in most cats who have clinical evidence of cardiac morbidity or mortality. Thus necropsy can help to characterize congenital and acquired cardiovascular disorders. This is particularly germane when seeking to discover heart disease in breeding animals, and when searching to discern cardiac cause in sudden, unexpected death. Interaction between practitioner and pathologist is essential to maximize clinical insight, confirm diagnosis, and determine pathological consequences of heart disease. Accordingly dissection techniques are best guided by clinical and imaging information.

CARDIOVASCULAR PATHOLOGY IN HEART FAILURE

Heart failure is not a disease but a clinical syndrome. It is the consequence of advanced pathophysiological progression from congenital or acquired cardiovascular disease, or cardiac injury. Heart disease may impose a pressure or volume overload, alter cardiac contractile or relaxation characteristics, cause abnormalities of heart rate and rhythm, or result in ion channel disruption.[5-7]

Compensatory hypertrophy represents a major cardiac adjustment to increased cardiac work.[5,6] Concentric hypertrophy is a typical response to pressure overloads such as aortic stenosis or arterial hypertension, and is related to increased ventricular systolic wall tension and increased afterload.[8] Sarcomeres are added in parallel with little change in chamber diameter. Eccentric hypertrophy causes a proportional increase in ventricular wall thickness and internal chamber diameter via synthesis of sarcomeres in series, and is a common adaptation in states of volume overload.[9]

Myocyte cell death can occur via necrosis or programmed death (apoptosis).[10,11] Cellular necrosis is a passive process resulting from lethal insult. It is characterized by cell membrane rupture and associated inflammation. Changes include cellular swelling, loss of membrane integrity and breakdown, nuclear chromatin clumping into poorly defined masses, swelling and disruption of sarcoplasmic reticulum and mitochondria, formation of granular mitochondrial matrix densities, and loss of calcium and electrolyte homeostasis. Apoptosis occurs in the absence of cell membrane rupture and inflammation; is an active, regulated, energy-requiring process under genetic control; and is characterized by nuclear DNA fragmentation. Nuclear chromatin becomes compacted and segmented into sharply delineated masses along the nuclear margins, the cytoplasm condenses, nuclear fragmentation occurs, and the cell surface develops pediculated protuberances and separates into membrane-bound apoptotic bodies that are phagocytized by adjacent cells.

Alterations of connective tissue play important roles in heart disease. The heart is composed of parenchyma and stroma. Parenchyma consists of cardiac myocytes, which are highly differentiated and perform specialized functions. Stroma contains cellular elements including fibroblasts and macrophages that are not well differentiated, and whose physiological behavior and phenotype are affected by circulating and local chemical mediators and signals.[12] Fibrosis represents disproportionate stromal growth with increased myocardial collagen content and may be reactive or reparative. Pathological myocardial remodeling results when either form of fibrosis occurs.

Myocytes are enmeshed in a stromal framework containing collagen, elastin, and other elements.[13] The interstitial matrix, of which collagen is the major component, represents networks of pericellular, interstitial, and fascicular connective tissue. Myocardial cells are diffusely interconnected by this connective tissue framework, which is composed of struts, pericellular weaves, and coiled perimysial fibers. This internal myocardial skeletal framework is thought to participate in myocardial function, integrate individual myocytes into three-dimensional conformational changes during systole, and contribute to myocardial compliance during diastole.[14,15] Matrix components can be visualized histologically by specialized staining techniques.

Pulmonary edema is the consequence of left-sided heart failure associated with diastolic dysfunction, myocardial failure, or volume overload. Edematous lungs are wet, heavy, and ooze edema fluid from cut sections. Edema fluid may appear pinkish and sometimes foamy. Microscopically, edema fluid is acidophilic or faintly granular, filling alveoli, interstitium, and lymphatics. Protein content is very low. Capillaries and lymphatics are distended. Intraalveolar hemorrhage may be apparent. Alveolar macrophages ("heart failure" cells) containing erythrocytes or hemosiderin may be present and increase with duration of edema. Chronic cardiogenic edema and associated pulmonary hypertension may cause muscular hypertrophy of small pulmonary arteries and fibrous thickening of pulmonary capillary walls. Occasionally in fulminant, terminal pulmonary edema, leukocytes accumulate in pulmonary capillaries, endothelial damage and alveolar type I epithelial cells are noted, and fibrin-rich fluid fills the alveoli.

Effusions (abdominal, pleural, and/or pericardial) generally are sterile, obstructive transudates early in right-sided heart failure, and can become modified transudates in chronic heart failure. They are characteristically modified transudates, pale yellow or serosanguineous, with 2 to 5 g/dL of protein. Cytological smears contain a mixture of blood cells and lymphocytes with a nucleated cell-to-red cell ratio roughly equal to blood, and some mesothelial cells. With time the effusion acquires greater numbers of inflammatory cells and increased protein. In long-standing effusions, mesothelial cells and macrophages may exhibit erythrophagia.[16] Occasionally chylous effusion may occur and appears milky white with mostly lymphocytes and variable numbers of neutrophils,

depending on duration and degree of pleuritis.[17] With long-standing pleural effusions of modified transudate or chyle, pleuritis may develop, cause lung lobe borders to become fibrotic, or even collapse. Chronic ascites or pericardial effusion may result in fibrin deposition.

MYOCARDIAL DISEASES (CARDIOMYOPATHIES)

Myocardial disorders constitute the majority of feline heart disease.[3,4,17a-22] They may be primary (idiopathic) or occur secondary to systemic or metabolic conditions.

IDIOPATHIC HYPERTROPHIC CARDIOMYOPATHY

Feline hypertrophic cardiomyopathy (HCM) is the most common form of cardiomyopathy. This heterogeneous disorder has diverse morphological features and broad clinical presentation.[3,4,17a-20,22]

Gross Pathology (Figure 43-1)

Most affected cats have diffuse but asymmetrical distribution of left ventricular (LV) hypertrophy involving

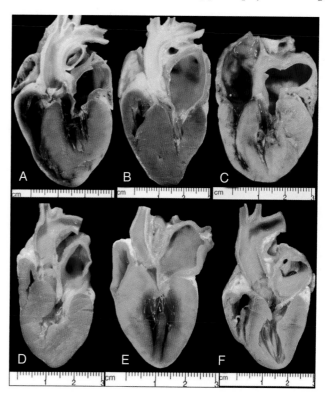

Figure 43-1 Hearts from cats with hypertrophic cardiomyopathy illustrating wide phenotypic variability characteristic of this disease. Notice substantial and diffuse left ventricular hypertrophy in **A** to **D** (concentric hypertrophy as indicated by all segments of the ventricular septum and LV caudal wall, which are similarly hypertrophied in **A** and **D**). Segmental left ventricular hypertrophy is associated predominantly with the basal ventricular septum in **E** and **F**. (From Fox PR: Hypertrophic cardiomyopathy: clinical and pathologic correlates, *J Vet Cardiol* 5:39, 2003.)

substantial portions of ventricular septum and LV free wall. Less commonly, segmental patterns of hypertrophy occur, often with abrupt transitions in wall thickness or involvement of noncontiguous segments. The LV cavity is reduced and the left atrium (LA) is enlarged and often hypertrophied. Absolute and relative heart weights are increased substantially. Heart weight in relation to body weight is significantly greater in cats (6.4 ± 0.1 g/kg) with HCM, compared with normal cats (mean, 4.8 ± 0.1 g/kg). Necropsy of 51 HCM cats recorded maximal ventricular septal thickness of 9.0 ± 0.2 mm (controls, 5.0 ± 0.2 mm) and anterolateral LV free wall thickness of 9.0 ± 0.1 mm (controls, 6.0 ± 0.3 mm). Focal, endocardial fibrosis is common. In cats with dynamic LV outflow obstruction, a fibrous, mural endocardial plaque is evident at the basal septum in apposition to the anterior mitral valve leaflet. The anterior mitral valve leaflet also is thickened in these cases. Pulmonary edema is present in more than half of necropsied cases and pleural effusion is evident in about 20 per cent. Arterial thromboembolism occurs in a high percentage of necropsied cases. Atrial or ventricular ball thrombi occasionally are present. Aneurysmal thinning of the LV apex is common.

Histopathology (Figures 43-2 and 43-3)

The most characteristic histological features include disorganized myocyte architecture, small intramural coronary arterial arteriosclerosis, and increased matrix or replacement fibrosis. Myocytes may be hypertrophied and have large, rectangular, hyperchromic nuclei. In a series of 51 HCM cats, ventricular septal myofiber disorganization was recorded from 15 (30 per cent); septal disorganization comprising 5 per cent or more of relevant tissue sections was present in 14 (27 per cent); and extensive myocyte disarray (≥25 per cent) was present in seven (14 per cent).[21] Cellular disorganization was predominantly type I pattern, which involved small foci of adjacent cardiac muscle cells. Abnormally thick intramural coronary arteries, usually with reduced lumens, were noted in 74 per cent of cats, and were most prevalent in sections with moderate or severe fibrosis. Medial and intimal thickening was associated with increased connective tissue elements (and much less commonly, smooth muscle cells). Interstitial myocardial fibrous tissue or replacement fibrosis was present in 53 per cent of cats. Myocyte fiber disarray also can be observed in the right ventricle of some affected patients.

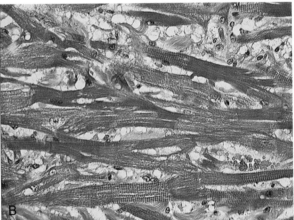

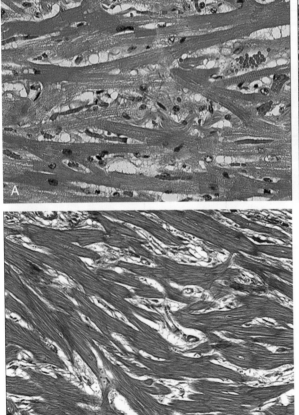

Figure 43-2 Cellular architecture from cats with hypertrophic cardiomyopathy illustrating myofiber disarray. **A** and **B,** Basal interventricular septum. **C,** RV wall. In **B** and **C,** interstitial fibrosis also is evident and marked. (H&E stain **[A]** and Masson trichrome **[B** and **C].** Magnification × 40.) (From Fox PR: Hypertrophic cardiomyopathy: clinical and pathologic correlates, *J Vet Cardiol* 5:39, 2003.)

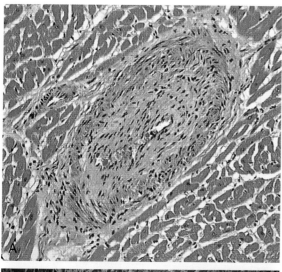

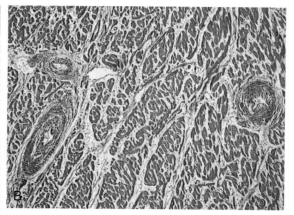

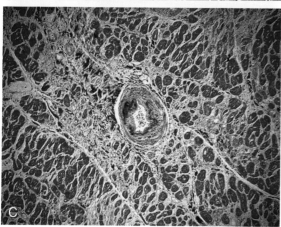

Figure 43-3 Arteriosclerosis (small vessel disease) of intramural coronary arteries in the left ventricle from three cats with hypertrophic cardiomyopathy. **A,** Abnormal intramural coronary artery with thickened wall and narrowed lumen caused by proliferation of smooth muscle and increased connective tissue elements. **B,** Arteriosclerosis with mild interstitial fibrosis. **C,** Region of replacement fibrosis surrounds arteriosclerotic arteriole. (From Fox PR: Hypertrophic cardiomyopathy: clinical and pathologic correlates, *J Vet Cardiol* 5:39, 2003.)

SECONDARY CAUSES OF LEFT VENTRICULAR HYPERTROPHY

Left ventricular hypertrophy can result from certain systemic and metabolic diseases, most notably hyperthyroidism[23] and systemic hypertension.[24-26] With thyrotoxicosis, symmetric LV hypertrophy can result, and untreated advanced cases may develop congestive heart failure.[27] Severe systemic hypertension can promote increased LV mass and hypertrophy, often with minimal left atrial enlargement. Congestive heart failure is rare. Hypersomatotropism (acromegaly) also has been associated with LV hypertrophy (see Chapter 29).[28]

DILATED CARDIOMYOPATHY

Dilated (congestive) cardiomyopathy (DCM) is an uncommon disorder whose etiology generally is unknown. Certain nutritional influences may impact myocardial structure and function. The most notable example is the association between feline taurine deficiency and DCM, and its reversibility with dietary taurine supplementation.[29] Although commercial diet reformulation largely eliminated this etiology by the early 1990s, taurine deficiency is still encountered occasionally. Idiopathic feline

myocardial failure is poorly characterized. A final, end-stage pathway for severe myocardial injury has been postulated for DCM,[30,31] which possibly may play a role in some affected cats.

Gross Pathology (Figure 43-4)

Pathological features are quite variable.[3,18,19,22] In classic taurine deficiency DCM, there is severe, generalized dilation of both ventricles and moderate biatrial dilation. Ventricular wall thinning, increased end-diastolic and end-systolic volumes, and biventricular heart failure commonly are present. Papillary muscles and ventricular trabeculae are flattened and atrophied. Heart weight of cats with DCM exceeds normal but is less than that of hearts with HCM. Mitral valve complex alterations occur in one-half of the cats and may include short and thick leaflets; short, stout, long, or thin chordae tendineae; and upward malposition of papillary muscles. Tricuspid valve complex alterations also may be observed, including adhesion of the septal leaflet to the ventricular septum, direct insertion of the lateral leaflet into papillary muscles, and short, stout, long, or thin chordae tendineae. These valvular complex changes often are similar to those observed in kittens with severe atrioventricular valvular dysplasia. Therefore it may be difficult in some younger animals to differentiate between primary myocardial disease and

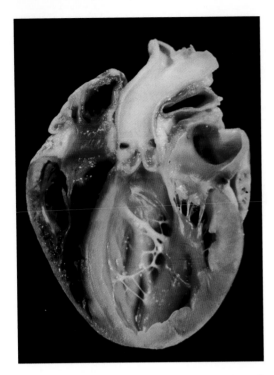

Figure 43-4 Gross heart specimen from a cat with idiopathic myocardial failure. Severe biventricular dilation is present. The ventricular septum is thin but the left ventricular free wall thickness is normal. Both atria are moderately large. Left ventricular papillary muscles are fused. (From Fox PR: Feline cardiomyopathies. In Fox PR, Sisson DD, Moïse NS, editors: *Textbook of canine and feline cardiology: principles and clinical practice,* ed 2, Philadelphia, 1999, Saunders, p 621.)

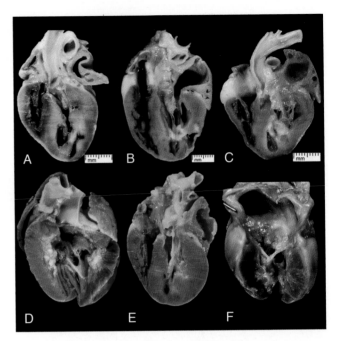

Figure 43-5 Hearts from cats with endomyocardial fibrosis illustrating extensive phenotypic variability of this disease. Gross hallmark features include marked left ventricular endocardial scar that bridges papillary muscles **(A),** ventricular septum and free wall **(B to D),** particularly involving the apex, septum, and/or free wall **(A to C).** When hypertrophy is present, it may involve the right and/or left ventricle and appear diffuse or focal. The left atrium generally is severely enlarged and right atrial enlargement also is prominent. (From Fox PR: Endomyocardial fibrosis and restrictive cardiomyopathy: pathologic and clinical features, *J Vet Cardiol* 6:25, 2004.)

end-stages of severe valvular dysplasia, or to determine the potential contribution of the latter condition. Endocardial fibrosis usually is mild and limited when present. Occasionally the myocardium will be diffusely fibrotic, or focal pale, gray areas representing myocardial infarction are observed. Lesions usually are greatest in the left ventricle. Arterial thromboembolism is common in cats, but does not occur in dogs.

Histopathology

There may be some endocardial fibroelastic thickening. Inflammatory reaction is absent or scanty. Myocardial cells appear thinner than normal and are separated by edematous, extracellular ground substances or connective tissue. Myocytolysis is common. Myocardial fibrosis ranges from mild and focal to extensive and diffuse.

RESTRICTIVE AND INFILTRATIVE CARDIOMYOPATHIES

Restrictive cardiomyopathy (RCM) is the most poorly characterized feline myocardial disorder.[3,18,22,32,33] Much has been extrapolated from human literature. The hallmark of RCM is abnormal diastolic function resulting from ventricular wall stiffness that impedes diastolic filling. A number of diseases have been associated with

RCM in human beings, including myocardial fibrosis, endomyocardial scarring, and infiltration.[34] These changes are encountered variably in cats. Two-dimensional and Doppler echocardiography reveal wide phenotypic heterogeneity, as well as variability in indices of diastolic function. Consequently the term *RCM* has become a loosely applied term for many forms of myocardial disease that have uncertain morphologies. At least two different morphological types of feline myocardial disease appear to qualify under the classification of RCM. One is characterized by left ventricular endomyocardial fibrosis and contains some features similar to those described in human patients with Löfflers's endocarditis and endomyocardial fibrosis. The other type is more obscure and represents a heterogeneous array of idiopathic, noninfiltrative RCM.

Gross Pathology (Figures 43-5 and 43-6)

In cats with endomyocardial fibrosis, the heart weight is greater than normal because of moderate LV hypertrophy. Dilation and hypertrophy of the right atrium (RA) and right ventricle (RV) are common. Extreme biatrial enlargement often occurs. The LA usually is most severely affected and may be hypertrophied. Pronounced, diffuse LV endocardial thickening with a whitish-gray, opaque, fibrous plaquelike scar is a pathological hallmark. This may occur in the left ventricular outflow and inflow

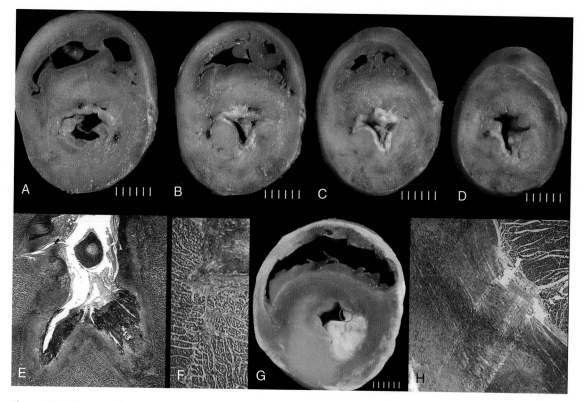

Figure 43-6 Patterns of endomyocardial fibrosis illustrated in cross-sectional view. **A** to **D,** Sequential sections from the mitral valve (**A**) to papillary muscle (**D**) taken at approximately 5 mm intervals. Diffuse, left ventricular endocardial scar is present in all sections. **E,** Panoramic left ventricular cross-sectional view at the papillary muscle level showing prominent circumferential endocardial scar (blue). Thrombus also is present. (Masson trichrome.) **F,** Replacement fibrosis is present in subendocardial regions and interstitial fibrosis is evident throughout mid-mural left ventricular myocardium. (Magnification × 200. Masson trichrome.) **G,** Cardiac section from another cat with severe endomyocardial fibrosis that partially obliterated the apical to mid-left ventricular cavity. Circle defines area of interest in **H. H,** Histological section demonstrating severe endocardial scar. (Magnification × 100. Masson trichrome.) Scales are in millimeters. (From Fox PR: Endomyocardial fibrosis and restrictive cardiomyopathy: pathologic and clinical features, *J Vet Cardiol* 6:25, 2004.)

tracts, over the papillary muscles, chordae tendineae, and left ventricular free wall. In cases in which endocardial scarring is severe, fibrous adhesions between papillary muscles and myocardium, distortion and fusion of chordae tendineae, mitral leaflets, and occasionally obliteration of the LV cavity, may occur. Mural, left atrial, or distal aortic thromboembolism is common.[32] In contrast, cats with idiopathic, noninfiltrative myocardial disease have more heterogeneous features and undoubtedly represent more than one disease process. It is characterized grossly by a relatively normal LV; the LA and often RA are moderately to severely enlarged in the absence of conditions causing volume overload or atrioventricular valve stenosis. The RV may become enlarged, depending on the presence and degree of pulmonary hypertension. There may be regional endocardial fibrosis, but not diffuse or severe endocardial scarring. Focal myocardial wall thinning associated with infarction can be present, and left ventricular apical aneurysmal thinning is common. Mural thrombosis may be present in some patients.[18]

Histopathology

With endomyocardial fibrosis (see Figure 43-6), extreme endocardial thickening results from hyaline, fibrous, and granulation tissue.[32,33] The surface is covered by a layer of hyaline tissue and collagenous fibers, occasionally displaying chondroid metaplasia. Underneath is loose, cellular, fibrous tissue. Adjacent to the myocardium is granulation tissue made up of histiocytes, lymphocytes, and plasma cells. Hypertrophy of myocytes and interstitial fibroplasia are common. Myocytolysis and arteriosclerosis in left ventricular free wall and ventricular septal intramural coronary arteries may accompany severe endomyocardial fibrosis in advanced cases. A spectrum of changes has been observed with idiopathic, noninfiltrative RCM. Myocytes may be hypertrophied or thin with varying degrees of necrosis. Myocardial fibrosis often is diffuse and may be focally or regionally severe. Endocardial fibrosis may be patchy but generally is relatively mild.

ARRHYTHMOGENIC RIGHT VENTRICULAR CARDIOMYOPATHY/DYSPLASIA

Arrhythmogenic right ventricular cardiomyopathy/dysplasia (ARVC) has been detected most commonly in domestic shorthair and Birman cats, although it occurs

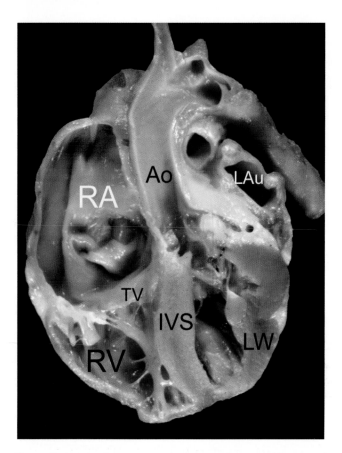

Figure 43-7 Heart from a cat with ARVC with severe dilatation of the right atrium (RA) and right ventricle (RV). *IVS,* Interventricular septum; *LW,* left ventricular free wall; *TV,* tricuspid valve; *Ao,* ascending aorta; *LAu,* left auricle. (From Fox PR: Arrhythmogenic right ventricular cardiomyopathy. In August JR, editor: *Consultations in feline internal medicine,* vol 5, St. Louis, 2006, Saunders, p 319.)

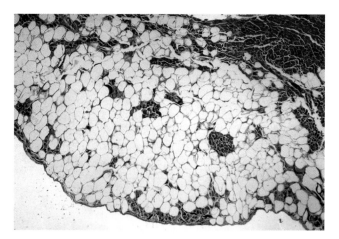

Figure 43-8 Fibrofatty variant of ARVC in a cat with ventricular tachycardia. Fatty replacement of the right ventricular wall is associated with residual myocytes embedded within or aborted by adipose cells. (Heidenhain trichrome stain.) (From Fox PR: Arrhythmogenic right ventricular cardiomyopathy. In August JR, editor: *Consultations in feline internal medicine,* vol 5, St. Louis, 2006, Saunders, p 319.)

in other breeds of domestic cats as well. Age at first detection ranges from 1 to 20 years old. There has been no documented gender predisposition.

Gross Pathology (Figure 43-7)

Typical findings include moderate-to-severe RV dilatation; RV wall thinning (diffuse or segmental); flattened appearance of RV wall trabeculae; and prominent RV septoparietal bands in the RV apex. Aneurysms in apical, subtricuspid, and infundibular regions of the RV wall may be small or extensive, and appear translucent. Severe right atrial cavity dilation usually is present and segments of the right atrial wall are markedly thinned. Mural thrombosis occasionally is observed in the RV.[19,35-37]

Histopathology (Figure 43-8)

Partial or virtually complete replacement of the RV free wall by fatty (25 per cent of cases) or fibro-fatty (75 per cent of cases) tissue is the hallmark histopathological feature.[8] The fibro-fatty pattern consists of focal or diffuse RV myocardial atrophy associated with adipose tissue and replacement-type fibrosis. The fatty pattern within the RV wall and trabeculae is characterized by multifocal or diffuse areas of adipose cell infiltration with only scant

interstitial fibrosis. Islands of myocytes often are surrounded by fat or fibro-fatty tissue. In both forms, residual surviving myocytes usually are scattered within the areas of fibrosis or fat, and fibro-fatty replacement usually extends from epicardium toward the endocardium. Focal or multifocal RV myocarditis is most prevalent in ARVC cats with the fibro-fatty pattern. It consists mostly of T lymphocytes associated with myocyte cell death and mild-to-severe fibrous tissue deposition. Similar findings also may be present in left and right atrial walls, as well as LV free wall and ventricular septum. Fatty infiltration occasionally is present in the LV free wall, but has not been described in the ventricular septum. Abnormal intramural small vessels with thickened walls (due primarily to medial hypertrophy) are uncommon. Apoptotic myocytes have been identified by terminal deoxynucleotidyl transferase dUTP nick end labeling (TUNEL) histochemical investigation in 75 per cent of affected cats.[19,35-37]

ABNORMAL, EXCESSIVE LEFT VENTRICULAR MODERATOR BANDS

Moderator bands (trabeculae septomarginalis) normally are present in the feline RV[38] and both canine ventricles. In cats abnormal diffuse networks of left ventricular moderator bands have been reported in association with congestive heart failure, ventricular dilation, and hypertrophy, without breed or gender predisposition.[39,40] Abnormal moderator band networks also have been identified in kittens as young as 1 day of age, suggesting a congenital origin. A causal relationship between these findings and cardiac impairment has not been established.

Gross Pathology (Figure 43-9)

Severely affected hearts are small with irregularly shaped contours, rounded apices, and occasionally, indentation

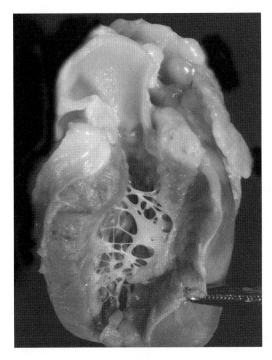

Figure 43-9 Heart from an adult cat who died of congestive heart failure. This gross specimen is transected through the left ventricular outflow tract and body of the left ventricle. There is an abnormal network of excessive and thickened moderator bands that bridge the ventricular septum and left ventricular free wall. The left ventricle was mildly hypertrophied. (From Fox PR: Feline cardiomyopathies. In Fox PR, Sisson DD, Moïse NS, editors: *Textbook of canine and feline cardiology: principles and clinical practice,* ed 2, Philadelphia, 1999, Saunders, p 621.)

of the mid-left ventricular epicardial surface. Heart weight is significantly lower than for hypertrophic, dilated, or restrictive cardiomyopathic hearts, but not significantly less than that of clinically normal hearts. The LV cavity may be narrowed irregularly in some affected hearts when excessive abnormal moderator band networks connect papillary muscles, LV free wall, or both to the ventricular septum.

Histopathology

The moderator bands consist of central Purkinje fibers and dense, parallel collagenous fibers covered by endothelium. There is loose, fibrous connective tissue between the endothelium and the collagenous fibers. Some moderator bands are composed of Purkinje fibers surrounded by loose fibrous connective tissue, adipose tissue, lymphocytes, and blood vessels, and are covered by endothelium.

THROMBOEMBOLIC DISEASE

Thrombus refers to clot formation (platelets, fibrin, coagulation factors, and cellular components) in the heart or vessels. An embolus results from migration of all or part of a clot or other material (e.g., tumor fragment, air, fat, bacteria, parasites, or foreign body). Thrombosis may

result from tissue (endothelial) injury, circulatory stasis or turbulence, or hypercoagulable state (see Chapters 37 and 58 in the fifth volume of this series). Arterial thromboembolism is a well-recognized complication of feline cardiomyopathies, and has been reported in up to 48 per cent of myopathic cats at necropsy. Distal aortic saddle emboli occur in more than 90 per cent of affected cats. Brachial, renal, and mesenteric arteries represent other recognized sites for emboli. Mural thrombi occasionally are present in the left atrium or ventricle.[3,18] Ischemic neuromyopathy results when distal arterial occlusion and vasoactive chemicals reduce collateral circulation.[41]

MISCELLANEOUS CARDIOVASCULAR DISEASES AND CONDITIONS

MYOCARDIAL INFARCTION

In cats myocardial infarction is observed frequently at necropsy examination associated with cardiomyopathies.[18,42-44] Cases of idiopathic myocardial failure, restrictive cardiomyopathy, and unclassified myocardial diseases have been observed with regions of infarcted LV posterior wall at the papillary muscle level. Less commonly, the ventricular septum or LV apex can be affected.

Gross Pathology

Infarction appears grossly as focal, dark gray, or pale myocardium. Atherosclerosis is a rare finding; however, affected animals may have yellow-white, dilated, and tortuous coronary arteries with adjacent irregular, dull foci of infarcted myocardium. Some patients with septicemia or vegetative endocarditis and coronary vasculitis will have coronary thromboembolism and hemorrhagic necrosis of adjacent myocardium.

Histopathology

In general, infarcted myocardium reveals myocyte streaking and waviness; sarcoplasmic coagulation, vacuolization, and fragmentation; contraction bands; myocytolysis; and fragmentation. There is excessive extracellular ground substance and occasional extravasation of erythrocytes separating affected myocytes. Atherosclerotic, thromboembolic, amyloid, or vasculitic coronary arteries usually are enclosed in adjacent necrotic myocardium. Contraction bands, fragmentation, and vacuolization of sarcoplasm, with or without extravasation of erythrocytes in and around the affected myocytes, are observed in circular myocardial necrosis with minimal coronary artery changes. In cases of severe feline hypertrophic cardiomyopathy, focal interstitial or massive myocardial fibrosis and acute vacuolar and/or coagulative necrosis may occur. Abnormal coronary arteries characterized by thickened walls and decreased luminal size occur in about one-third of affected hearts.

REFERENCES

1. Sonderegger-Iseli K, Burger S, Muntwyler J, et al: Diagnostic errors in three medical eras: a necropsy study, *Lancet* 355:2027, 2000.

2. Pelletier Jr LL, Klutzow F, Lancaster H: The autopsy: its role in the evaluation of patient care, *J Gen Intern Med* 4:300, 1989.

3. Liu SK, Fox PR: Cardiovascular pathology. In Fox PR, Sisson DD, Moïse NS, editors: *Textbook of canine and feline cardiology: principles and clinical practice*, ed 2, Philadelphia, 1999, Saunders, p 817.

4. Bishop S: Necropsy techniques for the heart and great vessels. In Fox PR, Sisson DD, Moïse NS, editors: *Textbook of canine and feline cardiology: principles and clinical practice*, ed 2, Philadelphia, 1999, Saunders, p 845.

5. Opie LH: *Heart physiology: from cell to circulation*, Philadelphia, 2004, Lippincott Williams & Wilkins.

6. Katz AM: The cardiomyopathy of overload: an unnatural growth response in the hypertrophied heart, *Ann Intern Med* 121:363, 1994.

7. Maron BJ, Towbin JA, Thiene G, et al: American Heart Association; Council on Clinical Cardiology, Heart Failure and Transplantation Committee; Quality of Care and Outcomes Research and Functional Genomics and Translational Biology Interdisciplinary Working Groups; Council on Epidemiology and Prevention, *Circulation* 113:1807, 2006.

8. Grossman W, Jones D, McLaurin LP: Wall stress and patterns of hypertrophy in the human left ventricle, *J Clin Invest* 56:56, 1975.

9. Ross J Jr: Adaptations of the left ventricle to chronic volume overload, *Circ Res* 35(Suppl 2):64, 1974.

10. Jennings RB, Ganote CE: Structural changes in myocardium during acute ischemia, *Circ Res* 35(Suppl 3):156, 1974.

11. Narula J, Haider N, Virmani R, et al: Apoptosis in myocytes in end-stage heart failure, *N Engl J Med* 335:1182, 1996.

12. Burlew BS, Weber KT: Connective tissue and the heart. Functional significance and regulatory mechanisms, *Cardiol Clin* 18:435, 2000.

13. Caulfield JB, Borg TK: The collagen network of the heart, *Lab Invest* 40:364, 1979.

14. Robinson TF: Structural arrangement of myocytes and fibrillar connective tissue in heart muscle. In Robinson TF, Kinne RKH, editors: *Cardiac myocyte-connective tissue interactions in health and disease, issues biomed*, vol 13, Basel, 1990, Karger, p 53.

15. Factor SM: Pathologic alterations of myocyte-connective tissue interactions in cardiovascular disease. In Robinson TF, Kinne RKH, editors: *Cardiac myocyte-connective tissue interactions in health and disease, issues biomed*, vol 13, Basel, 1990, Karger, p 130.

16. Wilkins RJ: Clinical pathology of feline cardiac disease, *Vet Clin North Am Small Anim Pract* 7:285, 1977.

17. Fossum TW, Forrester SD, Swenson CL, et al: Chylothorax in cats: 37 cases (1969-1989), *J Am Vet Med Assoc* 198:672, 1991.

17a. Fox PR, Liu SK, Maron BJ: Echocardiographic assessment of spontaneously occurring feline hypertrophic cardiomyopathy. An animal model of human disease, *Circulation* 92:2645, 1995.

18. Fox PR: Spontaneous animal models. In Marcus FI, Nava A, Thiene G, editors: *Arrhythmogenic RV cardiomyopathy/dysplasia recent advances*, 2007, Springer-Verlag Italia, p 69.

19. Fox PR: Feline cardiomyopathies. In Fox PR, Sisson DD, Moïse NS, editors: *Textbook of canine and feline cardiology: principles and clinical practice*, ed 2, Philadelphia, 1999, Saunders, p 621.

20. Fox PR: Hypertrophic cardiomyopathy. Clinical and pathologic correlates, *J Vet Cardiol* 5:39, 2003.

21. Liu SK, Roberts WC, Maron BJ: Comparison of morphologic findings in spontaneously occurring hypertrophic cardiomyopathy in humans, cats and dogs, *Am J Cardiol* 72:944, 1993.

22. Liu SK: Pathology of feline heart disease, *Vet Clin North Am Small Anim Pract* 7:322, 1977.

23. Liu SK, Peterson ME, Fox PR: Hypertrophic cardiomyopathy and hyperthyroidism in the cat, *J Am Vet Med Assoc* 185:52, 1984.

24. Littman MP: Spontaneous systemic hypertension in 24 cats, *J Vet Intern Med* 8:79, 1994.

25. Lesser M, Fox PR, Bond BR: Assessment of hypertension in 40 cats with left ventricular hypertrophy by Doppler-shift sphygmomanometry, *J Small Anim Pract* 33:55, 1992.

26. Carlos Sampedrano C, Chetboul V, Gouni V, et al: Systolic and diastolic myocardial dysfunction in cats with hypertrophic cardiomyopathy or systemic hypertension, *J Vet Intern Med* 20:1106, 2006.

27. Fox PR, Peterson ME, Broussard JD: Electrocardiographic and radiographic changes in cats with hyperthyroidism: comparison of populations evaluated during 1992-1993 vs. 1979-1982, *J Am Anim Hosp Assoc* 35:27, 1999.

28. Kittleson MD, Pion PD, DeLellis LA, et al: Increased serum growth hormone concentration in feline hypertrophic cardiomyopathy, *J Vet Intern Med* 6:320, 1992.

29. Pion PD, Kittleson MD, Rogers QR, et al: Myocardial failure in cats associated with low plasma taurine: a reversible cardiomyopathy, *Science* 237:764, 1987.

30. Baty CJ, Malarkey DE, Atkins CE, et al: Natural history of hypertrophic cardiomyopathy and aortic thromboembolism in a family of domestic shorthair cats, *J Vet Intern Med* 15:595, 2001.

31. Cesta MF, Baty CJ, Keene BW, et al: Pathology of end-stage remodeling in a family of cats with hypertrophic cardiomyopathy, *Vet Pathol* 42:458, 2005.

32. Fox PR: Endomyocardial fibrosis and restrictive cardiomyopathy: pathologic and clinical features, *J Vet Cardiol* 6:25, 2004.

33. Stalis IH, Bossbaly MJ, Van Winkle TJ: Feline endomyocarditis and left ventricular endocardial fibrosis, *Vet Pathol* 32:122, 1995.

34. Kushwaha SS, Fallon JT, Furster V: Medical progress: restrictive cardiomyopathy, *N Engl J Med* 336:267, 1997.

35. Fox PR, Maron BJ, Liu SK, et al: Spontaneously occurring arrhythmogenic right ventricular cardiomyopathy in the domestic cat: a new animal model similar to the human disease, *Circulation* 102:1863, 2000.

36. Fox PR: Right ventricular cardiomyopathy in cats. In Bonagura JD, Twedt DC, editors: *Kirk's current veterinary therapy XIV*, St. Louis, 2009, Saunders, p 815.

37. Fox PR: Arrhythmogenic right ventricular cardiomyopathy. In August JR, editor: *Consultations in feline internal medicine*, vol 5, St. Louis, 2006, Saunders, p 319.

38. Truex RC, Warshow LJ: The incidence and size of the moderator band in man and in mammals, *Anat Rec* 82:361, 1941.

39. Liu S, Fox PR, Tilley LP: Excessive moderator bands in the left ventricle of 21 cats, *J Am Vet Med Assoc* 180:1215, 1982.

40. Wray JD, Gajanayake I, Smith SH: Congestive heart failure associated with a large transverse left ventricular moderator band in a cat, *J Feline Med Surg* 9:56, 2007.

41. Griffiths I, Duncan ID: Ischaemic neuromyopathy in cats, *Vet Rec* 104:518, 1979.

42. Liu SK, Hsu FS, Lee RCT: *An atlas of cardiovascular pathology*, Taiwan, Republic of China, 1989, Pig Research Institute.

43. Liu SK: Myocardial infarction in animals. *Proceedings of the 2nd International Symposium on Pig Models for Biomedical Research*, Miaoli, Taiwan, Republic of China, 1992, Pig Research Institute.

44. Liu SK, Fox PR: Myocardial ischemia and infarction. In Kirk RW, Bonagura JD, editors: *Kirk's current veterinary therapy XI*, Philadelphia, 1992, Saunders, p 791.

44 Asthma

Philip Padrid

Asthma is a disorder of the lower airways causing airflow limitations that may resolve spontaneously or in response to medical treatment. Interestingly, asthma defined in this way is a rare disorder in the animal kingdom and likely occurs only in the feline and human species. "Airflow limitation" generally is the result of some combination of airway inflammation, accumulated airway mucus, and airway smooth muscle contraction. The clinical signs of asthma can be dramatic, including acute wheeze and respiratory distress. Sometimes, however, the only sign of asthma-induced airflow limitation is a daily cough. In human patients, this is referred to as "cough-variant" asthma.

Asthma may be considered a chronic bronchial disease in cats, with clinical signs similar to chronic bronchitis. Chronic bronchitis is defined as an inflammatory disorder of the lower airways that causes a daily cough, for which other causes of cough (including heartworm disease, pneumonia, lungworms, and neoplasia) have been excluded. In practice, a feline patient with a chronic cough who is otherwise healthy may suffer from one of a number of disorders, including bronchitis or asthma. The distinction between these latter two diseases is not made easily.

The definitive diagnosis of human asthma usually is based on specific pulmonary function studies that require patient cooperation. Clearly, this is not available for our patients seen in general practice. Because bronchitis and asthma both can cause a daily cough as the only clinical

sign, there are many times when it is not possible to distinguish bronchitis from asthma in the feline patient. Accordingly, the diagnosis, prognosis, and treatment options for both diseases overlap with great frequency. The purposes of this chapter are to (1) review our current understanding of the pathophysiology of asthma in cats, (2) review common clinical signs and diagnostic tests, (3) suggest rational and novel approaches for treating cats with this sometimes debilitating and life-threatening airway disorder, and (4) discuss reasonable expectations for long-term care.

PATHOPHYSIOLOGY

The potential causes of bronchitis and asthma are numerous; however, the airways are capable of responding to noxious stimuli in a limited number of ways. Airway epithelium may hypertrophy, undergo metaplastic change, erode, or ulcerate. Airway goblet cells and submucosal glands may hypertrophy and produce excessive amounts of viscid mucus. Bronchial mucosa and submucosa usually are infiltrated with variable numbers and types of inflammatory cells and may become edematous. Bronchial smooth muscle may remain unaffected, become hypertrophied, or spasm. In almost all cases, the unifying and underlying problem is chronic inflammation; however, the exact cause remains the subject of intense study without a current resolution.

The resulting clinical signs of cough, wheeze, and lethargy are due to limitation of airflow from excessive mucus secretions, airway edema, and airway narrowing from cellular infiltrates. Cats with asthma additionally may suffer acute airway narrowing from airway smooth muscle constriction. The diameter of an airway has a profound effect on the amount of air that can travel through that airway and on the speed with which that air travels. The Bernoulli principle and the Poiseuille-Hagen formula relate airflow, airspeed, and airway caliber through the following mathematical formulas:

$$p/pg + u^2/ug + x$$
$$= H \text{ (pressure decreases as velocity increases)}$$

$$F = DP\, p\, r^4/8\, h\, l \text{ (flow is directly proportional to radius}^4\text{)}$$

From these basic calculations, we can take away two related and clinically significant points. First, reduced airway diameter results in increased airflow velocity. This in turn causes a drop in airway pressure. Second, a 50 per cent reduction in the luminal size of an airway results in a sixteenfold reduction in the volume of air that flows across that airway. Thus small changes in airway diameter result in enormous changes in airflow or the amount of air that can pass through that airway. Importantly then, therapy that results in relatively small increases in airway size may cause a dramatic improvement in clinical signs.

Cough also may result from stimulation of mechanoreceptors located in inflamed and contracted airway smooth muscle. Inappropriate airway smooth muscle contraction in turn seems linked fundamentally to inflammation. Although many inflammatory cell types are found within asthmatic airways of human beings and cats, eosinophils appear to be primary effector cells in the development of asthmatic airway pathophysiology in both species. Highly charged cationic proteins within eosinophil granules are released into airways and cause epithelial disruption and sloughing. Additionally, these granular proteins can make airway smooth muscle more "twitchy" and prone to contraction after exposure to low levels of stimulation (airway hyperreactivity).

EOSINOPHIL AND T-LYMPHOCYTE INTERACTIONS

The pathogenesis of asthmatic airway hyperreactivity clearly is multifactorial. Numerous investigations suggest that the interaction between T lymphocytes and eosinophils within airways may play an important role in the generation of airway inflammation and airway hyperreactivity in human asthma.[1-3] Increased numbers of eosinophils and activated T lymphocytes are found in bronchoalveolar lavage specimens and bronchial mucosa of patients with asthma. The presence of these cells is correlated with disease severity. Activated T cells are recruited into the airways of asthmatic individuals when they are exposed to aeroallergens. These CD4-positive lymphocytes (among other cells) secrete interleukin-5 (IL-5) to promote eosinophilopoiesis, survival, activation, and recruitment into airways. A T helper 2–driven cytokine profile has been demonstrated in antigen-induced asthma models in the feline species.[4]

STUDIES IN NATURALLY OCCURRING DISEASE

Although coughing and wheezing cats have been identified by owners and veterinarians for almost a century, only in the last 15 years have we begun to study the disorder in earnest. Dye and associates identified pulmonary function abnormalities in cats with signs of chronic lower airway inflammation.[5] Some of these cats had increased pulmonary resistance that resolved after treatment with terbutaline, a β_2-agonist, indicating the presence of reversible bronchoconstriction in these patients. Additionally, some of these cats experience dramatic bronchoconstriction after exposure to low levels of methacholine, a drug with minimal effects on pulmonary function when used in equivalent doses in nonasthmatic cats. This was the first demonstration of spontaneous, naturally occurring airway hyperreactivity and reversible bronchoconstriction in a nonhuman species. Additionally, histological changes in airways from asthmatic cats include epithelial erosion, goblet cell and submucosal gland hyperplasia and hypertrophy, and an increased mass of smooth muscle, which are features of human asthmatic airways. Additional reviews have demonstrated the variation in clinical findings, radiographic patterns, and responses to therapy in cats with bronchial disease.[6,7] This likely is due to differences in staging these disorders, and the fact that other disorders, including pulmonary fibrosis and heartworm infection, can mimic the signs of bronchial disease in cats.[8,9]

EXPERIMENTALLY INDUCED FELINE ASTHMA

Studies of cats with naturally occurring asthma are critical to our understanding and formulation of rational treatment strategies. However, diagnostic studies required for definitive diagnosis use specialized equipment and often require an anesthetized patient. This has limited our ability to evaluate cats with spontaneous disease; our understanding of the pathogenesis and natural course of asthma in cats has been hampered as a result. Recent technological advances are allowing us now to study pulmonary function in awake, unsedated, or anesthetized cats and should yield new insights into the mechanisms of disease.

Experimental models of feline asthma have been developed to better understand the immunological mechanisms operative in the pathogenesis and perturbation of asthma and as a means to determine responses to therapy objectively. The first model of feline asthma involved antigen sensitization and chronic aerosol challenge with *Ascaris suum* as an antigen. These cats developed persistent airway eosinophilia and hyperresponsiveness to nebulized acetylcholine, with typical morphological changes observed in spontaneous bronchial disease of cats. These antigen-sensitized cats had elevated serum levels of soluble receptor for IL-2 found within 24 hours of antigen challenge and a decrease in the CD4+:CD8+ peripheral blood T-cell ratio compared to control values. These findings suggest T-cell activation in asthmatic cats similar to the findings in human beings with the disease.[10] In this experimental model, we found that treatment with cyclosporine A (CsA) dramatically inhibited the pathological changes in airway structure and function seen in cats not treated with CsA.[11] However, these findings should not be interpreted to mean that cyclosporine should be used to treat naturally occurring asthma in cats (see section on Treatment). The author has shown that serotonin is a primary mediator in feline mast cells that contribute to airway smooth muscle contraction in vitro.[12] This mediator is absent in human, equine, and canine airways. During an acute asthmatic attack, inhaled antigens within airways promote mast-cell degranulation acutely with release of preformed serotonin. These mediators cause sudden contraction of airway smooth muscle. Interestingly, it has long been assumed that histamine released from feline mast cells caused acute bronchoconstriction. This assumption has been challenged recently by the finding that histamine nebulized into cat airways has an unpredictable effect from one cat to another. Specifically, histamine may have no effect, it may cause bronchoconstriction, or it may actually dilate feline airways.

Norris Reinero et al developed an experimental model in which cats were sensitized and challenged chronically with either Bermuda grass allergen (BGA) or house dust mite to mimic well-recognized antigenic triggers of human asthma. These cats produce allergen-specific immunoglobin E (IgE), allergen-specific serum and bronchoalveolar lavage fluid (BALF) IgG and IgA, airway hyperreactivity, airway eosinophilia, an acute T helper 2 cytokine profile in peripheral blood mononuclear cells and BALF cells, and histological evidence of airway remodeling.[4] This model has been particularly helpful in evaluating specific immunomodulating treatment strategies. For example, cats sensitized and challenged with BGA to develop the asthmatic phenotype were treated with rush immunotherapy (parenteral high doses of BGA). These cats had significantly reduced eosinophil counts.[13] More recently, Reinero et al used CpG motifs (microbial oligodeoxynucleotide products that modulate activity in human and murine lymphocytes) in cats with BGA-induced airway inflammation and hyperreactivity to show that this approach dampened the eosinophilic response normally seen in these antigen-sensitized and challenged cats; however, the hyperactivity within airways was not affected.[14]

CLINICAL FINDINGS IN FELINE ASTHMA

INCIDENCE AND PREVALENCE

Currently, there are no reliable data regarding the incidence and prevalence of asthma in cats. The prevalence of lower airway disease in the general adult cat population is estimated to be approximately 1 per cent; prevalence in the Siamese breed may be 5 per cent or greater.[15] In 2000, a website (http://www.fritzthebrave.com) was developed to draw attention to the diagnosis and treatment of feline asthma. One result of this website was the generation of a "list-serve" with greater than 500

members, each of whom is the owner of one or more cats with asthma. A poll of these members revealed that more than 15 per cent of the owners represented by this relatively random sample had Siamese cats (Kathryn Hopper, personal communication).

CLINICAL SIGNS

Clinical signs are variable. Asthmatic cats may cough, wheeze, and struggle to breathe on a daily basis. In mild cases, clinical signs may be limited to occasional and brief coughing. Some cats with asthma may be asymptomatic between occasional episodes of acute airway obstruction. Severely affected cats may have a persistent daily cough and experience many episodes of life-threatening acute bronchoconstriction.

As outlined previously, a common problem for the practitioner is to distinguish between chronic bronchitis and asthma as the cause of a chronic cough in cats. Although these two disorders frequently are grouped together under the title of chronic bronchial disease or lower airway disease, the two disorders may require different therapeutic approaches and often have different prognoses. All cats with chronic bronchitis, by definition, have daily cough. Some cats with asthma may be asymptomatic between occasional episodes of acute airway obstruction. Other asthmatic cats may cough occasionally and demonstrate frequent tachypnea. Importantly, asthmatic cats but not bronchitic cats may benefit from bronchodilator treatment.

DIAGNOSIS

Reversible bronchoconstriction is one of the defining features of asthma and can be used to distinguish asthma from chronic bronchitis when the two diagnoses are not clearly separable by clinical means. However, demonstration of reversible bronchoconstriction via pulmonary function studies generally requires patient cooperation, and the equipment and expertise needed to perform these kinds of tests are not available in general veterinary practice. However, one maneuver can point the practitioner toward a diagnosis of asthma. If a patient is wheezing during the physical examination, the author will administer terbutaline by inhalation or parenterally (0.01 mg/kg IM) and reevaluate the patient in 5 to 10 minutes. Resolution of the wheezing implies bronchoconstriction that was reversible and the result of the bronchodilating effects of the medication. With the exception of this one maneuver, there are no specific practical tests that can be used in general practice for definitive diagnosis of asthma in cats. Therefore we generally rely on the following clinical criteria.

HISTORY

Cats with asthma display one or more of these clinical signs: cough, acute wheeze, tachypnea, or respiratory distress, including labored, open-mouth breathing. These signs usually are relieved quickly with some combination

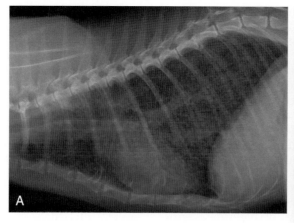

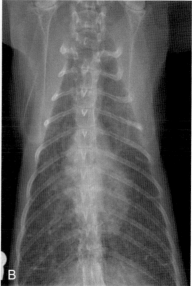

Figure 44-1 Lateral **(A)** and ventrodorsal **(B)** radiographs from a symptomatic asthmatic cat. Notice the prominent diffuse peribronchial pulmonary infiltrate. The size and contour of the cardiac silhouette are normal. The pulmonary vasculature is seen clearly and is normal in size.

of oxygen, bronchodilators, and corticosteroids. In some cases of asthma, the only clinical problem may be daily or intermittent chronic cough. *There are no other common diseases in cats that cause acute reversible wheeze or cough that comes and goes for long periods of time without worsening in severity or frequency.*

PHYSICAL EXAMINATION

There are no consistent physical examination findings on which to base a diagnosis of asthma. In fact, cats with asthma may have a normal physical examination at rest. Conversely, respiratory distress primarily during expiration is the hallmark of these disorders in cats. Adventitious sounds, including crackles, often are heard. Wheezes are only common in advanced disease or during acute worsening of signs.

FECAL EXAMINATION

Aelurostrongylus abstrusus or *Eucoleus aerophila* infections can cause cough and difficulty breathing in feline patients. In endemic areas, these lung parasites should be excluded by appropriate fecal testing, including flotation and Baermann examination.

THORACIC RADIOGRAPHS

Radiographs of the thorax of cats with asthma commonly demonstrate bronchial wall thickening, usually described as "doughnuts" and "tramlines" (Figure 44-1). Air trapping may be evidenced by hyperinflated airways. This is seen most prominently on the lateral view and can be appreciated by recognizing the position of the diaphragmatic crus at approximately the level of L1-L2.

In the author's experience, approximately 15 per cent of thoracic radiographs of cats with bronchial disease

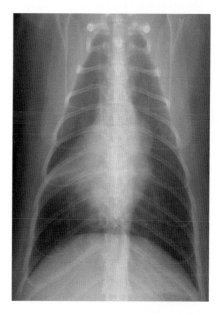

Figure 44-2 Dorsoventral radiograph from a cat with chronic asthma. Notice the mild mixed bronchial interstitial infiltrate. Additionally, there is apparent consolidation of the right middle lung lobe. This finding may be present in as many as 15 per cent of cats with chronic disease.

have increased density within the right middle lung lobe associated with a mediastinal shift to the right. This is evidence of atelectasis. It usually is easier to see this pattern on a dorsoventral or ventrodorsal exposure because the right middle lung lobe silhouettes with the cardiac silhouette on the lateral view (Figure 44-2). Atelectasis occurs most commonly in the right middle lung lobe because of mucus accumulation within the bronchus, and this airway is involved most frequently because it is the only airway that has a dorsal/ventral orientation within the bronchial tree and therefore subject to the effects of gravity. In more extreme cases, the clinician may appreciate fluffy, ill-defined heavy infiltrates in multiple lung lobes. The cause of these changes in cats with lower airway disease may be many small areas of atelectasis in several lung lobes resulting from multiple diffuse small mucus plugs. This presents a diagnostic challenge because this radiographic change is consistent with a number of disorders, including neoplasia and diffuse interstitial pneumonitis. Importantly, routine survey thoracic radiographs may be normal and should not cause the practitioner to abandon the diagnosis of asthma.

RESPONSE TO THERAPY AS A DIAGNOSTIC MEASURE

Cats with asthma may stop coughing or wheezing within 10 minutes after administration of a bronchodilator. The great majority of cats with asthma respond to high-dose corticosteroid therapy within 5 to 7 days, and a patient with a diagnosis of asthma who responds poorly should be reevaluated and the diagnosis revisited.

BRONCHOSCOPY

The author emphasizes that bronchoscopy is rarely required to make an accurate diagnosis of asthma in feline patients. Bronchoscopy in healthy cats is not a trivial undertaking. In cats with cough and respiratory compromise, bronchoscopy may be a life-threatening procedure[16] and only should be performed by persons adequately and formally trained in the technique (see Chapter 45). Instead, the previously described historical and physical examination findings and results of fecal and heartworm testing and thoracic radiography are sufficient to make a presumptive diagnosis. Definitive diagnosis usually can be made in these patients by a strongly positive response to therapy. In fact, in the author's experience, the primary indication for bronchoscopy in these patients occurs when there is not an otherwise predictable cessation or minimization of clinical signs after 6 to 7 days of aggressive corticosteroid treatment. Some clinicians prefer to obtain airway washings and culture before initiation of long-term respiratory therapy, although these points made here and in the next section should be considered before initiating bronchoscopy and interpreting the cytological and culture results.

TRACHEOBRONCHIAL CYTOLOGY

Asthmatic cats commonly have clinicopathological evidence of airway inflammation, including the finding of large numbers of eosinophils recovered from bronchial secretions. Until the 1980s, it generally was assumed that eosinophils played only a beneficial role in the immune system by protecting against parasite infestation. Within the last 20 years, however, it has become clear that the presence of these cells in the wrong place at the wrong time can result in significant cellular and tissue damage. It is therefore of great interest that eosinophils (often 20 to 25 per cent of total count) can be recovered in large numbers from the tracheobronchial washings of many healthy cats.[17] These cells appear to cause no damage to the local tissue environment, and their presence should not be assumed to indicate allergy or parasitism. For this reason, airway lavage fluid eosinophilia should not be used to diagnose asthma definitively in the feline species. Similarly, alveolar macrophages are a normal cell within the lung parenchyma and are the most common cell recovered from BALF obtained from healthy cats. These cells do not represent "granulomatous" or "histiocytic" inflammation reliably when obtained in airway lavage fluid from asthmatic cats.

TRACHEOBRONCHIAL CULTURE

The presence of a mixed population of aerobic bacteria in airways has been reported previously in cats with asthma. However, neither the lower airway nor lung parenchyma of healthy cats is sterile. Organisms usually considered as pathogens, such as *Klebsiella* and *Pseudomonas* spp., can be recovered from healthy feline airways.[17] Studies designed to correlate the clinical status of asthmatic cats with the presence or absence of bacteria within the airway have not been attempted or published, to the author's knowledge. In fact, one well-designed study showed that cats with signs of bronchial disease had fewer positive airway cultures than a cohort population of healthy cats.[5]

It is the author's experience that bacteria isolated from the asthmatic feline airway most commonly reflect colonization rather than true infection. The role of *Mycoplasma* may be an exception to this statement.[18] *Mycoplasma* (and certain viruses) can degrade neutral endopeptidase, which is an enzyme that is responsible for biodegradation of substance P, a protein capable of causing bronchoconstriction and edema in the feline airway. *Mycoplasma* then might prolong the effects of substance P on airway smooth muscle indirectly. It is tempting to speculate that *Mycoplasma* or viruses, such as herpesvirus, which can remain dormant in feline airways for an extended period of time, might be responsible for increasing the levels of substance P and contribute to spontaneous bronchoconstriction.

TREATMENT

The primary signs of asthma include cough and wheeze, and these signs frequently are the result of some degree of airway smooth muscle contraction. It is tempting to treat coughing cats with suspected asthma by using only bronchodilators to relax the airway smooth muscle contraction. Although this is a primary method of treatment when acute signs develop, it is critically important to understand that human (and likely feline) asthmatic airways show evidence of chronic ongoing inflammation whether the patient is symptomatic or not. Therefore treatment strategies are most successful if they are directed toward decreasing the underlying inflammatory component of the disease, in addition to addressing the acute clinical signs of cough, wheeze, and increased respiratory effort.

LONG-TERM CORTICOSTEROIDS

The most effective long-term treatment of asthma is systemically administered corticosteroids. This class of drugs is most likely to suppress airway inflammation, a process orchestrated by a network of proteins (cytokines) that act on circulating and structural airway cells. An important effect of corticosteroids is to inhibit the synthesis of genes for cytokines involved in generating airway inflammation.

The side effects of these medications are undesirable when given for long periods of time. Fortunately, inhaled corticosteroids are available that do not cause systemic side effects, and this therapeutic approach has greatly enhanced our ability to treat patients with asthma and will be discussed later. The author begins treatment of asthmatic cats with signs that occur more than once weekly (without medication) with prednisolone 1 to 2 mg/kg PO q12h for 5 to 7 days. At this point, the majority of newly diagnosed cats have greatly diminished clinical signs. The dose of corticosteroids then is tapered slowly, over at least 2 months. This approach is much more effective than giving low doses of prednisone for short periods in response to acute flare-ups.

Some cats are managed effectively and safely by administration of low-dose, alternate-day corticosteroids. However, most cats with asthma continue to wheeze/cough when treated in this conservative manner. For patients with a good response to higher doses of consistently administered systemic corticosteroids, inhaled corticosteroid therapy should be encouraged as an alternative to reduce adverse effects.

INJECTABLE CORTICOSTEROIDS

Parenteral administration of long-acting corticosteroids is limited to patients for whom no other method of drug administration is feasible. In this setting, injection of methylprednisolone acetate, 10 to 20 mg IM once every 4 to 8 weeks, often is effective. This therapy, when used chronically, commonly results in significant/serious side effects, including weight gain, diabetes mellitus (insulin resistance), and reduced immunity. This therapy is the treatment of last resort.

Patients with clinical signs that occur less than once weekly (without medication) generally are not considered to have chronic active inflammatory airways. These patients may be treated safely with bronchodilators when needed.

BRONCHODILATORS

The use of bronchodilators is based on the assumption that clinically significant bronchoconstriction is evident. Cats develop naturally occurring and clinically significant bronchoconstriction that can be life-threatening in severe cases.[19] Therefore bronchodilator drugs usually are beneficial to these patients. These drugs are classified generally as β-receptor agonists, methylxanthine derivatives, or anticholinergics.

Most adrenergic agonists have variable α- and β-receptor affinity. Nonselective β-receptor agonists, such as isoproterenol or mixed α- and β-receptor agonists such as epinephrine, are more likely to produce cardiovascular side effects than similarly administered selective β-agonists. Consequently, drugs with preferential affinity for β_2 receptors are likely to provide more effective bronchodilation with fewer side effects. The two principal β_2-agonists currently marketed in preparations that can be used readily and regularly in cats are terbutaline sulfate and albuterol sulfate.

Terbutaline Sulfate

Terbutaline is a selective β_2-receptor agonist that produces relaxation of the smooth muscle found principally in bronchial, vascular, and uterine tissues. The exact mechanism by which activation of β_2 receptors results in smooth muscle relaxation is not totally understood, but it likely involves intracellular cyclic adenosine monophosphate (cAMP)-induced suppression of the kinase controlling myosin and actin interaction.

Terbutaline is available as a tablet, elixir, and injectable preparation suitable for SQ or IM use. The dose rate has been reported to range from 0.01 mg/kg, given SQ or IM, to 0.1 to 0.2 mg/kg PO q8h. The major clinical indication for parenterally administered terbutaline is treatment of the patient with acute respiratory difficulty when inhaled albuterol therapy is not possible. Terbutaline also is prescribed as a chronic oral treatment for bronchodilation.

Many veterinarians use terbutaline as an emergency drug to treat asthmatic cats who present in respiratory distress. The home use of a rapid-acting bronchodilator, such as inhaled albuterol or injected terbutaline, can preclude the need for a stressful emergency room visit. The author teaches his clients to use an inhaler or to administer terbutaline to their asthmatic cats at a dose of 0.01 mg/kg SQ or IM. An obvious beneficial response generally occurs within 10 to 30 minutes. This may be repeated if a significant benefit is not observed after one dose. To determine if the drug has been absorbed and if a beneficial effect has occurred, heart rate and respiratory rate and effort are monitored before drug administration. A heart rate that approaches 240 beats per minute suggests that the drug has been absorbed. A respiratory rate or effort (or both) that declines by 50 per cent or more suggests a beneficial effect.

At usual doses, terbutaline has little effect on β_1 receptors; thus direct cardiostimulatory effects are unlikely. However, terbutaline always should be used with care in patients who may have increased sensitivity to adrenergic agents, in particular, cats with preexisting cardiac disease, diabetes mellitus, hyperthyroidism, hypertension, or seizure disorders. All β_2-agonists may lower serum potassium; thus it may be prudent to monitor serum potassium levels in at-risk patients receiving long-term terbutaline therapy. In clinical practice and experimentally, it is rare to find β_2-agonist–associated hypokalemia in cats.[20]

When terbutaline is used with other sympathomimetic drugs, the risk of adverse cardiovascular effects increases; similar risks occur when it is used concurrently with digoxin, tricyclic antidepressants, and monoamine oxidase inhibitors. These potential effects are more likely in patients with preexisting cardiac disease, especially hypertrophic cardiomyopathy. Use with various inhalation anesthetics may predispose patients to ventricular arrhythmias.

Albuterol Sulfate

Albuterol is a selective β_2-receptor agonist with pharmacological properties similar to terbutaline. Albuterol is available as a tablet or syrup and is contained in various inhalants. The author has only used the inhaled form of albuterol in feline patients. The inhaled form of albuterol comes as a single-strength 17 g metered-dose inhaler (MDI) that delivers 90 µg per actuation of the device. The pharmacokinetic profile of albuterol in cats has not been reported. When administered by inhalation to human beings, albuterol produces significant bronchodilation within 5 to 15 minutes that lasts for 3 to 4 hours. It also is well-absorbed orally and may have bronchodilatory effects for up to 8 hours. Anecdotal experience with this drug in clinical practice suggests a similar pharmacokinetic profile in cats.

Rarely, adverse effects include mild skeletal muscle tremors and restlessness, which generally subside after 2 to 3 days of chronic therapy. As with terbutaline, care must be exercised when administering albuterol to patients with preexisting cardiac disease, diabetes mellitus, hyperthyroidism, hypertension, and seizure disorders. Potential drug interactions are similar to those described previously for terbutaline.

Methylxanthines: Theophylline and Aminophylline

The methylxanthines relax smooth muscle, particularly bronchial smooth muscle, as well as stimulating the central nervous system (CNS) and acting as a weak cardiac stimulant and diuretic. Although the author does not use this class of drugs to treat feline patients with asthma, methylxanthines are used frequently in our profession and are addressed briefly.

Theophylline is considered a less potent bronchodilator than the β-agonists.[21] Theophylline has been shown in other species to produce centrally mediated increased respiratory effort for any given alveolar PCO_2, to improve diaphragmatic contractility with reduced diaphragmatic fatigue, to mildly increase myocardial contractility and heart rate, and to increase CNS activity, gastric acid secretion, and urine output. All of these effects *have not* been demonstrated in cats and should be understood to be an extrapolation from other species. Interestingly, at therapeutic concentrations of theophylline, only adenosine-receptor blockade has been demonstrated reliably. This has been suggested to explain the varied effects of theophylline.

Because of the relatively low therapeutic index and pharmacokinetic characteristics of theophylline, dose rates should be based on lean body mass. The dose depends on the preparation used. In standard preparations the recommended dose for cats is 4 mg/kg PO q8h-12h. When using sustained-release preparations, a dose of 25 mg/kg PO q24h should be considered. Although there have been reports of varied bioavailability with different proprietary forms of sustained-release

preparations, Theo-Dur and Diffumal both have been shown reliably to have bioavailability greater than 95 per cent in dogs. The dose rate of aminophylline in cats is 5 to 6 mg/kg PO q12h.

The pharmacokinetics of theophylline have been studied extensively in a number of species.[22] After oral administration, peak plasma rates occur within 1.5 hours. The rate of absorption is limited principally by dissolution of the dosage form in the gastrointestinal tract. Bioavailability in cats generally is greater than 90 per cent when non–sustained-release preparations are used; however, sustained-release preparations may have a more variable bioavailability. In general, the anhydrous theophylline tablet is preferred. A chronopharmacokinetic study in cats showed that evening administration is associated with better bioavailability and less fluctuation in plasma drug level.[23]

Although theophylline can produce CNS stimulation and gastrointestinal disturbances, these effects are associated most often with excessive dosing and resolve with dose adjustments. Seizures or cardiac arrhythmias may occur in severe toxicity. There are a number of known drug interactions with theophylline. The effects of theophylline may be diminished by phenytoin or phenobarbital and enhanced by cimetidine, allopurinol, clindamycin, and lincomycin. The effects of theophylline and β-adrenergic blockers may be antagonized if they are administered concurrently. Theophylline increases the likelihood of arrhythmias induced by adrenergic agonists and halothane and of seizures with ketamine.

Anticholinergics

There are cholinergic nerve fibers within the brainstem at the level of the nucleus ambiguus, as well as within the vagus nerve via the dorsal motor nucleus. Nervous impulses traverse through parasympathetic ganglia within the airway wall; postganglionic nerve fibers innervate the submucosal glands and airway smooth muscle. When activated, the endings of these nerve fibers release acetylcholine and can result in mucus secretion and smooth muscle contraction (bronchoconstriction).

In human beings, drugs that block cholinergic pathways are effective in the treatment of patients with chronic obstructive pulmonary disease (COPD). However, this class of drug has not demonstrated similar efficacy in treating cats with asthma. In the author's experience, the primary indication for anticholinergic drug therapy in veterinary respiratory medicine is to pretreat cats with existing asthma before anesthesia to decrease excessive mucoid secretions that otherwise might result from tracheal intubation. It also may be helpful as an adjunctive bronchodilator for patients with preexisting asthma for whom bronchoscopy is planned.[24]

ANTITUSSIVES

The cough reflex is complex, involving the central and peripheral nervous systems, as well as the smooth muscle of the bronchial tree. Chemical or mechanical irritation of the epithelium within bronchial mucosa causes bronchoconstriction, which in turn stimulates cough receptors located within the tracheobronchial tree. Afferent conduction from these receptors occurs via the vagus nerve to centers within the medulla that are distinct from the actual respiratory center.

Almost any respiratory tract disorder involving any level of the large and small airways can result in coughing. This normally should be viewed as a protective physiological process resulting in clearance of thick and tenacious secretions produced by chronic airway inflammation. Thus cough suppression as a single therapeutic agent is relatively contraindicated in patients with asthma, a disorder defined in part by the presence of chronic airway inflammation and hypersecretion of mucus.

MUCOLYTICS

Mucus is a normal protective coating of the respiratory system from the nasal cavity through to the larger bronchioles. It acts as a barrier to infectious and irritating particles. It also provides airway humidification and participates in maintaining an ideal environment for ciliary movement. Mucus is produced by submucosal glands and goblet cells within the surface epithelium of airways. Although submucosal glands produce a far greater volume of mucus than the goblet cells, both of these mucus-secreting tissues respond to direct contact with a variety of substances such as smoke, sulfur dioxide, and ammonia. Direct innervation is predominantly cholinergic.

The viscosity of pulmonary mucus secretions depends on the concentration of mucoproteins and deoxyribonucleic acid (DNA). Mucus chains are cross-linked by disulfide bonds, and it is this chemical bond that is affected by some mucolytic agents including N-acetylcysteine. The feline species is somewhat unique in forming sialic acid residues within the mucus strands, and this imparts a particularly viscous nature to feline mucus. While mucoprotein is the main determinant of viscosity in normal mucus, the concentration of DNA in mucus increases in purulent inflammation (because of increased cellular debris) and so does its contribution to viscosity. Importantly, although water is incorporated into the mucus gel matrix during mucus formation, topically applied water is not absorbed into the already formed mucus plug. Asthmatic cats produce large amounts of relatively viscous inflammatory exudate and mucus, which is firmly attached to the lining of bronchioles and bronchi. By effectively increasing bronchial-wall thickness, this thick adherent mucus can exacerbate the "lumen-narrowing" effects of bronchial constriction, enhance the overall inflammatory process, and potentiate persistent coughing. In this situation, mucolytic therapy has theoretical value in facilitating resolution of the inflammatory airway disease.

In general, mucolytic drugs act by altering mucus structure through changes in pH, direct proteolysis, and/or disruption of disulfide bond linkages. It also is worth remembering that normal saline, administered directly to the airways by nebulization, is an effective mucolytic and expectorant.

Bromhexine Hydrochloride

Bromhexine hydrochloride is a synthetic derivative of the alkaloid vasicine. Bromhexine decreases mucus viscosity by increasing lysosomal activity. This increased lysosomal activity enhances hydrolysis of acid mucopolysaccharide polymers, which contribute significantly to normal mucus viscosity. It should be remembered that, in purulent bronchial inflammation, bronchial mucus viscosity is more dependent on the large amount of DNA present. As bromhexine does not affect the DNA content, its mucolytic action is limited in these situations.

It also has been suggested that bromhexine increases the permeability of the alveolar–capillary barrier, resulting in increased concentrations of certain antibiotics in luminal secretions. Furthermore, over time (2 to 3 days), bromhexine results in a significant increase in immunoglobulin concentrations and in a decline in albumin and β-globulin concentrations in respiratory secretions. The increased immunoglobulins are IgA and IgG; IgM levels remain unchanged. It has been hypothesized that, because of these effects, concurrent administration of bromhexine and an antimicrobial agent will facilitate treatment of infectious tracheobronchitis.

The mucolytic dose of bromhexine hydrochloride in cats is 2 mg/kg PO q12h for 7 to 10 days, then 1 mg/kg PO q12h for a further 7 to 10 days. Bromhexine has been used safely by veterinarians outside the United States (David Church, personal observation). This author has never used this drug for this clinical application. After oral administration, bromhexine is absorbed rapidly, with peak plasma levels reached within 1 hour. Because it is lipophilic, it is redistributed rapidly, undergoes extensive hepatic metabolism, and is excreted via the urine and bile. Adverse effects to bromhexine reportedly are extremely uncommon.

Acetylcysteine

Acetylcysteine is the N-acetyl derivative of the naturally occurring amino acid l-cysteine. When administered directly into airways, acetylcysteine reduces viscosity of both purulent and nonpurulent secretions. This effect is thought to be a result of the free sulfhydryl group in acetylcysteine reducing the disulfide linkages in mucoproteins, which are thought to be at least partly responsible for the particularly viscid nature of respiratory mucus. The mucolytic activity of acetylcysteine is unaltered by the presence of DNA and increases with increasing pH.

For effective mucolytic activity, an acetylcysteine solution should be nebulized and administered directly to the respiratory mucosa as an aerosol. The dose rate in cats is 5 to 10 mg/kg for 30 min q12h. Additionally, there is at least one report of improved gas exchange in dogs with experimentally induced bronchoconstriction who were treated with oral acetylcysteine.[25]

Acetylcysteine is available as 10 and 20 per cent solutions of the sodium salt in various-size vials. This solution can be used readily in a nebulizer undiluted, although dilution with sterile saline will reduce the risk of reactive bronchospasm. When given orally, acetylcysteine is well absorbed; when given by nebulization directly into the respiratory tract, most acetylcysteine is involved in the sulfhydryl-disulfide reaction and the remainder is absorbed. The absorbed drug is metabolized via deacetylation to cysteine in the liver. Unfortunately, acetylcysteine appears to irritate respiratory tract epithelium, and cats develop cough and/or bronchoconstriction when acetylcysteine is administered directly into the respiratory tract. Consequently, its use in cats with asthma must be monitored carefully.

EXPECTORANTS

Expectorants are drugs used to produce an increased volume of respiratory secretions that theoretically can be coughed out more easily. Although drugs in this class are used in an enormous number of "over-the-counter" medications, a Food and Drug Administration (FDA) advisory review panel found no well-controlled studies that documented the effectiveness of expectorants in managing COPD in human patients. Likewise, there are no current data available to suggest that expectorants are effective adjunctive treatments for cats with disorders of the respiratory tract. However, because this class of drug is used and promoted with such regularity, a brief discussion is appropriate.

Guaifenesin

The most commonly prescribed expectorant is guaifenesin. An older name for this drug is glycerol guaiacolate; it was isolated from guaiac resin in 1826. When given in large amounts, guaifenesin acts as an emetic; it is likely that it stimulates a gastropulmonary vagal reflex. It also may be absorbed into bronchial mucosal glands and exert a direct mucotropic effect.

The dose required to stimulate production of mucus and respiratory tract secretions probably is equivalent to the dose needed to produce emesis; this is far higher than the 400 to 1600 mg/day range of dosing prescribed most commonly. Thus, at doses recommended to treat human beings with COPD, the effect of guaifenesin is likely equivalent to placebo.

ANTIBIOTICS

There is no objective evidence that bacterial infection plays a significant role in the cause or continuation of feline asthma. Similarly, there is no objective published evidence that antibiotic therapy has any effect on the duration or intensity of signs displayed by the cat with asthma. It is important to remember that the clinical signs of asthma in cats frequently wax and wane in severity, as well as in frequency of occurrence. There are many anecdotal reports describing the therapeutic effect of antibiotics in controlling asthmatic signs, but these reports are consistent with the "waxing and waning" nature of the clinical signs in nontreated cases.

A positive culture result obtained from a tracheobronchial wash does not necessarily imply the presence of a clinically significant airway infection and should not automatically prompt the clinician to initiate antibiotic therapy. In the author's opinion, antibiotics are rarely indicated for cats with asthma and are appropriate only when there is good evidence of superimposed airway infection. This may be inferred from the growth of a pure bacterial culture on a primary culture plate from material obtained from tracheobronchial secretions. This is because the concentration of aerobic bacteria recovered from the airways of healthy cats rarely exceeds 5×10^3 organisms/mL. In contrast, growth of a single organism recovered without the use of enrichment broth implies greater than 10^5 organisms/mL, which is consistent with an "infected" airway in human patients. Antibiotic therapy then is based on sensitivity data. Prophylactic or long-term therapy should be avoided unless there is documentation of a chronic airway infection, which is uncommon. In this context, we should remember that acute bacterial bronchitis occurs in cats and may resolve more quickly with antibiotic therapy. Chronic asthma should not be diagnosed on the finding of a cough that has developed within a few weeks of the patient presenting to the veterinarian.

One possible exception to these statements involves *Mycoplasma* species. *Mycoplasma* has been isolated from the airways of as many as 25 per cent of cats with signs of lower airway disease; however, *Mycoplasma* has not been cultured from the airways of healthy cats.[18,26] For this reason and because *Mycoplasma* has the potential to cause significant structural damage to airway epithelium, it may be prudent to treat any cat with a *Mycoplasma*-positive airway culture with an appropriate antibiotic (such as doxycycline 3 to 5 mg/kg PO q12h, with meals or followed by 10 mL of water).

CYPROHEPTADINE

Cyproheptadine (Periactin) is marketed as an antihistamine; however, it has been used for years as an appetite stimulant for depressed or anorectic cats because of its antiserotonin properties. As mentioned earlier, serotonin is a primary mediator released from activated mast cells into feline airways and causes acute smooth muscle contraction (bronchoconstriction) in cats but not in human beings. The author has shown that the ability of cyproheptadine to block serotonin receptors in muscle cells is effective in preventing antigen-induced airway smooth muscle constriction in vitro. Limited clinical observations in asthmatic cats *have not* supported these in vitro findings. The primary indication for this drug is a trial in the symptomatic asthmatic cat already receiving maximal doses of bronchodilators and corticosteroids. Cyproheptadine comes in both pill and liquid form and is dosed at 2 to 4 mg PO q12h.[22] A beneficial therapeutic response may not be seen for 4 to 7 days; however, depression, the primary side effect of this drug, may be observed 24 hours after administration. Depression is not life-threatening but may cause the owner to discontinue cyproheptadine therapy.

ANTI-LEUKOTRIENES

Leukotrienes belong to a family of inflammatory mediators that are derived from arachidonic acid and are known collectively as eicosanoids. The leukotrienes, LTC_4, LTD_4, and LTE_4, are known collectively as the cysteinyl leukotrienes and play an important role in airway inflammation. They produce mucus hypersecretion, increase vascular permeability and mucosal edema, induce potent bronchoconstriction, and act as chemoattractants to inflammatory cells, particularly eosinophils and neutrophils.

Orally administered anti-leukotriene drugs are competitive, highly selective, and potent inhibitors of the production or the function of LTC_4, LTD_4, and LTE_4. Specifically, zileuton blocks leukotriene biosynthesis by inhibiting production of the 5-lipoxygenase enzyme, whereas both montelukast and zafirlukast block adhesion of leukotrienes to their common leukotriene receptor (cys-LT1). In human patients, leukotrienes inhibit asthmatic responses to allergen, aspirin, exercise, and cold dry air. Additionally, leukotriene blockade has been shown in many clinical trials to decrease the amount and frequency of administration of corticosteroids in steroid-dependent human beings with asthma.

There have been few investigations regarding the role of leukotrienes in feline airway disease. Although LTE_4 is found in increased concentrations in urine of human beings with asthma, no such increase in urinary LTE_4 was found in 20 cats with signs of bronchial disease[27] or in cats with experimentally induced asthma in unpublished studies conducted by the author. More recently, in another experimental model of feline asthma, no increase in cysteinyl leukotrienes was found in either urine or BALF after challenge exposure to sensitizing antigen.[28] Additionally, zafirlukast did not inhibit airway inflammation or airway hyperreactivity in this feline asthma model.[29] Thus there is no current evidence that drugs that affect leukotriene synthesis or receptor ligation will play a significant role in the treatment of feline asthma. Having said that, there is at least one claim of efficacy using zafirlukast (1 to 2 mg/kg PO q12h) or montelukast (0.5 to 1.0 mg/kg PO q24h) for treatment of feline asthma.[30]

The pharmacokinetics of these drugs in cats has not been reported. In human beings, these drugs are well-absorbed orally, although the presence of food can reduce absorption by up to 60 per cent. They are highly protein-bound, metabolized extensively by the liver, and undergo biliary excretion predominantly. As only limited experience is available in the use of these drugs in cats, the prevalence, type, and severity of adverse reactions associated with their administration can not be easily or well documented.

In human beings, leukotriene-receptor antagonists occasionally have been associated with elevated hepatic enzyme levels, although active hepatic disease is uncommon. Human case reports also have suggested a rare association between the leukotriene-receptor antagonists and Churg-Strauss syndrome, which is a rare condition involving vasculitis-associated asthma, eosinophilia, and pulmonary infiltrates. The cause-and-effect association remains controversial because most of the affected patients were receiving corticosteroids before starting leukotriene-receptor–antagonist therapy. Consequently, it seems plausible that most of the cases were actually Churg-Strauss syndrome suppressed by the oral corticosteroids, which became unmasked when the corticosteroids were withdrawn.

AEROSOL DELIVERY OF CORTICOSTEROIDS AND BRONCHODILATORS

Aerosol administration of the corticosteroid fluticasone and the bronchodilator albuterol relies on delivery of the drug to the distal airways, which in turn depends on the size of the aerosol particles and various respiratory parameters such as tidal volume and inspiratory flow rate. Even in cooperative human patients, only approximately 10 to 30 per cent of the inhaled dose enters the lungs. Recent studies in cats have demonstrated that passive inhalation through a mask and spacer combination (Aerokat) is an effective method of delivering sufficient medication to be clinically effective.[30,32]

Drugs for inhalation typically come in a rectangular MDI or a round "diskus" form. At the present time, only the MDI form is practical for use in animals. The most effective means of using an MDI involves coordination between inhalation and actuation of the device, something that is not reliable in most infants, small children, or animals. For this reason, an alternative involves the use of a spacer device and a mask specifically designed for cats. A small, aerosol-holding chamber is attached to an MDI on one end and a face mask on the other. The spacer is approximately the size of the inner cardboard roll used for toilet paper. The MDI supplies precise doses of the aerosol drug, and the holding chamber contains the aerosol so that it can be inhaled when the patient inspires. The mask is designed to cover the nose of a cat. The designers of the Aerokat spacer have shown that a holding chamber with a length of 11 cm and a diameter of 3.5 cm or larger delivered almost all of a therapeutically "ideal" aerosol (i.e., aerosol of equivalent aerodynamic diameter ≤2.8 μm) produced by an MDI, and in some cases, delivery was enhanced because of evaporation of large, suspended particles. The choice of spacer is relevant because cats have a tidal volume of approximately 11 mL inspired air per kilogram of body weight. Currently, only the Aerokat brand spacers (Trudell Medical Inc, Ontario, CA) have been designed specifically based on the tidal volume characteristics of the cat. Using these spacer devices, cats will inhale the majority of drug propelled into the spacer by breathing seven to 10 times through the spacer-mask combination after actuation of the MDI. It is important to teach the owner to observe the pet actually breathing because cats initially may hold their breaths when introduced to this form of treatment.

The procedure is not time consuming, but it may be necessary to acclimate the cat to the mask. In the author's experience, 70 per cent of cats will allow use of the spacer mask immediately, 20 per cent can be conditioned to

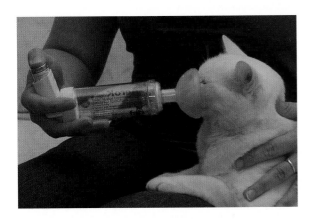

Figure 44-3 A feline patient with asthma who has been trained to receive corticosteroid and bronchodilator treatment using a metered-dose inhaler and a mask and spacer combination.

accept the apparatus within 1 week, and the remaining 10 per cent of patients likely will not tolerate this approach even with prolonged training.

When administering inhalation therapy, the MDI is first shaken to open an internal valve within the canister and then attached to the spacer. The mask attached to the other end of the spacer is placed snugly on the animal's nose or muzzle, and the MDI is pressed to release the medication into the spacer (Figure 44-3).

The most commonly used inhaled corticosteroid is fluticasone propionate (Flovent), a synthetic corticosteroid with an eighteenfold higher affinity for the corticosteroid receptor when compared to dexamethasone. Binding of the corticosteroid to this receptor results in a new molecular complex that leads to up- or down-regulation of the gene and its products. Fluticasone, like other corticosteroids, acts to inhibit mast cells, eosinophils, lymphocytes, neutrophils, and macrophages involved in the generation and exacerbation of allergic airway inflammation by transcriptional regulation of these target genes. Preformed and newly secreted mediators including histamine, eicosanoids, leukotrienes, and multiple cytokines also are inhibited.

Fluticasone is a large molecule and acts topically within the airway mucosa. Because there is poor absorption across gastrointestinal tract epithelium, there is minimal oral systemic bioavailability. Plasma levels do not predict therapeutic effects. This explains the lack of systemic side effects; however, it also suggests that clinically effective absorption into the airway mucosa is delayed. Optimal clinical effects therefore may not occur for 1 to 2 weeks.

Flovent has been used by the author to treat cats with bronchial asthma since 1993. Since then, a number of studies have demonstrated the clinical effectiveness of fluticasone for treatment of cats with allergic rhinitis, bronchitis, and asthma.[31,32] There have been no controlled published studies to determine the optimal dose or interval for use of Flovent in cats; however, there are anecdotal reports that reference more than 300 small animal patients treated with fluticasone during a period covering 1995 to 2006.[33] Dosage recommendations are based on these observations and recently published studies.

Flovent comes in three strengths; 44 µg, 110 µg, and 220 µg per actuation. The author has found that 44 µg dosing q12h almost never results in acceptable clinical responses. For cats with mild-to-moderate disease, 110 µg given q12h frequently results in clinical responses equivalent to that achieved by administration of prednisone 5 mg PO q12h. Cats with more serious disease may require 220 µg inhaled q12h. Administration of fluticasone more often than q12h has not resulted in additional clinical benefit in the author's experience. Administration of inhaled fluticasone q24h occasionally has been effective; administration less often than q24h has not been helpful.

The pharmacology of albuterol, a selective β_2-adrenergic bronchodilator, has been described previously. This drug is available through different manufacturers and is commonly prescribed as Ventolin or Proventil. Albuterol only comes in a single uniform strength (90 µg per actuation). Albuterol usually results in relaxation of airway smooth muscles within 1 to 5 minutes, so the effect is almost immediate. This drug should be used in animals with documented or assumed bronchoconstriction. Clinical signs that may indicate bronchoconstriction are wheeze, noisy lower airway breathing, prolonged expiratory phase of ventilation, and coughing. Albuterol can be used q24h before administering fluticasone or as needed for acute coughing and wheezing. In emergency cases, albuterol can be used every 30 minutes for up to 4 to 6 hours without serious side effects.

The use of inhaled medications to treat asthma and bronchitis is considered the standard of care in human beings and is now recommended widely for cats with asthma. This approach avoids many of the side effects seen previously in patients treated with systemic medications.

REASONABLE EXPECTATIONS

Asthma in human beings and cats is a chronic disorder without cure. The clinical signs may be constant or intermittent, mild, moderate, or severe, and the entire clinical course of asthma may change over time. Some patients require chronic daily oral medications, while others need only intermittent rescue inhaler medication.

In the author's experience, cats with well-controlled signs of asthma frequently have exacerbations of signs without any recognized cause. In these situations, it is important to evaluate the patient for other causes of cough, wheeze, and increased respiratory rate and effort. When no identifiable cause of exacerbation of signs is suspected, it is common for these patients to require a short course of intensive corticosteroid treatment. This may take 3 to 7 days before more serious clinical signs resolve. Some of these patients respond to antibiotic treatment for presumed respiratory *Mycoplasma* infections. The prognosis for asthmatic cats with clearly defined disease and with aggressive treatment usually is good to excellent for years of relatively comfortable stress-free living.

REFERENCES

1. Beasley R, Roche WR, Roberts JA, et al: Cellular events in the bronchi in mild asthma and after bronchial provocation, *Am Rev Respir Dis* 139:806, 1989.

2. Bradley BL, Azzawi M, Jacobson B, et al: Eosinophils, T lymphocytes, mast cells, neutrophils, and macrophages in bronchial biopsies from atopic asthma: comparison with atopic non-asthma and normal controls and relationship to bronchial hyper-responsiveness, *J Allergy Clin Immunol* 88:661, 1991.

3. US Department of Health and Human Services, National Institutes of Health, National Heart, Lung, and Blood Institute National Asthma Education and Prevention Program Expert Panel Report 3: Guidelines for the Diagnosis and Management of Asthma Full Report. Washington DC, 2007, p 2.

4. Norris Reinero CR, Decile KC, Berghaus RD, et al: An experimental model of allergic asthma in cats sensitized to house dust mite or Bermuda grass allergen, *Int Arch Allergy Immunol* 135:177, 2004.

5. Dye JA, McKiernan BC, Rozanski EA, et al: Bronchopulmonary disease in the cat: historical, physical, radiographic, clinicopathologic and pulmonary functional evaluation of 24 affected and 15 healthy cats, *J Vet Intern Med* 10:385, 1996.

6. Adamama-Moraitou KK, Patsikas MN, Koutinas AF: Feline lower airway disease: a retrospective study of 22 naturally occurring cases from Greece, *J Feline Med Surg* 6:227, 2004.

7. Foster SF, Allan GS, Martin P, et al: Twenty five cases of feline bronchial disease, *J Feline Med Surg* 6:181, 2004.

8. Reinero CR, Cohn LA: Interstitial lung diseases, *Vet Clin North Am Small Anim Pract* 37:937, 2007.

9. Dillon AR, Blagburn BL, Tillson DM, et al: Immature heartworm infection produces pulmonary parenchymal, airway, and vascular disease in cats. Proceedings of the ACVIM Forum, Seattle, WA, 2007.

10. Padrid PA, Snook S, Finucane T, et al: Persistent airway hyper-responsiveness and histological alterations after chronic antigen challenge in cats, *Am J Resp Crit Care Med* 151:184, 1995.

11. Padrid PA, Cozzi P, Leff AR: Cyclosporine A attenuates the development of chronic airway hyper-responsiveness and histological alterations in immune-sensitized cats, *Am J Respir Crit Care Med* 154:1812, 1996.

12. Padrid PA, Mitchell RW, Ndukwu IM, et al: Cyproheptadine-induced attenuation of type-I immediate hypersensitivity reactions of airway smooth muscle from immune-sensitized cats, *Am J Vet Res* 56:109, 1995.

13. Lee-Fowler TM, Cohn LA, Declue AE, et al: Evaluation of subcutaneous versus mucosal (intranasal) allergen-specific rush immunotherapy in experimental feline asthma, *Vet Immunol Immunopathol* 129:49, 2009.

14. Reinero CR, Cohn LA, Delgado C, et al: Adjuvanted rush immunotherapy using CpG oligodeoxynucleotides in experimental feline allergic asthma, *Vet Immunol Immunopathol* 121:241, 2008.

15. Padrid PA: Animal models of asthma. In Liggett SB, Meyers DA, editors: *The genetics of asthma: lung biology in health and disease*, New York, 1996, Marcel Dekker, p 211.

16. Johnson LR, Drazenovich TL: Flexible bronchoscopy and bronchoalveolar lavage in 68 cats (2001-2006), *J Vet Intern Med* 21:219, 2007.

17. Padrid PA, Feldman BF, Funk K, et al: Cytologic, microbiologic, and biochemical analysis of bronchoalveolar lavage fluid obtained from 24 healthy cats, *Am J Vet Res* 52:1300, 1991.

18. Chandler JC, Lappin MR: Mycoplasma respiratory infections in small animals: 17 cases (1988-1999), *J Am Anim Hosp Assoc* 38:111, 2002.

19. Padrid PA: Feline asthma, *Vet Clin North Am Small Anim Pract* 30:1279, 2000.

20. Petruska JM, Beattie JG, Stuart BO, et al: Cardiovascular effects after inhalation of large doses of albuterol dry powder in rats, monkeys, and dogs: a species comparison, *Fundam Appl Toxicol* 40:52, 1997.

21. Bjermer J: History and future perspectives of treating asthma as a systemic and small airways disease, *Respir Med* 95:703, 2001.

22. Boothe DM: Drugs affecting the respiratory system. In King LG, editor: *Textbook of respiratory disease in dogs and cats*, St Louis, 1994, Elsevier, p 236.

23. Dye JA, McKiernan BC, Jones SD, et al: Chronopharmacokinetics of theophylline in the cat, *J Vet Pharmacol Ther* 13:278, 1990.

24. Kirschvink N, Leemans J, Delvaux F, et al: Bronchodilators in bronchoscopy-induced airflow limitation in allergen-sensitized cats, *J Vet Intern Med* 19:161, 2005.

25. Ueno O, Lee LN, Wagner PD: Effect of N-acetylcysteine on gas exchange after methacholine challenge and isoprenaline inhalation in the dog, *Eur Respir J* 2:238, 1989.

26. Randolph JF, Moise NS, Scarlett JM, et al: Prevalence of mycoplasmal and ureaplasmal recovery from tracheobronchial lavages and of mycoplasmal recovery from pharyngeal swab specimens in cats with or without pulmonary disease, *Am J Vet Res* 54:897, 1993.

27. Mellema M, et al: Urinary leukotriene levels in cats with allergic bronchitis. Proceedings of the ACVIM Forum: 724, 1998.

28. Norris CR, Decile KC, Berghaus LJ, et al: Concentrations of cysteinyl leukotrienes in urine and bronchoalveolar lavage fluid of cats with experimentally induced asthma, *Am J Vet Res* 64:1449, 2003.

29. Reinero CR, Decile KC, Byerly JR, et al: Effects of drug treatment on inflammation and hyperreactivity of airways and on immune variables in cats with experimentally induced asthma, *Am J Vet Res* 66:1121, 2005.

30. Mandelker L: Experimental drug therapy for respiratory disorders in dogs and cats, *Vet Clin North Am Small Anim Pract* 30:1357, 2000.

31. Kirschvink N, Leemans J, Delvaux F, et al: Inhaled fluticasone reduces bronchial responsiveness and airway inflammation in cats with mild chronic bronchitis, *J Feline Med Surg* 8:45, 2006.

32. Padrid PA: Use of inhaled medications to treat dogs and cats in clinical practice, *J Am Anim Hosp Assoc* 42:165, 2006.

33. Padrid PA: Inhaled steroids to treat feline lower airway disease: 300 cases 1995-2007. Proceedings of the ACVIM Forum, San Antonio, TX: 2008.

CHAPTER
45 Bronchoscopy

Lynelle R. Johnson

Bronchoscopy is a valuable tool for investigation of lower respiratory tract disease. Direct visualization of the airways and bronchoalveolar lavage (BAL) of a specific airway segment can provide a definitive diagnosis of infectious, inflammatory, or neoplastic causes of cough and respiratory distress. Additionally, bronchoscopy allows therapeutic intervention and cure in cats with respiratory disease related to foreign body aspiration. Several factors make this procedure technically challenging in cats. Bronchoscopy requires general anesthesia, and this often is a concern in a patient with respiratory disease. The small size of the feline trachea does not allow intubation for ventilation and oxygenation throughout the procedure as is usually possible in dogs. In addition, small-diameter flexible endoscopes are preferred because of the small airways in cats, and these can be difficult to manipulate. Specific training and experience is needed to ensure proficiency and efficiency in completion of the endoscopic evaluation. Finally, cats are believed to develop bronchospasm during BAL, resulting in an increase in airway resistance[1] that could impact anesthetic recovery adversely. Nevertheless, bronchoscopy can be performed safely in most cats and can provide invaluable information on the etiology of disease and the need for specific therapy.

CASE SELECTION

Careful case selection and prior planning maximizes the likelihood of successful completion of a bronchoscopic procedure in the cat. Feline bronchial disease is the most common cause of acute or chronic cough, tachypnea, or respiratory distress, and these cats are all potential candidates for bronchoscopy. Bronchoscopy with BAL for cytological examination and culture can confirm inflammatory airway disease in the absence of *Mycoplasma* infection, airway parasites, or foreign body pneumonia that can cause clinical signs similar to bronchial disease. However, bronchoscopy should not be performed in any animal

unstable for anesthesia. Obese patients with increased respiratory effort may have difficulty recovering from anesthesia, although this is less common in cats than in dogs.

Surgical intervention may be required in a cat with an intraluminal airway mass, obstruction, or foreign body in a large airway. If a mass is present in the tracheal region, preparations should be made before anesthesia for a possible tracheotomy. Alternately, a foreign body or mass in the lower airways could require a thoracotomy. These procedures usually should be performed immediately because of the difficulty in recovering a cat with an airway obstruction. Cats with bullous or emphysematous lung disease evident on radiographs or computed tomography (CT) are at risk for pneumothorax during ventilation or during bronchoscopy, if the endoscope is wedged in a fragile airway.

COMPLICATIONS

Complications from bronchoscopy with BAL in the cat are relatively common and should be anticipated. In a recent report, over one-third of cats experienced some form of complication; however, the majority were minor and consisted of hemoglobin desaturation, abrupt termination of the procedure, or prolonged recovery from anesthesia.[2] These complications may not be a specific feature of bronchoscopy because nonbronchoscopic BAL via endotracheal tube collection in healthy cats also can result in dramatic reduction in arterial oxygenation.[3] In most situations, administration of supplemental oxygen results in rapid resolution of hypoxemia. Some cats may require recovery in an intensive care unit. Careful monitoring of respiratory rate, effort, and lung sounds always is advised in the immediate postoperative period. Although rare, pneumothorax has been reported as a complication of bronchoscopy in both cats and human beings.[2] Owners should be aware that bronchoscopy can result in mortality caused by worsened respiratory distress postprocedure or from an inability to restore ventilation and oxygenation after anesthesia.

ENDOSCOPES

A number of companies supply fiberoptic or video endoscopes that can be used in feline airways. A key component in the flexible endoscope is the presence of a channel through which to perform BAL. Although a rigid telescope can be used for laryngeal and tracheal investigation, it can not be maneuvered throughout the airways and does not have a channel for lavage. In addition to the flexible endoscope, a light source (xenon or halogen) is required. An imaging system is valuable for archiving the visual appearance of the airways. The following discussion details the author's experience with endoscopes used in feline bronchoscopy.

Feline bronchoscopy ideally should be performed with a flexible endoscope less than 5.0 mm in outer diameter that contains a channel for lavage and instrumentation. A pediatric bronchoscope commonly available in specialty veterinary hospitals or universities (Olympus P20D, Melville, NY) can be used in cats, although it is slightly larger in diameter than ideal at 5.0 mm × 55 cm in length. This endoscope provides good visualization of the carina and mainstem bronchi but is too large in most cats to pass into lobar bronchi other than the left and right caudal bronchi. When performing BAL with this endoscope, the relatively large diameter of the channel (2.0 mm) results in sampling of a larger bronchus rather than a bronchoalveolar segment. This endoscope is valuable for foreign body retrieval and biopsy of proximal lesions because of the relatively large channel and the availability of multiple instruments that can pass through this channel.

A specialized fiberoptic endoscope (Karl Storz 60003VB, Goleta, CA) designed for urethroscopy provides access to many of the segmental bronchi of the cat and therefore allows thorough examination of the airways. This 2.5 mm × 70 cm endoscope has a 1.2 mm channel that can be used for lavage or for obtaining small biopsy samples. The small diameter of the endoscope results in less light transmission down the airways, which can compromise image quality. Additional practice is required to maneuver this endoscope through the airways because of its small diameter and relatively long length. Recovering lavage fluid requires patience because of the small channel size, and gentle intermittent suction generally is most successful in recovering lavage fluid. A hybrid fiberoptic videoscope of similar diameter is now available from Olympus Medical.

Olympus also makes a number of smaller (3 to 3.8 mm diameter) fiberoptic or video endoscopes. The 3.8 mm × 55 cm video endoscope (Olympus BF3C160, Melville, NY) has a 1.2 mm channel and can access lobar bronchi and some segmental bronchi in most cats. The main advantage of this endoscope is improved maneuverability in the airways and better image quality, which allows superior assessment of epithelial changes associated with disease.

ANESTHESIA

A baseline pulse oximetry value should be taken before anesthesia. If a reading above 95 per cent can not be obtained, an arterial blood gas analysis should be considered. Although hypoxemia does not preclude anesthesia for bronchoscopy, knowledge of the oxygenation status before anesthesia is very important. A cat with a pulse oximetry reading of 100 per cent hemoglobin saturation should return to that level after the procedure. It is equally important to know that a cat with a hemoglobin saturation of only 92 per cent will likely be at a similar value after anesthesia.

In the 12 to 24 hours before bronchoscopy, premedication with terbutaline is recommended at 0.01 mg/kg SQ q8-12h or 0.625 mg/cat PO q12h to provide some bronchodilation before the procedure. In an experimental model of airway hyperresponsiveness, use of an inhaled bronchodilator was associated with a reduction in bronchoscopy-induced increase in airway resistance.[1] In addition, pretreatment with terbutaline reduced the complication rate associated with bronchoscopy in cats with naturally occurring respiratory disease.[2] Finally, cats should be oxygenated immediately before bronchoscopy.

Various anesthetic protocols can be used to induce and maintain a cat under anesthesia for bronchoscopy, and it is most important that the user is familiar with the side effects and actions of the drugs chosen. Use of a propofol infusion at 6 mg/kg/min and oxygenation via jet ventilation at 180 breaths/min provide a stable and predictable anesthetic plane. Repeated boluses of propofol can be given as needed to maintain anesthesia and are associated with relatively few cardiopulmonary side effects. When jet ventilation is not available, other means of providing oxygen include a red rubber catheter placed in the trachea, oxygen administered via the endoscopic channel, and laryngeal mask anesthesia. When using a tracheal catheter, careful monitoring is recommended because the cannula may not provide adequate exchange of gas at the alveolar level and hypoxemia may develop. Only oxygen at a low flow rate can be given via the endoscopic channel, and the operator must not wedge the endoscope in an airway when oxygen is supplemented in this fashion because it could result in a pneumothorax. The laryngeal mask provides an excellent means for providing gas anesthesia during bronchoscopy; however, the narrow and delicate endoscopes used for feline bronchoscopy can be damaged when passing through the orifice of the tube or an adapter that is required to provide anesthetic gas and collect exhaust. Pulse oximetry, electrocardiogram, and blood pressure should be monitored throughout the endoscopic procedure.

PROCEDURE

Bronchoscopy in small animal patients is routinely performed in sternal recumbency. A rolled-up towel is placed under the cat's chin to elevate the head and avoid occlusion of the larynx. In the cat, application of lidocaine to

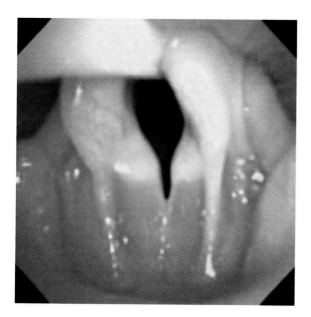

Figure 45-1 Endoscopic view of the larynx in a cat with chronic bronchitis and neutrophilic lower airway disease. A jet ventilator catheter is present at the top left of the image. The tissue surrounding the glottis is hyperemic, and the glistening appearance of the mucosa suggests edema. The region of the saccules and vocal folds appears swollen.

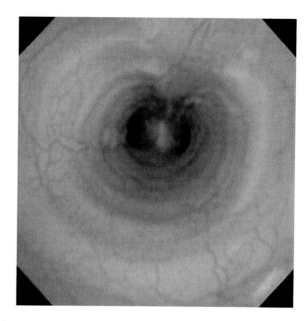

Figure 45-2 Trachea in a normal cat. Cartilage rings are visible under the mucosa as white C-shaped rings. The annular ligament between tracheal rings appears darker. The dorsal tracheal membrane is present at 12 o'clock on this image. Overall, the epithelial surface is pale pink, and submucosal vessels are readily apparent.

the larynx is helpful to prevent laryngospasm during intubation. Generally, two mouth gags are inserted between the canine teeth on either side of the jaw to keep the mouth open and protect the bronchoscope throughout the procedure. An assistant aids in monitoring anesthetic depth, maintaining patient position, and holding the mouth gags in place. If the cat approaches a light plane of anesthesia and swallows, gags, or exhibits an elevated respiratory rate, the endoscope should be withdrawn immediately until the cat returns to a stable plane of anesthesia. This will help avoid airway injury or expensive repairs to the endoscope if the cat should bite down on the outer sheath.

Examination of the airway begins with a direct assessment of the upper airway under a light plane of anesthesia to assess laryngeal structure and function. A fiberoptic or video endoscope generally is not used at this stage because of the risk of damage to the instrument; however, a rigid telescope can be used. Upper airway lesions in cats are much more subtle than in dogs; however, the larynx should be evaluated for normal function and the surrounding structures assessed for evidence of edema or inflammation. Some cats may have mild asymmetry of laryngeal motion on inspiration or expiration. Laryngeal paresis or paralysis is indicated by failure of the arytenoid cartilages to open on inspiration. In cats with lower respiratory tract inflammation, hyperemic, edematous, and swollen arytenoid cartilages are encountered commonly (Figure 45-1).

Examination of the trachea and lower airways is completed in a systematic fashion. The epithelial surface of normal feline airways is a pale yellowish pink (Figure 45-2). Submucosal vessels usually are apparent unless

edema or inflammation results in thickening of the mucosal surface. The tracheal cartilages are C-shaped rings that are connected on the dorsal surface by a very short strap of muscle, the dorsal tracheal membrane. Very rarely, cats will develop mild collapse of the trachea in association with chronic inflammatory disease, and in this situation, there generally is marked irregularity to the tracheal mucosa (Figure 45-3).

The lower airways of the cat follow a predictable monopodial branching pattern[4] (Figure 45-4). To ensure that all airways are analyzed systematically, a standard procedure should be followed to evaluate all accessible airways, record abnormal findings, and obtain respiratory samples. The first recognizable landmark is the carina, which bifurcates into the left and right principal bronchi (Figure 45-5). During the initial examination of the airways, the site and character of all abnormalities are recorded for comparison with radiographic changes and for contrast with future examinations. The principal left or right bronchus is entered and then lobar bronchi are followed caudally. The openings to the airway usually are round, smooth, and slightly moist in appearance. At regular intervals, smaller dorsal and ventral branches will be seen projecting from the main airway. Segmental and subsegmental airways should be entered when possible. Airway hyperemia or mucus accumulation is a sign of disease (Figure 45-6).

While performing the initial examination of the airways, a site for BAL should be chosen. Lavage for airway specimens usually is performed in an abnormal area, or if disease appears to be diffuse, lavage is performed in a middle lung lobe where disease processes often will result in pooling of secretions. After complete

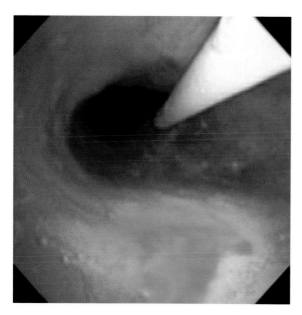

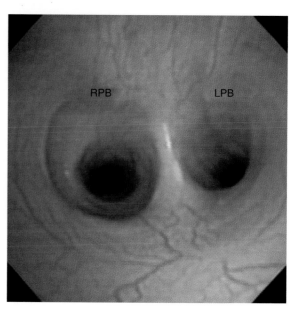

Figure 45-3 Hyperemic and irregular tracheal mucosa in a cat with mild tracheal collapse associated with chronic lower airway inflammatory disease. A jet ventilator is present at the right of the image. The tracheal mucosa appears thickened, vessels are poorly visible, and hemorrhage is noted, suggesting friability.

Figure 45-5 Carina of the cat showing the entrance into the left principal bronchus *(LPB)* and right principal bronchus *(RPB)*.

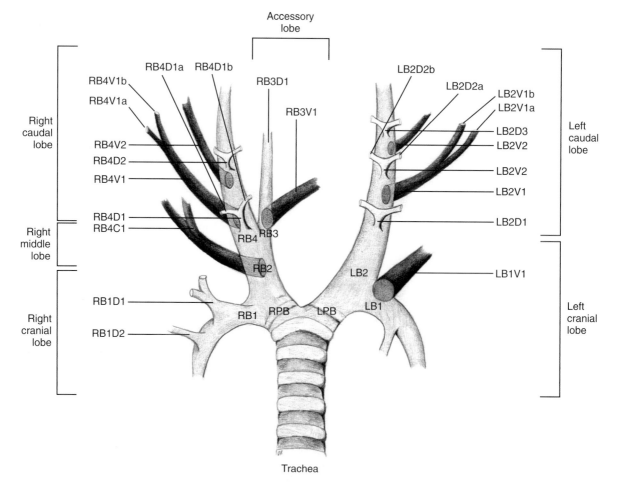

Figure 45-4 Map of the feline lower airways. This image represents a dorsal view of the airway branching pattern with the neck at the bottom of the image. (Reprinted with permission from Caccamo R, Twedt DC, Buracco P, et al: Endoscopic bronchial anatomy in the cat, *J Feline Med Surg* 9:140, 2007.)

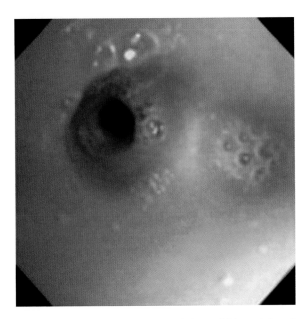

Figure 45-6 Segmental airways in the left caudal lung lobe of a cat with *Mycoplasma* pneumonia. Heavy mucoid impaction of the airways is present along with airway hyperemia.

visual examination and before BAL, the endoscope is withdrawn from the airways, the biopsy channel is flushed with sterile saline, and the outside of the instrument is wiped with saline-soaked sponges. On the second entry to the airway, the endoscope should be maintained within the center of the airway to prevent contact with the oral mucosa and airway epithelium. This will limit bacterial contamination of the tip of the bronchoscope when approaching the chosen site for lavage. The bronchoscope is wedged gently into the smallest bronchus possible, and warmed, nonbacteriostatic, sterile saline is instilled to flood the segment of alveoli supplied by that airway followed by 2 to 3 mL of air to clean the channel. The volume used for lavage depends on the diameter of the endoscope used and the ability to wedge within a certain size of airway. Generally, 3 to 5 mL of sterile saline per aliquot is used for BAL in cats. Retrieval of 50 to 75 per cent should be anticipated.[2] A frothy appearance to the fluid indicates the presence of surfactant. At least two different airway segments or lobes should be lavaged when possible to increase the likelihood that the disease process will be identified.

It is common for hemoglobin desaturation to occur during BAL; however, it usually is transient. If the desaturation is severe or sustained, the procedure should be aborted, the animal intubated, and hand ventilation performed until saturation returns to the prelavage level.

During the postanesthetic period, an oxygen-enriched environment should be provided. Intubation and ventilation can speed recovery. If postprocedure radiographs are performed, they typically reveal pulmonary infiltrates because of nonrecovered lavage fluid; however, this fluid usually is absorbed within 12 to 24 hours.

SAMPLE HANDLING

Samples obtained from bronchoscopy should be submitted for both cytological examination and culture. When more than one lung segment has been lavaged, the samples should be examined separately cytologically; however, a combined sample may be submitted for culture. Aerobic and *Mycoplasma* cultures should be submitted on every cat, and submission for anaerobic culture should be considered in patients with dense mucoid secretions. Consultation with the microbiology laboratory is recommended to ensure that the sample is handled properly during submission because some laboratories recommend special medium for transport. Although it has not yet been examined in lower respiratory tract samples, noncultivable *Mycoplasma* species can be detected occasionally in samples from the upper respiratory tract by polymerase chain reaction when culture is negative.[5] Therefore, in certain cases, submission of BAL fluid for molecular analysis may be helpful.

Cytological analysis should include an assessment of cellularity within the sample and a differential cell count to describe the inflammatory response. A cytocentrifuged sample provides a concentrated slide for assessing alterations in cell morphology and detection of organisms. BAL fluid from the normal cat is comprised of 300 to 400 cells/μL with 65 per cent macrophages, up to 25 per cent eosinophils, and 4 to 5 per cent lymphocytes and neutrophils.[6,7] Occasional mast cells also may be seen.

Neutrophilic inflammation usually is described as septic to indicate an infectious process or nonseptic, representing an inflammatory disease. Septic inflammation is associated most commonly with bacterial infection, and the presence of intracellular bacteria would support that diagnosis. Fungal organisms can stimulate an increase in neutrophils in a sample as well as activation of macrophages. Nonseptic inflammation is typical of chronic bronchitis in cats. Chronic, ongoing inflammation commonly leads to red blood cells in BAL fluid and/or hemosiderin-laden macrophages, an indicator of previous hemorrhage within the lung. Eosinophilic inflammation also is common in cats with bronchial disease and may suggest a hypersensitivity or allergic response, or an underlying parasitic disorder. Occasionally, neoplastic cells can be identified within BAL fluid.

SUMMARY

Although many lower respiratory diseases can be diagnosed accurately by cytological examination and culture of a transoral tracheal wash sample, bronchoscopy provides additional information on the various disease processes that can result in signs of lower airway disease. Additional training of both veterinarians and technicians is required to ensure the safety of the procedure for the patient and to maintain the equipment; however, the information obtained during bronchoscopy can be invaluable in achieving optimal patient care.

REFERENCES

1. Kirschvink N, Leemans J, Delvaux F, et al: Bronchodilators in bronchoscopy-induced airflow limitation in allergen-sensitized cats, *J Vet Intern Med* 19:161, 2005.
2. Johnson LR, Drazenovich TL: Flexible bronchoscopy in 68 cats: procedure and outcome (2001-2006), *J Vet Intern Med* 21:219, 2007.
3. Hawkins EC, DeNicola DB: Collection of bronchoalveolar lavage fluid in cats using an endotracheal tube, *Am J Vet Res* 50:855, 1989.
4. Caccamo R, Twedt DC, Buracco P, et al: Endoscopic bronchial anatomy in the cat, *J Feline Med Surg* 9:140, 2007.
5. Johnson LR, Drazenovich NL, Foley JE: Maximizing the sensitivity of *Mycoplasma* detection in nasal samples from cats, *J Vet Diagn Invest* 16:347, 2004.
6. Padrid PA, Feldman BF, Funk K, et al: Cytologic, microbiologic, and biochemical analysis of bronchoalveolar lavage fluid obtained from 24 healthy cats, *Am J Vet Res* 52:1300, 1991.
7. Hawkins EC, Stoskopf SK, Levy J, et al: Cytologic characterization of bronchoalveolar lavage fluid collected through an endotracheal tube in cats, *Am J Vet Res* 55:795, 1994.

SECTION
VII

Urinary System

India F. Lane, Section Editor

46 Commercial Pet Food–Related Nephrotoxicity

Joanne R. Smith and Richard E. Goldstein

Potential sites of toxicant introduction during pet food manufacture include contamination of bulk ingredients during growth, harvesting, or storage; incorrect formulation of additives (e.g., vitamin and mineral mix; errors in the manufacturing process; and accidental or malicious contamination of the finished product). Despite the protective measures and protocols to ensure safety of food components and accuracy of recipe preparation, commercial pet food contaminations have the potential for substantial morbidity and mortality, given the large distribution networks of the major pet food manufacturers. Therefore it is essential that every veterinarian can recognize a commercial food contamination and handle the situation promptly and capably. Early identification and proper notification of authorities, appropriate sample collection, and targeted analytical testing may minimize exposure to contaminated pet foods and ultimately reduce the morbidity and mortality of cats.

The kidney has a role in regulating water, electrolyte, osmolality, arterial pressure, and acid-base balance; excretion of metabolic waste products and foreign chemicals; the secretion, metabolism, and excretion of hormones; and gluconeogenesis. Unfortunately, because of the extensive reserve capacity of the kidneys, at least two-thirds of the nephrons must be damaged for this to become apparent clinically or with routine laboratory testing.

ETIOLOGY

Nephrotoxicants typically lead to acute kidney injury (AKI), although affected cats may develop chronic kidney disease (CKD) if they survive the initial episode. Acute injury is defined as a rapid decrease in the glomerular filtration rate (GFR). Acute injury can be classified into prerenal (functional response of structurally normal kidneys to hypoperfusion); intrinsic renal (involving structural damage to the renal parenchyma); or postrenal (urinary tract obstruction) causes. Glomerular, vascular, tubular, or interstitial injury may predominate in intrinsic injury. The kidneys are particularly susceptible to the effects of toxicants (Box 46-1); the organs receive 20 per cent of the cardiac output, and the renal cortex receives 90 per cent of total renal blood flow. Furthermore, their role in excretion means that various substances are concentrated in the kidneys as a result of tubular secretion or reabsorption.[1]

The most common mechanism of nephrotoxic damage is intrinsic renal injury caused by acute tubular necrosis (ATN), which leads to reabsorption of the glomerular filtrate. Other potential mechanisms include tubular epithelial damage and formation of casts with subsequent tubular blockage; renal vasoconstriction and ischemic necrosis; and changes in the glomerular ultrafiltration barrier.[2] In the context of pet food–related nephrotoxicity, recent episodes have included crystal nephropathy and hypercalcemic nephropathy.

PATHOGENESIS

The role of the proximal convoluted tubule (PCT) in concentrating and reabsorbing the glomerular filtrate renders it vulnerable to toxic injury. Cats may be susceptible to ATN because their small size predisposes them to this dose-dependent phenomenon. Toxic ATN may be caused by a wide variety of substances that potentially could contaminate pet foods, including heavy metals, organic solvents, mycotoxins,[3] and multiple classes of drugs.[4] The PCT contains enzymes that bioactivate agents (e.g., cytochrome P450); an increased transport of organic anions, cations, and heavy metals leading to their accumulation; and an increased susceptibility to ischemic injury. Toxins may damage the tubular epithelium by several subcellular mechanisms. The parent compound, or metabolites, may impair the normal function of mitochondria, disrupt lysosomal and cell membranes, shift ion gradients (i.e., intracellular calcium), and lead to free radical formation. Epithelial cells are sloughed into the tubular lumen and contribute to cast formation. The casts then increase intratubular pressure and decrease the GFR.

Box 46-1 Vulnerability of the Kidney to Toxicant Injury

Cardiac output ≈20%
High metabolic activity
Largest endothelial tissue by weight
Multiple enzyme systems
Transcellular transport
Concentration of substances
Protein unbinding
High oxygen consumption/delivery ratio in outer medulla

Loss of the epithelial barrier and the tight junctions between cells can result in back-leakage of the glomerular filtrate and further reduction in the effective GFR.[5]

Crystal nephropathy occurs when compounds precipitate in the intratubular lumen. The concentration of toxic crystals may be exacerbated further in cats with preexisting renal disease, in which remaining functional nephrons undergo compensatory solute diuresis. Crystal formation of specific compounds also is favored in the acidic urine typically produced by cats fed proprietary diets. A recent episode of pet food–related nephrotoxicity was attributed to contamination of wheat gluten, rice protein, and corn gluten with melamine and cyanuric acid.[6,7] It was presumed that melamine was added intentionally to increase the apparent protein content of the food and monetary value of these ingredients; cyanuric acid may have been a co-contaminant because it was used in melamine synthesis. Individually, melamine and cyanuric acid were relatively nontoxic; however, in combination they led to macroscopic and microscopic crystal deposition within the lumen of distal tubules and collecting ducts, severe interstitial edema, and hemorrhage at the corticomedullary junction (Figure 46-1).[8] Exposure to

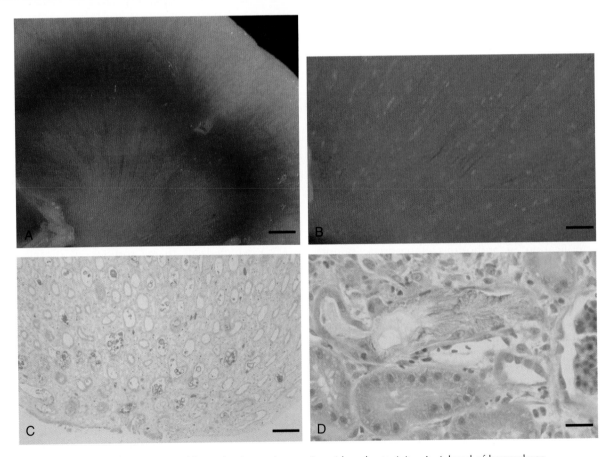

Figure 46-1 Renal lesions caused by melamine and cyanuric acid nephrotoxicity. **A,** A band of hemorrhage obscures the corticomedullary junction. Size bar = 0.3 cm. **B,** Pale yellow crystals seen within the renal medulla. Size bar = 0.1 cm. **C,** Multiple crystals distending the collecting tubules. Hematoxylin and eosin. Size bar = 200 μm. **D,** Fan-shaped crystals within the tubule; the tubular epithelium is attenuated and inflammatory cells are present in the adjacent interstitium. Hematoxylin-eosin. Size bar = 25 μm. (From Puschner B, Poppenga RH, Lowenstine LJ, et al: Assessment of melamine and cyanuric acid toxicity in cats, *J Vet Diagn Invest* 19:620, 2007 with permission.)

a *single* oral dose of melamine and cyanuric acid at dietary concentrations of 2000 mg/kg (0.2 per cent) was sufficient to cause acute renal failure. Concentrations of melamine in contaminated pet food samples ranged from 10 to 3200 mg/kg (0.001 to 0.32 per cent).[8] A survey performed by the American Association of Veterinary Laboratory Diagnosticians found that 347 animals were affected over a 2-month period; sixty-one per cent of the 235 cats died.

A third example of pet food–related nephrotoxicity is hypervitaminosis D and hypercalcemic nephropathy. Hypervitaminosis D may be caused by excess dietary cholecalciferol (vitamin D_3) or ergocalciferol (vitamin D_2). Hypercalcemia results from increases in intestinal absorption, osteoclastic bone resorption, and distal renal tubular reabsorption of calcium. It causes decreased urinary concentrating ability and polyuria by decreasing tubular reabsorption of sodium and by impairing the action of antidiuretic hormone on the tubular cells of the collecting duct. Hypercalcemia may cause azotemia by the following multiple mechanisms: prerenal reduction in extracellular fluid volume (anorexia, hypodipsia, vomiting, and polyuria); renal vasoconstriction caused by ionized hypercalcemia; decreased permeability of the glomerulus; and ATN from the ischemic and toxic effects of hypercalcemia (altered cell permeability and calcium pump activity, decreased cellular membrane permeability production and energy production, and cellular necrosis).[9] CKD may result from the ensuing nephron loss, nephrocalcinosis, tubulointerstitial inflammation, and interstitial fibrosis.[10]

All commercial cat foods provide vitamin D in excess of minimal requirements, and there is no regulated upper limit on the amount of vitamin D that may be included. Cats seem to be relatively resistant to cholecalciferol toxicity when the diet is otherwise complete and balanced; the effects of hypervitaminosis D may be modulated by increased dietary calcium and phosphorus and decreased dietary magnesium.[11] However, hypervitaminosis D in commercial pet foods has resulted in azotemia, nephrocalcinosis, and progressive renal disease and failure in cats.[12-15] Analysis of the diets showed the cholecalciferol concentrations exceeded dietary requirements by 30 to 100 times; renal failure occurred 4 to 14 months later.[13] In 2006, an episode of hypervitaminosis D and hypercalcemic nephropathy occurred after incorrect formulation of a mineral mix; the number of animals affected was not disclosed.[16]

CKD may be associated with long-term exposure to toxins and is mostly related to secondary pathological changes triggered by the initial injury. Different mechanisms are thought to cause the progressive nature of CKD: increases in single-nephron GFR and renal blood flow may promote intraglomerular hyperperfusion and hypertension, and/or systemic hypertension leading to glomerulosclerosis and proteinuria[17]; hypokalemia may cause tubulointerstitial inflammation and interstitial fibrosis nephropathy; and secondary renal hyperparathyroidism may cause nephrocalcinosis. Ultimately, these chronic changes may progress to an end-stage kidney. The initial insult usually is undetermined.

Box 46-2 Possible Risk Factors for Acute Kidney Injury

Preexisting renal disease
Advanced age
Volume depletion
Nephrotoxic drugs (e.g., NSAIDs)
Sepsis
Fever
Hypotension
Decreased cardiac output
Electrolyte imbalance (e.g., hypercalcemia, hypokalemia)
Metabolic acidosis
Trauma
Pigmenturia (e.g., hemoglobinuria)
Diabetes mellitus
Hepatic insufficiency
Vasculitis
Hyperviscosity syndrome
Dietary protein concentration

NSAIDs, Nonsteroidal antiinflammatory drugs.

CLINICAL SIGNS

Clinical signs associated with pet food–related nephrotoxicity depend on the dose of the toxic agent, the presence of associated diseases predisposing to renal injury (Box 46-2), and the severity of AKI. Acute renal dysfunction is characterized by rapid development of depression, anorexia, vomiting, and diarrhea. Nephrotoxicants may cause polyuria (>2 mL/kg/hr), oliguria (<0.27 mL/kg/hr), or anuria (<0.08 mL/kg/hr). Physical examination may demonstrate a good body condition score, dehydration, hypothermia, oral ulceration, uremic breath, tachycardia or bradycardia, and painful renomegaly. Important differential diagnoses for the latter physical findings include ureterolithiasis, renal lymphoma, and other toxicities (e.g., lily intoxication) (Box 46-3).

DIAGNOSIS

Confirming a diagnosis of pet food–related AKI relies initially on a thorough history and an index of suspicion. Geographical or temporal clustering of similar cases within the same household or region is suggestive of exposure to an infectious disease or toxin, although not all animals ingesting the affected diet may be symptomatic. Questions to include in a case history and the collection and handling methods of antemortem and postmortem samples in a case of suspected pet food–related toxicity are shown in Box 46-4.[18,19] The toxicology laboratory should be contacted before submitting samples; the consulting toxicologist will help refine the list of suspected toxins based on the case history, clinical signs, and available laboratory results. Testing then can be prioritized from most to least likely, allowing conservation of valuable tissues. The toxicologist also will be

Box 46-3 Differential Diagnoses For Acute Renal Injury

Common Nephrotoxic Agents	Common Ischemic Events	Other Events
NONTHERAPEUTICS	**SHOCK**	Ureteral obstruction
Heavy metals*	Hypovolemic	Urethral obstruction
Pesticides*	Cardiogenic	Lymphoma
Herbicides*	Distributive	Pyelonephritis
Lilies	Obstructive	Glomerulonephritis (including amyloidosis)
Ethylene glycol		Hypercalcemia
Envenomation	Decreased cardiac output	Systemic immune–mediated disease (e.g.,
Hemoglobin/myoglobin	Trauma	vasculitis secondary to pancreatitis)
	Hypotension	
THERAPEUTICS	Hyperthermia/hypothermia	
Aminoglycosides	Extensive cutaneous burns	
Cephalosporins	Renal vessel thrombosis	
Tetracyclines (outdated)	Hyperviscosity syndromes	
Cisplatin	NSAIDs inhibiting renal prostaglandins	
Acetaminophen		
Aspirin		
Ibuprofen		
Radiographic contrast agents		

NSAIDs, Nonsteroidal antiinflammatory drugs.
*Potential contaminants of bulk ingredients.

Box 46-4 Information Needed in a Case History of Suspected Pet Food Toxicity

- Animal signalment—breed, gender, age, and weight
- Previous medical history and routine medications
- Total number of animals in household/environment
- Number of animals potentially exposed
- Number of animals affected
- Type, chronology, duration, and severity of clinical signs

SPECIFIC INFORMATION TO INCLUDE IN THE FEEDING HISTORY

- Identify all food sources and determine the feeding amounts and availability of unintentional feeding sources.
- Identify the brand and type (dry/moist) of commercial foods, manufacturer, date codes or production lot numbers, and universal product code (UPC) number.
- Determine feeding method such as meal fed or ad lib, how long the food is left in the food bowl, and ambient temperature.
- Determine the length of time the animal has been eating that brand and from that specific container (bag/can) of food, as well as the consumption and palatability.
- Identify the method of pet food storage.

STANDARD ANTEMORTEM AND ENVIRONMENTAL SAMPLES TO COLLECT FOR TOXICOLOGICAL EXAMINATION

- Whole blood (anticoagulated with ethylenediaminetetraacetic acid [EDTA])
- Serum (separate serum before storage; red-top tubes contain zinc stearate)
- Urine
- Stomach contents from vomitus or lavage fluids
- Feces

- Hair
- Food—at least 4 cans or 1 kg dry food
- Water

STANDARD POSTMORTEM TISSUE SAMPLES TO COLLECT FOR TOXICOLOGICAL EXAMINATION

- Kidney and urine
- Liver and bile
- Gastrointestinal contents
- Abdominal fat
- Brain
- Eyeball
- Heart clot blood and serum

PROCEDURE FOR COLLECTION, TRANSFER, AND PRESERVATION OF EVIDENCE*

- Collect, package, and identify all samples.
- Log the time, place, description, and circumstances of all samples. Describe in detail how the samples were identified, processed, packaged, stored, and shipped.
- Log who has custody of any sample(s) and transfers of any sample(s).
- If possible, photograph any abnormalities (e.g., mold growth or foreign objects in the food), number these photographs consecutively, and describe each one in the written notes.
- Retain and store all relevant product labels in a safe place.
- Notify the diagnostic laboratory of the possibility of litigation.
- Use a shipping method that expedites delivery of samples to the laboratory; keep copies of shipping records and receipts of delivery.

*See Chapter 73 in the fifth volume of this series for recommendations about proper forensic procedures.

able to provide realistic time frames and the limitations of available tests and screens.

Multiple, duplicate food samples should be collected from different portions of the package or can for testing by an independent diagnostic laboratory and/or manufacturer. It is essential that the date codes or production lot numbers and the universal product code (barcode) number of the food are recorded whenever possible. Antemortem samples, including food, should be refrigerated and/or frozen in separate air-tight containers. Ideally, postmortem sampling should be performed by a board-certified pathologist; however, this may be unfeasible because of the distance to a diagnostic laboratory and financial constraints. Adequate amounts of appropriate tissues must be collected, properly stored, and labeled with the animal identification and owner's name, date of collection, and type of tissue. Samples for toxicological testing should be as large as possible and refrigerated or frozen. Formalin-fixed tissues are unsuitable for toxicological testing, but they should be collected for histopathological examination and sectioned and placed in an adequate volume of formalin (one part tissue to nine parts formalin). In addition to a log of the samples, case details, and communications, photographs of abnormal foodstuffs or postmortem lesions may be useful to the toxicologist. All samples should be triple-bagged and shipped as quickly as possible on ice or dry ice. Shipping should be avoided on weekends and holidays so that the samples do not sit for prolonged periods in warm conditions.

For cats who have ingested sufficient toxin to cause AKI, diagnosis of this condition is seldom a challenge. A complete blood count may show increased packed-cell volume and total protein caused by hemoconcentration or anemia, if gastrointestinal bleeding is present. Serum biochemistry findings include azotemia, hyperphosphatemia, hyperkalemia, and metabolic acidosis. Other variables that may be increased secondary to a decreased GFR include amylase and lipase. Urinalysis should allow differentiation of prerenal and renal azotemia based on the urine specific gravity. Glycosuria is consistent with tubular damage, stress hyperglycemia, or rarely, primary renal glycosuria. Findings on urinary sediment examination that indicate tubular damage include cylindruria, proteinuria, and pyuria. Crystalluria may be present; bacteriuria would be more consistent with pyelonephritis. Measurement of enzymuria, specifically the urinary γ-glutamyl transpeptidase:creatinine ratio, is one of the most sensitive methods for detection of early injury.[20]

Abdominal imaging (survey radiographs and ultrasound) may provide evidence of gross renal pathology (e.g., renal enlargement or distortion, parenchymal change, pyelectasia, and perirenal effusion). Imaging also permits exclusion of other insults, particularly obstructive urolithiasis. Excretory urography will not differentiate between filtration failure as a result of intrinsic renal injury or backpressure from ureteral obstruction; however, antegrade contrast nephropyelography (with direct injection of contrast into the renal pelvis) or contrast-enhanced computed tomography (CT) may confirm urolithiasis and may avoid the risk of contrast-induced nephropathy. To minimize further possible ischemic insult to the kidneys,

general anesthesia should be avoided until the patient is stabilized. Renal cytological examination may help to exclude lymphoma. Renal biopsy may help confirm the etiology but seldom gives prognostic information in AKI. The most common complication of renal biopsy is severe hemorrhage, so a coagulation profile always should be performed before the biopsy, although severe azotemia and improper technique also may influence the likelihood of postbiopsy hemorrhage.[21]

During a confirmed episode of pet food–related nephrotoxicity, potential cases should be screened using a complete history, with specific attention paid to the type and amount of diet consumed and water intake and urine output; physical examination; and the biochemistry profile and urinalysis (to include urine specific gravity and sediment examination). Unfortunately, an increase in serum creatinine always lags behind a reduction in GFR. Decreased creatinine clearance is an early marker of reduced renal function, and reliable estimations of GFR can be made from urine collections obtained over as little as 2 hours[22] or even 20 to 30 minutes,[23] rather than the traditional 24 hours. As previously mentioned, urinary enzymuria currently is the most sensitive test for renal tubular damage and may prove more practical; other biomarkers of early AKI have yet to be validated in cats.[24]

TREATMENT

A detailed discussion of treatment for acute azotemia is beyond the scope of this chapter. The goals of therapy are the prevention of further complications of renal failure, restoration of kidney function (if possible), and prevention of additional renal injury. Patient survival depends on meticulous patient monitoring in combination with appropriate diagnostic and therapeutic intervention to allow time for renal recovery in those patients most likely to survive.

Commonly recognized phases of acute intrinsic renal failure include initiation, extension, maintenance, and recovery.[25] The initiation phase occurs with exposure to the toxin and develops within minutes to hours. Extension occurs during the response to injury and subsequent renal damage that exacerbates the response to the initial insult; this occurs over hours to days. The maintenance phase consists of established tubular lesions and nephron dysfunction. The recovery phase occurs with nephron repair, for example, reestablishment of tubular epithelium, with compensatory hypertrophy of the remaining nephrons, occurring typically over weeks to months after establishment of renal failure. Initiation and extension represent the time during which damage might be prevented, discontinued, or minimized to alter the outcome of the acute insult. However, many patients present at the end of the initiation/extension phases or during the maintenance phase. Therapeutic intervention during the maintenance phase typically is ineffective in reducing existing renal lesions or improving renal dysfunction; however, it may permit the patient to live long enough to survive the reversible renal injury. Any initial improvement probably reflects correction of prerenal azotemia and not renal recovery. Even with incomplete renal functional recovery, sufficient renal function may be restored to allow a good quality of life. Mortality in AKI occurs when the patient succumbs from the consequences of acute uremia before recovery of the renal lesions could occur or when the renal damage was sufficiently severe to be irreversible. (See Chapter 48 for more information about recovery and survival from renal failure in cats.)

Some general guidelines for treatment of acute azotemia follow. Most cats with AKI are volume-depleted because of gastrointestinal fluid loss, in addition to the loss of urine-concentrating ability. Replacement of these losses corrects the prerenal component and protects against any additional ischemic renal tubular damage. The goal of fluid therapy is to correct water and solute imbalances. Parameters of volume status (skin turgor, mucous membrane moistness) and body weight should be evaluated at least q12h. Placement of a temporary indwelling, closed urinary catheter allows monitoring of hourly urine output. Using aseptic technique to withdraw urine from an injection port that caps the catheter facilitates quantification of small volumes of urine (as opposed to a long collection system). Strict asepsis at placement and routine maintenance (swabbing the exposed catheter with chlorhexidine tincture q8h) to avoid contamination is essential. Urine should be cultured q72h, and concurrent use of antibiotics should be avoided when the cat is catheterized to minimize selection for bacterial resistance. For nonrecumbent cats or those with polyuria, use of a preweighed litter tray or absorbent pads or nonabsorbent litter are alternate means of allowing quantification of urine output to guide fluid therapy. Caution is warranted to avoid acute volume overload, particularly in cats with azotemia and oliguric/anuric AKI. Chemosis, a nasal drip, and development of a gallop rhythm typically occur before pulmonary effusion or edema. The treatment for fluid overload is to supply only insensible losses (10 mL/kg/day); the extra fluid must be removed by dialysis because diuretics will only work if the kidneys can function. Additional conventional (nondialysis) therapy may be directed toward specific, expected metabolic and physiological derangements (e.g., hyperkalemia, metabolic acidosis, and hypertension). Pain management, antiemetic therapy, and aggressive nutritional support also are key components of overall patient management (see Chapters 12 and 21). Serial evaluation of physiological and biochemical parameters provides valuable information on the adequacy of management and evolution of disease.

More advanced renal replacement therapies, including peritoneal dialysis and hemodialysis, do allow for rapid correction of hydration and metabolic disturbances. Dialysis can remove nephrotoxins and therefore does have a direct effect on renal recovery, in addition to the indirect benefit of stabilization and improved clinical and nutritional status.[26] Although the availability of hemodialysis is limited, early referral of potential candidates is recommended to avoid the major costs and frustrations of restabilizing cats with AKI. Referral for dialytic therapy should be considered for acutely uremic patients who do not respond within 12 to 24 hours of appropriate and aggressive medical management and when it is a logistic option for clients. Clients need to be emotionally and financially prepared to undertake 2 to 4 weeks of dialytic therapy; 7 to 14 days is the earliest to expect resumption of renal function, although some patients may take months to recover. Alternatively, dialysis may be used to prepare a cat for renal transplantation.

Newer experimental therapies have shown benefit in improving renal recovery and tubular regeneration; however, they typically need to be administered before or with the insult.[27] Use of growth factors, free radical scavengers, or cytokine scavengers has not improved recovery once renal disease has been established. Treatment and monitoring of CKD also is beyond the scope of this chapter, but recent literature reviews and websites are available (see also Chapter 47).[28-30]

PROGNOSIS

The mortality rate for human beings with AKI is approximately 50 per cent, despite the availability of dialysis.[31] In a retrospective study of 32 cats with all types of AKI, 16 per cent died, 31 per cent were euthanized, 25 per cent had resolution of their azotemia, and 28 per cent were discharged with persistent azotemia.[32] This case series was divided into two groups: cats whose AKI was caused by nephrotoxicants (n = 18, or 56 per cent) and cats who suffered from all other causes (n = 14, or 44 per cent). Nine cats in the nephrotoxicant group survived, whereas eight cats in the "other causes" category survived. The nephrotoxicant group had a median survival time of 28 days, whereas the other group had a median survival time of 60 days. However, there was no statistical difference in survival times between the two groups. Urine production was a prognostic factor; all the cats who died were oliguric or anuric. For each unit (mEq/L) increase in the initial potassium concentration there was a 57 per cent decrease in survival. Additionally, hypoalbuminemia and acidosis at the time of presentation were negative prognostic indicators; initial concentrations of blood urea nitrogen and serum creatinine were not negative prognostic indicators[32] (see also Chapter 48).

CONTROL AND PREVENTION

Commercial pet food manufacturing techniques, such as extrusion and retorting, produce sufficient heat to destroy many pathogens and heat-labile toxins.[33] Proper warehousing and improved packaging materials (e.g., antioxidant-impregnated bags) help protect raw ingredients and finished products from moisture, contamination, and degradation during storage. Manufacturers use sensitive analytical methods to verify that separate components (bulk ingredients and vitamin/mineral formulations) and final products are free from contaminants. Palatability testing of pet foods also may indicate contamination or incorrect formulation.

Pet food and individual pet food ingredients are regulated by multiple governmental agencies in the United States. The Food and Drug Administration (FDA) legislates against toxins that might adulterate pet foods and also controls the permitted drug levels in pet food ingre-

Table 46-1 Websites in the United States to Use in a Case of Suspected Pet-Food Toxicity

Institution	Website
American Animal Hospital Association	www.aahanet.org
American Association of Veterinary Laboratory Diagnosticians	www.aavld.org
American College of Veterinary Internal Medicine	www.acvim.org
American College of Veterinary Pathologists	www.acvp.org
American Veterinary Medical Association	www.avma.org
Food and Drug Administration (FDA)	www.fda.gov
FDA Animal Food Safety System	www.fda.gov/cvm/AFSS.htm
FDA Center for Veterinary Medicine	www.fda.gov/cvm/default.html
FDA Center for Veterinary Medicine: Pet Foods	http://www.fda.gov/cvm/petfoods.htm#PetFoodContamination
FDA State Consumer Complaint Officer	www.fda.gov/opacom/backgrounders/complain.html
State Veterinary Associations	www.avma.org/statevma/
Veterinary Information Network	www.vin.com

dients in conjunction with the Association of American Feed Control Officials (AAFCO). The Environmental Protection Agency (EPA) established pesticide tolerances for animal commodities that are enforced jointly by the U.S. Department of Agriculture (USDA) and the FDA. Homeland Security legislation now dictates that each unit of pet food must be trackable from the manufacturer to the point of retail sale. This process makes prompt recall of specific, affected pet foods more feasible. Recent episodes of pet food contamination have exerted pressure to introduce legislation to improve regulatory oversight of pet foods. The American Association of Veterinary Laboratory Diagnosticians has proposed the formation of a National Animal Health Laboratory Veterinary Analytical Toxicology Response and Surveillance System. This central reporting system may use a network of sentinel veterinary hospitals for reporting and surveillance of animal health problems.[34]

In the United States, information about ongoing suspected pet food–related toxicities may be found on websites of the FDA; national, state, regional, or local veterinary associations; veterinary diagnostic laboratories[35]; colleges and schools of veterinary medicine and veterinary specialty college associations; pet food manufacturers; and media outlets (Table 46-1). Professional electronic mailing lists and consulting sites also have facilitated rapid flow of information (and sometimes misinformation) to veterinary practitioners. Generation of a hypothetical toxicant is based on toxins known to cause the clinical findings and appropriate documentation from toxicological testing of blood or tissues from affected cats. Once a toxin is identified, confirmation testing of the suspected food should be performed to establish a causal relationship.

Veterinarians who suspect a pet food contamination should contact the product manufacturer and their state FDA consumer complaint officer immediately[36]; there is no need to wait for results of laboratory testing to make the initial report. Accurate and thorough record-keeping in the veterinary hospital is essential. Attending veteri-

narians also should obtain written client authorization before release of specific medical information.

The FDA and manufacturer should perform additional testing to determine whether a product recall is warranted, and the media should be contacted to disseminate information about the potential contamination to consumers and the veterinary community. Recall procedures, recommendations for reporting potential cases, appropriate screening tests, and prophylactic and specific treatments need to be communicated promptly to minimize additional exposure and prevent unnecessary alarm. Current events suggest that additional foodborne toxicity or illness is likely in pet populations. Pet food retailers and veterinarians should educate pet owners to become aware of their pet's feeding practices. Pet owners should save pet food packaging and product labels, as well as samples of any food that appears suspect.

REFERENCES

1. Stokes JE, Bartges JW: Causes of acute renal failure, *Compend Contin Educ Pract Vet* 28:387, 2006.
2. Sebastian MM, Baskin SI, Czerwinski SE: Renal toxicity. In Gupta RC, editor: *Veterinary toxicology*, ed 1, New York, 2007, Elsevier, p 161.
3. Boermans HJ, Leung MCK: Mycotoxins and the pet food industry: toxicological evidence and risk assessment, *Int J Food Microbiol* 119:95, 2007.
4. Markowitz GS, Perazella MA: Drug-induced renal failure: a focus on tubulointerstitial disease, *Clinica Chimica Acta* 351:31, 2005.
5. Thadhani R, Pascual M, Bonventre JV: Acute renal failure, *New Engl J Med* 334:1448, 1996.
6. Jeong WI, Do SH, Jeong DH, et al: Canine renal failure syndrome in three dogs, *J Vet Sci* 7:299, 2006.
7. Brown CA, Jeong K-S, Poppenga RH, et al: Outbreaks of renal failure associated with melamine and cyanuric acid in dogs and cats in 2004 and 2007, *J Vet Diagn Invest* 19:525, 2007.
8. Puschner B, Poppenga RH, Lowenstine LJ, et al: Assessment of melamine and cyanuric acid toxicity in cats, *J Vet Diagn Invest* 19:616, 2007.

9. Morrow CM: Cholecalciferol poisoning, *Vet Med* December:905, 2001.

10. Schenk PA, Chew DJ, Nagode LA, et al: Disorders of calcium: hypercalcemia and hypocalcemia. In DiBartola S, editor: *Fluid, electrolyte, and acid-base disorders in small animal practice*, ed 3, St. Louis, 2006, Saunders Elsevier, p 122.

11. Sih TR, Morris JG, Hickman MA: Chronic ingestion of high concentrations of cholecalciferol in cats, *Am J Vet Res* 62:1500, 2001.

12. Haruna A, Kawai K, Takab T, et al: Dietary calcinosis in the cat, *J Anim Clin Res Found* 1:9, 1992.

13. Sato R, Yamagishi H, Naito Y, et al: Feline vitamin D toxicosis caused by commercially available cat food, *J Jpn Vet Med Assoc* 46:577, 1993.

14. Morita T, Awakura T, Shimada A, et al: Vitamin D toxicosis in cats: natural outbreak and experimental study, *J Vet Med Sci* 57:831, 1995.

15. Morris JG: Vitamin D synthesis by kittens, *Vet Clin Nutr* 3:88, 1996.

16. Elliott DA: *Product quality notice.* February 2, 2006, St. Charles, MO, 2006, Royal Canin USA Inc.

17. Brunker J: Protein-losing nephropathy, *Compend Contin Educ Pract Vet* 27:686, 2005.

18. Volmer PA, Meerdink GL: Diagnostic toxicology for the small animal practitioner, *Vet Clin North Am Small Anim Pract* 32:357, 2002.

19. Stenske KA, Smith, JR, Newman SJ, et al: Aflatoxicosis in dogs and dealing with suspected contaminated commercial foods, *J Am Vet Med Assoc* 228:1686, 2006.

20. Stockham SL, Scott MA: Enzymes. In Stockham SL, Scott MA, editors: *Fundamentals of veterinary clinical pathology*, ed 2, Ames, 2008, Blackwell, p 639.

21. Vaden S, Levine JF, Lees GE, et al: Renal biopsy: a retrospective study of methods and complications in 283 dogs and 65 cats, *J Vet Intern Med* 19:795, 2005.

22. Herrera-Gutierrez ME, Seller-Perez G, Banderas-Bravo E, et al: Replacement of 24-hour creatinine clearance by 2-hour creatinine clearance in intensive care units: a single center study, *Intensive Care Med* 33:1900, 2007.

23. Francey T: The specialist's approach to acute renal failure. Proceedings of the 17th ECVIM-CA Congress, Budapest, Hungary, 2007.

24. Honore PM, Joannes-Boyau O, Boer W: The early biomarker of acute kidney injury: in search of the Holy Grail, *Intensive Care Med* 33:1866, 2007.

25. Cowgill LD, Francey T: Acute uremia. In Ettinger SJ, Feldman EC, editors: *Textbook of veterinary internal medicine*, ed 6, St. Louis, 2005, Elsevier Saunders, p 1731.

26. Fischer JR, Pantaleo V, Francey T, et al: Veterinary hemodialysis: advances in management and technology, *Vet Clin North Am Small Anim Pract* 34:935, 2004.

27. Devarajan P: Cellular and molecular derangements in acute tubular necrosis, *Curr Opin Pediatr* 17:193, 2005.

28. May SN, Langston CE: Managing chronic renal failure, *Compend Contin Educ Pract Vet* 28:853, 2006.

29. Plotnik A: Feline chronic renal failure: long-term medical management, *Compend Contin Educ Pract Vet* 29:342, 2007.

30. *www.iris.com.* Accessed on June 10th, 2008.

31. Ympa YP, Sakr Y, Reinhart K, et al: Has mortality from acute renal failure decreased? A systematic review of the literature, *Am J Med* 118:827, 2005.

32. Worwag S, Langston C: Acute intrinsic renal failure in cats: 32 cases (1997-2004), *J Am Vet Med Assoc* 232:728, 2008.

33. Miller EP, Cullor JS: Food safety. In Hand MS, Thatcher CD, Remillard RL, editors: *Small animal clinical nutrition*, ed 4, Topeka, KA, 2000, Mark Morris Institute, p 183.

34. Burns K: Researchers examine contaminant in food, deaths of pets, *J Am Vet Med Assoc* 231:1636, 2007.

35. AAVLD Protocol for Suspected Pet Food Associated Nephrotoxicity: http://data.memberclicks.com/site/aavld/Protocol_Suspected_Pet_Food_Toxicity.pdf. Accessed June 10th, 2008.

36. FDA http://www.fda.gov/cvm/Documents/Pet_Food_Contamination.pdf. Accessed June 10th, 2008.

CHAPTER
47 Linking Treatment to Staging in Chronic Kidney Disease

Scott A. Brown

The International Renal Interest Society (IRIS) has proposed that the terms *chronic renal failure* and *chronic renal insufficiency* be replaced by *chronic kidney disease* (CKD) and that a staging system be used to facilitate the management of feline patients with CKD.[1] This classification scheme is based on a two-step process: (1) establish a diagnosis of CKD and (2) establish the stage of the disease. Stage of disease also can be linked to prognosis,[2] diagnostic approach, and treatment recommendations (Figure 47-1).[1]

The term CKD refers to any disease process in which there is a loss of renal function due to a prolonged (generally >2 months in duration) and, usually, progressive process. CKD generally will produce dramatic changes in renal structure as well, although the correlation between structural and functional changes in the kidney is imprecise. This is partly because of the tremendous renal functional reserve that allows cats to appear healthy for long periods of time with only a small fraction of initial renal tissue, perhaps less than 10 per cent. Thus a CKD often "smolders" for many months or years before becoming clinically apparent.

Most feline CKD is not reversible, and once acquired, rarely resolves. Although congenital disease causes a transient increase in incidence of CKD in cats less than 3 years of age, the prevalence of CKD increases with advancing age from 5 to 6 years upward. In aged populations at referral institutions, CKD affects up to 35 per cent of cats.[3,4] A reasonable estimate of the prevalence of CKD in the general feline population is 1 to 3 per cent.

ESTABLISHING A DIAGNOSIS OF CHRONIC KIDNEY DISEASE

The first step in the IRIS staging scheme is to establish a diagnosis of CKD. Any disease that affects the kidney of a cat is likely to alter both renal structure and function. It is the adequacy of renal function, however, that dictates the impact of this disease on the patient. Although the kidney has many biological functions of importance to a cat, the most basic and central renal function is filtration; the glomerular filtration rate (GFR) serves as the "gold standard" for assessment of kidney function in cats. It is generally fair to assume that changes in the level of most renal functions parallel changes in GFR in a clinical patient.

Confirmation of a reduced GFR is a highly reliable indicator of renal dysfunction, although it must be remembered that reductions of GFR (and elevations of serum creatinine) can be caused by renal, prerenal, and postrenal factors and that renal function may be lost due to acute kidney injury (also known as acute renal failure) or CKD. In the research laboratory, GFR is assessed as urinary clearance of marker substances, such as inulin or creatinine. In clinical patients, urinary clearance tests

475

Figure 47-1 Diagnostic and therapeutic emphases in different stages of feline chronic kidney disease (CKD). Once a diagnosis of CKD is established, the International Renal Interest Society (IRIS) recommends staging the disease on the basis of a measurement of serum creatinine concentration (Cr) in a cat that is hydrated with stable renal function. There are three sets of linked diagnostic and therapeutic considerations, with the importance of each set reflected by the thickness of the corresponding arrow in the diagram. See text for further details.

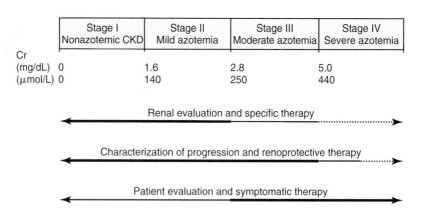

	Stage I Nonazotemic CKD	Stage II Mild azotemia	Stage III Moderate azotemia	Stage IV Severe azotemia
Cr (mg/dL)	0	1.6	2.8	5.0
(μmol/L)	0	140	250	440

Renal evaluation and specific therapy

Characterization of progression and renoprotective therapy

Patient evaluation and symptomatic therapy

Box 47-1 Establishing a Diagnosis of Renal Disease*

FINDINGS THAT ESTABLISH THE PRESENCE OF A RENAL DISEASE

Renal azotemia
Renal structural changes
Renal infection

FINDINGS SUGGESTIVE OF THE PRESENCE OF A RENAL DISEASE

Serial increases of serum creatinine concentration within normal range
Otherwise unexplained low urine specific gravity (<1.035)
Persistent renal proteinuria

*Distinguishing acute kidney injury (acute renal failure) from chronic kidney disease (CKD) generally is based on disease duration, with CKD being any renal disease present for 2 months or longer.

---

generally are not practical; however, the measurement of the disappearance from plasma of renally cleared marker substances such as creatinine, inulin, iohexol, or diethylenetriamine pentaacetic acid (DTPA), following intravenous administration, can provide an approximation of GFR.[5-9]

The IRIS recommendations recognize that in most clinical patients, GFR is assessed by the measurement of plasma or serum concentrations of creatinine (Cr) and/or blood urea nitrogen (BUN). The BUN is affected by several nonrenal factors, such as protein intake, liver function, and urine flow rate, making Cr a better index of GFR. Classically, CKD in cats was diagnosed (Box 47-1) as the presence of renal azotemia (elevated Cr) accompanied by low urine specific gravity (USG) (<1.035). The wide reference range for Cr has led to the oversimplified assertion that 75 per cent of nephrons must be destroyed before Cr (and BUN) rises out of the range. Unfortunately, although valid, these diagnostic criteria are insensitive, often failing to identify CKD until dramatic loss of functional renal mass has occurred. However, any structural damage that reduces GFR almost always will be reflected as an increase in Cr (or BUN), initially within the normal range. The IRIS recommends that serial measurements of Cr be interpreted with this relationship in mind, noting

that increases in Cr, even within the normal range, suggest a declining GFR and the presence of a renal disease.

Structural changes appreciated by palpation, radiography, ultrasonography, or histopathological examination generally are diagnostic of renal disease. In early feline CKD, when azotemia and clinical signs are absent, renal disease sometimes is discovered inadvertently as a result of imaging studies, laparotomy, or urinalyses conducted for other purposes.

The urinalysis may provide clues to the presence of a renal disease. A urinary tract infection localized to the kidney is one example. A potentially useful early indicator of the presence of CKD is a USG lower than 1.035 despite dehydration. Cats with early CKD often have a USG lower than 1.020. However, cats with early CKD, and some with CKD of any severity, may retain the ability to concentrate urine to a specific gravity greater than 1.035. Although USG is a simple and readily available test, interpretation of a low USG can be complicated by the presence of conditions that lead to retention of solute in tubular fluid (e.g., diuretic administration and diabetes mellitus), central diabetes insipidus, and nephrogenic diabetes insipidus (e.g., hyperadrenocorticism, hypercalcemia, and diseases causing septicemia).

Recently, tests for identification of proteinuria in cats that are both sensitive and specific have been developed.[10] These include the protein-creatinine ratio (UPC) and feline-specific albuminuria tests. The ability to identify persistent renal proteinuria with these tests offers promise for identifying early CKD.[10] The presence of persistent renal proteinuria in a cat is suggestive of renal disease.

Distinguishing acute kidney injury (AKI) from CKD is, in ideal circumstances, based on knowledge of disease duration, with CKD generally being defined as any renal disease that is present for 2 months or longer. History, physical examination, complete blood count, and renal imaging studies also are useful in distinguishing AKI and CKD. Although AKI may progress to CKD, it is generally identified soon (less than 2 weeks) after the insult. Staging and management of AKI and CKD differ; this chapter addresses the latter. Some findings that are suggestive of CKD, such as the presence of renal osteodystrophy and anemia, may assist in establishing a diagnosis of CKD but generally are not useful for identifying the presence of an otherwise masked case of CKD.

INITIAL EVALUATION OF CATS WITH CHRONIC KIDNEY DISEASE

For all patients with CKD, a thorough history and physical examination should be accompanied by complete clinical pathology testing, which includes a serum biochemical panel, hematology, and urinalysis with specific proteinuria tests and aerobic bacterial culture. Survey radiography, abdominal ultrasonography when available, and blood pressure measurements also should be performed (see Chapter 49). This initial battery of tests (best conducted while the disease is stable) allows the veterinarian to stage the disease and to choose proper therapeutic and diagnostic strategies.

STAGING OF CHRONIC KIDNEY DISEASE

CKD in cats often progresses along a continuum from an initial nonazotemic stage to end-stage uremia. In many cats with CKD, the rate of progression is remarkably slow. As veterinarians, we are obligated to address the specific problems and patient needs that characterize the animal's disease, and these vary from stage to stage. Staging of an animal with an established diagnosis of CKD is based on measurement of Cr in a well-hydrated patient with stable renal function (Table 47-1).[1] This classification system employs four stages: Stage I: nonazotemic CKD disease; Stage II: mild renal azotemia; Stage III: moderate renal azotemia; and Stage IV: severe renal azotemia.

SUBSTAGING CHRONIC KIDNEY DISEASE ON BASIS OF BLOOD PRESSURE

Cats with CKD frequently exhibit elevations of systemic arterial blood pressure (BP)[11] (see Chapter 49). The American College of Veterinary Internal Medicine Consensus Statement[11] and IRIS[1] define systemic hypertension as any elevation of BP that leads to target-organ damage (TOD) and defined blood pressure ranges associated with minimal, low, moderate, and severe risk of TOD (Table 47-2). The target organs of concern in cats are the kidneys (TOD: progression of CKD, proteinuria); eyes (TOD: blindness, intraocular hemorrhage, retinal detachment, retinal vessel tortuosity); brain (TOD: seizures, depression); and cardiovascular system (TOD: congestive heart failure, vessel rupture). Left ventricular hypertrophy (LVH) is observed commonly in hypertensive cats, although there is controversy as to whether this constitutes true TOD or is simply an adaptive change. Nonetheless, the presence of LVH in a cat with CKD should be taken as presumptive evidence of clinically significant hypertension unless proven otherwise. The IRIS recommends that BP be measured using a device and method individualized for each clinical practice in every cat with CKD and that target organs be evaluated carefully for the presence of TOD, which is referred to as a complication. Although some devices provide both systolic and diastolic BP, staging most often is done on the basis of systolic BP measurements; recent evidence suggests that systolic hypertension is the most important determinant of TOD in other species.[11] Additional information about

Table 47-1 IRIS* Staging of Feline Chronic Kidney Disease (CKD)

Stage	I: Nonazotemic CKD	II: Mild Renal Azotemia CKD	III: Moderate Renal Azotemia CKD	IV: Severe Renal Azotemia CKD
Creatinine:				
(µmol/L)	<140	140-250	251-440	>440
(mg/dL)	<1.6	1.6-2.8	2.9-5.0	>5.0

*IRIS: International Renal Interest Society

Table 47-2 Blood Pressure: Substaging of Feline Chronic Kidney Disease (CKD)

	Risk of Future Target Organ Damage*			
	Minimal or No Risk (N)	Low Risk (L)	Moderate Risk (M)	High Risk (H)
BLOOD PRESSURE (mm Hg)				
Systolic	<150	150-159	160-179	≥180
Diastolic	<95	95-99	100-119	≥120
SUBSTAGE				
No complications present†	Nnc	Lnc	Mnc	Hnc
Complications present	Nc	Lc	Mc	Hc

*If blood pressure is not measured, the patient is classified as risk not determined (RND).
†Complications include any evidence of target organ damage in eyes (e.g., intraocular hemorrhage or retinal detachment), central nervous system (e.g., seizures or profound otherwise unexplained depression), cardiovascular system (e.g., congestive heart failure), or kidneys (e.g., proteinuria).

Table 47-3 Proteinuria: Substaging of Feline Chronic Kidney Disease (CKD)

Substage	Nonproteinuric (NP)	Borderline Proteinuric (BP)	Proteinuric (P)
Urine protein-to-creatinine ratio	<0.2	0.2-0.4	>0.4

blood pressure measurement and feline hypertension can be found in Chapter 49.

SUBSTAGING CHRONIC KIDNEY DISEASE ON BASIS OF PROTEINURIA

Recent findings have suggested that renal protein leak is not only a marker of severity of renal disease but also of prognosis; proteinuria itself potentially is a cause of renal injury.[10,12] We now recognize that proteinuria is associated with increased risk of developing end-stage CKD in cats[12] and that there is an increased risk of mortality in aged cats when proteinuria is present. Further, studies have shown that therapies that reduce the magnitude of proteinuria are often renoprotective.

Proper substaging based on proteinuria mandates following a multistep paradigm (Table 47-3).[1,10] A positive finding of proteinuria in a urinalysis with routine dipstick evaluation should trigger further investigation. Because of frequent false positives and postrenal causes of proteinuria, a positive dipstick reaction should lead the clinician to carefully evaluate the urine sediment findings to determine if inflammation or infection may be the cause. The result should be confirmed by a more specific test for proteinuria, such as a sulfosalicylic acid test, measurement of the UPC, or assessment of albuminuria. It is important to localize the source of the protein as prerenal, postrenal, or renal. When monitoring a feline patient with renal proteinuria, it is important to determine if the proteinuria is transient or persistent (at least two tests at 2-week intervals). If persistent renal proteinuria is present in a patient with CKD, further management generally is based on the UPC.

RENAL EVALUATION AND SPECIFIC THERAPY

Every CKD is caused by a primary renal disease. In cats with early CKD (stages I and II), identification of the primary renal disease is an important focus (see Figure 47-1). Examples of renal evaluation that may be appropriate at these early stages include renal imaging (survey with or without contrast radiographic studies, ultrasonography), urinalysis with specific tests for proteinuria and urine culture, and renal biopsy. Known causes of CKD that may be diagnosed through this approach include diseases of the macrovascular compartment (e.g., systemic hypertension, coagulopathies, chronic hypoperfusion), microvascular compartment (e.g., systemic and glomerular hypertension, glomerulonephritis, developmental disorders, congenital collagen defects, amyloidosis), interstitial compartment (e.g., pyelonephritis, neoplasia, neoplastic, obstructive uropathy, allergic and immune-mediated nephritis), and tubular compartment (e.g., tubular reabsorptive defects, chronic low-grade nephrotoxicity, obstructive uropathy). These conditions may be acquired or heritable. A variety of breeds are afflicted with heritable CKD that may give rise to pathognomonic clinical and histopathological findings, including the Abyssinian (medullary amyloidosis) and Persian (polycystic kidney disease) cats.

Specific therapy is defined as a treatment that is directed at elimination of the primary renal disease. The goal of specific therapy is to reduce injury caused by the primary renal disease in order to prevent progression of CKD to the later stages. Examples of specific therapy (Table 47-4) include antibiotic therapy in cases of pyelonephritis, antihypertensive medications for cats with hypertensive nephropathy, dietary calcium restriction for animals with hypercalcemic nephropathy, immunosuppressive drugs for immune complex glomerulonephritis, and surgery for obstructive uropathy.

Interstitial fibrosis and alterations in renal shape and size occur in most patients with stage III and IV CKD, regardless of inciting primary renal disease. The severity of interstitial fibrosis is correlated positively with the magnitude of decline in GFR and correlated negatively with prognosis. Chronic interstitial nephritis, also known as *chronic tubulointerstitial fibrosis,* describes the morphological appearance of kidneys with stage III or IV CKD of any cause; invasive renal evaluation (e.g., biopsy) at these stages is unlikely to yield clues as to the identity of the primary disease. Consequently, for cats in stages III and IV, renal evaluation and specific therapy are a lower priority.

EVALUATION OF PROGRESSION AND RENOPROTECTIVE THERAPY

A critical consideration in the treatment of cats with CKD is the progressive nature of the disease. Because effective therapy for end-stage uremia (i.e., intensive fluid therapy, renal transplantation, and/or dialysis) often is prohibitively expensive, a goal of management is to prevent progression of CKD to end-stage failure. There are several reasons that renal function will deteriorate progressively in an animal with CKD. As outlined above, in treating cats in stage I and early stage II, it is important to use a specific therapy to minimize renal damage that occurs as a manifestation of the primary renal disease process. However, in stages II to IV there are two additional general processes that contribute to progressive destruction of renal tissue in the middle stages of CKD: (1) abnormalities caused by a disruption of renal homeostatic mechanisms (e.g., complications of kidney disease such as systemic hypertension and hyperphosphatemia); and (2) maladaptive changes in remnant renal tissue (e.g., glomerular hypertension). These two processes lead to a vicious cycle of self-perpetuating renal injury referred to as *inherent progression.* Therapeutic intervention can

Table 47-4 Diagnostic and Therapeutic Focus of Staged Management of Feline Chronic Kidney Disease (CKD)

Process	Primary Focus in Stage(s)	Diagnostic Assessment	Therapeutic Considerations
Primary renal disease	I-II	**Renal Evaluation** Renal palpation Radiography Ultrasonography Urinalysis Renal biopsy	**Specific Therapy (Examples)** Antibiotics for pyelonephritis Antihypertensive drugs for hypertensive nephropathy Immunosuppressive drugs for immune complex glomerulonephritis
Progressive loss of kidney function	II-III	**Evaluation of Progression** Serial measurements of creatinine	**Renoprotective Therapies** Dietary phosphorus restriction, intestinal phosphorus binders Antihypertensive therapy (see below) Antiproteinuric therapy Dietary n-3 PUFA supplementation Calcitriol (2.5-3.5 ng/kg PO q24h)
Uremia	III-IV	**Patient Evaluation** History Physical examination Body condition scoring Hematology Serum biochemical panel Urinalysis Urine culture	**Symptomatic Therapies** Renal diet formulated for feline renal disease Manage acid-base and electrolyte disorders Antiemetics Erythropoietin Fluid therapy Calcitriol (2.5-3.5 ng/kg PO q24h) Treat postrenal factors, such as uroliths, when identified Feeding tube placement Renal replacement therapy
Elevated blood pressure	I-IV	Serial measurements of blood pressure	**Antihypertensive Therapy** Calcium channel blocker (e.g., amlodipine 0.25 mg/kg PO q24h) Angiotensin-converting enzyme inhibitor (e.g., enalapril or benazepril 0.5-1.0 mg/kg PO q12-24h)
Proteinuria	I-IV	Urinalysis Urine culture Urine protein-to-creatinine ratio Albumin specific tests	**Antiproteinuric Therapies:** Angiotensin-converting enzyme inhibitors (dosage as above) Dietary protein restriction (renal diet) Dietary n-3 PUFA supplementation (renal diet ± 0.25 g n-3 PUFA–containing fish oil/kg)

modify renal adaptations and limit the extent of the complications of kidney disease, theoretically limiting progressive renal injury by interrupting the vicious cycle described.

Although the rate of progressive decline of renal function varies, studies to date suggest that inherent progression occurs in all animals with IRIS stages II to IV, albeit very slowly in many cats. Characterization of the rate of progression of CKD through serial determinations of Cr is a high priority at this time. Measures that may slow inherent progression, referred to as *renoprotective therapies* (see Table 47-4), include dietary phosphorus restriction,[13,14] antihypertensive agents in animals with high blood pressure,[15-18] antiproteinuric therapy,[19,20] and fish oil supplementation.[21,22] There is evidence that calcitriol administration slows progression in dogs with CKD,[23] and this approach often is recommended in cats as well. When given, calcitriol is administered at a dosage of 2.5

to 3.5 ng/kg PO q24h separately from meals (ensure that the cat is normocalcemic with a serum phosphorus < 6.0 mg/dL).

Control of hyperphosphatemia is widely accepted to be renoprotective in cats with CKD. Adjustments of therapy are based on measurement of serum phosphorus concentration; therapeutic targets vary by IRIS stage (Table 47-5).[1] Cats with IRIS stage I CKD generally do not require therapeutic intervention for hyperphosphatemia. If necessary, the addition of an intestinal phosphorus binder to a feline maintenance diet or the use of a specially formulated ("renal") diet usually is effective in reducing phosphorus concentrations in this population. In stage II to IV CKD, a special renal diet is definitely indicated.[24] If dietary restriction of phosphorus is unsuccessful in maintaining the target level of serum phosphorus within 2 to 3 months, phosphate-binding gels containing calcium acetate, calcium carbonate, or

Table 47-5 Therapeutic Targets for Management of Hyperphosphatemia in Cats with CKD

Iris Stage	Target Serum Phosphorus	Management Options
I	2.5-4.5 mg/dL (0.81-1.45 mmol/L)	Normal ration ± intestinal phosphorus binder *or* Dietary phosphorus restriction
II	2.5-5 mg/dL (0.81-1.61 mmol/L)	Dietary phosphorus restriction ± intestinal phosphorus binder
III	2.5-4.5 mg/dL (0.81-1.45 mmol/L)	Dietary phosphorus restriction plus intestinal phosphorus binder
IV	2.5-6 mg/dL (0.81-1.94 mmol/L)	Dietary phosphorus restriction plus intestinal phosphorus binder

[handwritten: throwinapets.com 100mg/kg/day divided w/ meals]

aluminum hydroxide should be administered with meals (initial dosage of 30 mg/kg PO with dosage increased as needed to achieve desired effect). Calcium-containing phosphate-binding agents should be used with caution in cats receiving calcitriol. By late stage II and in stages III and IV, the addition of an intestinal phosphorus-binding agent generally is required to reach the target serum phosphorus concentration.

Approximately 20 per cent of cats with CKD exhibit elevations of BP.[25] Hypertension may be observed in any IRIS stage and is not controlled effectively by feeding a low-salt diet (see Chapter 49). In cats with BP measurements in the moderate- or high-risk substage (M or H; see Table 47-2) and those with a low risk of exhibiting complications (substage Lc), antihypertensive therapy is appropriate. Unless emergency therapy is required (e.g., in cases of acute blindness due to retinal detachment), it is important to document elevated BP on at least two occasions because this therapy often is lifelong. Because of the importance of maintaining renal perfusion in animals with CKD, first-choice antihypertensive medications are vasodilatory agents. The most commonly employed agents are calcium channel blockers such as amlodipine besylate (0.25 to 0.5 mg/kg PO q24h) or angiotensin-converting enzyme inhibitors (ACEI) such as benazepril or enalapril (0.5 to 1 mg/kg PO q12-24h). Although these antihypertensive drugs may be coadministered at the recommended dosages, a calcium channel blocker usually is recommended as initial therapy in cats (particularly in substage H),[11,26] and an ACEI (e.g., benazepril or enalapril) may be added if the highest recommended dosage of amlodipine is ineffective. The institution of antihypertensive therapy and any dosage adjustments should be followed in 5 to 10 days with a reevaluation of Cr, BP, and UPC. The best markers of antihypertensive therapy efficacy are a reduction in BP (preferably by at least one risk category; see Table 47-2)[1] and a reduction in the UPC (preferably to <0.4).[12,18]

Proteinuria (UPC >0.4) is associated with worsening prognosis in CKD cats. If renal proteinuria of this magnitude is persistent in an animal with CKD, the clinician should consider antiproteinuric therapy (e.g., angiotensin-converting enzyme inhibitor, low-protein renal diet, and/or n-3 PUFA supplementation). In this situation, antiproteinuric therapy is considered renoprotective and is thus a high priority in IRIS stages II and III. Specially formulated renal diets are moderately low in protein and supplemented with n-3 PUFA. If the above measures do not reduce the magnitude of proteinuria to the target UPC of 0.4, the diet may be further supplemented with 0.25 g/kg body weight of n-3 PUFA–containing fish oil. Serial determinations of the level of proteinuria using complete urinalyses and UPC measurements should be performed to evaluate the success of this approach. The therapeutic goal is a UPC less than 0.4. The reader is referred to Chapter 45 in the fifth volume of this series for an in-depth discussion of proteinuria.

In dogs[22,23] and perhaps cats,[24,27] there is evidence to support the inclusion of dietary n-3 PUFA in IRIS stages II and III, regardless of the level of BP or UPC. This may be accomplished with the use of renal diets with supplemental n-3 PUFA (as above). Although renoprotective therapy is a high priority in IRIS stages II and III, it becomes increasingly less important in late stage IV as the focus of therapy becomes management of the complications of uremia (see next section).

PATIENT EVALUATION AND SYMPTOMATIC THERAPY

Patient evaluations, which include efforts to identify developing complications (e.g., systemic hypertension, disorders of potassium homeostasis, metabolic acidosis, proteinuria, anemia, and bacterial urinary tract infections) should be pursued aggressively and prospectively during all routine visits, regardless of IRIS stage.

As CKD progresses into IRIS stage IV, clinical consequences of the reduction of GFR become apparent; thorough patient evaluations followed by appropriate adjustments in symptomatic therapy (see Table 47-4) become increasingly important. Initially, uremia causes occasional vomiting and lethargy. As CKD progresses within stage IV (generally over many months or years in cats), anorexia, weight loss, dehydration, oral ulceration, vomiting, and diarrhea may become fully manifest. Loose teeth, deformable maxilla and mandible, or pathological fractures may be seen with renal secondary osteodystrophy, but these are uncommon in cats. Physical examination and imaging studies of animals in IRIS stages III to IV usually reveal small, irregular kidneys, although normal to large kidneys can be observed in cats with neoplasia, hydronephrosis, or glomerulonephritis. Mucous membranes are pale in IRIS stages III and IV due to the presence of a nonregenerative, normocytic, normochromic anemia.

Symptomatic therapy is a high priority at this time. As dietary restriction of protein may relieve some of the signs of uremia, a high-quality protein (e.g., egg protein) should be fed at a level of 2.8 to 3.8 g/kg body wt/day for cats. Commercial diets formulated for cats with CKD generally meet this recommendation. Cats with stage IV CKD often exhibit acid-base and electrolyte disorders; these should be treated aggressively. Although commercial renal diets are supplemented with potassium and alkali, hypokalemia and acidemia are common observations in cats with IRIS stage IV CKD. Potassium citrate or sodium bicarbonate, given PO to effect, may be indicated if the patient is acidemic (plasma bicarbonate <18 mEq/L). Potassium supplementation (1 to 3 mEq/kg/day) may be required to maintain normokalemia, particularly in polyuric or inappetent cats.

Administration of an H-2 receptor antagonist such as famotidine (2.5 mg PO q24h) may decrease gastric acidity and vomiting. Anabolic steroids, such as oxymetholone or nandrolone, have been administered to stimulate RBC production in animals that are anemic, but this approach is not effective. Human recombinant erythropoietin (50 to 100 IU/kg SQ 2 to 3 times weekly initially, dosed to effect after hematocrit reaches the target range of 30 to 35 per cent with supplemental iron administration and weekly hematocrit determinations)[28] generally is effective in stimulating RBC production; however, antierythropoietin antibodies develop in a significant percentage of animals treated with the human protein, and these may result in refractory anemia. Until a feline-specific product becomes widely available, erythropoietin administration is now recommended only for patients showing clinical signs of anemia (e.g., weakness, marked lethargy not attributable to other factors), which generally occurs at a hematocrit of less than 20 per cent. (See Chapter 66 for a discussion of erythropoietin therapy.)

In latter stage III and stage IV, fluid therapy with polyionic solutions, given IV or SQ in the hospital or SQ by owners at home (10 to 50 mL/kg SQ q24-72h), often is beneficial. Renal secondary hyperparathyroidism may contribute to uremia in cats, and calcitriol may be a useful adjunct to dietary phosphorus restriction and intestinal phosphorus binders to manage this condition.[23,29] Placement of feeding tubes, such as nasogastric or percutaneous endoscopic gastrostomy (PEG) tubes, can be an effective approach to the management of the chronically inappetent cats in late stage IV (see Chapter 12). Cats with CKD may develop ureteroliths, and obstructive uropathy should be considered in any cat with CKD who develops a sudden, unexpected increase in Cr. (See Chapter 52 in this volume, and Chapters 41 and 43 in the fifth volume of this series, for a discussion on upper tract uroliths.) Renal replacement therapy (renal transplantation and/or dialytic therapy) should be discussed with owners in early stage IV with implementation considered in late stage IV.

ADDITIONAL PATIENT EVALUATIONS

Scheduled evaluations of cats with CKD should include a thorough history and physical examination, BP measurement, complete serum biochemical panel, hematology, urinalysis, UPC, and aerobic bacterial urine culture. It should be noted that systemic hypertension, proteinuria, and urinary tract infections may be observed in any IRIS stage. In IRIS stages I and II, annual evaluations may suffice. Evaluations should be done on a semiannual basis

in stage III, regardless of the health of the animal. Uremic animals in IRIS stage IV should be evaluated at 1- to 2-month intervals. Cats with unstable renal function, complications of hypertension, or undergoing adjustments to therapy also should be seen more frequently.

SUMMARY

The proper management of a cat with CKD requires a clear understanding of the diagnostic and therapeutic priorities in the stage of disease during which the patient is being managed. Early in the disease process (IRIS stage I), a careful evaluation of the kidney is critical to identify the primary disease process and specific therapy to eliminate this disease. In the middle stages (II and III), inherent progression and renoprotective therapy are paramount. In the final stage of CKD, IRIS stage IV, more frequent and thorough evaluations of the patient with institution of appropriate symptomatic therapy become the primary consideration of the veterinarian. Attention to these key needs is likely to extend quality and quantity of life in affected cats.

REFERENCES

1. Elliott J, Watson ADJ: Chronic kidney disease: staging and management. In Bonagura JD, Twedt DC, editors: *Current veterinary therapy XIV*, St Louis, 2009, Elsevier Saunders, p 883.
2. Boyd LM, Langston C, Thompson K, et al: Survival in cats with naturally occurring chronic kidney disease, *J Vet Intern Med* 22:1111, 2008.
3. Polzin DJ, Osborne CA: Update—conservative medical management of chronic renal failure. In Kirk RW, editor: *Current veterinary therapy IX*, Philadelphia, 1986, WB Saunders, p 1167.
4. Krawiec D, Gelberg H: Chronic renal disease in cats. In Kirk RW, editor: *Current veterinary therapy X*, Philadelphia, 1989, WB Saunders, p 1170.
5. Moe L, Heiene R: Estimation of glomerular filtration rate in dogs with 99M-Tc-DTPA and iohexol, *Res Vet Sci* 58:138, 1995.
6. Brown SA, Finco DR, Boudinot D, et al: Evaluation of a single injection method, using iohexol, for estimating glomerular filtration rate in cats and dogs, *Am J Vet Res* 57:105, 1996.
7. Finco D, Braselton W, Cooper T: Relationship between plasma iohexol clearance and urinary exogenous creatinine clearance in dogs, *J Vet Intern Med* 215:368, 2001.
8. Gleadhill A, Michell AR: Evaluation of iohexol as a marker for the clinical measurement of glomerular filtration rate in dogs, *Res Vet Sci* 60:117, 1996.
9. Van Hoek I, Vandermeulen E, Duchateau L, et al: Comparison and reproducibility of plasma clearance of exogenous creatinine, exo-iohexol, endo-iohexol, and 51Cr-EDTA in young adult and aged healthy cats, *J Vet Intern Med* 21:950, 2007.
10. Lees GE, Brown SA, Elliott J, et al: Assessment and management of proteinuria in dogs and cats: 2004 ACVIM Forum Consensus Statement. *J Vet Intern Med* 19:377, 2005.
11. Brown S, Atkins C, Bagley R, et al: Guidelines for the identification, evaluation, and management of systemic hypertension in dogs and cats, *J Vet Intern Med* 21:542, 2007.

12. Syme HM, Markwell PJ, Pfeiffer D, et al: Survival of cats with naturally occurring chronic renal failure is related to severity of proteinuria, *J Vet Intern Med* 20:528, 2006.

13. Ross LA, Finco DR, Crowell WA: Effect of dietary phosphorus restriction on the kidneys of cats with reduced renal mass, *Am J Vet Res* 43:1023, 1982.

14. Brown SA, Finco DR, Crowell WA, et al: Beneficial effects of dietary mineral restriction in dogs with marked reduction in functional renal mass, *J Am Soc Nephr* 1:1169, 1991.

15. Jacob F, Polzin DJ, Osborne CA, et al: Association between initial systolic blood pressure and risk of developing a uremic crisis or of dying in dogs with chronic renal failure, *J Am Vet Med Assoc* 222:322, 2003.

16. Mathur S, Brown CA, Dietrich UM, et al: Evaluation of a technique of inducing hypertensive renal insufficiency in cats, *Am J Vet Res* 65:1006, 2004.

17. Mathur S, Syme H, Brown CA, et al: Effects of the calcium channel antagonist amlodipine in cats with surgically induced hypertensive renal insufficiency, *Am J Vet Res* 63:833, 2002.

18. Jepson RE, Elliott J, Brodbelt D, et al: Effect of control of systolic blood pressure on survival in cats with systemic hypertension, *J Vet Intern Med* 21:402, 2007.

19. Grauer G, Greco D, Getzy D, et al: Effects of enalapril versus placebo as a treatment for canine idiopathic glomerulonephritis, *J Vet Intern Med* 14:526, 2000.

20. King JN, Gunn-Moore DA, Tasker S, et al: Tolerability and efficacy of benazepril in cats with chronic kidney disease, *J Vet Intern Med* 20:1054, 2006.

21. Brown SA, Brown CA, Crowell WA, et al: Beneficial effects of chronic administration of dietary omega-3 polyunsaturated fatty acids in dogs with renal insufficiency, *J Lab Clin Med* 131:447, 1998.

22. Brown SA, Brown CA, Crowell WA, et al: Effects of dietary polyunsaturated fatty acid supplementation in early renal insufficiency in dogs, *J Lab Clin Med* 135:275, 2000.

23. Polzin DJ, Ross S, Osborne CA: Calcitriol. In Bonagura JD, Twedt DC, editors: *Current veterinary therapy XIV*, St Louis, 2009, Elsevier Saunders, p 892.

24. Ross SJ, Osborne CA, Kirk CA, et al: Clinical evaluation of dietary modification for treatment of spontaneous chronic kidney disease in cats, *J Am Vet Med Assoc* 229:949, 2006.

25. Syme HM, Barber PJ, Markwell PJ, et al: Prevalence of systolic hypertension in cats with chronic renal failure at initial evaluation, *J Am Vet Med Assoc* 220:1799, 2002.

26. Elliott J, Barber PJ, Syme HM, et al: Feline hypertension: clinical findings and response to antihypertensive treatment in 30 cases, *J Small Anim Pract* 42:122, 2001.

27. Plantinga EA, Everts H, Kastelein AMC, et al: Retrospective study of the survival of cats with acquired chronic renal insufficiency offered different commercial diets, *Vet Rec* 157:185, 2005.

28. Cowgill LD, James KM, Levy JK, et al: Use of recombinant human erythropoietin for management of anemia in dogs and cats with renal failure, *J Am Vet Med Assoc* 212:521, 1998.

29. Nagode LA, Chew DJ, Podell M: Benefits of calcitriol therapy and serum phosphorus control in dogs and cats with chronic renal failure, *Vet Clin North Am Small Anim Pract* 26:1293, 1996.

48 Survival and Outcome of Kidney Disease

Cathy E. Langston

Disorders of the kidney are encountered commonly in cats. The prevalence of chronic kidney disease (CKD) is estimated at 1.6 per cent in the cat population.[1] The incidence of indicators of potential kidney disease (polyuria, polydipsia, poorly concentrated urine, increased serum urea nitrogen, increased serum creatinine concentration) was 20 per cent in one study.[2] If there are 84 million pet cats in the United States (Pet Food Institute, Washington, DC, 2006*), 16 million have some degree of kidney dysfunction. A substantial commitment is required to care for a cat with CKD, including time and financial and emotional components. Acute kidney injury also is a big challenge for pet owners, both financially and emotionally, especially during the initial hospitalization. Knowing about the potential outcomes allows cat owners to better prepare emotionally and make appropriate decisions about care.

CHRONIC KIDNEY DISEASE

FACTORS AFFECTING SURVIVAL

Stage of Kidney Disease

Recent studies have shown that the International Renal Interest Society (IRIS) stage of kidney disease predicts survival.[3,4] The IRIS stage is based on serum creatinine, with subcategories for blood pressure and proteinuria (Table 48-1) (see Chapters 47 and 49). The IRIS staging system is intended for use with cats who have been diagnosed already with CKD and are clinically stable. In one study that applied IRIS staging criteria to cats at initial diagnosis and after stabilization, 30 per cent of cats cat-

egorized initially as stage IV were classified in a lower stage after they had been stabilized.[3] It is likely that the prerenal component of azotemia in several of the cats caused them to be categorized initially in a more advanced stage. The prerenal component of azotemia is rapidly reversible with fluid therapy. Median survival time for cats with stage IIb CKD (after rehydration) in that study was 3.1 years (1151 days), compared to 1.9 years (679 days) for cats with stage III CKD, and 35 days for cats with stage IV CKD.[3] These results are similar to a study evaluating survival of 50 cats with CKD based on IRIS stage at diagnosis.[4] In that study, survival times of cats in stage IIb kidney disease were reported as 1.4 years (504 days) in normotensive patients, but only 187 days in stage IIb cats with hypertension. Stage III cats had a reported survival time of 154 days (normotensive patients) and 281 days (hypertensive patients); because of the small number of cats in this group, there was not a statistically significant difference in survival times between normotensive and hypertensive cats. Cats in stage IV CKD were found to have a survival time of 57 days (normotensive patients) and 21 days (hypertensive patients).[4]

A prospective study determined that an increased serum creatinine was associated with a shorter survival time.[5] In that study, the relative risk of reaching a renal endpoint, defined as death or euthanasia from renal failure or need for parenteral fluid therapy, was 2.3 times higher in cats with stage III CKD than for those in stage II (p = not significant), 3.8 times higher for those in stage IV than for those in stage III, and 9.3 times higher for those in stage IV than for those in stage II.[5] Median survival times estimated from a Kaplan Meier survival curve were 60 days for cats in stage IV CKD and 475 days for cats in stage III disease.[5] A study comparing cats who survived to those who did not survive for more than 1

---

*http://www.petfoodinstitute.org/reference_pet_data.cfm.

Table 48-1 IRIS Staging System*

	Stage I	Stage II†	Stage III	Stage IV
Creatinine (mg/dL)	<1.6	1.6-2.8	2.9-5.0	>5.0

*Substages based on urine protein:creatinine (<0.2 = nonproteinuric, 0.2-0.4 = borderline proteinuric, >0.4 = proteinuric) and blood pressure (see Tables 47-2 and 47-3).

†Some studies include Stage IIb, which includes only those cats with a serum creatinine above the reference of the laboratory.

month from diagnosis found that patients with a higher serum creatinine concentration at diagnosis were more likely to die of kidney disease within the first month after diagnosis.[6] At diagnosis, the surviving cats had a median serum creatinine concentration of 2.7 mg/dL and the nonsurvivors had a median serum creatinine concentration of 5.5 mg/dL.[6]

Median survival time in one study was 123 days once the serum creatinine concentration exceeded 4 mg/dL and 44 days when the creatinine exceeded 5 mg/dL.[3] In another study, cats who developed a serum creatinine concentration greater than 4.5 mg/dL died within 5 to 63 days and typically presented 3 weeks after the increase in serum creatinine with dehydration and complete anorexia.[7] Another study found the serum creatinine concentration at the time of diagnosis to be a poor predictor of survival time in uremic cats.[8] In that study, 10 per cent of the cats were assessed as being dehydrated at diagnosis. Mean serum creatinine concentration in those cats at diagnosis was 3.6 mg/dL.[8]

The results of these studies indicate that IRIS stage of kidney disease, based on serum creatinine concentration, is associated with survival in cats. Cats discharged in IRIS stage IIb kidney disease have only a 42 per cent chance of dying of renal disease, compared to a 68 per cent chance for cats in stage III and an 86 per cent chance for cats in stage IV CKD.[3] Thus more than one half of cats with stage IIb CKD develop another disease process that leads to death. This is not surprising considering that the mean age at diagnosis of CKD in all cats is 12.3 years and the mean survival time from that point is 2.3 years.[3] However, this information can be valuable when counseling owners on what to expect once their cat is diagnosed with CKD.

Proteinuria

The urine protein:creatinine ratio (UPC) is a spot measurement of urinary protein excretion that predicts 24-hour urine protein excretion accurately without the inconvenience of trying to collect urine from a cat for a full 24 hours. Urine albumin-to-creatinine ratio is no more accurate than UPC and is not readily available.[4,9] A rapid and easy semiquantitative assay is available for microalbuminuria in cats, defined as urinary albumin concentration of less than 30 mg/dL, which is the lower limit of detection of standard urine dipsticks. Although microalbuminuria testing may prove to be an early predictor of renal damage, at this time we lack clinical cor-

relates of microalbuminuria. In one study of more than 300 feline urine samples, more than 100 tested positive for microalbuminuria but only 16 had a UPC higher than 0.4.[9] Thus the role of testing for microalbuminuria in feline CKD remains to be clarified.

Significant proteinuria is not a common finding in cats with CKD. From 50 to 66 per cent of affected cats have UPCs lower than 0.2 and only 20 per cent or less have UPCs higher than 0.4.[4,5] Multiple studies have shown that proteinuria is associated with a shorter survival time.[4-6] An increased UPC was the most likely variable to be associated with increased mortality in cats with CKD.[6] Cats with CKD and UPCs higher than 0.4 had a fivefold higher risk of reaching a renal endpoint than cats with UPCs below 0.2, and median survival time of cats with UPCs higher than 0.4 is about 1 year, compared to a median survival time of about 3 years in cats with UPCs lower than 0.2.[4,5] The results of survival analyses of cats with CKD and UPCs between 0.2 and 0.4 vary; one study showed no difference in survival between this group and cats with UPCs below 0.2, while another study showed survival times intermediate between survival in cats with UPCs lower than 0.2 or higher than 0.4.[4,5] From these findings, we can conclude that a UPC over 0.4 is detrimental but values from 0.2 to 0.4 remain equivocal.

Angiotensin-converting enzyme (ACE) inhibitors, such as enalapril and benazepril, are known to decrease proteinuria, and benazepril has been found to decrease proteinuria in cats with naturally occurring CKD.[10-12] In a study of surgically induced CKD, benazepril did not decrease proteinuria; however, the degree of proteinuria at the start of treatment was small.[13] Despite its antiproteinuric effects, benazepril did not improve survival times in cats with CKD when compared to placebo.[10] That study also did not find a survival advantage from benazepril in a subset of cats with UPCs above 1; however, there were only 13 cats in that group. Because of day-to-day variation, the UPC must change by more than 80 per cent in dogs with UPCs around 0.5 to represent an actual change in value.[14] Similar data are not available for cats. Although side effects of ACE inhibitors are uncommon in stable, well-compensated cats, complications include worsening azotemia, hyperkalemia, and a decrease in blood pressure, and these parameters should be monitored shortly after starting therapy or following dose adjustments. (See Chapter 45 in the fifth volume of this series for further discussion on proteinuria.)

Hypertension

Hypertension is a poor prognostic indicator in dogs with CKD. Dogs with a systolic blood pressure above 160 mm Hg were three times more likely to develop a uremic crisis or die than dogs with a systolic blood pressure less than 143 mm Hg. Survival times were shorter and progression of azotemia was more rapid in the hypertensive dogs. However, blood pressure remained above 160 mm Hg in 10 of 11 dogs treated with antihypertensive medications.[15]

Although systolic blood pressure in cats is correlated to magnitude of proteinuria, cats treated for hypertension did not have a reduced survival time compared to cats without hypertension.[4] This may have occurred because cats with hypertension treated with amlodipine had a significant reduction in blood pressure over the follow-up period.[4] (See Chapter 49 for further discussion of hypertension.)

Biochemical Parameters

Serum phosphorus concentration was correlated to survival in several studies.[3,5,6] In one study, serum phosphorus was considered a dependent variable because the increase in phosphorus concentration was correlated to the independent variable serum creatinine.[5] In another study, serum phosphorus was predictive of survival in a multivariate model. For each 1 mg/dL increase in serum phosphorus, there was an 11.8 per cent increase in the risk of death.[3] Other commonly measured biochemical parameters are not correlated consistently with survival. Serum urea concentration was correlated to survival in two studies[5,6] but not in a third.[3] However, in one study serum urea was considered a dependent variable correlated to serum creatinine and not a separate indicator.[5] Serum concentrations of potassium, calcium, bicarbonate, and albumin were not predictive when evaluated.[3,5,6]

Anemia

Hematocrit was correlated with a shorter renal survival time in several studies.[5,6,8] Hematocrit is correlated negatively to serum creatinine and thus is not an independent variable in predicting survival in cats with CKD.[5,16] The hematocrit value was not significant in the multivariate analysis in one study (e.g., anemia was not a significant predictor of an increased risk of death); however, 30 per cent of the anemic cats in that study received some therapy specific for anemia, which may have affected outcome.[3]

Clinical Parameters

Weight loss and/or progressive azotemia in the face of medical management have been suggested as possible indicators of clinical decompensation and signal the ideal time to recommend a renal transplant.[17-20] One study found that weight loss was the most reliable indicator of clinical deterioration in cats with CKD.[7] Of 135 cats in one study who reached clinical decompensation (determined subjectively), median survival time was 40 days from that point.[3]

TREATMENT

Despite the high prevalence of CKD in cats, surprisingly few studies have evaluated the impact of treatment on survival. (See Chapter 47 for further discussion on linking treatment with staging in CKD.)

Diet

Ross et al showed that a renal diet improves survival and delays uremic crisis in cats with CKD. No cats with CKD who were fed the renal diet (n = 22) died of renal disease or developed a uremic crisis during the 2-year study period, whereas 6 of 23 cats with CKD who were fed an adult maintenance diet developed a uremic crisis and 5 died of renal disease.[21] Feeding renal diets to dogs with CKD produced similar improvements in survival times and the times to developing a uremic crisis.[22]

Benazepril Therapy

ACE inhibitors are used routinely in proteinuric and non-proteinuric renal disease in human beings.[23] They have been shown to decrease proteinuria and improve survival in dogs with glomerulonephritis.[24] ACE inhibitors, specifically benazepril, also have been shown to decrease proteinuria in cats.[10-12] One study did not find an antiproteinuric effect of benazepril in a surgical mode of CKD; however, the baseline level of proteinuria was mild.[13]

Several studies have evaluated the effect of benazepril on survival in cats with CKD. In one of the largest studies (involving 192 cats), survival times (637 ± 480 days) were not significantly different between the group treated with benazepril and the placebo group (520 ± 323 days, $p = 0.47$).[10] In another placebo-controlled study of 61 cats, benazepril did not improve survival.[11]

In 11 cats with spontaneously occurring CKD, patients receiving benazepril (n = 6) had a significantly decreased serum creatinine concentration (2.6 mg/dL) after 24 weeks of treatment, compared to 3.4 mg/dL pretreatment ($p < 0.05$). Cats in the control group (not receiving benazepril) showed no improvement in serum creatinine concentration (3 mg/dL at 24 weeks of treatment, compared to 2.8 mg/dL pretreatment).[12] Two other studies did not find a difference in creatinine before and after treatment or between control cats and cats treated with benazepril.[10,11]

In the study that demonstrated a significant effect of benazepril on serum creatinine concentration, cats who were treated had 2+ to 3+ proteinuria prior to treatment.[12] Urine protein:creatinine measurements were not provided. In the BENRIC study, cats who were treated with benazepril had a mean pretreatment UPC of 0.39, and in the study by Mizutani et al, mean pretreatment UPC was approximately 0.2.[10,11] In the BENRIC study, a subgroup analysis was performed comparing survival times of cats with UPCs higher than 1. Benazepril-treated cats with initial UPCs of 1 or higher (n = 4) had a median renal survival time of 484 days, compared with 124 days in the placebo-treated group (n = 9). This difference was not statistically significant ($p = 0.27$); however, the number of cats was low.[10]

Although the current evidence suggests that benazepril does not prolong survival time in the majority of cats with CKD, further investigation of its use is warranted, specifically in proteinuric cats.

Renal Transplantation

Renal transplantation is a method of treating end-stage CKD in cats. Perioperative mortality (within the first month) is approximately 23 per cent.[20,25,26] The 6-month survival rate is 60 to 70 per cent, and the 3-year survival rate is approximately 40 to 50 per cent.[20,26] Age over 10 years predicts a worse outcome, particularly in the first 6 months postoperatively; however, in one study, these deaths were not attributed to age-related diseases.[27]

DISEASE-SPECIFIC SURVIVAL

Nephrolithiasis and ureterolithiasis are found commonly in cats with CKD, and the incidence appears to have increased in the past 2 decades. Ross et al reported that 47 per cent of cats with CKD have upper urinary tract uroliths. A retrospective case-controlled study showed no difference in rate of disease progression, incidence of uremic crisis, or death between cats with CKD with nephrolithiasis and those without nephrolithiasis.[28]

Ureterolithiasis can present as an acute or chronic disease. An increasingly common presentation is an acute uremic crisis in a previously asymptomatic cat. Some patients are managed medically, and some affected cats undergo surgical intervention (ureterotomy, ureteral resection and anastomosis, ureteronephrectomy, renal transplantation) (see Chapter 52). In a retrospective series of 153 cats with ureteral calculi, 57 per cent of patients treated medically survived more than 1 month after diagnosis, compared to 80 per cent of cats treated with ureteral surgery. Of those cats surviving for more than 1 month, the 6-month and 24-month survival rates for cats treated medically were 72 per cent and 66 per cent, respectively, compared with 91 per cent and 88 per cent for cats treated with ureteral surgery. In both groups, approximately one half of the patients had persistent azotemia.[29]

ACUTE KIDNEY INJURY

MEDICAL MANAGEMENT

Although multiple case reports or case series of specific causes of acute renal failure (ARF) in cats have been published, few studies have reported the outcome of cats with acute kidney failure from a variety of causes. In one study of 32 cats with ARF, the overall mortality rate was 47 per cent.[30] Excluding cats treated with hemodialysis, the mortality rate was 37 per cent. In that study four cats were euthanized within the first 24 hours of diagnosis. It is likely that these cats were euthanized due to financial reasons and their negative outcome might have confounded the survival rates. When excluding these four patients from the study, the mortality decreases to 39 per cent overall, or 20 per cent of those cats treated medically.[30] The mortality rate was 56 per cent in a study of 99 dogs with ARF and was 62 per cent in a study of hospital-acquired renal failure in 29 dogs.[31,32] The mortality rate in human beings with ARF is approximately 50 per cent.[33-35]

Decreased urine production (<0.5 mL/kg/hr) is a poor prognostic factor in cats with ARF.[30] In a study of dogs with hospital-acquired ARF, the initial urine production was significantly associated with survival, with an odds ratio of mortality of 20.[32]

No association has been found between the severity of azotemia and outcome in cats with ARF.[30,36,37] In contrast, the severity of azotemia was not predictive of outcome in dogs with hospital-acquired ARF, although an initial severe increase in serum creatinine concentration was associated with failure to recover from ARF in another

study of community-acquired ARF in dogs.[31,32] In the study of cats with ARF,[30] blood urea nitrogen and serum creatinine concentrations were evaluated at initial presentation, before any prerenal contribution to the azotemia had been corrected. After correction of the prerenal component, a more accurate assessment of the intrinsic renal function might have been possible, but the retrospective nature of the study prevented such evaluation.[30]

The initial serum potassium concentration is a prognostic factor. For each unit increase (mEq/L) in serum potassium concentration, there was a 57 per cent decrease in chance of survival.[30] Serum albumin also was a prognostic factor for survival, with nonsurvivors having lower albumin concentrations.[30] This finding also has been noted in cats with CKD and in several studies of human patients with ARF.[30,38,39]

Disease etiology is a prognostic factor with ARF. In one study, 50 per cent of cats with ARF due to nephrotoxic or other causes survived, whereas 75 per cent of cats with ARF due to ischemia survived.[30] In dogs with hospital-acquired ARF, 43 per cent of patients with nephrotoxicant exposure survived, although no association between type of renal insult and outcome was found in that study.[32]

Approximately one half of cats who survived the episode of ARF were discharged with normal serum creatinine concentrations. The remaining one half of the survivors had persistent azotemia.[30] Twenty four of 99 dogs with ARF developed chronic renal failure (24 of 43 survivors).[31] One half of the cats with ischemic causes had normal serum creatinine concentrations at discharge, compared to 28 per cent of cats with nephrotoxic causes and 10 per cent of those with miscellaneous causes of ARF. Despite this low percentage of affected cats who returned to normal in the miscellaneous group, it remains notable that three of those four cats lived more than 2 years. Only one cat who had a normal serum creatinine concentration at discharge died during the follow-up period, and the cause of death was not renal related.[30]

HEMODIALYSIS

In studies of cats with ARF who were treated with hemodialysis, 35 to 40 per cent of patients with ARF due to nephrotoxic causes survived.[36,37] In one study of 15 cats with ARF treated with hemodialysis, no cat with an ischemic cause was included, and all 5 cats with suspected pyelonephritis or unknown causes survived.[36] In another study of cats with acute uremia who were treated with hemodialysis, 72 per cent of patients with hemodynamic or metabolic causes survived, compared to a survival rate of 58 per cent for cats with ARF due to infectious causes, and 29 per cent for cats with ARF due to unknown causes (Table 48-2).[37,40] In dogs treated with hemodialysis, 70 per cent of patients with ARF due to infectious diseases survived, compared to 18 to 20 per cent with ARF due to toxic causes and 40 to 56 per cent of dogs with ARF due to hemodynamic or other causes.[41,42] Because hemodialysis generally is reserved for patients who have failed to

Table 48-2 Survival Rates* for Patients with Acute Renal Failure Treated with Intermittent Hemodialysis

Category	Survival Rate (%)
Obstructive (cats)	70-75
Infectious	58-86
Metabolic/Hemodynamic	56-72
Other	29-56
Toxic	18-35

*Based on survival of more than 30 days without need for ongoing dialysis.

respond satisfactorily to medical management and who are presumed to have more severe renal injury, direct comparisons to outcomes with medical management are not possible.

Of the nonsurviving patients, approximately one half die or are euthanized due to extrarenal conditions (e.g., pancreatitis, respiratory complications). About one third of nonsurvivors are euthanized due to failure of recovery of renal function. Ongoing uremic signs, dialysis complications, and unknown causes account for the remaining patient deaths. Of the surviving patients, approximately one half regain normal renal function (defined by normal serum creatinine concentration) and the remaining patients develop persistent CKD.

PERITONEAL DIALYSIS

Extracorporeal renal replacement therapies such as intermittent hemodialysis or continuous renal replacement therapies are becoming more readily available but are still quite limited in distribution. Extracorporeal techniques require specialized equipment, whereas peritoneal dialysis uses equipment and supplies that are readily available in many veterinary hospitals. In one report of the use of peritoneal dialysis in treatment of six cats with acute renal failure, five cats survived, all having normal renal function after 1 year. All of the surviving cats had complications associated with peritoneal dialysis, including subcutaneous edema, dialysate retention, and hypoalbuminemia; however, these complications were managed successfully.[43]

REFERENCES

1. Lund EM, Armstrong PJ, Kirk CA, et al: Health status and population characteristics of dogs and cats examined at private veterinary practices in the United States, *J Am Vet Med Assoc* 214:1336, 1999.
2. Watson ADJ: Indicators of renal insufficiency in dogs and cats presented at a veterinary teaching hospital, *Aust Vet Practit* 31:54, 2001.
3. Boyd LM, Langston CE, Thompson K, et al: Survival in cats with naturally occurring chronic kidney disease (2000-2002), *J Vet Intern Med* 22:1111, 2008.
4. Syme HM, Markwell PJ, Pfeiffer D, et al: Survival of cats with naturally occurring chronic renal failure is related to severity of proteinuria, *J Vet Intern Med* 20:528, 2006.
5. King J, Tasker S, Gunn-Moore D, et al: Prognostic factors in cats with chronic kidney disease, *J Vet Intern Med* 21:906, 2007.
6. Kuwahara Y, Ohba Y, Kitoh K, et al: Association of laboratory data and death within one month in cats with chronic renal failure, *J Small Anim Pract* 47:446, 2006.
7. Elliott J, Syme HM, Reubens E, et al: Assessment of acid-base status of cats with naturally occurring chronic renal failure, *J Small Anim Pract* 44:65, 2003.
8. Elliott J, Barber PJ: Feline chronic renal failure: clinical findings in 80 cases diagnosed between 1992 and 1995, *J Small Anim Pract* 39:78, 1998.
9. Whittemore JC, Gill VL, Jensen WA, et al: Evaluation of the association between microalbuminuria and the urine albumin-creatinine ratio and systemic disease in dogs, *J Am Vet Med Assoc* 229:958, 2006.
10. King JN, Gunn-Moore DA, Tasker S, et al: Tolerability and efficacy of benazepril in cats with chronic kidney disease, *J Vet Intern Med* 20:1054, 2006.
11. Mizutani H, Koyama H, Watanabe T, et al: Evaluation of the clinical efficacy of benazepril in the treatment of chronic renal insufficiency in cats, *J Vet Intern Med* 20:1074, 2006.
12. Watanabe T, Mishina M: Effects of benazepril hydrochloride in cats with experimentally induced or spontaneously occurring chronic renal failure, *J Vet Med Sci* 69:1015, 2007.
13. Brown SA, Brown CA, Jacobs G, et al: Effects of the angiotensin converting enzyme inhibitor benazepril in cats with induced renal insufficiency, *Am J Vet Res* 62:375, 2001.
14. Nabity MB, Boggess MM, Kashtan CE, et al: Day-to-day variation of the urine protein:creatinine ratio in female dogs with stable glomerular proteinuria caused by X-linked hereditary nephropathy, *J Vet Intern Med* 21:425, 2007.
15. Jacob F, Polzin DJ, Osborne CA, et al: Systemic hypertension in dogs with spontaneous chronic renal failure: prevalence, target-organ damage and survival (abstract), *J Vet Intern Med* 13:253, 1999.
16. Cowgill LD: Management of anemia associated with renal failure. In August JR, editor: *Consultations in feline internal medicine*, vol 2, Philadelphia, 1994, WB Saunders, p 331.
17. Gregory CR: Renal transplantation, In Bojrab MJ, editor: *Current techniques in small animal surgery*, ed 4, Philadelphia, 1998, Williams & Wilkins, p 434.
18. Bernsteen L, Gregory CR, Kyles AE, et al: Renal transplantation in cats, *Clin Tech Small Anim Pract* 15:40, 2000.
19. Katayama M, McAnulty JF: Renal transplantation in cats: patient selection and preoperative management, *Compend Contin Educ Pract Vet* 24:868, 2002.
20. Katayama M, McAnulty JF: Renal transplantation in cats: techniques, complications, and immunosuppression, *Compend Contin Educ Pract Vet* 24:874, 2002.
21. Ross SJ, Osborne CA, Kirk CA, et al: Clinical evaluation of dietary modification for treatment of spontaneous chronic kidney disease in cats, *J Am Vet Med Assoc* 229:949, 2006.
22. Jacob F, Polzin DJ, Osborne CA, et al: Clinical evaluation of dietary modification for treatment of spontaneous chronic renal failure in dogs, *J Am Vet Med Assoc* 220:1163, 2002.
23. Hou FF, Zhang H, Zhang GH, et al: Efficacy and safety of benazepril for advanced chronic renal insufficiency, *N Engl J Med* 354:131, 2006.
24. Grauer GF, Greco DS, Getzy DM, et al: Effects of enalapril versus placebo as a treatment for canine idiopathic glomerulonephritis, *J Vet Intern Med* 14:526, 2000.
25. Case JB, Kyles AE, Nelson RW, et al: Incidence of and risk factors for diabetes mellitus in cats that have undergone

renal transplantation: 187 cases (1986-2005), *J Am Vet Med Assoc* 230:880, 2007.

26. Schmiedt CW, Holzman G, Schwarz T, et al: Survival, complications, and analysis of risk factors after renal transplantation in cats, *Vet Surg* 37:683, 2008.

27. Adin CA, Gregory CR, Kyles AE, et al: Diagnostic predictors of complications and survival after renal transplantation in cats, *Vet Surg* 30:515, 2001.

28. Ross SJ, Osborne CA, Lekcharoensuk C, et al: A case-control study of the effects of nephrolithiasis in cats with chronic kidney disease, *J Am Vet Med Assoc* 230:1854, 2007.

29. Kyles AE, Hardie EM, Wooden BG, et al: Management and outcome of cats with ureteral calculi: 153 cases (1984-2002), *J Am Vet Med Assoc* 226:937, 2005.

30. Worwag S, Langston CE: Feline acute intrinsic renal failure: 32 cats (1997-2004), *J Am Vet Med Assoc* 232:728, 2008.

31. Vaden SL, Levine J, Breitschwerdt EB: A retrospective case-control study of acute renal failure in 99 dogs, *J Vet Intern Med* 11:58, 1997.

32. Behrend E, Grauer GF, Mani I, et al: Hospital-acquired acute renal failure in dogs: 29 cases (1983-1992), *J Am Vet Med Assoc* 208:537, 1996.

33. Lane IF, Grauer GF, Fettman MJ: Acute renal failure. Part I. Risk factors, prevention, and strategies for protection, *Compend Contin Educ Pract Vet* 16:15, 1994.

34. Brady MA, Janovitz EB: Nephrotoxicosis in a cat following ingestion of Asiatic hybrid lily (*Lilium* sp.), *J Vet Diagn Invest* 12:566, 2000.

35. Ympa YP, Sakr Y, Reinhart K, et al: Has mortality from acute renal failure decreased? A systematic review of the literature, *Am J Med* 118:827, 2005.

36. Langston CE, Cowgill LD, Spano JA: Applications and outcome of hemodialysis in cats: a review of 29 cases, *J Vet Intern Med* 11:348, 1997.

37. Pantaleo V, Francey T, Fischer JR, et al: Application of hemodialysis for the management of acute uremia in cats: 119 cases (1993-2003) (abstract), *J Vet Intern Med* 18:418, 2004.

38. Obialo CI, Okonofua EC, Nzerue MC, et al: Role of hypoalbuminemia and hypocholesterolemia as copredictors of mortality in acute renal failure, *Kidney Int* 56:1058, 1999.

39. Mahajan S, Tiwari S, Bharani R, et al: Spectrum of acute renal failure and factors predicting its outcome in an intensive care unit in India, *Ren Fail* 28:119, 2006.

40. Fischer JR, Pantaleo V, Francey T, et al: Clinical and clinicopathological features of cats with acute ureteral obstruction managed with hemodialysis between 1993 and 2004: a review of 50 cases (abstract), *J Vet Intern Med* 18:418, 2004.

41. Francey T: Outcomes of hemodialysis [CD]. Advanced Renal Therapies Symposium, New York City, 2006.

42. Francey T, Cowgill LD: Use of hemodialysis for the management of ARF in the dog: 124 cases (1990-2001) (abstract), *J Vet Intern Med* 16:352, 2002.

43. Dorval P, Boysen SR: Management of acute renal failure in cats using peritoneal dialysis: a retrospective study of six cases (2003-2007), *J Feline Med Surg* 11:107, 2009.

49 Managing and Monitoring Systemic Hypertension

Harriet M. Syme

Successful management of hypertension in cats relies on routine blood pressure measurement to identify patients in need of treatment. However, it is important to recognize that the decision to treat a patient for hypertension should never be made on the basis of blood pressure measurements alone. In any clinical situation in which antihypertensive therapy is contemplated, consideration should be given to the pretest probability that the cat has hypertension. For example, a young cat without any evidence of an underlying disease that would predispose to hypertension or any signs of end-organ damage (Box 49-1) is extremely unlikely to be hypertensive. If blood pressure is measured in such a cat, it should be done to provide a baseline to monitor as the cat gets older; antihypertensive therapy would be inappropriate no matter how high the result. Conversely, an old cat with chronic kidney disease (CKD), subtle areas of subretinal fluid accumulation, and moderate blood pressure elevation should receive immediate antihypertensive therapy because the pretest probability of hypertension is very high and there is evidence that end-organ damage is occurring.

EPIDEMIOLOGY OF HYPERTENSION

These case examples illustrate how awareness of the epidemiology of hypertension influences treatment decisions, especially in the absence of end-organ lesions. One epidemiological factor to consider when deciding whether a patient should be treated for hypertension is age. In published case series of cats with hypertensive ocular lesions, it is evident that most affected cats are old, with an average age at presentation of 15 years. There are very few documented cases of systemic hypertension in cats less than 10 years of age.[1] Cats with primary hyperaldosteronism may be slightly younger at presentation (mean age 10 years in one study), but this disease is relatively uncommon[2] (see Chapter 24). Thus any potential diagnosis of systemic hypertension in a young cat should be considered tenuous; if there is no evidence of end-organ damage, the patient should be considered to have white-coat hypertension (see White-Coat Effect, below) until proven otherwise.

CKD has been associated with the development of systemic hypertension in cats and in other species. Published studies have shown fairly consistently that about two thirds of cats who are diagnosed with hypertension are azotemic,[1,3] but estimates of the proportion of azotemic cats who are hypertensive are much less consistent, ranging from 19 to 65 per cent.[4,5] These widely differing estimates probably are due to differences in the populations studied and differences in the cut-off points used to define hypertension. Contrary to expectation, cats do not appear to be more likely to become hypertensive the more azotemic that they become but usually are only

Box 49-1   Hypertension in Cats: Predisposing Clinical Conditions and Potential Target Organ Damage

Evidence of Possible Target Organ Damage Resulting from Hypertension	Clinical Problems Associated with Hypertension
OCULAR	**COMMON**
Hyphema	Renal dysfunction
Blindness	Azotemia
Retinal detachment	Proteinuria
Hypertensive retinopathy/ choroidopathy	Hyperthyroidism
	At diagnosis and after instituting treatment
NEUROLOGICAL	
Seizures	**UNCOMMON**
Altered mentation	Hyperadrenocorticism
Focal neurological deficits (brain or spinal cord)	Primary hyperaldosteronism
	Pheochromocytoma
CARDIOVASCULAR	Drug therapy
Murmur	Glucocorticoids
Arrhythmia	
Gallop	
Left ventricular hypertrophy	
Asymmetric septal hypertrophy	
Aortic dilation	
Epistaxis	

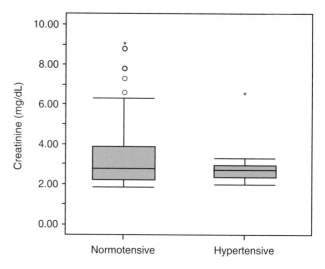

Figure 49-1 Relationship between severity of azotemia and blood pressure status. Data are taken from a cross-sectional study of 103 cats (20 of whom were hypertensive) diagnosed with azotemic chronic kidney disease in first-opinion practices.[4]

mildly azotemic when hypertension is diagnosed. This fact is illustrated in Figure 49-1, which shows the creatinine concentrations in a group of 103 cats with azotemic CKD; although overall there was no difference in creatinine concentration between hypertensive and normotensive cats, the cats who were hypertensive generally were not severely azotemic. There are a couple of possible explanations for these findings. First, cats who were severely azotemic may have been hypovolemic, which reduced their blood pressure; second, hypertensive cats were often presented due to development of blindness or hyphema, not due to clinical signs associated with renal failure (e.g., polydipsia, vomiting). Therefore, when using epidemiological evidence to select patients for blood pressure measurement or to assess the likelihood that a patient is truly hypertensive, it is important to recognize that any degree of azotemia, no matter how mild, should be considered as a risk factor.

Interestingly, in reports of larger series of hypertensive cats published to date, about 20 to 25 per cent of the cats have been nonazotemic and nonhyperthyroid.[6] Although some of these cats may have had less common causes of hypertension (see Box 49-1), it seems unlikely that rare disorders would account for this many patients. Nonazotemic, nonhyperthyroid cats have been described as having "idiopathic hypertension." In these cats, hypertension may actually be primary—unassociated with any underlying disease process. Others have suggested that

affected cats may have nonazotemic CKD. Practitioners should be aware that an identifiable cause will not be found in all hypertensive patients.

Hyperthyroidism often is cited as a common cause of hypertension in cats. However, the relationship between the two conditions is complex, not least because of the common association of both hypertension and hyperthyroidism with CKD. Experimental studies in human beings and rodents have shown that hyperthyroidism induces a reduction in total peripheral resistance (TPR) that offsets the increase in cardiac output and results in very little change in mean arterial pressure.[7] This adaptation may be the reason that relatively few hyperthyroid cats have hypertensive ocular lesions[8] and that similarly few cats presented for hypertensive ocular lesions have hyperthyroidism.[1] Nonetheless, hyperthyroidism is the disease second most commonly associated with hypertension in cats; therefore measurement of blood pressure in all hyperthyroid cats is recommended. Hyperthyroid cats can develop hypertension following treatment, so it is important to measure blood pressure both before and after therapy.[9]

END-ORGAN DAMAGE

One determinant of whether to treat a cat with antihypertensive drugs is evidence that the patient has end-organ damage or will likely develop it if treatment is not implemented. It is thus worth reviewing the clinical signs that may be associated with systemic hypertension and also the blood pressure measurements that have been obtained from these patients, in order to derive guidelines for when hypertension should be treated.

Blindness due to retinal detachment and/or intraocular hemorrhage is found commonly in cats presented with signs referable to hypertension. Less severe changes include focal retinal detachments and small intraretinal hemorrhages, areas of retinal edema, and localized narrowing of retinal arterioles. An excellent review of the ocular lesions that may be found in hypertensive cats has been published.[10] One study compared oscillometric blood pressure measurements in cats with hypertensive retinopathy with measurements in healthy, nonaffected cats; more than 90 per cent of the hypertensive cats had systolic blood pressure (SBP) measurements above 168 mm Hg, while 90 per cent of the healthy cats had SBP measurements below 168 mm Hg.[11] These results support clinical studies that have used SBP measurements of between 160 and 170 mm Hg, in association with compatible ocular lesions, to define hypertensive retinopathy/choroidopathy.[1,5,12]

Neurological signs also have been reported in cats with spontaneous systemic hypertension. The signs are variable and may include focal deficits referable to the brain or spinal cord, seizures, coma, or sudden death. Development of neurological signs has been well documented in cats following renal transplantation or sub–total nephrectomy; in these patients the acuteness of the blood pressure rise may make them particularly vulnerable to injury.[13,14] Anecdotally, owners report that many cats who present with severe hypertension become brighter and more active following the instigation of treatment, which may be due to resolution of neurological depression.

Cardiac changes that have been reported in hypertensive cats include auscultation of a murmur or a gallop, hypertrophy of the left ventricular free wall, asymmetric septal hypertrophy, or dilation of the aortic root (detected by echocardiography).[15-17] It is important to note, however, that none of these findings are limited to cats with systemic hypertension and there is considerable overlap in echocardiographic findings in hypertensive and normotensive cats. This lack of specificity means that cardiac evaluation rarely is helpful in deciding whether a patient should be started on antihypertensive treatment. Similarly, studies of tissue Doppler imaging have shown that myocardial velocity gradients are altered to a similar degree in cats with left ventricular hypertrophy attributed to systemic hypertension and in cats with idiopathic hypertrophic cardiomyopathy.[18] Heart failure has been reported in hypertensive cats but appears to be relatively uncommon.[1,12,19]

MEASUREMENT OF BLOOD PRESSURE

Reliable measurement of blood pressure is required for the appropriate management of patients with hypertension, both to identify cats in need of antihypertensive therapy and to monitor response to treatment. Although invasive measurement, obtained by the direct insertion of a catheter into an artery, is the most accurate method for determining blood pressure, it is rarely practical outside of anesthetic or critical care settings. Noninvasive measurement of blood pressure has limited accuracy but is more practical than direct measurement in most clinical settings.

Various noninvasive methods of blood pressure measurement have been described. Unfortunately, none have been shown to measure blood pressure consistently and

accurately in cats, particularly nonsedated cats. Arguably, it is more important that blood pressure measurement devices be precise, rather than accurate; however, most evaluations of the performance of blood pressure measuring devices have focused on accuracy. Using a target analogy, the different meaning of the terms *accuracy* and *precision* are represented visually in Figure 49-2. Precise measurements are reproducible, although there may be a significant bias from the "true" value. Measurement bias may not be important if it is consistent. For example, if it is known that systolic blood pressure measurements of 170 mm Hg made with a particular device predict those cats who are at risk of target organ damage, it is of no consequence if the "true" measurements are actually much greater or less than this value provided that the same device is always used for measurement. Estimates of the accuracy and/or precision of several different blood

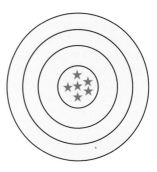

Accurate and precise

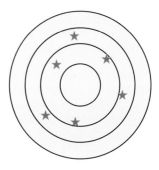

Accurate but not precise

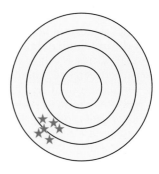

Precise but not accurate

Figure 49-2 Target analogy for considering accuracy and precision.

pressure measuring devices usually have been obtained in anesthetized patients. A study that compared indirect and direct blood pressure measurements in awake and anesthetized cats found that the correlation between the measurements was much stronger in anesthetized patients. This was particularly true for the oscillometric measurement device, which had a coefficient of determination (R^2 value) of only 0.362 to 0.550 in conscious cats when compared with direct measurements.[20] The correlation was considerably better (0.602 to 0.853) when the cats were anesthetized. Although far from ideal, the correlation between Doppler and direct measurements in awake cats was much stronger ($R^2 = 0.822$ to 0.826) than with the oscillometric method. In a different study, measurement of blood pressure made by the Doppler method predicted the presence of end-organ damage, while those made by oscillometric methods did not.[21]

An additional disadvantage of the oscillometric method is the amount of time that it can take to obtain blood pressure measurements and the number of cats for which measurement is not achieved successfully. One study of 28 cats reported successful measurement in just 115 of 223 (52 per cent) attempts to measure blood pressure by the oscillometric method; in 55 per cent of cases, it took longer than 10 minutes to achieve five measurements.[21] By comparison, Doppler measurement of systolic blood pressure was successful for all attempts (280) and was much faster.[21] Another report describing blood pressure measurement by the oscillometric method in 203 cats also suggested that considerable time (15 to 60 minutes) be allowed for measurement.[22] Blood pressure measurements were only obtained successfully using the oscillometric method in 41 of 54 (76 per cent) hypertensive cats in another study.[11]

For these reasons, it is the author's opinion that blood pressure measurement in awake cats should be performed using a Doppler technique, while readily acknowledging that this method has its limitations. With practice, it usually is possible to obtain five measurements of systolic blood pressure by the Doppler method in less than 5 minutes (excluding the time allowed for acclimatization). A description of this method of blood pressure measurement is provided in Figure 49-3.

MEASUREMENT OF BLOOD PRESSURE BY THE DOPPLER METHOD

Figure 49-3 shows blood pressure being measured in the forelimb, although the hindlimb or tail also may be used. The site that is used probably is not important, provided that it is consistent between measurements; ideally, an identical method should be used by all personnel who measure blood pressure within a veterinary practice. The cat in the photographs lost his eye due to an iris melanoma, not from systemic hypertension (see Figure 49-3, A).

Ideally, cats should be restrained minimally by their owner for blood pressure measurement as shown in the figure. Measurements are made after 10 minutes of acclimatization and before any stressful procedures are performed. The circumference of the limb is measured

initially to enable selection of a cuff width that is 30 to 40 per cent of the limb's circumference. The length of the cuff is not important provided it is sufficient to encircle the limb (see Figure 49-3, B). The cuff is fitted snugly to the limb midway between the elbow and carpus. This should be done before attaching the cuff to the sphygmomanometer (Figure 49-3, C).

Various approaches can be taken to maximize acoustic coupling between the Doppler probe and the cat's skin. The fur may be clipped, and this may be essential in cats with very dense haircoats. However, the sound of the clippers can be stressful, and clipping is not necessary in most cats. Instead, an alcohol-soaked swab may be used to wet the hair in the area to which the probe is to be applied, as shown in the figure. A small amount of ultrasound coupling gel also can be rubbed gently into the fur (see Figure 49-3, D).

Before the probe is applied to the limb, a liberal amount of ultrasound coupling gel should be placed onto the Doppler probe. The clinician/nurse should ensure that either the amplifier is turned off or the volume turned to zero before the probe is applied to the limb; otherwise, very loud "static" noise will result, which will likely upset the cat. Once the probe is in direct contact with the skin, the volume setting is increased and the probe moved gently around without losing contact with the skin until arterial pulsations are detected. The pulse usually can be found close to the carpal pad and slightly to the medial aspect of the limb. With practice, it is not necessary to look at where the probe is being placed, so the pulse can be found with the minimum of limb manipulation.

The pressure in the cuff is increased to about 20 mm Hg above the point at which the pulse can no longer be heard and then is deflated slowly while the clinician/nurse listens for the point at which the pulsations resume and views the dial of the sphygmomanometer so that this pressure can be recorded. This is the systolic blood pressure. The cuff is then deflated fully so that blood flow to and from the limb is unimpeded and the process is repeated several times. The first measurement is disregarded, and then between three and five consecutive measurements of blood pressure are made in the same manner. Ideally, they should all be within 10 mm Hg of each other. If there is a downward progression in the series of measurements, the process should be repeated until the measurements become consistent (see Figure 49-3, E and F).

WHITE-COAT EFFECT

The term *white-coat effect* has been used to describe the transient increase in blood pressure caused by anxiety that may occur when a patient is examined in a clinical setting. It is presumed that this is an effect of sympathetic stimulation. Transient increases in blood pressure have been demonstrated in cats subjected to a mock visit to a veterinary clinic; documented increases in blood pressure were as great as 75 mm Hg.[23] The increases in blood pressure did tend to dissipate, and blood pressure was within 20 mm Hg of baseline by the end of a 10-minute waiting

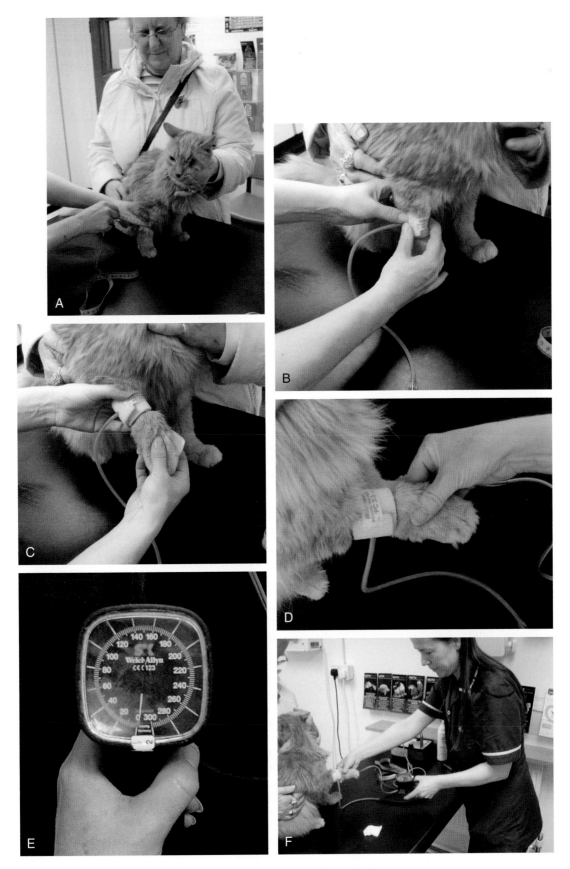

Figure 49-3 A to **F,** Measurement of blood pressure by the Doppler method.

period in most, but not all, of the cats. Most concerning was the observation that the cats showing the greatest white-coat effect could not be predicted from their demeanor or from considering other clinical parameters; there was no statistically significant association between the magnitude of the white-coat effect and heart rate, for example.[23] The white-coat effect may result in an erroneous diagnosis of systemic hypertension and unnecessary treatment. There is no evidence to support the widely held clinical assumption that the white-coat effect is greater in cats that are acting in an aggressive manner than in those that are more tractable.

Although greater emphasis has been placed on transient increases in blood pressure, it is important to recognize that blood pressure also can be reduced due to conditions such as sedation, hypovolemia, and parasympathetic overactivity, potentially resulting in a diagnosis of systemic hypertension being overlooked.

DECIDING TO TREAT FOR SYSTEMIC HYPERTENSION

The decision to treat a cat who has definitive evidence of end-organ damage (most often ocular changes) as a result of systemic hypertension usually is straightforward. For asymptomatic cats, treatment decisions must weigh the consequences of providing unnecessary treatment (i.e., for white-coat hypertension) against those of not treating a cat who is truly hypertensive and at risk for developing end-organ damage. The decision will rest, in part, on the severity of the blood pressure elevation, as reflected in the American College of Veterinary Internal Medicine's consensus statement guidelines (outlined in Table 49-1).

In the author's practice, antihypertensive therapy is instituted in any cat with systolic blood pressure measurements over 170 mm Hg and compatible ocular lesions. If no ocular lesions are present, the cat is not started on therapy on the basis of measurements made at a single visit (irrespective of how high these are), but the owner is asked to return the cat to the clinic in 1 to 2 weeks for blood pressure measurement to be repeated. Therapy is instituted only if blood pressure again also is

Table 49-1 American College of Veterinary Internal Medicine Consensus Statement: Risk of Target-Organ Damage According to Blood Pressure[46]

Risk Category*	Systolic Blood Pressure (mm Hg)	Diastolic Blood Pressure (mm Hg)	Risk of Target Organ Damage
I	<150	<95	Minimal
II	150-159	95-99	Mild
III	160-179	100-119	Moderate
IV	≥180	≥120	Severe

*In patients in whom both systolic and diastolic measurements are made, the risk category assigned is whichever of the two is the highest.

high on this second visit. Screening for hypertension in asymptomatic cats is performed only if they are over 9 years of age, unless they are azotemic or have some other identifiable risk factor for development of hypertension.

TREATMENT OF SYSTEMIC HYPERTENSION

SODIUM INTAKE

Although a reduction in dietary sodium intake often is recommended as an initial step in the management of systemic hypertension in human beings, there is no evidence that this intervention is of any benefit in the management of hypertension in cats. Restriction of dietary sodium intake had no effect on blood pressure in cats with normal renal function or with surgically induced renal failure in one study.[24] Reduction in sodium intake did, however, result in potentially deleterious effects, including activation of the renin-angiotensin system. Therefore, although excess sodium intake should be avoided in hypertensive cats, restricting salt intake is not advisable for the sole purpose of hypertensive management. Pharmacological management is thus the mainstay of treatment for systemic hypertension in cats.

CALCIUM CHANNEL BLOCKERS

The calcium channel blocker amlodipine has been demonstrated in numerous studies to be a safe and effective treatment for systemic hypertension in cats.[3,15,24-27] An initial dose of 0.625 mg/cat (¼ of a 2.5 mg tablet) is recommended; if the reduction in blood pressure is inadequate, the dose is doubled to 1.25 mg/cat (½ of a 2.5 mg tablet). Reduction in systolic blood pressure of 40 to 70 mm Hg is typical when implementing therapy, with the greatest decreases seen in cats with the highest pretreatment blood pressure measurements; clinically significant hypotension is uncommon.[26-28] Amlodipine is classified as a second-generation dihydropyridine calcium channel blocker. It exerts its actions through the L-type (long-lasting) voltage-operated channels that are located in many tissues but are present at highest concentrations in blood vessels, atria, and skeletal muscle. Calcium channel blockers of the dihydropyridine class act predominantly on the smooth muscle of the arterial vasculature, resulting in vasodilation and a corresponding decrease in blood pressure. This drug is tolerated very well; side effects are reported rarely. Although the dosing is imprecise when commercially available tablets are split into quarters, treatment cost is low and tablet fragments can be hidden in food easily. Crushing the tablets and resuspending the powder does not alter bioavailability of the drug when administered to human beings.[29] The half-life of amlodipine is known to be long (35 hours in human beings and 30 hours in dogs).[30] Although the half-life in cats has not been measured, its duration of effect seems to be maintained for longer than 24 hours, making it suitable for q24h dosing. Further, the lack of precision in daily dosing rarely presents a clinical problem.[27,30]

The use of a transdermal formulation of amlodipine in hypertensive cats also has been reported.[28] Bioavailability of the transdermal formulation was reported to be only about 30 per cent of that of the orally administered drug, and it is possible that bioavailability reached this level only because cats ingested the product from the pinnae while grooming. Given the ease with which amlodipine can be administered orally, the requirement for a transdermal formulation seems debatable.

In an experimental model of induced renal insufficiency and hypertension in cats, diltiazem was shown to decrease blood pressure; however, the effect was not maintained for 24 hours, indicating that the drug would need to be given at least q12h for effective blood pressure control.[31] Diltiazem is a member of the benzothiazepine class of calcium channel blockers and would be anticipated to have more cardiac effects than drugs of the dihydropyridine class, such as amlodipine. The primary cardiac effect of calcium channel blockers is inhibition of the spontaneous diastolic depolarization of cardiac myocytes (phase 4 of the cardiac action potential), which may cause slowing of sinoatrial depolarization and delayed conduction through the atrioventricular node. Diltiazem administration has been reported in a small number of cats with spontaneous hypertensive disorders; although some improvement in blood pressure was noted, amlodipine was found to be more efficacious.[1]

ANGIOTENSIN-CONVERTING ENZYME INHIBITORS AND ANGIOTENSIN RECEPTOR BLOCKERS

Angiotensin-converting enzyme inhibitors (ACE inhibitors) are used frequently for the treatment of hypertension in human beings. These drugs also are known to be safe and well tolerated in cats. However, numerous lines of evidence show that this class of drugs is not suitable for primary treatment (at least as monotherapy) of hypertension in cats because the change in blood pressure that occurs is simply too small. Reported changes in blood pressure have been less than 15 mm Hg in experimental studies using implanted blood pressure transponders to enable accurate and continuous measurement of blood pressure.[30,32,33] The response to ACE inhibitor administration also has been unsatisfactory in cases of spontaneous feline hypertension.[1,12,34]

Clinical experience with angiotensin receptor blockers (ARBs [e.g., losartan]) in feline practice is limited. In one experimental study of cats who had undergone subtotal nephrectomy, administration of losartan in combination with enalapril did not result in significant blood pressure reduction.[31] These agents are not recommended currently for management of systemic hypertension in cats.

BETA-BLOCKERS

Beta-blockers have the potential to reduce blood pressure by decreasing heart rate and stroke volume and also by inhibiting the release of renin. Selective beta-1 blockers such as atenolol are preferred, because they prevent the undesirable side effect of bronchoconstriction mediated via beta-2 receptors. However, beta-blockers have not been found to be effective in management of cats with hypertension associated with CKD.[25,34] It has been proposed that beta-blocker therapy may be appropriate in cats with hyperthyroidism because the hypertension is mediated, in part, by adrenergic mechanisms and the increase in heart rate. In a recent study, however, atenolol was effective in reducing heart rate in hypertensive hyperthyroid cats, yet a satisfactory decline in systolic blood pressure (posttreatment SBP <160 mm Hg) was evident in only six of the 20 (30 per cent) cats treated.[35] Therefore amlodipine remains the treatment of choice for management of systemic hypertension in cats, even when associated with hyperthyroidism.

ALDOSTERONE RECEPTOR ANTAGONIST

Spironolactone is a mineralocorticoid (aldosterone) receptor antagonist. Its primary indication in the management of hypertension therefore lies in the treatment of cats with primary hyperaldosteronism (see Chapter 24). In affected cats spironolactone also moderates hypokalemic myopathy, with the majority of treated cats showing an increase in potassium concentration (although rarely reaching normal levels).[2] Many hypertensive cats with hyperaldosteronism require treatment with amlodipine in addition to spironolactone. Amlodipine may exert some antialdosterone activity as well. In addition to their vasodilatory effects, calcium channel blockers may reduce aldosterone synthesis and secretion by adrenal cortical cells directly. However, recent work indicates that T-type calcium channel blockers are more effective in this regard than L-type blockers such as amlodipine.[36] It also has been shown that some calcium channel blockers, including amlodipine, may be competitive inhibitors of aldosterone binding to mineralocorticoid receptors.[37] The effect of amlodipine on aldosterone secretion has not been studied directly in cats.

The recommended dose of spironolactone is 1 to 2 mg/kg PO q12h. Given that the smallest available tablet size is 25 mg, most cats receive a total dose of 6.25 mg (one quarter tablet) per cat. In a recent study of cats with heart disease, four of 13 cats treated with spironolactone developed a cutaneous drug reaction.[38] Lesions included an ulcerative dermatitis in the preauricular area between the eye and the ear, not dissimilar to that observed occasionally in cats as an adverse reaction to methimazole or carbimazole.

EMERGENCY HYPERTENSIVE THERAPY

Hydralazine has been used for the emergency treatment of systemic hypertension in cats following renal transplant procedures.[14] The drug was administered subcutaneously, typically at a dose of 2.5 mg/cat, resulting in a reduction in blood pressure within 15 minutes of its administration. Hydralazine is a direct-acting vasodilator with more effect on arteriolar than venous vessels. The rapid reduction in blood pressure that occurs in response to treatment with this drug may cause reflex tachycardia; combined treatment with a beta-blocker may be necessary to prevent this complication.

Although hydralazine apparently is very effective in reducing blood pressure rapidly in cats, emergency treatment for hypertension in most clinical patients is simply not necessary. Emergency therapy is indicated in patients in whom the increase in blood pressure is known to be acute, usually following high-risk surgeries such as renal transplantation and some neurological procedures. In these scenarios, blood pressure should be monitored frequently in an intensive care setting. In most instances in which hypertension is diagnosed in cats, urgent treatment, rather than emergency treatment, is required. Even in cats presented for sudden blindness (although arguably it is the recognition of blindness by the owner that is acute rather than the blindness per se), the elevation in blood pressure invariably is chronic. These patients should be started on amlodipine treatment immediately. There is no evidence that more rapidly acting therapies will be any more likely to preserve or restore the cat's vision, and the risk of side effects will be increased with their use.

THERAPEUTIC END-POINTS

Having decided that a patient should be treated with antihypertensive agents, one should then consider the desired goals of therapy: By how much should blood pressure be lowered, and what clinical response can be expected to this reduction? The lesions that can be monitored most easily are those in the eye. Reducing blood pressure below about 160 mm Hg (into risk category I or II; see Table 49-1) apparently is effective at preventing cats from developing new ocular lesions.[1,10] With a reduction in blood pressure, there also will be improvement of existing lesions; retinal hemorrhage and hyphema will resolve slowly, subretinal exudates will reabsorb, and the retina may reattach. Retinal edema may resolve relatively quickly. Unfortunately, these improvements often are not associated with restoration of vision. Even if vision is restored following reattachment of the retina, improvement usually is temporary and subsequent retinal degeneration results in permanent vision loss.

Amlodipine treatment has been reported to reduce left ventricular hypertrophy in hypertensive cats, with 11 of 14 and six of 14 cats in one study meeting criteria for left ventricular hypertrophy before and after treatment respectively.[15] However, in the same study, there was no statistically significant difference in any of the measured cardiac dimensions when compared before and after treatment, making the relevance of this finding questionable. A separate study, which compared the survival of hypertensive cats with (33 of 39) and without (six of 39) evidence of left ventricular hypertrophy, found no difference between the two groups.[17] None of the deaths in that study were attributed to heart failure. In contrast, left ventricular hypertrophy is an independent risk factor for both cardiovascular events and all-cause mortality in hypertensive human patients.[39] Cardiac causes of death have been reported in a few cases of poorly controlled

feline hypertension,[26] but to date it appears that hypertension is not the significant risk factor for fatal cardiac disease in cats that it is in human beings.

Renal disease is reported to be the most common cause of death in cats with hypertension, with six of 19 cats in one study[26] and seven of 18 cats in another[17] dying or being euthanized due to progressive CKD. Hypertension also is known to worsen the prognosis in human beings and dogs with CKD.[40,41] However, it is currently unclear whether hypertension results in more rapid progression of CKD in cats. In one study of 136 cats that evaluated risk factors of importance in the progression of CKD, a diagnosis of systemic hypertension was not independently related to survival.[42] However, cats with higher blood pressure were more proteinuric, and that in turn was related to their survival time; therefore hypertension could still be of prognostic significance indirectly. A potential limitation of that study was that all of the cats who had been diagnosed with hypertension were treated subsequently with amlodipine, reducing their blood pressure and potentially confounding the analysis. In an attempt to address that limitation, a subsequent study evaluated the survival of hypertensive cats treated with amlodipine specifically.[3] In addition to evaluating factors shown previously to predict progression of CKD—such as severity of azotemia, proteinuria, hyperphosphatemia, and age—the study used a composite value for all systolic blood pressure measurements obtained during the follow-up period to evaluate the effect of blood pressure control on survival time. Surprisingly, other than proteinuria, none of the evaluated variables was associated independently with survival time. The association between proteinuria and the survival of the hypertensive cats in that study is shown in Table 49-2.

In theory treatment with amlodipine in hypertensive cats could cause or exacerbate proteinuria, because this drug causes greater dilation of the afferent than the efferent renal arterioles, potentially allowing the transmission of high systemic pressures to the glomerular capillaries. However, worsening of glomerular hypertension does not appear to happen in hypertensive cats because treatment with amlodipine tends to cause a reduction in proteinuria as shown in Figure 49-4. This presumably is because of

Table 49-2 Survival Time of Hypertensive Cats Treated with Amlodipine, Stratified by Severity of Proteinuria

UPC	IRIS Category	Number of Cats	Median Survival Time (days)*
<0.2	Nonproteinuric	36	490 (range 217-1169)
0.2-0.4	Borderline proteinuric	34	313 (range 124-607)
>0.4	Proteinuric	48	162 (range 73-406)

UPC, Urine protein-to-creatinine ratio; *IRIS*, International Renal Interest Society.
*Data from Jepson RE, Elliott J, Brodbelt D, et al: Effect of control of systolic blood pressure on survival in cats with systemic hypertension, *J Vet Intern Med* 21:402, 2007.

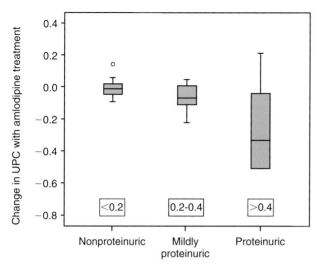

Figure 49-4 Change in proteinuria with amlodipine treatment of cats with systemic hypertension. (From Syme HM et al: Proteinuria in cats: prognostic marker or mediator? *J Feline Med Surg* 11(3):211-218, 2009.)

the profound decrease in systemic blood pressure that occurs when treatment with amlodipine is initiated.

The importance of proteinuria as a prognostic indicator in cats with hypertension has led to the recommendation that hypertensive treatments in cats be adjusted based on urine protein-to-creatinine (UPC) ratios. Cats who are proteinuric (UPC >0.4) may be treated with an ACE inhibitor in addition to amlodipine. The rationale for this proposal is that these drugs dilate the efferent arteriole preferentially, reducing pressure across the glomerulus and reducing proteinuria. Treatment with ACE inhibitors has been shown to be beneficial in slowing progression of renal damage in human patients with naturally occurring kidney disease.[43] Published studies of ACE-inhibitor treatment in cats with azotemic CKD have demonstrated that these drugs significantly reduce proteinuria, but they have not been able to demonstrate a statistically significant survival benefit, although favorable trends were evident.[44,45] However, these studies did not include patients with hypertension, so the effect of ACE-inhibitor treatment in the hypertensive CKD population currently is unknown.

FOLLOW-UP EVALUATIONS

Cats with serious or rapidly progressive clinical signs of hypertension should be re-evaluated within 1 to 3 days of initiating pharmacological treatments. Other patients should be evaluated 7 to 10 days after instituting or changing therapy and thereafter at 1- to 4-month intervals dependent on stability.[46] In addition to clinical examination, measurement of blood pressure, creatinine concentration, urinalysis, and fundic examination should be included in the patient re-assessment protocol. Other specific assessments should be performed as indicated by

initial evidence of target organ damage and concurrent disease. Intermittent monitoring of serum or plasma potassium concentration also may be advisable because concentrations tend to decline with amlodipine therapy.[25,26]

SUMMARY

Effective antihypertensive therapy will reduce the risk of blindness and other ocular signs of hypertension in cats. It also is likely to prevent the development of cardiac changes, although these are less often the cause of clinical signs. It does not appear currently that hypertension contributes directly to the progression of renal disease, but there may be an indirect effect due to an association with proteinuria. In the great majority of clinical situations amlodipine is the antihypertensive agent of choice in cats.

REFERENCES

1. Maggio F, DeFrancesco TC, Atkins CE, et al: Ocular lesions associated with systemic hypertension in cats: 69 cases (1985-1998), *J Am Vet Med Assoc* 217:695, 2000.
2. Ash RA, Harvey AM, Tasker S: Primary hyperaldosteronism in the cat: a series of 13 cases, *J Feline Med Surg* 7:173, 2005.
3. Jepson RE, Elliott J, Brodbelt D, et al: Effect of control of systolic blood pressure on survival in cats with systemic hypertension, *J Vet Intern Med* 21:402, 2007.
4. Syme HM, Barber PJ, Markwell PJ, et al: Prevalence of systolic hypertension in cats with chronic renal failure at initial evaluation, *J Am Vet Med Assoc* 220:1799, 2002.
5. Stiles J, Polzin DJ, Bistner DI: The prevalence of retinopathy in cats with systemic hypertension and chronic renal failure or hyperthyroidism, *J Am Anim Hosp Assoc* 30:654, 1994.
6. Elliott J, Fletcher MG, Syme HM: Idiopathic feline hypertension: epidemiological study, *J Vet Intern Med* 17:754, 2003.
7. Syme HM: Cardiovascular and renal manifestations of hyperthyroidism, *Vet Clin North Am Small Anim Pract* 37:723, 2007.
8. van der Woerdt A, Peterson ME: Prevalence of ocular abnormalities in cats with hyperthyroidism, *J Vet Intern Med* 14:202, 2000.
9. Syme HM, Elliott J: The prevalence of hypertension in hyperthyroid cats at diagnosis and following treatment, *J Vet Intern Med* 17:754, 2003.
10. Crispin SM, Mould JR: Systemic hypertensive disease and the feline fundus, *Vet Ophthalmol* 4:131, 2001.
11. Sansom J, Rogers K, Wood JL: Blood pressure assessment in healthy cats and cats with hypertensive retinopathy, *Am J Vet Res* 65:245, 2004.
12. Littman MP: Spontaneous systemic hypertension in 24 cats, *J Vet Intern Med* 8:79, 1994.
13. Brown CA, Munday JS, Mathur S: Hypertensive encephalopathy in cats with reduced renal function, *Vet Pathol* 42:642, 2005.
14. Kyles AE, Gregory CR, Wooldridge JD, et al: Management of hypertension controls postoperative neurologic disorders after renal transplantation in cats, *Vet Surg* 28:436, 1999.
15. Snyder PS, Sadek D, Jones GL: Effect of amlodipine on echocardiographic variables in cats with systemic hypertension, *J Vet Intern Med* 15:52, 2001.
16. Nelson L, Reidesel E, Ware WA, et al: Echocardiographic and radiographic changes associated with systemic hypertension in cats, *J Vet Intern Med* 16:418, 2002.

17. Chetboul V, Lefebvre HP, Pinhas C, et al: Spontaneous feline hypertension: clinical and echocardiographic abnormalities, and survival rate, *J Vet Intern Med* 17:89, 2003.

18. Sampedrano C, Chetboul V, Gouni V, et al: Systolic and diastolic myocardial dysfunction in cats with hypertrophic cardiomyopathy or systemic hypertension, *J Vet Intern Med* 20:1106, 2006.

19. Wey AC, Atkins CE: Aortic dissection and congestive heart failure associated with systemic hypertension in a cat, *J Vet Intern Med* 14:208, 2000.

20. Brown S, Haberman C, Morgan J: Evaluation of doppler ultrasonic and oscillometric estimates of blood pressure in cats, *J Vet Intern Med* 15:281, 2001.

21. Jepson RE, Hartley V, Mendl M, et al: A comparison of CAT Doppler and oscillometric Memoprint machines for non-invasive blood pressure measurement in conscious cats, *J Feline Med Surg* 7:147, 2005.

22. Bodey AR, Sansom J: Epidemiological study of blood pressure in domestic cats, *J Small Anim Pract* 39:567, 1998.

23. Belew AM, Barlett T, Brown SA: Evaluation of the white-coat effect in cats, *J Vet Intern Med* 13:134, 1999.

24. Buranakarl C, Mathur S, Brown SA: Effects of dietary sodium chloride intake on renal function and blood pressure in cats with normal and reduced renal function, *Am J Vet Res* 65:620, 2004.

25. Henik RA, Snyder PS, Volk LM: Treatment of systemic hypertension in cats with amlodipine besylate, *J Am Anim Hosp Assoc* 33:226, 1997.

26. Elliott J, Barber PJ, Syme HM, et al: Feline hypertension: clinical findings and response to antihypertensive treatment in 30 cases, *J Small Anim Pract* 42:122, 2001.

27. Snyder PS: Amlodipine: a randomized, blinded clinical trial in 9 cats with systemic hypertension, *J Vet Intern Med* 12:157, 1998.

28. Helms SR: Treatment of feline hypertension with transdermal amlodipine: a pilot study, *J Am Anim Hosp Assoc* 43:149, 2007.

29. Lyszkiewicz DA, Levichek Z, Kozer E, et al: Bioavailability of a pediatric amlodipine suspension, *Pediatr Nephrol* 18:675, 2003.

30. Stopher DA, Beresford AP, Macrae PV, et al: The metabolism and pharmacokinetics of amlodipine in humans and animals, *J Cardiovasc Pharmacol* 7(suppl 12):S55, 1988.

31. Mathur S, Brown CA, Dietrich UM, et al: Evaluation of a technique of inducing hypertensive renal insufficiency in cats, *Am J Vet Res* 65:1006, 2004.

32. Brown SA, Brown CA, Jacobs G, et al: Effects of the angiotensin converting enzyme inhibitor benazepril in cats with induced renal insufficiency, *Am J Vet Res* 62:375, 2001.

33. Miller RH, Lehmkuhl LB, Smeak DD, et al: Effect of enalapril on blood pressure, renal function, and the renin-angiotensin-aldosterone system in cats with autosomal dominant polycystic kidney disease, *Am J Vet Res* 60:1516, 1999.

34. Jensen J, Henik RA, Brownfield M, et al: Plasma renin activity and angiotensin I and aldosterone concentrations in cats with hypertension associated with chronic renal disease, *Am J Vet Res* 58:535, 1997.

35. Henik RA, Stepien RL, Wenholz LJ, et al: Efficacy of atenolol as a single antihypertensive agent in hyperthyroid cats, *J Feline Med Surg* 10:577, 2008.

36. Tanaka T, Tsutamoto T, Sakai H, et al: Comparison of the effects of efonidipine and amlodipine on aldosterone in patients with hypertension, *Hypertens Res* 30:691, 2007.

37. Dietz JD, Du S, Bolten CW, et al: A number of marketed dihydropyridine calcium channel blockers have mineralocorticoid receptor antagonist activity, *Hypertension* 51:742, 2008.

38. MacDonald KA, Kittleson MD, Kass PH: Effect of spironolactone on diastolic function and left ventricular mass in Maine Coon cats with familial hypertrophic cardiomyopathy, *J Vet Intern Med* 22:335, 2008.

39. Levy D, Garrison RJ, Savage DD, et al: Prognostic implications of echocardiographically determined left ventricular mass in the Framingham Heart Study, *N Engl J Med* 322:1561, 1990.

40. Jacob F, Polzin DJ, Osborne CA, et al: Association between initial systolic blood pressure and risk of developing a uremic crisis or of dying in dogs with chronic renal failure, *J Am Vet Med Assoc* 222:322, 2003.

41. Jafar TH, Stark PC, Schmid CH, et al: for the AIPRD Study Group: Progression of chronic kidney disease: the role of blood pressure control, proteinuria, and angiotensin-converting enzyme inhibition: a patient-level meta-analysis, *Ann Intern Med* 139:244, 2003.

42. Syme HM, Markwell PJ, Pfeiffer D, et al: Survival of cats with naturally occurring chronic renal failure is related to severity of proteinuria, *J Vet Intern Med* 20:528, 2006.

43. Maschio G, Alberti D, Janin G, et al: Effect of the angiotensin-converting-enzyme inhibitor benazepril on the progression of chronic renal insufficiency. The Angiotensin-Converting-Enzyme Inhibition in Progressive Renal Insufficiency Study Group, *N Engl J Med* 334:939, 1996.

44. King JN, Gunn-Moore DA, Tasker S, et al: Tolerability and efficacy of benazepril in cats with chronic kidney disease, *J Vet Intern Med* 20:1054, 2006.

45. Mizutani H, Koyama H, Watanabe T, et al: Evaluation of the clinical efficacy of benazepril in the treatment of chronic renal insufficiency in cats, *J Vet Intern Med* 20:1074, 2006.

46. Brown S, Atkins C, Bagley R, et al: Guidelines for the identification, evaluation, and management of systemic hypertension in dogs and cats, *J Vet Intern Med* 21:542, 2007.

CHAPTER
50 Purine Uroliths

Josephine S. Gnanandarajah, Jody P. Lulich,
Hasan Albasan, and Carl A. Osborne

Between January 1, 2007 and December 31, 2007, the Minnesota Urolith Center performed quantitative mineral analysis on uroliths from 11,174 cats. Five hundred fifty cats (4.92 per cent) had uroliths composed of purines. Of these 550 cats, uroliths from 520 (94.5 per cent) were composed of ammonium acid urate (47 per cent were female, and 53 per cent were male; median age, 6 years); uroliths from 27 were composed of xanthine (37 per cent were female and 63 per cent were male; median age, 2 years); uroliths from two cats were composed of uric acid monohydrate; and uroliths from one cat were composed of sodium acid urate. During the same time period eight of these cats with uroliths composed of ammonium acid urate were evaluated at the Veterinary Medical Center, University of Minnesota. Of these eight cats three were female and five were male, and their median age was 6 years. The only specific breeds identified were a Birman and Maine Coon. All purine uroliths were retrieved from the urinary bladder or urethra.

WHAT ARE PURINES?

Purines are heterocyclic aromatic nitrogen-containing bases that form the building blocks of nucleic acid. Purines are a six-membered pyrimidine ring fused to five-membered imidazole rings (Figure 50-1). Naturally occurring ring purines belong to three major classes of purine compounds: aminopurines (adenine and guanine), oxypurines (hypoxanthine, xanthine, uric acid, and allantoin), and methylpurines (caffeine, theophylline, and theobromine).[1]

Animal proteins and purine-rich diets are the major sources of exogenous purines for mammals. In addition to the exogenous sources, purines also are synthesized de novo in the liver from nonpurine precursors. During de novo synthesis of purines, molecules such as glycine, aspartate, glutamine, N^{10}-formyltetrahydrofolate, carbon dioxide, glucose, and adenosine triphosphate (ATP) contribute to the formation of the purine ring (see Figure 50-1).[2,3]

Purine bases also can be salvaged and recycled endogenously from degrading nucleic acids. Preformed free purines that are derived from diet and nucleic acid degradation react with 5-phosphoribosyl-1-pyrophosphate (PRPP) in a reaction catalyzed by phosphoribosyltransferases (adenine phosphoribosyltransferase or hypoxanthine-guanine phosphoribosyltransferase) and form adenosine monophosphate (AMP), guanosine monophosphate (GMP), and inosine monophosphate (IMP). The detailed purine metabolic pathway is illustrated in Figures 50-2 and 50-3.[2,4,5]

WHAT IS URIC ACID?

Uric acid is an organic intermediate metabolite that arises in the purine metabolic pathway. Xanthine oxidase catalyzes the final step in uric acid synthesis. In most mammals uric acid is metabolized further into soluble allantoin. The degradation of uric acid is initiated by urate oxidase (uricase). The first intermediary metabolite of oxidative conversion of uric acid is 5-hydroxy isourate (HIU). HIU hydrolase catalyzes the hydrolysis of HIU

499

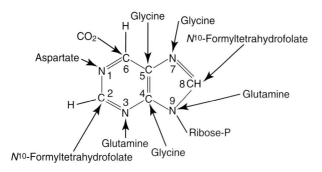

Figure 50-1 Structure of the purine and sources of atom in the purine rings during de novo synthesis are indicated.[7,42] The atoms are numbered according to the international system.

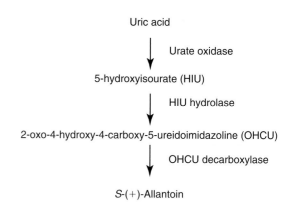

Figure 50-3 Uric acid degradation pathway.[41]

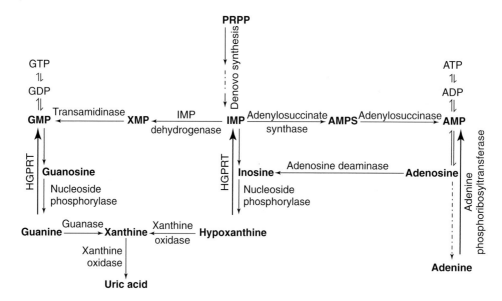

Figure 50-2 Schematic diagram of purine metabolic pathway.[7,42,49] During de novo purine synthesis, bases are constructed on 5-phosphoribosyl-1-pyrophosphate (PRPP) in multiple steps. Hypoxanthine-guanine phosphoribosyltransferase (HGPRT) is a crucial enzyme involved in the salvage pathway.[7,42,49] *IMP,* Inosine monophosphate; *AMP,* adenosine monophosphate; *GMP,* guanosine monophosphate.

to form 2-oxo-4-hydroxy-4-carboxy-5-ureidoimidazoline (OHCU).[4] OHCU is decarboxylated by OHCU decarboxylase into dextrorotatory allantoin (S-(+)-allantoin)[4] (see Figure 50-3). However, in human beings and primates the uric acid is the end product of purine catabolism.

In serum at physiological pH, uric acid is circulated in the form of monosodium urate. In mammals renal excretion is the major route of uric acid excretion although residual amounts of uric acid also are eliminated via the intestine. During renal clearance blood urate is filtered completely through the glomerulus, followed by reabsorption of the majority (≈90 per cent) of urates by the proximal tubules back into the circulation. Urate transporters in epithelia of the proximal tubules are essential for urate reabsorption (see the following).[6] The reabsorbed uric acid is metabolized further in liver, with a fraction that is not catabolized going through the glomerular filtration-reabsorption cycle.[7] This process leaves only 10 per cent of the plasma urate for excretion in urine.[8]

WHAT ARE THE PATHOPHYSIOLOGICAL METHODS OF URATE UROLITH FORMATION?

Supersaturation of uric acid in urine is essential for urate urolithiasis. Excess production, increased renal excretion, increased renal secretion, and decreased renal tubular reabsorption of uric acid promote hyperuricosuria. However, studies in human beings and dogs have demonstrated that urine supersaturation of uric acid alone is not sufficient to cause urate stones.[1] In addition, other physiochemical characteristics of the urine, such as pH, urine volume, cation concentration, and macromolecules, also play a critical role in regulating urate stone formation.

Molecular mechanisms of urate urolithiasis in cats have not been identified clearly. Renal tubular reabsorptive defect and portal vascular anomalies are the two postulated mechanisms thought to be involved in the pathogenesis of urate urolithiasis in this species.[7] However, no systematic studies have been carried out to prove the aforementioned hypotheses. Analyzing the comparative pathophysiological mechanisms involved in urate stone formation in human beings, dogs, and cats will provide the preliminary information to design systematic explorative studies in cats.

Again, uric acid is generated from purine catabolism, which takes place in the liver (see Figure 50-2). The final step in uric acid synthesis is catalyzed by xanthine oxidase. Although uric acid metabolism takes place primarily in the liver,[9] in human beings xanthine oxidase also is expressed in the jejunum. In cats and dogs the tissue distribution of xanthine oxidase is not known. Interestingly, human beings lack urate oxidase activity in the liver, because the urate oxidase gene was lost in primate ancestors about 15 million years ago. Therefore uric acid is the end product of purine catabolism in human beings.[10,11]

Comparative analysis of plasma concentration of urate in cats and Dalmatian dogs suggests that the urate oxidase enzyme is present in cats.[12,13] Evidence of urate oxidase in the peroxisomes of hepatic parenchymal cells in cats[14] may account for the relatively low prevalence of urate uroliths in this species. It would be worthwhile to investigate the urate oxidase activity in cats with urate stones to determine if stone-forming cats possess a functional urate oxidase.

Dalmatian dogs excrete mainly uric acid in their urine and are highly likely to develop hyperuricosuria. In the Dalmatian dog it is believed that hyperuricosuria is inherited as an autosomal recessive condition and regulated by a single gene.[15] Phylogenetic genome comparison and other studies indicate that urate oxidase is expressed in dogs.[4] In addition, Safra et al revealed that the urate oxidase gene is not responsible for the hyperuricosuria phenotype in Dalmatian dogs, based on the cDNA sequence identity and negative LOD scores.[15] However, uric acid levels are high in serum and urine of Dalmatian dogs compared with other breeds. It also has been shown that both stone-forming and non–stone-forming Dalmatian dogs have comparable levels of uric acid in plasma.[16,17] Liver and kidney transplantation studies in Dalmatian dogs have enabled investigators to localize the cause of hyperuricosuria to the liver.[18-23] Before this study, it was believed that Dalmatian dogs had a defect in the mechanism of urate reabsorption at the proximal tubules.[24,25] Simkin postulates that normal dogs (non–stone-formers) express promoters that facilitate the uric acid transport across the hepatocyte and proximal tubular cells, although no studies have been carried out to test this hypothesis.[26]

However, in vitro studies revealed that functional urate oxidase is present in liver homogenates of Dalmatian dogs. In contrast, liver slices from Dalmatian dogs were unable to metabolize uric acid.[27] The findings of these in vitro studies enabled the investigators to localize the cause of defective urate metabolism specifically to the membrane transporters in hepatocytes. Further investigations attempted to identify specific urate transporters in hepatocytes. Galectin-9, one of the putative urate transporters, was found to have no role in hyperuricosuria.[28] Reports on other urate transporters and their role in hyperuricosuria in Dalmatian dogs are not available.

However, Safra et al have shown that the locus CFA03 in the canine genome is linked to hyperuricosuria in Dalmatian dogs.[29] Surprisingly, none of the candidate genes of this locus are known to be associated with purine metabolism or urate transport.[29] However, follow-up studies on the other candidate genes of locus CFA03 have not been published to date.

In non-Dalmatian dogs, urate stone formation often is found in conjunction with a portal vascular anomaly.[30,31] In portovascular shunts, liver functions are impaired significantly, resulting in inefficient hepatic conversion of ammonia to urea and uric acid to allantoin.[30]

The cellular mechanisms involved in hyperuricemia and hyperuricosuria have not been investigated in cats. In light of the findings from other species, it is likely that a defective purine metabolism is one of the causes. It is possible that consumption of a purine-rich diet and increased nucleic acid catabolism as a result of extensive tissue damage or tissue proliferation (for example, lymphoma or leukemia) will lead to hyperuricemia and hyperuricosuria by simply increasing the purine pool of the body.[1] This leads to the hypothesis that the feline urate oxidase is unable to cope with a high load of uric acid generated from a high purine pool.

Reports indicate that a hepatic portal vascular anomaly also could contribute to hyperuricemia and hyperuricosuria in cats.[32] Because purine metabolism primarily is taking place in the liver, purine metabolism also would be affected, resulting in limited uric acid production. In the event of a hepatic portovascular shunt, urate uroliths would be seen predominantly in young cats, rather than in older animals. However, there is no significant correlation between the age of cats and urate stone formation. Therefore extensive serum chemistry analysis (purine metabolites, ammonia levels, liver function tests) needs to be performed to address the role of hepatic portovascular shunt in urate urolithiasis in cats.

In serum at physiological pH, uric acid is circulated in the form of monosodium urate. In mammals renal excretion is the major route of uric acid excretion, although residual levels of uric acid also are eliminated via the intestine. During renal clearance, blood urate is filtered completely through the glomerulus, followed by the majority (≈ 90 per cent) of the urate fraction being reabsorbed back into the circulation at the proximal tubules. This mechanism leaves only 10 per cent of the plasma urate for excretion in the urine.[8] The reabsorbed uric acid is metabolized further in the liver, with a fraction that is not catabolized going through the glomerular filtration-reabsorption cycle.[7] Postglomerular renal handling of uric acid varies among species, mainly at the level of proximal tubule reabsorption and secretion.[8,33,34]

In cats, the net urate reabsorption has been observed.[12] Dogs also exhibit net reabsorption of urate. In Dalmatian dogs the urate excreted in urine is higher than the filtered uric acid. This indicates that Dalmatian dogs have either a defect in renal urate reabsorption or abnormal tubular secretion of urate, or both. Studies that explored the renal physiology of this phenomenon confirmed that Dalmatian dogs have deficient proximal tubular urate reabsorption.[35] However, later studies involving kidney and liver transplants implicated defective transport mechanisms in hepatocytes as the etiology of the hyperuricosuria in Dalmatian dogs. Specific cellular transporters involved in the pathogenesis of this condition in Dalmatian dogs have not been identified.

Urate transporters in epithelia of the proximal tubules are essential for urate reabsorption.[6] Various membrane-associated urate transporters have been identified in human beings. Human beings reabsorb 90 per cent of the filtered urate through the sodium couple anion exchanger (Uric Acid Transporter-1, URAT1) located on the apical brush border of the proximal tubule epithelium.[36] Studies have shown that a mutation in the URAT1 gene is manifested as hyperuricosuria and hypouricocemia.[36]

Another urate transporter, UAT1 (also known as galectin-9) is expressed on the apical and basolateral membrane of proximal tubular cells as well as in other tissues. UAT1 is postulated to be functioning as a bidirectional transporter of urate across the tubular epithelia.[37] Urate also is transported into the proximal tubular epithelial cells via two other anion exchangers, known as OAT1 and OAT3. These transporters are located primarily at the basolateral membrane of the epithelia.[38-40] In addition, multidrug-resistance–associated protein 4 (MRP4), an organic anion transporter, was reported to mediate the secretion of urate into the lumen from the tubular cells. MRP4 also is expressed in the liver.[41]

Recently another potential urate transporter, SLC2A9 (a fructose transporter), was reported in human beings by Vitart et al.[42] The gene SLC2A9 encodes two protein isoforms with different lengths, each carrying around 10 different single nucleotide polymorphisms (SNPs). The causal role of these genetic variabilities on serum uric acid levels in human beings has yet to be identified.

The presence and the functions of the aforementioned urate transporters in dogs and cats have not been investigated.

WHY DO CATS FORM URATE UROLITHS?

Imbalances between uric acid synthesis and excretion lead to an increase in the uric acid pool in blood and urine (the possible mechanisms of the imbalance have been discussed previously). Three major risk factors that lead to formation of uric acid stones in human beings are hypovolumic urine, hyperuricosuria, and acidic urine.[43] In cats, highly concentrated acidic urine was associated with consumption of a purine precursor-enriched diet. However, this observation was made only in few cases.[44]

URIC ACID EXCRETION

At physiological pH, uric acid circulates in blood as urate. The concentration of the uric acid in feline plasma is around 0.223 ± 0.007 mg/dL.[12] In non-Dalmatian dogs and Dalmatian dogs the serum uric acid concentrations are ≤ 0.5 mg/dL and ≥ 1 mg/dL, respectively. Human serum uric acid concentration is reported as 3.36 mg/dL to 8.4 mg/dL, relatively higher compared with that in other

mammals (0.0336 to 2.016 mg/dL).[45] A healthy, non-Dalmatian dog excretes 55.2 ± 2.7 mg of uric acid per day,[1,30] whereas a Dalmatian dog excretes 439 ± 50.2 mg of uric acid per day.[22,30] Concentrations of uric acid and xanthine in the urine of cats with xanthine stones are 3.4 mg/dL and 54 mg/dL respectively.[32]

In addition to imbalances in synthesis and excretion, urine volume also contributes to supersaturation of salts in urine. In the event of intravascular volume depletion, urine volume is reduced to conserve more water, and as a result, cation concentration will be increased.

URINE pH

Solubility of uric acid depends on its concentration and the pH of the solution. Urinary pH is the major physiological factor that determines the crystallization of uric acid. Uric acid is a less soluble weak organic acid compared with its base, urate. Physiologically relevant ionization constant of uric acid is 5.5 (pKa). When urine pH is greater than 5.5, uric acid is converted into urate. Under conditions of low urine pH, uric acid becomes less soluble. Uric acid stones are more likely to form when the urine is supersaturated with uric acid under low pH (5.5).[43,46,47] At physiological pH, 98 per cent of the uric acid is in the form of urate.

In dogs and cats the association of urine pH to uric acid stone formation has not been studied extensively. In a few cases of urate stone formers among cats, urine was found to be highly acidic and concentrated.[32] Although the average pH of cat urine is 6.3, the type of diet highly influences the pH of the urine, making diet another potential factor associated with uric acid stone formation in cats.[48] It is essential to conduct systematic studies to determine whether the lower pH of urine in cats makes them susceptible to uric acid stone formation in the presence of urine supersaturation.

Because ammonia acts as a buffer in human urine, lower urinary ammonia concentration was hypothesized to be one of the reasons for low urine pH.

CATION CONCENTRATIONS IN URINE

Supersaturation of cations also influences the solubility of uric acid in the urine. Monosodium urate tends to form less soluble stones in the urine.[49] In cats most of the urate stones are in the form of ammonium acid urate.[32] In an aqueous solution ammonia exists as nonionized NH_3 and monovalent cation NH_4^+.[48] It has been reported that supersaturation of urate and ammonium leads to crystallization of ammonium acid urate stone formation at high urine pH.[8] However, there are no reports that compare ammonium ion levels in urine from stone-forming cats with normal cats. It is likely that ammonium supersaturation, in the presence of other aggravating factors, can promote ammonium acid urate formation in cats. Consumption of excess dietary protein will increase the urea load, resulting in excess ammonia production. Additionally, conversion of glutamine into glutamate and α-ketoglutarate in the proximal tubule of the kidney also will generate ammonia.

Aciduria and hypokalemia contribute to increased urinary excretion of ammonia (hyperammonuria).[48] Unlike in dogs and human beings, metabolic acidosis in cats does not alter the renal excretion of ammonia.[50-52] During urinary tract infections, urease-producing bacteria in urine also can convert urea into NH_3 and NH_4^+, and these in turn can act as promoters of uric acid stone formation.

URINARY MACROMOLECULES

Macromolecules such as proteins and glycosaminoglycan (GAG) in urine are known to play a critical role in urolithiasis, either as promoters or inhibitors of stone formation.[53] Tamm-Horsfall protein (also known as uromodulin) levels were found to be significantly ($p = 0.03$) higher in non–stone-forming Dalmatian dogs than in stone-forming Dalmatian dogs, suggesting an inhibitor role for this protein.[16] According to Carvalho et al, there were no statistical differences in the levels of GAG and nephrocalcin between the non–stone-forming and stone-forming Dalmatian dogs.[16] In cats, no studies have been carried out to investigate the role of the macromolecules in urate urolithiasis. However, even in other species the precise role of these macromolecules in urate urolithiasis has not been investigated systematically.

OTHER PATHOLOGICAL CONDITIONS

Other pathophysiological conditions enhance urate urolith formation because of their pathological effects. In human beings a high prevalence (28.5 per cent) of urate stone formation is observed among patients with Type 2 diabetes mellitus.[54-56] A similar trend also has been observed in obese human patients.[57-59] In dogs and cats, no reports are available to support such trends.

HOW ARE URATE STONES DIAGNOSED IN CATS?

Of the eight cats diagnosed with purine uroliths at the University of Minnesota in 2007, seven presented for signs referable to the urinary tract. Four male cats were evaluated for urethral obstruction. Inappropriate urination and dysuria were reported in two female cats and one male cat. One female cat did not present with clinical signs related to the urinary tract; however, this cat was anorectic. In seven cats for whom urinalysis results were available, neither urate nor amorphous crystals were observed. Struvite crystals were detected in one cat.

Results of liver enzyme analysis and liver function tests were available in some of these urate stone–forming cats. Three cats had serum concentrations of bile acids performed (Table 50-1). One cat was diagnosed with a hepatic portosystemic shunt; there were no abnormalities in the serum concentrations of albumin or liver enzymes in this patient. In one cat with normal postprandial serum bile acids, the albumin concentration was low (2.3 g/dL). Potential indicators of liver disorders also were detected in two cats who presented for urethral obstruction. One cat had a low serum albumin level, and the other had moderate elevations in serum concentrations of alanine aminotransferase (ALT) (210 U/L) and aspartate aminotransferase (AST) (98 U/L). In both of these cats serum concentrations of these enzymes were within the normal range 3 months later. These findings indicate that serum concentrations of routine tests to evaluate liver function are not sufficiently sensitive to identify cats with abnormal liver function. Likewise, liver function is normal in some cats with urate urolithiasis.

Survey radiography was performed in six cats to investigate a cause for urinary tract disease. In two cats, uroliths were sufficiently radiopaque to arrive at a diagnosis of urolithiasis (Figures 50-4 and 50-5). In these two patients the smallest identifiable urolith was 4 and 3.2 mm in diameter. In the remaining cases contrast

Table 50-1 Serum Concentrations of Liver Enzymes in Eight Cats with Urate Urolithiasis

	Bile Acid mg/dL (Fasting)	Bile Acid mg/dL (Postprandial)	ALT U/L	ALP U/L	AST U/L	Albumin mg/dL	Glucose mg/dL	Total Bilirubin mg/dL
1	11	40	34	24	21	2.6	98	0.2
2	ND	ND	31	8	70	2.2	111	0.2
3	9.8	17.2	32	22	ND	3.2	102	0.2
4	1.8	2.2	45	19	20	3.8	166	0.3
5	ND	ND	33	25	21	3.0	116	0.1
6	ND	ND	201	51	98	3.5	166	0.2
7	ND	ND	ND	ND	ND	2.7	90	ND
8	ND	1.7	40	24	44	2.3	180	0.1
Normal range	0-15	5-20	16-127	2-88	14-42	2.4-4.1	74-143	0-0.3

ALT, Alanine aminotransferase; *ALP,* alkaline phosphatase; *AST,* aspartate aminotransferase; *ND,* not done.

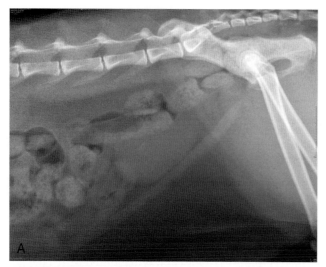

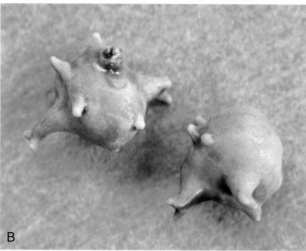

Figure 50-4 A, Lateral survey abdominal radiograph of a 6-year-old male cat with two uroliths in the urinary bladder. **B,** Surgically removed uroliths were composed of 100 per cent ammonium acid urate.

cystography and/or ultrasonography (Figure 50-6) were required to detect uroliths.

ONCE STONES ARE DETECTED, HOW SHOULD THEY BE MANAGED?

Medical protocols have not been developed that promote dissolution of ammonium urate uroliths in cats consistently. We have completed medical dissolution of an ammonium urate urocystolith in a 3-year-old neutered male cat with a combination of allopurinol (15 mg/kg PO q12h) and a diet relatively low in purines. Similarly we also have dissolved ammonium urate uroliths in a 6-year-old female cat with a lower dose of allopurinol (15 mg/kg PO q24h) and a diet relatively low in purines.

Uroliths small enough to pass through the urethra may be removed with the aid of a urinary catheter, or by voiding urohydropropulsion. In female cats laser lithotripsy can be used to fragment uroliths to sizes that can be extracted through the urethra (see Chapter 52). However, surgery remains the most reliable method to remove larger, active uroliths from the urinary tract of male cats.

HOW CAN URATE UROLITH RECURRENCE BE PREVENTED?

In one retrospective study, urate uroliths recurred in approximately 11 per cent of cats over a 5-year period.[60] During this same period approximately 2.3 per cent of patients had their second recurrence. This may underestimate the true recurrence rate, because most urate stones will be missed by conventional methods of medical imaging. Of the eight cats described in this chapter, only one patient had previous urate uroliths.

CONTROLLING RISK FACTORS

Several factors have been identified as contributing causes for urate urolith formation. A high incidence of urate uroliths has been identified in dogs with portovascular shunts. However, concomitant liver disease and urate urolithiasis is reported infrequently in cats. In our series one cat was diagnosed with a hepatic vascular shunt. The defect was repaired with an ameroid constrictor ring. At 2 and 10 months following placement of the ameroid ring, the serum concentrations of bile acids remained elevated (preprandial and postprandial bile acid concentrations were 8.5 mg/dL and 52 mg/dL at 2 months, and 7.0 mg/dL and 79 mg/dL at 10 months; normal values are below 15 mg/dL and below 20 mg/dL, respectively). Ultrasound of the urinary bladder did not reveal recurrence of urocystoliths at the later follow-up period. The predisposition of cats with portal vascular anomalies to form ammonium urate probably is associated with concomitant hyperuricemia, hyperammonemia, hyperuricuria, and hyperammonuria.

For those cats in whom an underlying correctable cause has not been identified, prevention relies primarily on dietary modification. To minimize the risk of urolith formation, we recommend feeding diets with reduced quantities of purines. Likewise, diets should not be formulated to promote formation of highly acidic urine. Because amino acids provide nitrogen and carbon for endogenous production of purines, it is desirable to restrict dietary protein to maintenance levels. In addition to reducing dietary protein, consider feeding diets that are formulated from nutrient sources derived from low purine foods (Table 50-2).

The therapeutic benefit of xanthine oxidase inhibitors such as allopurinol is unknown. Because of the potential for adverse side effects (gastrointestinal upset, skin rashes, leukopenia, thrombocytopenia, hepatitis, and kidney failure), we reserve the use of allopurinol for cats with highly recurrent disease. Because of the potential for adverse effects, consider conservative dosing at 5 to 10 mg/kg PO q24h.

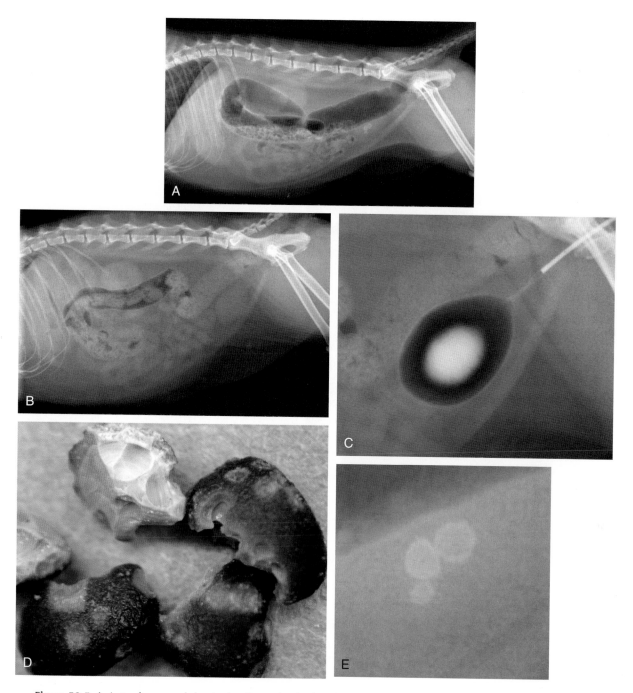

Figure 50-5 A, Lateral survey abdominal radiograph of a female cat with several urocystoliths composed of ammonium acid urate prior to laser lithotripsy. **B,** Following laser lithotripsy. **C,** The postlithotripsy double-contrast cystogram verified that all uroliths and urolith fragments were removed completely and that the urinary bladder wall remained contiguous. **D,** Uroliths, once fragmented into smaller pieces, were removed by a combination of basket retrieval and voiding urohydropropulsion. These uroliths were visible on survey radiographs (**E,** Enlargement of uroliths from **A**) because a shell of radiopaque calcium oxalate monohydrate surrounded the ammonium acid urate stone.

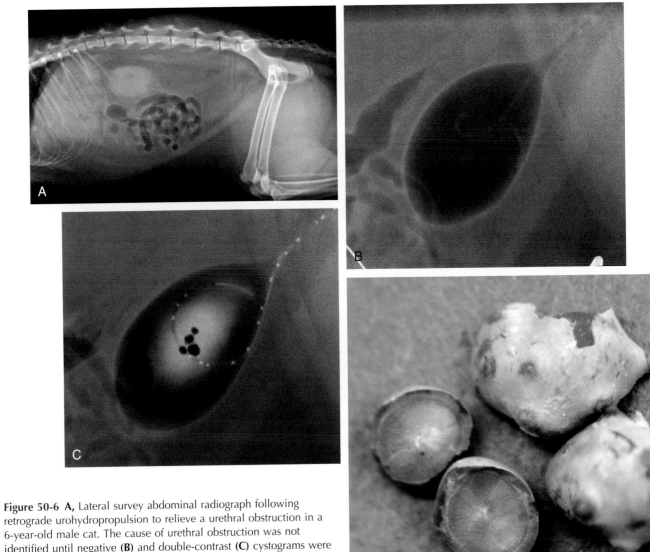

Figure 50-6 A, Lateral survey abdominal radiograph following retrograde urohydropropulsion to relieve a urethral obstruction in a 6-year-old male cat. The cause of urethral obstruction was not identified until negative **(B)** and double-contrast **(C)** cystograms were performed. **D,** Surgically removed uroliths were composed of 100 per cent ammonium acid urate.

Table 50-2 Relative Purine Content of Foods

	Foods to Avoid (High Purine Content)	Foods to Use Sparingly (Moderate Purine Content)	Foods Permissible to Feed (Negligible Purine Content)
Fish	Anchovies, herring, mackerel, mussels, roe, sardines, scallops, oysters	Fish and shellfish not listed in the foods to avoid	
Meats	Organ meats (brains, heart, kidney, liver) Game meats (duck, goose) Meat broths	Chicken, beef, lamb, pork	Gelatin
Fruits and Vegetables		Beans, cauliflower, green peas, lentils, mushrooms, cauliflower, spinach	Nuts, and fruits and vegetables not listed in the other two columns
Egg/Dairy		Oats, wheat germ	Eggs, cheese, milk, ice cream, butter
Pasta /Rice		Whole grain breads and cereals	Rice, pasta, macaroni, breads and cereals from refined grains
Miscellaneous	Baker's and brewer's yeast		

REFERENCES

1. Bartges JW, Osborne CA, Lulich JP, et al: Canine urate urolithiasis. Etiopathogenesis, diagnosis, and management, *Vet Clin North Am Small Anim Pract* 29:161, 1999.
2. Berg JM, Tymoczko JL, Stryer L: Nucleotide biosynthesis. In *Biochemistry*, New York, 2007, WH Freeman and Company, p 709.
3. Rodwell VW: Metabolism of purine & pyrimidine nucleotides. In Murray RK, Granner DK, Rodwell VW, editors: *Harper's illustrated biochemistry*, ed 27, New York, 2006, Lange Medical Books/McGraw-Hill, p 301.
4. Ramazzina I, Folli C, Secchi A, et al: Completing the uric acid degradation pathway through phylogenetic comparison of whole genomes, *Nat Chem Biol* 2:144, 2006.
5. Simoni RE, Gomes LN, Scalco FB, et al: Uric acid changes in urine and plasma: an effective tool in screening for purine inborn errors of metabolism and other pathological conditions, *J Inherit Metab Dis* 30:295, 2007.
6. Terkeltaub R, Bushinsky DA, Becker MA: Recent developments in our understanding of the renal basis of hyperuricemia and the development of novel antihyperuricemic therapeutics, *Arthritis Res Ther* 8(Suppl 1):S4, 2006.
7. Jackson OF, Sutor DJ: Ammonium acid urate calculus in a cat with a high uric acid excretion possibly due to a renal tubular reabsorption defect, *Vet Rec* 86:335, 1970.
8. Shekarriz B, Stoller ML: Uric acid nephrolithiasis: current concepts and controversies, *J Urol* 168:1307, 2002.
9. Kooij A, Schijns M, Frederiks WM, et al: Distribution of xanthine oxidoreductase activity in human tissues—a histochemical and biochemical study, *Virchows Arch B Cell Pathol Incl Mol Pathol* 63:17, 1992.
10. Oda M, Satta Y, Takenaka O, et al: Loss of urate oxidase activity in hominoids and its evolutionary implications, *Mol Biol Evol* 19:640, 2002.
11. Yeldandi AV, Yeldandi V, Kumar S, et al: Molecular evolution of the urate oxidase-encoding gene in hominoid primates: nonsense mutations, *Gene* 109:281, 1991.
12. Kim YK, Jung DK, Jung JS, et al: Urate excretion by the cat kidney, *Comp Biochem Physiol Comp Physiol* 102:735, 1992.
13. Truszkowski R, Goldmanowna C: Uricase and its action: distribution in various animals, *Biochem J* 27:612, 1933.
14. Usuda N, Reddy MK, Hashimoto T, et al: Tissue specificity and species differences in the distribution of urate oxidase in peroxisomes, *Lab Invest* 58:100, 1988.
15. Safra N, Ling GV, Schaible RH, et al: Exclusion of urate oxidase as a candidate gene for hyperuricosuria in the Dalmatian dog using an interbreed backcross, *J Hered* 96:750, 2005.
16. Carvalho M, Lulich JP, Osborne CA, et al: Role of urinary inhibitors of crystallization in uric acid nephrolithiasis: Dalmatian dog model, *Urology* 62:566, 2003.
17. Porter P: Urinary calculi in the dog. II. Urate stones and purine metabolism, *J Comp Pathol* 73:119, 1963.
18. Appleman RM, Hallenbeck GA, Shorter RG: Effect of reciprocal allogeneic renal transplantation between Dalmatian and non-Dalmatian dogs on urinary excretion of uric acid, *Proc Soc Exp Biol Med* 121:1094, 1966.
19. Benedetti E, Kirby JP, Asolati M, et al: Intrasplenic hepatocyte allotransplantation in dalmatian dogs with and without cyclosporine immunosuppression, *Transplantation* 63:1206, 1997.
20. Dunn TB, Kumins NH, Raofi V, et al: Multiple intrasplenic hepatocyte transplantations in the dalmatian dog, *Surgery* 127:193, 2000.
21. Kocken JM, Borel Rinkes IH, Bijma AM, et al: Correction of an inborn error of metabolism by intraportal hepatocyte transplantation in a dog model, *Transplantation* 62:358, 1996.
22. Kuster G, Shorter RG, Dawson B, et al: Uric acid metabolism in Dalmatians and other dogs. Role of the liver, *Arch Intern Med* 129:492, 1972.
23. Takeda T, Kim TH, Lee SK, et al: Hepatocyte transplantation in biodegradable polymer scaffolds using the Dalmatian dog model of hyperuricosuria, *Transplant Proc* 27:635, 1995.
24. Duncan H, Wakim KG, Ward LE: The effects of intravenous administration of uric acid on its concentration in plasma and urine of Dalmatian and non-Dalmatian dogs, *J Lab Clin Med* 58:876, 1961.
25. Harvey AM, Christensen HN: Uric acid transport system: apparent absence in erythrocytes of the Dalmatian coach hound, *Science* 145:826, 1964.
26. Simkin PA: The Dalmatian defect: a hepatic endocrinopathy of urate transport, *Arthritis Rheum* 52:2257, 2005.
27. Giesecke D, Tiemeyer W: Defect of uric acid uptake in Dalmatian dog liver, *Experientia* 40:1415, 1984.
28. Bannasch DL, Ryun JR, Bannasch MJ, et al: Exclusion of galectin 9 as a candidate gene for hyperuricosuria in the Dalmatian dog, *Anim Genet* 35:326, 2004.
29. Safra N, Schaible RH, Bannasch DL: Linkage analysis with an interbreed backcross maps Dalmatian hyperuricosuria to CFA03, *Mamm Genome* 17:340, 2006.
30. Kruger JM, Osborne CA: Etiopathogenesis of uric acid and ammonium urate uroliths in non-Dalmatian dogs, *Vet Clin North Am Small Anim Pract* 16:87, 1986.
31. Marretta SM, Pask AJ, Greene RW, et al: Urinary calculi associated with portosystemic shunts in six dogs, *J Am Vet Med Assoc* 178:133, 1981.
32. Osborne CA, Lulich JP, Thumchai R, et al: Feline urolithiasis. Etiology and pathophysiology, *Vet Clin North Am Small Anim Pract* 26:217, 1996.
33. Gutman AB, Yu TF: A three-component system for regulation of renal excretion of uric acid in man, *Trans Assoc Am Physicians* 74:353, 1961.
34. Steele TH, Boner G: Origins of the uricosuric response, *J Clin Invest* 52:1368, 1973.
35. Mudge GH, Cucchi J, Platts M, et al: Renal excretion of uric acid in the dog, *Am J Physiol* 215:404, 1968.
36. Enomoto A, Kimura H, Chairoungdua A, et al: Molecular identification of a renal urate anion exchanger that regulates blood urate levels, *Nature* 417:447, 2002.
37. Lipkowitz MS, Leal-Pinto E, Rappoport JZ, et al: Functional reconstitution, membrane targeting, genomic structure, and chromosomal localization of a human urate transporter, *J Clin Invest* 107:1103, 2001.
38. Cha SH, Sekine T, Fukushima JI: Identification and characterization of human organic anion transporter 3 expressing predominantly in the kidney, *Mol Pharmacol* 59:1277, 2001.
39. Hediger MA, Johnson RJ, Miyazaki H, et al: Molecular physiology of urate transport, *Physiology (Bethesda)* 20:125, 2005.
40. Sekine T, Watanabe N, Hosoyamada M, et al: Expression cloning and characterization of a novel multispecific organic anion transporter, *J Biol Chem* 272:18526, 1997.
41. Van Aubel RA, Smeets PH, van den Heuvel JJ, et al: Human organic anion transporter MRP4 (ABCC4) is an efflux pump for the purine end metabolite urate with multiple allosteric substrate binding sites, *Am J Physiol Renal Physiol* 288:F327, 2005.
42. Vitart V, Rudan I, Hayward C, et al: SLC2A9 is a newly identified urate transporter influencing serum urate concentration, urate excretion and gout, *Nat Genet* 40:437, 2008.
43. Cameron MA, Sakhaee K: Uric acid nephrolithiasis, *Urol Clin North Am* 34:335, 2007.
44. Osborne CA, Polzin DJ, Kruger JM, et al: Relationship of nutritional factors to the cause, dissolution, and prevention

of feline uroliths and urethral plugs, *Vet Clin North Am Small Anim Pract* 19:561, 1989.

45. Johnson RJ, Segal MS, Srinivas T, et al: Essential hypertension, progressive renal disease, and uric acid: a pathogenetic link? *J Am Soc Nephrol* 16:1909, 2005.

46. Coe FL, Parks JH: Stone disease in hereditary distal renal tubular acidosis, *Ann Intern Med* 93:60, 1980.

47. Emmerson BT: The management of gout, *N Engl J Med* 334:445, 1996.

48. Allen TA: Measurement of the influence of diet on feline urinary pH, *Vet Clin North Am Small Anim Pract* 26:363, 1996.

49. Wilcox WR, Khalaf A, Weinberger A, et al: Solubility of uric acid and monosodium urate, *Med Biol Eng* 10:522, 1972.

50. Lemieux G, Lemieux C, Duplessis S, et al: Metabolic characteristics of cat kidney: failure to adapt to metabolic acidosis, *Am J Physiol* 259:R277, 1990.

51. Sartorius OW, Roemmelt JC, Pitts RF, et al: The renal regulation of acid-base balance in man. IV. The nature of the renal compensations in ammonium chloride acidosis, *J Clin Invest* 28:423, 1949.

52. Vinay P, Allignet E, Pichette C, et al: Changes in renal metabolite profile and ammoniagenesis during acute and chronic metabolic acidosis in dog and rat, *Kidney Int* 17:312, 1980.

53. Khan SR, Kok DJ: Modulators of urinary stone formation, *Front Biosci* 9:1450, 2004.

54. Daudon M, Lacour B, Jungers P: High prevalence of uric acid calculi in diabetic stone formers, *Nephrol Dial Transplant* 20:468, 2005.

55. Pak CY, Sakhaee K, Moe O, et al: Biochemical profile of stone-forming patients with diabetes mellitus, *Urology* 61:523, 2003.

56. Taylor EN, Stampfer MJ, Curhan GC: Diabetes mellitus and the risk of nephrolithiasis, *Kidney Int* 68:1230, 2005.

57. Cameron MA, Maalouf NM, Adams-Huet B, et al: Urine composition in type 2 diabetes: predisposition to uric acid nephrolithiasis, *J Am Soc Nephrol* 17:1422, 2006.

58. Daudon M, Lacour B, Jungers P: Influence of body size on urinary stone composition in men and women, *Urol Res* 34:193, 2006.

59. Ekeruo WO, Tan YH, Young MD, et al: Metabolic risk factors and the impact of medical therapy on the management of nephrolithiasis in obese patients, *J Urol* 172:159, 2004.

60. Albasan H, Osborne CA, Lulich JP: Urolith recurrence in cats, *J Vet Intern Med* 20:786, 2006.

CHAPTER
51 Urinary Tract Tumors

Ruthanne Chun and Heather M. Wilson

Although tumors of the urinary tract are rare in cats, the treatment and prognosis vary considerably depending on tumor type. Thus, if cancer is on the list of differential diagnoses, an evaluation—including a minimum database of complete blood count (CBC), serum chemistry profile, and urinalysis, followed by abdominal imaging—is warranted, as is cytological examination or biopsy of the mass to obtain a diagnosis. The following chapter discusses what is known about the diagnosis and management of feline urinary tract neoplasms in greater detail.

RENAL TUMORS

INCIDENCE

Primary renal tumors are rare in cats. Lymphoma is the neoplasm that affects the kidneys of cats most commonly; other reported tumors include renal adenoma, renal adenocarcinoma, and transitional cell carcinoma.[1-3] Less common considerations are nephroblastoma or hemangiosarcoma.[1] Involvement of both kidneys does not exclude neoplasia, because bilateral disease has been reported with both lymphoma and renal adenocarcinoma.[4,5] Other differential diagnoses for enlarged kidneys, especially for cats with bilateral disease, include polycystic kidney disease or perirenal pseudocysts. It is possible, albeit rare, for cats to have concurrent polycystic kidney disease or perirenal cysts and cancer involving the kidneys.[6,7]

HISTORY AND PHYSICAL EXAMINATION FINDINGS

Lymphoma involving the kidneys in cats typically is high grade and therefore is a rapidly progressive disease.[2,3] Owners may report inappetence or anorexia, lethargy, vomiting, and weight loss in affected cats. Other renal cancers are more slowly progressive and have a more insidious history of gradual weight loss, inappetence, and progressive lethargy. Signs of paraneoplastic syndromes occasionally manifest first; for example, seizures secondary to tumor-associated polycythemia.[8]

On physical examination the kidneys may be enlarged unilaterally or bilaterally. Renal tumors are nonpainful, smooth to lobulated, soft to firm masses. Although rare, polycythemia secondary to renal tumors may be associated with dark red gingival membranes and/or a heart murmur.[1,8]

DIAGNOSTIC EVALUATION

The diagnostic evaluation of suspected renal tumors is divided into an assessment of the kidney mass and investigation of whether the tumor has spread elsewhere in the body. Although abdominal radiography and compression radiography may help to localize a lesion to the kidney, ultrasonography is the noninvasive diagnostic tool used most commonly for cats with renal masses.[9,10] The finding of hypoechoic subcapsular thickening on ultrasound examination is strongly supportive, but not definitive for, a diagnosis of lymphoma.[10] Diagnosis of lymphoma or carcinoma may be obtained through cytological evaluation of a fine-needle aspirate sample[11]; either ultrasound-guided core biopsy or surgical biopsy of the mass may be required for definitive diagnosis in some cases.

Evaluation for systemic involvement includes a CBC, serum chemistry profile, urinalysis, thoracic radiographs (e.g., pulmonary metastasis check), and a complete abdominal ultrasound. All cats with renal lymphoma should be tested for feline leukemia virus (FeLV), because up to 50 per cent are reported to be positive.[12] Typically renal tumors are associated with anemia; however, polycythemia has been reported in cats with renal tumors.[1,8] The most likely causes of this interesting paraneoplastic

509

syndrome are excessive erythropoietin production by tumor cells or renal hypoxia. The serum chemistry profile, in conjunction with urine specific gravity, is used primarily to assess the degree of azotemia because this may affect how well cats tolerate surgical or chemotherapeutic intervention. Although a urine sediment examination is recommended, tumor cells rarely exfoliate into the urine. Assessment of contralateral renal function by scintigraphy or pyelography often is recommended prior to nephrectomy.

Greater than 50 per cent of cats with renal or transitional cell carcinoma have metastatic disease to the regional lymph nodes or lungs, and it is unusual for cats with renal lymphoma to have disease localized solely to the kidneys.[1,12] Furthermore, renal lymphoma is associated with central nervous system (CNS) involvement, and it is reported that 40 per cent of the deaths in cats with renal lymphoma are as a result of CNS involvement.[12]

TREATMENT AND PROGNOSIS

Renal Adenoma

Because these are benign tumors, treatment with complete surgical excision should be curative.

Renal Carcinoma/Adenocarcinoma/Transitional Cell Carcinoma

The treatment of choice for renal adenocarcinoma is surgical excision. Although the percentage of cats who go on to develop metastatic disease is not known, pulmonary metastasis following surgical excision has been reported.[8] Further, the disease also has been reported to affect both kidneys simultaneously.[5] Therefore chemotherapy is indicated but the drug, or drug combination, with best efficacy is not known. Human beings with renal carcinoma are treated with a combination of surgery, cisplatin chemotherapy, immunotherapy with either interleukin-2 or interferon alpha, and tyrosine kinase receptor inhibitors.[13] Because cisplatin is fatal to cats, carboplatin therapy (240 mg/m^2 IV q21d)[14] could be considered.

In dogs with transitional cell carcinoma, treatment recommendations are combination therapy of piroxicam with either doxorubicin or carboplatin. Although the use of nonsteroidal antiinflammatory drugs (NSAIDs) is avoided in animals with renal failure, piroxicam may be considered for nonazotemic cats with renal transitional cell carcinoma. Limited long-term data are available for cats treated with piroxicam; a conservative dosing recommendation would be to start at 0.3 mg/kg PO q24h for 7 to 10 days, then taper to q48h therapy.

It is difficult to provide accurate survival data because of the paucity of available literature describing this disease. Reported survival times range from 8 months to longer. If significant metastatic disease is identified at the time of initial presentation, survival time is likely to be only weeks to months.

Nephroblastoma

Although reported very rarely in cats and dogs, this tumor arises from embryonal tissues and typically is well encapsulated although metastases may occur.[15] Malignant nephroblastoma, reported in one cat, is treated surgically. The effect of chemotherapy is unknown, and prognosis depends on extent of disease and ability to remove the tumor surgically.

Hemangiosarcoma

Although less common than in dogs, visceral hemangiosarcoma in cats often is associated with hemorrhage, metastasis, and a short survival time.[16-18] The ability to excise the tumor completely is associated with a better outcome.[18] Chemotherapy with carboplatin has been associated with complete remission of short duration (<168 days) in one cat with subcutaneous hemangiosarcoma.[14] For dogs with visceral hemangiosarcoma, treatment with a doxorubicin-based chemotherapy protocol prolongs survival.[19-21]

Lymphoma

Because of the systemic nature of the disease, cats with renal lymphoma are treated with chemotherapy. A combination chemotherapy protocol utilizing vincristine, cyclophosphamide, doxorubicin, and prednisone ± L-asparaginase (CHOP) is recommended.[22] Although median survival times of 266 days have been reported in cats with various forms of lymphoma treated with cyclophosphamide, prednisone, and vincristine,[23] other reports support the addition of doxorubicin to lymphoma chemotherapy protocols.[24] Furthermore, because of the common association of renal lymphoma with CNS involvement, many oncologists recommend that cyclophosphamide be substituted out for cytosine arabinoside, because this drug reaches cytotoxic concentrations within the CNS.

Along with the chemotherapy protocol utilized, prognostic factors for cats with lymphoma include clinical substage (e.g., whether the animal is ill or well at the time of diagnosis), FeLV status, and response to therapy.[24] Although there are no recent case series of cats with renal lymphoma treated with a doxorubicin-based combination chemotherapy protocol, it is the opinion of these authors that FeLV-negative cats with a good response to chemotherapy can have a median survival of 12 months or longer.

LOWER URINARY TRACT NEOPLASIA

BLADDER TUMORS

Incidence and Risk Factors

Neoplasia of the feline lower urinary tract represents a very small portion of lower urinary tract disease. Incidence rates for primary bladder tumors vary from 0.07 per cent to 0.38 per cent of all tumors in cats.[25-27] This is far lower than that reported for human beings and dogs. One possible reason for the lower incidence observed in cats is the difference in tryptophan metabolism among the species. Unlike dogs and human beings, cats produce very small quantities of the renally excreted tryptophan metabolites, ortho-aminophenol in particular, which can accumulate in the bladder and act as a carcinogen.[25,28]

In other species environmental toxins and exposure to chemicals such as herbicides and insecticides play a large role in the development of transitional cell carcinoma (TCC).[27,29] TCC is the most common form of bladder cancer found in the human being, dog, and cat.[25-27,29] There is no known association between exposure to these carcinogens and bladder tumor development in cats. However, there are very few cases reported in the literature, so evidence for or against these risk factors is lacking. Associations between bladder cancer and neuter status, body condition score, and exposure to cyclophosphamide can not be made in cats for the same reasons.

Nevertheless, a few risk factors can be determined using the information that has been published to date. Like human beings, male cats are at an increased risk of developing TCC.[27,29,30] Older cats are affected routinely. The average age of affected cats typically is over 9 years of age.[27,29-31]

Cyclooxygenase-2 (Cox-2) overexpression has been identified in cats with TCC of the bladder. Reports of four fishing cats *(Prionailurus viverrinus)* diagnosed with TCC indicated Cox-2 overexpression in most samples tested.[32,33] Another study looking at various tumors of domestic cats revealed that seven of 19 cats with TCC of the bladder had Cox-2 overexpression.[34] Whether Cox-2 overexpression is related to malignant transformation or progression of the tumor remains to be seen.

Other reported primary bladder tumors in the cat include non–TCC (squamous cell carcinoma, undifferentiated carcinoma, and adenocarcinoma), leiomyoma, leiomyosarcoma, hemangiosarcoma, lymphoma, and fibroma.[27,31] These tumors all are extremely rare. No information regarding incidence or risk factors for these tumors is available in the literature.

Biological Behavior and Pathology

TCC of the urinary bladder in cats tends to be an aggressive disease that often has already invaded into the muscle layer of the bladder wall by the time a diagnosis is made (Stage T_2 or higher based on the World Health Organization staging system for dogs, applied here to cats as well) (Box 51-1).[35] Additionally, 20 to 29 per cent of cats present with metastasis at the time of diagnosis.[26,29] Interestingly, the majority of metastatic lesions appear to be in organs other than the locoregional lymph nodes.[26,29] Of the nine cats described with antemortem metastasis, only one reportedly had lymph node metastasis. Other areas of reported metastases include the lungs, mesentery, abdominal wall, liver, peritoneum, and spleen.[26,29] As in human beings and dogs, it is possible to transplant tumor cells from the bladder mass to the abdominal wall after a fine-needle aspirate (FNA).[29] Therefore care must be taken when deciding which diagnostic tests to pursue.

In the literature there are two case reports of cats with lymphoma of the urinary bladder for whom clinical history is provided. One of these cats was euthanized because of an inoperable bladder mass and uroabdomen. The other was treated with chemotherapy; however, there was a strong suspicion that lymphoma progressed to the CNS. As noted previously there is an association with renal lymphoma and CNS lymphoma in cats, and it may be that other areas of the urinary tract have a similar propensity.[36,37]

History and Clinical Signs

Lower urinary tract signs are commonly associated with tumors of the bladder. Cats may present with one or many of the following clinical signs: hematuria, stranguria, dysuria, pollakiuria, tenesmus, rectal prolapse, inappropriate urination, and incontinence.[26,38] It also is common to palpate a mass in the caudal abdomen on physical examination. Greater than 50 per cent of cats present with a bladder mass in the apex of the bladder or in the bladder wall.[29] Therefore urinary obstruction is not a consistent presenting sign. Secondary infections also are common. Therefore a history of short-term response to various antibiotics also is common. Other less common clinical signs include weight loss and anorexia, particularly with lymphoma of the urinary bladder (Table 51-1).[36,37]

Box 51-1 WHO Staging System for Canine Bladder Tumors—Applied to Cats

T	**PRIMARY TUMOR**
T_{is}	Carcinoma in situ
T_0	No evidence of primary tumor
T_1	Superficial papillary tumor
T_2	Tumor invading the bladder wall with induration
T_3	Tumor invading neighboring organs (prostate, uterus, vagina, and pelvic canal)
N	**REGIONAL LYMPH NODE (INTERNAL AND EXTERNAL ILIAC LYMPH NODES)**
N_0	No regional lymph node involvement
N_1	Regional lymph nodes involved
N_2	Regional and juxtaregional lymph nodes involved
M	**DISTANT METASTASIS**
M_0	No evidence of metastasis
M_1	Distant metastasis present

Modified from Owen LN: TNM Classification of Tumours of Domestic Animals, Geneva, 1980, World Health Organization.

Table 51-1 Clinical Signs Associated with Transitional Cell Carcinoma of the Bladder in 20 Cats[29]

Sign	Number of Cats	Percentage of Group ($n = 20$)
Hematuria	16	76
Stranguria	9	42.9
Pollakiuria	8	38
Urinary obstruction	3	14.3
Inappropriate urination	3	14.3
No clinical signs	1	4.7

Table 51-2 Differential Diagnoses for Lower Urinary Tract Tumors in Cats

Tumor Location	Possible Neoplastic Differential Diagnoses	Possible Nonneoplastic Differential Diagnoses
Urinary bladder	Transitional cell carcinoma Other carcinomas (squamous cell carcinoma, adenocarcinoma, and undifferentiated carcinoma) Leiomyoma Lymphoma Hemangiosarcoma Leiomyosarcoma Fibroma	Feline lower urinary tract disease—idiopathic Urinary calculi Bacterial cystitis Pyogranulomatous inflammation Inappropriate urination—behavioral
Urethra	Transitional cell carcinoma Leiomyoma Leiomyosarcoma Squamous cell carcinoma	Granulomatous disease Inflammation Urethral calculi
Prostate	Prostatic carcinoma Transitional cell carcinoma	Prostatic abscess[44] Paraprostatic cyst[44] Prostatic cyst

Diagnosis and Staging

Because of the extremely low incidence of primary bladder neoplasia in cats, it is prudent to exclude other common causes of lower urinary tract signs first. Cystitis, whether bacterial or sterile, is more common in cats. Additionally, urinary calculi and behavioral causes of lower urinary signs are common. Baseline laboratory data such as a CBC, serum chemistry profile, retroviral testing, urinalysis (including urine sediment exam), and urine culture and sensitivity all are part of the diagnostic evaluation for the differential diagnoses listed in Table 51-2. Profound hypereosinophilia, as a paraneoplastic syndrome, has been documented in one cat with TCC of the urinary bladder.[39] Inflammation within the bladder can lead to significant changes in the morphology of uroepithelium seen on the urine sediment. Urine sediment examination alone is never a definitive way to diagnose TCC in any species, although it may raise suspicion for a neoplastic process. Cytological examination is considered diagnostic when used in conjunction with the demonstration of a bladder mass and an otherwise quiet urine sediment. Bladder masses are readily revealed by ultrasonography (Figures 51-1 and 51-2); abdominal ultrasound examination also can be used to evaluate other organs and lymph nodes within the peritoneal cavity as part of the staging process. It is best to examine the bladder when it is distended, because inflammation can cause significant thickening of the bladder wall.

Contrast studies also are valuable tools for imaging bladder masses, especially if ultrasound is not available. Retrograde pneumocystography, positive contrast cystography, or double contrast cystography can be helpful for delineating a bladder mass as well as urethral involvement. Advanced imaging using computed tomography (CT) or magnetic resonance imaging (MRI) also may be helpful if contrast studies are inconclusive. Cystoscopic examination and biopsy of the urinary tract is being used more commonly in feline medicine. For all urinary tract cancers, three-view thoracic radiographs are an important part of staging because lung metastasis is common.

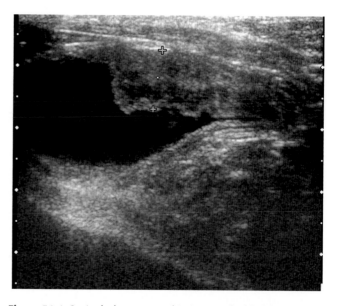

Figure 51-1 Sagittal ultrasonographic image of a bladder mass in a cat. This mass is located near the trigone and is indicated by the white crosses. This mass was biopsied and determined to be a transitional cell carcinoma.

A definitive diagnosis of TCC in the bladder can be difficult to achieve. Because it is possible to seed the abdominal wall with a FNA, and many cats have potentially resectable tumors, percutaneous tumor aspiration for cytological examination is not recommended. It may be difficult in many cats, especially female cats, to use traumatic catheterization because of the small diameter of the urethra and catheter. Traumatic catheterization may be more feasible in larger male cats. Often, laparotomy with surgical biopsy of the bladder mass is required for a definitive diagnosis.

Although lymphoma is diagnosed easily on cytological examination, FNA is not recommended for any bladder mass. If urine sediment examination is unable to secure a diagnosis, biopsy (surgical or other) is necessary.

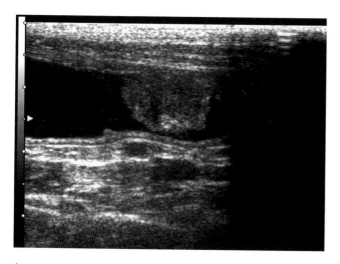

Figure 51-2 Sagittal ultrasonographic image of a bladder mass in a cat. This mass is associated with the bladder wall and is not located in the trigone region of the bladder. This mass was biopsied and determined to be a transitional cell carcinoma.

Treatment and Prognosis

Few recommendations exist regarding the therapy for primary bladder tumors in cats. Often tumors are diagnosed at an advanced stage, limiting the available therapeutic options. However, some general recommendations can be made.

Surgery alone or in combination with chemotherapy is ideal whenever possible. Even if not curative, tumor debulking for masses located away from the trigone may resolve clinical signs and reduce the tumor to microscopic disease, which allows for a better chance for response to chemotherapy. Hemangiosarcoma of the bladder may carry a worse prognosis than other mesenchymal tumors of the bladder; consequently, adjunct chemotherapy with doxorubicin may be prudent, although no published data exist to support this recommendation.

In a study of 20 cats with TCC of the urinary bladder, 11 cats underwent surgery alone or in combination with chemotherapy. Those cats who survived the initial postoperative period went on to live longer than other cats managed medically; however, there was not a significant difference in overall survival, likely because of the small number of cats.[29]

Surgery is not recommended for cats with trigonal masses. Gastrocystoplasties, ureteroileostomy, trigonal colonic anastomoses, ureterocolocolostomies, ileocystoplasties, jejunal pouches, and ureterocolonic anastomoses are fraught with serious complications and typically provide only short-term relief in the face of high morbidity and high local recurrence rates.[30]

There are few reports of medical management including chemotherapy and NSAIDs in cats with TCC and lymphoma of the bladder. There are too few cases to determine if chemotherapy is an effective treatment for this disease; however, anticancer drugs that have been administered include doxorubicin, cyclophosphamide, mitoxantrone, carboplatin, piroxicam, and meloxicam.[29] NSAIDs should be reserved for nonazotemic cats. There

is a case report of one cat diagnosed with lymphoma of the bladder treated with the CHOP protocol; progressive disease occurred before completing the protocol.[37] Finally, most bladder tumors often are too invasive and large for intravesicular therapies.

Radiation therapy in the area of the bladder generally is not recommended. The acute and late effects to the bladder often are unacceptable. The inability of external beam radiation therapy to avoid structures such as the colon, ureters, intestine, and urethra also make radiation therapy a poor choice.

Palliative measures, such as cystostomy tubes, are an option for some cats in order to maintain urine flow. However, there is a 49 per cent complication rate, with complications including secondary infections (up to 85 per cent of cases), inadvertent tube removal, patient destruction of tubes, tube breakage into the bladder, inflammation of the stoma, hematuria, urine leakage around the tube, inadvertent removal of the collection bag, and, in one cat, uroperitoneum.[40] In one study, the tubes were in place for only 83 days before being removed because of complications or by the patient.

URETHRAL TUMORS

Urethral tumors are extremely rare in cats. No information exists regarding their incidence or risk factors. There are reports of only three cats with urethral tumors; two with TCC and one with a leiomyoma.[31,41] Cats also can have extension of a trigonal TCC extending into the urethra.[29] Clinical signs associated with these tumors are similar to those of bladder tumors. Urinary obstruction is a common finding with these tumors.

Diagnosis and staging of urethral tumors is similar to that of primary bladder tumors. However, contrast studies or advanced imaging (CT or MRI) are essential because ultrasound often can not acquire images inside the pelvic cavity.

The available treatment options for urethral tumors in cats are few. Surgery often is not possible given the location and invasiveness of the mass. When attempted, incomplete surgical margins are common and dehiscence or rapid recurrence is likely.[41] Palliative urine diversion again may be possible using a cystostomy tube. Radiation therapy also is not likely to produce long-term responses and the side effects may be quite severe.[41]

The prognosis for urethral tumors in cats is poor. Cats often are euthanized shortly after diagnosis because of progression of local disease and a poor quality of life.

TUMORS OF THE PROSTATE

These tumors also are extremely rare in cats. There are only eight reports of prostatic tumors in cats in the literature. The average age at diagnosis for these cats is around 10 years.[42] The majority of these cats were neutered males with the exception of one, who was neutered after diagnosis.[42,43] Neutering did not slow the progression of the tumor in this cat. The clinical signs associated with prostatic carcinoma in these cats were consistent with lower urinary tract signs. There is one report of obstipation and urethral obstruction secondary to a prostatic carcinoma in a cat.[43] Other prostatic diseases also are rare in cats. One report in the literature of a prostatic abscess in a neutered male cat indicated that the prostate was not painful; therefore pain on palpation does not rule out nonneoplastic causes of prostamegaly.[44]

Metastasis was reported in three of the eight cats (37.5 per cent) with prostatic carcinomas.[42] Full staging including CBC, serum biochemistry analysis, urinalysis, urine culture and antimicrobial sensitivity, abdominal ultrasound, and three-view thoracic radiographs is recommended. A diagnosis usually is made with a surgical biopsy, although ultrasound-guided FNA may be possible with sedation. Contrast studies also may be helpful in determining the extent of the tumor within the pelvic canal.

Therapeutic options for cats with prostatic carcinoma are very limited. The average survival time is less than 3 months in most patients.[42] Surgical resection and anastomosis has been attempted; however, recurrence or metastasis often is rapid.[43]

REFERENCES

1. Henry CJ, Turnquist SE, Smith A, et al: Primary renal tumours in cats: 19 cases (1992-1998), *J Feline Med Surg* 1:165, 1999.
2. Clark WR, Wilson RB: Renal adenoma in a cat, *J Am Vet Med Assoc* 193:1557, 1988.
3. Valli VE, Jacobs RM, Norris A, et al: The histologic classification of 602 cases of feline lymphoproliferative disease using the National Cancer Institute working formulation, *J Vet Diagn Invest* 12:295, 2000.
4. Gabor LJ, Malik R, Canfield PJ: Clinical and anatomical features of lymphosarcoma in 118 cats, *Aust Vet J* 76:725, 1998.
5. Steinberg H, Thomson J: Bilateral renal carcinoma in a cat, *Vet Pathol* 31:704, 1994.
6. Podell M, DiBartola SP, Rosol TJ: Polycystic kidney disease and renal lymphoma in a cat, *J Am Vet Med Assoc* 201:906, 1992.
7. Raffan E, Kipar A, Barber PJ, et al: Transitional cell carcinoma forming a perirenal cyst in a cat, *J Small Anim Pract* 49:144, 2008.
8. Klainbart S, Segev G, Loeb E, et al: Resolution of renal adenocarcinoma-induced secondary inappropriate polycythaemia after nephrectomy in two cats, *J Feline Med Surg* 10:264, 2008.
9. Armbrust LJ, Biller DS, Hoskinson JJ: Compression radiography: an old technique revisited, *J Am Anim Hosp Assoc* 36:537, 2000.
10. Valdes-Martinez A, Cianciolo R, Mai W: Association between renal hypoechoic subcapsular thickening and lymphosarcoma in cats, *Vet Radiol Ultrasound* 48:357, 2007.
11. Burkhard MJ, Meyer DJ: Invasive cytology of internal organs. Cytology of the thorax and abdomen, *Vet Clin North Am Small Anim Pract* 26:1203, 1996.
12. Mooney SC, Hayes AA, Matus RE, et al: Renal lymphoma in cats: 28 cases (1977-1984), *J Am Vet Med Assoc* 191:1473, 1987.
13. Schrader AJ, Hofmann R: Metastatic renal cell carcinoma: recent advances and current therapeutic options, *Anticancer Drugs* 19:235, 2008.
14. Kisseberth WC, Vail DM, Yaissle J, et al: Phase I clinical evaluation of carboplatin in tumor-bearing cats: a Veterinary Cooperative Oncology Group study, *J Vet Intern Med* 22:83, 2008.
15. Bryan JN, Henry CJ, Turnquist SE, et al: Primary renal neoplasia of dogs, *J Vet Intern Med* 20:1155, 2006.
16. Scavelli TD, Patnaik AK, Mehlhaff CJ: Hemangiosarcoma in the cat: retrospective evaluation of 31 surgical cases, *J Am Vet Med Assoc* 187:817, 1985.
17. Culp WT, Drobatz KJ, Glassman MM, et al: Feline visceral hemangiosarcoma, *J Vet Intern Med* 22:148, 2008.
18. Johannes CM, Henry CJ, Turnquist SE, et al: Hemangiosarcoma in cats: 53 cases (1992-2002), *J Am Vet Med Assoc* 231:1851, 2007.
19. Wood CA, Moore AS, Gliatto JM, et al: Prognosis for dogs with stage I or II splenic hemangiosarcoma treated by splenectomy alone: 32 cases (1991-1993), *J Am Anim Hosp Assoc* 34:417, 1998.
20. Ogilvie GK, Powers BE, Mallinckrodt CH, et al: Surgery and doxorubicin in dogs with hemangiosarcoma, *J Vet Intern Med* 10:379, 1996.
21. Hammer AS, Couto CG, Filppi J, et al: Efficacy and toxicity of VAC chemotherapy (vincristine, doxorubicin, and cyclophosphamide) in dogs with hemangiosarcoma, *J Vet Intern Med* 5:160, 1991.
22. Zwahlen CH, Lucroy MD, Kraegel SA, et al: Results of chemotherapy for cats with alimentary malignant lymphoma: 21 cases (1993-1997), *J Am Vet Med Assoc* 213:1144, 1998.
23. Teske E, van Straten G, van Noort R, et al: Chemotherapy with cyclophosphamide, vincristine, and prednisolone (COP) in cats with malignant lymphoma: new results with an old protocol, *J Vet Intern Med* 16:179, 2002.
24. Vail DM, Moore AS, Ogilvie GK, et al: Feline lymphoma (145 cases): proliferation indices, cluster of differentiation 3 immunoreactivity, and their association with prognosis in 90 cats, *J Vet Intern Med* 12:349, 1998.
25. Brearly MJ, Thatcher C, Cooper JE: Three cases of transitional cell carcinoma in the cat and a review of the literature, *Vet Rec* 118:91, 1986.
26. Wimberly HC, Lewis, RM: Transitional cell carcinoma in the domestic cat, *Vet Pathol* 16:223, 1979.
27. Knapp DW: Tumors of the urinary system. In Withrow S, Vail D, editors: *Small animal clinical oncology*, ed 4, Philadelphia, 2007, Saunders, p 649.
28. Beatty JA, Martin P, Kendall K, et al: Haematuria in a geriatric cat, *Aust Vet J* 77:160, 1999.
29. Wilson HM, Chun R, Larson VS, et al: Clinical signs, treatments, and outcome in cats with transitional cell carcinoma of the urinary bladder: 20 cases (1990-2004), *J Am Vet Med Assoc* 231:101, 2007.
30. Schwartz PD, Willer RL: Urinary bladder neoplasia in the dog and cat, *Probl Vet Med* 1:128, 1989.
31. Schwartz PD, Green RW, Patnaik AK: Urinary bladder tumours in the cat: a review of 27 cases, *J Am Anim Hosp Assoc* 21:237, 1985.
32. Landofli JA, Terio KA: Transitional cell carcinoma in fishing cats (*Prionailurus viverrinus*): pathology and expression of cyclooxygenase-1, -2 and p53, *Vet Pathol* 43:674, 2006.
33. Southerland-Smith M, Harvey C, Campbell M, et al: Transitional cell carcinoma in four fishing cats (*Prionailurus viverrinus*), *J Zoo Wildlife Med* 35:370, 2004.
34. Beam SL, Rassnick KM, Moore AS, et al: An immunohistochemical study of cyclooxygenase-2 expression in various feline neoplasms, *Vet Pathol* 40:496, 2003.
35. Owen LN: *TNM Classification of tumours of domestic animals*, Geneva, 1980, World Health Organization.
36. Benigni L, Lamb CR, Corzo-Menendez N, et al: Lymphoma affecting the urinary bladder in three dogs and a cat, *Vet Radiol Ultrasound* 47:592, 2006.

37. Bennett SL, Holland JA, Meehan MC: Mural lymphoma associated with the urinary bladder of a cat, *Aust Vet Pract* 33:155, 2003.

38. Barrand KR: Rectal prolapse associated with urinary bladder neoplasia in a cat, *J Small Anim Pract* 40:222, 1999.

39. Sellon RK, Rottman JB, Jordan HL, et al: Hypereosinophilia associated with transitional cell carcinoma in a cat, *J Am Vet Med Assoc* 201:591, 1992.

40. Beck AL, Grierson JM, Ogden DM, et al: Outcome of and complications associated with tube cystotomy in dogs and cats: 76 cases (1995-2006), *J Am Vet Med Assoc* 230:1184, 2007.

41. Takagi S, Kadosawa T, Ishiguro T, et al: Urethral transitional cell carcinoma in a cat, *J Small Anim Pract* 46:504, 2005.

42. Fan TM, de Lorimier LP: Tumors of the male reproductive system. In Withrow S, Vail D, editors: *Small animal clinical oncology*, ed 4, Philadelphia, 2007, Saunders, p 637.

43. LeRoy BE, Lech ME: Short communication: Prostatic carcinoma causing urethral obstruction and obstipation in a cat, *J Feline Med Surg* 6:397, 2004.

44. Mordei A, Liptak JM, Hofstede T, et al: Case report: prostatic abscess in a neutered cat, *J Am Anim Hosp Assoc* 44:90, 2008.

52 Urological Interventional Techniques in the Feline Patient

Allyson C. Berent

Interventional radiology and interventional endoscopy (IR/IE) involve the use of fluoroscopy (IR) and other contemporary imaging modalities, such as ultrasound or endoscopy (IE), to perform diagnostic and therapeutic procedures in virtually any part of the body (e.g., vasculature, lymphatics, gastrointestinal tract, biliary tract, respiratory tract, or urinary tract). These techniques facilitate minimally invasive approaches to the diagnosis and treatment of complicated problems.

Currently an expanding investigation of the use of some novel techniques in veterinary medicine has been undertaken, particularly pertaining to the upper and lower urinary tract. The relatively common incidence of urinary tract obstruction, urolithiasis, ureteral ectopia, neoplasia, and stricture, along with the invasiveness and morbidity associated with traditional surgical techniques, make the use of these minimally invasive procedures very appealing. Such interventional techniques have been considered standard-of-care practice in human medicine for the last few decades; similar procedures are now being applied in veterinary medicine with increasing popularity.

This chapter provides an overview of some of the minimally invasive urological procedures being performed in our feline veterinary patients. The chapter also will present some promising future endourological and IR applications under investigation.

BACKGROUND—INTERVENTIONS IN HUMAN UROLOGY

In human urology the development and improvements in ureteroscopy, ureteral stenting, extracorporeal shockwave lithotripsy (ESWL), laser lithotripsy, laparoscopy, and percutaneous nephroureterolithotomy (PCNUL) have almost eradicated the need for open urinary surgery for stone disease, strictures, trauma, or neoplasia. Currently, ureteroscopy is the first-line evaluation of ureteral neoplasia, upper tract essential hematuria, ureteral calculi larger than 5 mm, and evaluation for ureteral obstructions. Cystoscopy is the standard diagnostic tool for human patients with dysuria because it can provide both diagnostic and treatment options. Ureteroliths smaller than 5 mm have a 98 per cent chance of spontaneous passage with medical management alone.[1,2] For larger stones, or those that do not pass spontaneously, ESWL is effective in 50 to 81 per cent of cases, although most of the literature suggests that this number is closer to 50 to 67 per cent.[1,2] Ureteroscopy has a near 100 per cent success rate when Holmium:YAG laser lithotripsy is used.[3-7] PCNUL has been successful for large proximal impacted ureteral stones.[8] Ureteral stenting was first introduced in 1967 for evaluation of human patients with malignant ureteral obstructions.[9] Stents still are widely used to treat both benign and malignant obstructive disease and this is considered standard-of-care.[9-15] Ureteral stenting for stone disease typically is done after ureteroscopy for postscoping spasm and edema, and in children, it has been performed routinely prior to ureteroscopy to allow for passive ureteral dilation in anticipation of immediate ureteral bypass, spontaneous stone passage, and the ease of extracorporeal shockwave lithotripsy.[9-15] Ureteral stenting also has been shown to ease a future ureteroscopy dramatically in a small pediatric ureter.[15] Percutaneous cystolithotomy (PCCL) often is the treatment of choice for large cystic stone burdens, in which repetitive urethral trauma is a concern for transurethral lithotripsy.[16]

EQUIPMENT

ENDOSCOPES

Various flexible and rigid endoscopes are used for traditional interventional endosurgical procedures. Rigid cystoscopy is performed commonly in female cats for urethral, bladder, and ureteral access. The recommended diameter is the 1.9 mm rigid scope (with the largest diameter actually measuring nearly 11 French) with a 30-degree lens angle. Flexible ureteroscopes are used for urethral and bladder access if the rigid scope does not fit in a female cat's urethra and for the percutaneous, antegrade approach through the bladder wall. Rigid nephroscopes (1.9 to 7.3 mm diameter) can be used for PCNUL when performed in an antegrade fashion. This might be used for proximal ureterolith or nephrolith retrieval or evaluation of a renal pelvis for essential renal hematuria when necessary.

LITHOTRIPSY

Multiple types of intracorporeal lithotrites and lasers are available including ultrasonic, pneumatic, electrohydraulic, and holmium:YAG lasers, which can be used for stone fragmentation, and a diode laser that is used most often for tissue coagulation or resection (i.e., lasering intramural ureteral ectopia). Extracorporeal shock wave lithotripsy (ESWL) also has application for small to moderate size ureteral calculi in cats, but success has been variable with stone passage in feline patients, when compared with dogs.[17-19]

IMAGING

For many of the more commonly performed IR procedures, a traditional fluoroscopy unit is sufficient. A C-arm fluoroscopy unit has the advantage of mobility of the image intensifier, permitting various tangential views without moving the patient. Ultrasonography is useful for percutaneous needle access into the renal pelvis or urinary bladder.

URINARY ACCESS (GUIDEWIRES, CATHETERS, AND STENTS)

Guidewires of various sizes, shapes, and stiffness are needed for each procedure. Urinary catheters and stents can be used for various purposes to divert urine throughout the entire urinary collection system. Catheters are defined as flexible or rigid hollow tubes employed to drain fluids from body cavities. Most catheters in the urinary system are used for temporary drainage of the renal pelvis (nephrostomy tubes), ureter, or urinary bladder (cystostomy tubes). Urinary catheters are classically soft, comfortable, polyurethane type tubes with an open lumen, permitting temporary drainage. Stents are defined as small tubes, often expandable, inserted across a blocked lumen to restore patency. Urinary stents typically are used for permanent or long-term diversion in the kidney, ureter, bladder, or urethra. Stents most often are completely indwelling tubes that can be placed for various purposes, most commonly to bypass a malignant obstruction, stricture, or embedded stone (i.e., ureterolithiasis). Stents come in different materials (e.g., metal, polyurethane, plastic, rubber), shapes, and sizes (Figure 52-1).

DISEASES OF THE UPPER URINARY COLLECTION SYSTEM: RENAL PELVIS AND URETER

Ureteral disease can create a significant dilemma in our feline patients and is far more common than disease of the renal pelvis. The relatively common incidence of ureteral disease, combined with the invasiveness and morbidity associated with traditional surgical techniques, makes the use of minimally invasive alternatives (IR/IE) appealing.

Feline ureterolithiasis is the most common upper urinary tract frustration that requires immediate intervention. Other causes for ureteral obstruction include ureteral strictures/stenosis and ureteral neoplasia. Greater than 98 per cent of feline ureteroliths were recently documented to be composed of calcium oxalate, which is a trend from earlier decades. This means that these stones will not dissolve medically, and either need to pass spontaneously, remain in place, or be removed. Once medical management fails (traditionally: intravenous fluid therapy, mannitol CRI [constant rate infusion], and alpha-adrenergic blockade ± amitriptyline), partial obstructions often are monitored and left in the ureter, considering the risk-benefit ratio of attempted surgical removal. If there is a complete ureteral obstruction, decompression of the renal pelvis becomes imperative in order to preserve renal function to the ipsilateral kidney. After a ureteral obstruction, studies in dogs have shown

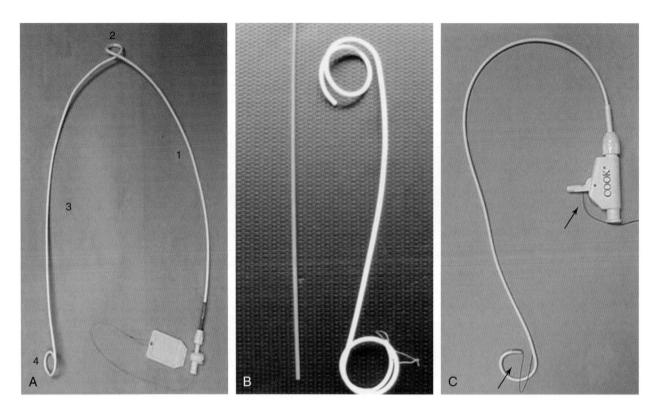

Figure 52-1 Three different types of ureteral stents/catheters. All are made of polyurethane material. **A,** An 8-Fr nephroureteral stent. This stent (1) exits the body wall from the nephrostomy side and traverses the renal parenchyma until it reaches the renal pelvis at the proximal loop (2). The shaft of the stent sits in the ureter (3) and the distal loop (4) remains in the urinary bladder for complete collection system drainage. **B,** A 3-Fr variable length (8-20 cm) double pigtail ureteral stent that remains indwelling. The proximal loop remains in the renal pelvis and the distal loop in the urinary bladder. The blue tubing is a pushing catheter that is used to push the ureteral stent over the guidewire. **C,** A 5-Fr locking loop pigtail catheter. The string is used to lock the loop so that the catheter will not be dislodged.

the ureteral pressures increase immediately and can take over 24 hours after obstruction relief for the pressure to decline.[20] After a transient increase in pressure the renal blood flow diminishes to 40 per cent of normal over the first 24 hours, but drops to 20 per cent of normal by 2 weeks.[21,22] This increase in pressure generated by the ureteral obstruction is transmitted to the entire nephron and a decrease in glomerular filtration rate (GFR) occurs via concurrent vasoactive mediator release, leukocyte influx, and subsequent fibrosis.[21] The longer the ureter remains obstructed, the more damage occurs, which is irreversible. In a study of normal dogs it was found that after 7 days of obstruction, the GFR was permanently diminished by 35 per cent, and when the obstruction lasted for 14 days, the GFR was diminished by 54 per cent.[21,23-25] These numbers were in a dog model without preexisting azotemia, chronic interstitial nephritis, or chronic obstructions, so extrapolation of a worse outcome might be expected in our feline patients, making aggressive and timely intervention worth considering.

Traditional intervention has been accomplished surgically via ureterotomy, neoureterocystostomy, ureteronephrectomy, and renal transplantation. Kyles et al recently reported two retrospective studies in a large number of cats.[26,27] There were high procedure-associated complications (over 30 per cent) and mortality (18 to 39 per cent

depending on the type of management) documented. This study was from two universities with extensive experience with ureteral surgery. The morbidity and mortality may be even higher in environments in which operating microscopes and microsurgical experience are not as available. Many of the associated complications with surgery are caused by site edema, recurrence of stones that pass from the renal pelvis to the surgery site, stricture formation, and ureterotomy-associated or nephrostomy tube–associated urine leakage.[26,27] Over 10 per cent of cats who survived their complications required a second surgical procedure during the same visit, and 30 per cent of those cats subsequently were euthanized or died for serial complications associated with their ureteral stones/surgeries.[26] Of the large number of cats in that study, a relatively small number had long-term imaging follow-up, and 40 per cent of those who underwent subsequent imaging had evidence of ureteral stone recurrence, of whom 85 per cent had evidence of nephrolithiasis at the time of the first ureteral surgery.[26] The number of cats who did not have stone recurrence with prior nephrolithiasis was not evident in that study. Chronic renal failure is common at the time of diagnosis (>75 per cent were azotemic with a unilateral obstruction), and persistent azotemia is a widespread problem after a successful intervention (over 50 per cent of cats).[26,27] However, in spite of all of the surgical concerns, the survival rates were dramatically higher for cats who had intervention performed, when compared with those patients treated with medical management alone. Medical management has been shown to be effective in a minority of cases,[26] but should be considered prior to any intervention, particularly for stones in the distal one-third of the ureter, and for stones smaller than 2 to 3 mm. Finding a less invasive alternative that results in immediate decompression and stabilization of associated azotemia, and allows patency to be established concurrently would be ideal, and in human beings minimally invasive treatments have replaced open surgery.[1-15] The placement of a double pigtail ureteral stent, either minimally invasively (IR technique) or surgically, could potentially circumvent the complications of surgery alone (e.g., leakage, stricture, re-obstruction), and quickly and efficiently stabilize the patient while decreasing renal pelvic pressure and stopping the cycle of pressure-induced nephron death and renal fibrosis.

URETERAL STENTING

Ureteral stenting has been performed for a variety of disorders in dogs and cats.[28,29] The goals of ureteral stenting include (1) to divert urine from the renal pelvis into the urinary bladder to bypass a ureteral obstruction (e.g., ureterolithiasis, obstructive neoplasia, ureteral stricture/stenosis), (2) to encourage passive ureteral dilation (for ureteral stenosis/strictures or future stone passage), (3) to decrease surgical tension on the ureter after/during surgery (i.e., resection and anastomosis or proximal ureteral re-implantation) and prevent postoperative leakage or edema, and (4) to aid in extracorporeal shockwave lithotripsy for large obstructive ureteroliths or nephroliths that could result in serial ureteral obstructions if the stones do not pass completely down the ureter (steinstrasse).[1]

The first report of ureteral stent placement was in 1967 in a human patient for malignant obstruction.[9] Since that time nonresectable trigonal or ureteral tumors are treated similarly, with an indwelling double pigtail ureteral stent used to bypass the obstruction. These tumors are accessed more easily through an antegrade percutaneous approach, in order to gain access down the ureter, an observation we have appreciated in veterinary patients as well. In human beings there is a 96 to 98 per cent success rate in stent placement with this antegrade approach.[9-12] It was not until 1977 that a report of ureteral stenting for benign disease was published, for a ureteral stricture.[12] Then, in 2005 ureteral stenting was described in pediatric urology as a means to facilitate ureteroscopic procedures.[15] Stents encouraged passive dilation of the ureter, a finding that has been reproduced in dogs.[13] The stent is left in place for several weeks, enabling spontaneous voiding of ureteroliths or the subsequent passage of a ureteroscope in such small patients.[13,15] However, few reports of clinical investigation or application of ureteral stents in dogs or cats have been published.[27,28] At the author's institution, over 90 dog or cat ureters have been stented for various clinical purposes.

Ureteral stents are used classically to bypass obstructions from ureterolithiasis, malignant obstructive neoplasia, trauma, and ureteral stenosis or stricture. A ureteral stent can be placed after interventional procedures (such as ureteroscopy, ureteral balloon dilation, or lithotripsy) in order to prevent temporary obstruction from ureteral edema or spasm; following surgical ureterotomy, ureteral resection, and anastomosis; when there is a ureteral tear; to provide tension relief and healing; to prevent postoperative ureteral leaking; and to prevent ureteral stricture formation while the surgical site heals. Some people believe ureteral stents also are ideal in patients with large nephroliths (>10 to 15 mm) or ureteroliths (>4 to 5 mm) who are undergoing ESWL to aid in ureteral stone localization and stone fragment passage after the ESWL treatment.[13,14,17,18] Ureteral stenting has been performed in cats with large numbers of obstructive nephroliths, in order to maintain urine flow and to prevent entry of nephroliths into the proximal ureter.

Ureteral Stents

There are three main types of ureteral stents/catheters: (1) an indwelling double pigtail ureteral stent (vet stent, double pigtail ureteral stent, Infiniti Medical LLC, Malibu, CA), which is the most common type used in veterinary and human medicine, (2) a nephroureteral stent (nephroureteral catheter, Cook Medical, Bloomington, IN), and (3) locking loop pigtail catheter (Dawson-Meuller drainage catheter, 5 Fr, Cook Medical, Bloomington, IN; Infiniti 6 Fr locking loop drainage catheter, Infiniti Medical LLC, Malibu, CA) (see Figure 52-1). The double pigtail stent, which is the stent of choice in cats, is completely intracorporeal and can remain in place for months or years if necessary (recommended for <6 months, but the author has experience with >2 years of stent patency in cats and dogs). Each loop of the pigtail is curled (one in the bladder and one in the renal pelvis), allowing for direct urinary diversion from the kidney to the urinary bladder, around the stones, or through the stricture (Figure 52-2).

In female cats ureteral stents most often are placed either cystoscopically or via a cystotomy; in retrograde manner, the stent can be advanced through the ureteral orifice at the ureterovesicular junction. Retrograde placement also can be accomplished during surgical cystotomy. Ureteral stents also can be placed antegrade through the renal pelvis (percutaneously or surgically), or surgically during ureterotomy. Under general anesthesia the retrograde technique uses cystoscopy and concurrent fluoroscopy. An angle-tipped hydrophilic guidewire (0.018″ Weasel wire) (Weasel Wire [0.035″, 0.025″, 0.018″] hydrophilic angle-tipped guidewire, Infiniti Medical LLC, Malibu, CA) is advanced into the distal ureter from the ureterovesicular junction. The wire is advanced up the length of the ureter and curled into the renal pelvis. Care is taken to bypass the obstruction carefully without perforating the ureter (see Figure 52-2). An open-ended ureteral catheter (open-ended ureteral catheter, 3 French, Cook Medical, Bloomington, IN) then is advanced over the wire under fluoroscopic guidance, and the guidewire is removed. A retrograde contrast ureteropyelogram is performed to help identify any lesions, stones, or filling

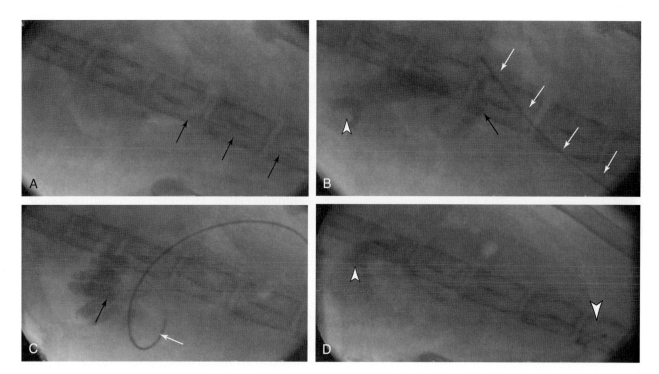

Figure 52-2 Fluoroscopic images of a placement of a double pigtail ureteral stent in a female cat. **A,** A 0.018″ angle-tipped hydrophilic guidewire *(black arrows)* is advanced up the right ureter to the level of the obstruction under endoscopic and fluoroscopic guidance. **B,** A 3-Fr open-ended ureteral catheter *(white arrows)* is advanced over the guidewire and the wire is removed prior to a retrograde ureteropyelogram. This helps document the obstructed area of the ureter and to guide the catheter and stent into the renal pelvis. **C,** The guidewire *(black arrow)* is re-advanced into the renal pelvis to create a curl and the stent *(white arrow)* is pushed over the guidewire so the proximal end forms a pigtail inside the pelvis. **D,** The wire is then removed and the pigtails form proximally within the renal pelvis and distally inside the urinary bladder *(arrowheads)*.

defects in the ureter or renal pelvis. The wire is re-advanced through the catheter into the renal pelvis and the catheter is withdrawn. An indwelling double pigtail ureteral stent (vet stent, double pigtail ureteral stent, Infiniti Medical LLC, Malibu, CA) is placed over the guidewire under fluoroscopic guidance, with one curl remaining in the renal pelvis in front of the obstruction and the other in the urinary bladder. In cats this typically is a 12 cm, 3-Fr double pigtail multifenestrated stent (vet stent, double pigtail ureteral stent, Infiniti Medical LLC, Malibu, CA).

Retrograde ureteral access can be utilized for imaging purposes as well. Retrograde ureteropyelography, in which contrast media is infused up the ureter from its distal end, provides advantages over other methods of contrast urography. The retrograde procedure provides more accurate visualization of the ureter than does intravenous pyelography (IVP), because adequate ureteral filling and distension can be ensured. The retrograde approach also eliminates the risk of contrast-induced nephropathy, because the contrast agent remains in the renal collection system and is not injected intravascularly. Furthermore, when performed cystoscopically the procedure is less invasive than antegrade pyelography, eliminating the need for renal needle puncture.

As described for retrograde placement of a ureteral stent, a guidewire is advanced up the ureteral orifice using

cystoscopic and fluoroscopic guidance. An open-ended ureteral catheter is advanced over the wire and the wire subsequently is removed. Contrast media then is injected through the catheter to create mild ureteral distension and adequate visualization. Injections of contrast media can be repeated safely to confirm subtle lesions (see Figure 52-2).

The antegrade technique, the preferred technique for male cats, requires percutaneous renal access with a renal access needle (21-gauge) (disposable trocar needle, 21 g × 7 cm, Cook Medical, Bloomington, IN) or over-the needle catheter (22-gauge). This can be done with either ultrasound or fluoroscopy. The guidewire is passed down the ureter, into the urinary bladder and out the urethra to have through-and-through access ("flossed"). This approach also is employed for ureteral obstruction by a bladder mass, when the ureteral orifice can not be identified cystoscopically (Figure 52-3). The stent then is placed in a retrograde fashion over the wire, as described above, to keep the hole in the kidney as small as possible (Figure 52-4).

Nephroureteral Stents

The nephroureteral (NU) stent (nephroureteral catheter, Cook Medical, Bloomington, IN) is used classically for a combination of maintaining a tract into the renal pelvis, down the ureter, and into the bladder after PCNUL

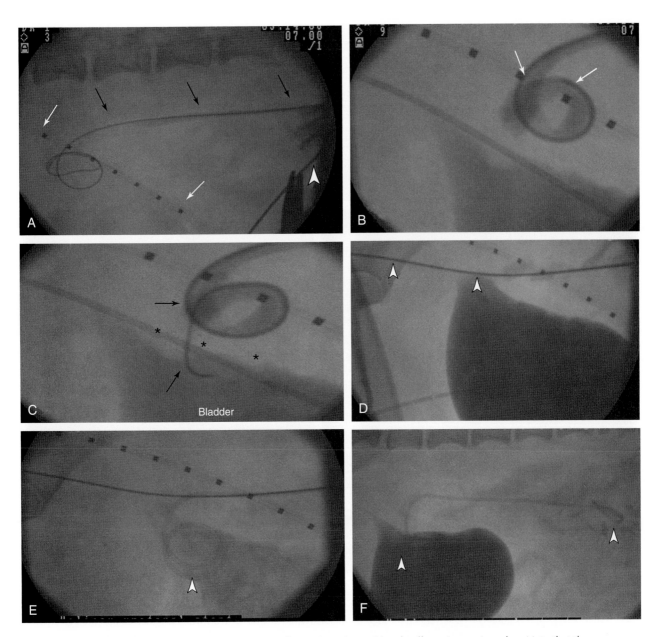

Figure 52-3 Antegrade ureteral stent placement for a trigonal transitional cell carcinoma in a dog. Note that these images are oriented with cranial to the left and caudal to the right. **A,** Antegrade pyelography is performed using ultrasound guidance with a renal access needle *(arrowhead)*. A guidewire is advanced down the needle and directed to the level of the ureterovesicular junction *(black arrows)*. A marker catheter is in the colon to allow for measurements of the ureteral length *(white arrows)*. **B,** Closer image of the ureterovesicular junction as the guidewire and catheter *(white arrows)* are maneuvering through the tumor. A concurrent ureterogram and cystogram are visualized. **C,** The guidewire *(black arrows)* is being advanced through the tumor *(black asterisks)* and into the urinary bladder. **D,** The guidewire is directed out of the urethra so that "through and through" access is obtained *(arrowheads)*. **E,** Over a guidewire the ureteral stent is passed into the renal pelvis with one curl in the pelvis and the other in the urinary bladder *(arrowhead)*. **F,** Fluoroscopic image of the ureteral stent curled in the bladder *(arrowheads)* after wire removal.

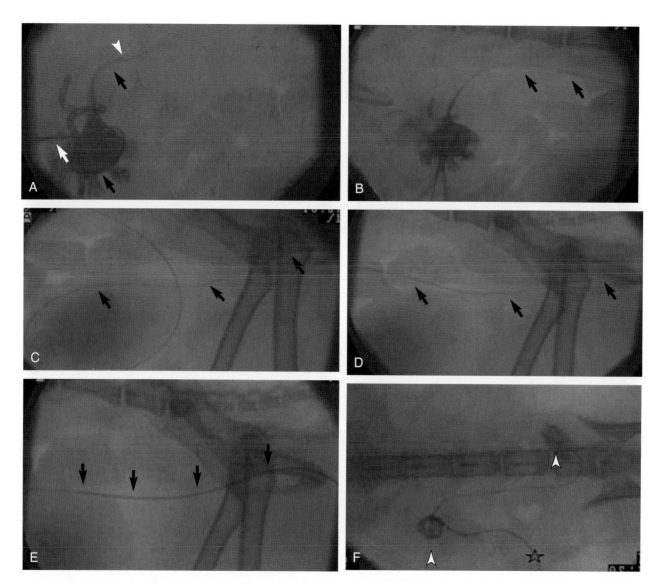

Figure 52-4 Antegrade ureteral stent placement in a male cat. **A,** Fluoroscopic image of an antegrade pyelogram; both the renal pelvis and ureter are filled with contrast media *(black arrows)*. The catheter is in place within the renal pelvis while a guidewire is advanced through the pelvis *(white arrow)*. The *arrowhead* indicates the point of obstruction. **B,** The guidewire is directed distally in the ureter *(black arrows)*, past the ureteroliths. **C,** Lateral orientation. The guidewire is advanced from the kidney, down the ureter, and into the urinary bladder and then out of the urethra. **D,** Lateral orientation. The guidewire is straightened, creating direct ureteral access. **E,** The ureteral stent is being passed over the guidewire from the urethra and into the ureter *(black arrows)*. **F,** The ureteral stent is in place with one curl in the renal pelvis and the other in the urinary bladder *(arrowheads)*. A percutaneous nephrostomy tube is in place within the renal pelvis and exiting the body wall *(star)*.

procedures (see the following). This stent is partially indwelling and partially external. It protects the ureter after lithotripsy from a PCNUL, allowing any ureteral edema to subside and residual stone fragments to pass (see Figure 52-1, *A*). In order for a seal to form from the kidney to the body wall after a larger sheath is placed in the renal pelvis, the catheter must exit the body wall from the renal pelvis and maintain a tight seal. The catheter forms a loop in the renal pelvis with multiple fenestrations for drainage, and then passes down the ureter and into the urinary bladder. This maintains a draining tract from the renal pelvis to the bladder, bypassing the ureter temporarily, as well as allowing a seal to form to the body

wall from the kidney. It usually remains in place for 2 to 4 weeks after PCNUL. This stent is used more commonly in dogs than in cats, because the stent size required for cats is so small that microcatheters, rather than typical NU stents, are required.

For patients in whom minimally invasive stent placement is very difficult, we have had greater success in a majority of cases (~90 per cent) with surgical placement via cystotomy and/or ureterotomy. Once the stent is in place, the concern about multiple ureteroliths, nephroliths, or postoperative leakage is eliminated, because the stent will dilate the ureter, bypass the stones, prevent nephrolith travel, and avert any leakage from occurring.

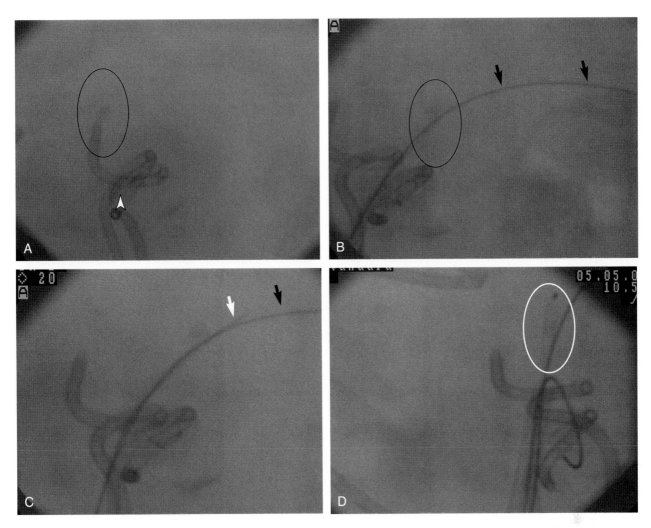

Figure 52-5 Fluoroscopic images of a cat undergoing PCNUL for bilateral ureteral obstruction. **A,** A urolith is visualized in the proximal ureter *(inside circle)*. Nephrostomy tubes are in place within the renal pelves *(arrowhead)*. **B,** A guidewire *(black arrows)* is advanced past the urolith *(circle)* and down the ureter. **C,** A stone basket *(white arrow)* is ensheathed and advanced through the renal access sheath and beyond the stone next to the guidewire *(black arrow)*. **D,** The stone basket is opened and the stone is entrapped *(circle)*.

PERCUTANEOUS NEPHROURETEROLITHOTOMY

Nephroliths in cats are rarely a direct clinical problem unless they result in ureteral obstruction, chronic infection, or progressive azotemia. Proximal ureteroliths or nephroliths can be accessed by nephroureteroscopy. This approach is used more commonly in dogs, but can be attempted in cats if the ureter and pelvis are sufficiently dilated to accommodate the ureteroscope (2.7 mm). A renal access needle is advanced into the renal pelvis through the parenchyma under ultrasound or fluoroscopic guidance, as described for antegrade ureteral stents. A guidewire is advanced through the needle, down the ureter, into the urinary bladder, and out the urethra. A renal balloon dilator or serial vascular dilators are then advanced over the wire, preloaded with an access sheath that is large enough to fit the cystoscope (11 Fr) or ureteroscope (8 Fr). The balloon is inflated through the renal parenchyma and the sheath then is advanced over the balloon for a smooth transition into the renal pelvis. The balloon is deflated and removed over the wire. The endoscope then is advanced over the wire toward the stone. Once the stone is identified, a stone basket can be used to remove the stone through the access sheath (Figure 52-5) or the stone can be fragmented with the laser lithotrite.

EXTRACORPOREAL SHOCKWAVE LITHOTRIPSY FOR URETEROLITHIASIS

ESWL is another minimally invasive alternative for the removal of ureteral calculi. ESWL delivers external shockwaves through a water medium directed under fluoroscopic guidance in two planes. The stone is shocked anywhere from 1000 to 3500 times at different energy levels to allow for implosion and powdering. The debris then is left to pass down the ureter into the urinary bladder over a 1- to 2-week period. This procedure can be performed safely for ureteroliths smaller than 5 mm in dogs and 3 to 5 mm in cats. For larger stone burdens an indwelling double pigtailed ureteral stent is placed prior to ESWL to aid in stone debris passage, ureteral imaging, and immediate relief of the ureteral obstruction prior to ESWL treatment. For stones of larger sizes or those imbedded in the ureteral mucosa, PCNUL may be necessary. In cats ureteral stent placement prior to lithotripsy is ideal to aid in stone identification and passage. ESWL has been effective in only a small number of feline cases and is ideal for very distal ureteroliths, or stones smaller than 3 mm in diameter. Reports from a small number of cases suggest that this technique is effective in a minority of cases for ureterolithiasis.[18,19] Increased application of ureteral stents may improve the success rate.

PERCUTANEOUS NEPHROSTOMY TUBE PLACEMENT

Ureteral obstructions secondary to ureteroliths or malignancy can result in severe hydronephrosis or life-threatening azotemia. Whereas some patients can be managed medically until a ureterolith passes, others require aggressive support to avoid permanent damage. Surgical or other corrective procedures can be relatively prolonged and complicated procedures in these debilitated patients with an unclear outcome of residual renal function. Another temporary strategy for these challenging cases involves nephrostomy tube placement. Nephrostomy tube drainage can be used to relieve obstruction rapidly and help determine whether adequate renal function remains before proceeding to interventional procedures.

Historically nephrostomy tubes have been met with much resistance because of the high risk of postplacement complications (over 50 per cent).[26,30] These complications usually were caused by premature removal or dislodgement, urine leakage, or poor drainage. With the advent of sturdy, multifenestrated tubes that form a loop within the renal pelvis, these complications seem to have declined dramatically. A 5-Fr or 6-Fr locking loop pigtail catheter (Infiniti 6 Fr locking loop drainage catheter, Infiniti Medical LLC, Malibu, CA; Weasel Wire [0.035", 0.025", 0.018"] hydrophilic angle-tipped guidewire, Infiniti Medical LLC, Malibu, CA) is recommended (see Figure 52-1, C).

Nephrostomy tube placement is initiated under ultrasound guidance with a renal access needle, as used for pyelocentesis and ureteropyelography. After imaging is completed, a guidewire is passed through the needle under fluoroscopic guidance and coiled into the dilated renal pelvis (Figure 52-6). In some cases, the guidewire can be maneuvered down the ureter, bypassing the obstruction. With through-and-through access, a nephroureteral stent may be placed instead. For nephrostomy tube placement, the renal pelvis should be larger than 0.8 to 1 cm to allow the pigtail to curl easily within the pelvic space. The locking loop pigtailed catheter

then is advanced over the guidewire into the renal pelvis and the curl is formed. Once the curl in the renal pelvis is made, the pigtail is "locked," the access needle is removed, and the catheter is secured to the body wall. The catheter is secured externally using a "Chinese finger trap" suture tying method. The nephrostomy catheter should remain in place for 2 to 4 weeks in order for the tract to seal. Alternatively, the catheter can be removed and the tract closed surgically, once the obstruction is relieved.

Nephrostomy tube drainage provides time for patient stabilization and resolution of azotemia prior to definitive treatment of the ureteral obstruction. External drainage also creates immediate decompression of the renal pelvis, which may improve filtration and protect renal function. Hemodialysis, in contrast, allows for immediate patient stabilization but does not alleviate renal pelvic pressure.

MANAGEMENT OF RENAL HEMATURIA

Idiopathic renal hematuria is a rare condition in which a focal area of bleeding in the upper urinary tract results in long-term hematuria, iron deficient anemia (chronically), and the potential for clot formation.[31,32] In human beings, vascular malformations have been visualized ureteroscopically and cauterized through the instrument's working channel.[31] Ureteroscopic cauterization also has been performed in a small number of dogs to date.[33] The diagnosis of renal hematuria is made by visualizing frank blood exiting the ureteral orifice. Visualization can be done via cystoscopy (retrograde in a female cat or percutaneous antegrade in a male cat) or via cystotomy. Once the source of bleeding is identified, either ureteronephrectomy or pyeloscopy with cauterization, or selective renal arterial embolization are performed. Focal vascular lesions are rare in cats; however, procedures that preserve renal function and avoid nephrectomy are ideal in this species.

DISEASES OF THE LOWER URINARY COLLECTION SYSTEM: URINARY BLADDER AND URETHRA

LASER LITHOTRIPSY

Laser lithotripsy is an innovative technique for intracorporeal fragmentation of uroliths.[7] The holmium:YAG (yttrium, aluminum, garnet) laser is a solid-state pulsed laser that emits light at an infrared wavelength of 2100 nm.[5] The energy is absorbed in less than 0.5 mm of fluid, making it safe to fragment uroliths in tight locations, such as the urethra, ureter, renal pelvis, or urinary bladder, with limited risk to urothelial damage.[5] It combines both tissue cutting and coagulation properties, as well as the ability to fragment stones on contact.[5] Laser lithotripsy has been applied in multiple animal species including dogs, pigs, human beings, horses, goats, and steers,[33-39] and it has become widely used in clinical practice for both dogs and cats.

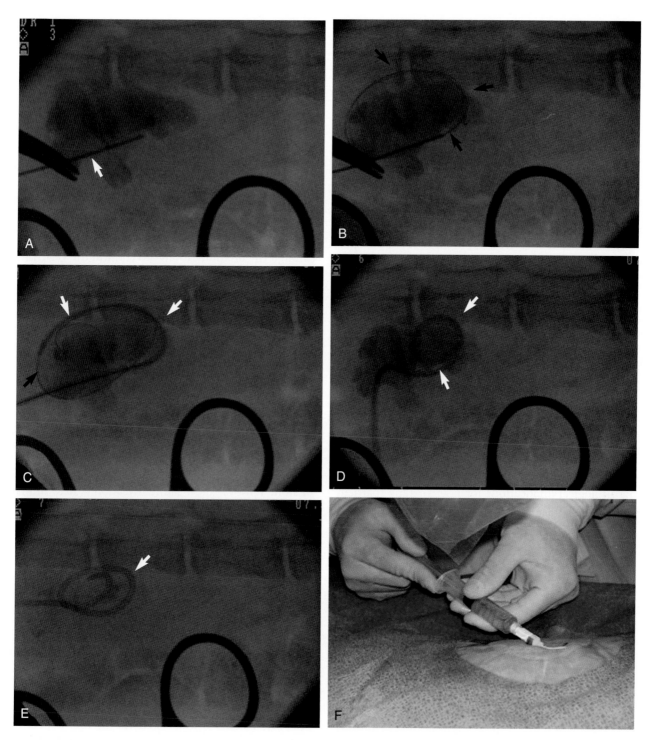

Figure 52-6 Fluoroscopic images of percutaneous nephrostomy tube placement in a cat with a ureteral obstruction. **A,** Renal access is obtained using a renal access needle *(white arrow)* and an antegrade pyelogram is performed. **B,** A guidewire *(black arrows)* is advanced through the needle and coiled in the dilated renal pelvis. **C,** A locking loop pigtail catheter *(white arrows)* is advanced over the guidewire *(black arrow)* and coiled inside the dilated renal pelvis. **D,** The string is pulled on the catheter for the loop to form a tight lock. **E,** The pelvis is drained with the catheter. **F,** The catheter is secured to the body wall for urine drainage.

Small diameter fibers (200, 365, 550 microns) are guided through the working channel of a small diameter cystoscope or ureteroscope. Although the various commercial models of lithotrites vary slightly, the pulse duration of the holmium laser ranges from 250 to 750 microseconds, the pulse energy from 0.2 to 4 J/pulse, and the frequency from 5 to 45 Hz. Power generated ranges from 3 to 100 watts, depending on the type of procedure.

The laser energy is focused on the urolith surface. Pulsed laser energy is absorbed by water inside the urolith, resulting in a photothermal effect and subsequent urolith fragmentation. A vapor bubble is created when the pulse of laser energy traveling through water from the tip of the fiber is trapped within a bubble (Moses effect). If the fiber tip is 0.5 mm or more away from tissue, the vapor bubble collapses, the water absorbs the energy, and no impact is made. As the fiber tip is advanced less than 0.5 mm from the calculus, the vapor bubble impacts the stone. The closer the fiber tip is to the target, the larger the effect.[6] Uroliths are fragmented until the pieces are small enough to be removed normograde through the urethral orifice, either via voiding urohydropropulsion or with the assistance of a stone basket.

Laser lithotripsy is useful for cystic and urethral calculi in cats, as well as for renal and ureteral calculi in dogs. All stone types are able to be fragmented using laser lithotripsy. In female cats lithotripsy is performed via transurethral cystoscopy. The male cat urethra, however, can not accommodate a cystoscope large enough to have a working channel for the laser; percutaneous or keyhole cystoscopic approaches are required (see next section). Other urological applications for laser therapy (particularly a 980 nm wavelength diode laser) include incision of urethral and ureteral strictures, ablation of superficial transitional cell carcinoma within the urethral lumen, and laser ablation of urinary polyps.

PERCUTANEOUS CYSTOLITHOTOMY/KEYHOLE TRANSVESICULAR CYSTOURETHROSCOPY

Traditionally, lower urinary tract calculi in small animal patients have been removed by cystotomy. More recently minimally invasive procedures have shown success in stone removal including laser lithotripsy[38,39] and laparoscopic-assisted cystotomy.[40,41] However, the use of lithotripsy is limited by patient size, gender, species, stone size, and stone number. Laparoscopic-assisted cystotomy requires two incisions, a pneumoperitoneum, and investment in additional equipment. Another minimally invasive technique, termed PCCL, allows cystourethrolith retrieval in any size, gender, or species, and is easy to perform in cats.

In children the treatment of choice for bladder stone retrieval is PCCL.[16] The urinary bladder is filled with contrast material, and a needle and guidewire are used to access the bladder. Serial dilations over the wire allow for a transvesicular cystoscopy sheath to be placed. Stones are visualized and retrieved transvesicularly. After the procedure a suprapubic cystostomy catheter is left in

place for 24 hours, and a urethral catheter is left in place for 48 hours.

For human beings with large cystolith burdens, PCCL (± lithotripsy) is now recommended over transurethral lithotripsy, and has been shown to be safe, minimally invasive, and effective. This model has been adapted for application in animals. The procedure is performed under general anesthesia with the patient positioned in dorsal recumbency. A urethral catheter (3.5 to 5 Fr) is placed and sterile saline infused into the urinary bladder to palpate the location of the apex accurately. A small ventral midline skin incision approximately 1.5 to 2 cm in length is made over the bladder apex. A 1 to 1.5 cm incision is made into the abdominal cavity to accept one finger. The caudal abdomen is palpated digitally until the bladder is identified. The urinary bladder is deflated through the urethral catheter to confirm the vesicle location during digital palpation. The bladder apex is grasped atraumatically with Babcock forceps. Once the bladder is brought to the incision, three stay sutures (one apical and two lateral) are placed using 3-0 polydioxanone (PDS). The bladder is held to the abdominal incision and packed to reduce urine leakage into the abdomen. A stab incision is made into the bladder lumen between the stay sutures. A 6-mm metal screw trocar with a diaphragm is advanced from the stab incision into the bladder lumen angled toward the urethra. A rigid (1.9 integrated, 30-degree lens) cystoscope is advanced through the trocar into the urinary bladder. The entire mucosal surface of the bladder and proximal urethra are visualized and the location and number of uroliths are identified. This technique can be used for evaluation of bladder polyps, ureteral bleeding, or stone retrieval. Slow saline irrigation is used to maintain bladder distension and visibility. A stone retrieval basket is advanced through the working channel of the cystoscope and guided to remove the uroliths. For any small remaining fragments that do not fit in the basket, suction is applied through the trocar as saline is irrigated through the urethral catheter. The entire urethra then is visualized using a small rigid cystoscope in an antegrade manner to identify and remove any urethroliths and confirm a patent urethra. Stones larger than the 6-mm sheath are entrapped in the basket; at the end of the procedure they can be removed through the cystotomy incision (after sheath removal), or fragmented with the laser lithotrite. If necessary the incision is extended slightly to accommodate larger uroliths. The scope and trocar are removed and the incision is closed using 3-0 PDS. The bladder is leak-tested via the urethral catheter and the stay sutures are removed. The abdominal incision is closed routinely in three layers.

URETHRAL BALLOON DILATION OR METALLIC STENTING FOR BENIGN/MALIGNANT OBSTRUCTIONS

Malignant obstructions of the urethra can cause severe discomfort, dysuria, and life-threatening azotemia. Transitional cell carcinoma is the most common tumor of the trigone and urethra in cats and is reported rarely when compared with dogs (see Chapter 51).[42-44] Chemotherapy and nonsteroidal antiinflammatory therapy have been successful in slowing tumor growth but complete cure is uncommon.[43,44] When signs of obstruction occur, more aggressive therapy is indicated. Placement of a cystostomy tube,[45-47] transurethral resection,[48] and surgical diversion[49,50] have been described in dogs; however, these procedures are invasive, require manual drainage, and are associated with significant morbidity.[48] Transurethral placement of a self-expanding metallic urethral stent can be a fast, reliable, and safe alternative to establish urethral patency in such patients.[51] This technique has been performed in over 70 canine patients at the author's institution, but in only a few feline patients. Urethral stenting also may be useful in patients with benign urethral strictures when traditional treatments have failed, or when surgery is refused or not indicated. Benign urethral strictures may resolve with urethral balloon dilation alone, which has been performed in a small number of cats (Figure 52-7).

A marker catheter is placed inside the colon to allow for maximal urethral measurement and determination of stent size. The bladder is distended maximally with contrast agent and a pull-out urethrogram is performed to allow for maximal distension of the urethra with a urethral access sheath in place to prevent urinary leakage out of the urethral papilla/orifice. Measurements of the normal urethral diameter and the length of obstruction are obtained, and an appropriately sized self-expanding metallic urethral stent (SEMS) (vet stent-urethra, Infiniti Medical, Malibu, CA) or balloon-expandable metallic stent (BEMS) (balloon-expandable metallic stent, Infiniti Medical, Malibu, CA) is chosen (approximately 10 to 15 per cent greater than the normal urethral diameter and 3 to 5 mm longer than the obstruction on both the cranial and caudal ends). The stent is deployed under fluoroscopic guidance and a repeat contrast cystourethrogram is performed to document restored urethral patency. In cats a BEMS is more likely to be used because of the small diameter and short length of the urethra. SEMS typically are wider and longer. BEMS also are used classically for short strictures when balloon dilation fails. The author typically applies a topical solution of 0.1 per cent Mitomycin C (MMC) to a stricture after it is broken with a balloon, in a similar manner as described for stenting above. After dilatation, approximately 2 to 3 mL of solution is left to dwell on the stricture site for 5 minutes and then flushed with saline. MMC is an antibiotic that is produced by *Streptomyces caespitosus* and also exhibits antineoplastic and antiproliferative activities.[52-54] It is used most commonly for topical treatment of upper and lower tract transitional cell carcinoma. As an antiproliferative agent, MMC inhibits fibroblast proliferation and decreases scar tissue formation. MMC has been shown in rats, dogs, and human beings to be effective in reducing stricture recurrence in the urinary, respiratory, and gastrointestinal tracts.[52-54]

PERCUTANEOUS CYSTOSTOMY TUBE PLACEMENT

If stenting is not available or indicated, percutaneous cystostomy tubes may be placed to bypass a urethral obstruction or "buy time" while a urethral/trigonal lesion is healing. Cystostomy tubes can be placed either percutaneously or surgically. With the locking loop pigtail catheter (see Figure 52-1, *C*), percutaneous cystostomy tube placement has become a relatively fast and easy technique when necessary. As described previously for nephrostomy tubes, an 18-gauge over-the-needle catheter is advanced into the urinary bladder as for a cystocentesis (paramedian). The stylet is removed and the hydrophilic guidewire is advanced though the catheter and into the urinary bladder. The wire is curled within the bladder two to three times. Fluoroscopic guidance is helpful for appropriate placement, but is not necessary. A locking loop catheter then is advanced over the wire with the stylet still in place (and the trocar removed). Once the entire loop of the catheter is well within the urinary bladder, the stylet is removed. The loop is locked by applying traction to the string at the distal end of the catheter. The catheter is secured tightly to the body wall as described above, and is left in place for at least 2 to 4 weeks prior to removal. Other tubes, such as latex mushroom-tipped catheters, Foley catheters, or low profile tubes can be placed with open or laparoscopic-assisted surgical techniques.[45,46] A cystopexy usually is performed at the same time; tubes should remain in place for approximately 2 weeks after placement.

Cystostomy tubes are associated commonly with secondary infections (at least 86 per cent in one study) owing to the external nature of the tube, and complications with the tubes have been reported in as high as 49 per cent of patients, involving inadvertent tube removal, eating of the tube by the patients, fistulous tract formation, and mushroom tip breakage during removal.[47] This is not ideal in circumstances in which chemotherapy (for malignant obstructions) or immunosuppressive therapy (for proliferative urethritis) is being used.

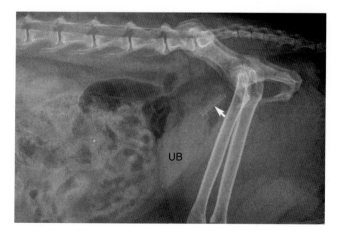

Figure 52-7 Lateral radiograph of a cat with a balloon expandable metallic urethral stent *(arrow)* placed to bypass a malignant obstruction. *UB,* Urinary bladder. (Courtesy Dr. Marilyn Dunn.)

ANTEGRADE URETHRAL CATHETERIZATION

Urethral catheterization is performed routinely in veterinary practice in order to alleviate urinary obstruction, monitor urine output, or maintain urethral patency. Occasionally, retrograde catheterization can be difficult, particularly in small patients or in obstructed cats. In these scenarios antegrade urethral catheterization, using fluoroscopic assistance, can be performed rapidly, easily, and safely. The procedure is particularly useful in male cats with urethral tears, allowing atraumatic catheter placement for long-term management.[55]

Under general anesthesia, cystocentesis is performed using an over-the-needle catheter as described above for cystostomy tube placement. Contrast agent is injected to define the urinary bladder and urethra (Figure 52-8). Under fluoroscopic guidance, a guidewire is advanced antegrade into the bladder and down the urethra until exiting the penis or vulva. For a 5-Fr urinary catheter, an 0.018″ or 0.035″ guidewire and an 18-gauge over-the-needle catheter are recommended. For a 3.5-Fr catheter, an 0.018″ guidewire can be placed through a 22-gauge set. A urinary catheter (open-end or pig-tail) then is advanced over-the-wire in a retrograde fashion into the urinary bladder and the guidewire is removed. Closed-end catheters can be used as well, but the tip must be cut to allow advancement. The urinary catheter is secured in place in routine fashion.

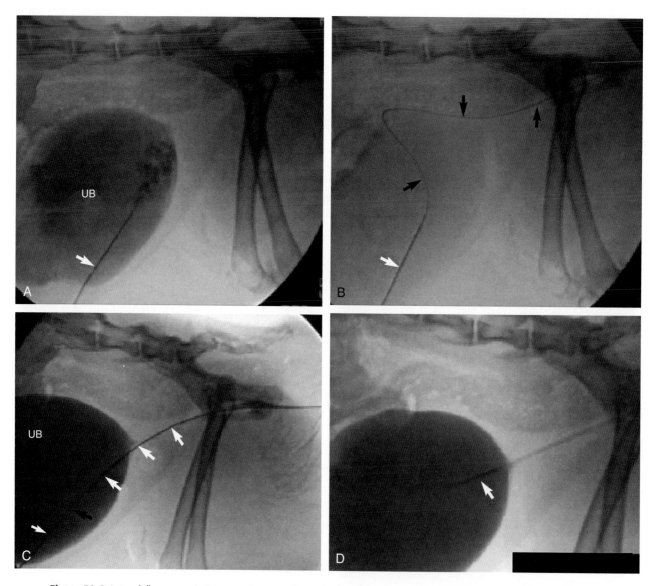

Figure 52-8 Lateral fluoroscopic images of antegrade urethral catheterization in a male cat with a urethral tear. **A,** An 18-gauge over-the-needle catheter is used to perform a cystocentesis *(white arrow)*, and contrast is injected through the needle to highlight the bladder during fluoroscopy. **B,** A guidewire (0.035″) *(black arrows)* is passed through the catheter, into the bladder, and out through the urethra in an antegrade manner. **C,** An open-ended urethral catheter (5-Fr red rubber catheter) is advanced over the guidewire through the urethral lumen *(thick white arrows)* into the urinary bladder and sutured in place at the prepuce. **D,** The guidewire then is removed from the urethral catheter *(white arrow)* and the catheter remains in place in the urethral lumen. (Courtesy Dr. Chick Weisse.)

REFERENCES

1. Al-Awadi KA: Steinstrasse: a comparison of incidence with and without J stenting and the effect of J stenting on subsequent management, *BJU Int* 84:618, 1999.

2. Coe FL, Evan A, Worcester E: Kidney stone disease, *J Clin Invest* 115:2598, 2005.

3. Matsuoka K, Iida S, Nakanami M, et al: Holmium:yttrium-aluminum-garnet laser for endoscopic lithotripsy, *Urology* 45:947, 1995.

4. Bagley DH: Expanding role of ureteroscopy and laser lithotripsy for treatment of proximal ureteral and intrarenal calculi, *Curr Opin Urol* 12:277, 2002.

5. Wollin TA, Denstedt JD: The holmium laser in urology, *J Clin Laser Med Surg* 16:13, 1998.

6. Bagley DH, Das A: *Endourologic use of the holmium laser.* Jackson, WY, 2001, Tenton NewMedia.

7. Denstedt, JD, Razvi, HA, Sales JL, et al: Preliminary experience with holmium:YAG laser lithotripsy, *J Endourol* 9:255, 1995.

8. Al-Shammari AM, Al-Otaibi K, Leonard MP, et al: Percutaneous nephrolithotomy in the pediatric population, *J Urol* 162:1721, 1999.

9. Zimskind PD: Clinical use of long-term indwelling silicone rubber ureteral splints inserted cystoscopically, *J Urol* 97:840, 1967.

10. Yossepowitch O: Predicting the success of retrograde stenting for managing ureteral obstruction, *J Urol* 166:1746, 2001.

11. Uthappa MC: Retrograde or antegrade double-pigtail stent placement for malignant ureteric obstruction? *Clinical Rad* 60:608, 2005.

12. Goldin AR: Percutaneous ureteral splinting, *Urology* 10:165, 1977.

13. Lennon GM: Double pigtail ureteric stent versus percutaneous nephrostomy: effects on stone transit and ureteric motility, *Eur Urol* 31:24, 1997.

14. Mustafa M: The role of stenting in relieving loin pain following ureteroscopic stone therapy for persisting renal colic with hydronephrosis, *Int Urol Nephrol* 39:91, 2007.

15. Hubert KC: Passive dilation by ureteral stenting before ureteroscopy: eliminating the need for active dilation, *J Urol* 174:1079, 2005.

16. Salah MA, Holman E, Munim Khan A, et al: Percutaneous cystolithotomy for pediatric endemic bladder stone: experience with 155 cases from 2 developing countries, *J Pediatr Surg* 40:1628, 2005.

17. Block G, Adams LG, Widmer WR, et al: Use of extracorporeal shock wave lithotripsy for treatment of nephrolithiasis and ureterolithiasis in five dogs, *J Am Vet Med Assoc* 208:531, 1996.

18. Adams LG, Senior DF: Electrohydraulic and extracorporeal shock-wave lithotripsy, *Vet Clin North Am Small Anim Pract* 29:293, 1999.

19. Lane IF: Lithotripsy: an update on urologic applications in small animals, *Vet Clin North Am Small Anim Pract* 34:1011, 2004.

20. Wen JG, Frokiaer J, Jorgensen TM, et al: Obstructive nephropathy: an update of the experimental research, *Urol Res* 27:29, 1999.

21. Coroneos E, Assouad M, Krishnan B, et al: Urinary obstruction causes irreversible renal failure by inducing chronic tubulointerstitial nephritis, *Clin Nephrol* 48:125, 1997.

22. Wilson DR: Renal function during and following obstruction, *Ann Rev Med* 28:329, 1977.

23. Fink RW, Caradis DT, Chmiel R, et al: Renal impairment and its reversibility following variable periods of complete ureteric obstruction, *Aust NZ J Surg* 50:77, 1980.

24. Kerr WS: Effect of complete ureteral obstruction for one week on kidney function, *J Appl Physiol* 6:762, 1954.

25. Vaughan DE, Sweet RE, Gillenwater JY: Unilateral ureteral occlusion: pattern of nephron repair and compensatory response, *J Urol* 109:979, 1973.

26. Kyles A, Hardie E, Wooden E, et al: Management and outcome of cats with ureteral calculi: 153 cases (1984-2002), *J Am Vet Med Assoc* 226:937, 2005.

27. Kyles A, Hardie EM, Wooden BG, et al: Clinical, clinicopathologic, radiographic, and ultrasonographic abnormalities in cats with ureteral calculi: 163 cases (1984-2002), *J Am Vet Med Assoc* 226:932, 2005.

28. Berent A, Weisse C, Bagley D, et al: Ureteral stenting for benign and malignant disease in dogs and cats. Proceedings of the ACVS Forum, Chicago, IL, 2007.

29. Berent A: Ureteral stenting in cats: a minimally invasive alternative. Proceedings of the ACVS Forum, San Diego, CA, 2008.

30. Hardie EM, Kyles AE: Management of ureteral obstruction, *Vet Clin North Am Small Anim Pract* 34:989, 2004.

31. Tawfiek ER, Bagley DH: Ureteroscopic evaluation and treatment of chronic unilateral hematuria. *J Urol* 160:700, 1998.

32. Mishina M, Watanabe T, Yugeta N, et al: Idiopathic renal hematuria in a dog: the usefulness of a method of partial occlusion of the renal artery, *J Vet Med Sci* 59:293, 1997.

33. Weisse C, Berent A: Interventional radiology and endosurgery of the urinary system. In Bonagura JD, Twedt DC, editors: *Current veterinary therapy XIV*, St. Louis, 2009, Saunders, p 965.

34. Howard RD, Pleasant RS, May KA: Pulsed dye laser lithotripsy for treatment of urolithiasis in two geldings, *J Am Vet Med Assoc* 212:1600, 1998.

35. Streeter RN, Washburn KE, Higbee RG, et al: Laser lithotripsy of a urethral calculus via ischial urethrotomy in a steer, *J Am Vet Med Assoc* 219:640, 2001.

36. Davidson EB, Ritchey JW, Higbee RD, et al: Laser lithotripsy for treatment of canine uroliths, *Vet Surg* 33:56, 2004.

37. Halland SK, House JK, George LW: Urethroscopy and laser lithotripsy for the diagnosis and treatment of obstructive urolithiasis in goats and pot-bellied pigs, *J Am Vet Med Assoc* 220:1831, 2002.

38. Adams LG, Berent AC, Moore GE, et al: Use of laser lithotripsy for fragmentation of uroliths in dogs: 73 cases (2005-2006), *J Am Vet Med Assoc* 323:1680, 2008.

39. Grant DC, Were SR, Gevedon ML: Holmium:YAG lithotripsy for urolithiasis in dogs, *J Vet Intern Med* 22:534, 2008.

40. Rawlings CA, Mahaffey MB, Barsanti JA, et al: Use of laparoscopic-assisted cystoscopy for removal of urinary calculi in dogs, *J Am Vet Med Assoc* 222:759, 2003.

41. Miller DC, Park JM: Percutaneous cystolithotomy using a laparoscopic entrapment sac, *Urol* 62:333, 2003.

42. Wilson HM, Chun R, Larson VS, et al: Clinical signs, treatments, and outcome in cats with transitional cell carcinoma of the urinary bladder: 20 cases, *J Am Vet Med Assoc* 231:101, 2007.

43. Knapp DW, Glickman NW, Widmer WR, et al: Cisplatin versus cisplatin with piroxicam in a canine model of human invasive urinary bladder cancer, *Cancer Chemother Pharmacol* 46:221, 2000.

44. Norris AM, Laing EJ, Valli VEO, et al: Canine bladder and urethral tumors: a retrospective study of 115 cases (1980-1985), *J Vet Intern Med* 16:145, 1992.

45. Smith JD: Placement of a permanent cystostomy catheter to relieve urine outflow obstruction in dogs with transitional cell carcinoma, *J Am Vet Med Assoc* 206:496, 1995.

46. Stiffler KS, McCrackin Stevenson MA, et al: Clinical use of low-profile cystostomy tubes in four dogs and a cat, *J Am Vet Med Assoc* 223:325, 2003.

47. Beck AL, Grierson JM, Ogden DM, et al: Outcome of and complications associated with tube cystostomy in dogs and cats: 76 cases (1995-2006), *J Am Vet Med Assoc* 230:1184, 2007.

48. Liptak JM, Brutscher SP, Monnet E, et al: Transurethral resection in the management of urethral and prostatic neoplasia in 6 dogs, *Vet Surg* 33:505, 2004.

49. Fries CL, Binnington AG, Valli VE, et al: Enterocystoplasty with cystectomy and subtotal intracapsular prostatectomy in the male dog, *Vet Surg* 20:104, 1991.

50. Stone EA, Withrow SJ, Page RL, et al: Ureterocolonic anastomosis in ten dogs with transitional cell carcinoma, *Vet Surg* 17:147, 1988.

51. Weisse C, Berent A, Solomon J, et al: Evaluation of palliative stenting for management of malignant urethral obstructions in dogs, *J Am Vet Med Assoc* 229:226, 2006.

52. Ayyildiz A, Nuhoglu B, Gulerkaya B, et al: Effect of intraurethral mitomycin-C on healing and fibrosis in rats with experimentally induced urethral stricture, *J Urol* 11:1122, 2004.

53. Mazdak H, Meshki I, Ghassami F: Effect of mitomycin C on anterior urethral stricture recurrence after internal urethrotomy, *Eur Urol* 51:1089, 2006.

54. Daher P, Riachy E, Goerges B, et al: Topical application of mitomycin C in the treatment of esophageal and tracheobronchial stricture: a report of 2 cases, *J Pediatr Surg* 42:E9, 2007.

55. Meige F, Sarrau S, Autefage A: Management of traumatic urethral rupture in 11 cats using primary alignment with a urethral catheter, *Vet Comp Orthop Traumatol* 21:76, 2008.

SECTION
VIII

Neurology

Joan R. Coates, Section Editor

53 Intervertebral Disk Disease

John H. Rossmeisl, Jr.

Compared with dogs, feline intervertebral disk disease (IVDD) appears to be uncommon. However, as demonstrated by numerous case reports of IVDD in cats, it should be a differential diagnostic consideration in cats with clinical signs of transverse myelopathy or radiculopathy.[1-9] The veterinary literature represents feline IVDD most commonly in domesticated *(Felis catus)* cats; however, IVDD also has been documented in exotic, nondomesticated felids, such as Bengal *(Panthera tigris tigris)* and Malayan *(Panthera tigris jacksoni)* tigers, leopards *(Panthera pardus),* and the African lion *(Panthera leo).*[10]

ANATOMY OF THE INTERVERTEBRAL DISK

The intervertebral disk is a complex biochemical structure that lies between each vertebra from C2 caudally to the sacrum and coccygeal vertebrae, thus forming the amphiarthrodial joints that serve to structurally link and allow for vertebral column motion in multiple planes while resisting applied biomechanical forces.[11] Each intervertebral disk consists of three anatomical components: the innermost located nucleus pulposus, an outer annulus fibrosus, and cartilaginous endplates.

The nucleus pulposus is a notochordal remnant that functions as a scaffold for development of the sclerotome into the vertebral column.[11] Water is the principal biochemical component of the nucleus pulposus, and is bound within the disk matrix by proteoglycan components within the ground substance. Proteoglycan monomers of the disk are each composed of a single protein core to which numerous polysaccharide subunits, called glycosaminoglycans, are bound covalently. The annulus fibrosus is a fibrous structure that encompasses the nucleus pulposus circumferentially. Transverse sectioning of the annulus fibrosus reveals multiple lamellae of collagen fibers arranged in an eccentric fashion, such that the ventrally positioned lamellar bands are thicker and more numerous than dorsal layers. Similar to the variability reported in other species, craniocaudal disk thickness and the ratio of ventral to dorsal annular thickness in cats differs between regions of the vertebral column.[12,13] In cats the contribution of the intervertebral disks to the total length of the vertebral column ranges from 12 to 18 per cent, with disk thickness being greatest in the cervical region and least in the thoracic area.[12] The specific regional contributions of disk thickness to feline vertebral column length have been reported as 14 per cent in the cervical, 15 per cent in the thoracic, and 6 per cent in the lumbar regions, respectively.[12] The ratio of ventral to dorsal annular thickness in cats is highest (3.2:1) in the lumbar area, intermediate in the cervical region (1.8:1), and lowest in the thoracic spine (1.3:1).[13]

The cartilaginous endplates define the cranial and caudal limits of the disk relative to adjoining vertebral epiphyses. Fibers from both the annulus and nucleus are interwoven intimately with collagenous constituents of the endplate as well as osseous elements of the adjacent vertebrae, which imparts additional strength to each disk.[13] The thin, central-most aspect of the cartilaginous endplate also participates in the nutrition of the disk, allowing for diffusion of water and solutes.[11]

EPIDEMIOLOGY AND PATHOGENESIS

Current incidence of clinically significant IVDD in the feline population is unknown. Previous estimates of incidence in cats with clinical signs of IVDD have ranged between 0.02 and 0.12 per cent.[4,7,9] In a retrospective, postmortem study of 205 cats with spinal cord disease, the prevalence rate of IVDD was 4 per cent (eight of 205 cats).[3]

Both chondroid and fibroid disk degeneration occur in cats.[4-7,14-18] Hansen type I IVDD is associated with chondroid metaplasia of the disk, and Hansen type II IVDD is associated with fibroid metaplasia, a normal aging process of the disk. Recent literature suggests that the majority of cats with clinically significant compressive myelopathy or radiculopathy have Hansen type I IVDD (Figure 53-1), characterized by herniation of nucleus pulposus through torn annular fibers with subsequent extrusion of nuclear material into the spinal canal (Figure 53-2, A).[4,6-8] Published reports and clinical experience indicate that clinically significant thoracolumbar spinal cord dysfunction resulting from IVDD affects middle-aged cats predominantly, with the mean age of 7 years, although the age range (1 to 18 years) is quite variable.[4] There does not appear to be a gender predilection.

Secondary spinal cord dysfunction can occur over any disk space in the spinal column. The caudal lumbar and lumbosacral areas are predisposed. Nearly two thirds (20 of 32) of the cases in the literature reported IVD extrusions involved the L4-L5, L5-L6, L6-L7, or L7-S1 disk interspaces (see Figure 53-1).[6-9] The disk interspaces between T11-T12 and L2-L3 were involved frequently, occurring in 31 per cent (10 of 32) of clinically affected cats (see Figure 53-1).[4,6,7] The proclivity for cats to jump onto objects, thereby applying increased biomechanical loads on their lumbar spines, has been suggested as a mechanism for the observed predilection for caudal lumbar disk extrusions.[7,9] One study reported that the body weight of cats with L4-L5 IVDD was greater than that of cats with IVDD involving the thoracolumbar junction. This further supported the hypothesis of increased biomechanical strain on the lumbar vertebral column as a possible risk factor for IVDD of the caudal lumbar region.[7]

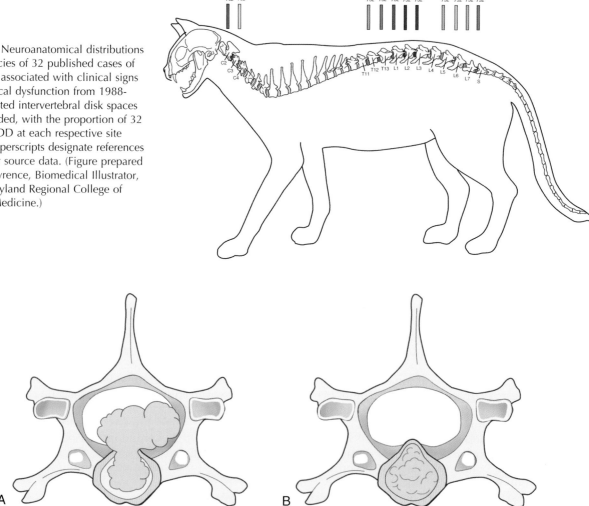

Figure 53-1 Neuroanatomical distributions and frequencies of 32 published cases of feline IVDD associated with clinical signs of neurological dysfunction from 1988-2008.* Affected intervertebral disk spaces are color-coded, with the proportion of 32 cats with IVDD at each respective site provided. Superscripts designate references compiled for source data. (Figure prepared by Terry Lawrence, Biomedical Illustrator, Virginia-Maryland Regional College of Veterinary Medicine.)

Figures 53-2 Schematic representations of Hansen type I **(A)** and II **(B)** IVDD, respectively. (Figures prepared by Terry Lawrence, Biomedical Illustrator, Virginia-Maryland Regional College of Veterinary Medicine.)

*References 1,2,5-9,25-27,29,32.

Postmortem studies suggest that degeneration of the intervertebral disk is a common incidental finding in aged cats; concurrent clinical signs of spinal cord dysfunction are rare.[14-19] In these studies a significant increase in the incidence and severity of intervertebral disk degeneration was noted in cats between 11 and 14 years of age. Another study reported disk protrusions in all cats who were older than 15 years of age at the time of examination.[14,15] The likelihood of multiple disk protrusions also increased with age in old cats.[15] Hansen type II disk protrusions (see Figure 53-2, *B*) are characterized by protrusion of dorsal annular elements into the spinal canal, and account for approximately 80 per cent of disk-associated necropsy lesions reported in asymptomatic cats.[14-19] This was in contrast to symptomatic cats with spinal cord dysfunction with Hansen type II disk protrusions that involved the cervical spine predominantly.[17,19]

Clinical signs of radiculopathy or myelopathy caused by cervical IVDD is uncommon, with a total of four cats reported.[1,5,20,21] Two of these cats had acute histories associated with Hansen type I IVDD localized to the C1 to C5 spinal cord region (see Figure 53-1),[1,5] and two cats had chronic Hansen type II IVDD localized to the C6 to T2 spinal cord region.[20,21] Clinical signs associated with cervical IVDD may be less obvious because of the higher likelihood of Hansen type II than Hansen type I IVDD, and because of the fact that the ratio of the spinal canal diameter to spinal cord diameter is greatest in the cervical spinal canal region.[1,7,17]

In cats with IVDD, protrusion or extrusion of disk material into the vertebral canal is a primary event that incites concussive, contusive, or compressive types of injury processes to the spinal cord tissue. These mechanical forces initiate a cascade of vascular, biochemical, and inflammatory mediators that subsequently cause secondary tissue injury to the spinal cord. Ischemia is postulated to be a principal contributor to acute spinal cord injury by perpetuating the secondary injury processes, such as free radical generation and cellular excitotoxicity.[22] Spinal cord ischemia also can be secondary to physical destruction or thrombotic obstruction of the microcirculation, functional vasospasm induced by numerous biochemical mediators associated with the secondary injury cascade, or exacerbated by systemic hypotension resulting from loss of autoregulation.[22]

CLINICAL SIGNS

Clinical signs associated with feline IVDD are variable and dependent on the neuroanatomical location of the affected disk(s), as well as the severity and extent of the accompanying spinal cord injury. Spinal cord function is assessed during gait analysis and postural reaction testing during the neurological examination. (The reader is referred to Chapter 49 in the fifth volume of this series for a full discussion of the neurological examination.) The final neuroanatomical localization within the spinal cord is determined by evaluation of segmental spinal reflexes, muscle mass and tone, and by determining a discrete area of hyperpathia on palpation of the spinal column.

Onset of clinical signs in cats with clinically significant spinal cord dysfunction secondary to IVDD can be static or progressive.[4] This author utilizes a functional classification scheme (Table 53-1), modified from those described in dogs with spinal cord injuries, to determine the severity of neurological dysfunction in cats with IVDD.[23,24] Clinical signs in cats with mild IVDD also may be nonspecific, such as reluctance to jump or climb into litter pans, lethargy, and anorexia.[4,9]

DIFFERENTIAL DIAGNOSIS

The differential diagnosis for cats with clinical signs of spinal cord dysfunction should include traumatic injury of the spine (fracture or subluxation), meningomyelitis (feline infectious peritonitis, feline leukemia virus–associated myelopathy, cryptococcosis, toxoplasmosis, feline immunodeficiency virus), diskospondylitis, vertebral (osteosarcoma, multiple myeloma) or spinal cord (lymphoma, meningioma, glioma) neoplasia, and

Table 53-1 Functional Classification of Clinical Severity of Neurological Dysfunction in Cats with IVDD

Clinical Grade and Severity*	Description of Neurological Dysfunction (C1-T2 Spinal Cord Segments)	Description of Neurological Dysfunction (T3-S3 Spinal Cord Segments)
0	Clinically normal	Clinically normal
1	Pain only	Pain only
2	Proprioceptive ataxia and/or ambulatory tetraparesis/hemiparesis[†]	Proprioceptive ataxia and/or ambulatory paraparesis[†]
3	Nonambulatory tetraparesis/hemiparesis[†]	Nonambulatory paraparesis[†]
4	Tetraplegia/hemiplegia[†]	Paraplegia with intact nociception ± urinary and fecal incontinence[†]
5	Tetraplegia with neurogenic respiratory failure ± absent nociception[†]	Paraplegia with absent nociception ± urinary and fecal incontinence[†]

*The scale goes from 0, which is normal, to 5, which is severe.
[†]Evidence of spinal hyperpathia may or may not be present.

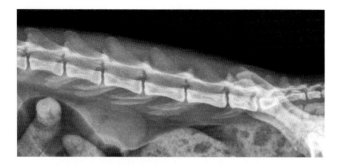

Figure 53-3 Lateral survey radiograph of a cat with an acute onset of paraparesis. Note the narrowing of the L5-L6 disk space.

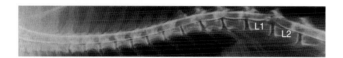

Figure 53-4 Lateral myelogram of a cat with a 1-week history of progressive pelvic limb ataxia and paraparesis. There is a ventral extradural compressive lesion at L1 to L2, confirmed as Hansen type I disk extrusion at surgery.

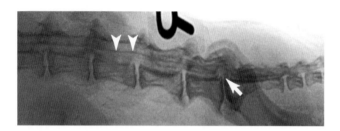

Figure 53-5 Right lateral myelogram of a cat with a flaccid tail, and urinary and fecal incontinence. Between L7 and S1 there is spondylosis, narrowing of the disk space, and ventral extradural attenuation of the contrast columns overlying this space *(arrow)*. Contrast was injected iatrogenically into the epidural space and inadvertently into the central canal during the procedure *(arrowheads)*. An L7-S1 dorsal laminectomy and diskectomy were performed and confirmed Hansen type II IVD extrusion.

ischemic myelopathy (fibrocartilaginous embolism, aortic thromboembolism).

DIAGNOSIS

Spinal radiographic findings of IVDD include narrowing of the affected disk interspace (Figure 53-3), mineralized opacity within the vertebral canal or intervertebral foramen, and in situ mineralization of intervertebral disks. Cats with lumbosacral IVDD also may have evidence of transitional vertebrae.[9] Spinal radiography also may be within normal limits.

Other imaging modalities such as myelography, computed tomography (CT), and magnetic resonance imaging (MRI) have been used to diagnose IVD extrusions in cats. These imaging techniques are indispensable tools for excluding diagnosis of other possible causes of spinal

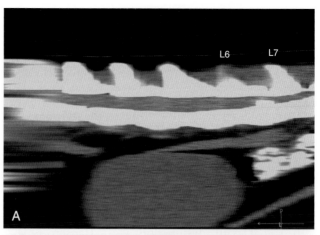

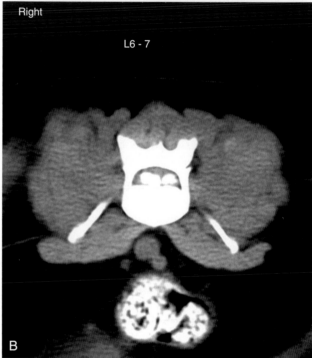

Figures 53-6 Sagittal **(A)** and transverse **(B)** CT images of the lumbar spine of a cat with an acute onset of caudal lumbar hyperpathia and paraparesis. Note the hyperattenuating, extruded disk material within the vertebral canal overlying the L6-L7 disk space.

cord dysfunction and for providing more precise localization of extruded disks for surgical planning. Myelography has been used successfully for localizing extruded disks.[1,4-9] In acutely symptomatic cats myelography can show a single ventral or ventrolateral, extradural compressive lesion, often with marked attenuation of the contrast columns (Figures 53-4 and 53-5), although multiple sites of IVDD have been reported occasionally.[6] On CT examination of the spine, extruded disks appear as extradural hyperattenuating material within the spinal canal, often associated with compression or displacement of the adjacent neural parenchyma (Figure 53-6).[7] Spinal MRI is being used more frequently in diagnosis of IVDD in cats.[5] Abnormalities on MRI include loss of the normal hyperintense signal of the nucleus pulposus at the disk interspace on T2-weighted images, attenuation of the ventral subarachnoid space by hypointense material within the spinal canal, and extradural compression and displacement of the spinal cord (Figures 53-7 and 53-8). Magnetic resonance imaging using a T2-weighted image in cats with acute onset IVD extrusion may show a diffuse hyperintensity in the spinal cord reflective of spinal cord edema or focal area hyperintensity suggestive of contusive injury.[5]

Cerebrospinal fluid (CSF) analysis in cats with IVDD usually is nonspecific and includes albuminocytologic dissociation, mild suppurative pleocytosis, and iatrogenic blood contamination.[6,7] Still, CSF analysis is an important test for diagnosis of other pathological changes that are not attributable to IVDD. Collection of CSF is recommended in all cats prior to myelography, and ideally should be performed caudal to the area of neuroanatomical localization.

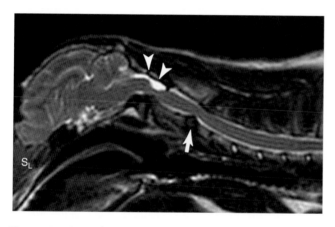

Figure 53-7 Sagittal T2-weighted MR image of a cat with a 1-month history of progressive ataxia of all limbs and tetraparesis. There is signal hypointensity within the C2-C3 and C3-C4 disk spaces, compared with the normal high signal in the nucleus pulposus regions of the more caudally located disks. Ventral extradural, disk-associated spinal cord compression is apparent at C2-C3 *(arrow)*, as well as an arachnoid-like cystic lesion in the dorsal C1-C2 area *(arrowheads)*.

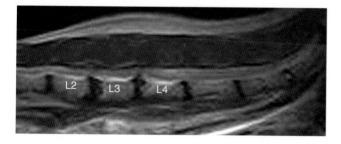

Figure 53-8 Sagittal T2-weighted MR image of the lumbar spine of a cat with a 2-year history of recurrent paraparesis. Multifocal lumbar disk degeneration is present, as suggested by the reduced in situ T2 signal intensity within all disks in the scan field. At L3-L4, there is moderate spinal cord compression overlying the disk. Mild, disk-associated spinal cord compression also is evident at L2-L3.

TREATMENT AND PROGNOSIS

Intervertebral disk extrusion in cats may be managed conservatively or surgically. There are insufficient data in the literature to predict recovery rates based on severity of neurological dysfunction and whether or not to pursue medical or surgical treatment. Results in small numbers of cats suggest that conservative management may be associated with a poor outcome.[7,20,21] Other disadvantages of conservative treatment include incomplete recovery of neurological function, significant risk of future recurrence of clinical signs, and prolonged recovery times.[5,7,20,21] Still, conservative treatment has been used successfully in cats with clinical signs of IVDD. Conservative management includes strictly enforced cage confinement for a defined time, analgesia, administration of antiinflammatory agents, and urinary bladder management (Table 53-2).

Similar to what has been described in dogs with signs of IVDD, conservative management is indicated in mildly affected cats with grade 1 or 2 deficits (see Table 53-1), or in patients for whom owner-dictated constraints preclude further diagnostic or surgical interventions. Although the optimal period of cage confinement is unknown, 4 weeks generally is recommended. Weekly clinical reevaluations during the conservative management period, especially in those cats with neurogenic urinary bladder dysfunction, also should be performed to assess the effects of conservative treatment and monitor for complications (i.e., urine retention, urinary tract infection, chemical dermatitis). Physical rehabilitation also may benefit the recovery of cats with spinal cord dysfunction.

Surgical intervention is indicated in cats with grade 2 deficits with progression of paresis, cats classified as grade 3 to 5 (see Table 53-1), or if clinical signs are refractory to conservative therapy. Surgery allows for definitive histopathological diagnosis of lesions, and more rapid and complete clinical resolution of observed neurological dysfunction.[25,26] A variety of techniques have been used in the surgical treatment of feline IVD extrusion, including hemilaminectomy, dorsal laminectomy, and mechanical disk fenestration. Prognosis for cats undergoing decompressive surgery is good to excellent in patients with thoracolumbar and lumbosacral IVD extrusion and intact nociception.[4,9,27] If we consider only cats with spinal pain who show improvement or resolution, or cats who initially were nonambulatory and showed sufficient improvement, as surrogate measures of surgical success, then 83 per cent (24 of 29) of reported cats with thoracolumbar and lumbosacral IVD extrusion treated surgically had successful postoperative outcomes.[2,6-9,25-31] Residual neurological deficits (ataxia, paresis, and urinary and fecal incontinence) remained in 41 per cent (12 of 29) of surgically treated cats during postoperative follow-up periods that ranged from 1 month to 4.5 years.[6-9,29,31] Recurrence rates of clinical signs of feline IVDD are unknown.

Presumed high-velocity, low-volume explosive thoracolumbar disk extrusions resulting in severe spinal cord contusion or intramedullary penetration of disk material and spinal cord laceration are often accompanied by loss

Table 53-2 Oral Drugs Used in the Symptomatic Treatment of Feline IVDD

Drug	Drug Type	Dose	Adverse Effects	Indication
Ketoprofen	NSAID	1 mg/kg PO q24h	GI distress; nephrotoxicity	Disk-related inflammation or pain
Meloxicam	NSAID	0.1 mg/kg PO q24h for 2-4 days; then 0.1 mg/cat PO q24h	GI distress; nephrotoxicity	Disk-related inflammation or pain
Prednisone	Corticosteroid	0.5 mg/kg/day PO	GI distress, polydipsia/polyuria, polyphagia	Disk-related inflammation or pain
Butorphanol	Opioid	0.5-2.0 mg/kg PO q4-6h	Sedation, anorexia	Disk-related pain
Buprenorphine	Opioid	0.01-0.03 mg/kg buccal/sublingual q8h	Sedation, GI distress, dysphoria	Disk-related pain
Gabapentin	Anticonvulsant	2.5-10 mg/kg PO q12-24h	Sedation, ataxia, anorexia	Chronic neuropathic pain
Prazosin	α-adrenergic antagonist	0.25-0.5 mg/cat PO q12-24h	Hypotension, GI distress	Urinary retention from UMN bladder; decrease urethral resistance
Diazepam	Benzodiazepine	1-2.5 mg/cat PO q8-12h	Sedation, paradoxical excitement, polyphagia, hepatotoxicity	As for prazosin
Tramadol	Mixed-action analgesic	12.5 mg/cat PO q12-24h	Ptyalism, sedation	Disk-related pain

NSAID, Nonsteroidal antiinflammatory drug; *GI,* gastrointestinal; *UMN,* upper motor neuron bladder characterized physically by a turgid, distended bladder that is difficult to impossible to express manually because of an increase in urethral outlet resistance; associated most commonly with severe T3-L3 spinal cord injury.

of deep pain perception and myelomalacia.[26,32] However, neither the presence of *focal* myelomalacia nor the loss of nociception completely preclude the possibility of recovery.[6,26]

The available literature suggests that the prognosis for cats with clinical evidence of cervical spinal cord dysfunction secondary to IVD extrusion is considered guarded when compared with spinal cord dysfunction that involves other areas of the spinal cord.[1,5,20,21] The most recent report describes a tetraparetic cat with type I IVDD at C2-C3 that was treated surgically with ventral slot decompression, but died in the acute postoperative period.[1] Another hemiparetic cat with MRI evidence of a disk extrusion at C3-C4 improved with conservative therapy, but the rate of improvement was slow over the ensuing 6 months, and the cat remained hemiparetic.[5] The remaining two cats with recurrent episodes of tetraparesis after conservative treatment had Hansen type II IVDD in the caudal cervical region diagnosed at necropsy.[20,21]

NEUROPATHOLOGICAL FINDINGS

Gross pathological changes that may be observed at surgery or necropsy in cases of IVDD are numerous. Overlying the site of disk extrusion or protrusion, the compressed spinal cord may appear indented, flattened, or otherwise deformed. Epidural hemorrhage or organized hematomas may be visualized in instances in which the disk extrudes into or through the venous sinus; in some cases, this epidural hemorrhage can extend several seg-

ments cranial and caudal to the lesion site. Acute spinal cord contusion from IVDD also may result in grossly visible subdural hemorrhage. In subacute to chronic cases there may be visible adhesions between disks within the vertebral canal and the dura. Nerve roots compressed by lateral or intraforaminal extruded disks may appear swollen and edematous.

Microscopic lesions that develop in the spinal cord following intervertebral disk extrusion or protrusion are characterized commonly as compressive myelopathy. Observed abnormalities in the spinal cord typically are most severe immediately overlying the site of the disk extrusion, but can extend cranially or caudally for several segments. Acute and severe concussive spinal cord injury resulting from disk extrusion can cause nonselective liquefactive necrosis of gray and white matter. The white matter of the dorsal, lateral, and ventral funiculi may appear rarified as a result of ballooning of myelin sheaths and axonal swelling or dropout. Gray matter lesions include neuronal loss with subsequent replacement of neurons with foci of microglia. Wallerian degeneration can be observed in ascending and descending tracts cranial and caudal to the site of the lesion.[33]

REFERENCES

1. Maritato KC, Colon JA, Mauterer JV: Acute nonambulatory tetraparesis attributable to cranial cervical intervertebral disc disease in a cat, *J Feline Med Surg* 9:494, 2007.
2. Smith PM, Jeffery ND: What is your diagnosis? A case of intervertebral disc protrusion in a cat, *J Small Anim Pract* 47:104, 2006.

3. Marioni-Henry K, Vite CH, Newton AL, et al: Prevalence of diseases of the spinal cord of cats, *J Vet Intern Med* 18:851, 2004.

4. Rayward R: Feline intervertebral disc disease: a review of the literature, *Vet Comp Ortho Trauma* 15:137, 2002.

5. Lu D, Lamb CR, Wesselingh K, et al: Acute intervertebral disc extrusion in a cat: clinical and MRI findings, *J Feline Med Surg* 4:65, 2002.

6. Knipe MF, Vernau KM, Hornof WJ, et al: Intervertebral disc extrusion in six cats, *J Feline Med Surg* 3:161, 2001.

7. Munana KR, Olby NJ, Sharp NJ, et al: Intervertebral disk disease in 10 cats, *J Am Anim Hosp Assoc* 37:384, 2001.

8. Kathmann I, Cizinauskas S, Rytz U, et al: Spontaneous lumbar intervertebral disc protrusion in cats: literature review and case presentations, *J Feline Med Surg* 2:207, 2000.

9. Harris JE, Dhupa S: Lumbosacral intervertebral disk disease in six cats, *J Am Anim Hosp Assoc* 44:109, 2008.

10. Kolmstetter C, Munson L, Ramsay EC: Degenerative spinal disease in large felids, *J Zoo Wildl Med* 31:15, 2000.

11. Bray JP, Burbidge HM: The canine intervertebral disk part one: structure and function, *J Am Anim Hosp Assoc* 34:55, 1998.

12. Hansen HJ: A pathologic-anatomical study on disc degeneration in dogs, *Acta Orthop Scand Suppl* 11:1, 1952.

13. Butler WF: Comparative anatomy and development of the mammalian disc. In Ghosh P, editor: *The biology of the intervertebral disc*, Boca Raton, 1988, CRC Press, p 83.

14. King AS, Smith RN: Degeneration of the intervertebral disc in the cat, *Acta Orthop Scand* 34:139, 1964.

15. King AS, Smith RN: Disc protrusions in the cat: age incidence of dorsal protrusions, *Vet Rec* 72:381, 1960.

16. King AS, Smith RN: Disc protrusions in the cat: ventral protrusions and radial splits, *Res Vet Sci* 1:301, 1960.

17. King AS, Smith RN: Disc protrusions in the cat: distribution of dorsal protrusions along the vertebral column, *Vet Rec* 72:335, 1960.

18. Butler WF: Histological age changes in the ruptured intervertebral disc of the cat, *Res Vet Sci* 9:130, 1968.

19. King AS, Smith RN: Protrusion of the intervertebral disc in the cat, *Vet Rec* 70:509, 1958.

20. Heavner JE: Intervertebral disc syndrome in the cat, *J Am Med Vet Assoc* 159:425, 1971.

21. Littlewood, JD, Herrtage ME, Palmer AC: Intervertebral disc protrusion in a cat, *J Small Anim Pract* 25:119, 1984.

22. Olby N: Current concepts in the management of acute spinal cord injury, *J Vet Intern Med* 13:399, 1999.

23. Griffiths IR: Spinal disease in the dog, *In Pract* 4:44, 1982.

24. Rossmeisl JH, Lanz OI, Inzana KD, et al: A modified lateral approach to the canine cervical spine: procedural description and clinical application in 16 dogs with lateralized compressive myelopathy or radiculopathy, *Vet Surg* 34:436, 2005.

25. Bagley RS, Tucker RL, Moore MP, et al: Radiographic diagnosis: intervertebral disc extrusion in a cat, *Vet Radiol Ultrasound* 36:380, 1995.

26. Salisbury SK, Cool JR: Recovery of neurological function following focal myelomalacia in a cat, *J Am Anim Hosp Assoc* 24:227, 1988.

27. Jaegar GH, Early PJ, Munana KR, et al: Lumbosacral disc disease in a cat, *Vet Comp Orthop Traumatol* 17:104, 2004.

28. Seim HB, Nafe LA: Spontaneous intervertebral disk extrusion with associated myelopathy in a cat, *J Am Anim Hosp Assoc* 17:201, 1981.

29. Sparkes AH, Skerry TM: Successful management of a prolapsed intervertebral disc in Siamese cat, *Fel Pract* 18:7, 1990.

30. Gilmore DR: Extrusion of a feline intervertebral disk, *Vet Med Small Anim Clin* 78:207, 1983.

31. Wheeler SJ, Clayton Jones DG, Wright JA: Myelography in the cat, *J Small Anim Pract* 30:685, 1985.

32. McConnell JF, Garosi LS: Intramedullary intervertebral disk extrusion in a cat, *Vet Radiol Ultrasound* 45:327, 2004.

33. Griffiths IR: Some aspects of the pathology and pathogenesis of the myelopathy caused by disc protrusion in the dog, *J Neurol Neurosurg Psychiatry* 35:403, 1972.

54 Novel Anticonvulsant Therapies

Kerry Smith Bailey and Curtis W. Dewey

A seizure is the clinical manifestation of hypersynchronous abnormal neuronal activity originating in the cerebral cortex. Seizure disorders are a well recognized neurological problem in cats.[1-5] Much of what is known regarding the etiology and diagnosis of feline seizure disorders can be extrapolated from dogs; however, caution should be taken when comparing treatment options between the two species.

There are various classification schemes for seizure disorders and types. One scheme classifies seizure disorders as primary and secondary. Seizure types can be classified as focal or generalized.[1,5] Focal seizures originate from a discrete epileptogenic focus within the cerebral cortex. Clinical features of focal seizures in cats are variable, including drooling, facial movements, hippus, excessive vocalization/growling, random skittish behavior, and abnormal head, neck, or limb movements.[1,6] Focal seizures can progress into generalized seizures, although they occur more commonly as isolated episodes. Generalized seizures originate from both cerebral hemispheres and usually manifest as tonic-clonic movements. These may be particularly violent in cats, and often are accompanied by salivation, urination, defecation, and pupillary dilation.[6]

Primary seizure disorders are those conditions that have no underlying cause. Cats who are determined to have a primary seizure disorder are diagnosed as idiopathic epileptics. Typically these seizures are generalized; however, focal seizures also may be a feature of idiopathic epilepsy. Historically, focal seizures have been associated with structural lesions of the forebrain; however, in the authors' experiences the presence of focal seizures does not exclude a diagnosis of idiopathic epilepsy. Secondary seizure disorders are classified as conditions in which an underlying structural lesion, such as neoplasia, trauma, hydrocephalus, infection, ischemia, or metabolic disease has been identified (Figure 54-1). Differentiating between the two classification schemes of seizure disorders is critical for determining a prognosis, as well as for devising an appropriate treatment plan. In both situations, anticonvulsants are needed to treat the seizure activity; additional therapies may be necessary for treating secondary seizure disorders.

PRINCIPLES OF ANTICONVULSANT THERAPY

Initial seizures are associated with either a single or a limited number of epileptic foci within the cerebral hemisphere. The number of cells with the ability to fire spontaneously (a focus of pacemaker cells) increases with progressive seizure activity. A similar focus also may develop in the same location in the opposite hemisphere with continuous or recurrent seizure activity causing the number of foci to multiply rapidly. Therefore an increase in the number or severity of seizures is accompanied by an increase in neurons that fire spontaneously and propagate seizure activity.[7] The severity of seizures in cats is not a good prognostic indicator; this is in contrast to response to therapy.[3] Aggressive, safe, and effective anticonvulsant therapy is critical for achieving a therapeutic response.

The major inhibitory neurotransmitter in the brain is gamma-aminobutyric acid (GABA) and the major excitatory neurotransmitter is glutamate. Imbalance between these neurotransmitters can lead to seizure activity. Additionally, within an epileptic focus there are periods of

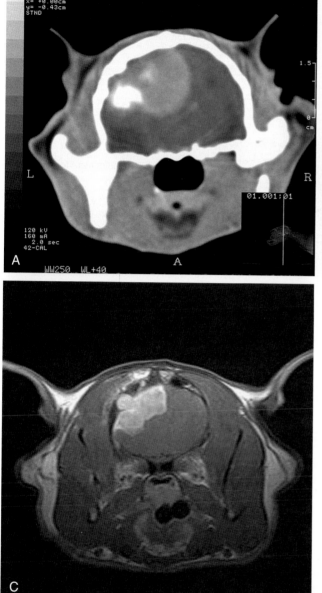

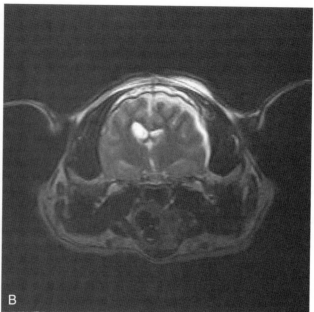

Figure 54-1 A, Computed tomography postcontrast transverse image at the level of the thalamus. There is a large extraaxial contrast-enhancing mass in the right temporal lobe; a portion of the mass is calcified. The mass was removed and diagnosed as a meningioma. **B,** T2-weighted transverse image at the level of the interthalamic adhesion causing a midline shift and edema in the left cerebral hemisphere. A hyperintensity also is present on the periphery of the left cerebral hemisphere. This cat was diagnosed with intracranial empyema at surgery, the result of a dog bite wound of the cranium. **C,** A postcontrast transverse T1-weighted image of the brain. There is a large extraaxial contrast-enhancing mass in the right parietal lobe that was removed surgically and diagnosed as a meningioma.

exaggerated depolarization known as a paroxysmal depolarization shift (PDS).[7] The PDS originates in the dendritic zone of the neuron. Both influx of calcium through voltage-gated calcium channels and influx of sodium through non-NMDA and NMDA receptor channels are theorized to give rise to the PDS. Channelopathies or mutations within the ion channels can be responsible for the generation of seizures. Following brain and/or neuronal injury, changes occur in the inherent excitability of glutaminergic neurons. These voltage-gated calcium channels become abnormally sensitive, and there is morphological and functional loss of the inhibitory neurons and synapses such as GABA.

Knowledge of the pathogenesis of seizures allows for a better understanding of the general mechanism of action

of anticonvulsants. Anticonvulsant drugs often are characterized based on their anticonvulsant activity against single seizures induced by maximal electrical or chemical stimulation in experimental animal models that use a maximal electroshock seizure and the pentylenetetrazol seizure tests. Most conventional antiepileptic drugs have anticonvulsant activity in at least one of these two models.[8] Three standard mechanisms currently accepted for most of the established anticonvulsant drugs include conventional GABA facilitation, inhibition of sodium channels, or modulation of low-voltage-activated calcium currents.[9]

Pharmacokinetic properties must be considered for an ideal anticonvulsant drug. The drug should have rapid intestinal absorption after oral administration, good bioavailability, and should achieve a steady state within a reasonable period of time. In addition, the drug should have linear kinetics that produce predictable drug concentrations with minimal to no protein binding and limited drug-to-drug interactions. Last, the ideal anticonvulsant would have minimal to no hepatic metabolism, especially in patients with hepatopathy.[10]

INDICATIONS FOR ANTICONVULSANT THERAPY

Maintenance anticonvulsant therapy is recommended when a cat presents with more than one seizure (either generalized or focal) within a 6-month time period, when a cat has more than one cluster event (a cluster is defined as more than one seizure in a 24-hour time period), or when a seizure presents in status (continuous seizure activity that lasts more than 5 minutes or the presence of multiple seizures without returning to normal in between the seizures). Anticonvulsant therapy also may be recommended with seizures occurring after a traumatic brain injury. Seizure caused by structural forebrain disease (neoplasia, inflammation, anomaly) also is an indication for treatment with anticonvulsants.

ASSESSMENT OF THERAPY

Successful seizure control begins with thorough client education. First and foremost, the client needs to understand that anticonvulsant therapy potentially is a lifelong commitment. Although seizure elimination is a goal, a more realistic goal is to decrease the frequency and severity of seizures. Approximately 30 per cent of dogs will become seizure free; however, such data are not available for cats. Each cat responds differently to anticonvulsants and therapy should be tailored to the individual feline patient. Initially, therapy is considered trial and error until the correct drug and dose combination is attained. The expense of therapy should take into account not only the cost of drugs, but also office visits, monitoring of drug levels and laboratory evaluations, and the unexpected cost of potential emergency therapy/hospitalization for breakthrough seizures. Clients should be made aware of any reported drug side effects and should be encouraged to be cognizant of their cat's health, appetite, and behavior. Clients need to be assured that their cat's quality of life is paramount, and that effective drug therapy balances potential drug side effects with therapeutic success.

All clients should be encouraged to maintain a seizure log (Figure 54-2), detailing the number of seizures as well as unique features of the seizure (i.e., length of ictal and postictal periods, seizure type, events that may affect the environment). The log is reviewed during recheck visits. Physical and neurological examinations, monitoring of anticonvulsant drug concentrations, and laboratory evaluation should be performed about every 6 months, and may be more frequent in the initial stages of therapy.

Defining successful response to an anticonvulsant drug is based on the individual cat. Therapeutic effective-

---

Kitty's Seizure Log

January 1:   Had family over for the New Year

January 18: 1 generalized seizure (30 seconds; ate immediately after)

January 19: 2 short seizures (face twitched; ears back, growling, responded to her name being called)

January 19: Went to Dr. Smith – phenobarbital level checked – 21

February: No seizures!

March 29:   1 generalized seizure (1 minute; slept for 2 hours after)

April 11:   Recheck with Dr. Smith – bloodwork and urine test performed (CBC, Chemistry – all OK; Phenobarbital level checked – 23)

             No seizures in April!

May 1:   1 generalized seizure (about 1 minute; normal immediately after)

May 2:   1 generalized seizure (1-2 minutes, took about 2 hours to get back to normal, seemed blind)

May 3:   3 short facial twitching seizures; growling and drooling

May 5:   2 generalized seizures (7:30 am – 30 seconds; ate after; 11 am – 1 minute – took to Dr. Smith)

May 6:   Levetiracetam added to phenobarbital

Figure 54-2 Example of a seizure log, indicating the number of seizures, distinguishing characteristics, any change in the normal routine of the cat, and any changes in medication administered.

---

ness of an anticonvulsant drug is considered when there is a reduction of number of seizures by 50 per cent or more. For example, a cat who had a seizure six times each month prior to therapy, and three times or less each month after therapy is considered to have had a favorable response to medication. When therapy is not effective, the treatment plan is reevaluated (Figure 54-3). Treatment failures are the result of progressive disease, refractory seizures, poor client compliance, inadequate drug dosing, and drug side effects and interactions. The first step in investigating reasons for treatment failure is to confirm the dose of the drug that is being administered. The drug dosage is reassessed and the treatment schedule is verified. The physical and neurological examinations are performed to ascertain underlying disease. If not already performed, diagnostic procedures are discussed with the client. Changes in anticonvulsant drug dosing are based on drug concentration within the therapeutic target range and associated side effects. If the drug concentration is low in the target range and side effects are minimal, increasing the dosage is a viable option. If the drug concentration is on the higher end of the target

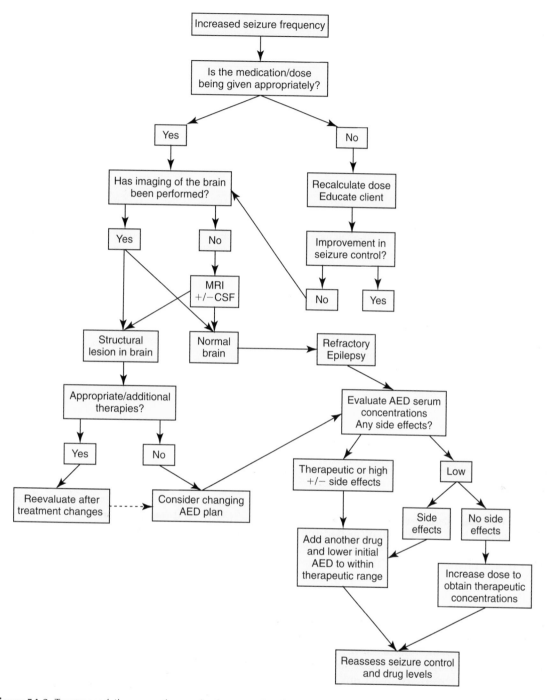

Figure 54-3 Treatment failures are the result of progressive disease, refractory seizures, poor client compliance, or inadequate drug dosing.

range or side effects are present, addition of another anticonvulsant is considered.

When cats become seizure free, clients often inquire about discontinuing medication(s). Discontinuation of an anticonvulsant drug is considered when the cat is seizure free for 6 months. "Withdrawal seizures" may occur if the anticonvulsant is stopped abruptly. This is seen more commonly with phenobarbital, owing to development of physical drug dependence.[11] Slow weaning over weeks to months is recommended. Rarely

cats will experience an idiosyncratic drug reaction or severe drug side effects, which may necessitate rapid withdrawal of the drug.

DRUG DOSING

Accurate drug dosing for some of the newer anticonvulsants is best achieved by calculating the exact dose and having the drug compounded (Table 54-1).

Table 54-1 Maintenance Anticonvulsant Therapy in Cats

Drug	Formulation	Elimination Half-Life	Dose	Therapeutic Range	Major Side Effects	Other
Phenobarbital	PO, IV	40-50 hr	2.5 mg/kg q12h	10-20 µg/mL	Sedation, polyuria, polydipsia, polyphagia, weight gain, blood dyscrasias	Silicon in blood tubes binds PB
Levetiracetam	PO, IV	2.9 hr	20 mg/kg q8h	5-45 µg/mL	None	May be useful as an emergency anticonvulsant
Zonisamide	PO	33 hr	5 mg/kg q12h, 10 mg/kg q12h (when on PB)	UD (neurotoxicity appears to occur with trough levels >46.3 µg/mL)	Anorexia, diarrhea, vomiting, somnolence, and locomotor ataxia	Side effects were noted at a 20 mg/kg/day dose. May be dosed q24h
Gabapentin	PO	UD	5-10 mg/kg/day (anecdotal information)	UD	Sedation, ataxia	Pregabalin is the next generation of gabapentin, proposed dose is 2-4 mg/kg q8-12h in dogs

PO, Per os; *IV,* intravenous; *PB,* phenobarbital; *UD,* undetermined.

TRADITIONAL ANTICONVULSANT THERAPIES

PHENOBARBITAL

Phenobarbital is the current drug of choice in cats with multiple seizure episodes.[4,12] The elimination half-life in cats is 34 to 50 hours, and when given at a dose of 2.5 mg/kg PO q12h, phenobarbital is an effective anticonvulsive drug. Side effects associated with phenobarbital use in cats are minimal and include sedation and ataxia, weight gain secondary to polyphagia, and polydipsia and polyuria. Hepatotoxicity, a complication well recognized in dogs, has not been reported in cats.[13,14] Rarely cats treated with phenobarbital have developed leukopenia and thrombocytopenia. These are considered immune-mediated hypersensitivity reactions and are reversible with removal of the drug.[12,15] Phenobarbital is available in both oral and parenteral formulations. Serum drug concentrations should be measured 2 to 3 weeks after starting the drug. Therapeutic levels are similar to those reported in dogs (25 to 40 µg/mL). The ideal therapeutic range in cats is approximately 23 to 30 µg/mL. Serum drug concentrations should be monitored every 6 months, and 2 to 3 weeks after any change in dosage.[2,5] A complete blood count, serum biochemistry profile, and serum bile acid assay are monitored every 6 months.

ORAL DIAZEPAM

Oral diazepam has a longer elimination half-life in cats (15 to 20 hours) than dogs (3 to 4 hours), and can be an effective anticonvulsant for cats.[2] Cats also will not develop tolerance to diazepam. Diazepam has been a drug of choice for treatment of feline seizures.[16] Although rare, use of diazepam in cats has been associated with a potentially fatal hepatopathy.[17,18] Cats with this idiosyncratic drug reaction display lethargy, sedation, and anorexia within the first 5 to 7 days of initiating drug therapy. Signs can progress to fulminant hepatic failure and death. Therefore use of oral diazepam should be limited, with diligent monitoring of clinical signs. Serum alanine transaminase and aspartate transaminase activity can be used to monitor for acute hepatoxicity. Still, oral diazepam is used with caution in cats. Intravenous diazepam has not been associated with hepatotoxicity and is discussed in the emergency therapy section of this chapter.

BROMIDE

Bromide initially was thought to be a safe anticonvulsant in cats because of its lack of hepatic metabolism. With its long elimination half-life (approximately 11 days) and availability of therapeutic drug monitoring, bromide was considered to be a potentially promising anticonvulsant in cats.[16] However, an allergic pneumonitis developed in 35 to 42 per cent of cats to whom bromide was administered.[19,20] The clinical signs are consistent with a life-threatening bronchial asthma and abate with the discontinuation of bromide. Moreover, seizure control was obtained in only 35 per cent of cats treated with bromide.[19]

NOVEL ANTICONVULSANT THERAPIES

LEVETIRACETAM

Levetiracetam is a novel anticonvulsant with a mechanism of action not entirely understood, but that is substantially different from that of the more conventional anticonvulsant drugs (Figure 54-4).[8,21,22] In vitro and in vivo recordings of epileptiform activity from the hippocampus have shown that levetiracetam inhibits burst firing without affecting normal neuronal excitability, suggesting that the drug may selectively prevent hypersynchronization of epileptiform burst firing and propagation of seizure activity. Levetiracetam appears to be able to retard electrical kindling, a property that persists even after the drug has been discontinued. Therefore levetiracetam may have antiepileptogenic properties and may assist in preventing the progression of epilepsy in at-risk patients.[8,21] The synaptic vesicle protein SV2A is the binding site for levetiracetam.[23] SV2A is present in high concentrations in the synaptic plasma membranes within the central nervous system. The molecular action of SV2A is unknown, but it may be involved in transporting calcium or adenosine triphosphate (ATP).[24] Levetiracetam is considered an ideal anticonvulsant drug with regard to its pharmacokinetics.[10] It is absorbed rapidly following oral administration, and has an oral bioavailability of approximately 100 per cent.[25] Peak plasma concentrations are achieved at 2 hours in the majority of cats.[26] Food does not affect the extent of absorption of levetiracetam, allowing it to be administered safely independent of feeding schedule, which eases the task of giving the drug q8h.[10,27] The majority of levetiracetam is excreted unchanged in the urine, and approximately 24 per cent is excreted in the urine as an inactive metabolite. Renal elimination occurs primarily by glomerular filtration and correlates well with creatinine clearance. Therefore the dose should be decreased accordingly in patients with impaired renal function. Levetiracetam is not significantly protein bound (<10 per cent) and therefore will not displace highly protein-bound drugs.[22]

At a dose of 20 mg/kg PO q8h, levetiracetam is a safe and effective anticonvulsant when given as an adjunct to phenobarbital in cats with suspected idiopathic epilepsy.[26] The half-life is approximately 3 hours.[25,26] Side effects are rare and may include transient inappetence and lethargy. In addition to treating suspected epileptics, the authors have used levetiracetam in two cats with intracranial meningiomas that were removed surgically, in whom seizure control was not adequate with phenobarbital alone. Both cats had a reduction in their seizures' frequency and severity and did not experience any side effects related to the levetiracetam.

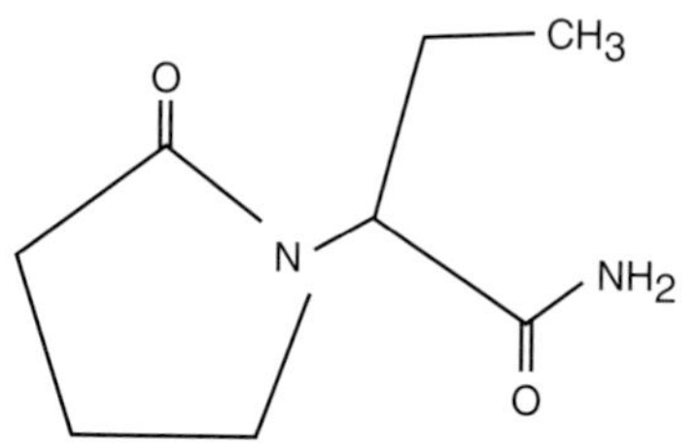

Levetiracetam also seems to be a promising sole anticonvulsant, and has been used by the authors on occasions when phenobarbital was not a viable option. Side effects were not noted in either of the cats treated solely with levetiracetam and the drug appeared to be effective in reducing the seizure frequency and severity.

Although a therapeutic range has not been determined specifically for cats, it appears to be similar to that in human beings (5 to 45 µg/mL). Monitoring is recommended approximately 1 week after starting the medication, and then every 6 to 12 months. The goal with monitoring is more to aid in adjusting the drug dose, rather than avoiding side effects, because of levetiracetam's high margin of safety. We have found that increasing the dose in 2 mg/kg increments is useful when the drug does not appear to be effective. In addition, monitoring routine laboratory tests is recommended approximately every 6 to 12 months, as in all cats treated with anticonvulsant medications.

ZONISAMIDE

Zonisamide is a sulfonamide-based anticonvulsant drug that has been used successfully in dogs as an add-on anticonvulsant.[28,29] Suspected mechanisms of action include blockage of T-type calcium- and voltage-gated sodium channels in the brain, facilitation of dopaminergic and serotonergic neurotransmission in the central nervous system, scavenging free radical species, enhancing GABA in the brain, inhibition of glutamate-mediated neuronal excitation in the brain, and inhibition of carbonic anhydrase activity.[12] Zonisamide is metabolized by hepatic microsomal enzymes, and the half-life of zonisamide is significantly shorter in patients receiving phenobarbital or other drugs that increase the hepatic microsomal enzyme, p450.[30] The half-life of zonisamide in cats is 33 hours.[31] The dose for dogs not receiving phenobarbital is 5 mg/kg PO q12h, and 10 mg/kg PO q12h in dogs receiving phenobarbital; however, this dosing scheme has not been confirmed for cats. Approximately one half of cats receiving the higher dose of zonisamide experience adverse reactions such as anorexia, diarrhea, vomiting, somnolence, and ataxia.[31] The authors have used zonisamide in two cats who experienced seizures refractory to phenobarbital; one cat had severe side effects necessitating the removal of the drug and the other patient responded very well and had a dramatic reduction in seizure frequency. Additional studies are indicated to determine the efficacy of zonisamide as an anticonvulsant. However, because of the high likelihood of side effects, zonisamide does not appear to be an ideal add-on anticonvulsant in cats at this time. The use of zonisamide may be more successful as a sole drug in situations when the lower dose can be utilized, or possibly as a q24h dosing regimen based on its long elimination half-life of 33 hours.

Figure 54-4 Chemical structure of levetiracetam.

GABAPENTIN AND PREGABALIN

Pregabalin is a new anticonvulsant drug considered to be the "next generation" of gabapentin. Its mechanism of action appears to be related to interaction with the a2d subunit of neuronal voltage-gated calcium channels. Reducing calcium influx leads to reduction of the synaptic release of glutamate, an excitatory neurotransmitter. In dogs treated with 4 mg/kg PO q8-12h, pregabalin has a half-life of 6.8 hours; this dose appeared well-tolerated.[32] The major side effect noted in dogs is sedation and the dose must be increased gradually from 2 mg/kg PO to 4 mg/kg PO q8-12h as needed for effectiveness.[33]

Although information is not available regarding the use of pregabalin in cats, it will likely prove to be an effective anticonvulsant for this species. The authors recently used this drug in a cat who experienced seizures refractory to phenobarbital and levetiracetam. It is too soon to determine the efficacy of this drug in this particular patient. Its predecessor, gabapentin, has been used with limited success in cats; anecdotally, the dose is 5 to 10 mg/kg PO q12h. Sedation is the most common side effect noted with gabapentin therapy, and is likely a side effect associated with pregabalin in cats as well. The half-life and therapeutic range for both gabapentin and pregabalin are unknown in cats.

EMERGENCY ANTICONVULSANT THERAPY

Status epilepticus has been associated with a significantly shorter mean survival time in dogs and therefore it is important to recognize and treat this condition quickly.[34] Status epilepticus is considered a medical emergency. Continued seizures can lead to hyperthermia, hypoxia, hypotension, renal failure, disseminated intravascular coagulation, aspiration pneumonia, and cardiopulmonary failure.

TRADITIONAL EMERGENCY THERAPY

Intravenous diazepam (0.5 to 1 mg/kg) is considered first-line emergency therapy because of its safety and rapid onset of action. If bolus administration is unsuccessful in ceasing seizures, additional boluses or a continuous rate infusion (CRI) may be administered. Suggested CRI rates are 0.5 to 2 mg/kg/hr IV. If the cat remains seizure free for 12 to 24 hours, diazepam CRI should be tapered and discontinued, while monitoring carefully for additional seizure activity.

If diazepam is unsuccessful in ceasing seizures, other traditional options include pentobarbital, phenobarbital, and propofol. Pentobarbital is a barbiturate that is useful in treating intractable seizures at a dose of 2 to 15 mg/kg IV to effect.[12,35] It is not an anticonvulsant drug, but ceases the motor activity that is associated with seizure activity. A complicating factor when using pentobarbital is that animals tend to paddle when recovering, which can be confused easily with seizure activity. Pentobarbital can cause severe respiratory depression and hypothermia.

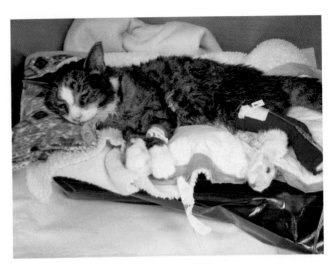

Figure 54-5 Intubation often is necessary with use of propofol CRI. This cat is lying on an air mattress with head elevated—all part of diligent nursing care associated with a patient in status epilepticus.

Phenobarbital is another viable emergency drug to treat status epilepticus. A recommended bolus dose is 2 to 6 mg/kg IV to effect. The effect is not immediate and can take 15 to 25 minutes, so potential exists for overdosing. Using phenobarbital as an emergency drug is useful when it is also used as the maintenance drug. Phenobarbital also can be administered as a CRI at a rate of 2 to 4 mg/kg/hr IV.

Propofol is an injectable anesthetic agent that has been shown to have GABA agonist activity in the central nervous system, and lowers intracranial pressure and overall metabolic activity in the brain.[12] The drug is administered as a slow IV bolus (1 to 6 mg/kg) to prevent respiratory apnea.[36] Intubation may be necessary should this occur (Figure 54-5). Propofol can be administered as a CRI at a rate of 0.1 to 0.6 mg/kg/min IV.

NOVEL THERAPY

Drugs used for treatment of status epilepsy can cause varying degrees of sedation. This side effect may be undesirable in cases of postoperative craniotomy procedures, making a patient prone to aspiration pneumonia. In these situations, intravenous levetiracetam is a viable option. An injectable formulation has been developed for use in human beings with partial-onset (focal) seizures and is well-tolerated by people, dogs, and cats. Pharmacokinetic properties for intravenous use are similar to those for oral administration.[25,37] Side effects have not been noted in dogs and cats, although human patients report dizziness, somnolence, fatigue, and headaches.[38] The authors have bolus-administered levetiracetam 20 mg/kg IV in cats with success in ceasing seizure activity. The anticonvulsant effect is rapid and is maintained for several hours, longer than a single intravenous dose of diazepam. Sedation effects are minimal and cats appear to recover from the seizure episode more rapidly than with diazepam administration.

REFERENCES

1. Barnes HL, Chrisman CL, Mariani CL, et al: Clinical signs, underlying cause and outcome in cats with seizures: 17 cases (1997-2002), *J Am Vet Med Assoc* 225:1723, 2004.
2. Platt SR: Feline seizure control, *J Am Anim Hosp Assoc* 37:515, 2001.
3. Quesnel AD, Parent JM, McDonell W: Clinical management and outcome of cats with seizure disorders: 30 cases (1991-1993), *J Am Vet Med Assoc* 210:72, 1997.
4. Thomas WB, Dewey CW: Seizures and narcolepsy. In Dewey CW, editor: *A practical guide to canine and feline neurology*, ed 2, Ames, IA, 2008, Wiley-Blackwell, p 193.
5. Shell LG: Seizures in cats, *Vet Med* 93:541, 1998.
6. Quesnel AD, Parent JM, McDonell W: Diagnostic evaluation of cats with seizure disorders: 30 cases (1991-1993), *J Am Vet Med Assoc* 210:65, 1997.
7. March PA: Seizures: classification, etiologies, and pathophysiology, *Clin Tech Small Anim Pract* 13:119, 1998.
8. Klitgaard H, Matagne A, Gobert J, et al: Evidence for a unique profile of levetiracetam in rodent models of seizures and epilepsy, *Eur K Pharmacol* 353:191, 1998.
9. Lukyanetz EA, Shkryl VM, Kostyuk PG: Selective blockade of N-type calcium channels by levetiracetam, *Epilepsia* 43:9, 2002.
10. Patsalos PN: Pharmacokinetic profile of levetiracetam: toward ideal characteristics, *Pharmacol Ther* 85:77, 2000.
11. Podell M: Seizures. In Platt SR, Olby NJ, editors: *BSAVA manual of canine and feline neurology*, Gloucester, 2004, British Small Animal Veterinary Association, p 97.
12. Dewey CW: Anticonvulsant therapy in dogs and cats, *Vet Clin North Am Small Anim Pract* 36:1107, 2006.
13. Dayrell-Hart B, Steinberg SA, VanWinkle RJ, et al: Hepatotoxicity of phenobarbital in dogs:18 cases (1985-1989), *J Am Vet Med Assoc* 199:1060, 1991.
14. Gaskill CL, Miller LM, Mattoon JS, et al: Liver histopathology and liver and serum alanine aminotransferase and alkaline phosphatase activities in epileptic dogs receiving phenobarbital, *Vet Pathol* 42:147, 2005.
15. Ducote JM, Coates JR, Dewey CW, et al: Suspected hypersensitivity to phenobarbital in a cat, *J Feline Med Surg* 1:123, 1999.
16. Boothe DM: Anticonvulsant therapy in small animals, *Vet Clin North Am Small Anim Pract* 28:411, 1998.
17. Center SA, Elston TH, Rowland PH, et al: Fulminant hepatic failure associated with oral administration of diazepam in 11 cats, *J Am Vet Med Assoc* 209:618, 1996.
18. Hughes D, Moreau RE, Overall KL, et al: Acute hepatic necrosis and liver failure associated with benzodiazepine therapy in six cats, *J Vet Emerg Crit Care* 6:13, 1996.
19. Boothe DM, George KL, Couch P: Disposition and clinical use of bromide in cats, *J Am Vet Med Assoc* 221:1131, 2002.
20. Wagner SO: Lower airway disease in cats on bromide therapy for seizures, *J Vet Intern Med* 15:562, 2001.
21. Hovinga CA: Levetiracetam: a novel antiepileptic drug, *Pharmacotherapy* 21:1375, 2001.
22. Leppik IE: The place of levetiracetam in the treatment of epilepsy, *Epilepsia* 42:44, 2001.
23. Lynch BA, Lambeng N, Nocka K, et al: The synaptic vesicle protein SV2A is the binding site for the antiepileptic drug levetiracetam, *Proc Natl Acad Sci U S A* 101:9861, 2004.
24. Gillard M, Chatelain P, Fuks B: Binding characteristics of levetiracetam to synaptic vesicle protein 2A (SV2A) in human brain and in CHO cells expressing the human recombinant protein, *Eur J Pharmacol* 536:102, 2006.
25. Carnes MB, Boothe DM, Axlund TW: Disposition of levetiracetam in cats, *J Vet Intern Med* 22:765, 2008.
26. Bailey KS, Dewey CW, Boothe DM, et al: Levetiracetam as an adjunct to phenobarbital treatment in cats with suspected idiopathic epilepsy, *J Am Vet Med Assoc* 232:867, 2008.
27. Shorvon SD, van Rijckevorsel K: A new antiepileptic [editorial], *J Neurol Neurosurg Psychiatry* 72:426, 2002.
28. Dewey CW, Guiliano R, Boothe DM, et al: Zonisamide therapy for refractory idiopathic epilepsy in dogs, *J Am Anim Hosp Assoc* 40:285, 2004.
29. von Klopmann T, Rambeck B, Tipold A: Prospective study of zonisamide therapy for refractory idiopathic epilepsy in dogs, *J Small Anim Pract* 48:134, 2007.
30. Orito K, Saito M, Fukunaga K, et al: Pharmacokinetics of zonisamide and drug interaction with phenobarbital in dogs, *J Vet Pharmacol Ther* 31:259, 2008.
31. Hasegawa D, Kobayashi M, Kuwabara T, et al: Pharmacokinetics and toxicity of zonisamide in cats, *J Feline Med Surg* 10:418, 2008.
32. Salazar V, Dewey CW, Schwark WS, et al: Pharmacokinetics of single-dose oral pregabalin administration in dogs, *J Vet Intern Med* 22:765, 2008.
33. Dewey CW, Cerda-Gonzalez S, Levine JM, et al: Pregabalin therapy for refractory idiopathic epilepsy in dogs, *J Vet Intern Med* 22:765, 2008.
34. Saito M, Munana KR, Sharp NJ, et al: Risk factors for development of status epilepticus in dogs with idiopathic epilepsy and effects of status epilepticus on outcome and survival time: 32 cases (1990-1996), *J Am Vet Med Assoc* 219:618, 2001.
35. Platt SR, McDonnell JJ: Status epilepticus: patient management and pharmacologic therapy, *Compend Contin Educ Pract Vet* 22:722, 2000.
36. Steffen F, Grasmueck S: Propofol for treatment of refractory seizures in dogs and a cat with intracranial disorders, *J Small Anim Pract* 41:496, 2000.
37. Dewey CW, Bailey KS, Boothe DM, et al: Pharmacokinetics of single-dose intravenous levetiracetam administration in normal dogs, *J Vet Emerg Crit Care* 18:153, 2008.
38. Ramael S, Daoust A, Otoul C, et al: Levetiracetam intravenous infusion: a randomized, placebo-controlled safety and pharmacokinetic study, *Epilepsia* 47:1128, 2006.

55 Brain Tumors: Clinical Spectrum

Mark T. Troxel

With the advent of advanced imaging such as magnetic resonance imaging (MRI) and computed tomography (CT), along with increasing availability of these diagnostic tools in veterinary hospitals, intracranial lesions are being diagnosed more than ever. As a result veterinary practitioners are better able to diagnose brain tumors, to provide definitive treatment for the patient, and to better estimate the prognosis. This chapter discusses the diagnosis and treatment of feline brain tumors and provides details regarding individual tumor types.

INCIDENCE AND ETIOLOGY

The true incidence of feline brain tumors is unknown. Estimates from several studies suggest that feline brain tumors are relatively uncommon, ranging from 3.5 per 100,000 cases (0.0035 per cent) to as high as 4.6 per cent.[1-3] However, data from these studies must be interpreted cautiously because they are derived from analyses of necropsy records, and may not reflect the true incidence in the population at large.

The etiology currently is unknown for most tumor types. With the exception of increased incidence of meningioma in young cats with mucopolysaccharidosis I,[4] there are no studies in veterinary medicine that correlate genetic or environmental risk factors with intracranial neoplasia (see Chapter 56).

In fact, there have been few large-scale studies regarding feline brain tumors published in the veterinary literature. Most reports have been small retrospective case series on meningiomas, and occasional case reports detailing diagnostic and treatment strategies for other tumor types. Many of these reports describe histopathological findings with little information concerning clinical data.

A recent retrospective study analyzed the frequency of different tumor types in a large cohort of cats with intracranial tumors.[5] The medical records of 160 cats with an intracranial neoplasm identified at necropsy were analyzed (Table 55-1). The neoplasm was considered a primary brain tumor in 70 per cent of the cats, and classified as a secondary brain tumor in the remaining 30 per cent. As with other studies,[1,3,6-12] meningioma was the most common tumor type identified, occurring in 58 per cent of the cats. The most common secondary tumors were lymphoma (16 per cent) and pituitary tumors (9.3 per cent). Metastatic brain tumors were identified in only nine of the 160 cats (5.6 per cent), whereas only six cats (3.8 per cent) had direct extension of a tumor into the brain.[5] Compared with other tumor types, multiple meningiomas are fairly common in cats.[3,10] Two or more discrete intracranial tumors of the same type (primarily meningiomas) were found in 16 of the cats (10 per cent). Another 16 cats (10 per cent) had two different histological types of intracranial tumors.[5]

Tumor location appears to be predictive of tumor type.[5] In addition to expected relationships (e.g., meningioma in the meninges, pituitary tumor in the pituitary gland), third ventricular tumors are most likely to be meningiomas. Lymphoma was identified in all cats with either diffuse cerebral or diffuse brainstem involvement.

Table 55-1 Top 10 Brain Tumors Identified in 228 Cats with 244 Brain Tumors*

Tumor Type	Number	Frequency (%)
PRIMARY BRAIN TUMORS		
Astrocytoma	7	2.8
Ependymoma	7	2.8
Meningioma	144	59.0
Olfactory neuroblastoma	2	0.8
Oligodendroglioma	6	2.4
SECONDARY BRAIN TUMORS		
Hemangiosarcoma	2	0.8
Lymphoma	39	16.0
Nasal (adeno) carcinoma	3	1.2
Pituitary	22	9.0
Pulmonary adenocarcinoma	3	1.2

*Adapted from Troxel MT, Vite CH, Van Winkle TJ, et al: Feline intracranial neoplasia: retrospective review of 160 cases (1985-2001), *J Vet Intern Med* 17:850, 2003.

SIGNALMENT

Brain tumors have been reported in all ages and breeds of cats.[5] Although there is a wide variation in age at presentation, most affected cats are older than 10 years of age.[1,5-7,13-16] Male cats are affected more often by meningioma or pituitary tumor than female cats; however, a statistically significant difference has not been detected. No gender bias has been identified for other brain tumors.

CLINICAL SIGNS

Clinical signs of brain tumors are caused by primary or secondary effects of the lesion. Primary effects include direct compression of surrounding brain parenchyma or invasion into adjacent brain tissue. Secondary effects include edema, obstructive hydrocephalus, and hemorrhage.[7,8]

The duration of clinical signs is variable.[7,13,14,16,17] Many cats are brought to a veterinarian for examination following an insidious onset of clinical signs with a chronic, progressive course, but an acute onset of clinical signs is possible. One study reported that an acute onset of clinical signs occurred in 15 per cent of affected cats,[14] whereas another reported an overall median duration of clinical signs of only 21 days.[5] A wide variety of clinical signs have been reported by owners, but the abnormalities reported most commonly include behavior changes, locomotor deficits (e.g., circling, pacing), and ataxia.[5,7,13-15,17]

Seizures reportedly are uncommon in cats with brain tumors compared with dogs.[15] Two recent studies, however, found that seizures are among the most commonly recognized abnormalities noted by owners prior to presentation, with a frequency of 14 to 22.5 per cent.[5,18]

In one of these studies one third of the cats with a forebrain (cerebrum, thalamus) tumor had experienced seizures.[18] Seizures were the first clinical sign observed by owners in 64 per cent of all cats with a brain tumor who had experienced seizures.[18] It also was thought previously that cats with a structural brain lesion were more likely to have partial or complex partial seizures, whereas cats with metabolic or toxic diseases were more likely to have generalized seizures.[19] A retrospective study of 61 cats with intracranial tumors found that 14 cats (23 per cent) had experienced seizure activity at the time of presentation. Ten of these 14 cats (71 per cent) had either generalized seizures only or both generalized and partial seizure activity. An additional cat experienced partial seizures with secondary generalization. Only three of the 14 cats (21.4 per cent) experienced partial seizures alone.[18] These findings suggest that cats with brain tumors commonly experience generalized seizures.

Cats with nonspecific clinical signs are fairly common.[1,5] One study found that 21 per cent of cats had no specific neurological signs at the time of presentation.[5] The most commonly reported nonspecific signs are lethargy (20 per cent) and inappetence or anorexia (18 per cent).[1,5]

DIAGNOSIS

The following section describes common methods used to diagnose intracranial tumors, as well as brief descriptions of some techniques that are less sensitive and specific or are not utilized routinely. Histopathological examination remains the gold standard for diagnosis.[7,8]

NEUROLOGICAL EXAMINATION

A thorough and systematic neurological examination, as well as a complete general physical examination, should be performed on all cats who present with clinical signs referable to the nervous system. A description of the neurological examination can be found elsewhere.[20] (See Chapter 49 in the fifth volume of this series for a discussion of the neurological examination of cats.) Goals of the neurological examination are twofold: (1) to determine whether the patient likely has neurological disease, and (2) to determine the likely location of disease. The clinical signs displayed by the cat and the results of the neurological examination reflect lesion location, rather than specific etiology (Table 55-2). Based on the patient's signalment, history, and neurological examination findings, the practitioner then can formulate a differential diagnosis list and diagnostic plan.

MINIMUM DATABASE

The minimum database for diagnosis of neurological disease in cats includes a complete blood count, serum biochemical analyses, urinalysis, serum total T_4, feline leukemia virus (FeLV) and feline immunodeficiency virus (FIV) testing, thoracic radiographs, and systolic blood pressures.[6-9,15] These tests rarely provide a definitive

Table 55-2 Clinical Signs Commonly Observed in Cats Based on Lesion Location

Lesion Location	Possible Clinical Signs
Cerebrum, thalamus	Seizure, behavior change, altered mental status, circling, pacing, head pressing, head turn, contralateral postural reaction deficits, blindness
Brainstem	Altered mental status, circling, head tilt, nystagmus, ataxia, hemiparesis or tetraparesis, postural reaction deficits (contralateral most common, ipsilateral if rostral midbrain), dysphagia, cranial nerve deficits (III-XII possible), irregular respiration
Cerebellum	Cerebellar ataxia, truncal ataxia, hypermetria, intention tremors, broad-based stance, ipsilateral menace response deficit with normal vision and palpebral reflex, opisthotonus, vestibular signs

diagnosis for intracranial neoplasia. However, these tests help to exclude systemic or metabolic diseases that lead to secondary neurological signs. In addition, they are important preanesthetic screening tools, because many of the diagnostic methods used to diagnose brain tumors and other central nervous system (CNS) disorders require general anesthesia. Unlike cats with spinal lymphoma, cats with brain tumors, including lymphoma, have a low incidence of FeLV infection. In a recent retrospective study, less than 4 per cent of 160 cats with brain tumors tested positive for either FeLV or FIV.[5] Abdominal radiographs or ultrasound should be performed if there are clinical signs or physical examination findings referable to the abdominal cavity.

ADVANCED IMAGING

Magnetic Resonance Imaging

The physics of MRI has been described in numerous publications and details can be found elsewhere.[21] Briefly, MRI involves placing a patient in a scanner that has a large magnet. The protons (hydrogen nuclei) that are found in water molecules in the body align themselves with the magnetic field. Another electromagnetic field oscillates at specific radiofrequencies perpendicular to the main magnetic field, which pushes some of the protons out of alignment with the main magnetic field. As these protons return to their normal alignment with the main magnetic field, they emit a radiofrequency signal that is detected by a receiver. Protons in different tissue types throughout the body realign at different speeds. A computer analyzes these differences, and images are created based on the location and speed of realignment.[21]

Several MRI pulse sequences are performed routinely that take advantage of natural physical characteristics of tissues to highlight different features. The most common sequences utilized are T2-weighted images (T2WI), pre-

contrast and postcontrast T1-weighted images (T1WI), and fluid-attenuated inversion recovery (FLAIR) images. Fluid is hyperintense (bright) on T2WI; therefore cerebrospinal fluid (CSF) in the ventricular system is white. This pulse sequence is excellent for detection of pathology, because many CNS diseases will lead to increased fluid in the brain, either via intracellular fluid from cells (e.g., inflammatory or neoplastic cells) or from edema. The delineation between gray and white matter is clearly identifiable on T2WI. Fluid is hypointense (dark) on T1WI, so CSF in the ventricular system is black. Precontrast T1WI studies are performed to evaluate the brain for normal anatomical structures and to compare with T1WI images obtained after administration of contrast agent (gadolinium), which appears as a hyperintense (white) signal on postcontrast T1WI. Contrast enhancement indicates breakdown in the blood-brain barrier (BBB). Possible causes include neoplasia, inflammatory disease, infection, vasculitis, and hemorrhage. Several areas within the brain contrast enhance routinely because of high vascularity and/or lack of BBB. These include the meninges (mild), pituitary gland, choroid plexus, and pineal gland. The FLAIR sequence is used primarily for detection of pathology in periventricular regions and near the surface of the brain. FLAIR images are T2WI in which the signal for "pure" fluids (e.g., CSF) is suppressed. As a result CSF is black on FLAIR image, whereas impure fluids such as cerebral edema remain hyperintense and are detected more easily in the periventricular and subarachnoid regions where they can be overlooked on T2WI.

MRI is the imaging modality of choice for detection of CNS lesions in human patients. The sensitivity for detection of brain tumors has been shown to be 98 to 99 per cent for human beings, dogs, and cats.[22-24] MRI provides superior resolution of intracranial lesions compared with CT, and is more sensitive for detection of primary and secondary brain tumors, infarction, white matter diseases, subacute to chronic hemorrhage, and neurodegenerative diseases.[25] Advantages of MRI over CT include the ability to produce high resolution images of soft-tissue structures, the acquisition of images in multiple planes without having to move the patient, lack of ionizing radiation, the ability to visualize edema easily, and lack of "beam-hardening" artifacts surrounding the brainstem and cerebellum that can obscure small lesions.[21,25] Relative disadvantages compared with CT include increased cost, lower sensitivity in identifying bone lesions, calcification, acute hemorrhage, and longer scan time.[21,25]

MRI features of individual brain tumors have been described for several tumor types and will be discussed in additional detail below. Findings that appear to aid in the differentiation of neoplastic from nonneoplastic lesions include single lesion, regular shape (spheroid or ovoid), contact with the meninges, presence of a dural tail (extension of hyperintense signal or contrast enhancement along the meninges beyond the boundary of the lesion), lesions that affect the adjacent bone, and the presence of contrast enhancement.[26]

Computed Tomography

Computed tomographic images essentially are cross-sectional "slices" of the body utilizing x-ray technology.

However, photon detection is much higher with CT compared with conventional radiographs; therefore slight differences in attenuation lead to improved contrast resolution.* Advantages of CT compared with MRI include shorter scan times; higher sensitivity for detection of bone lesions, calcification, and acute hemorrhage; and reduced cost.[21,29] Disadvantages compared with MRI include exposure of the patient to large doses of radiation; decreased sensitivity for soft tissue structures; presence of bone artifacts created by thick bone surrounding the caudal fossa (brainstem and cerebellum), which can lead to inability to visualize lesions; and inability to easily obtain images in all planes without moving the patient.[21,29] Description of CT features of large numbers of feline brain tumors primarily has been limited to meningioma,[13,14,28,30,31] but small case series or case reports have described the use of CT for pituitary tumors,[32-34] lymphoma,[35-37] ependymoma,[38] intracerebral plasma cell tumor,[39] and middle-ear tumors extending into the brainstem.[40]

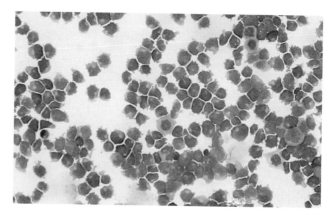

Figure 55-1 Cerebrospinal fluid obtained from a 4-year-old neutered male cat with a 2-week history of ataxia and seizures. Cytological examination revealed a lymphocytic pleocytosis characterized by a large number of lymphoblasts.

HISTOPATHOLOGICAL AND CYTOLOGICAL EXAMINATIONS

Although neurological examination findings and advanced imaging may lead to a strong presumptive diagnosis of intracranial neoplasia,[5,24] histopathological examination remains the gold standard for definitive diagnosis.[9] Tissue biopsy can be made via surgical or stereotactic techniques. Cytological examination of tissue specimens obtained at surgery or necropsy also may be useful in rapid diagnosis.[41,42]

ANCILLARY DIAGNOSTIC TESTS

Cerebrospinal Fluid Analysis

CSF analysis rarely provides a definitive diagnosis for brain tumor.[16,43] It is used to aid in the diagnosis of CNS disease, but may not be necessary based on results of MRI or CT imaging.[6] In general, CSF collection is very safe. However, space-occupying masses can lead to increased intracranial pressure (ICP), and the subsequent alteration of ICP with CSF drainage may lead to brain herniation.[22] CSF collection should be performed after imaging whenever possible to evaluate potential risks versus benefits.[6]

CSF analysis is very sensitive for identification of CNS disease, but is not specific to etiology with the exception of the occasional detection of lymphoblasts with CNS lymphoma (Figure 55-1), rare identification of tumor cells on CSF cytology, and identification of infectious organisms (e.g., *Cryptococcus neoformans*).[5,37,43,44] There is a wide range of reported CSF results for various tumor types.† For example, one study found normal CSF in 3 of 10 cats with meningioma.[17] CSF analysis was performed in 28

cats in a retrospective study of 160 cats with brain tumors. The median total protein was 38 mg/dL (range, 16 to 427; normal, <25) and the median nucleated cell count was 5 cells/μL (range, 0 to 162; normal, <5).[5] Similar findings were reported in a retrospective study of CSF analyses of cats with noninflammatory CNS disease.[44] Albuminocytologic dissociation (increased total protein without a concomitant increase in nucleated cell count) has been reported to occur with intracranial neoplasia. This abnormality was identified in eight (28.6 per cent) cats.[5] However, albuminocytologic dissociation has been reported with other CNS disorders, including noninflammatory degeneration with tissue necrosis, vascular lesions with hemorrhage, and certain types of viral encephalitis.[43]

Skull Radiographs

In general, skull radiographs have limited value in the diagnosis of brain tumors, but may be of some assistance if advanced imaging is not available or cost-prohibitive to the owner. Routine views should include lateral and ventrodorsal (VD) or dorsoventral (DV) views. The closed-mouth VD view is best for evaluation of the frontal and prefrontal regions, whereas the open-mouthed VD view is best for evaluation of the nasal cavity. Open-mouth frontal view is best for evaluation of the foramen magnum and cerebellar region.[27] Dorsoventral and right and left oblique DV views can be used to evaluate the tympanic bullae to rule out otitis media and ear tumors (see Chapter 31).[15,27] Meningiomas lead frequently to thickening of the overlying calvaria (hyperostosis) that can be detected on skull radiographs, as well as with CT and MRI.[5,17,28] Varying degrees of calcification within the tumor, enlargement of the middle meningeal artery, and rare invasion of the calvaria with localized destruction of bone also may be detected on routine skull radiographs.[17]

Electroencephalography

Electroencephalography (EEG) is the recording of spontaneous electrical activity from the cerebral cortex via subcutaneous or surface electrodes. A study analyzing

---

*References 6, 7, 9, 15, 27, 28.
†References 5, 17, 35-37, 39, 44-46.

EEG results from 201 dogs and six cats thought to have space-occupying lesions found that EEG recordings from all of the patients had abnormalities in at least one lead. However, there was no correlation between the side of the brain affected on EEG and lesion location in the 27 dogs that underwent necropsy (none of the cats underwent necropsy). A major limitation of the study was that none of the patients appeared to undergo advanced imaging, and only a small proportion of the patients underwent necropsy.[47] Another smaller study of 10 cats with meningioma found that only 50 per cent of the cats had EEG abnormalities over the appropriate cerebral hemisphere. Two cats had normal EEG recordings, two cats had changes contralateral to lesion location, and one cat had abnormalities only on the right side despite a massive tumor distorting both sides of the brain. These studies suggest that EEG is sensitive for detecting a cerebral lesion, but not specific to lesion location.[17]

Ultrasound

Brain imaging with ultrasound is limited because of bone interference. However, it can be directed through an open fontanelle (primarily to diagnose hydrocephalus), or intraoperatively through a craniotomy window to assist with locating an intraparenchymal lesion and for ultrasound-guided biopsy.[27]

Other Diagnostic Tests

Many other diagnostic tools have been described in the literature, including magnetic resonance spectroscopy,[27,48] electromyography (EMG),[16] cerebral angiography,[16,27] cavernous sinus venography,[16,27] optic thecography,[16,27] scintigraphy,[16,27] and others. Many of these are performed infrequently because of the widespread availability and increased sensitivity of MRI and CT. Others (EMG) are performed uncommonly or are still in the early stages of use in veterinary neurology (MR spectroscopy).

TREATMENT

Treatment options generally fall into two categories: (1) symptomatic treatment and (2) definitive treatment. The goal of symptomatic treatment is to alleviate secondary effects of the brain tumor, whereas definitive treatment is aimed at eliminating the tumor or reducing tumor volume.[49] There are few large scale studies describing treatment options for individual tumor types with the exception of meningioma. Additional information regarding treatment for individual tumor types is presented later in this chapter.

SYMPTOMATIC TREATMENT

Corticosteroids

Corticosteroids are the mainstay of symptomatic treatment.[6-9,15] They are used primarily to reduce peritumoral edema and decrease CSF production, both of which help to lower ICP, alleviating clinical signs temporarily. Prednisone or prednisolone is used most commonly. The typical dose is 0.5 mg/kg PO q12h for 1 to 2 weeks, followed by tapering to the lowest effective dose. Once daily dosing may be required long term to control clinical signs.

Anticonvulsants

Phenobarbital is the first-line anticonvulsant in cats and should be started if seizures occur. The standard starting dose is 1 to 2 mg/kg PO q12h.[7] Serum phenobarbital levels should be measured 2 weeks after initiating treatment or after any change in dose. The "therapeutic range" is 15 to 40 µg/mL. Although hepatotoxicity appears to be less common in cats compared with dogs, many neurologists prefer not to exceed 35 µg/mL to decrease the risk of inducing liver damage. Phenobarbital induces synthesis and release of liver enzymes, particularly alkaline phosphatase (ALP). Bile acid assays should be performed every 6 months to differentiate hepatotoxicity from normal increases in liver enzyme values. Bile acid assays, and possibly abdominal ultrasound and liver biopsy, also should be performed when there are clinical signs of liver dysfunction, compatible blood value alterations (e.g., increased liver enzymes, decreased blood urea nitrogen, decreased cholesterol, decreased albumin), or increasing serum phenobarbital levels without increasing doses of phenobarbital.

Potassium bromide (KBr) can be used if needed; however, a recent study found that almost 40 per cent of cats developed a cough and had clinical and radiographic features similar to those seen in feline asthma. One of the cats was euthanized because of the severity of coughing.[50] Potassium bromide should be discontinued at the first sign of coughing in the feline patient.

Diazepam is a very effective anticonvulsant and at one time was the second choice for oral anticonvulsant therapy until several reports described acute, fulminant hepatic necrosis in some cats treated with oral diazepam.[51-53] Oral diazepam can be used, but with extreme caution. Serum liver enzymes should be monitored at 1 week and at 1 month after initiation of treatment.[54]

A recent study evaluated levetiracetam (Keppra; 20 mg/kg PO q8h) as an adjunct to phenobarbital in a small group of cats with suspected idiopathic epilepsy. A good response (greater than 50 per cent reduction of seizures) was observed in seven of 10 cats. Side effects were transient and included lethargy and inappetence in two cats.[55] Limited information is available regarding other anticonvulsants; however, there is anecdotal use of zonisamide (Zonegran; 5 to 10 mg/kg PO q12h) in cats with seizures and it appears to be well tolerated. (See Chapter 54 for further discussion of novel anticonvulsant therapies.)

DEFINITIVE TREATMENT

Surgery

Excision of meningioma and other tumors that are surgically accessible is considered the gold standard for definitive treatment and should be performed whenever possible.[7,15] Multiple studies have been published describing the surgical removal of meningioma in small case

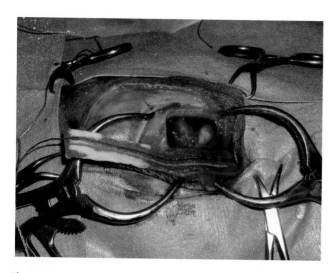

Figure 55-2 Intraoperative photograph of a 12-year-old neutered male cat undergoing a left lateral rostrotentorial craniectomy. The cat's nose is to the left. An extraaxial mass is visible through the cranial portion of the craniectomy window. Normal brain tissue is visible at the caudal end of the window. Histopathological examination confirmed the mass to be a meningioma. The cat survived 3 years before being euthanized for an unrelated illness.

series, as well as individual case reports.[5,13,14,17,30] In general, meningiomas (Figure 55-2) in cats are less invasive than in dogs and, as a result, they usually are easily excised.[49] Sporadic case reports describe surgical excision of lymphoma,[37] ependymoma,[38,56] medulloblastoma,[57,58] and aural tumors that extended into the brain.[40] A recent report also describes the technique of transsphenoidal hypophysectomy for removal of pituitary gland tumors.[34]

Radiation Therapy

Along with surgical excision, radiation therapy (RT) can be an effective definitive treatment option for cats, and is becoming more widely available in veterinary medicine. Despite this, there are few reports describing its use in cats. Most of these reports describe use of RT in cats with pituitary tumors or intracranial lymphoma.[32,33,37,59] Typically RT consists of 15 to 20 fractions of radiation to the tumor, requiring a brief (10 to 15 minute) anesthetic procedure each time. Administration of photons or electrons via linear accelerator is the most common form of RT in veterinary medicine, but some institutions use Cobalt-60 gamma radiation. DNA is damaged by the radiation in the targeted tissue. When the tumor cells attempt to divide, they are unable to replicate themselves and undergo cell death. For tumors that are dividing rapidly, the tumor will shrink sooner and a clinical effect is seen more quickly, whereas slow-growing tumors may take up to 3 to 4 months before clinical benefit is noted. Oral corticosteroids are often started prior to RT to help alleviate clinical signs. In general, patients who do not respond to corticosteroids prior to starting RT may not be acceptable candidates for RT, because it may take too long to see the beneficial effects.

Most patients tolerate radiation treatment very well as long as there are no concurrent systemic medical diseases (e.g., heart murmur, diabetes mellitus). The most common side effect is radiation-induced inflammation in the brain; however, this usually resolves quickly with a short course of oral corticosteroids. Long-term adverse effects are uncommon because the natural remaining life span after diagnosis of a brain tumor usually is too short for long-term effects to occur.

Radiosurgery

Radiosurgery, also known as stereotactic radiosurgery, is a new medical procedure in which a single, high dose of radiation is applied precisely to a tumor or other lesion that is inaccessible for surgical excision. This treatment option has been described in dogs, but not in cats.[60] The primary disadvantage of the technique is that a frame must be attached to the patient's skull. To circumvent this requirement in human medicine, a new device called the CyberKnife has been developed, incorporating a frameless robotic radiosurgery system that is able to track patient movement and adjust the linear accelerator accordingly. This eliminates the need for a head frame leading to increased patient comfort during the procedure. A frameless system would be beneficial for veterinary patients owing to the size of the skull and variations in skull size across breeds. Patient movement would be minimal because of the requirement for anesthesia in veterinary patients, making it easier to perform the procedure. To date, use of the CyberKnife has not been reported in veterinary medicine. However, because a frame is not required, it may be of more practical benefit in veterinary medicine in the future for patients with tumors that are not surgically accessible and for patients who are poor anesthetic risks for traditional RT. Stereotactic RT tends to be expensive, but is comparable to the combined cost of surgery and traditional RT.

Chemotherapy

To date there are no published reports detailing the use of chemotherapeutic agents for treatment of feline brain tumors. Chemotherapy typically is not very helpful for brain tumors and few chemotherapeutic agents are capable of crossing the blood-brain barrier. The exceptions are cyclohexyl-chloroethyl-nitrosourea (CCNU; Lomustine, as well as other nitrosourea compounds) and cytosine arabinoside (cytarabine, Cytosar), both of which are tolerated fairly well by cats. The most commonly reported side effects with CCNU are neutropenia and thrombocytopenia.[61]

Hormone Therapy

Many meningiomas express progesterone receptors.[62,63] In vitro studies have shown that the receptors might be functional and could be a target for treatment using antiprogesterone drugs.[64,65] Clinical studies have shown some efficacy in human patients,[66,67] but no clinical trials have been performed in veterinary patients at this time. This may be a future mode of treatment for feline meningioma when the tumor is not surgically accessible or owner financial constraints are encountered.

PROGNOSIS

Limited information is available in the veterinary literature regarding long-term prognosis for individual tumor types with the exception of meningioma. The average survival time following surgical removal of meningioma in cats is approximately 2 years.[5,13,14] Patients who are treated with supportive measures alone often are euthanized or die within 3 to 6 months owing to progression of clinical signs.[7] Information regarding the survival time for individual tumor types can be found below.

CLASSIFICATION OF TUMORS

Intracranial tumors are classified based on origin. Primary brain tumors arise from cells that normally are found in the brain parenchyma or meninges.[8] Secondary brain tumors are those that invade the brain by hematogenous metastasis, local invasion, or extension from adjacent nonneural tissues.[8] Lymphoma can occur as a primary CNS neoplasm, but typically is classified as a secondary tumor by reason of the high prevalence of lymphoma in extraneural tissues.[8] Primary tumors are significantly more common than secondary tumors, and account for 70 per cent of all intracranial tumors.[5]

PRIMARY BRAIN TUMORS

Meningeal

Meningioma

Meningioma is the most common primary brain tumor of cats, accounting for approximately 60 per cent of all intracranial tumors.[5-9] They can arise from any of the three meningeal layers, but are thought to arise most frequently from the arachnoid mater.[68] Although they are cytologically benign, they often have malignant biological behavior caused by compression of the underlying brain parenchyma.[6,9] Most are supratentorial (rostral to the tentorium cerebelli, affecting the cerebrum, thalamus, or midbrain), but they have been reported in all locations within the calvaria.* In cats meningiomas arise frequently from the tela choroidea of the third ventricle.[5,10] In one study tumors of the third ventricle were more likely to be a meningioma than any other tumor type.[5] They occur most commonly as a solitary mass, but multiple meningiomas are fairly common in cats (Figure 55-3).[3,5,11,71] Meningiomas are frequent incidental findings. It is not uncommon to identify one or more meningiomas at necropsy.[5,10,11]

Meningiomas occur most frequently in middle-aged to older cats, although cats with MPS I may be predisposed to development at a young age (see Chapter 56).[4-9,14] Male cats are affected more often than females (1.5:1 ratio).[4,5,11] No breed predisposition has been identified.

---

*References 5-7, 10, 11, 17, 31, 69, 70.

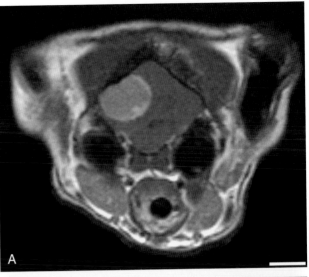

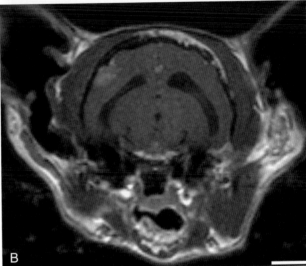

Figure 55-3 Postcontrast transverse MRI images from a 9-year-old neutered male cat at the level of the tympanic bullae (**A**), and junction between the thalamus and midbrain (**B**), demonstrating two discrete extraaxial contrast-enhancing masses, both of which have a broad base along the overlying calvaria. There is marked compression of the underlying right cerebellum (**A**) as the cause of the cat's presenting complaint of cerebellar/vestibular ataxia. The mass over the right parietal lobe (**B**) is causing mild compression of the brain and right lateral ventricle and was considered an incidental finding. Both of these masses are meningiomas.

CT and MRI most often show an extraaxial mass (i.e., outside the brain parenchyma) that is strongly contrast-enhancing (Figures 55-4 and 55-5).[5,17,24,28,72] The mass commonly has a broad base along the skull. Varying degrees of compression of the brain, shifting of midline structures, and herniation are possible. Hyperostosis (thickening of the overlying skull) is a relatively common finding of feline meningioma. Although not pathognomonic for meningioma, hyperostosis is rare with other lesions. Invasion into, or destruction of, the overlying calvaria is rare in cats, but has been reported.[69]

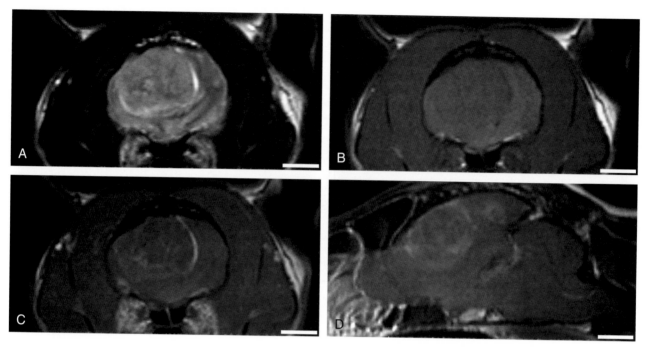

Figure 55-4 Magnetic resonance images of an 11-year-old spayed female domestic shorthair cat with a sudden onset of seizures and behavior change. A very large extraaxial mass is visible overlying the right frontal lobe with extension across midline to the left. The mass is hyperintense on transverse T2-weighted images **(A),** isointense on T1-weighted images **(B),** and has moderate, heterogeneous contrast enhancement **(C).** Both transtentorial and cerebellar herniation are apparent on the sagittal image **(D).** Despite aggressive medical treatment, the cat died of complications related to increased intracranial pressure and herniation prior to surgery.

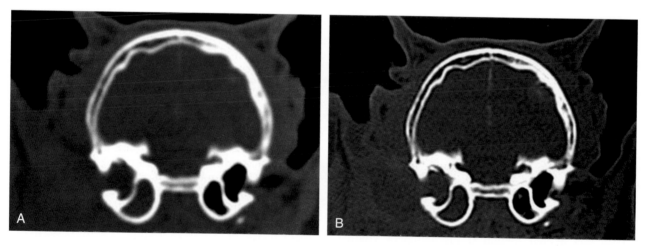

Figure 55-5 Computed tomographic scan obtained from a 13-year-old spayed female Norwegian Forest Cat to evaluate orbital and facial swelling. These transverse images at the level of the tympanic bullae show a small area of mineralization over the left parietal lobe on precontrast images **(A)** and moderate homogeneous contrast enhancement **(B).** This mass is a presumed incidental meningioma. The cat has concurrent right otitis media. The tympanic bulla is filled with soft tissue and/or fluid. (Courtesy Dr. Matt Wright [http://www.dvminsight.com].)

If the mass is accessible, surgery is considered the treatment of choice. Many studies have reported an average survival time of approximately 2 years, which is significantly longer than with symptomatic treatment (Figure 55-6).[5,13,14,17] Complete surgical excision may be curative. RT and chemotherapy are utilized infrequently because meningioma tends not to be very responsive to these treatment modalities; however, these therapies can be attempted if the tumor is not surgically accessible. As described above, several studies have demonstrated that meningioma cells express progesterone receptors. This may be a target for therapy in the future.[62,63]

Gliomas

Glioma is a type of neoplasm that arises from glial cells, which include astrocytes, oligodendrocytes, and

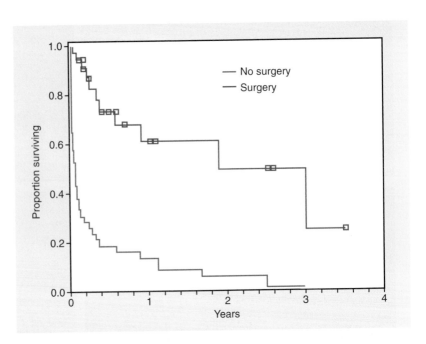

Figure 55-6 Kaplan-Meier curve showing survival times of cats with meningiomas following surgery, compared with all cats in which surgery was not performed (regardless of treatment). Cats who had surgery survived a significantly longer time (*p* < 0.0001). (Reprinted with permission from Troxel MT, Vite CH, Van Winkle TJ, et al: Feline intracranial neoplasia: retrospective review of 160 cases (1985-2001), *J Vet Intern Med* 17:850, 2003.)

microglial cells.[68] Glial cells (neuroglia) comprise a network of cells and fibers that support the function of neurons in the CNS.

Astrocytoma

An astrocytoma is a type of glioma that arises from astrocytes. Most of the information currently available comes from case reports or small case series with a description of clinical signs and pathological findings. As a result, little information is available regarding treatment and prognosis.

Astrocytoma is the second most common primary brain tumor identified in cats, accounting for 2.8 per cent of all brain tumors in cats in one recent study.[5] Cats with astrocytoma typically are older (12.9 ± 3.1 years in one study); however, the reported age range in several case reports was from 1 to 16 years of age.[5,45,46,72-75] Astrocytomas have been reported to occur in all regions of the brain, but they appear to be more common in the supratentorial compartment of the calvaria. Common clinical signs include altered mental status, behavior change, pacing, circling, and seizures. Cerebrospinal fluid analysis has been reported for several cases, but results were not specific to astrocytoma.[5,45]

Computed tomographic imaging has been described in two cats. One cat had a uniformly contrast-enhancing mass in the thalamus,[76] whereas the other cat had a ring-enhancing mass in the rostral cerebrum.[72] MRI findings were reported in one study for gliomas but were grouped together (one astrocytoma, three oligodendrogliomas), so specific MRI features for astrocytoma have not been reported to date.[24] All of the gliomas were intraaxial, hyperintense on T2WI, and hypointense on T1WI. Contrast enhancement was variable, but all four tumors were ring-enhancing. Mass effect was noted in two cats. Cystic regions were identified in three of four gliomas.

Treatment and survival times have been reported for only two cats with astrocytoma.[5] After surgical debulking with inconclusive histopathological findings, one cat had a second surgery at day 39 followed by megavoltage RT (linear accelerator with unspecified dosing scheme) and survived for 179 days. Histopathological examination indicated that the mass was a glioblastoma multiforme (grade IV astrocytoma). The other cat died the first day after surgery.

Oligodendroglioma

Oligodendroglioma is a tumor arising from oligodendrocytes, the myelin-producing cells of the CNS.[68] This is an uncommonly reported tumor of cats. One study found that it was the third most common primary brain tumor in cats, accounting for 2.4 per cent of all intracranial tumors.[5] The tumor appears to affect the supratentorial and infratentorial compartments equally, with reports identifying the tumors in all locations of the brain.[5,77,78] Affected cats typically are middle-aged to older, with a median age of 9.3 years (range, 3.4 to 14 years).[5] No gender or breed predispositions have been identified. Clinical signs are variable and are reflective of lesion location, with seizures, behavior change, circling, aggression, and ataxia reported most frequently.[5,77,78]

CSF analysis is nonspecific, but most often shows mild to moderate increases in total protein and nucleated cell counts.[5,77] Neoplastic cells were identified on cytological examination of CSF in two cats, but were not specific for oligodendrocytes.[77]

CT imaging findings have been described for one cat in whom a mildly contrast-enhancing, intraaxial mass was found in the cerebrum.[28] MRI typically demonstrates an intraaxial mass that is hyperintense on T2WI, hypointense on T1WI, and shows variable peripheral ring enhancement (Figure 55-7).[24,77]

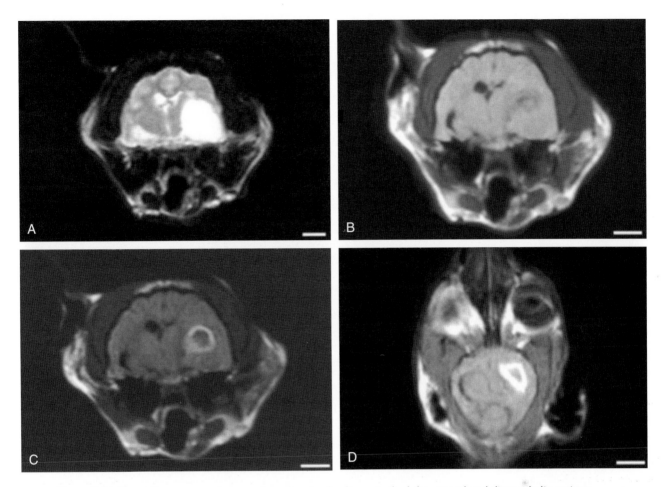

Figure 55-7 Magnetic resonance images of an oligodendroglioma in the left temporal and diencephalic regions. There is mass effect with a compression of the left lateral ventricle and deviation of midline structures from left to right. A cyst appears to be present in the center of the tumor. Moderate peritumoral edema is present. The tumor has a hyperintense, homogeneous signal on transverse T2-weighted images **(A);** a hypointense, heterogeneous signal on transverse T1-weighted images **(B);** and shows marked ring enhancement on the transverse **(C)** and dorsal **(D)** postcontrast images. (Reprinted with permission from Troxel MT, Vite CH, Massicotte C, et al: Magnetic resonance imaging features of feline intracranial neoplasia: retrospective analysis of 46 cats, *J Vet Intern Med* 18:176, 2004.)

Neuroepithelial Tumors

Ependymoma

Ependymomas arise from the epithelial lining (ependymal cells) of the ventricular system.[68] Typically considered uncommon tumors, ependymomas were identified in one study with the same frequency (2.8 per cent) as astrocytomas, the second most common primary brain tumor.[5] Most of the reported ependymomas have been supratentorial, but they can occur anywhere in the brain.[5,38,79-82] In one study approximately 70 per cent of all ependymomas occurred in the third ventricle (Figures 55-8 and 55-9).[5]

Choroid Plexus Tumor

The choroid plexus is an epithelial structure within each of the ventricles that is responsible for production of much of the CSF. Choroid plexus tumor is a rare neoplasm that originates from the choroid plexus. There are only three reports of choroid plexus tumor in the veterinary literature; however, none of them described spinal fluid analysis or treatment.[5,83,84] Reported clinical signs included seizures, blindness, and vestibular dysfunction. MRI of one cat revealed a mass in the left lateral ventricle; however, imaging details were not available.[5]

Primitive Neuroectodermal Tumors

Olfactory Neuroblastoma

This is an uncommon tumor of the nasal cavity that can invade the brain, orbit, and sinuses.[85] The cell of origin is controversial, which has led to a variety of names (e.g., olfactory esthesioneuroblastoma, esthesioneurocytoma, olfactory neuroepithelioma, intranasal neuroblastoma, olfactory placode tumor).[85] Three cats were found to have type C retroviral particles within the tumor cells, and viral budding was identified in one cat.[86] This suggests that FeLV infection may be linked to olfactory neuroblastomas in some cats; however, not all cats with olfactory neuroblastoma are FeLV-positive.

Several case reports and small case series exist in the veterinary literature. Clinical signs often relate to nasal

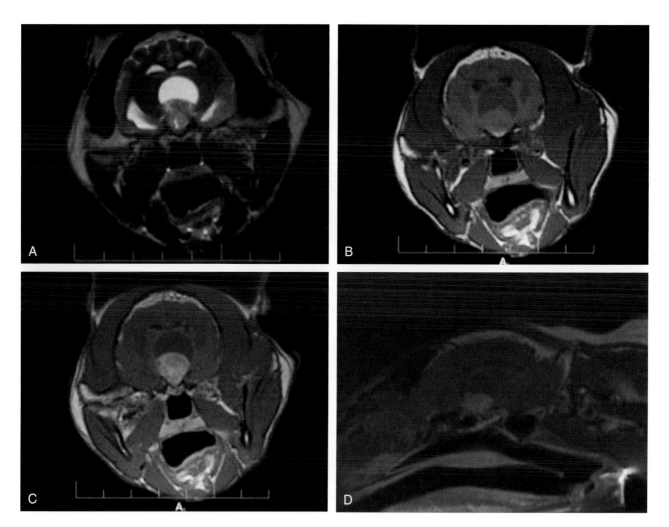

Figure 55-8 Magnetic resonance images from a cat with a mass in the ventral diencephalon in the region of the pituitary gland and third ventricle. The mass is hyperintense and heterogeneous on T2-weighted images (**A**), isointense on T1-weighted images (**B**), and shows marked homogeneous contrast enhancement on the transverse (**C**) and sagittal (**D**) postcontrast images. Obstructive hydrocephalus of the third ventricle is visible dorsal to the mass. (Courtesy Dr. Joan Coates, Department of Veterinary Medicine and Surgery, College of Veterinary Medicine, University of Missouri.)

disease, such as nasal and/or ocular discharge, sneezing, dyspnea, swelling of the frontal sinus, and protrusion of the eye.[5,85-88] The tumors commonly invade the calvaria through the cribriform plate, leading to seizures, behavior change, altered mental status, staggering/ataxia, circling, and disorientation. Neurological signs may be the only changes noted by the owner.[88]

MRI findings have been reported in two cats (Figure 55-10).[24] The tumor was located in the ventral frontal lobe with extension through the cribriform plate. Both tumors were extraaxial with apparent compression of the brain parenchyma leading to marked peritumoral cerebral edema and mass effect. The masses were variable in intensity on both T1WI and T2WI with marked, heterogeneous contrast enhancement.

Treatment details have been reported for one cat with olfactory neuroblastoma. The tumor was diagnosed by excisional biopsy and the cat was treated with palliative corticosteroids; however, the patient was lost to follow-up after its initial 30-day recheck examination.[5]

Medulloblastoma

Medulloblastoma is a rare primitive neuroectodermal tumor thought to arise from the external germinal layer of the cerebellum.[68] Medulloblasts are not an identifiable cell; they are thought to exist within the germinal cells of the developing cerebellum.[68] Two case reports exist in the veterinary literature. A 2-year-old male crossbred cat with vomiting, progressive ataxia, and a tendency to lean to the left underwent MRI and surgical excision of the mass.[58] The cat reportedly recovered uneventfully, but there was no information on survival time in the report. Another 2-year-old neutered male crossbred cat was described with a 1-month history of leaning to the left, truncal ataxia, and tendency to fall while going down the stairs.[57] A cerebellar mass with well-defined margins was visualized on MRI that had variable intensity on both T2WI and T1WI. The mass showed marked, slightly heterogeneous contrast enhancement. Two weeks after the initial medical examination, the mass was excised

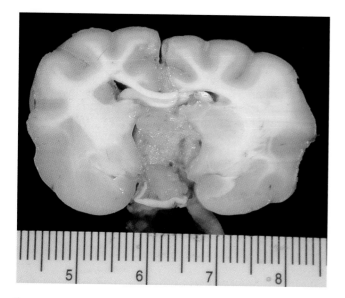

Figure 55-9 Transverse section of the brain of the cat in Figure 55-8. A large, nodular mass is present in the third ventricle. The histological diagnosis was ependymoma. (Courtesy Dr. Joan Coates, Department of Veterinary Medicine and Surgery, College of Veterinary Medicine, University of Missouri; and Dr. Kei Kuroki, Department of Veterinary Pathobiology, College of Veterinary Medicine, University of Missouri.)

surgically through a suboccipital craniectomy. The cat was discharged 5 days after surgery with persistent truncal ataxia and intention tremor, but deteriorated and died 23 days later.

SECONDARY BRAIN TUMORS

Lymphoma

Lymphoma reportedly is rare in the CNS, with the exception of spinal lymphoma.[3,68] However, it was the second most common intracranial neoplasm in one study, accounting for 16 per cent of all feline brain tumors.[5] It can occur in any region of the brain, with diffuse brainstem, diffuse cerebral, and meningeal involvement being most common.[5] Lymphoma often is a multisystemic disease. As such, intracranial lymphoma generally is categorized as a secondary brain tumor. However, primary intracranial lymphoma, in which malignant lymphoid cells are detected only in the brain, was identified in 35 per cent of cats with lymphoma in one study.[5]

The median age for cats affected by lymphoma was 10.5 years; however, there was a very wide range of reported ages (0.4 to 19.4 years).[5,35-37,89-91] Most of the reported cases have occurred in domestic shorthair cats, but the disease also has been reported in a Siamese,

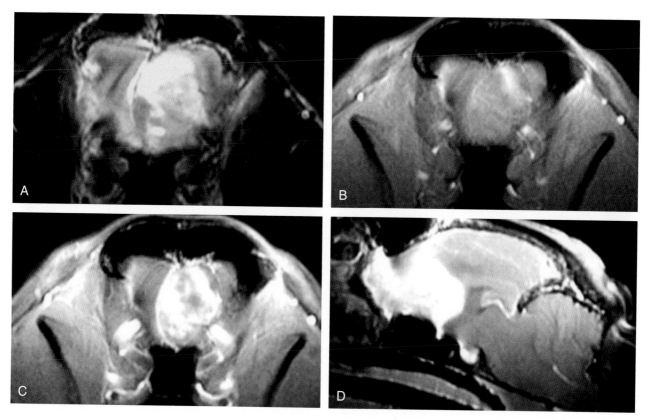

Figure 55-10 Olfactory neuroblastoma in the left olfactory bulb and frontal lobe of a cat. Marked mass effect with deviation of midline structures from left to right is visible. The mass has a hyperintense, heterogeneous signal on transverse T2-weighted images **(A)**; a hyperintense, homogeneous signal on transverse T1-weighted images **(B)**; and a marked, heterogeneous contrast enhancement on transverse **(C)** and sagittal **(D)** postcontrast images. The region of hyperintense signal noted on both the T2WI and T1WI is suggestive of subacute hemorrhage. (Reprinted with permission from Troxel MT, Vite CH, Massicotte C, et al: Magnetic resonance imaging features of feline intracranial neoplasia: retrospective analysis of 46 cats, *J Vet Intern Med* 18:176, 2004.)

Persian, and Japanese domestic cat. No gender predisposition has been found. Unlike spinal lymphoma, in which 32 of 36 cats in two studies were FeLV-positive,[92,93] FeLV does not appear to be linked to intracranial lymphoma in cats.[5] Similarly, FIV infection does not appear to be correlated with intracranial lymphoma.[5]

CSF analysis results have been reported for only a small number of cases.[5,36,91] CSF shows a variable increase in total protein and nucleated cell counts. In one study CSF results in four cats showed a median total protein of 54.5 mg/dL (range, 35 to 404) and nucleated cell count of 14.5 cells/μL (range, 0 to 162).[5] Differential cell counts were performed in an additional two cats, which showed a large number of neutrophils (median 76 per cent), and smaller numbers of lymphocytes (median 4 per cent) and monocytes (10 per cent). Lymphoblasts accounted for 20 per cent of the differential cell counts for one of the cats, but were not observed in the other cat. Eosinophils were identified in the CSF in one case report.[91]

CT and MRI characteristics have been reported for several cats with intracranial lymphoma.[24,35-37,91] Results are inconsistent because of the variable nature of the disease, occurring as a solitary mass or diffuse disease, and in both intraaxial and extraaxial locations (Figures 55-11 and 55-12). Solitary ring-enhancing lesions were identified on CT imaging in one study.[37] In a recent retrospective study detailing the MRI features of feline brain tumors, MRI was performed on six cats with lymphoma.[24] One cat had a normal MRI scan and was later found to have lymphoma isolated to the cerebral meninges at necropsy. The remaining five cats had solitary masses, of which three were extraaxial and two were intraaxial. Tumor shape and margins were variable. In general, the mass was hyperintense and heterogeneous on T2WI, isointense or hypointense on T1WI, and displayed marked contrast enhancement without ring enhancement. Mass effect was noted in all three cats with an extraaxial mass, and a dural tail was identified in one cat. In one report CT showed no precontrast brain abnormalities; however, postcontrast enhancement of the falx cerebri was noted on two contiguous slices. Subsequent MRI showed diffuse enhancement of the meninges and falx cerebri.[36] MRI of another cat showed a hyperintense right cerebrum with thickened cortex and poorly defined gyri.[91]

Data concerning treatment and survival times are lacking in the veterinary literature. In general the long-term prognosis for intracranial lymphoma is considered guarded to poor. If a surgically accessible mass is identified on MRI or CT, and there are no other systemic signs of neoplasia, surgical excision followed by RT and/or chemotherapy would likely provide the longest disease-free interval. Surgical excision, followed by oral corticosteroid therapy, has been reported in three cats who survived for 30, 65, and 97 days postoperatively.[5,37] RT has been described in two cats.[37] One cat had primary intracranial lymphoma based on CT imaging and excisional biopsy. This cat received three doses of radiotherapy (eight Gy/treatment) and cyclic combination chemotherapy, and survived 210 days from the onset of neurological signs. Another cat, already undergoing systemic chemotherapy

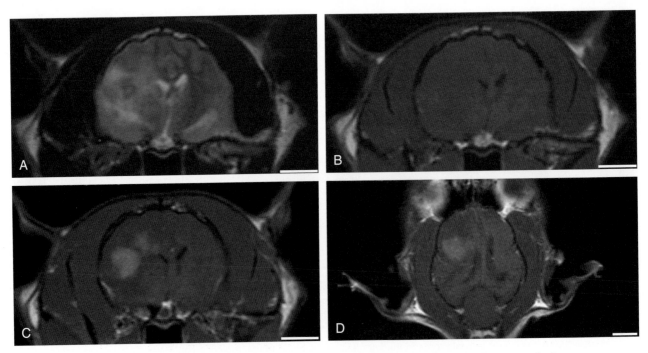

Figure 55-11 Magnetic resonance images from a 4-year-old indoor/outdoor cat with a sudden onset of seizures, behavior change, and circling. MRI revealed an abnormal region in the right cerebral hemisphere, primarily involving the parietal and temporal lobes. There is an amorphous region of hyperintense signal on T2-weighted images **(A)** that is hypointense on T1-weighted images **(B).** There is moderate patchy contrast enhancement on postcontrast transverse images **(C),** but a more discrete region is visible on dorsal views **(D).** Moderate perilesional cerebral edema is visible, along with midline shift from right to left.

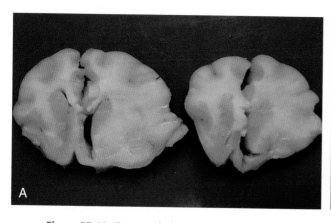
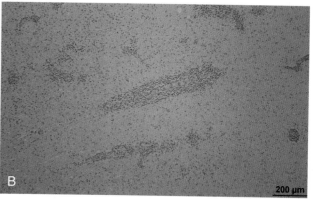

Figure 55-12 Gross pathology (**A**) and histopathology (**B**) from the cat in Figure 55-11. Gross examination of the right frontal lobe revealed widening of the corona radiata (white matter) with loss of distinction between the gray and white matter, as well as a soft, gelatinous region in the right ventral frontal lobe. Histopathological examination revealed a perivascular infiltrate of lymphocytes. The lymphocytes extended into the neuropil and were found in the meninges (not shown). Immunohistochemistry identified these changes as B-cell lymphoma. (Courtesy Dr. Elizabeth Buckles, Department of Biomedical Sciences, College of Veterinary Medicine, Cornell University.)

for generalized lymphoma, including the use of cytosine arabinoside because of the recent onset of neurological signs, lived an additional 40 days after RT. It is unclear from the report how long the cat was being treated prior to the development of CNS signs. Palliative treatment with corticosteroids alone yielded median survival time of only 21 days (range, 9 to 270) for nine cats in one study,[5] and a median survival time of 34 days (range, 3 to 70) in another study describing six cats.[37]

Pituitary Tumors

Pituitary tumors reportedly are an uncommon cause of neurological signs in cats[3]; however, they were the third most common tumor identified in the cranial vault in one study, accounting for 9.3 per cent of all intracranial tumors.[5] Pituitary tumors can arise from the neurohypophysis or adenohypophysis. Characterization of cell type is described infrequently in the literature, making it difficult to separate tumor types with regard to clinical presentation, treatment, and prognosis.

As with other brain tumors, affected cats typically are older, with a median age of approximately 10 years.[5,33,34] Although a greater number of cats are male (3.7:1), this has not been found to be a statistically significant difference.[5] No breed disposition has been noted.

Clinical signs at presentation often manifest as an endocrine dysfunction.[5,32-34,94] Polyuria/polydipsia, lethargy, inappetence, and weight loss are frequent historical complaints. Cats with pituitary tumors commonly have concurrent pituitary-dependent hyperadrenocorticism (PDH), acromegaly (see Chapter 29), or insulin-resistant diabetes (Figure 55-13). Hypoadrenocorticism and hyperthyroidism also have been reported.[5]

Neurological signs are more common in cats compared with dogs. Seizures, aggression, and visual deficits occur in less than 10 per cent of affected dogs.[95] However, in cats blindness appears to be common, and in one study it was reported in 35.7 per cent of cats with pituitary tumors.[5,96] Altered mental status, circling, and ataxia also

are noted frequently in affected cats.* Seizures appear to be uncommon in cats with pituitary tumors, but can occur.[97]

CT imaging and MRI features of pituitary tumors have been published.[24,34,98] The average size of the pituitary gland in normal cats is 5.4 mm long, 5 mm wide, and 3.2 to 3.4 mm in height, based on MRI measurements.[98] Normal pituitary glands enhance on both CT and MRI after administration of contrast agent. As such, small pituitary tumors may be difficult to visualize until the pituitary gland is larger than published reference ranges. Published CT and MRI reports of pituitary tumor imaging generally describe the tumor as variable in intensity on precontrast imaging, but they usually enhanced strongly after administration of intravenous contrast (Figures 55-14 and 55-15).[24,34,94,97,99]

Therapeutic options for pituitary tumors include medical treatment for endocrine disorders if present, symptomatic control of neurological signs, RT, and surgery. The veterinary literature contains many case reports and small case series describing medical treatment of PDH and acromegaly[97,100-105] (see Chapter 29). Medical treatment for PDH in cats has been unrewarding to date. Medication options include mitotane, trilostane, and ketoconazole.

RT has shown promise for alleviating clinical signs and increasing survival time, even though the decrease in tumor size may be minimal.[32,33,97] RT utilizing [60]cobalt in three cats with pituitary tumors, insulin-resistant diabetes mellitus, and acromegaly led to resolution of diabetes and insulin requirement in two cats and a reduction in insulin dose for the other cat.[32] RT with a linear accelerator led to survival times from 5 to 20 months in one study of five cats with pituitary tumors (four adenomas, one carcinoma).[32,33] In a more recent study eight cats irradiated with a linear accelerator had a median survival time

---

*References 5, 32-34, 59, 94, 96.

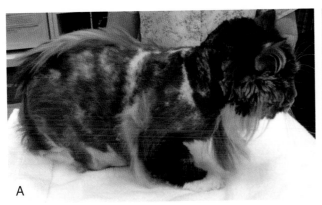

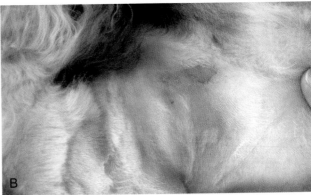

Figure 55-13 A 10-year-old spayed female cat with a recent onset of polyphagia (previously finicky eater), poor regrowth of hair following grooming, and mild mental dullness. On presentation the cat had a very poor hair coat **(A)** and thin, friable skin **(B).** Low-dose dexamethasone suppression testing was abnormal, suggestive of pituitary-dependent hyperadrenocorticism. See Figure 55-14 for CT images of this cat. (Courtesy Dr. Joan Coates, Department of Veterinary Medicine and Surgery, College of Veterinary Medicine, University of Missouri.)

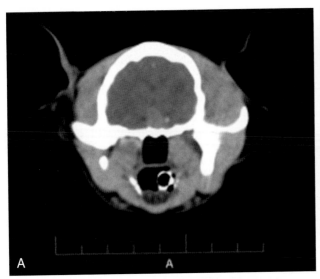

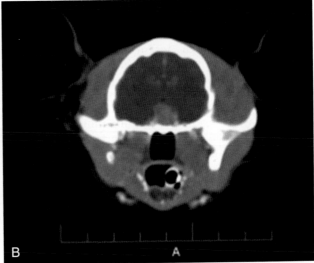

Figure 55-14 Computed tomographic images of the cat in Figure 55-13 with a presumptive pituitary macroadenoma. Precontrast images **(A)** show a large hyperdense mass originating from the pituitary gland that enhanced markedly following administration of intravenous contrast **(B).** (Courtesy Dr. Joan Coates, Department of Veterinary Medicine and Surgery, College of Veterinary Medicine, University of Missouri.)

of 523 days (range, 252 to 1,894 days) regardless of cause of death.[94] Six of the cats were still alive at 1 year, whereas three cats were alive at 2 years after treatment. Resolution of neurological signs occurred in all five cats who presented for that problem.

Surgical treatment options include bilateral adrenalectomy and hypophysectomy.[34,99,106] Both surgical procedures are not performed routinely in veterinary medicine. Although case numbers are limited, hypophysectomy has shown some promise in increasing disease-free survival times. Transsphenoidal hypophysectomy was reported for the treatment of seven cats with PDH.[34] Two cats died within 1 month of surgery as a result of unrelated disease. The remaining five cats went into clinical and biochemical remission; however, one cat had a recurrence of PDH at 19 months and died 28 months after surgery. This cat had pituitary remnants detected during its 6-month follow-up CT examination. Two of the five cats were euthanized at 6 and 8 months, respectively. One cat had an undefined anemia unrelated to the surgery, and the other cat had recurrent rhinitis and otitis media as a complication of the surgery. The remaining two cats were still alive at the time of writing with remission periods of 46 and 15 months. The most common complications were oronasal fistula, dehiscence of the soft palate, and transient decreased tear production.

Tumors that Affect the Brain via Direct Extension

Potentially any tissue within the head can give rise to a neoplasm that invades the calvarium and affects the brain secondarily.

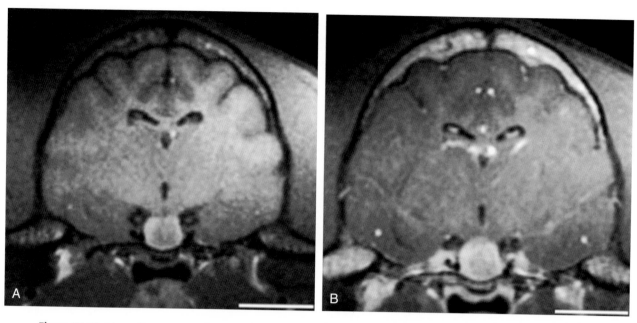

Figure 55-15 Magnetic resonance images of a pituitary tumor in a cat. The tumor is round with a distinct margin, and has isointense, heterogeneous signal characteristics on T1-weighted images **(A)**. There is moderate, heterogeneous, ring-enhancing contrast enhancement **(B)**. (Adapted and reprinted with permission from Troxel MT, Vite CH, Massicotte C, et al: Magnetic resonance imaging features of feline intracranial neoplasia: retrospective analysis of 46 cats, *J Vet Intern Med* 18:176, 2004.)

Nasal Tumors

Nasal tumors are uncommon in cats compared with dogs. A variety of histological types have been described in the veterinary literature. Olfactory neuroblastoma is discussed earlier in this chapter. Nasal tumors occur more commonly in male cats (2:1). Most of them are malignant and locally invasive. However, invasion through the cribriform plate into the cranial vault has been reported. Some cats present initially with signs of upper respiratory disease, whereas neurological signs are the primary initial complaint in other patients.[5,88] A recent retrospective study of 32 cats with tumors of the nose and paranasal sinuses described four cats who had extension of disease into the brain (two undifferentiated carcinomas, two olfactory neuroblastomas).[87] Reported neurological signs include circling, mental dullness, and seizures.[5,87,88]

Aural Tumors

Two cats have been described in the literature that had middle ear tumors extending into the brainstem. One cat had a papillary adenoma and the other cat had an adenocarcinoma. Both cats underwent ventral bulla osteotomy and craniectomy. One cat lived for 630 days, whereas the other cat was alive but lost to follow-up after 840 days.[10] (See Chapter 69 for a full discussion of tumors of the ear canal.)

Osteosarcoma

Osteosarcoma of the calvarium is rare in cats (Figure 55-16). It is much more common in the orbit, mandible, and maxilla. Only one report exists, which describes a 13-year-old spayed female cat with a compulsive gait, circling, absent menace response bilaterally, and postural

reaction deficits.[107] A giant cell osteosarcoma was identified at necropsy.

Miscellaneous Tumors

Plasmacytoma

One case report exists describing a 6-year-old neutered male domestic shorthair cat with a 1-week history of an acute onset of behavior change, staring into corners, and compulsively circling to the left. A 1-cm focal, contrast-enhancing mass associated with the left lateral ventricle was discovered on CT imaging, along with marked contrast enhancement of the ependymal lining of the left lateral ventricle. A midline shift to the right and cerebral edema also were observed. CSF analysis was performed. The total protein and nucleated cell counts both were mildly elevated (protein 69 mg/dL; nucleated cell count, 25 cells/µL). The nucleated cells were comprised primarily of small lymphocytes and macrophages, along with 20 per cent unidentifiable cells that in hindsight may have been plasma cells. The cat was treated symptomatically with prednisone, but deteriorated and died 2 weeks later. Histopathological examination was performed and the tumor mass was determined to be an intracranial plasmacytoma.[39] (See Chapter 65 for a full discussion of plasma cell disorders.)

Teratoma

Teratoma is a well differentiated germ cell tumor arising from two or three embryonic germ layers.[108] One published case report exists in the literature.[109] A 4-month-old female domestic shorthair cat was presented for evaluation with multiple facial deformities and

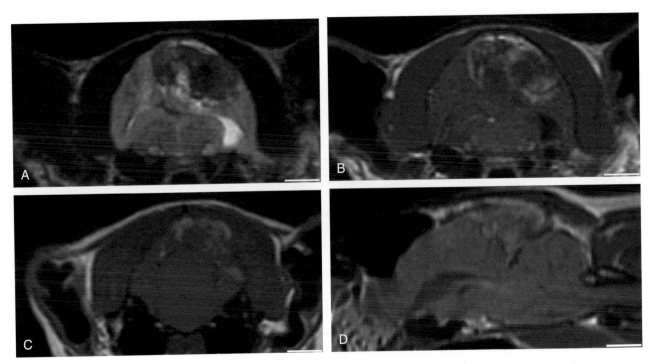

Figure 55-16 Brain MRI of a 6-year-old cat with a 2-week history of circling to the left, head pressing, altered mental status, and seizures. MRI showed a large extraaxial mass over the left parietal and occipital lobes. The mass has variable signal intensity with large areas of hypointensity on both T2-weighted images **(A)** and T1-weighted images (not shown). There is marked heterogeneous contrast enhancement **(B).** At the level of the occipital lobe **(C)** the mass is clearly either originating from or involving the skull. The mass also invades the overlying temporalis muscle. The mass is causing marked ventral displacement of the brain with marked compression of both lateral ventricles **(A and B),** transtentorial herniation, and cerebellar herniation **(D).** The cat was euthanized after the MRI and the mass was identified as osteosarcoma on histopathological examination.

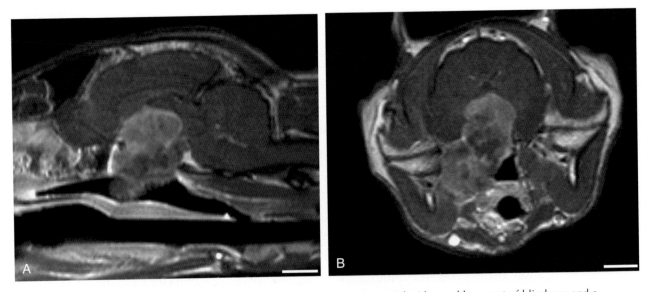

Figure 55-17 Brain MRI of a 14-year-old spayed female cat who presented with a sudden onset of blindness and a several-week history of gagging/retching. Postcontrast sagittal image **(A)** and transverse image at the level of the thalamus **(B)** are shown. A large mass was identified in the nasopharynx predominantly on the right side extending through the calvaria into the cranial vault at the left of the pituitary gland and optic chiasm. The cat was euthanized after the MRI and a postmortem biopsy of the mass was performed. Histopathological examination showed the mass to be an anaplastic carcinoma.

progressive pelvic limb incoordination, visual impairment, and seizures. The cat was euthanized. At necropsy, a teratoma was identified in the thalamus and a dermoid cyst was found in the ventral frontal lobe.

Metastatic Neoplasia

Metastasis to the brain is relatively uncommon, occurring in just over 5 per cent of cats with brain tumors (Figure 55-17).[5] Published reports have described metastasis of pulmonary adenocarcinoma, unclassified adenocarcinoma, squamous cell carcinoma, malignant fibrous histiocytoma, fibrosarcoma, unclassified sarcoma, hemangiosarcoma, sweat gland carcinoma, mammary adenocarcinoma, endometrial adenocarcinoma, and malignant melanoma.[5,110-113]

REFERENCES

1. Engle GC, Brodey RS: A retrospective study of 395 feline neoplasms, *J Am Anim Hosp Assoc* 5:21, 1969.
2. Vandevelde M: Brain tumors in domestic animals: an overview. In *Brain tumors in man and animals*, Research Triangle Park, NC, 1984, National Institute of Environmental Sciences.
3. Zaki FA, Hurvitz AI: Spontaneous neoplasms of the central nervous system of the cat, *J Small Anim Pract* 17:773, 1976.
4. Haskins ME, McGrath JT: Meningiomas in young cats with mucopolysaccharidosis I, *J Neuropathol Exp Neurol* 42:664, 1983.
5. Troxel MT, Vite CH, Van Winkle TJ, et al: Feline intracranial neoplasia: retrospective review of 160 cases (1985-2001), *J Vet Intern Med* 17:850, 2003.
6. Adamo PF, Forrest L, Dubielzig R: Canine and feline meningiomas: diagnosis, treatment, and prognosis, *Compend Contin Educ Pract Vet* 26:951, 2004.
7. Dewey CW, Coates JR, Bahr A, et al: Primary brain tumors in dogs and cats, *Compend Contin Educ Pract Vet* 22:756, 2000.
8. LeCouteur RA: Brain tumors of dogs and cats, *Vet Med Rep* 2:332, 1990.
9. LeCouteur RA: Current concepts in the diagnosis and treatment of brain tumours in dogs and cats, *J Small Anim Pract* 20:411, 1999.
10. Luginbuhl H: Studies on meningiomas in cats, *Am J Vet Res* 22:1030, 1961.
11. Nafe LA: Meningiomas in cats: a retrospective clinical study of 36 cases, *J Am Vet Med Assoc* 174:1224, 1979.
12. Nafe LA: The clinical presentation and diagnosis of intracranial neoplasia, *Semin Vet Med Surg (Small Anim)* 5:223, 1990.
13. Gallagher JG, Berg J, Knowles KE, et al: Prognosis after surgical excision of cerebral meningiomas in cats: 17 cases (1986-1992), *J Am Vet Med Assoc* 203:1437, 1993.
14. Gordon LE, Thacher C, Matthiesen DT, et al: Results of craniotomy for the treatment of cerebral meningioma in 42 cats, *Vet Surg* 23:94, 1994.
15. Kraus KH, McDonnell J: Identification and management of brain tumors, *Semin Vet Med Surg (Small Anim)* 11:218, 1996.
16. Moore MP, Bagley RS, Harrington ML, et al: Intracranial tumors, *Vet Clin North Am Small Anim Pract* 26:759, 1996.
17. Lawson DC, Burk RL, Prata RG: Cerebral meningioma in the cat: diagnosis and surgical treatment of ten cases, *J Am Anim Hosp Assoc* 20:333, 1984.
18. Tomek A, Cizinauskas S, Doherr M, et al: Intracranial neoplasia in 61 cats: localisation, tumour types and seizure patterns, *J Feline Med Surg* 8:243, 2006.
19. Quesnel AD, Parent JM, McDonell W, et al: Diagnostic evaluation of cats with seizure disorders: 30 cases (1991-1993), *J Am Vet Med Assoc* 210:65, 1997.
20. Coates JR, Levine JM: Performing the neurological examination. In August JR, editor: *Consultations in feline internal medicine*, vol 5, St. Louis, 2006, Saunders, p 449.
21. Grossman RI, Yousem DM: Techniques in neuroimaging. In *Neuroradiology: the requisites*. ed 2, St. Louis, 1994, Mosby-Year Book, p 1.
22. Thomas WB, Wheeler SJ, Kramer R, et al: Magnetic resonance imaging features of primary brain tumors in dogs, *Vet Radiol Ultrasound* 37:20, 1996.
23. Kraft SL, Gavin PR, DeHaan C, et al: Retrospective review of 50 canine intracranial tumors evaluated by magnetic resonance imaging, *J Vet Intern Med* 11:218, 1997.
24. Troxel MT, Vite CH, Massicotte C, et al: Magnetic resonance imaging features of feline intracranial neoplasia: retrospective analysis of 46 cats, *J Vet Intern Med* 18:176, 2004.
25. Gilman S: Imaging the brain. First of two parts, *N Engl J Med* 338:812, 1998.
26. Cherubini GB, Mantis P, Martinez TA, et al: Utility of magnetic resonance imaging for distinguishing neoplastic from nonneoplastic brain lesions in dogs and cats, *Vet Radiol Ultrasound* 46:384, 2005.
27. Bailey MQ: Diagnostic imaging of intracranial lesions, *Semin Vet Med Surg (Small Anim)* 5:232, 1990.
28. LeCouteur RA, Fike JR, Cann CE, et al: X-ray computed tomography of brain tumors in cats, *J Am Vet Med Assoc* 183:301, 1983.
29. Gilman S: Imaging the brain. Second of two parts, *N Engl J Med* 338:889, 1998.
30. Fingeroth JM, Hansen B, Myer CW: Diagnosis and successful removal of a brain tumor in a cat, *Companion Anim Pract* 2:6, 1988.
31. Kaldrymidou E, Polizopoulou ZS, Koutinas AF, et al: Papillary meningioma in the cerebellum of a cat, *J Comp Pathol* 123:222, 2000.
32. Goossens MM, Feldman EC, Nelson RW, et al: Cobalt 60 irradiation of pituitary gland tumors in three cats with acromegaly, *J Am Vet Med Assoc* 213:374, 1998.
33. Kaser-Hotz B, Rohrer CR, Stankeova S, et al: Radiotherapy of pituitary tumours in five cats, *J Small Anim Pract* 43:303, 2002.
34. Meij BP, Voorhout G, Van Den Ingh TS, et al: Transsphenoidal hypophysectomy for treatment of pituitary-dependent hyperadrenocorticism in 7 cats, *Vet Surg* 30:72, 2001.
35. Morozumi M, Miyahara K, Sato M, et al: Computed tomography and magnetic resonance findings in two dogs and a cat with intracranial lesions, *J Vet Med Sci* 59:807, 1997.
36. Morozumi M, Sasaki N, Oyama Y, et al: Computed tomography and magnetic resonance findings of meningeal syndrome in a leukemic cat, *J Vet Med Sci* 55:1035, 1993.
37. Noonan M, Kline KL, Meleo K: Lymphoma of the central nervous system: a retrospective study of 18 cats, *Compend Contin Educ Pract Vet* 19:497, 1997.
38. Simpson DJ, Hunt GB, Tisdall PL, et al: Surgical removal of an ependymoma from the third ventricle of a cat, *Aust Vet J* 77:645, 1999.
39. Greenberg MJ, Schatzberg SJ, deLahunta A, et al: Intracerebral plasma cell tumor in a cat: a case report and literature review, *J Vet Intern Med* 18:581, 2004.
40. Lucroy MD, Vernau KM, Samii VF, et al: Middle ear tumours with brainstem extension treated by ventral bulla osteotomy and craniectomy in two cats, *Vet Comp Oncol* 2:234, 2004.

41. Long SN, Anderson TJ, Long FH, et al: Evaluation of rapid staining techniques for cytologic diagnosis of intracranial lesions, *Am J Vet Res* 63:381, 2002.

42. Vernau KM, Higgins RJ, Bollen AW, et al: Primary canine and feline nervous system tumors: Intraoperative diagnosis using the smear technique, *Vet Pathol* 38:47, 2001.

43. de Lahunta A: *Veterinary neuroanatomy and clinical neurology*, ed 2, Philadelphia, 1983, Saunders.

44. Rand JS, Parent J, Percy D, et al: Clinical, cerebrospinal fluid, and histological data from thirty-four cats with primary noninflammatory disease of the central nervous system, *Can Vet J* 35:103, 1994.

45. Komarnisky MD: Astrocytoma in a cat, *Can Vet J* 26:237, 1985.

46. Sarfaty D, Carrillo JM, Patnaik AK: Cerebral astrocytoma in four cats: clinical and pathologic findings, *J Am Vet Med Assoc* 191:976, 1987.

47. Croft PG: Electroencephalography and space-occupying lesions in small animals, *J Small Anim Pract* 13:175, 1972.

48. Shores A, Warber-Matich S, Cooper TG: The role of magnetic resonance spectroscopy in neuro-oncology, *Semin Vet Med Surg (Small Anim)* 5:237, 1990.

49. Dewey CW: Encephalopathies: disorders of the brain. In Dewey CW, editor: *A practical guide to canine and feline neurology*, ed 1, Ames, 2003, Iowa State Press, p 99.

50. Boothe DM, George KL, Couch P: Disposition and clinical use of bromide in cats, *J Am Vet Med Assoc* 221:1131, 2002.

51. Center SA, Elston TH, Rowland PH, et al: Fulminant hepatic failure associated with oral administration of diazepam in 11 cats, *J Am Vet Med Assoc* 209:618, 1996.

52. Levy JK, Cullen JM, Bunch SE, et al: Adverse reaction to diazepam in cats, *J Am Vet Med Assoc* 205:156, 1994.

53. Hughes D, Moreau RE, Overall LL, et al: Acute hepatic necrosis and liver failure associated with benzodiazepine therapy in six cats, 1986-1995, *J Vet Emerg Crit Care* 6:13, 1996.

54. Thomas WB: Seizures and narcolepsy. In Dewey CW, editor: *A practical guide to canine and feline neurology*, ed 1, Ames, 2003, Iowa State Press, p 193.

55. Bailey KS, Dewey CW, Boothe DM, et al: Levetiracetam as an adjunct to phenobarbital treatment in cats with suspected idiopathic epilepsy, *J Am Vet Med Assoc* 232:867, 2008.

56. Niebauer GW, Dayrell-Hart BL, Speciale J: Evaluation of craniotomy in dogs and cats, *J Am Vet Med Assoc* 198:89, 1991.

57. Kitagawa M, Koie H, Kanayamat K, et al: Medulloblastoma in a cat: clinical and MRI findings, *J Small Anim Pract* 44:139, 2003.

58. Kuwabara M, Kitagawa M, Sato T, et al: Early diagnosis of feline medulloblastoma in the vermis, *Vet Rec* 150:488, 2002.

59. Chastain CB, Panciera D, Kaser-Hotz B, et al: Radiotherapy of pituitary tumors in cats, *Small Anim Clin Endocrinol* 13:8, 2002.

60. Lester NV, Hopkins AL, Bova FJ, et al: Radiosurgery using a stereotactic headframe system for irradiation of brain tumors in dogs, *J Am Vet Med Assoc* 219:1562, 2001.

61. Fan TM, Kitchell BE, Dhaliwal RS, et al: Hematological toxicity and therapeutic efficacy of lomustine in 20 tumor-bearing cats: critical assessment of a practical dosing regimen, *J Am Anim Hosp Assoc* 38:357, 2002.

62. Adamo PF, Cantile C, Steinberg HS: Evaluation of progesterone and estrogen receptor expression in 15 meningiomas of dogs and cats, *Am J Vet Res* 64:1310, 2003.

63. Speciale J, Koffman BM, Bashirelahi N, et al: Identification of gonadal steroid receptors in meningiomas from dogs and cats, *Am J Vet Res* 51:833, 1990.

64. Olson JJ, Beck DW, Schlechte J, et al: Hormonal manipulation of meningiomas in vitro, *J Neurosurg* 65:99, 1986.

65. Olson JJ, Beck DW, Schlechte JA, et al: Effect of the anti-progesterone RU-38486 on meningioma implanted into nude mice, *J Neurosurg* 66:584, 1987.

66. Grunberg SM, Weiss MH, Spitz IM, et al: Treatment of unresectable meningiomas with the antiprogesterone agent mifepristone, *J Neurosurg* 74:861, 1991.

67. Sharif S, Brennan P, Rawluk D: Nonsurgical treatment of meningioma: a case report and review, *Br J Neurosurg* 12:369, 1998.

68. Summers BA, Cummings JF, de Lahunta A: Tumours of the central nervous system. In Summers BA, Cummings JF, de Lahunta A, editors: *Veterinary neuropathology*, St. Louis, 1995, Mosby-Year Book, p 351.

69. Hague PH, Burridge MJ: A meningioma in a cat associated with erosion of the skull, *Vet Rec* 84:217, 1969.

70. Mandara MT, Ricci G, Sforna M: A cerebral granular cell tumor in a cat, *Vet Pathol* 43:797, 2006.

71. McGrath JT: Morphology and classification of brain tumors in domestic animals. In *Brain tumors in man and animals*, Research Triangle Park, NC, 1984, National Institute of Environmental Sciences.

72. Fuchs C, Meyer-Lindenberg A, Wohsein P, et al: Computer tomographic characteristics of primary brain tumors in dogs and cats, *Berl Munch Tierarztl Wochenschr* 116:436, 2003.

73. Cusick PK, Parker AJ: Brain stem gliomas in cats, *Vet Pathol* 12:460, 1975.

74. Duniho S, Schulman FY, Morrison A, et al: A subependymal giant cell astrocytoma in a cat, *Vet Pathol* 37:275, 2000.

75. Sant'Ana FJ, Serakides R, Graca DL: Pilocytic astrocytoma in a cat, *Vet Pathol* 39:759, 2002.

76. Kornegay JN: Altered mental attitude, seizures, blindness, circling, compulsive walking. Forebrain diseases, *Probl Vet Med* 3:391, 1991.

77. Dickinson PJ, Keel MK, Higgins RJ, et al: Clinical and pathologic features of oligodendrogliomas in two cats, *Vet Pathol* 37:160, 2000.

78. Smith DA, Honhold N: Clinical and pathological features of a cerebellar oligodendroglioma in a cat, *J Small Anim Pract* 29:269, 1988.

79. Fox JG, Snyder SB, Reed C, et al: Malignant ependymoma in a cat, *J Small Anim Pract* 14:23, 1973.

80. Ingwersen W, Groom S, Parent J: Vestibular syndrome associated with an ependymoma in a cat, *J Am Vet Med Assoc* 195:98, 1989.

81. McKay JS, Targett MP, Jeffery ND: Histological characterization of an ependymoma in the fourth ventricle of a cat, *J Comp Pathol* 120:105, 1999.

82. Tremblay C, Girard C, Quesnel A, et al: Ventricular ependymoma in a cat, *Can Vet J* 39:719, 1998.

83. Knowlton FP: A case of tumor of the floor of the fourth ventricle with cerebellar symptoms in a cat, *Am J Physiol* 13:xx, 1905.

84. Verlinde JD, Ojemann JG: Eenige aangeboren misvormingen van het central zenuwstelsel, *Tijdschrift Voor Diergeneeskunde* 7:557, 1946.

85. Cox NR, Powers RD: Olfactory neuroblastomas in two cats, *Vet Pathol* 26:341, 1989.

86. Schrenzel MD, Higgins RJ, Hinrichs SH, et al: Type C retroviral expression in spontaneous feline olfactory neuroblastomas, *Acta Neuropathol* 80:547, 1990.

87. Cox NR, Brawner WR, Powers RD, et al: Tumors of the nose and paranasal sinuses in cats: 32 cases with comparison to a national database (1977 through 1987), *J Am Anim Hosp Assoc* 27:339, 1991.

88. Smith MO, Turrel JM, Bailey CS, et al: Neurologic abnormalities as the predominant signs of neoplasia of the nasal cavity in dogs and cats: seven cases (1973-1986), *J Am Vet Med Assoc* 195:242, 1989.

89. Barker J, Greenwood AG: Intracranial lymphoid tumor in a cat, *J Small Anim Pract* 14:15, 1973.

90. Fondevila D, Vilafranca M, Pumarola M: Primary central nervous system T-cell lymphoma in a cat, *Vet Pathol* 35:550, 1998.

91. Lapointe JM, Higgins RJ, Kortz GD, et al: Intravascular malignant T-cell lymphoma (malignant angioendotheliomatosis) in a cat, *Vet Pathol* 34:247, 1997.

92. Lane SB, Kornegay JN, Duncan JR, et al: Feline spinal lymphosarcoma: a retrospective evaluation of 23 cats, *J Vet Intern Med* 8:99, 1994.

93. Spodnick GJ, Berg J, Moore FM, et al: Spinal lymphoma in cats: 21 cases (1976-1989), *J Am Vet Med Assoc* 200:373, 1992.

94. Mayer MN, Greco DS, LaRue SM: Outcomes of pituitary tumor irradiation in cats, *J Vet Intern Med* 20:1151, 2006.

95. Ihle SL: Pituitary corticotroph macrotumors, *Vet Clin North Am Small Anim Pract* 27:287, 1997.

96. Davidson MG, Nasisse MP, Breitschwerdt EB, et al: Acute blindness associated with intracranial tumors in dogs and cats: eight cases (1984-1989), *J Am Vet Med Assoc* 199:755, 1991.

97. Peterson ME, Taylor RS, Greco DS, et al: Acromegaly in 14 cats, *J Vet Intern Med* 4:192, 1990.

98. Wallack ST, Wisner ER, Feldman EC: Mensuration of the pituitary gland from magnetic resonance images in 17 cats, *Vet Radiol Ultrasound* 44:278, 2003.

99. Abrams-Ogg AC, Holmberg DL, Stewart WA, et al: Acromegaly in a cat: diagnosis by magnetic resonance imaging and treatment by cryohypophysectomy, *Can Vet J* 34:682, 1993.

100. Daley CA, Zerbe CA, Schick RO, et al: Use of metyrapone to treat pituitary-dependent hyperadrenocorticism in a cat with large cutaneous wounds, *J Am Vet Med Assoc* 202:956, 1993.

101. Myers NC, Bruyette DS: Feline adrenocortical diseases: Part I—hyperadrenocorticism, *Semin Vet Med Surg (Small Anim)* 9:137, 1994.

102. Neiger R, Witt AL, Noble A, et al: Trilostane therapy for treatment of pituitary-dependent hyperadrenocorticism in 5 cats, *J Vet Intern Med* 18:160, 2004.

103. Nelson RW, Feldman EC, Smith MC: Hyperadrenocorticism in cats: seven cases (1978-1987), *J Am Vet Med Assoc* 193:245, 1988.

104. Schwedes CS: Mitotane (o,p'-DDD) treatment in a cat with hyperadrenocorticism, *J Small Anim Pract* 38:520, 1997.

105. Skelly BJ, Petrus D, Nicholls PK: Use of trilostane for the treatment of pituitary-dependent hyperadrenocorticism in a cat, *J Small Anim Pract* 44:269, 2003.

106. Watson PJ, Herrtage ME: Hyperadrenocorticism in six cats, *J Small Anim Pract* 39:175, 1998.

107. Negrin A, Bernardini M, Diana A, et al: Giant cell osteosarcoma in the calvarium of a cat, *Vet Pathol* 43:179, 2006.

108. Horowitz MB, Hall WA: Central nervous system germinomas. A review, *Arch Neurol* 48:652, 1991.

109. Chenier S, Quesnel A, Girard C: Intracranial teratoma and dermoid cyst in a kitten, *J Vet Diagn Invest* 10:381, 1998.

110. Atasever A, Kul O: Metastasis of a mammary carcinoma in the central nervous system of a cat, *Dtsch Tierarztl Wochenschr* 103:472, 1996.

111. O'Rourke MD, Geib LW: Endometrial adenocarcinoma in a cat, *Cornell Vet* 60:598, 1970.

112. Roels S, Ducatelle R: Malignant melanoma of the nictitating membrane in a cat *(Felis vulgaris)*, *J Comp Pathol* 119:189, 1998.

113. Moïse NS, Riis RC, Allison NM: Ocular manifestations of metastatic sweat gland adenocarcinoma in a cat, *J Am Vet Med Assoc* 180:1100, 1982.

CHAPTER

56 Gene Therapy for Lysosomal Storage Diseases

Charles H. Vite

Lysosomes and their enzymes degrade glycoproteins, polysaccharides, and complex lipids that have been taken into the cell by endocytosis or autophagy.[1] Diseases resulting from defective lysosomal function and from the lysosomal accumulation of their substrates are known as lysosomal storage diseases (LSDs). In most cases a genetic deficiency of a specific lysosomal enzyme's activity results in the accumulation of its specific substrate, causing cell swelling or cell death (Figure 56-1). In a small number of LSDs substrate storage occurs without defective lysosomal enzyme activity. In these cases a genetic deficiency of a structural protein, transporter protein, enzyme cofactor, or recognition marker is present, resulting in abnormal lysosomal function.

LSDs are inherited predominantly as autosomal recessive traits with the exception of two X-linked diseases: mucopolysaccharidosis II and Fabry disease.[2] Abnormalities of multiple organ systems occur. Central nervous system (CNS) dysfunction and neuropathology are common. In the majority of cases swollen neurons and/ or swollen glia can be identified histologically.[3,4] Evidence of neurodegeneration (Figure 56-2), including cell loss, ubiquitin and neurofilament inclusions, and astrogliosis may be found.[5,6] In some diseases toxic metabolites accumulate, resulting in large areas of necrosis.[7] In LSDs with secondary changes in ganglioside metabolism, meganeurites, neurite sprouting, and abnormal synaptic connections develop.[4,8-12] It remains unclear what effect cell swelling, neuronal degeneration and necrosis, sec-

ondary changes in gangliosides and other metabolites, and abnormal synaptic connections have on the development of the clinical signs of CNS dysfunction.

Over 45 different LSDs have been described in various species and no effective therapy exists to treat the majority of these diseases. A large number of murine and large animal models of LSDs have been identified with 12 described in cats.[13-15] All cats described thus far have been under 1 year of age. A brief review of clinical signs associated with these diseases in the cat is provided in the following and a detailed review of the specific LSDs also is provided in Chapter 51 in the fourth volume of this series.

ALPHA-MANNOSIDOSIS

Alpha-mannosidosis (AMD) is caused by deficient activity of lysosomal α-mannosidase (LAMAN) that results in defective glycoprotein degradation and the intracellular accumulation of mannose-rich oligosaccharides.[16,17] Disease in cats is characterized by progressive signs of cerebellar dysfunction, corneal and lenticular opacities, gingival hyperplasia, skeletal abnormalities, thymic aplasia, hepatomegaly, and polycystic kidneys (Figure 56-3).[18-22] The cDNA encoding lysosomal α-mannosidase (MANB) has been cloned, and disease in Persian cats is caused by a four base pair deletion in the α-mannosidase gene resulting in a frameshift and

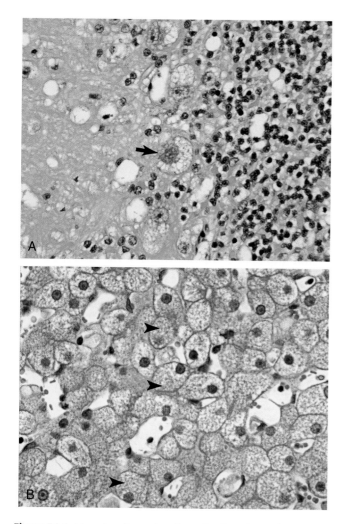

Figure 56-1 Hematoxylin and eosin–stained sections of cerebellum (**A**) and liver (**B**) showing severe dilatation of Purkinje cells *(arrow)* seen in feline alpha-mannosidosis and hepatocytes *(arrowheads)* seen in feline Niemann-Pick type C disease.

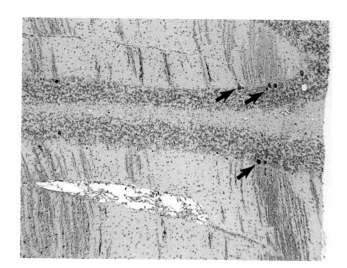

Figure 56-2 Calbindin-stained section of cerebellum of cat with Niemann-Pick type C. The number of Purkinje cell staining brown *(arrows)* is decreased greatly because of apoptotic cell loss.

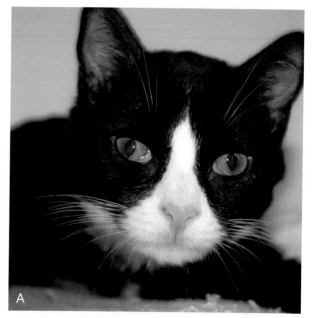

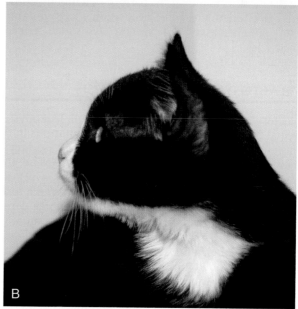

Figure 56-3 A and **B,** Cat with alpha-mannosidosis showing narrowed palpebral fissure, shortened nose, and corneal and lenticular opacities. **A** demonstrates the tremor seen evidenced by the lack of focus of the ear tips and whiskers.

premature termination.[23] The mutation in affected domestic longhair cats and in domestic shorthair cats has not been determined.[24,25] Neuropathological findings include vacuolated neurons, glial cells, and endothelial cells throughout the brain and spinal cord; Purkinje cell loss; and myelin deficiency of the CNS and peripheral nervous system (PNS).[18,19,21,22,24] Meganeurite, neurite sprouting, and axonal spheroids also are described.[26] Hepatocellular swelling occurs. The disease is diagnosed by assaying LAMAN activity in serum, white blood cells, or fibroblasts, or by testing for the known mutation.

NEURONAL CEROID LIPOFUSCINOSIS

Neuronal ceroid lipofuscinoses (NCL) are a group of at least eight distinct disorders (including Batten disease) caused by mutations in CLN genes (which produce both lysosomal enzymes and membrane-associated proteins) or the cathepsin D gene. The molecular and biochemical mechanisms leading to disease are not well understood.[27] NCL has been described in Siamese cats, Japanese domestic cats, and domestic shorthair cats in Europe.[28,29] Clinical signs included visual defects, ataxia, postural reaction deficits, myoclonus, and seizures in cats under 1 year of age. Brain atrophy, dilated cerebral ventricles, gliosis of the cerebral cortex and cerebellum, and loss of Purkinje cells are found. Cytoplasmic accumulation of autofluorescent material containing protein, lipid, and carbohydrate, occurs in the brain and other organs. Subunit C of mitochondrial ATP synthase is a major protein component of the stored material in most forms of NCL. The mutation resulting in NCL in cats has not been identified and diagnosis is made on the basis of signalment, clinical signs, electron microscopic evaluation of tissue, and—when present—assays of specific lysosomal enzyme deficiencies.

GALACTOSYLCERAMIDE LIPIDOSIS

Galactosylceramide lipidosis (globoid cell leukodystrophy [GLD]; Krabbe disease) is caused by mutations in the gene encoding galactosylceramidase (GALC) leading to accumulation of the toxic metabolite psychosine that results in destruction of oligodendroglia.[30,31] GLD has been described in domestic shorthair kittens and a longhaired kitten.[32-34] Clinical signs include dysmetria, generalized tremors, and paraplegia. Histological evaluation of the brain and spinal cord showed bilateral and symmetrical loss of myelin and axons, PAS-positive mononuclear cells (globoid cells), and astrogliosis. Globoid cells also may be found in the cerebrospinal fluid. Disease in cats has not been characterized enzymatically or genetically, and the diagnosis is made by clinical signs and measuring GALC activity in leukocytes or cultured fibroblasts.

GANGLIOSIDOSES

GM1 gangliosidosis is caused by a mutation in the gene encoding lysosomal acid beta-galactosidase resulting in the storage of the GM1 ganglioside and oligosaccharides. The disease has been described in Siamese cats, domestic shorthair cats, and Korat cats.[35-39] Affected kittens developed generalized tremors, dysmetria, spastic quadriplegia, blindness, and seizures. Microscopic analysis of the nervous system shows vacuolization of neurons in brain, retina, spinal cord, and ganglia; cerebellar Purkinje cell and granular cell loss; the development of meganeurites and abnormal synaptic connections; and diminished myelination. Hepatocellular vacuolation also occurs. The disease is diagnosed by measuring decreased enzyme activity in leukocytes, or by identification of the recently identified mutation of the GLB1 gene.[40]

GM2 gangliosidosis is caused by mutations in the genes encoding beta-hexosaminidase, HEXA and HEXB, or in the gene encoding the cofactor necessary for hydrolysis of GM2 ganglioside (GM2A). Defects in any of these three genes may result in the storage of GM2 ganglioside and associated disease. Three forms of GM2 gangliosidoses are described in human patients: Tay-Sachs disease (mutation in HEXA), Sandhoff disease (mutation in HEXB), and GM2 activator deficiency (caused by a mutation in GM2A).[41] GM2 gangliosidosis is homologous to Sandhoff disease and has been described in shorthaired cats and Korat cats.[42-46] Clinical signs in affected cats include corneal clouding, hypermetria, head tremors, seizures, and paralysis. Histological examination shows vacuolization of neurons and hepatocytes, and the development of meganeurites and abnormal synaptic connections.[47] Diagnosis is made by confirming decreased enzyme activity, or by identification of mutations that have been identified in both cat breeds.[45,48]

GLYCOGENOSES

Glycogen storage disease type II (acid maltase deficiency; Pompe disease) is caused by a mutation in the gene encoding acid alpha-glucosidase leading to the accumulation of glycogen in skeletal and cardiac muscle, as well as in other tissue.[49] Glycogen storage disease type II has been described in one cat.[50] No clinical abnormalities were described in this report. Histological evaluations showed cytoplasmic storage of glycogen in spinal cord neurons (the brain was not examined). Disease in cats has not been characterized enzymatically or genetically.

MUCOLIPIDOSIS

Mucolipidosis II (MLII; I-Cell disease) is caused by a defect in N-acetylglucosamine-1-phosphotransferase (GNPTA), which is responsible for the posttranslational addition of the mannose 6-phosphate recognition marker to lysosomal enzymes, a necessity for targeting the lysosomal enzyme to the lysosome. In MLII, lysosomal enzymes are not internalized in the lysosome and instead are secreted into the extracellular space. Affected cats show mental dullness, facial dysmorphia, retinal degeneration, skeletal abnormalities, paraparesis, and ataxia.[51-53] Light microscopic changes include widespread storage of material in fibroblasts, endothelial cells, cartilage, and heart valves. A missense point mutation in the GNPTA gene has been identified that results in a stop codon leading to premature termination of the coding sequence.[54]

MUCOPOLYSACCHARIDOSES

The mucopolysaccharidoses (MPS) are a group of lysosomal storage diseases caused by deficiencies of enzymes involved in the degradation of glycosaminoglycans (mucopolysaccharides). Multisystemic disease with or without nervous system dysfunction is described. Preliminary diagnosis of MPS disease is made by finding increased urinary excretion of glycosaminoglycans, and confirmed by finding decreased serum or tissue concentrations of the individual lysosomal enzymes.[55]

MPS I (Hurler, Scheie, and Hurler/Scheie syndromes) is caused by alpha-L-iduronidase (IDUA) deficiency resulting in storage of dermatan and heparan sulfates. MPS I cats show growth retardation, dysostosis multiplex, facial deformity, lameness, corneal opacity, and cardiac murmurs (Figure 56-4).[56-58] No measurable neurological dysfunction is present. Pathology includes multiple epiphyseal dysplasia, mitral valve thickening, and cytoplasmic vacuolization of neurons, hepatocytes, and other cell types. The diagnosis is made by finding low enzyme activity in leukocytes, or confirming the presence of the causative mutation, a three base pair deletion in the IDUA gene.[59]

MPS VI (Maroteaux-Lamy syndrome) is caused by deficient activity of N-acetylgalactosamine 4-sulfatase (arylsulfatase B) resulting in the storage of dermatan sulfate. Affected cats are dwarfed with facial deformity, corneal opacity, joint laxity and swelling, lameness, and fusion of the cervical and lumbar spine (Figure 56-5).[60-64] Histological findings include epiphyseal dysplasia and cytoplasmic vacuolization of many tissues. The CNS is not

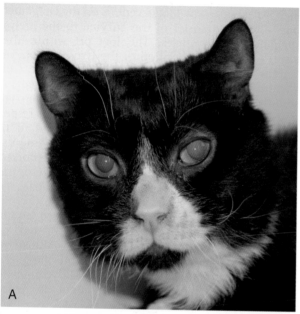

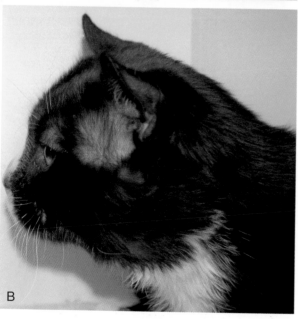

Figure 56-4 Cats with MPS I are similar to cats with other types of mucopolysaccharidosis, including small ears, widely-spaced eyes, shortened nose, and corneal clouding.

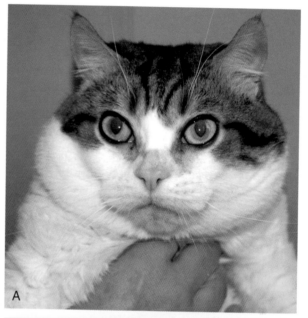

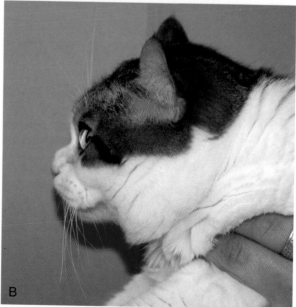

Figure 56-5 Cats with MPS VI are similar to cats with other types of mucopolysaccharidosis, including small ears, widely-spaced eyes, shortened nose, and corneal clouding. In this cat a depressed bridge of the nose, frontal bossing, and tearing caused by nasolacrimal duct occlusion also are evident.

involved. The causative mutation is a point mutation in the arylsulfatase B gene.

MPS VII (Sly syndrome) is caused by deficient beta-glucuronidase (GUSB) activity resulting in the storage of dermatan sulfate, heparan sulfate, and chondroitin 4-, 6-sulfates.[55] Clinical signs include growth retardation, facial and thoracic deformity, corneal opacity, joint swelling, lameness, and cardiac murmurs.[65] The gene encoding GUSB has been cloned in cats and the point mutation identified.[66]

SPHINGOMYELINOSES

Sphingomyelinoses types A and B (Niemann-Pick disease type A and B) are both caused by deficient activity of acid sphingomyelinase and the accumulation of sphingomyelin.[67] Affected Siamese cats with Niemann-Pick type A show tremors, ataxia, and pelvic limb weakness. Histopathological examination shows vacuolization of neurons, hepatocytes, and cells of the reticuloendothelial system.[68] Molecular characterization of the disease in cats has not been performed.

Niemann-Pick type C (sphingomyelinosis type C) is caused by a mutation in either the NPC1 or NPC2 gene.[69,70] The proteins NPC1 and NPC2 are critical for the movement of unesterified cholesterol and glycosphingolipids from the endosomal/lysosomal compartment to the Golgi apparatus, plasma membrane, and endoplasmic reticulum. NPC1 is a membrane-bound protein and NPC2 a soluble protein. Mutations in either gene result in the lysosomal accumulation of unesterified cholesterol and glycosphingolipids. Cats with NPC disease have a spontaneously-occurring missense mutation in NPC1 and show progressive signs of cerebellar dysfunction and hepatic disease (Figure 56-6).[71-76] Histological evaluation

shows Purkinje cell loss and storage of lipid in neurons, hepatocytes, and macrophages; ectopic dendritogenesis and axonal spheroid formation also occur.[77] Diagnosis is made by molecular testing for the known mutation, by identification of the intralysosomal storage of unesterified cholesterol, and/or biochemical evidence of impaired LDL-induced cholesterol esterification.

THERAPY OF LYSOSOMAL STORAGE DISEASES

Lysosomal hydrolases are synthesized as pre-proenzymes on endoplasmic reticulum–bound ribosomes, and modified to their functional form in the endoplasmic reticulum and Golgi apparatus. In the Golgi apparatus a mannose 6-phosphate (M6P) recognition marker is added, which is recognized by M6P receptors on the Golgi membrane, allowing transfer of the enzyme to the prelysosomal/endosomal vesicles. The low pH within these vesicles results in dissociation of the lysosomal enzyme from the receptor. The receptor recycles to the Golgi apparatus and the lysosomal enzyme is packaged into lysosomes.[78,79] A portion of the M6P-modified enzyme also is released into the extracellular space and is responsible for the lysosomal enzyme activity found in the extracellular space and in serum. Secreted enzyme may be endocytosed by cells expressing M6P receptors on their cell membrane. Intracellularly, the lysosomal enzyme dissociates from the receptor and is packaged into lysosomes.[79-81]

Therapeutic approaches for LSDs are based on this knowledge that lysosomal enzymes are secreted and endocytosed by neighboring cells, and can be transferred by direct cell-to-cell exchange.[82-84] Therefore the goal of therapy has been to deliver functioning M6P-conjugated enzyme to the enzyme-deficient patient in whom

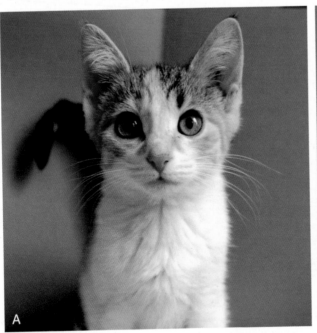
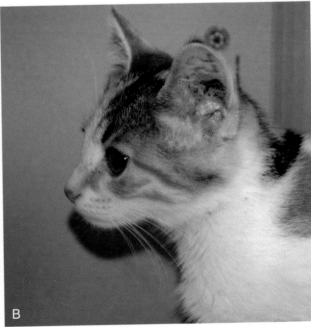

Figure 56-6 Cat with Niemann-Pick type C showing no evidence of facial dysmorphism.

receptor-mediated uptake of the normal lysosomal enzyme by diseased cells will result in correction of pathology. Three general treatment strategies have been developed: enzyme replacement therapy, heterologous cell or organ transplantation, and somatic gene transfer.

ENZYME REPLACEMENT THERAPY

Enzyme replacement therapy with recombinant glucocerebrosidase injections is a clinical success in the major form of human Gaucher disease, an LSD without CNS involvement.[85] However, in LSDs in which signs of CNS dysfunction are the predominant feature, intravenously administered enzyme appears incapable of crossing the blood-brain barrier in concentrations necessary to sufficiently treat the brain.[86] The drawbacks for enzyme replacement therapy include the need to produce the recombinant protein, the need for lifelong therapy, high cost, the development of antibodies to the enzyme, and incomplete response to therapy.

Enzyme replacement therapy with N-acetylgalactosamine-4-sulfatase has been used in the therapy of feline MPS VI and MPS I.[87-91] Affected MPS VI cats treated weekly from birth showed a reduction in urinary glycosaminoglycan concentrations and improvement in lysosomal storage in heart, aorta, skin, dura, liver, and perivascular cells of the brain. Therapy also resulted in improvement of bone pathology, improved mobility of the cervical spine, and less spinal cord compression. Treatment of six MPS I cats resulted in diminished glycosaminoglycan storage in liver and spleen and improvement in histological abnormalities. There was no improvement in CNS pathology.

HETEROLOGOUS CELL OR ORGAN TRANSPLANTATION

The rationale for treating LSD patients with cell or organ transplantation is based on the hypothesis that transplanted cells producing normal enzyme in enzyme-deficient recipients will provide a permanent, possibly self-replicating source of enzyme-producing cells that will secrete enzyme continuously into the extracellular space where it can be taken up by mutant cells. Treatment of neurological disease may occur from either small quantities of enzyme that cross the blood-brain barrier, or more likely from transplanted cells that establish themselves in the CNS and secrete lysosomal enzymes to treat neighboring cells.[92]

Two kinds of transplantation that have been examined are hematopoietic stem cell transplantation and direct intracranial implantation of neural progenitor cells, fibroblasts, and amniotic epithelial cells. Benefits compared with enzyme replacement include the need to potentially treat only one time and the expected correction of CNS disease through the ability of normal donor-derived monocytes to cross the blood-brain barrier and become microglia where they can secrete lysosomal enzymes to cross-correct mutant cells. Drawbacks to the use of transplantation to treat LSDs include the need for matched donor-recipient cells, high morbidity and mortality associated with the procedure, incomplete response to therapy, and high cost.

The most commonly performed method of hematopoietic stem cell transplantation is bone marrow transplantation (BMT). Several factors affect the success of BMT in patients with LSD including the type of disorder, the age of the recipient at the time of transplantation, the genotype of the donor and recipient, the degree of clinical disease at the time of transplant, the failure to achieve stable engraftment in some patients, and the development of graft-versus-host disease.[55] In general, therapy earlier in life is more effective than later in life, and CNS and bone disease are difficult to improve. In the feline model of AMD, BMT in three affected cats prevented the progression of neurological signs successfully, increased lifespan significantly, improved lysosomal α-mannosidase levels in the CNS, and corrected lysosomal storage in neurons throughout the brain.[93,94] In feline MPS I, BMT resulted in improved mobility, less severe skeletal deformities, and less pronounced facial dysmorphism. Increased iduronidase activity in liver and spleen; reduced GAG concentrations throughout the body including the brain; reduced ganglioside accumulation in the brain; and reduced storage in mononuclear cells of the brain, liver, kidney, and myocardium were seen.[95] In feline MPS VI, BMT resulted in some improvement in bone and joint lesions but did not have significant effect on the mechanical testing properties of bone.[96,97] Urinary glycosaminoglycan excretion was decreased.[98]

SOMATIC GENE TRANSFER

Somatic gene transfer involves placing a copy of a normal enzyme's cDNA into diseased cells thereby providing a source of normal enzyme to the cells.[99] Because lysosomal enzymes are secreted, transduced cells release normal enzyme into the extracellular space where nearby untransduced cells may internalize the protein through receptor-mediated endocytosis. Gene transfer may be performed using an ex vivo approach, in which cells are genetically modified outside of the body prior to transplantation in the patient, or by an in vivo approach in which cDNA is delivered directly into the patient's cells using a viral or liposomal vector. For CNS gene therapy in vivo vector-mediated gene transfer requires delivery of the vector across the blood-brain barrier.

Using a variety of viral vectors, including adenovirus, adeno-associated virus, lentivirus, and herpesvirus, several investigators have achieved significant enzyme expression in the brains of murine models by direct injection of these vectors into the brain.[99,100] The advantages of gene therapy include the potential for lifelong correction of disease following gene transfer. Drawbacks include the potential for immunologic reaction to the vector or protein, and the possibility of insertional mutagenesis.[101] Recently an increased incidence of hepatocellular carcinoma has been reported in several mouse studies following systemic administration.[99]

Recombinant adeno-associated virus (AAV) vectors are excellent for in vivo gene transfer to the CNS. They are nonpathogenic, can be produced in high titers, can infect the nondividing cells of the brain, and can result in long-term gene expression in the murine brain.[101] At least 12 primate AAV serotypes have been identified.[102] Specific AAV serotypes differ in the composition of their capsid proteins and in their ability to transduce different tissues. A comparison of the ability of three AAV serotypes (AAV1, AAV2, and AAV5) to transduce cells of the brain with the cDNA of beta-glucuronidase under the control of the human GUSB promoter was examined in the cat.[103] This study showed that AAV2 was capable of transducing cells of the gray matter, while the AAV1 vector resulted in greater transduction of the gray matter than AAV2 while also transducing cells of the white matter. Interestingly, in contrast to the mouse brain, AAV5 did not transduce cells of the cat brain. This study indicated that some AAV serotypes are more effective than others at transducing the cat brain, and that what may be most effective in mice may not be similarly effective in cats.

Six 8-week-old cats with AMD received six intracerebral injections of an AAV1 vector carrying the normal alpha-mannosidase cDNA (MANB) into each cerebral hemisphere and two injections into the cerebellum.[104] The treated cats were indistinguishable from age-matched untreated cats until approximately 12 weeks of age when treated cats stabilized or showed improvement in neurological function. Three cats did not develop a loss of balance, four did not develop a resting nystagmus, and none developed coarse whole body tremors. Surprisingly, all treated cats showed some improvement in clinical signs from 12 to 18 weeks of age. Intention tremor and truncal ataxia improved in three cats, and the fine whole body tremor improved in all treated cats. Although all 18-week-old treated cats were markedly improved compared with untreated age-matched cats, all treated cats continued to have a very mild truncal ataxia, a mild intermittent fine whole body tremor, and a short-strided gait. Untreated cats generally are euthanized at 18 weeks of age because of concerns for quality of life, and four treated cats were similarly euthanized at 18 weeks of age to compare histological changes. Of the two remaining treated cats, one was evaluated weekly until 30 weeks of age and one until 1 year of age. These two cats maintained the ability to walk with remarkably little tremor and ataxia (Figure 56-7).

Histological analysis of the brains of treated cats showed complete resolution of storage in neurons, glia, and endothelial cells up to 4.5 mm from the injection track, and up to 2 mm from cells producing MANB messenger RNA. While lysosomal storage increased as the distance from the needle track increased, no regions of the treated cat brain showed lysosomal storage as severe as that found in untreated AMD cats. Even in regions of the brain distant from the injection tracks, such as the occipital cortex, cells were not as swollen as those seen in untreated AMD cats. Myelination abnormalities also improved through the brains of treated cats. Finally, resolution of storage also could be seen in cells of the choroid plexus, ependyma, and meninges. Although disease was not cured in the treated cats, these studies suggested that

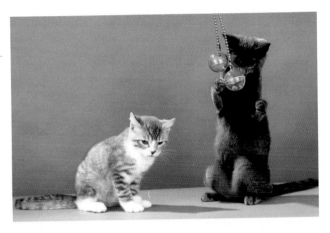

Figure 56-7 Untreated cat with alpha-mannosidosis on the left showing small stature, dropped carpi, and inactivity. AAV-MANB treated age-matched cat with alpha-mannosidosis on the right showing larger size and improved ability to play.

direct gene therapy to the brain could delay, ameliorate, or even improve disease in the cat.

Studies using AAV vectors to treat feline GM2 gangliosidoses and MPS VI also are reported. Recombinant AAV vectors carrying the cDNA of human beta-hexosaminidase alpha and beta subunit genes were delivered to the brain of affected cats, resulting in measurable enzyme expression in the injected hemisphere as well as in the contralateral hemisphere.[105] Therapy also resulted in decreased GM2 levels in the brain. Neonatal MPS VI cats injected intravenously or intramuscularly with AAV vectors containing feline aryl-sulfatase B cDNA showed high serum levels of enzyme, skeletal improvements, decreased glycosaminoglycan storage, as well as decreased inflammation and apoptosis.[106] Subretinal or intravitreal injection of an AAV vector containing feline 4-sulfatase resulted in significant improvement in retinal pigment epithelium inclusions and swelling.[107]

Retroviral vectors are capable of transducing dividing cells, can be pseudotyped, and integrate into the genome resulting in long-term transgene expression.[100] In veterinary medicine, the most substantial evidence of the efficacy of gene therapy is the intravenous administration of retroviral vectors to transfer the canine beta-glucuronidase cDNA into neonatal MPS VII dogs.[108] Therapy resulted in high serum GUSB activity, as well as marked improvement in growth and bone and joint abnormalities, resulting in the ability of treated MPS VII dogs to continue walking years after untreated dogs have lost this ability. Retroviral therapy of neonatal MPS I cats with canine alpha-iduronidase cDNA resulted in serum concentration of iduronidase up to eight times that of normal cats; however, this level dropped over time.[109] The decrease in enzyme activity over time likely was caused by a CTL response to transduced hepatocytes.[110] In vitro gene therapy using retroviral vectors also has been performed in cats. Treatment of MPS VI by transplantation of retrovirally transduced bone marrow (into the blood) and skin fibroblasts (into the renal capsule) has been attempted, but did not result in clinical improvement.[111,112]

Retroviral therapy is unlikely to be effective in transducing the nondividing cells of the brain. However, retroviral-mediated gene therapy of MPS VII dogs resulted in significantly decreased storage of glycosaminoglycan in CNS neurons, which is hypothesized to be caused by the very high serum activity of enzymes (eight times normal) that occurred in treated dogs (Haskins, personal communication). Additionally, in one study in MPS I dogs, neonatal intravenous administration of a retroviral vector carrying the canine IDUA cDNA resulted in marked reduction of glycosaminoglycan storage in the brain. Reduction in CNS storage in this study was postulated to be caused by very high serum IDUA activity (28 times normal) with the ability of a small amount of serum enzyme to cross the blood-brain barrier and correct neurons, or because of low gene expression in the brain.[113]

Integrating recombinant lentiviral vectors, using human immunodeficiency virus and feline immunodeficiency virus, and nonintegrating herpes virus vectors show promise for the therapy of CNS disease in murine models, with both successfully transducing neurons in murine models with expression of enzyme persisting over time. To date, however, there are no published data concerning their efficacy in the cat brain.

In summary, successful therapy of the CNS components of lysosomal storage diseases will require improved methods to deliver functioning enzyme to the brain. This may be possible through extraordinarily high serum concentrations of lysosomal enzyme or intrathecal administration/production of lysosomal enzyme. Additionally, methods to increase the ability of lysosomal enzymes or gene therapy vectors to cross the blood-brain barrier also are being developed.[99,114] It is hoped that the development of therapies for the lysosomal storage diseases may result in improved therapy of many other single gene disorders affecting the CNS. It is clear that at this time a tempered optimism for the future treatment of inherited CNS disease in patients is warranted.

ACKNOWLEDGMENT

Thanks to Dr. Mark Haskins for his critical review of the manuscript. Financial support was provided by Ara Parseghian Medical Research Foundation, Dana's Angels Research Trust, RR02512.

REFERENCES

1. Sabatini DD, Adesnik MB: The biogenesis of membranes and organelles. In Scriver CR, Beaudet AL, Sly WS, et al, editors: *Metabolic and molecular bases of inherited disease*, ed 8, New York, 2001, McGraw-Hill, p 3369.
2. Scriver CR, Beaudet AL, Sly WS, et al: *Metabolic and molecular bases of inherited disease*, ed 8, New York, 2001, McGraw-Hill.
3. Jolly RD, Walkley SU: Lysosomal storage diseases of animals: an essay in comparative pathology, *Vet Pathol* 34:527, 1997.
4. Walkley SU: Cellular pathology of lysosomal storage disorders, *Brain Path* 8:175, 1998.
5. Walkley SU, Baker HJ, Rattazzi MC, et al: Neuroaxonal dystrophy in neuronal storage disorders: evidence for major GABAergic neurons involvement, *J Neurol Sci* 104:1, 1991.
6. Heuer GG, Passini MA, Jiang K, et al: Selective neurodegeneration in murine mucopolysaccharidosis VII is progressive and reversible, *Ann Neurol* 52:762, 2002.
7. D'Agastino AN, Sayre GP, Hayles AB: Krabbe's disease, *Arch Neurol* 8:98, 1963.
8. Purpura DP, Suzuki K: Distortion of neuronal geometry and formation of aberrant synapses in neuronal storage disease, *Brain Res* 116:1, 1976.
9. Purpura DP, Baker HJ: Meganeurites and other aberrant processes of neurons in feline GM1-gangliosidosis: a Golgi study, *Brain Res* 143:13, 1978.
10. Walkley SU: Pathobiology of neuronal storage disease, *Intl Rev Neurobiol* 29:191, 1988.
11. Walkley SU, Wurzelmann S, Rattazzi MC, et al: Distribution of ectopic neurite growth and other geometrical distortions of CNS neurons in feline GM2 gangliosidosis, *Brain Res* 510:63, 1990.
12. Siegel DA, Walkley SU: Growth of ectopic dendrites on cortical pyramidal neurons in neuronal storage diseases correlates with abnormal accumulation of GM2 ganglioside, *J Neurochem* 62:1852, 1994.
13. Suzuki K, Mannson JE: Animal models of lysosomal storage disease: an overview, *J Inherit Metab Dis* 21:540, 1998.
14. Watson DJ, Wolfe JH: Lentiviral vectors for gene transfer to the central nervous system: applications in lysosomal storage disease animal models. In Machida C, editor: *Viral vectors for gene therapy: methods and protocols*, Totowa, NJ, 2002, Humana Press, p 383.
15. Ellinwood NM, Vite CH, Haskins ME: Gene therapy for lysosomal storage diseases: the lessons and promise of animal models, *J Gene Med* 6:481, 2004.
16. Michalski JC, Klein A: Glycoprotein lysosomal storage disorders: alpha-mannosidosis and beta-mannosidosis, fucosidosis, and alpha-N-acetylgalactosaminidase deficiency, *Biochim Biophys Acta* 1455:69, 1999.
17. Thomas GH: Disorders of glycoprotein degradation and structure: alpha-mannosidosis, beta-mannosidosis, fucosidosis, and sialidosis. In Scriver CR, Beaudet AL, Sly WS, et al, editors: *Metabolic and molecular bases of inherited disease*, ed 8, New York, 2001, McGraw-Hill, p 3507.
18. Vandevelde M, Fankhauser R, Bichsel P, et al: Hereditary neurovisceral mannosidosis associated with alpha-mannosidase deficiency in a family of Persian cats, *Acta Neuropathol* 58:64, 1982.
19. Jezyk PF, Haskins ME, Newman LR: Alpha-mannosidosis in a Persian cat, *J Am Vet Med Assoc* 189:1483, 1986.
20. Alroy J, Schunk KL, Ranghavan SS, et al: Alpha-mannosidase deficiency in Persian cats: a model of human alpha-mannosidosis. In Salvayre R, Douste-Blazy L, Gatt S, editors: *Lipid storage disorders*, 1988, Plenum Publishing, p 649.
21. Maenhout T, Kint JA, Dacremont G, et al: Mannosidosis in a litter of Persian cats, *Vet Rec* 122:351, 1988.
22. Vite CH, McGowan JC, Braund KG, et al: Histopathology, electrodiagnostic testing, and magnetic resonance imaging show significant peripheral and central nervous system myelin abnormalities in the cat model of alpha-mannosidosis, *J Neuropathol Exp Neurol* 60:817, 2001.
23. Berg T, Tollersrud OK, Walkley SU, et al: Purification of feline lysosomal alpha-mannosidase, determination of its cDNA sequence and identification of a mutation causing alpha-mannosidosis in Persian cats, *Biochem J* 328:863, 1997.
24. Cummings JF, Wood PA, de Lahunta A, et al: The clinical and pathologic heterogeneity of feline alpha-mannosidosis, *J Vet Intern Med* 2:163, 1988.
25. Blakemore WF: A case of mannosidosis in the cat: clinical and histopathological findings, *J Small Anim Pract* 27:447, 1986.

26. Walkley SU, Blakemore WF, Purpura DP: Alterations in neuron morphology in feline alpha-mannosidosis: a Golgi study, *Acta Neuropathol* 53:75, 1981.

27. Peltonen L, Hoffman SL: The neuronal ceroid lipofuscinoses. In Scriver C et al, editors: *Metabolic and molecular bases of inherited disease (OMMBID)*, New York, 2005, McGraw-Hill. Available at www.ommbid.com

28. Green PD, Little PB: Neuronal ceroid-lipofuscin storage in Siamese cats, *Can J Comp Med* 38:207, 1974.

29. Weissenbock H, Rossel C: Neuronal ceroid-lipofuscinosis in a domestic cat: clinical, morphological and immunohistochemical findings, *J Comp Path* 117:17, 1997.

30. Miyatake T, Suzuki K: Globoid cell leukodystrophy: additional deficiency of psychosine galactosidase, *Biochem Biophys Res Commun* 48:539, 1972.

31. Wenger DA, Suzuki K, Suzuki Y, et al: Galactosylceramide lipidosis: globoid cell leukodystrophy (Krabbe Disease). In Scriver CR, Beaudet AL, Sly WS, et al editors: *Metabolic and molecular bases of inherited disease*, ed 8, New York, 2001, McGraw-Hill, p 3669.

32. Johnson KH: Globoid leukodystrophy in the cat, *J Am Vet Med Assoc* 157:2057, 1970.

33. Salvadori C, Modenato M, Corlazzoli DS, et al: Clinicopathological features of globoid cell leukodystrophy in cats, *J Comp Pathol* 132:350, 2005.

34. Sigurdson CJ, Basaraba RJ, Mazzaferro EM, et al: Globoid cell-like leukodystrophy in a domestic longhaired cat, *Vet Pathol* 39:494, 2002.

35. Baker HJ Jr, Lindsey JR, McKhann GM, et al: Neuronal GM1 gangliosidosis in a Siamese cat with beta-galactosidase deficiency, *Science* 174:838, 1971.

36. Blakemore WF: GM-1 gangliosidosis in a cat, *J Comp Pathol* 82:179, 1972.

37. Purpura DP, Pappas GD, Baker HJ: Fine structure of meganeurites and secondary growth processes in feline GM1-gangliosidosis, *Brain Res* 143:1, 1978.

38. Purpura KP, Baker HJ: Neurite induction in mature cortical neurones in feline GM1-ganglioside storage disease, *Nature* 266:553, 1977.

39. Baker HJ, Mole JA, Lindsey JR, et al: Animal models of human ganglioside storage diseases, *Fed Proc* 35:1193, 1976.

40. Martin DR, Rigat BA, Foureman P, et al: Molecular consequences of the pathogenic mutation in feline GM1 gangliosidosis, *Mol Genet Metab* 94:212, 2008.

41. Gravel R, Kaback MM, Proia RL, et al: The GM2. In Scriver C et al, editors: *Metabolic and molecular bases of inherited disease (OMMBID)*, New York, 2005, McGraw-Hill. Available at *www.ommbid.com*

42. Cork LC, Munnell JF, Lorenz MD, et al: GM2 ganglioside lysosomal storage disease in cats with beta-hexosaminidase deficiency, *Science* 196:1014, 1977.

43. Cork LC, Munnell JF, Lorenz MD: The pathology of feline GM2 gangliosidosis, *Am J Pathol* 90:723, 1978.

44. Baker HJ, Reynolds GD, Walkley SU, et al: The gangliosidoses: comparative features and research applications, *Vet Pathol* 16:635, 1979.

45. Muldoon LL, Neuwelt EA, Pagel MA, et al: Characterization of the molecular defect in a feline model for type II GM2-gangliosidosis (Sandhoff disease), *Am J Pathol* 144:1109, 1994.

46. Neuwelt EA, Johnson WG, Blank NK, et al: Characterization of a new model of GM2-gangliosidosis (Sandhoff's disease) in Korat cats, *J Clin Invest* 76:482, 1985.

47. Walkley SU, Wurzelmann S, Rattazzi MC, et al: Distribution of ectopic neurite growth and other geometrical distortions of CNS neurons in feline GM2 gangliosidosis, *Brain Res* 510:63, 1990.

48. Martin DR, Krum BK, Varadarajan GS, et al: An inversion of 25 base pairs causes feline GM2 gangliosidosis variant, *Exp Neurol* 187:30, 2004.

49. Hirschhorn R, Reuser AJJ: Glycogen storage disease type II: acid a-glycosidase (acid maltase) deficiency. In Scriver C et al, editors: *Metabolic and molecular bases of inherited disease (OMMBID)*. www.ommbid.com. New York, 2005, McGraw-Hill.

50. Sandstrom B, Westman J, Ockerman PA: Glycogenosis of the central nervous system in the cat, *Acta Neuropathol* 14:194, 1969.

51. Bosshard NU, Hubler M, Arnold S, et al: Spontaneous mucolipidosis in a cat: an animal model of human I-cell disease, *Vet Pathol* 33:1, 1996.

52. Hubler M, Haskins ME, Arnold S, et al: Mucolipidosis type II in a domestic shorthair cat, *J Small Anim Pract* 37:435, 1996.

53. Mazrier H, van Hoeven M, Wang P, et al: Inheritance, biochemical abnormalities and clinical features of feline mucolipidosis II: the first animal model of human I-Cell disease, *J Heredity* 94:363, 2003.

54. Giger U, Tcherneva E, Caverly J, et al: A missense point mutation in N-acetylglucosamine-1-phosphotransferase causes mucolipidosis II in domestic shorthair cats, *J Vet Intern Med* 20:781, 2006.

55. Neufeld E, Muenzer E: The mucopolysaccharidoses. In Scriver C, et al, editors: *Metabolic and molecular bases of inherited disease (OMMBID)*. www.ommbid.com. New York, 2005, McGraw-Hill.

56. Haskins ME, Jezyk PF, Desnick RJ, et al: Alpha-L-iduronidase deficiency in a cat: a model of mucopolysaccharidosis I, *Pediatr Res* 13:1294, 1979.

57. Haskins ME, Jezyk PF, Desnick RJ, et al: Mucopolysaccharidosis in a domestic short-haired cat—a disease distinct from that seen in the Siamese cat, *J Am Vet Med Assoc* 175:384, 1979.

58. Haskins ME, McGrath JT: Meningiomas in young cats with mucopolysaccharidosis I, *J Neuropathol Exp Neurol* 42:664, 1983.

59. He X, Li CM, Simonaro CM, et al: Identification and characterization of the molecular lesion causing mucopolysaccharidosis type I in cats, *Mol Genet Metab* 106:67, 1999.

60. Cowell KR, Jezyk PF, Haskins ME, et al: Mucopolysaccharidosis in a cat, *J Am Vet Med Assoc* 169:334, 1976.

61. Di Natale P, Annella T, Daniele A, et al: Animal models for lysosomal storage diseases: a new case of feline mucopolysaccharidosis VI, *J Inherit Metab Dis* 15:17, 1992.

62. Haskins ME, Jezyk PF, Desnick RJ, et al: Animal model of human disease: mucopolysaccharidosis VI Maroteaux-Lamy syndrome, arylsulfatase B-deficient mucopolysaccharidosis in the Siamese cat, *Am J Pathol* 105:191, 1981.

63. Haskins ME, Jezyk PF, Patterson DF: Mucopolysaccharide storage disease in three families of cats with arylsulfatase B deficiency: leukocyte studies and carrier identification, *Pediatr Res* 13:1203, 1979.

64. Jezyk PF, Haskins ME, Patterson DF, et al: Mucopolysaccharidosis in a cat with arylsulfatase B deficiency: a model of Maroteaux-Lamy syndrome, *Science* 198:834, 1977.

65. Gitzelmann R, Bosshard NU, Superti-Furga A, et al: Feline mucopolysaccharidosis VII due to beta-glucuronidase deficiency, *Vet Pathol* 31:435, 1994.

66. Fyfe JC, Kurzhals RL, Lassaline ME, et al: Molecular basis of feline beta-glucuronidase deficiency: an animal model of mucopolysaccharidosis VII, *Genomics* 58:121, 1999.

67. Schuchman EH, Desnick RJ: Niemann-Pick disease types A and B: acid sphingomyelinase deficiencies. In Scriver C et al, eds: *Metabolic and molecular bases of inherited disease*

(OMMBID), New York, 2005, McGraw-Hill. Available at www.ommbid.com

68. Wenger DA, Sattler M, Kudoh T, et al: Niemann-Pick disease: a genetic model in Siamese cats, *Science* 208:1471, 1980.

69. Vanier MT, Millat G: Niemann-Pick disease type C, *Clin Genet* 64:269, 2003.

70. Carstea ED, Morris JA, Coleman KG, et al: Niemann-Pick C1 disease gene: homology to mediators of cholesterol homeostasis, *Science* 277:228, 1997.

71. Brown DE, Thrall MA, Walkley SU, et al: Feline Niemann-Pick disease type C, *Am J Pathol* 144:1412, 1994.

72. Lowenthal AC, Cummings JF, Wenger DA, et al: Feline sphingolipidosis resembling Niemann-Pick disease type C, *Acta Neuropathol* 81:189, 1990.

73. March PA, Thrall MA, Brown DE, et al: GABAergic neuroaxonal dystrophy and other cytopathological alterations in feline Niemann-Pick disease type C, *Acta Neuropathol* 94:164, 1997.

74. Somers KL, Royals MA, Carstea ED, et al: Mutation analysis of feline Niemann-Pick C1 disease, *Mol Genet Metab* 79:99, 2003.

75. Munana KR, Luttgen PJ, Thrall MA, et al: Neurological manifestations of Niemann-Pick disease type C in cats, *J Vet Intern Med* 8:117, 1994.

76. Vite CH, Ding W, Bryan C, et al: Clinical, electrophysiological, and serum biochemical measures of progressive neurological and hepatic dysfunction in feline Niemann-Pick type C disease, *Ped Res* 64:544, 2008.

77. Zervas M, Dobrenis K, Walkley SU: Neurons in Niemann-Pick disease type C accumulate gangliosides as well as unesterified cholesterol and undergo dendritic and axonal alterations, *J Neuropathol Exp Neurol* 60:49, 2001.

78. Waheed A, Hasilik A, von Figura K: Processing of phosphorylated recognition marker in lysosomal enzymes. Characterization and partial purification of a microsomal alpha-N-acetylglucosaminyl phosphodiesterase, *J Biol Chem* 256:5717, 1981.

79. Kornfeld S, Sly WS: Disorders of lysosomal enzyme phosphorylation and localization. In Scriver CR, Beaudet AL, Sly WS, et al, editors: *Metabolic and molecular bases of inherited disease*, ed 8, New York, 2001, McGraw Hill, p 3469.

80. Natowicz MR, Chi MM, Lowry OH, et al: Enzymatic identification of mannose 6-phosphate on the recognition marker for receptor-mediated pinocytosis of beta-glucuronidase by human fibroblasts, *Proc Natl Acad Sci USA* 76:4322, 1979.

81. Distler J, Hieber V, Sahagian G, et al: Identification of mannose 6-phosphate in glycoproteins that inhibit the assimilation of beta-galactosidase by fibroblasts, *Proc Natl Acad Sci USA* 76:4235, 1979.

82. Fratantoni JC, Hall CW, Neufeld EF: Hurler and Hunter syndromes: mutual correction of the defect in cultured fibroblasts, *Science* 162:570, 1968.

83. Sando GN, Neufeld EF: Recognition and receptor-mediated uptake of a lysosomal enzyme, alpha-L-iduronidase, by cultured human fibroblasts, *Cell* 12:619, 1977.

84. Olsen I, Dean MF, Harris G, et al: Direct transfer of a lysosomal enzyme from lymphoid cells to deficient fibroblasts, *Nature* 219:244, 1981.

85. Brady RO, Barton NW: Enzyme replacement therapy for Gaucher disease: critical investigations beyond demonstration of clinical efficacy, *Biochem Med Metab Biol* 52:1, 1994.

86. Sly WS, Vogler C: Brain-directed gene therapy for lysosomal storage disease: going well beyond the blood-brain barrier, *Proc Natl Acad Sci USA* 99:5760, 2002.

87. Crawley A, Niedzielski, K, Isaac EL, et al: Enzyme replacement therapy from birth in a feline model of mucopolysaccharidosis type VI, *J Clin Invest* 99:651, 1997.

88. Byers S, Nuttall JD, Crawley AC: Effect of enzyme replacement therapy on bone formation in a feline model of mucopolysaccharidosis type VI, *Bone* 21:425, 1997.

89. Bielicki J, Crawley A, Davey R: Advantages of using same species enzyme for replacement therapy in a feline model of mucopolysaccharidosis type VI, *J Biol Chem* 274:36335, 1999.

90. Auclair D, Hopwood JJ, Brooks DA, et al: Replacement therapy in mucopolysaccharidosis type VII: advantages of early onset of therapy, *Mol Genet Metab* 78:163, 2003.

91. Kakkis ED, Schuchman EH, He X, et al: Enzyme replacement therapy of feline mucopolysaccharidosis I, *Mol Genet Metab* 72:199, 2001.

92. Krivit W, Lockman LA, Watkins PA, et al: The future for treatment by bone marrow transplantation for adrenoleukodystrophy, metachromatic leukodystrophy, globoid cell leukodystrophy and Hurler syndrome, *J Inherit Metab Dis* 18:398, 1995.

93. Walkley SU, Thrall MA, Dobrenis K, et al: Bone marrow transplantation corrects the enzyme defect in neurons of the central nervous system in a lysosomal storage disease, *Proc Natl Acad Sci USA* 91:2970, 1994.

94. Thrall MA, Haskins ME: Bone marrow transplantation. In August JR, editor: *Consultations in feline internal medicine*, vol 3, Philadelphia, 1997, Saunders, p 514.

95. Ellinwood N, Colle M-A, Weil MA, et al: Bone marrow transplantation for feline MPSI, *Mol Genet Metab* 91:239, 2007.

96. Norrdin RW, Moffat KS, Thrall MA, et al: Characterization of osteopenia in feline mucopolysaccharidosis VI and evaluation of bone marrow transplantation therapy, *Bone* 14:361, 1993.

97. Norrdin RW, Simske SJ, Gaarde S, et al: Bone changes in mucopolysaccharidosis VI cats and the effects of bone marrow transplantation: mechanical testing of long bones, *Bone* 17:485, 1995.

98. Dial SM, Byrne T, Haskins M, et al: Urine glycosaminoglycan concentrations in mucopolysaccharidosis VI-affected cats following bone marrow transplantation or leukocyte infusion, *Clin Chim Acta* 263:1, 1997.

99. Sands MS, Haskins ME: CNS-directed gene therapy for lysosomal storage disease, *Acta Pediatrica* 97:22, 2008.

100. Ellinwood NM, Vite CH, Haskins ME: Gene therapy for lysosomal storage disease: the lessons and promise of animal models, *J Gene Med* 6:481, 2004.

101. Schultz BR, Chamberlain JS: Recombinant adeno-associated virus transduction and integration, *Mol Ther* 16:1189, 2007.

102. Gao G, Vandenberghe LH, Wilson JM: New recombinant serotypes of AAV vectors, *Cur Gene Ther* 5:285, 2005.

103. Vite CH, Passini MA, Haskins M, et al: AAV vector-mediated gene transfer for the cat brain, *Gene Ther* 10:1874, 2003.

104. Vite CH, McGowan JC, Niogi SN, et al: Effective gene therapy for an inherited CNS disease in a large animal model, *Ann Neurol* 57:355, 2005.

105. Martin DR, Baker HJ, Cox NR, et al: Gene therapy of feline gangliosidosis with AAV vectors, *Mol Genet Metab* 92:S14, 2007.

106. Tessitore A, Faella A, O'Malley T, et al: Biochemical, pathological, and skeletal improvement of mucopolysaccharidosis VI after gene therapy to liver but not muscle, *Mol Ther* 16:30, 2008.

107. Ho TT, Maguire AM, Aguirre GD, et al: Phenotypic rescue after adeno-associated virus-mediated delivery of 4-sulfatase to the retinal pigment epithelium of feline mucopolysaccharidosis VII, *J Gene Med* 4:613, 2002.

108. Ponder KP, Melniczek JR, Xu L, et al: Therapeutic neonatal hepatic gene transfer in mucopolysaccharidosis VII dogs, *Proc Natl Acad Sci USA* 99:13102, 2002.

109. Liu Y, Xu L, Ellinwood NM, et al: Neonatal retroviral-mediated gene therapy for MPSI mice and cats. 2004.

110. Ponder KP, Wang B, Wang P, et al: Mucopolysaccharidosis I cats mount a cytotoxic T lymphocyte response after neonatal gene therapy that can be blocked with CTLA4-Ig, *Mol Ther* 14:5, 2006.

111. Yogalingam G, Crawley A, Hopwood JJ, et al: Evaluation of fibroblast-mediated gene therapy in a feline model of mucopolysaccharidosis type VII, *Biochim Biophys Acta* 1453:284, 1999.

112. Simonaro CM, Haskins ME, Abkowitz JL, et al: Autologous transplantation of retrovirally transduced bone marrow or neonatal blood cells into cats can lead to long-term engraftment in the absence of myeloablation, *Gene Ther* 6:107, 1999.

113. Traas AM, Wang P, Ma X, et al: Correction of clinical manifestations of canine mucopolysaccharidosis I with neonatal retroviral vector gene therapy, *Mol Ther* 15:1423, 2007.

114. Shi N, Pardridge WM: Noninvasive gene targeting to the brain, *Proc Natl Acad Sci USA* 97:7567, 2000.

57 Tremor Syndromes

Joan R. Coates and Danielle M. Eifler

Tremor is a movement disorder characterized as involuntary hyperkinesias of regular repetitive movement oscillations around a joint.[1] Tremors can occur at rest or during voluntary movement and typically cease with sleep. Most tremors in animals occur during movement and are associated with diseases of cerebellum and basal nuclei and related pathways, or with a diffuse disease process affecting myelin.[2-4] However, lesions that cause tremor can be located in any region within the nervous and musculoskeletal systems (Figure 57-1). Often the cause of tremor in animals is related to an underlying systemic or neurological disease process and can be a hallmark clinical sign to a specific disease process.[5] Rarely in cats are tremors a stand-alone clinical entity, which brings forth the importance of performing complete physical and neurological examinations of cats. Tremor disorders in dogs are not uncommon and have been described in past reviews.[2,3,6] Tremors in cats have been characterized sporadically with specific disease processes in the veterinary literature. This chapter reviews tremor in cats with respect to classification, pathophysiology, and specific diseases and disorders. Clinical disease presentations for tremor are emphasized, as well as employing a systematic approach when determining an underlying cause of tremor.

CLASSIFICATION OF TREMOR

Tremors are characterized as repetitive, rhythmic, oscillatory, involuntary movements of the entire body or part of the body with regular amplitude and frequency.[7,8] Tremors occur as synchronous contractions of agonist and antagonist muscle groups. An important clinical feature of tremor is that the movement ceases during sleep.[1] As long as the dominant feature of the movement disorder is rhythmicity, it should be labeled as tremor.[7] Electromyography defines tremor as exhibiting biphasic, rhythmic bursts of electrical activity. There are many different classification schemes for tremor. Variables used when classifying tremor include rhythm, amplitude, frequency, anatomical localization, and relation to movement activity. In human beings the gold standard for tremor research still remains through clinical presentations and phenomenology.[7,8] Clinical disease entities associated with tremor are further separated based on the condition from which the tremor is elicited, additional findings on neurological examination, medical and family history, and tremor frequency.[9] However, tremor classification in animals still remains enigmatic. Tremor in animals is classified according to its anatomical distribution as well as frequency and amplitude during rest, posture maintenance, movement, and performance of specific tasks.[2,3,10] A recent article on classification of involuntary contractions in domestic animals categorized tremor as *repetitive myoclonus*.[11]

ANATOMICAL

Anatomically, tremors in domestic animals are localized (focal) or generalized.[6] A localized tremor in animals can involve the head or one limb or region. Head bob originates from the neck muscles and consists of rapid tremors of the head and neck that are motioned in a horizontal or vertical direction and often are idiopathic in nature in

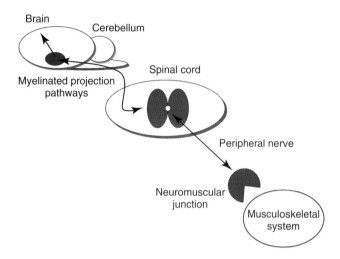

Figure 57-1 Schematic representation of the major components of the nervous system depicting structures involved in tremor generation.

dogs.[2] This tremor syndrome may have some similarity to a benign postural tremor in human beings referred to as essential tremor.[11] Limb tremors in animals more often are associated with neuromuscular disease weakness. Generalized tremors are caused by systemic disease processes related to degenerative diseases, myelin abnormalities, toxins, encephalitides, electrolyte disturbances, and idiopathic causes.

PHYSIOLOGICAL VERSUS PATHOLOGICAL

Founded on etiology, tremor types in human beings also are categorized as normal (physiological) or abnormal (pathological).[8] Physiological tremors occur in all contracting muscle groups and persist throughout the waking and sometimes sleep states. The movement is very fine and barely perceptible. Physiological tremor is elicited by holding the limb outstretched and can be a normal phenomenon. Physiological tremor may be caused by the influence of muscle spindle input, motor neurons, and muscle inertia. It is higher in frequency, in the range of 8 to 13 Hz.[8] Physiological tremor can be enhanced by fear or anxiety, drug effects, metabolic disturbances, and epinephrine. Enhanced physiological tremor also is included in the category of essential tremor. Mechanisms include stimulation of beta-adrenergic receptors by increased circulating levels of catecholamines.[12,13] Synchronization of motor units is influenced by central and peripheral nervous systems.

Abnormal or pathological tremor is used clinically and often affects specific muscle groups, and is classified based on electromyographic changes. Tremors in animals that are pathological are characterized by impairment of normal motor function.[2,6] During activation of a muscle group, the motor unit discharges independently in an attempt to maintain a posture or regulate the movement of a limb or body part. In a pathological state, the motor unit discharges become synchronized, the result being tremor. This rhythmic synchronization determines the

tremor amplitude and characteristic electromyographic pattern. Pathological tremor usually is preferential to certain muscle groups and the rate in most forms ranges between 4 and 7 Hz. Pathological tremors can be differentiated from physiological tremors by a greater amount of synchronization, thus greater amplitude and slower frequency.[8]

Pathological tremors are defined broadly as tremors at rest and during movement (action) (Table 57-1). Resting tremor is an involuntary rhythmic oscillation of part of the body that is not activated voluntarily and is supported against gravity.[1] In people, resting tremor usually is a manifestation of Parkinson syndrome and other diseases associated with the basal nuclei. Resting tremor will tend to decrease during voluntary movement. These tremors are low-amplitude oscillations with midrange frequency (3 to 5 Hz). Resting tremor is characterized electromyographically as alternating activity in agonist and antagonist muscles. Resting tremor has not been recognized in domestic animals. Horses with degeneration of the substantia nigra and globus pallidus caused by ingesting the toxin present in yellow star thistle, and the Kerry Blue Terrier and Chinese Crested dog with a neurodegenerative disease that affects the substantia nigra and caudate nuclei, have action-related tremor but not resting tremor.[14,15] This type of neurodegeneration has not been reported in cats.

An action tremor occurs during voluntary contraction of skeletal muscle. Action tremor refers to a tremor that is present when the limbs are actively maintained in certain positions and persists throughout active movement.[1] Action tremor is absent when limbs are relaxed and becomes evident when muscles become active. Action tremors often can appear as fine and fast oscillatory movements (5 to 8 Hz). In veterinary patients fine tremor more often is associated with diffuse neuromuscular disease weakness. Action tremor also is characterized by relatively rhythmic bursts of grouped motor neuron discharges that are not quite synchronous.

Action tremor is subclassified according to the activity produced by voluntary muscle contraction: postural, isometric, and kinetic tremor.[7] Types of action tremor also have been subdivided as postural tremor and intention tremor.[8] Postural-related tremors occur while any part of the body is maintained voluntarily against gravity. Essential tremor is a postural tremor characteristically present during maintenance of a position.[16-18] This tremor occurs as an alternating flexion-extension movement. In human beings essential tremor is the most common hyperkinetic movement disorder. Orthostatic tremor is highly dependent on posture especially during standing, causing cramping and uncontrollable shaking in the limbs.[19] Diagnostic criterion depends on confirmation of a high-frequency electromyographic recording pattern. The tremor activity will cease once the patient is lifted off the ground. Orthostatic tremor has been well described in dogs, but not recognized in cats.[20] Action tremors that are kinetic in nature occur during any voluntary movement. Kinetic tremor is subclassified as intention tremor or nonintention (simple kinetic) tremor.[7] Nonintention tremor occurs during any voluntary movement, but is not accentuated during goal-directed movements. Intention tremor

Table 57-1 Terminology for Tremor with Subclassification

Tremor Type	Definition	Frequency Hz
REST TREMOR	Tremor in a body part that is not voluntarily activated and completely supported against gravity	3-5
ACTION TREMOR	Tremor that is produced by voluntary muscle contraction—including postural, isometric, and kinetic	
Postural	Tremor that is present while voluntarily maintaining a position against gravity	5-8
Physiological	Present in normal joints or muscle that can oscillate	Distal joint: >7; Proximal joint: <4
Enhanced physiological	Postural tremor elicited by endogenous or exogenous causes	8-12
Essential	Postural tremor of hands and head	4-12
Orthostatic	Postural induced tremor of limbs during standing	>12
Kinetic	Tremor occurring during voluntary movement—including simple, intention and task specific	
Unspecified kinetic (simple)	Tremor that occurs during voluntary movements not target directed	3-10
Isometric	Tremor occurring as a result of muscle contraction against a stationary object	3-10
Intention	Tremor when amplitude increases during visually guided movements toward target at termination of movement	2-4
Task specific	Tremor may appear or become exacerbated during specific activities	3-10

Adapted from Deuschl G, Bain P, Brin M: Consensus statement of the Movement Disorder Society on Tremor, *Mov Disord* 13(Suppl 3):2, 1998.

is one of the most well-defined types of tremor in our veterinary patients. This type of kinetic action tremor occurs during purposeful voluntary movement,[21] becomes apparent during goal-directed movements, and is greatest at the termination of movement.[22] Intention tremors exhibit a high amplitude that fluctuates from beat to beat as the target goal is approached and a low frequency (<5 Hz) that is coarse. Afferent or efferent pathways of the cerebellum are the origin of the intention tremor. Some kinetic tremors may become exacerbated during specific activities; this is known as task-specific tremor. Isometric tremor occurs when muscles contract against a stationary object.

PATHOPHYSIOLOGY

The underlying basis for generation of tremor is spontaneous neuronal or axonal discharges in the central nervous system (CNS) and/or peripheral nervous system.[6] This increased excitability in animals often is caused by any disorder that interferes with normal myelination, ion channel function, electrolyte concentrations, and neurotransmission.[10] Systems that produce rhythmic activity are called oscillators; such nomenclature has been adapted for human research.[9] Oscillatory modes of neuronal behavior occur at all levels of the neuraxis that involve sensorimotor integration, motor timing, muscle coordination, and sympathetic control.[23] Pathological tremors are subclassified according to several oscillatory mechanisms that relate to generation of the tremor: mechanical oscillator of an extremity, reflex oscillators,

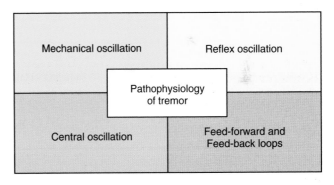

Figure 57-2 Schematic for four basic modes of oscillators involved in pathophysiology of tremor.

central oscillators, and feed-forward or feed-back loops[9] (Table 57-2 and Figure 57-2). Some disease processes may involve a combination of these mechanisms.

MECHANICAL OSCILLATION

Mechanical tremor occurs in the extremity muscles maintained against gravity and depends on the integrity of sensorimotor loops and limb mechanics.[21] This can be elicited as the limb is held in extension. The limb will oscillate with a resonance frequency caused by activation of muscle spindles and rhythmic contraction of motor units necessary to maintain limb position. Mechanical oscillators are influenced by cardioballistic (vibration secondary to cardiac activity) oscillations, unsteady

Table 57-2 Potential Pathophysiological Mechanisms of Diseases That Cause Tremors in Cats

Disease Category	Mechanical Oscillation of an Extremity	Reflex Oscillations	Central Oscillators	Feed-Forward or Feed-Back Loops
Degenerative	Motor neuron disease, hypertrophic polyneuropathy, Storage disease (Niemann-Pick disease), Devon Rex myopathy, Nemaline rod myopathy			Storage disorders—globoid cell leukodystrophy, alpha-mannosidosis, GM1 and GM2 gangliosidosis, glycogen storage disease type IV, Niemann-Pick disease type A and C, Lafora's disease; lysosomal storage disease in Abyssinian cats; cerebellar cortical abiotrophies; hypomyelination; dysmyelinopathies
Metabolic		Hyperthyroidism, hypoglycemia	Hypocalcemia (puerperal hypocalcemia, vitamin D-dependent rickets, hypoparathyroidism) Hypercalcemia (hyperparathyroidism) Hypokalemia (hyperthyroidism, renal failure, nutritional) Hyperkalemia	
Neoplasia				Primary and secondary intracranial tumors that involve the cerebellum
Immune	Myasthenia gravis			
Inflammatory	Polyradiculoneuritis; rabies			Feline infectious peritonitis; parvovirus; spongiform encephalopathy; toxoplasmosis
Toxic	Black widow spider envenomation; Nitenpyram toxicity	Methylphenidate toxicity	Pyrethrin toxicity; ivermectin toxicity; piperazine toxicity; D-limonene?; DEET?; 5-fluorouracil?	Bromethalin toxicity Mercury toxicity Metronidazole

postural innervations, and unfused contractions of single motor units. Mechanical oscillation is caused by any disease process that alters the motor unit resulting in weakness and tremors (neuropathic tremor). Neuropathic tremor occurs as an irregular postural and kinetic tremor presumably caused by loss of input from muscle-spindle afferents.[24,25] An action tremor of fast frequency can occur with some polyneuropathies. Neuropathy needs to be considered in patients presenting with isolated tremor along with abnormalities in electrophysiological studies.

Pathology of any part of the motor unit may manifest tremors as part of the clinical disease spectrum. Motor neuronopathies are disorders of the ventral horn cells that cause generalized weakness. Motor neuron loss results in progressive weakness with muscle atrophy. A characteristic feature of motor neuron disease that differs from peripheral neuropathy is muscular weakness and fasciculation with muscle atrophy, but preservation of

reflexes until the late stage of the disease.[26] Tremors are progressive and involve the head musculature predominately.[27] Peripheral neuropathies consist of disorders that affect the axon, axonopathies; the Schwann cells or myelin directly, myelinopathies (demyelinating diseases); or both the axons and Schwann cells, mixed axonal and demyelinating diseases. Neuropathic tremor is associated most frequently with demyelinating neuropathies.[1] The pathogenesis for generation of tremor is poorly understood. Myelin is essential for normal conduction of the nerve action potential. Axons lacking myelination may discharge spontaneously, associated with presence of high extracellular potassium levels and depolarization.[4] Another explanation may be abnormalities in cerebellar Purkinje cells in animals with myelin abnormalities.[4] Myelin deficiency most likely is seen as an action tremor and if severe, intention tremor. (Specific polyneuropathies in cats are described in detail in Chapter 50 of the fifth volume in this series.) Some storage diseases with predominant clinical and pathological findings of peripheral neuropathy will manifest tremor.[28] (See Chapter 51 in the fourth volume of this series, and Chapter 56 in this volume.)

REFLEX OSCILLATION

Tremors can be generated through reflex activation of oscillators in the CNS.[9,21] Any movement in one direction (i.e., flexion) will stretch the extensor muscles and cause a reflex activation of antagonistic muscles. This allows for smooth flexion of a joint so that there is no overshooting of the movement. Tremors can occur when the reflexively activated antagonistic muscle groups become synchronized excessively. This most often is because of situations or disease processes that cause activation of the sympathetic nervous system.[12] Tremors associated with mechanism of reflex oscillation are activated by posture movement. Hyperthyroidism can manifest tremor in cats through this mechanism.[29] A retrospective study reported 18 per cent of hyperthyroid cats exhibited signs of muscle tremor.[30,31] Thyroid hormone and epinephrine can upregulate the sensitivity of muscle spindles and enhance the rhythmic afferent activity leading to greater synchronization and enhanced reflex activity.[12] Cats with hyperthyroidism also may have hypocalcemia and hypokalemia that too can accentuate tremor-associated neuromuscular weakness.[32,33]

Hypoglycemia causes release of norepinephrine to stimulate gluconeogenesis.[34,35] The adrenergic response thereby increases synchronization of muscle spindles, resulting in tremor.[36] Adrenergic manifestations are evident when the onset of hypoglycemia is rapid. Other adrenergic signs include mydriasis, tachycardia, irritability, vocalization, and nervousness. Methylphenidate is a CNS stimulant used to treat hyperactivity in children, and its mechanism of action is to increase the release and decrease reuptake of norepinephrine and dopamine. Methylphenidate toxicity has been reported to cause tremor in a cat.[37] The cat presented with generalized tremor, vocalization, agitation, and hypersensitivity to external stimuli. The cat was treated symptomatically with diazepam and supportive care and clinical signs resolved within 24 hours.

CENTRAL OSCILLATION

Central oscillators have frequencies that are independent of limb mechanics.[21] Central oscillators are groups of cells in the CNS that have the capacity to fire repetitively. Two hypotheses have been proposed for mechanisms underlying central oscillations. The first is the rhythmic activity of a group of neurons within a nucleus. The second is that oscillations are generated within loops consisting of neuronal populations and their axonal connections. These connections promote neuronal activity through synapses that promote inhibitory or excitatory influences. Mechanisms that affect membrane conductance can result in tremor by activating central oscillators. Normally neurons fire randomly, but if their membrane conductance is altered so that their activity is synchronized, tremors can result.[8]

The resting membrane and threshold potential of a neuron is maintained by balances between sodium, potassium, calcium, and chloride.[38] Excess or depletion of these electrolytes can alter membrane conductance and influence central oscillators. Hyperchloridemia causes membrane hyperpolarization, lessening the likelihood for generation of an action potential. Hypercalcemia (>14 mg/dL) increases membrane threshold (increases necessary depolarization) resulting in hypoexcitability of the muscle membrane. Hypocalcemia (<7.5 mg/dL) causes membrane hyperexcitability by decreasing the membrane threshold (decreases amount of depolarization necessary for action potential). Hypokalemia (<3 mEq/L) increases the resting membrane potential, making the myofiber refractory to depolarization. Hyperkalemia (>6.5 mEq/L) decreases the resting membrane potential, resulting in hyperexcitability. Neurotransmitters also modulate membrane properties and the interactions among oscillating neurons.[21]

FEED-FORWARD AND FEED-BACK LOOPS

A fourth mechanism is malfunction of the feed-forward loops within the CNS, especially involving the cerebellum and feed-back information from the periphery.[9] The cerebellum is important in modulating control of fine motor activity. Cerebellar dysfunction can produce static and kinetic tremor within the classification of postural and intention tremor, respectively. Normally, rapid limb movements generated toward a goal-directed target are stopped by short burst muscle contractions from antagonist muscle groups.[39] If there are delays in loops controlling these actions, goal-directed movements also will be delayed and overshoot in an attempt to compensate.[40] These movements result in a coarse tremor generated at the proximal joints known as intention tremor. Cats with cerebellar dysfunction may exhibit this activity during eating or playing. The resting posture of an animal with cerebellar dysfunction may show broad-based stance with the thoracic and pelvic limbs and truncal ataxia. Titubation refers to forward and backward or side-to-side swaying motions (postural tremor) that occur with rostral cerebellar lesion involvement.[41] Fine tremors also may occur in the head and neck in animals with pure cerebellar dysfunction.[42,43] Tremor of cerebellar origin in cats may be associated with lateral cerebellar zone and vermal lesions.[43,44] Cerebellar dysfunction results from a number of primary cerebellar disorders (Box 57-1).

Unconscious proprioceptive feedback also is vital for cerebellar control of motor function. This information is conveyed by rapid conduction of heavily myelinated fibers. Moreover, any process that interferes with these heavily myelinated pathways can result in tremor that is activated by posture and goal-directed movements. During action the tremor at times may be so coarse as to resemble intention tremor of cerebellar disease.[4,45] Disorders of the peripheral nervous system that result in myelination may result from congenital, inherited, metabolic, inflammatory, and toxic etiologies.

Box 57-1 Primary Cerebellar Disorders in Cats Associated with Tremor

DEGENERATIVE
Lysosomal storage diseases, motor neuronopathy, myelinopathies, cerebellar cortical degeneration

ANOMALOUS
Cerebellar hypoplasia (parvovirus), epidermoid cysts

METABOLIC
Endocrine
Hyperthyroidism, hypoglycemia
Electrolyte Disturbances
Hypokalemia and hyperkalemia, hypocalcemia and hypercalcemia, hyponatremia and hypernatremia, hepatic encephalopathy

NEOPLASTIC
Meningioma, ependymoma, choroid plexus tumor

INFLAMMATORY (INFECTIOUS AND NONINFECTIOUS)
Feline panleukopenia, feline infectious peritonitis (noneffusive form), fungal disease, toxoplasmosis, polioencephalomyelitis, feline spongiform encephalopathy, idiopathic encephalomyelitis

TOXIC
Hexachlorophene, organophosphates, pyrethrins, metaldehyde, bromethalin, 5-fluorouracil, theobromine, strychnine, metronidazole, ivermectin

TRAUMA
Traumatic brain injury

VASCULAR
Thromboembolic disease

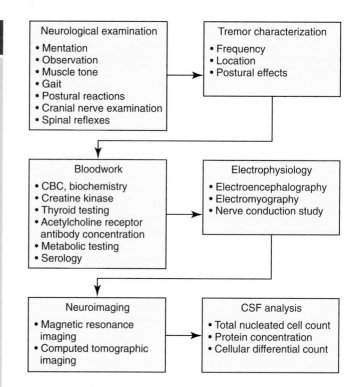

Figure 57-3 Flow diagram of the diagnostic approach for a patient with tremor.

DIAGNOSTIC APPROACH

Diagnosis of the underlying cause of tremor in cats requires thorough patient evaluation and a systematic approach (Figure 57-3).[10] Neurological examination will determine presence or absence of neurological disease and possible neuroanatomical localization (see Chapter 49 in the fifth volume of this series). It is important to exclude underlying causes of generalized weakness that may show clinical signs of tremor.[46] The patient is evaluated at rest, during maintenance of a static posture during standing and recumbency, and at gait (action). Muscle tone is evaluated at rest and during changes with posture and activity. Muscle tone represents the resistance to passive movement of a joint as seen in spasticity (increased tone in extensor muscles) and rigidity (increased tone in extensor and flexor muscles). Cats with neuromuscular weakness will manifest a plantigrade stance, and in severe weakness the thoracic limbs will be palmigrade. The muscles are visibly observed for any rippling or other spontaneous movements.

The character of the tremor is observed to determine rate and coarseness. Tremor is described according to its frequency: low (<4 Hz), medium (4 to 7 Hz), and high (>7 Hz).[7] Regions of the body are described based on localization: head, axial (proximal) musculature, and appendicular (distal) musculature. Fine tremors are high frequency and low amplitude, and are seen commonly with neuropathic tremor and neuromuscular weakness. Coarse tremors are low frequency and high amplitude, and are associated more commonly with intention tremor and cerebellar dysfunction. The tremor also is observed during voluntary movement for evidence of action tremor. With a stethoscope applied to the affected regions, the tremor can be auscultated for pitch and sound.[20] Tremors can be observed as the cat is lifted off the ground while relieving muscle contraction.

Gait integrates many of the neuroanatomical systems. The steppage is observed for dysmetria with relation to hypermetria and hypometria. The stride length is observed; long stride is characteristic of upper motor neuron dysfunction, whereas shortened stride is associated commonly with neuromuscular weakness. Postural reactions and cranial nerve examination further assist with determining functional impairment. Reflexes involving spinal and cranial nerves will assist with localization. Neuroanatomical localization is determined with careful consideration given to neuromuscular and cerebellar systems.

Results of complete blood count, serum biochemistry (including creatine kinase activity), and urinalysis are useful for screening other metabolic and systemic disease processes.[47] Electrolyte disturbances involving sodium,

Table 57-3 Documented Diseases in Cats Associated with Tremor and Elevated Creatine Kinase Activity

Disease	Severity of Creatine Kinase Elevation
DEGENERATIVE	
Inherited motor neuron disease	++
Nemaline rod myopathy	Normal to +
Niemann-Pick disease type A and phenotypic variant of type A	+
Glycogen storage disease type IV	+ to ++
Late-onset cerebellar abiotrophy	?
METABOLIC	
Hyperthyroidism	+ to ++
Hypoparathyroidism	++ to +++
Periparturient hypocalcemia	++ to +++
Hypokalemia	+ to +++
IMMUNE	
Myasthenia gravis	+ to ++
INFECTIOUS	
Toxoplasmosis	?
Feline immunodeficiency virus	+++
TOXIC	
Black widow spider envenomation	+++
Metronidazole toxicity	+++

+, Mild; ++, moderate; +++, severe; ?, elevated enzyme activity but degree not reported.

potassium, chloride, and calcium can result in neuromuscular weakness and tremor. Creatine kinase (CK) activity is useful for evaluating for evidence of myopathic disease and muscle damage (Table 57-3). CK activity may be elevated by muscle damage secondary to other underlying problems.[47] Elevations in CK may be mild to severe with some tremor disorders depending on the causative source of the myopathy.[48] Normal reference range for cats is less than 580 IU/L. Large increases or persistent increases are considered to be of clinical significance. In degenerative conditions the CK may be normal or only mildly elevated. Specific blood tests are used to evaluate for adrenal and thyroid dysfunction. Increased serum thyroxine (T_4) concentration will confirm hyperthyroidism. Acetylcholine receptor antibody concentration is a specific test for myasthenia gravis.[49] Exercise evaluation for underlying metabolic myopathy is conducted with serum lactate and pyruvate concentrations, but significance with myopathy in cats is unknown. Serology is performed for infectious disease testing.

Electrophysiological techniques are important in characterizing tremor and excluding other movement disorders. Electroencephalography can determine if the movement disorder is associated with a cortical event like seizure. Electrodiagnostic testing (see Chapter 50 in the third volume of this series) also supports disease associated with myopathy or neuropathy. Electromyography and nerve conduction studies assess function of the motor unit.[50] Electromyography evaluates muscle for spontaneous electrical discharge activity that can occur with primary myopathic disease or secondary to neuropathic disease. Motor nerve conduction studies evaluate for evidence of axonopathy and/or myelinopathy. Slow nerve conduction velocity occurs in demyelinating neuropathies. Histopathological examination of nerve and muscle is important in determining whether the underlying weakness is neurogenic or myopathic in origin.

Magnetic resonance imaging of the brain and cerebrospinal fluid analysis are performed to exclude structural brain abnormality as a potential cause of the tremor. Neuroimaging may show evidence of cerebellar atrophy or hypoplasia and abnormalities associated with demyelination in the CNS. Primary and secondary tumors that affect the basal ganglia or white matter pathways have been associated with tremor. Cerebrospinal fluid analysis will guide differential diagnoses toward inflammatory or infectious causes.

DIFFERENTIAL DIAGNOSIS

It often is helpful to approach differential diagnoses in a systemic way. The *D*egenerative, *A*nomalous, *M*etabolic, *N*eoplastic/*N*utritional, *I*atrogenic/*I*nflammatory/*I*diopathic/*I*mmune, *T*oxic/*T*raumatic, *V*ascular (DAMNITV) classification scheme has been used to categorize etiological diagnoses.[51] Signalment and regions of tremor involvement in cats will facilitate establishing a list of differential diagnoses (Figure 57-4). Major disease categories to consider for tremor in cats are degenerative, anomalous, metabolic, inflammatory, and toxic.

DEGENERATIVE

Motor Neuron Disease
Motor neuron disease is rare and usually occurs in young growing animals with an insidious and progressive clinical disease course of neuromuscular weakness. Cats show ventroflexion of the neck, dysphagia, progressive tetraparesis, and diffuse muscle atrophy. Inherited forms have been described in the Maine Coon cat[52] and an adult form has been reported in cats.[27] Spinal muscular atrophy in Maine Coon cats has been described as autosomal recessive disease, with onset of clinical signs at 4 months of age that include tremors and proximal muscle weakness.[52] A fine muscle tremor is most noticeable in the pelvic limbs. On histopathological examination, there was loss of motor neurons confined to the ventral horn of the spinal cord and Wallerian degeneration in the ventral roots. Adult-onset spinal muscular atrophy has age of onset between 6 and 12 years of age with a progressive course over months to years. Head tremor and tongue fasciculation were present in two cats. Diagnosis was confirmed at necropsy with the predominant pathology showing loss of motor neurons.[27]

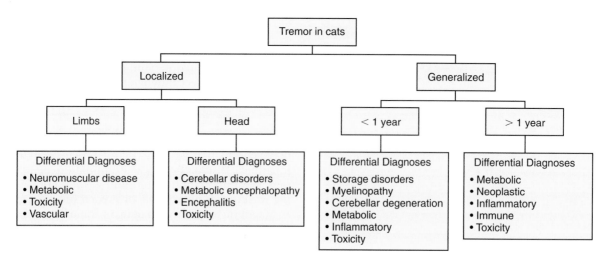

Figure 57-4 Differential diagnostic considerations for cats with tremor based on location and age.

Some degenerative myopathies in cats manifest tremor as a clinical sign of weakness.[53] Hereditary myopathy of Devon Rex cats manifests with generalized weakness and fatigue.[54] A localized head tremor develops during exercise. Cats with nemaline rod myopathy have shown continuous generalized tremor or localized tremor in the limbs and tail during ambulation.[55] These muscle disorders are described in more detail in Chapter 59.

Lysosomal Storage Diseases

Lysosomal storage diseases are characterized by accumulation of sphingolipids, glycolipids, oligosaccharides, or mucopolysaccharides within lysosomes.[56,57] Some lysosomal storage diseases can generate tremor from pathologies within the peripheral and central nervous systems. Peripheral nerve pathology in cats has been demonstrated in globoid cell leukodystrophy, Niemann-Pick type A, alpha-mannosidosis, and glycogen storage disease type IV.[57] Niemann-Pick disease, also called sphingomyelinosis or sphingomyelin lipidosis, is a group of lysosomal storage diseases characterized by accumulations of sphingomyelin caused by defect in the enzyme sphingomyelinase.[56] Type A, phenotypic variant of type A, and type C cause tremor via multiple mechanisms. Cuddon et al reported a phenotypic variant of Niemann-Pick disease type A with peripheral neuropathy in Siamese cats.[58] Phenotypic variant of type A is likely to cause tremor through mechanical oscillation. Fine, generalized muscle tremors are most pronounced during ambulation in the pelvic limbs and tail, and to a lesser extent in the thoracic limbs.[58] A mild head tremor also developed as the neurological signs progressed. Lower motor neuron weakness is evident on neurological examination. Electrodiagnostic studies reveal evidence of myelinopathy and axonopathy. Peripheral nerve changes on histopathological examination include widespread demyelination with many vacuolated macrophages, and the CNS also is mildly affected.

Type A and type C Niemann-Pick disease manifest clinical signs and pathological changes associated with the cerebellum. Tremor most likely is generated through the feed-forward and feed-back loop oscillation mecha-

nisms. However, because multiple areas of the nervous system are affected, other mechanisms could be responsible for tremor generation. Niemann-Pick disease type A has been reported in several cats including domestic shorthair, Siamese, and Balinese cats.[59-61] Affected cats show clinical signs between 3 and 7 months of age.[59,61] Continuous head bobbing has been noted, as well as conscious proprioceptive deficits, ataxia, hypermetria, loss of balance, and visual deficits. Neurological changes are most severe in the cerebellar Purkinje cells and ventral funiculi of the spinal cord.

Niemann-Pick disease type C is an autosomal recessive disorder that has been documented in domestic shorthair cats.[62-64] Signs are predominantly cerebellar in nature, with the first signs being an intention tremor of the head beginning between 6 and 12 months of age.[62] These tremors initially are not present at rest and involve only the head. The tremor progresses to generalized body tremor within 6 months of disease onset.[62,63] As the clinical signs progress to predominate as cerebellar and spinal cord dysfunction, the cats become more reluctant to ambulate. Histopathological findings include distension and vacuolation of neurons in the cerebellar nuclei, cerebral cortex, basal nuclei, red nuclei, vestibular nuclei, and spinal cord dorsal ventral ganglia and ventral horns. Presence of eosinophilic axonal spheroids (neuroaxonal dystrophy) is especially prominent in the cerebellar folia, and is considered the neurological hallmark of this disease.[63] Myelin loss also is noted in the spinocerebellar tracts in some cats, and this myelin loss most likely contributes to tremors in addition to the direct effects of substrate accumulation in the cerebellum. GABAergic neuroaxonal dystrophy may contribute to brain dysfunction.[65]

The GM1 and GM2 gangliosidoses are lysosomal storage diseases caused by accumulations of ganglioside resulting from a defect in the enzyme hexosaminidase A in GM1 gangliosidosis and β-hexosaminidase in GM2 gangliosidosis.[56] Although the clinical signs may vary depending on the type of gangliosidosis, tremors are a common feature as well as other signs of cerebellar dysfunction.[66] GM2 gangliosidosis variant O occurred in a family of Japanese cats[67] and a different form may have been observed in Korat and domestic cats in the United States.[68] In GM2 gangliosidosis variant O, there is a generalized body and head tremor. Histopathological examination reveals mild cerebral cortical atrophy and dilation of the lateral ventricles, and neurons in the cerebral cortex and cerebellum are distended with membranous cytoplasmic bodies.

A lysosomal storage disease has been described in Abyssinian cats that results in body tremors, incoordination, and occasionally seizures.[69,70] Affected cats have accumulations of phospholipid in lysosomes, although the exact nature of the storage disease has not been elucidated.

Lafora's disease has been documented in a 5-month-old spayed female Maine Coon cat.[71] This cat presented initially with brief and infrequent episodes of whole-body tremors and head bobbing. These episodes increased in frequency and severity to also include mentation changes. Histologically, Lafora bodies, which are deposits of polyglucosan, were found predominantly in the cerebellar Purkinje cells.

Glycogen Storage Diseases

Glycogen storage diseases are a heterogeneous group of inherited disorders characterized by deficient metabolism of glycogen, and by deposition of abnormal forms and quantities of glycogen.[72] Signs of peripheral nerve and muscle disease are common in the initial clinical course. Glycogen storage disease type IV is an inherited autosomal recessive disease seen in Norwegian Forest cats, caused by a deficiency in the glycogen branching enzyme α-1,4-D-glucan: α-1,4 glucan 6-glucosyl transferase.[73] Affected cats develop fever, fine generalized muscle tremors, bunny-hopping gait, and weakness at 5 months of age. The tremors may be very fine at rest, but can increase with exercise or cease with sleep.[74] Clinical signs progress to tetraplegia, muscle atrophy and joint contracture, and CNS involvement by 8 months of age. Hypoglycemia and seizure occur in the latter disease stage.[74] Tremor probably is generated through mechanical and feed-forward oscillation mechanisms. Elevated creatine kinase activity and abnormalities on electromyography support myopathic disease. Stored PAS-positive material is found in neurons of the CNS and peripheral nervous system. Nerve changes are characterized by severe axonal degeneration, presence of enlarged and vacuolated macrophages, fiber loss, and endoneurial fibrosis. Neurogenic atrophy is present with PAS-positive inclusions observed in muscle fibers, endomysium, and perimysium. Glycogen accumulation occurs in the Purkinje cells of the cerebellum, motor nuclei of the brainstem, spinal cord, and retinal ganglion cells.[75]

Abnormalities of Myelination

Abnormalities associated with congenital tremor have been reported in a number of domestic animals.[4] During development, axons may be thinly myelinated with normal myelin, known as hypomyelination, or myelin is abnormal with nonmyelinated axons, referred to as dysmyelination. Demyelination refers to breakdown and loss of normal myelin. Myelin is formed by oligodendrocytes in the CNS and Schwann cells in the peripheral nervous system. Severe myelin deficiency will manifest intention tremor and most often is congenital in origin.[4,76] Hypomyelination has been observed in two 4-week-old Siamese kittens.[77] These kittens developed progressive signs of whole-body action tremors and frenzied behavior with indiscriminate biting. The kittens were euthanized and postmortem examination revealed marked hypomyelination of the spinal cord. The ventral and lateral funiculi were affected most severely. Hypertrophic polyneuropathy in affects causes peripheral myelinopathy and pathology in spinal cord funiculi.[78,79] Clinical signs of hypertrophic polyneuropathy begin between 7 and 12 months of age and are progressive over several weeks. Cats have a generalized tremor that worsens with activity. Gait is described as ataxia and hypermetria. The pelvic limbs show a plantigrade stance and reduced spinal reflexes. Facial and limb sensation also are decreased. Postmortem findings include peripheral nerve thickening with sub-perineurial masses of mucoid material. Demyelination is present with normal axonal architecture. A defect in Schwann cells is suspected that results in an inability to form and maintain stable myelin.[78]

ANOMALOUS

Cerebellar Cortical Degeneration

Cerebellar cortical degeneration refers to degeneration and loss of Purkinje and granular cells within the cerebellar cortex that affect the architecture and function of the cerebellum.[80] Although there are several reports of cerebellar cortical degeneration and tremor in cats, the age of onset can vary. Early onset has been described in cats from Japan, with clinical signs observed initially between 6 to 8 weeks of age.[81,82] Tremors are observed as head and intention tremor.[81] Postmortem examination revealed cerebellar atrophy with loss of Purkinje cells. Early-onset cerebellar signs also were reported in three full-sibling kittens.[83] The kittens displayed intention tremors. The cerebellum was normal in size but there was loss of Purkinje cells. Later-onset progressive cerebellar cortical abiotrophy has been reported in a domestic shorthair cat[84] and Siamese cat[85] at 1.5 years of age. Intention tremor of the head was observed in the Siamese cat and more generalized tremor observed in the domestic shorthair cat. Depressed menace response and other central cerebellovestibular signs were present. Interestingly, in the domestic shorthair cat there was retinal degeneration that consisted of severe loss of both rod and cone photoreceptors.[84] Histopathological examination in both breeds revealed loss of Purkinje cells in the cerebellar cortex.

Feline parvovirus, also called feline panleukopenia virus, results in cerebellar hypoplasia in developing fetuses and in kittens infected or exposed to vaccination late in gestation or early in postnatal life while the cerebellum is developing.[86] Intention tremor involving the head is common. Other cerebellar signs include a broad-based stance and ataxia that are nonprogressive. Severity of clinical signs can vary among kittens in the litter. On postmortem examination, the cerebellum is hypoplastic. The hemispheres and dorsal portion of the vermis are the areas affected most commonly.[87-89] There often is loss of the external germinal cell layer and Purkinje cells. Other brain malformations such as hydrocephalus and hydranencephaly have been noted in some instances.[90] Affected kittens with less severe clinical signs can compensate over time.

Descriptions of other degenerative cerebellar disease–induced tremor are reviewed elsewhere and in Chapter 53 of the fourth volume of this series.[91,92]

METABOLIC

Tremors associated with metabolic conditions tend to be episodic and of irregular frequency.[6] Electrolyte, glucose, and acid-base imbalances can cause tremor for which underlying causes need to be investigated. Clinical signs of tremor can predominate with hypocalcemia along with fasciculation and tetany. Cats who undergo bilateral thyroidectomy and iatrogenic removal of the parathyroid glands are susceptible to hypocalcemia.[93] Eclampsia (hypocalcemia) is thought to occur most commonly at peak lactation in queens nursing large litters, but it also can occur during pregnancy within 3 to 17 days of parturition.[94] Rare disorders that cause hypocalcemia in cats include primary hypoparathyroidism and vitamin D–dependent rickets type 2.

Hypokalemia can result from a variety of diseases, and although it does alter nerve membrane conductance, it also can result in a primary polymyopathy (see Chapter 59). Decreased serum levels of potassium caused by several underlying conditions can result in generalized muscle weakness and tremors in cats. Decreased extracellular potassium causes a reduction in membrane sensitivity by increasing the resting membrane potential.[33] One of the most common clinical signs of hypokalemia is ventroflexion of the neck (see Figures 59-1, *A* and *B*). Hypokalemia can occur secondary to underlying diseases such as hyperthyroidism and renal failure.[32,33] Cats fed a vegetarian diet presented with muscle tremors of head and pinnae presumed to be caused by hypokalemia.[95] Clinical signs associated with hypokalemia often resolve after potassium supplementation.

Endocrine disease can cause tremor by affecting central and mechanical oscillators. Tremors have been described in association with several endocrine disorders in cats.[29] Hyperthyroidism in cats causes tremors and other clinical signs of neuromuscular weakness.[30,96] Clinical signs resolve after return to a euthyroid state. Hypoglycemia is a secondary complication of insulin overdose in management of diabetes mellitus in cats.[97] Rapid decreases of blood glucose result in adrenergic response with signs that include tremor. Glycogen depletion can be observed in kittens.[36]

NEOPLASTIC

Neoplasia of any area of the CNS has the potential to cause tremor. Specifically, neoplasia of the cerebellum will manifest intention tremor more commonly. Common cerebellar neoplasms in cats include meningioma, lymphosarcoma, and ependymoma (see Chapter 55).

INFLAMMATORY

Tremor as a clinical presentation has been reported in an 18-month-old female Siamese cat with polyradiculoneuritis.[97a] The cat presented with a 6-month history of pseudohypermetria, ataxia, muscle twitching, and sensory loss. Muscle twitching was evident in the head and limbs. Generalized fine tremors developed and waxed and waned in severity. On necropsy examination, polyradiculoneuritis involved both ventral and dorsal nerve roots. Mechanical oscillation is suspected in tremor generation.

There have been various reports of tremors in cats infected with feline infectious peritonitis (FIP) virus. Neurological abnormalities are seen in 12.5 per cent of cats with FIP and are seen more commonly in cats with the noneffusive form.[98,99] Ataxia related to vestibular dysfunction is the most common neurological sign. Intention tremor and fine head tremor have been associated with cerebellar and meningeal disease. The FIP-inducing coronavirus induces a vasculitis involving the meninges, ependymal lining, and choroid plexus. Focal facial seizures also may be mistaken for muscle tremors in cats with FIP.[98,100]

Neurological abnormalities are a predominant feature of cats infected with feline immunodeficiency virus (FIV), in approximately 5 per cent of cases.[101] Tremors associated with FIV include intention tremors as well as twitching movements of the face and tongue.[101] Behavioral changes such as fearful behavior, aggression, loss of house training, and compulsive roaming are manifested most frequently. Other neurological signs include seizures, myopathy, paresis, and disruption of sleep patterns.[102]

Although rabies is not associated commonly with tremors, they may be observed in infected cats. Cats most often present with the furious form of rabies and they may appear anxious, may stare, attempt to bite or scratch, run continuously, and can show weakness or incoordination. Generalized shaking, trembling, and muscle tremors may be seen in addition to these clinical signs.[103]

Toxoplasmosis usually results in subclinical disease in cats, but can result in neurological abnormalities and other systemic signs.[104,105] Clinical signs will vary depending on the organ affected. Tremors have been reported, as well as ear twitching and head bobbing. Central nervous system infection can be manifested as blindness, behavioral changes, incoordination, mentation changes, anisocoria, and seizures.

Spongiform encephalopathy has been reported to cause tremor in cats. A 7-year-old spayed female domestic shorthair cat presented for a 4-month history of progressive aggressive behavioral changes.[106] The cat had persistent tremors and severe ataxia in the pelvic limbs. Muscle tremors were abolished with supportive care, but abnormal behavior persisted. The cat continued to deteriorate and developed hypermetria in the pelvic limbs. Intention tremor of the head also developed. Histopathological examination revealed diffuse vacuolation of the neuropil and neuronal cell bodies most marked in the frontal lobe of the cerebral cortex. Because of the lack of plaques that are associated with transmissibility, it is unclear if this is a true example of transmissible spongiform encephalopathy. Spongiform encephalopathy also was reported in an 8-month-old female domestic shorthair cat who presented with a 2-week history of generalized ataxia and lethargy.[107] Head tremors were observed. Neurological examination also revealed head tilt, cervical spine ventroflexion, tetraparesis, and visual deficits. Histopathological examination revealed generalized vacuolation of the grey matter of the brain and spinal cord. (See Chapter 8 in the fourth volume of this series for further discussion of the spongiform encephalopathies.)

IMMUNE-MEDIATED

Myasthenia gravis is a common neuromuscular junction disease in cats.[49] Myasthenia gravis is characterized by failure of neuromuscular transmission caused by reduction in nicotinic cholinergic receptors on the postsynaptic membrane. Both congenital and acquired forms have been reported. Acquired myasthenia gravis is caused by production of antibodies directed against acetylcholine receptors. Tremor has been recognized in cats with myasthenia gravis and presumably is caused by muscle weakness.[108] Affected cats also can show short choppy stride, voice change, cervical spinal ventroflexion, and regurgitation. Myasthenia gravis in cats has been reviewed previously in Chapter 48 of the fourth volume of this series.

TOXIC

Exogenous toxins can generate tremor through multiple mechanisms.[109] Toxins may exert effects at the neuromuscular junction through increased release of acetylcholine and increased receptor stimulation and subsequent muscular fatigue. Other toxins can cause imbalances of neurotransmitters in the CNS to cause tremor. In particular, neurotoxic agents that stimulate the CNS will manifest signs of hyperactivity, hyperesthesia, muscle tremor and fasciculation, and behavioral changes. Toxicants affecting the autonomic nervous system induce clinical signs by interference with cholinergic neurotransmission. Stimulation of the cholinergic neurotransmission will result in bronchoconstriction, muscle tremors, exocrine gland stimulation, bradycardia, and other CNS effects. Blockade of cholinergic neurotransmission depends on the type of cholinergic receptor involved. Muscarinic receptor blockade causes salivation, lacrimation, bronchial secretion, vomiting, and diarrhea. Nicotinic blockage results in skeletal muscle paralysis and often tremor. Mixed signs also include CNS depression, seizures, miosis, and hyperactivity. Toxins like bromethalin and hexachlorophene affect myelin, causing intramyelinic edema and altering conduction of the action potential.

Toxins that have effects at the neuromuscular junction and autonomic nervous system activate tremor by mechanical oscillation mechanisms. Central nervous system stimulants such as chocolate, amphetamines, and caffeine are phosphodiesterase inhibitors and often will cause clinical signs of tremor. Organophosphates potentiate effects of acetylcholine at the neuromuscular junction by binding acetylcholinesterase. Tremor and fascicula-

tion associated with muscle weakness occur as depolarizing neuromuscular junction blockade effects take place.[110] Delayed distal symmetrical neuropathy associated with organophosphate toxicity in cats can occur 1 to 4 weeks after exposure as a result of neuronal esterase.[111-113] Atropine is used to counteract the muscarinic effects of the organophosphate. Diphenhydramine has been used as an adjunctive therapy to counteract the neuromuscular nicotinic effects although its use has been considered controversial.[114] Another case involving a cat with chronic organophosphate toxicity reported worsening of tremor intensity with diphenhydramine administration that resolved with discontinuation of the drug.[115] Enzyme reactivators and muscle relaxants can help to reduce signs of tremor. Determination of reduced cholinesterase activity in cats is of questionable prognostic value owing to presence of the pseudocholinesterase enzyme comprising a large portion of the total blood esterase activity.

Black widow spider envenomation causes clinical signs characterized initially by spasticity and later (12 to 24 hours) by profound muscle weakness and flaccidity.[116] The neurotoxin α-latrotoxin exerts its effects at the neuromuscular junction through release of acetylcholine and norepinephrine from nerve terminals of the autonomic and somatic nervous systems. The initial spasm and pain is associated with excessive release of acetylcholine and continuous end-plate potentials. Tremor may be generated from both reflex and mechanical oscillation mechanisms. The flaccid paralysis is a result of irreversible neuromuscular junction blockade and destruction of motor endplates. Biochemical abnormalities can include hypokalemia, hyperglycemia, hypocalcemia, and azotemia. Muscle enzyme elevations are observed with aspartate aminotransferase and creatine kinase.

Pyrethrins and pyrethroid insecticides alter both sodium and chloride conductance causing tremor. Class I and II pyrethrins and pyrethroid compounds act on gated sodium channels in nerve and muscle causing persistent depolarization and failure of membrane repolarization.[117,118] Class II pyrethroids inhibit binding of GABA to the $GABA_A$ receptor, which prevents influx of chloride. This causes further membrane depolarization and blockade of action potential and failure of membrane repolarization. Young cats are affected more frequently. Clinical signs include hyperexcitability, seizures, and muscle weakness manifesting as tremors and fasciculation.[119,120] Permethrin is a synthetic pyrethroid insecticide and neurotoxicant. Cats are deficient in glucuronyl transferase and lack the glucuronidation mechanism to metabolize permethrins, making them particularly sensitive. Hyperesthesia, generalized tremors, muscle fasciculations, hyperthermia, and seizures are common signs observed in affected cats.[121] A study reported that 34 per cent of cats with permethrin toxicity had tremors lasting up to 32 hours.[122] Respiratory distress can ensue secondary to muscle weakness.

Tremor also may be mediated by overstimulation of the GABA-related chloride channel. Ivermectin is an anthelmintic agent that stimulates the $GABA_A$ channel to enhance chloride conductance causing neuromuscular blockade in parasites. Large dosage of ivermectin in cats can cause generalized tremor and other clinical signs including vocalization, ataxia, anorexia, dementia, bradycardia, and death.[123] Piperazine, an anthelmintic, also is a GABA agonist enhancing chloride conductance and membrane hyperpolarization. Toxic effects in cats include head and neck tremors, muscular weakness, seizures, hyperesthesia, tetany, myoclonus, and mydriasis.[123] Metronidazole is an antibiotic, antiprotozoal agent that is lipophilic readily penetrating the blood-brain barrier. Metronidazole toxicity can cause tremor in cats, although more common neurological signs include ataxia, blindness, hyperactivity, vestibular signs, altered mentation, and seizures.[124] The exact mechanism by which metronidazole exerts its toxic effects on the CNS are poorly understood, but may include binding of ribonucleic acid (RNA) and inhibition of protein synthesis leading to axonal degeneration. Metronidazole also may exert its effects through the GABA receptors within the cerebellum and vestibular systems.[125] Histopathological examination in a cat with metronidazole administration revealed multifocal areas of necrosis in the brainstem.[126]

Toxins can alter CNS myelination and generate tremor through feed-forward and feed-back loop oscillation mechanisms resulting in postural and intention tremor. Both bromethalin and hexachlorophene are toxins that result in intramyelinic edema and demyelination.[127,128] Bromethalin is a rodenticide that uncouples oxidative phosphorylation depleting cellular adenosine triphosphate (ATP).[109] Cats mainly exhibit facial tremors.[128] Other clinical signs in cats include ataxia, conscious proprioceptive deficits, paresis/paralysis, depression that can progress to stupor, focal or generalized seizures, decerebrate posture, and vocalization.[129] Histopathological findings are present in the central nervous system, and consist of hypertrophied astrocytes and oligodendrocytes with diffuse spongiosis of the white matter, mild microgliosis, and optic nerve vacuolization.[130] Hexachlorophene toxicity has been reported in a 2-week-old female kitten who received undiluted topical hexachlorophene over a 2-week period.[127] After 14 days the kitten developed hypothermia, tachycardia, tachypnea, dyspnea, white mucous membranes, and muscle tremors. Histopathological examination revealed spongiosis in the cerebral and cerebellar white matter.

Experimentally, mercury has been demonstrated to result in intention tremors and fine tremors of the ears in cats.[131] Other signs of toxicity included anorexia, apprehension, ataxia, hypermetria, jaw chomping, mydriasis, and generalized seizures. Pathological changes include neuronal degeneration and perivascular cuffing in the cerebral cortex, loss of cerebellar granular and Purkinje cells, and demyelination in the dorsal funiculus.[131,132]

Other toxins known to cause tremor in cats with mixed mechanisms include D-limonene, diethyltoluamide (DEET), toluene and chlorophen-based anthelmintics, and 5-fluorouracil. Adverse effects of 5-fluorouracil in animals can include seizures, hyperesthesia, hyperexcitability, nervousness, muscle tremors, and cerebellar ataxia.[133] Toluene and dichlorophen-based anthelmintics cause tremor in cats by unknown mechanisms of toxicity.[134]

TREATMENT

Potential clinical complications associated with prolonged tremor include hyperthermia, hypoglycemia, dehydration, and anorexia. The goal for the control of tremors in animals is to determine the cause, remove any inciting cause, and provide immediate and prolonged symptomatic treatment for acquired diseases.[10] Toxic, metabolic, and iatrogenic causes are important differential diagnoses for acute-onset tremor. Electrolyte imbalances and other metabolic disorders are treated symptomatically and by managing the underlying disease process.

Treatment for tremor-induced neurotoxicity primarily involves basic life support, seizure control, modification of toxicant kinetics (absorption, distribution, metabolism, and excretion), and antagonism of pharmacological effects.[135,136] Specific pharmacological therapeutic regimens for use in cats often are extrapolated from those used in dogs. The affected cat should be removed from inciting environmental toxins. Often a dark, quiet room is necessary to remove external stimuli associated with CNS stimulants (e.g., strychnine, bromethalin). Bathing is indicated if there has been topical exposure. Toxins causing spasticity can be counterbalanced with use of muscle relaxants. Diazepam (0.25 to 1.0 mg/kg IV or per rectum) is a centrally acting muscle relaxant and can relieve acute-onset tremor disorders. However, diazepam should be avoided in cats with organophosphate toxicity because it may potentiate muscle tremor, and other muscarinic signs.[110] Methocarbamol, also a centrally acting muscle relaxant, can be administered. Phenobarbital (1 to 2 mg/kg PO q12h) is an anticonvulsant that can counterbalance disorders that alter the GABA receptor in central pathways and also manage associated seizures. Use of β-adrenergic blocking agents may alleviate reflex oscillation caused by hyperthyroidism and other enhanced physiological tremor. Adrenergic β2 receptors are located on both intrafusal and extrafusal muscle fibers and in central pathways.

Frequent patient monitoring and other measures of supportive care are important. Fluid therapy maintains electrolyte concentration and normovolemia. Oxygenation, blood pressure, electrolytes, and glucose should be monitored. In severe cases of respiratory muscle weakness, assisted ventilation may be necessary.

MOVEMENT DISORDERS THAT MIMIC TREMOR

Other hyperkinetic movement disorders may mimic tremor syndrome. *Shivering-shuddering* is a temporary disturbance occurring under conditions such as hypothermia and emotional stress.[137] *Fasciculation* is visible as irregular movements over the surface of the affected muscle caused by spontaneous contractions of individual motor units suggestive of a lower motor neuron lesion.[1] Muscle fasciculations do not produce rhythmic limb or body movements as seen with tremor. Fasciculation is common in motor neuron disease. *Myoclonus* is an involuntary jerk-like movement caused by a muscle contraction or inhibition in one area of the body and does not stop during sleep. Myoclonus is caused by lesions at various areas of the CNS that alter pattern generation and can be focal or generalized.[11] *Seizure* is a paroxysmal disorder that is a positive movement defect that must be differentiated from tremor and myoclonus.

Some movement disorders are associated with increased muscle tone. *Myokymia* refers to involuntary spontaneous, localized, transient, or persistent movements that affect a few muscle bundles within a single muscle.[1] These movements usually are coarser, slower, more prolonged, and involve a wider area than fasciculations. Movements associated with myokymia have been described as rippling and vermicular (worm-like) and also may appear as tremor. Myokymia is not affected by motion and can persist during sleep. Myokymia can be generalized or focal. *Neuromyotonia* is characterized by muscle stiffness and persistent contraction.[1] Recent studies link myokymia and neuromyotonia to antibodies directed against the voltage-gated potassium channels that result in prolonged depolarization and hyperexcitability. As more calcium enters the nerve terminal, it causes release of more acetylcholine and interference with repolarization. Myokymia and neuromyotonia have been reported in a domestic shorthair cat.[138] *Spasms* are involuntary contractions of a muscle or group of muscles. Prolonged spasm may cause reflex rigidity or may be followed by muscle contracture. Prolonged and severe muscle spasms occur in tetany and tetanus.[139] *Tetany* is a period of sustained muscular contraction without periods of relaxation.[1] The term tetanus is associated with the toxic effects of *Clostridium tetani*. *Myotonia* is a sustained contraction of muscles caused by ion channel defects in the muscle membrane. Congenital myotonia has been described in domestic shorthaired kittens.[140,141]

REFERENCES

1. Ropper AH, Brown RH: Tremor, myoclonus, focal dystonias, and tics. In Ropper AH, Brown RH, editors: *Adams and Victor's principles of neurology*, New York, 2005, McGraw-Hill, p 80.
2. Bagley RS: Tremor syndromes in dogs: diagnosis and treatment, *J Small Anim Pract* 33:485, 1991.
3. Cuddon PA: Tremor syndromes, *Prog Vet Neurol* 1:285, 1990.
4. Duncan ID: Abnormalities of myelination of the central nervous system associated with congenital tremor, *J Vet Intern Med* 1:10, 1987.
5. Wagner SO, Podell M, Fenner WR: Generalized tremors in dogs: 24 cases, *J Am Vet Med Assoc* 211:731, 1997.
6. Bagley RS: Tremor and involuntary movements. In Platt SR, Olby NJ, editors: *BSAVA manual of canine and feline neurology*, ed 3, Gloucester, 2004, British Small Animal Veterinary Association, Woodrow House, p 189.
7. Deuschl G, Bain P, Brin M: Consensus statement of the movement disorder society on tremor, *Mov Disord* 13:2, 1998.
8. Jankovic J, Fahn S: Physiologic and pathologic tremors, *Ann Intern Med* 93:460, 1980.
9. Deuschl G, Raethjen J, Lindemann M: The pathophysiology of tremor, *Muscle Nerve* 24:716, 2001.
10. Podell M: Tremor, fasciculations, and movement disorders, *Vet Clin North Am Small Anim Pract* 34:1435, 2004.
11. de Lahunta A, Glass EN, Kent M: Classifying involuntary muscle contractions, *Compend Contin Educ Pract Vet* 28:516, 2006.
12. Marsden CD, Meadows JC: The effect of adrenaline on the contraction of human muscle—one mechanism whereby adrenaline increases the amplitude of physiological tremor, *J Physiol (Lond)* 194:70P, 1968.
13. Marsden CD, Foley TH, Owen DAL, et al: The influence of noradrenaline, tyramine and activation of sympathetic nerves on physiologic tremor in man, *Clin Sci* 33:53, 1967.
14. de Lahunta A, Averill DRJ: Hereditary cerebellar cortical and extrapyramidal nuclear abiotrophy in Kerry Blue Terriers, *J Am Vet Med Assoc* 168:1119, 1976.
15. O'Brien DP, Johnson GS, Schnable RD, et al: Genetic mapping of canine multisystem degeneration and ectodermal dysplasia loci, *J Heredity* 96:727, 2005.
16. Metzer WS: Essential tremor: an overview, *J Ark Med Soc* 90:587, 1994.
17. Deuschl G, Wezelburger R, Raethjen J: Tremor, *Curr Opin Neurol Neurosurg* 13:437, 2000.
18. Lorenz D, Deuschl G: Update on pathogenesis and treatment of essential tremor, *Curr Opin Neurol* 20:447, 2007.
19. Thompson PD, Rothwell JC, Day BL, et al: The physiology of orthostatic tremor, *Arch Neurol* 43:584, 1986.
20. Garosi LS, Rossmeisl JH, de Lahunta A, et al: Primary orthostatic tremor in Great Danes, *J Vet Intern Med* 19:606, 2005.
21. Elble RJ: Central mechanisms of tremor, *J Clin Neurophysiol* 13:133, 1996.
22. Sanes JN, Le Witt PA, Mauritz KH: Visual and mechanical control of postural and kinetic tremor in cerebellar system disorders, *J Neurol Neurosurg Psychiatry* 51:933, 1998.
23. Welsh JP, Lang EJ, Sugihara I, et al: Dynamic organization of motor control within the olivocerebellar system, *Nature* 374:453, 1995.
24. Adams RD, Shahani BT, Young RR: Tremor in association with polyneuropathy, *Trans Am Neurol Assoc* 97:44, 1972.
25. Shahani BT, Young RR, Adams RD: Neuropathic tremor: evidence on the site of the lesion, *Electroencephalogr Clin Neurophysiol* 34:800, 1973.
26. Olby N: Motor neuron disease: inherited and acquired, *Vet Clin North Am Small Anim Pract* 34:1403, 2004.
27. Shelton GD, Hopkins AL, Ginn PE, et al: Adult-onset motor neuron disease in three cats, *J Am Vet Med Assoc* 212:1271, 1998.
28. Coates JR, O'Brien DP: Inherited peripheral neuropathies in dogs and cats, *Vet Clin North Am Small Anim Pract* 34:1361, 2004.
29. LeCouteur RA, Dow SW, Sisson AF: Metabolic and endocrine myopathies of dogs and cats, *Semin Vet Med Surg (Small Anim)* 4:146, 1989.
30. Peterson ME, Kintzer PP, Cavanagh PG: Feline hyperthyroidism: pretreatment, clinical and laboratory evaluation of 131 cases, *J Am Vet Med Assoc* 183:103, 1983.
31. Peterson ME, Gamble DA: Effect of nonthyroidal illness on serum thyroxine concentrations in cats: 494 cases (1988), *J Am Vet Med Assoc* 197:1203, 1990.
32. Dow SW, Fettman MJ, Curtis CR, et al: Hypokalemia in cats: 186 cases (1984-1987), *J Am Vet Med Assoc* 194:1604, 1989.
33. Nemzek JA, Kruger JM, Walshaw R, et al: Acute onset of hypokalemia and muscular weakness in four hyperthyroid cats, *J Am Vet Med Assoc* 205:65, 1994.
34. Braund KG: Endogenous causes of neuropathies in dogs and cats, *Vet Med* Aug:740, 1996.
35. Walters PC, Drobatz KJ: Hypoglycemia, *Compend Contin Educ Pract Vet* 14:1150, 1992.

36. Howerton TL, Shell LG: Neurologic manifestations of altered serum glucose, *Prog Vet Neurol* 3:57, 1992.

37. Gustafson BW: Methylphenidate toxicosis in a cat, *J Am Vet Med Assoc* 208:1052, 1996.

38. Shelton GD: Disorders of neuromuscular transmission, *Semin Vet Med Surg (Small Anim)* 4:126, 1989.

39. Hallett M, Berardelli A, Matheson J, et al: Physiological analysis of simple rapid movements in patients with cerebellar deficits, *J Neurol Neurosurg Psychiatry* 54:124, 1991.

40. Findley LJ: Classification of tremors, *J Clin Neurophysiol* 13:122, 1996.

41. Mauritz KH, Dichgans J, Hufschmidt A: Quantitative analysis of stance in late cortical cerebellar atrophy of the anterior lobe and other forms of cerebellar ataxia, *Brain* 102:461, 1979.

42. Botterell EH, Fulton JF: Functional localization in the cerebellum of primates: III. Lesion of hemispheres (neocerebellum), *J Comp Neurol* 69:63, 1938.

43. Holliday TA: Clinical signs of acute and chronic experimental lesions of the cerebellum, *Vet Sci Comm* 3:259, 1980.

44. Kornegay JN: Cerebellar vermian hypoplasia in dogs, *Vet Pathol* 23:374, 1986.

45. Victor M, Ropper AH: Diseases of the peripheral nerves. In Victor M, Ropper AH, editors: *Adams and Victor's principles of neurology*, ed 8, New York, 2005, McGraw-Hill, p 1110.

46. Dickinson PJ, LeCouteur RA: Feline neuromuscular disorders, *Vet Clin North Am Small Anim Pract* 34:1307, 2004.

47. Platt SR, Garosi LS: Neuromuscular weakness and collapse, *Vet Clin North Am Small Anim Pract* 34:1281, 2004.

48. Cardinet GH III: Skeletal muscle function. In Kaneko JJ, editor: *Clinical biochemistry of domestic animals*, San Diego, 1997, Academic Press, p 407.

49. Shelton GD, Ho M, Kass PH: Risk factors for acquired myasthenia gravis in cats: 105 cases (1986-1998), *J Am Vet Med Assoc* 216:55, 2000.

50. Cuddon PA: Electrophysiology in neuromuscular disease, *Vet Clin North Am Small Anim Pract* 32:31, 2002.

51. Lorenz MD, Kornegay JN: Localization of lesions in the nervous system. In Lorenz MD, Kornegay JN, editors: *Handbook of veterinary neurology*, ed 4, Philadelphia, 2004, Elsevier Science, p 45.

52. He Q, Lowrie C, Shelton GD, et al: Inherited motor neuron disease in domestic cats: a model of spinal muscular atrophy, *Pediatr Res* 57:324, 2005.

53. Shelton GD, Engvall E: Canine and feline models of human inherited muscle diseases, *Neuromuscul Disord* 15:127, 2005.

54. Malik R, Mepstead K, Yang F, et al: Hereditary myopathy of Devon Rex cats, *J Small Anim Pract* 34:539, 1993.

55. Cooper BJ, de Lahunta A, Gallagher EA: Nemalin myopathy of cats, *Muscle Nerve* 9:618, 1986.

56. Jolly RD, Walkley SU: Lysosomal storage disease of animals: an essay in comparative pathology, *Vet Pathol* 34:527, 1997.

57. March PA: Neuronal storage disorders. In August JR, editor: *Consultations in feline internal medicine*, vol 4, Philadelphia, 2001, Saunders, p 393.

58. Cuddon PA, Higgins RJ, Duncan ID, et al: Polyneuropathy in feline Niemann-Pick disease, *Brain* 112:1429, 1989.

59. Baker HJ, Wood PA, Wenger DA, et al: Sphingomyelin lipidosis in a cat, *Vet Pathol* 24:386, 1987.

60. Wenger DA, Sattler M, Kudoh T, et al: Niemann-Pick disease: a genetic model in Siamese cats, *Science* 208:1471, 1980.

61. Snyder SP, Kingston RS, Wenger DA: Animal model of human disease. Niemann-Pick disease. Sphingomyelinosis of Siamese cats, *Am J Pathol* 108:252, 1982.

62. Lowenthal AC, Cummings JF, Wenger DA, et al: Feline sphingolipidosis resembling Niemann-Pick disease type C, *Acta Neuropathol (Berl)* 81:189, 1990.

63. Muñana KR, Luttgen PJ, Thrall MA, et al: Neurological manifestations of Niemann-Pick disease type C in cats, *J Vet Intern Med* 8:117, 1994.

64. Brown DE, Thrall MA, Walkley SU, et al: Feline Niemann-Pick disease type C, *Am J Pathol* 144:1412, 1994.

65. March PA, Thrall MA, Brown DE, et al: GABAergic neuroaxonal dystrophy and other cytopathological alterations in feline Niemann-Pick disease type C, *Acta Neuropathol* 94:164, 1997.

66. Baker HJ, Walkley SU, Rattazzi MC, et al: Feline gangliosidoses as models of human lysosomal storage diseases. In Desnick RJ, Patterson DF, Scarpelli DG, editors: *Animal models of inherited metabolic diseases*, New York, 1982, Alan R. Liss Inc, p 203.

67. Yamato O, Matsunaga S, Takata K, et al: GM2-gangliosidosis variant 0 (Sandhoff-like disease) in a family of Japanese domestic cats, *Vet Rec* 155:739, 2004.

68. Neuwelt EA, Johnson WG, Blank NK, et al: Characterization of a new model of GM$_2$-gangliosidosis (Sandhoff's disease) in Korat cats, *J Clin Invest* 76:482, 1985.

69. Berg PB, Baker MK, Lange AL: A suspected lysosomal storage disease in Abyssinian cats. Part I. Genetic, clinical and clinical pathological aspects, *J South Afr Vet Assoc* 48:195, 1997.

70. Lange AL, Berg PB, Baker MK: A suspected lysosomal storage disease in Abyssinian cats. Part II. Histopathological and ultrastructural aspects, *J South Afr Vet Assoc* 48:201, 1977.

71. Hall DG, Steffens WL, Lassiter L: Lafora bodies associated with neurologic signs in a cat, *Vet Pathol* 35:218, 1998.

72. Hers HG, Van Hoof F, de Barsy T: Glycogen storage disease. In Scriver CR, Beaudet AL, Sly WS, et al, editors: *The metabolic basis of inherited disease*, New York, 1989, McGraw-Hill.

73. Fyfe JC, Giger U, Van Winkle TJ, et al: Glycogen storage disease type IV: inherited deficiency of branching enzyme activity in cats, *Pediatr Res* 32:719, 1992.

74. Coates JR, Paxton R, Cox NR, et al: A case presentation and discussion of Type IV glycogen storage disease in a Norwegian Forest cat, *Prog Vet Neurol* 7:5, 1996.

75. Fyfe JC, Van Winkle TJ, Haskins ME, et al: Animal model of human disease. Glycogen storage disease type IV, *Comp Path Bulletin* 26:3, 1994.

76. Mayhew IG, Blakemore WF, Palmer AC, et al: Tremor syndrome and hypomyelination in Lurcher pups, *J Small Anim Pract* 25:551, 1984.

77. Stoffregen DA, Huxtable CR, Cummings JF, et al: Hypomyelination of the central nervous system of two Siamese kitten littermates, *Vet Pathol* 30:388, 1993.

78. Summers BA, Cummings JF, de Lahunta A, editors: *Veterinary neuropathology*, St. Louis, 1995, Mosby, p 402.

79. Dahme E, Kraft W, Scabell J: Hypertrophische polyneuropathie bei der Katze, *J Vet Med* 34:271, 1987.

80. de Lahunta A: Abiotrophy in domestic animals: a review, *Can J Vet Res* 54:65, 1990.

81. Inada S, Mochizuki M, Izumo S, et al: Study of hereditary cerebellar degeneration in cats, *Am J Vet Res* 57:296, 1996.

82. Taniyama H, Takayanagi S, Izumisawa Y, et al: Cerebellar cortical atrophy in a kitten, *Vet Pathol* 31:710, 1994.

83. Willoughby K, Kelly DF: Hereditary cerebellar degeneration in three full sibling kittens, *Vet Rec* 151:295, 2002.

84. Barone G, Foureman P, de Lahunta A: Adult-onset cerebellar cortical abiotrophy and retinal degeneration in a domestic shorthair cat, *J Am Anim Hosp Assoc* 38:51, 2002.

85. Shamir M, Perl S, Sharon L: Late onset of cerebellar abiotrophy in a Siamese cat, *J Small Anim Pract* 40:343, 1999.

86. Csiza CK, Scott FW, de Lahunta A, et al: Pathogenesis of feline panleukopenia virus in susceptible newborn kittens. I. Clinical signs, hematology, serology, virology, *Infect Immun* 3:833, 1971.

87. Csiza CK, de Lahunta A, Scott FW, et al: Pathogenesis of feline panleukopenia virus in susceptible newborn kittens. II. Pathology and immunofluorescence, *Infect Immun* 3:838, 1971.

88. Kilham L, Margolis G, Colby ED: Congenital infections of cats and ferrets by feline panleukopenia virus manifested by cerebellar hypoplasia, *Lab Invest* 17:465, 1967.

89. Langheinrich KA, Nielsen SW: Histopathology of feline panleukopenia: a report of 65 cases, *J Am Vet Med Assoc* 158(Suppl 2):863, 1971.

90. Greene CE, Gorgasz EJ, Martin CL: Hydranencephaly associated with feline panleukopenia, *J Am Vet Med Assoc* 180:767, 1982.

91. Kornegay JN: Ataxia of the head and limbs: cerebellar diseases in dogs and cats, *Prog Vet Neurol* 1:255, 1990.

92. de Lahunta A: Diseases of the cerebellum, *Vet Clin North Am Small Anim Pract* 10:91, 1980.

93. Meric SM: Diagnosis and management of feline hyperthyroidism, *Compend Contin Educ Pract Vet* 11:1053, 1989.

94. Fascetti AJ, Hickman MA: Preparturient hypocalcemia in four cats, *J Am Vet Med Assoc.* 215:1127, 1999.

95. Leon A, Bain SAF, Levick WR: Hypokalaemic episodic polymyopathy in cats fed a vegetarian diet, *Aust Vet J* 69:249, 1992.

96. Joseph RJ, Peterson ME: Review and comparison of neuromuscular and central nervous manifestations of hyperthyroidism in cats and humans, *Prog Vet Neurol* 3:114, 1992.

97. Whitley NT, Drobatz KJ, Panciera DL: Insulin overdose in dogs and cats: 28 cases (1986-1993), *J Am Vet Med Assoc* 211:326, 1997.

97a. Flecknell PA, Lucke VM: Chronic relapsing polyradiculoneuritis in a cat, *Acta Neuropathol* 41:81, 1978.

98. Kline KL, Joseph RJ, Averill DR: Feline infectious peritonitis with neurologic involvement: clinical and pathological findings in 24 cats, *J Am Anim Hosp Assoc* 30:111, 1994.

99. Rand JS, Parent JM, Percy D, et al: Clinical, cerebrospinal fluid and histological data from twenty-seven cats with primary inflammatory disease of the central nervous system, *Can Vet J* 35:103, 1994.

100. Timmann D, Cizinauskas S, Tomek A, et al: Retrospective analysis of seizures associated with feline infectious peritonitis in cats, *J Feline Med Surg* 10:9, 2008.

101. Pedersen NC, Yamamoto JK, Ishida T, et al: Feline immunodeficiency virus infection, *Vet Immunol Immunopathol* 21:111, 1989.

102. Podell M, Chen E, Shelton GD: FIV-associated inflammatory myopathy in adult cats, *J Vet Intern Med* 12:206, 1998.

103. Greene CE, Rupprecht CE: Rabies and other lyssavirus infections. In Greene CE, editor: *Infectious diseases of the dog and cat,* ed 3, St. Louis, 2006, Elsevier, p 167.

104. Dubey JP, Carpenter JL: Neonatal toxoplasmosis in littermate cats, *J Am Vet Med Assoc* 203:1546, 1993.

105. Dubey JP, Carpenter JL: Histologically confirmed clinical toxoplasmosis in cats: 100 cases (1952-1990), *J Am Vet Med Assoc* 203:1556, 1993.

106. Leggett MN, Dukes J, Pirie HM: A spongiform encephalopathy in a cat, *Vet Rec* 127:586, 1990.

107. Vidal E, Montoliu P, Anor S, et al: A novel spongiform degeneration of the grey matter in the brain of a kitten, *J Comp Pathol* 131:98, 2004.

108. Joseph RJ, Carrillo JM, Lennon VA: Myasthenia gravis in the cat, *J Vet Intern Med* 2:75, 1988.

109. Dorman DC, Parker AJ, Buck WB: Bromethalin toxicosis in the dog. Part I: clinical effects, *J Am Anim Hosp Assoc* 26:589, 1990.

110. Jaggy A, Oliver JE: Chlorpyrifos toxicosis in two cats, *J Vet Intern Med* 4:135, 1990.

111. Fikes JD, Zachary JF, Parker AJ: Clinical, biochemical, electrophysiologic, and histologic assessment of chlorpyrifos induced delayed neuropathy in the cat, *Neurotoxicology* 13:663, 1992.

112. Bouldin TW, Cavanagh JB: Organophosphorous neuropathy. I. A teased-fiber study of the spatio-temporal spread of axonal degeneration, *Am J Pathol* 94:241, 1979.

113. Bouldin TW, Cavanagh JB: Organophosphorous neuropathy. II. A fine-structural study of the early stages of axonal degeneration, *Am J Pathol* 94:253, 1979.

114. Clemmons RM, Meyer DJ, Sundlof SF, et al: Correction of organophosphate-induced neuromuscular blockade by diphenhydramine, *Am J Vet Res* 45:2167, 1984.

115. Levy JK: Chronic chlorpyrifos toxicosis in a cat, *J Am Vet Med Assoc* 203:1682, 1993.

116. Twedt DC, Cuddon PA, Horn TW: Black widow spider envenomation in a cat, *J Vet Intern Med* 13:613, 1999.

117. Vijverberg HPM, van den Bercken J: Action of pyrethroid insecticides on the vertebrate nervous system, *Neuropathol Appl Neurobiol* 8:421, 1982.

118. de Wille JR, Brown LD, Narahashi T: Pyrethroid modifications of the activation and inactivation kinetics of the sodium channels in squid axons, *Brain Res* 512:26, 1990.

119. Whittem T: Pyrethrin and pyrethroid insecticide intoxication in cats, *Compend Contin Educ Pract Vet* 17:489, 1995.

120. Hansen SR, Stemme KA, Villar D, et al: Pyrethrins and pyrethroids in dogs and cats, *J Am Anim Hosp Assoc* 16:707, 1994.

121. Richardson JA: Permethrin spot-on toxicoses in cats, *J Vet Emerg Crit Care* 10:103, 2000.

122. Sutton NM, Bates N, Campbell A: Clinical effects and outcome of feline permethrin spot-on poisonings reported to the veterinary poisons information service (VPIS), London, *J Feline Med Surg* 9:335, 2007.

123. Lovell RA: Ivermectin and piperazine toxicoses in dogs and cats, *Vet Clin North Am Small Anim Pract* 20:453, 1990.

124. Caylor KB, Cassimatis MK: Metronidazole neurotoxicosis in two cats, *J Am Anim Hosp Assoc* 37:258, 2001.

125. Dow SW, LeCouteur RA, Poss ML, et al: Central nervous system toxicosis associated with metronidazole treatment of dogs: five cases (1984-1987), *J Am Vet Med Assoc* 195:365, 1989.

126. Olson EJ, Morales SC, McVey AS, et al: Putative metronidazole neurotoxicosis in a cat, *Vet Pathol* 42:665, 2005.

127. Thompson JP, Senior DF, Pinson DM, et al: Neurotoxicosis associated with the use of hexachlorophene in a cat, *J Am Vet Med Assoc* 190:1311, 1987.

128. Dorman DC, Parker AJ, Dye JA, et al: Bromethalin neurotoxicosis in the cat, *Prog Vet Neurol* 1:189, 1990.

129. Murphy MJ: Toxin exposures in dogs and cats: drugs and household products, *J Am Vet Med Assoc* 205:557, 1994.

130. Dorman DC, Zachary JF, Buck WB: Neuropathologic findings of bromethalin toxicosis in the cat, *Vet Pathol* 29:139, 1992.

131. Gruber TA, Costigan P, Wilkinson GT, et al: Chronic methylmercurialism in the cat, *Aust Vet J* 54:155, 1978.

132. Khera KS: Teratogenic effects of methylmercury in the cat: note on the use of this species as a model for teratogenicity studies, *Teratology* 8:293, 1973.

133. Harvey HJ, MacEwen EG, Hayes AA: Neurotoxicosis associated with use of 5-fluorouracil in five dogs and one cat, *J Am Vet Med Assoc* 171:277, 1977.

134. Lovell RA, Trammel HL, Beasley VR, et al: A review of 83 reports of suspected toluene/dichlorophen toxicoses in cats and dogs, *J Am Anim Hosp Assoc* 26:652, 1990.

135. Dorman DC, Fikes JD: Diagnosis and therapy of neurotoxicological syndromes in dogs and cats: selected syndromes induced by pesticides, part 2, *Prog Vet Neurol* 4:111, 1993.

136. Dorman DC: Diagnosing and treating toxicoses in dogs and cats, *Vet Med* p 273, 1997.

137. Denny-Brown D, Gaylor JB: Note on the nature of the motor discharge in shivering, *Brain* 58:233, 1935.

138. Galano HR, Olby NJ, Howard JF Jr, et al: Myokymia and neuromyotonia in a cat, *J Am Vet Med Assoc* 227:1608, 2005.

139. Killingsworth C, Chiapella A, Veralli P, et al: Feline tetanus, *J Am Anim Hosp Assoc* 13:209, 1977.

140. Toll J, Cooper B, Altschul M: Congenital myotonia in 2 domestic cats, *J Vet Intern Med* 12:116, 1998.

141. Hickford EH, Jones BR, Gething MA, et al: Congenital myotonia in related kittens, *J Small Anim Pract* 39:281, 1998.

58 Metabolic Encephalopathy: Organic Acidurias

Dennis P. O'Brien and Rebecca A. Packer

The organic acidurias are a heterogeneous group of diseases characterized by excretion of abnormal organic acids in the urine.[1-3] Organic acids can be either excessive amounts of a metabolite found normally in the urine, or one that would not be expected in the urine of a normal cat. The abnormal organic acid in the blood and/or the underlying metabolic disease that produced it can lead to altered brain function and signs of metabolic encephalopathy. In this chapter we will review the role of organic acids in metabolism, and the pathogenesis, recognition, and treatment of organic acidurias.

ORGANIC ACIDS

The organic acids are vital compounds in intermediate metabolism—the intermediate steps in conversion of nutrients into cellular components and energy (Figure 58-1). At the center of intermediate metabolism is the Krebs cycle. Fats, carbohydrates, and proteins in the diet are broken down into organic acids that enter the Krebs cycle at various points and sometimes are conjugated with coenzyme A (CoA). Hydrogen molecules generated from the metabolism of these acids in the mitochondria are fed into the respiratory chain to yield adenosine triphosphate (ATP) needed to supply the energy needs of cells. In addition to their role in energy production, the organic acids of intermediate metabolism can be crucial steps in the synthesis of cellular components such as neurotransmitters. For example, gamma aminobutyric acid (GABA) and glutamate, respectively the most important inhibitory and excitatory neurotransmitters in the brain, are synthesized from α-ketoglutarate in the "GABA shunt" (Figure 58-2).

Several of the B-vitamins are significant cofactors in intermediate metabolism. Thiamin (vitamin B_1) is a cofactor for several dehydrogenase reactions, most importantly the conversion of α-ketoglutarate to succinyl CoA in the Krebs cycle.[4] Neonates are particularly sensitive to biotin (vitamin B_7) deficiency, which is essential to activate a number of carboxylases necessary for normal gluconeogenesis, fatty acid synthesis, and amino acid catabolism.[5] Cobalamin (vitamin B_{12}) is necessary for conversion of methylmalonyl CoA to succinyl CoA, the entry to the Krebs cycle for cholesterol and some fatty acids and amino acids (see below).[4]

Anything that obstructs the flow through these metabolic pathways can lead to an abnormal accumulation of the organic acids upstream from the obstruction. Alternatively, excessive levels of organic acids absorbed from the gastrointestinal tract can overload the metabolic capabilities of the system. Clinical signs result from either the accumulation of abnormal levels of organic acids or from downstream effects of a blockage in the metabolic pathway.

DIAGNOSING ORGANIC ACID DISORDERS

Because they are small molecules, the organic acids are excreted readily in the urine. This is in contrast to other errors of metabolism such as the lysosomal storage dis-

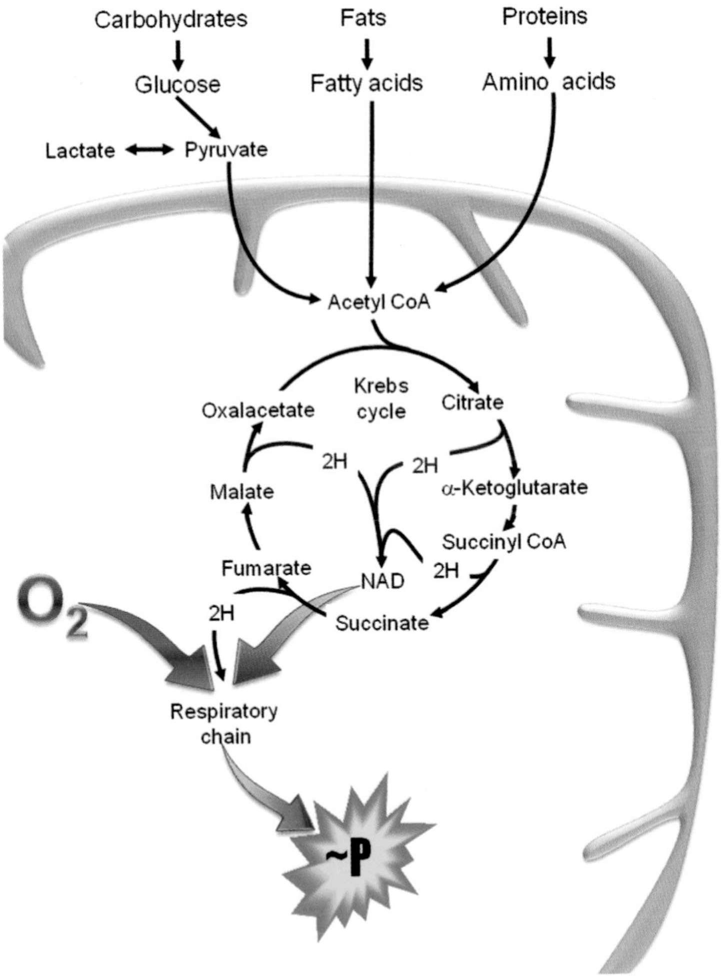

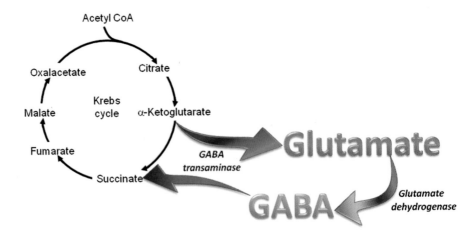

Figure 58-1 Carbohydrates, fats, and proteins are metabolized to simple organic acids, which can be fed into the Krebs cycle within the mitochondria. In turn, hydrogen ions liberated in the metabolism of the organic acids in the Krebs cycle provide the fuel for oxidative phosphorylation in the respiratory chain and the generation of high energy phosphates (~P). In anaerobic metabolism, pyruvate is converted to lactate within the cytoplasm.

Figure 58-2 Organic acids also are substrates for synthesis. Glutamate and GABA, the most important excitatory and inhibitory neurotransmitters respectively, are produced from α-ketoglutarate in the GABA shunt.

eases in which the byproduct is a large macromolecule that accumulates within the cell. Specialized laboratories can detect the abnormal organic acids in urine by gas chromatography/mass spectroscopy. The pattern of organic acids found indicates the nature of the disturbance and sometimes can indicate a specific enzyme or vitamin deficiency as the source of the disorder. Although routine clinical pathology tests typically do not detect organic acids, they may contain clues that should lead to a urine organic acid assay (Box 58-1). An unexplained

metabolic acidosis should raise suspicion of an organic acid disorder. The unknown acid could produce a high anion gap or low bicarbonate or total CO_2 on a serum biochemistry panel, and a blood gas analysis would reveal a metabolic acidosis with respiratory compensation. Interference with energy production or utilization could produce hypoglycemia or ketosis, which would be detected on urinalysis. If the urea cycle is affected, increased blood ammonia could result without other signs of liver disease.

Clinical signs of organic acidurias will vary; however, because the brain is the most metabolically demanding organ in the body, disorders of metabolism often can present with signs of encephalopathy. A large portion of the body's energy utilization goes to fuel brain functions such as generation of the resting membrane potential and neurotransmitter cycling. The cerebral cortex is the most sensitive to such disturbances. Therefore altered consciousness, behavior changes, seizures, and loss of vision and postural reactions would be common signs. In some cases, such as thiamin deficiency, brainstem areas are more sensitive and central vestibular signs and motor disturbances predominate. Signs often will wax and wane, and because the pathway affected may only be utilized by specific nutrients, diet sometimes can alter the signs. If the organic acids produce a significant metabolic acidosis, the cat may have Kussmaul breathing as it attempts to compensate by eliminating CO_2. Other organs may be involved, and congenital disturbances can affect growth, resulting in a kitten who is small and developmentally delayed. When the organic aciduria is secondary, signs of the primary disease also will be apparent.

The brain also is the prime target of endogenous toxins that accumulate with liver failure. A history of waxing and waning encephalopathy that is affected by diet would be highly suggestive of hepatic encephalopathy, and elevated blood ammonia levels would support the diagnosis. If no portosystemic shunt is found and the liver appears normal on biopsy, then a urine organic acid profile would be indicated.

Box 58-1 Clues to an Organic Aciduria

Alterations on routine clinical pathology tests that should raise suspicion of an organic aciduria if there is no obvious explanation such as diabetes mellitus or liver failure.

- Decreased total CO_2 or bicarbonate
- Increased anion gap
- Metabolic acidosis on blood gas analysis
- Ketonuria
- Hypoglycemia
- Hyperammonemia

D-LACTIC ACIDOSIS WITH GASTROINTESTINAL DISEASE

We have seen two cats with encephalopathy associated with gastrointestinal disease and profound metabolic acidosis. Serum lactate levels, as measured by routine benchtop assay, were normal, and yet very high levels of lactate were detected in the urine.[6] This presented a quandary about the discrepancy between the serum and urine tests and about the source of the lactate elevation. Neither cat was in shock or otherwise hypoxemic, and both cats had been clinically normal for years making an inborn error of metabolism unlikely.

Lactic acid can exist as one of two stereoisomers, L-lactate and D-lactate (Figure 58-3), and enzymes can only metabolize one isoform or the other. In mammals L-lactate dehydrogenase in the cytoplasm converts L-lactate efficiently to pyruvate, which enters the mitochondria to fuel the Krebs cycle. When there is insufficient oxygen for aerobic metabolism such as hypoxemia, shock, or extreme muscle activity, this reaction can be reversed resulting in the lactic acidosis. The traditional concept that neurons rely exclusively on glucose for energy has been challenged by the "lactate shuttle" hypothesis.[7] In this paradigm, L-lactate provides up to 75 per cent of the energy requirements of neurons. The excitatory neurotransmitter glutamate is taken up from the synapse by astrocytes to be recycled, but it also stimulates conversion of pyruvate to L-lactate within the astrocyte. This lactate is shuttled to neurons through specific lactate transporters, where it is metabolized readily to pyruvate and then through the Krebs cycle to produce the energy needed to maintain the resting membrane potential. Therefore this system links energy supply with demand produced by excitation.

Normally, little D-lactate is produced in mammals. In diseases such as diabetes mellitus or propylene glycol toxicity, D-lactate can be produced through the methylglyoxal pathway.[8,9] D-lactate dehydrogenase is found only in the mitochondria where it is less efficient, and the enzyme is expressed poorly in brain tissue.[10] Although elevations of L-lactate or unrelated acidosis have little effect on brain function, D-lactic acidosis results in profound encephalopathy, probably because of interference

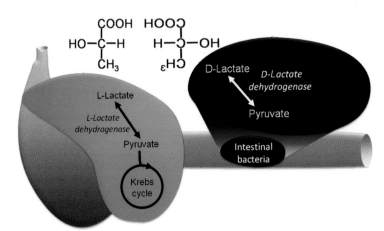

Figure 58-3 Lactate forms two stereoisomers, the L and D isoforms, which are mirror-image structures. L-lactate dehydrogenase in mammals metabolizes the L isoform in the liver and other organs including the brain. D-lactate dehydrogenase in intestinal bacteria produces the D isoform, which can cause encephalopathy.

with the lactate shuttle.[11,12] Bacteria can produce both the D and L isoforms of lactate through fermentation of carbohydrates. Therefore D-lactate is found commonly in foods that have undergone bacterial fermentation such as pickles and yogurt. Conditions that alter gastrointestinal bacterial flora, such as short-bowel syndrome in human beings or grain overload in cattle, can lead to excessive D-lactate production in the intestine and encephalopathy.[11,12]

The two cats with D-lactate encephalopathy had pancreatic exocrine insufficiency or pancreatitis, which presumably altered their gastrointestinal flora. Although both patients had cobalamin deficiency and methylmalonic acid elevation (see the following), the degree of methylmalonic acid elevations could not explain the acidosis, and signs improved with correction of the acidosis prior to cobalamin administration.[6] Serum lactate levels measured within normal reference range on routine bench-top lactate assay because the enzyme-based test used detects only the L isoform, whereas the gas chromatography/mass spectroscopy performed on the urine detects both isoforms. Research currently is being conducted to determine the prevalence of D-lactic acidosis in cats with gastrointestinal disease and whether it correlates with signs of encephalopathy or bacterial overgrowth.

Correction of the acidosis with intravenous bicarbonate resulted in clinical improvement in both cases, but treating the underlying disease was necessary for long-term improvement. The cat with pancreatic exocrine insufficiency was treated with oral pancreatic enzyme supplementation (see Chapter 20). The appetite and fecal consistency normalized, and the cat showed no further episodes of encephalopathy. Cobalamin levels remained low, however, and the cat ultimately was treated with parenteral cyanocobalamin. The cat with pancreatitis showed similar improvement with therapy.

METHYLMALONIC ACIDURIA AND COBALAMIN DEFICIENCY

Cobalamin (vitamin B_{12}) is a cofactor for the enzyme that converts methylmalonyl CoA to succinyl CoA, which can then enter the Krebs cycle (Figure 58-4). This is an essential step in the metabolism of odd chain fatty acids, cholesterol, and branch chain amino acids. Cobalamin also is essential for the conversion of homocysteine to methionine.[13,14] Cobalamin has a complex system for absorption and transport. Dietary cobalamin is bound to intrinsic factor, which is produced exclusively by the pancreas in cats and promotes cobalamin absorption in the ileum.[15] This absorption depends on a receptor in the ileal enterocytes, cubilin.[16] In the blood stream cobalamin is bound to transcobalamin, which mediates absorption of the vitamin by the target cells.[17] A portion of the cobalamin taken up by hepatocytes is excreted in the bile, creating enterohepatic recirculation of the vitamin.[14] Dietary deficiency or disturbances at any stage of the processing of cobalamin can lead to signs of deficiency, including encephalopathy.[18,19]

Gastrointestinal disease can cause cobalamin deficiency in cats in several ways.[13,14] Pancreatic disease can lead to deficient intrinsic factor, whereas biliary disease could decrease availability of recirculated cobalamin. Infiltrative bowel disease such as intestinal lymphoma or inflammatory bowel disease can interfere with absorption of cobalamin by the enterocytes. With insufficient cobal-

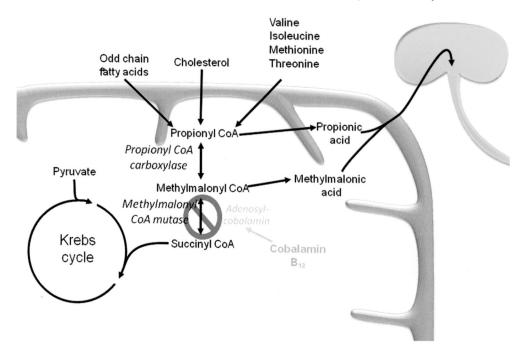

Figure 58-4 In cobalamin deficiency, the enzyme that depends on this vitamin as a cofactor can not function. The metabolism of cholesterol, odd chain fatty acids, and branch chain amino acids through this pathway is obstructed. This leads to an accumulation of the organic acids immediately upstream from the obstruction (methylmalonic and propionic acid), which then are excreted in the urine.

amin, there is accumulation of methylmalonic acid, and to a lesser extent the immediately upstream metabolite propionic acid, which are detected in the urine.

Treatment of the underlying gastrointestinal disease can result in improvement in cobalamin absorption, but parenteral administration still may be necessary. Although the exact requirement of cobalamin in cats is not known, supplementation with parenteral cyanocobalamin at a rate of 1 mg every 2 weeks has been recommended.[14] (The reader is referred to Chapter 13 in the fifth volume of this series for a complete discussion of the relationship of cobalamin with chronic gastrointestinal disease.)

CONGENITAL COBALAMIN DEFICIENCY

Two cases have been reported of young cats with cobalamin deficiency not related to gastrointestinal disease.[18,19] One cat presented at 11 months of age with repeated episodes of disorientation, imbalance, and blindness. Although the serum chemistry profile showed a decrease in total CO_2 (8 mmol/L; reference interval, 16 to 25 mmol/L) and an increase in anion gap (36 mmol/L; reference interval, 10 to 23 mmol/L), a blood gas analysis was not performed at that time. Brain computed tomographic (CT) imaging and cerebrospinal fluid (CSF) analysis were unremarkable. The postprandial blood ammonia level and preprandial and postprandial bile acid levels were within normal limits, and abdominal ultrasound did not reveal any hepatic disease; however, the cat had been started on a low-protein diet as empirical treatment for possible hepatic encephalopathy. She improved dramatically with diet change and supportive intravenous fluids, and continued to show no clinical signs while on the low-protein diet.[18]

Three years later, however, her owners elected to switch her to a seafood-based "natural" diet. Within 2 months of the diet change she presented with a 2-day history of behavior change, excessive grooming, weakness, and imbalance progressing to stupor. At that time a venous blood gas analysis revealed a metabolic acidosis with respiratory compensation (pH 7.239; HCO_3^- 6 mmol/L; pCO_2 15.1 mm Hg), and urinalysis showed ketonuria. In spite of intensive therapy, she died within 8 hours of admission. Subsequent organic acid analysis of the urine showed elevated methylmalonic and propionic acid in addition to the ketones, and serum cobalamin levels were undetectable.[18]

The other patient was a 9-month-old male cat with a history of lethargy, anorexia, cold intolerance, and failure to thrive since a young age. He also had low total CO_2, methylmalonic aciduria, and low serum cobalamin. In addition, serum hypoglycemia and hyperammonemia were detected. The cat was euthanized, and the only abnormality detected in the liver was a biochemical change consistent with cobalamin deficiency.[19]

Neither of these cats had signs of gastrointestinal disease. Both presumably had a congenital defect in cobalamin metabolism, although the exact nature of the defect was not determined in either case. They also illustrate the similarity in clinical signs between the organic acidurias and hepatic encephalopathy. Either syndrome could present with signs of waxing and waning encephalopathy. The amount of nutrients that need to be metabolized through the deficient pathway can influence the severity of clinical signs. Therefore decreasing protein in the diet would have decreased the amount of branch chain amino acids that had to be metabolized through the methylmalonyl CoA pathway. Unfortunately these amino acids are found in high concentrations in seafood, and the dietary increase in branch chain amino acids precipitated a fatal crisis when the diet was changed in the older cat.

In some organic acidurias, increased levels of the organic acid in the cell can interfere with the function of other enzymes. The enzyme carbamyl phosphate synthase combines ammonia with bicarbonate to produce carbamyl phosphate, which enters the urea cycle (Figure 58-5). Methylmalonic acid inhibits the activity of this enzyme. Therefore cobalamin deficiency also can prevent entry of ammonia into the urea cycle and mimic the effects of hepatic insufficiency on ammonia metabolism.

Both cases presented with clues suggestive of an organic aciduria. They both had low total CO_2 and increased anion gap because of the presence of the organic

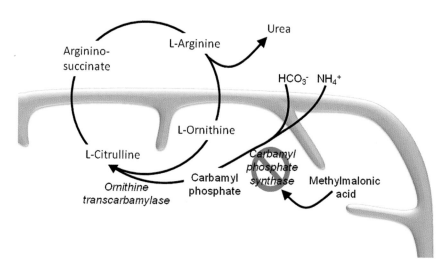

Figure 58-5 Abnormal organic acid levels can interfere with other functions. For example, elevated methylmalonic acid can inhibit the enzyme that mediates entry of ammonia into the urea cycle, causing hyperammonemia.

acid in the blood. In addition, the first cat had an unexplained ketonuria, and the second patient an unexplained hyperammonemia. Early recognition of the nature of the disorder and administration of parenteral cyanocobalamin may have helped.

INBORN ERRORS OF METABOLISM

The cases of congenital cobalamin deficiency discussed above most likely were caused by a mutation in the gene for one of the crucial factors in cobalamin uptake or transport. Mutations occur in chromosomes constantly because of the effects of radiation, mutagenic toxins, or errors in DNA replication. Many of these mutations will be of no functional consequence. Rarely such a mutation could provide a desirable change in function of the protein produced. Then natural or human selection can act to increase the incidence of that gene in the population. Mutations that interfere with the protein function, however, can lead to disease. In some cases the gene is deleted completely and no protein is produced.

Function also may be lost if a change in the nucleic acid sequence leads to a premature stop codon. The stop codon consists of three nucleic acids in the DNA that signals the end of the sequence to be translated into a protein. If a mutation produces a stop codon early in the sequence of the gene, a truncated protein is produced that may be lacking a critical element and be nonfunctional. Alternatively, the mutation can change the sequence of amino acids produced. This could alter the three-dimensional structure of the protein or directly affect an active site such as the substrate binding site of an enzyme. In this situation, the protein is produced but the function is decreased or abolished. When such mutations alter the activity of an important enzyme in the metabolic pathways and produce disease, they are called inborn errors of metabolism.

Washizu and colleagues described an 18-month-old female cat with stunted growth and postprandial depression.[20] She had elevated liver enzymes and ammonia with normal preprandial and postprandial bile acids. A low-protein diet improved the liver enzyme values, but not the elevated ammonia. Contrast portography showed normal portal circulation and a liver biopsy was normal. A urine organic acid profile showed elevated orotic acid and uracil.

The enzyme ornithine transcarbamylase combines carbamyl phosphate with ornithine as ammonia enters the urea cycle (see Figure 58-5). A deficiency in this enzyme would prevent ammonia metabolism one step down from where methylmalonic acid blocked the pathway, resulting in accumulation of carbamyl phosphate as well as ammonia. Orotic acid and uracil are byproducts of carbamyl phosphate metabolism by an alternative pathway.[20]

Although inborn errors of metabolism have been reported rarely in cats, we have seen an increasing incidence of hereditary diseases in cats as pure breed cats become more popular, and an increased index of suspicion is leading to better recognition of such diseases. With the mapping of the feline genome, researchers can apply the techniques of molecular biology that have been used successfully in other species to identify the genes responsible for hereditary diseases in cats. In the organic acidurias, the presence of an abnormal organic acid in the urine can point toward a specific enzyme, or at least a specific metabolic pathway, as being affected. The genes involved then are considered candidates for the one responsible for causing disease. By comparing the sequence of these candidate genes between normal and affected cats, the disease causing mutation can be identified. Such an approach has been used successfully in cats with the related inborn errors of metabolism, the lysosomal storage diseases (see Chapter 56).[21]

If there are no clear candidate genes or no mutation is found in the candidates, then a whole genome mapping strategy is needed to identify the disease locus, the location on the feline chromosome where the defective gene resides. Fine mapping techniques then can narrow down the region of the chromosome where the mutant gene resides until the locus contains a small number of known genes. These genes then become candidates to be sequenced based on their location as well as their function. This approach was used successfully by Fyfe and colleagues to identify the mutation responsible for spinal muscular atrophy in Maine Coon cats.[22]

Once a mutation has been identified, a DNA test can be developed to permit breeders to identify carriers of the condition. Breeders then can avoid producing affected kittens by not breeding two carriers of a recessive trait. Equally importantly, they can decrease the frequency of the mutant allele in the population through wise breeding strategies without further limiting what already may be a limited gene pool. The DNA test also can be used as a diagnostic test in cats showing clinical signs compatible with the disease in question.

THERAPY FOR ORGANIC ACIDURIAS

Gene-based therapies one day may be available to treat the hereditary diseases[21] (see Chapter 56). Until then symptomatic therapy is necessary. In patients with profound metabolic acidosis, sodium bicarbonate should be administered to restore a more normal pH. Carnitine is an amino-acid derivative that plays an important role in the transport of organic acids across the mitochondrial membrane and in removal of these acids from the body.[23] Oral L-carnitine may help to replace carnitine lost in the urine and thus promote more efficient excretion of the organic acids. When the organic aciduria is secondary to a vitamin deficiency or another disease such as intestinal bacterial overgrowth, correcting the underlying problem will resolve the organic aciduria. Although dietary deficiencies are uncommon in cats who are fed quality commercial foods, administration of parenteral vitamin B-complex should be considered once samples have been collected for testing. In some cases altering the diet can sidestep a deficient enzyme by avoiding production of the organic acid that must be metabolized through the deficient pathway.[24] Consultation with a nutritionist may be necessary to formulate a diet that can shift metabolism away from the impaired pathway without creating a nutritional deficiency.

SUMMARY

Although the organic acidurias could be viewed as academic oddities, the true incidence of disease can not be determined until an index of suspicion permits recognition when the cases are presented to the clinic. The outcome of an unrecognized and untreated organic aciduria can be brain damage and death. Although some organic acidurias may not be treatable, others can be managed readily with simple dietary changes or vitamin supplementation. Urine organic acid assays are becoming more readily available, and should be considered for any feline patient in whom an unexplained metabolic acidosis, ketonuria, or other metabolic disturbance raises the suspicion of an organic aciduria.

REFERENCES

1. Haan EA, Scholem RD, Croll HB, et al: Malonyl coenzyme A decarboxylase deficiency: clinical and biochemical findings in a second child with a more severe enzyme defect, *Europ J Pediatr* 144:567, 1986.
2. Ozand PT, Gascon GG: Organic acidurias: a review. Part 2, *J Child Neurol* 6:288, 1991.
3. Ozand PT, Gascon GG: Organic acidurias: a review. Part 1, *J Child Neurol* 6:196, 1991.
4. Butterworth RF: Metabolic encephalopathies. In Siegel GJ, Albers RW, Brady ST, et al, editors: *Basic neurochemistry*, Amsterdam, 2006, Elsevier, p 593.
5. Pacheco-Alvarez D, Solorzano-Vargas RS, Del Rio AL: Biotin in metabolism and its relationship to human disease, *Arch Med Res* 33:439, 2002.
6. Packer RA, Cohn LA, Wohlstadter DR, et al: D-lactic acidosis secondary to exocrine pancreatic insufficiency in a cat, *J Vet Intern Med* 19:106, 2005.
7. Pellerin L, Bouzier-Sore AK, Aubert A: Activity-dependent regulation of energy metabolism by astrocytes: an update, *GLIA* 55:1251, 2007.
8. Christopher MM, Broussard JD, Fallin CW, et al: Increased serum D-lactate associated with diabetic ketoacidosis, *Metab Clin Exp* 44:287, 1995.
9. Christopher MM, Eckfeldt JH, Eaton JW: Propylene glycol ingestion causes D-lactic acidosis, *Lab Invest* 62:114, 1990.
10. Flick MJ, Konieczny SF: Identification of putative mammalian D-lactate dehydrogenase enzymes, *Biochem Biophys Res Commun* 295:910, 2005.
11. Abeysekara S, Naylor JM, Wassef AW, et al: D-Lactic acid-induced neurotoxicity in a calf model, *Am J Physiol—Endocrin Metabol* 293:E558, 2007.
12. Ewaschuk JB, Naylor JM, Zello GA: D-lactate in human and ruminant metabolism, *J Nutr* 135:1619, 2005.
13. Ruaux CG, Steiner JM, Williams DA: Metabolism of amino acids in cats with severe cobalamin deficiency, *Am J Vet Res* 62:1852, 2001.
14. Simpson KW, Fyfe J, Cornetta A, et al: Subnormal concentrations of serum cobalamin (vitamin B12) in cats with gastrointestinal disease, *J Vet Intern Med* 5:26, 2001.
15. Fyfe JC: Feline intrinsic factor (IF) is pancreatic in origin and mediates ileal cobalamin (CBL) absorption, *J Vet Intern Med* 7:133, 1993.
16. Fyfe JC, Giger U, Hall CA, et al: Inherited selective intestinal cobalamin malabsorption and cobalamin deficiency in dogs, *Ped Res* 29:24, 1991.
17. Linnell JC, Collings L, Down MC, et al: Distribution of endogenous cobalamin between the transcobalamins in various mammals, *Clin Sci* 57:139, 1979.
18. Kelmer E, Shelton GD, Williams DA, et al: Organic acidemia in a young cat associated with cobalamin deficiency, *J Vet Emerg Crit Care* 17:299, 2007.
19. Vaden SL, Wood PA, Ledley FD, et al: Cobalamin deficiency associated with methylmalonic acidemia in a cat, *J Am Vet Med Assoc* 200:1101, 1992.
20. Washizu T, Washizu M, Zhang C, et al: A suspected case of ornithine transcarbamylase deficiency in a cat, *J Vet Med Sci* 66:701, 2004.
21. Ellinwood NM, Vite CH, Haskins ME: Gene therapy for lysosomal storage diseases: the lessons and promise of animal models, *J Gene Med* 6:481, 2004.
22. Fyfe JC, Menotti-Raymond M, David VA, et al: An approximately 140-kb deletion associated with feline spinal muscular atrophy implies an essential LIX1 function for motor neuron survival, *Genome Res* 16:1084, 2006.
23. Hass RH, Nyhan WL: Disorders of organic acids. In Berg B, editor: *Neurologic aspects of pediatrics*, Boston, 1992, Butterworth-Heinemann, p 37.
24. O'Brien DP, Barshop BA, Faunt KK, et al: Malonic aciduria in Maltese dogs: normal methylmalonic acid concentrations and malonyl-CoA decarboxylase activity in fibroblasts, *J Inherit Metab Dis* 22:883, 1999.

59 Myopathic Disorders

Debbie S. Ruehlmann

Feline skeletal muscle is distinctively different from skeletal muscle in dogs. Skeletal muscle in dogs is composed of slow- and fast-twitch fatigue-resistant myofibers, whereas muscle in cats also includes fast-twitch fatigable myofibers. This fiber type enables cats to be superior sprinters while utilizing energy from glycogen in anaerobic pathways for intense exercise. Slow- and fast-twitch fatigue-resistant fibers utilize mitochondrial fatty acid oxidation primarily, which is ideal for endurance or sustained exercise.[1]

Diseases affecting normal skeletal muscle function in cats can be categorized as acquired or inherited (Box 59-1). The hallmark clinical sign of any disorder affecting muscle function is weakness. Exercise-induced weakness often is characteristic. The primary gait manifestation for most feline myopathic disorders is a stiff, short-strided, or stilted gait with decreased ability to jump. Somewhat unique to cats affected with myopathic disease, as well as other neuromuscular diseases, is a tendency to develop weakness of the cervical paraspinal extensor muscles, causing cervical spinal ventroflexion or inability to elevate the head and neck (Figure 59-1). Lateral movement of the head and neck seems to be spared. Generalized muscle atrophy may be apparent in some cats affected with myopathies. In contrast, muscle hypertrophy is an abnormality specific to feline dystrophin-deficient muscular dystrophy. Myalgia may be present with myopathy.

In general, distinguishing myopathies clinically from other neuromuscular diseases that involve the motor unit may be difficult based on physical and neurological examinations. Typically, general proprioception and spinal reflexes are not affected in muscle disease. Muscle

tone may or may not be decreased. Peripheral neuropathy and radiculopathy often result in hyporeflexia and hypotonia. Diseases involving the neuromuscular junction may or may not affect muscle tone and spinal reflexes. Myasthenia gravis often presents very similarly to myopathy, and affected cats have intact spinal reflexes and muscle tone. Diseases of the motor unit considered as differential diagnoses for generalized weakness in cats are shown in Box 59-2. Further diagnostic testing will assist with establishing a more definitive diagnosis.

The minimum database in cats presenting with generalized weakness consistent with myopathic disease includes a complete blood count, serum chemistry profile, urinalysis, and serum creatine kinase (CK) activity.

Electrodiagnostic evaluation and muscle biopsy are the mainstays of achieving a diagnosis for myopathy. Electromyography (EMG) often is abnormal in many myopathies. Normal resting muscle generally is electrically silent. Electromyographic abnormalities described for myopathic disease include prolongation of insertional activity, presence of spontaneous activity including fibrillation potentials, positive sharp waves, complex repetitive discharges, and myotonic discharges. The presence of these abnormalities on EMG studies is not specific for primary myopathy. Nerve conduction studies will further assist with confirming or excluding neuropathy and neuromuscular junction disease. Although the waveform for the compound muscle action potential can show reduced amplitudes, nerve conduction velocities are normal in myopathic disease. Muscle biopsy will further support electrodiagnostic findings and provide a primary diagnosis more definitively. A 1 cubic centimeter core sample is ideal for evaluation. Frozen and formalin fixed specimens

Box 59-1 Feline Myopathies

ACQUIRED
Inflammatory
    Infectious
    Idiopathic/immune
    Paraneoplastic
Toxins and drugs
Metabolic
    Hypokalemia
    Hyperthyroidism
    Hypernatremia
    Endocrine
Ischemic
Neoplastic
Fibrotic and contractures
Nutritional

INHERITED
Muscular dystrophy
    Dystrophin deficiency
    Laminin alpha 2 deficiency
Myotonia congenita
Hypokalemic paralysis
    Burmese kittens
Nemaline rod myopathy
Glycogen storage disease type IV
    Norwegian forest cats
Devon Rex myopathy

MISCELLANEOUS
Tubulin reactive inclusion myopathy
Myositis ossificans
Feline hyperesthesia syndrome
    Possible inclusion body myopathy

Box 59-2 Feline Neuromuscular Diseases

Myopathic Disorders
Neuropathies
    Polyradiculoneuritis/neuritis (infectious/idiopathic)
    Diabetic polyneuropathy
    Ischemic neuromyopathy
    Lymphoma involving nerve roots/peripheral nerves
    Feline motor neuron diseases
    Trauma (brachial plexus, cauda equina, peripheral
        nerve)
    Feline dysautonomia
Inherited Polyneuropathies
    Sphingomyelinase-deficiency polyneuropathy
    Birman cat distal neuropathy
    Hypertrophic polyneuropathy
    Hyperoxaluric peripheral neuropathy
    Hyperchylomicronemia-associated neuropathy
Neuromuscular Junction Disorders
    Myasthenia gravis (congenital and acquired)
    Organophosphate toxicity
    Tick paralysis
    Botulism
    Toxins/drugs/envenomation
Tetanus (spinal cord interneurons)

ACQUIRED MYOPATHIES

INFLAMMATORY MYOPATHIES

Infectious

Protozoal

Infections resulting in clinical signs of polymyositis in cats most commonly are parasitic and involve toxoplasmosis. Although kittens can be affected, most affected cats are at least 1 year of age.[2] Clinical signs vary among weakness, reluctance to move, and muscle hyperesthesia. Clinical signs of systemic infection often predominate to include anterior uveitis, chorioretinitis, central nervous system dysfunction, respiratory signs, and gastrointestinal disease. Fever and weight loss are common. Hematological and serum chemistry abnormalities typically are present and may include mild nonregenerative anemia, neutrophilia, lymphocytosis, eosinophilia, hyperglobulinemia, and elevations in bilirubin and hepatic enzyme activity. CK activity may be normal or mildly to moderately elevated. Presumptive diagnosis is based on history, clinical signs, serological testing, and response to therapy. In a retrospective study of 15 cats with toxoplasmosis, serum IgM titers were positive in 14 cats, and serum IgG titers were positive in nine of the affected cats.[2] In the convalescent phase of the disease, nine cats still had positive IgM titers. Four cats did not develop IgG titers in either the acute or convalescent phases of infection. Definitive diagnosis is based on identification of encysted parasites within muscle biopsy sections; parasites are found in bradyzoite form, and usually are associated with a mild to moderate granulomatous inflammatory reaction (Figure 59-2). Multifocal disease distribution of parasitic migration makes microscopic localization difficult,

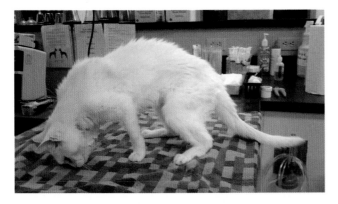

Figure 59-1 Twelve-year-old domestic shorthair cat with hypokalemic myopathy. Weakness of the cervical epaxial muscles and inability to extend the head and neck is apparent. (Courtesy Dr. Christine Rutter, Tufts University College of Veterinary Medicine.)

are recommended for evaluation by most laboratories. Prior to performing the procedure, it is imperative to contact the laboratory that will be processing and interpreting the biopsies to ensure proper sample submission.

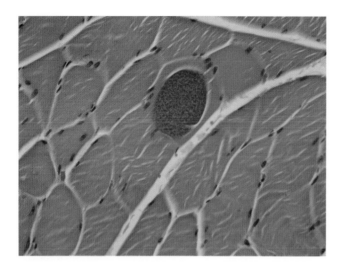

Figure 59-2 Transverse section of feline skeletal muscle showing *Toxoplasma gondii* cyst. Organism is in bradyzoite form with no inflammatory response present. (H&E stain. Magnification 400×.) (Courtesy the Armed Forces Institute of Pathology.)

and the decision to initiate treatment should not be based on absence of organisms in muscle tissue. Clindamycin, 10 mg/kg PO q8h for a minimum of 4 weeks, is the treatment of choice in cats with clinical toxoplasmosis.[3] Response to therapy and prognosis is considered to be good if treatment is initiated early in the disease course. Cats with concurrent feline immunodeficiency virus (FIV) or feline leukemia virus (FeLV) infection, however, may be more difficult to manage, with likely recurrences. A compromised immune system is a likely factor in disease pathogenesis in cats with FeLV and FIV infection.

Sarcocystosis has been reported sporadically in immunocompromised cats with cancer and in those patients receiving chemotherapy.[4] Although infection with *Neospora caninum* has been induced experimentally, natural infection involving this organism in cats has not been reported.[5]

Bacterial

Clostridial myopathy often is associated with muscle injury, penetrating wounds, surgical procedures, and muscular injections. Cats generally are resistant to the effects of tetanus toxin. Development of tetanus secondary to infection with *Clostridium tetani*, focal or generalized, can be delayed for as long 3 weeks after the inciting wound or injury. Although most infections are focal, the infection can be disseminated.[6] The predominant clinical sign is severe pain. Physical examination findings may include crepitus, swelling, and hyperesthesia of affected regions. Radiography may reveal subcutaneous gas. Histopathological findings include extensive muscle necrosis and the presence of gram-positive bacteria. Diagnosis is confirmed with positive results on anaerobic cultures. *C. tetani*, *C. sporogenes*, *C. septicum*, and *C. chauvoei* have been isolated from affected cats.[6,7]

If not treated early, infection often is fatal. Treatment involves aggressive surgical débridement and appropriate antibiotic therapy. Depending on the wound location, flushing with hydrogen peroxide can inhibit clostridial growth. Penicillin G is considered the treatment of choice; however, metronidazole may be more effective.[8] (The reader is referred to Chapter 8 in the fifth volume of this series for a complete discussion of localized and generalized tetanus.)

Viral

Myopathic abnormalities including perivascular and pericapillary lymphocytic infiltration and myofiber necrosis, phagocytosis, and regeneration have occurred with FIV infection in a research setting.[9] Clinical signs of myopathy did not develop in infected cats; however, periodic elevations in CK were reported during the study. Histopathological abnormalities in these cats were comparable to HIV-1–associated polymyositis reported in human beings.

Idiopathic Polymyositis

Idiopathic polymyositis, presumed to be immune-mediated in origin, has been reported sporadically in cats.[10-13] Histopathological examination of muscle specimens from affected cats shows a lymphocytic polymyositis. Similar findings in cats with thymoma and myasthenia gravis raise an index of suspicion for an immune-mediated basis.[11,12] Some affected cats respond to corticosteroid therapy and spontaneous remission has been reported in others.

The reported age of onset of clinical signs varies ranging from 3 months to 13 years. There is no apparent breed or gender predilection.[10] Clinical signs include weakness, exercise intolerance, and anorexia and dysphagia in a smaller number of cases. Neurological examination findings include generalized weakness manifested as a stiff, stilted gait affecting all limbs, cervical spinal ventroflexion, generalized muscle atrophy, and muscle hyperesthesia. Fever is reported in a few cases. The onset of signs typically is subacute. In the majority of cases the duration of clinical signs prior to presentation is less than 1 week, but can range from 1 day to 4 weeks.[10] Serum CK activity can be as high as tenfold above the normal range (26 to 141 IU/L). Liver enzyme (aspartate aminotransferase and alanine aminotransferase) activities can be mildly to moderately increased.[3,10] Mild decreases in serum potassium have been reported to occur in some affected cats; however, this is not thought to be associated with the primary disease process. Radiographic abnormalities may include changes consistent with the presence of a thymoma and evidence of decreased esophageal motility.

Electromyographic findings are typical for myopathic disease. Although there are few reports of electrodiagnostic evaluation in cats affected with polymyositis, it is the author's experience, based on a limited number of cases, that changes are most prominent in the proximal appendicular muscle groups and epaxial muscles.

Histopathological findings on muscle sections include a multifocal distribution of interstitial infiltration of mononuclear cells, consisting predominantly of lymphocytes and macrophages with infrequent neutrophils, and rare eosinophils and plasma cells. Perivascular, endomysial, and perimysial distribution has been observed.

Associated myofiber necrosis, regeneration, and internal nuclei also are prominent features.[10,12] Of the three patients with thymoma reported to have polymyositis, two of the cats also had myocarditis.

Early reports suggest a fair to guarded prognosis with incomplete response to prednisone and a high likelihood of recurrence of signs. An initial immunosuppressive dose of prednisone (4 mg/kg/day PO) with subsequent taper has been recommended for the treatment of idiopathic polymyositis of cats and dogs.[3,14] In the author's experience, treatment with prednisone at an initial dose of 2 mg/kg PO q12h for 2 to 4 days followed by a tapering course over 4 to 6 months often results in complete remission of clinical signs. The long-term prognosis is good.

Paraneoplastic

Polymyositis also has been described in association with some tumors in cats and dogs. This has been described in greater detail in dogs with malignant tumors including carcinomas and myeloid leukemias.[15,16] Thymomas have been associated with paraneoplastic polymyositis in cats. Pathogenesis is thought to be immune-mediated, involving T-cell proliferation against an antigen of the sarcolemma or other muscle component. Thoracic and abdominal radiography and abdominal ultrasound are recommended as part of the diagnostic evaluation when paraneoplastic polymyositis is presumed. This author has observed polymyositis in a cat in association with hepatocellular carcinoma, in addition to polymyositis in association with thymoma.

TOXIN- AND DRUG-INDUCED MYOPATHIES

Several toxins and drugs may induce myopathy. Penicillamine and cimetidine have been associated with polymyositis in the veterinary and human literature.[3] Medications such as azathioprine and the somatostatins can result in metabolic myopathic disturbances. Snake and insect toxins, and monensin (ionophore antibiotic) have direct effects on the muscle membrane by affecting transport of sodium and potassium.[17] Diuretics, insulin overdose, theophylline, amphotericin B, and glycyrrhetinate can cause hypokalemic myopathy (see the hypokalemic myopathy section of this chapter).

METABOLIC MYOPATHIES

Hypokalemic Myopathy

Severe muscle weakness secondary to hypokalemia is a well-recognized disease in cats. Muscle weakness is one of the earliest signs of potassium depletion, which is attributable to a disproportionately higher loss from muscle compared with other tissues. Hypokalemia can occur from systemic loss, reduced intake, or from a shift of potassium from the extracellular to intracellular space. Although hypokalemic myopathy can affect cats at any age, older cats with some degree of chronic kidney disease are at higher risk. In a review of 186 cats with hypokalemia, cats with severe hypokalemia (< 3.0 mEq/L) were 3.5

times more likely to have chronic kidney disease.[18] Other causes of hypokalemia include chronic vomiting, chronic diarrhea, potassium-deficient diets, hyperaldosteronism, metabolic acidosis, metabolic alkalosis, hyperthyroidism, and renal tubular acidosis. Drug-induced hypokalemia has been associated with administration of diuretics, insulin overdose, theophylline, amphotericin B, and glycyrrhetinate.[17-19]

Muscle weakness associated with hypokalemia results initially from increase in the membrane potential of the myocyte, rendering the cells refractory to depolarization. The membrane eventually becomes permeable to sodium ions, and membrane hypopolarization occurs resulting in rapid onset and severe muscle weakness.[20] In addition, muscle glycogen metabolism and blood flow during exercise become impaired secondary to hypokalemia.[21]

Affected cats typically present with acute onset of severe generalized weakness, although in retrospect owners may have observed some degree of lethargy and exercise intolerance weeks prior to onset of clinical signs. Limb weakness typically is manifested as a stiff and stilted gait. Cats are easily fatigued and sudden collapse is not uncommon. Persistent ventroflexion of the neck is a hallmark feature of the disease. Pain on muscle palpation can be elicited in some cats.

Serum potassium levels usually are severely low, reported to be less than 3.1 mEq/L.[21] The actual potassium depletion within muscle is more severe than what is reflected in the serum level. In a normal physiological state, serum potassium concentration represents whole body potassium stores. However, as potassium is lost from the body or intake is reduced, there is a disproportionately higher loss from muscle compared with other tissues. Moreover, there also is a disproportionately higher loss from extracellular fluid when compared with tissue. In human beings, serum potassium levels less than 2.0 mEq/L have been correlated with muscle necrosis and rhabdomyolysis.[22] Serum CK is mildly to moderately elevated in these cats. In six cats reported as having hypokalemic myopathy, serum potassium values ranged from 2.0 to 3.1 mEq/L (normal, 4.1 to 5.3 mEq/L), and the average serum CK value was 6418 IU/L (normal, 0 to 156 IU/L).[21] In a review of 186 hypokalemic cats, 20 patients had serum potassium values below 3.1 mEq/L (normal, 4.1 to 5.3 mEq/L); the average serum CK value of those cats was 2337 IU/L with the highest reported value of 6410 IU/L (normal, 0 to 156 IU/L).[18] When potassium levels were restored, serum CK levels returned to within the normal reference range.

Electromyographic findings in affected cats showed increased insertional activity, and abnormal spontaneous activity to include positive sharp waves and fibrillation potentials and bizarre high frequency discharges.[21] Muscle biopsies usually were normal; a few cases showed evidence of myofiber necrosis with secondary inflammatory changes.

The most important treatment strategy for hypokalemic myopathy is to normalize the serum potassium level. Oral administration is the safest route. Potassium gluconate at a dose of 2.5 to 5 mEq PO q12h should be administered initially with daily measurements of serum potassium levels.[21] Dilution of the potassium gluconate

50 per cent with water is helpful to avoid vomiting. Once the serum potassium normalizes, continued dietary supplementation with 2 to 4 mEq PO q12h in cats with significant renal potassium losses is necessary to prevent recurrence.[21] Chronic oral potassium chloride supplementation may cause metabolic acidosis and contribute to further potassium depletion. Long-term management should entail regular monitoring of serum potassium and urinary losses. Cats with severe hypokalemia who are too moribund to receive oral medication should be administered potassium chloride intravenously at a rate of 0.5 to 1 mEq/kg/hr[21] until a serum concentration of 3.5 mEq/L is reached. Potassium chloride for IV infusion should be diluted in a balanced electrolyte solution such as lactated Ringer's. Careful infusion is imperative to avoid phlebitis and fatal heart arrhythmias or asystole.[21] Continuous electrocardiographic monitoring is recommended in addition to frequent serum potassium level evaluations. Improvement in strength following treatment is rapid and observed typically within 2 to 5 days. Recovery generally is complete with appropriate therapy. Prognosis is considered good, depending on the underlying cause and/or severity of renal failure.

A unique condition has been reported in young Burmese cats 2 to 12 months of age involving hypokalemic-associated episodic weakness.[23-25] This disease is thought to be an inherited channelopathy, and is described in the section on inherited myopathies of this chapter.

Hyperthyroidism

Hyperthyroidism has been associated with muscle weakness. Generalized weakness as a historical complaint is estimated to occur in 12 to 17 per cent of cases, characterized as decreased ability to jump and fatigue associated with exercise.[26,27] Cervical spinal ventroflexion has occurred in 1 to 3 per cent of these cases. Extreme muscle weakness usually is associated with concurrent hypokalemia. The prognosis for the weakness is good with treatment of the underlying hyperthyroidism.

Hypernatremia

There is one case report of signs of polymyopathy associated with hypernatremia in a 7-month-old kitten.[28] Clinical signs were of 5 days duration and included reluctance to move and cervical ventroflexion. The serum sodium level at presentation was 215 mEq/L (normal, 148 to 165 mEq/L). Signs resolved with correction of the electrolyte imbalance and recurred in association with relapse of the hypernatremia. Long-term management with a low sodium diet was effective in controlling clinical signs.

Hypoadrenocorticism

Muscle weakness occurs frequently in association with hypoadrenocorticism in cats.[29] The weakness typically is generalized, although cervical spinal ventroflexion has not been reported. The cause of myopathy appears to be multifactorial. Hyperkalemia develops with depletion of muscle intracellular potassium, decreased membrane sodium-potassium adenosine triphosphate (ATP) activity, and diminished β-adrenergic stimulation of the sodium-potassium adenosinetriphosphatase (ATPase) pump. Adrenal insufficiency also impairs muscle carbohydrate metabolism, and muscle blood flow.[30]

Corticosteroid-Induced Myopathy

Corticosteroid-induced myopathy is well recognized in dogs and human beings as a cause of profound weakness and loss of muscle mass. The predominant effects of glucocorticoids on muscle are increase in protein catabolism and inhibition of synthesis of myofibrillar proteins. Type II myofiber atrophy is a consistent finding in affected dogs. Although this form of Cushing's myopathy has not been reported in cats, muscle wasting is a prominent finding, and histopathological abnormalities, primarily atrophy of fast twitch type II fibers, have been demonstrated in cats after receiving long-acting glucocorticoid therapy.[30] These observations would suggest that clinical myopathies associated with glucocorticoid excess do exist in cats. In suspected cases of weakness attributable to corticosteroid administration, dosage reduction to alternate-day therapy and using a nonfluorinated corticosteroid preparation may be of benefit.[30]

ISCHEMIC MYOPATHY

Ischemic myopathy and neuropathy in cats often occurs due to embolism of the terminal aorta as a secondary consequence of cardiomyopathy. Clinical signs are peracute to acute in onset, and include severe pain of the pelvic limb musculature and varying degrees of paresis or paralysis. Clinical signs can be symmetric or asymmetric. Muscles distal to the stifle are affected more severely by the ischemia. The gastrocnemius and cranial tibial muscles are often firm, and the distal limbs may be cool to touch. Patellar and flexor withdrawal reflexes may remain intact; however, limb rigidity may occur due to ischemic muscle contracture. Anesthesia of the digit and tarsal region can occur in the more severe cases. CK levels are markedly elevated. Diagnosis is further supported by weak to absent femoral pulses. Nail beds may appear cyanotic. Definitive diagnosis is made by color Doppler ultrasound–directed flow studies of the aorta and its terminal branches. Cardiomyopathy is diagnosed by echocardiography. Treatment includes pain management, thrombolytic agents, and management of the underlying heart disease. The prognosis is guarded. Although cats may regain motor function within weeks to months, most will suffer recurrence or die of heart failure within 6 months.[8] (The reader is referred to Chapters 37 and 58 in the fifth volume of this series for a complete discussion of thromboembolic disease.)

NEOPLASIA

Primary skeletal muscle tumors are rare.[12,13] Benign rhabdomyomas account for one third of striated muscle tumors and are congenital tumors originated from cardiac muscle (see Chapter 68).[31] Malignant rhabdomyosarcomas arise from muscle and nonmuscle tissues and do not involve the heart. Typically they are firm, spherical masses located deep within muscle tissue of the limbs, neck, and head. They tend to outgrow their blood supply and become necrotic. Rhabdomyosarcomas in all species typically are locally aggressive into adjacent muscles and along fascial planes. Tumor metastasis occurs by lymphatic routes to regional lymph nodes, and by hematogenous routes to lungs, viscera, and bones.[31]

Tumors involving other tissues such as lipomas, fibromas, fibrosarcomas, and other bone sarcomas may metastasize locally into skeletal muscle and represent the most common neoplasms affecting skeletal muscle.[12,31] Distant metastasis to skeletal muscle has been reported with malignant melanomas, angiosarcomas, and lymphoid tumors.[31]

FIBROTIC MYOPATHY AND CONTRACTURES

Fibrotic myopathy is a condition in which muscle is replaced by dense collagenous connective tissue resulting in a taut fibrous band. It occurs in various muscles of dogs including the gracilis, semitendinosus, and infraspinatus muscles. The resulting gait abnormality typically is a nonpainful mechanical lameness. Surgical intervention in an attempt to relieve the fibrous band can be considered in severe disabling cases; however, recurrence is likely within several months. Fibrotic myopathy of the right semitendinosus muscle has been reported in an adult neutered male Himalayan cat.[32] The cause was unknown. The cat presented with a nonpainful lameness characterized by marked flexion of the hip, stifle, and hock with an abruptly shortened anterior stride. Surgery, entailing a Z-plasty lengthening procedure, resolved the lameness. Clinical signs of lameness recurred within weeks of the surgery, but were milder in comparison with the initial lameness.

Quadriceps muscle contracture occurs commonly in dogs, usually following fractures of the distal femur in which there is inadequate repair or prolonged immobilization of the limb. Contractures also can be congenital or acquired as a complication of osteomyelitis of the femur or toxoplasmosis.[8,32] The affected limb becomes progressively fixed in abduction and extension. This results in secondary muscle atrophy and periarticular fibrosis.[8] Prognosis for recovery is guarded. Surgical intervention often is not successful. Quadriceps muscle contracture has been reported in a cat associated with a malunion of a femoral fracture and in a cat with congenital quadriceps muscle contracture.[33]

NUTRITIONAL MYOPATHIES

A myopathy has been reported in a 2-year-old cat whose diet consisted of boiled Norwegian coley (a saltwater fish).[34] Clinically the cat presented with swollen and painful muscles of both thoracic and pelvic limbs, with the proximal musculature affected more severely. Histopathological changes of the muscle showed various stages of degeneration and necrosis that included pale swollen myofibers, hyaline degeneration, necrosis, and fibrovascular reaction with macrophages and myophagia. Mild

hemorrhage and hemosiderosis were present. It was concluded to be a nutritional myopathy based on histopathological changes. Vitamin E deficiency with a low level of unsaturated fats was thought to be primarily responsible, although other deficiencies, including selenium, may have played a role. Analysis of boiled Norwegian coley showed 1.9 mg vitamin E per 400 kcal, and 2.4 grams unsaturated fats per 400 kcal. The NRC recommendations were 80 mg vitamin E and 9 grams of unsaturated fat per 400 kcal. Dietary management with vitamin supplementation including 100 mg vitamin E daily and a multivitamin supplement resulted in complete recovery within 2 weeks.

Dietary factors that contribute significantly to nutritionally induced myopathy include diets that are potassium-depleted, acidifying, and magnesium-restricted. These factors have been problematic in the past; however, quality pet food manufacturers now ensure that their diets are properly balanced.

INHERITED MYOPATHIES

MUSCULAR DYSTROPHY

Dystrophin-Deficient Muscular Dystrophy

Of all the inherited feline myopathic disorders, dystrophin-deficient muscular dystrophy is the best documented and studied. In human beings this disease is known as Duchenne muscular dystrophy and has its highest prevalence in young boys, affecting one in 3,500 to 4,000 worldwide.[34,35] Case reports of spontaneously occurring disease in cats have been sporadic; however, affected domestic shorthair cats have been described in the United States and Europe.[36-41]

The most common underlying molecular basis for muscular dystrophy in all species reported to date including human beings, mice, dogs, and cats is deficiency in the intracellular protein, dystrophin. Dystrophin is a large rod-shaped protein, highest in concentration in skeletal and smooth muscle directly underlying the sarcolemma. Dystrophin deficiency in cats with clinical and histopathological muscle disease has been documented by immunohistochemical techniques in several reports.[37-41] Lin et al demonstrated dystrophin levels in affected cats to be less than 10 per cent of that in normal cats.[35]

Although dystrophin does not span the entire cell membrane, it is tightly associated with transmembrane proteins, referred to as dystrophin-associated proteins. These connect dystrophin to the extracellular matrix protein, laminin alpha 2.[35] Dystrophin also is intimately associated with actin filaments, which form part of the scaffolding that links myofibrils to the cytoskeleton. Functionally, dystrophin is thought to play a role in regulation of cell membrane permeability, mechanical protection against sheer forces that occur during myofiber contraction, and regulation of calcium influx and efflux.[42] The dystrophin associated proteins are thought to be integral to the function of dystrophin .[35]

In Duchenne muscular dystrophy, dystrophin deficiency results in destabilization of the entire complex formed by dystrophin, dystrophin-associated proteins, and laminin alpha 2.[35] There are secondary decreases in concentrations of dystrophin-associated proteins, and of laminin alpha 2 in some cases, although to a lesser degree than deficiency of dystrophin.[31]

Duchenne muscular dystrophy is inherited as an X-linked recessive disorder. Dystrophin is a highly conserved protein, found to be encoded on the X chromosome of all placental mammals.[37] These genetic mutations lead to deficiency of the normally functioning protein and to the phenotypic appearance of myopathic disease. Variations of these mutations result in different clinical presentations of muscular dystrophy. Duchenne muscular dystrophy, the most prevalent, causes severe skeletal muscle weakness and atrophy, and cardiac disease, although few patients die of cardiac failure. Becker's muscular dystrophy is a milder variant in which dystrophin is present although truncated and partially functional. X-linked dilated cardiomyopathy is caused by the absence of dystrophin in cardiac muscle, and the presence of dystrophin expression in skeletal muscle. Homology of muscular dystrophy in dogs and genetically modified mice to the human diseases is well-documented.[36]

Other forms of muscular dystrophy have been described in human beings that involve primary deficiencies in laminin alpha 2 associated with genetic mutations in the laminin alpha 2 gene or a result of mutation in other genes.[43] Interestingly, laminin alpha 2 deficiency has been described in cats, in whom the clinical presentation differs from that in feline dystrophin-deficient muscular dystrophy.

Early reports of dystrophin-deficient muscular dystrophy in male cats suggested an X-linked dystrophin deficiency. The earliest report was described by Carpenter in 1989, describing two affected males in a litter of four cats.[37] Other reports of spontaneously occurring cases that followed also were young males. Female cats have been reported who were clinically affected by the disease with demonstrated lack of dystrophin in immunohistochemical stained muscle sections; these cats were from a research colony breeding to a single affected male.[42] Presumed heterozygote females are asymptomatic, but still develop histopathological abnormalities and decrease in dystrophin staining in skeletal and cardiac muscle, although they have not been shown to develop clinical signs of disease.[36] In 1994 a large deletion within the X chromosome of the dystrophin and Purkinje promoter was identified in a cat affected by muscular dystrophy. The deletion resulted in lack of specific protein isoforms in cardiac and skeletal muscle. A dystrophin isoform within skeletal muscle expressed by the cortical promoter of the gene was present in low quantities in these cats, but not at concentrations adequate to prevent clinical disease.[44]

In cases reported to date the phenotypic expression of dystrophin-deficient feline muscular dystrophy is unique compared with other species, with hallmark clinical signs of muscle stiffness and hypertrophy. Because of the marked muscle hypertrophy in affected cats, the disease also has been termed feline hypertrophic muscular dystrophy.[35,36,39,45] In human beings severe skeletal muscle atrophy and weakness are the predominant clinical signs.

In Duchenne muscular dystrophy, the onset of progressive weakness occurs typically at 5 years of age, often becoming crippling by 10 to 12 years of age when the patient becomes wheelchair-bound. Affected patients succumb to the disease in their mid 20's due to respiratory and/or cardiac failure.[36,41,46] Clinical signs reported in dogs are comparable to Duchenne muscular dystrophy, involving progressive muscle atrophy and weakness, which occurs at 3 months of age, followed by cardiac or respiratory failure at 2 to 3 years of age.[36] In feline dystrophin-deficient muscular dystrophy, the age of onset of signs typically is 3 to 6 months of age, but has been reported to be as late as 21 months.[37,38,40,41] All muscles including the limb, trunk, head, and neck show symmetrical hypertrophy (Figure 59-3).[37,38,41] In one cat the hypertrophied neck muscles prevented neck flexion and the ability to eat. Tongue hypertrophy in affected cats has led to subsequent renal failure and hyperosmolar syndrome due to impaired water intake.[37,40] Exercise intolerance and dyspnea are more common clinical signs than overt weakness. Death associated with respiratory distress has been reported.[41] Of 12 cats affected with muscular dystrophy, two developed heart failure, one of whom died at 6 months of age.[36]

Regurgitation is a common clinical sign.[38,40,41] Gross pathology in affected cases has shown esophageal stenosis at the esophageal hiatus secondary to hypertrophy of the diaphragm and/or associated megaesophagus.[37,38,40,41]

A stiff gait with adduction of the hocks, bunny hopping while running, and decreased ability to jump are typical locomotory signs.[37,41] Gross sublingual calcification may be apparent on physical examination. Rhabdomyolysis and malignant hyperthermia syndromes associated with general anesthesia are reported occasionally in Duchenne

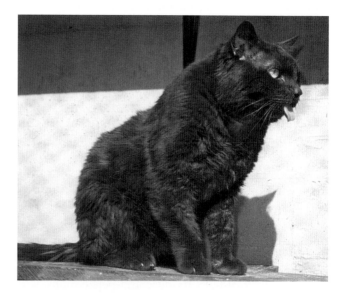

Figure 59-3 Adult Domestic Shorthair cat with dystrophin-deficient muscular dystrophy. Marked hypertrophy of the muscles of the head, neck, and shoulders is apparent, as well as protrusion of the tongue secondary to glossal hypertrophy. (Courtesy Dr. Frederic P. Gaschen. Copyright 2005 Elsevier B.V.)

muscular dystrophy.[42,44] Serum biochemical abnormalities in dystrophin-deficient cats are comparable to those that occur in Duchenne muscular dystrophy. CK levels have been reported to range from over 200 to greater than 200,000 IU/L,[37,38,40] and typically are greater than 10,000. Mild to moderate elevations in aspartate aminotransferase (AST), lactate dehydrogenase (LDH), and alanine transaminase (ALT) also are typical, and are presumed to be of muscle origin, although liver disease may occur.[37,38,40,41] Leakage of cytosolic enzymes is caused by sarcolemma membrane instability or myofiber necrosis.[40] Histopathological examination of the liver in affected cats has shown centrolobular hepatocyte necrosis, centrilobular and midzonal swelling attributable to congestive heart failure, and lipidosis.[37]

Abdominal radiography reveals hepatosplenomegaly and mild peritoneal effusion.[40] Thoracic radiography shows megaesophagus, irregular shape or scalloping of the diaphragm, cardiomegaly, and increased pulmonary vasculature.[36,40]

Although clinical signs of heart failure are uncommon, the disease does cause cardiac change to varying degrees in affected and presumed heterozygous carrier cats.[36] Radiographic abnormalities include mild to moderate cardiomegaly, usually nonprogressive, from 6 to 9 months of age.[36] Echocardiographic changes in affected cats with subclinical heart disease include concentric left ventricular wall hypertrophy and decreased left ventricular internal diameter.[36] Hyperechoic myocardial lesions observed echocardiographically in dystrophin-deficient cats have correlated with mineralization of the myocardium on histopathological examination. Doppler imaging has shown more pronounced alterations in longitudinal myocardial fibers.[45] In dystrophin-deficient cats, dystrophin has been documented to be absent from the myocardium.[36] Electrocardiographic abnormalities are found in a smaller percentage of dystrophin-deficient cats with subclinical heart disease. When present, abnormal findings include increased R wave in lead II, notching of the R wave, and shifted mean electrical axis.[36,40]

Electromyographic abnormalities in dystrophin-deficient cats have been reported to include the presence of myotonic discharges, fibrillation potentials, complex repetitive discharges, positive sharp waves, and prolonged insertional activity more severe in the proximal limb muscles.[37-40] Nerve conduction studies have been reported to be normal.

Characteristic histopathological changes observed in feline dystrophin-deficient muscular dystrophy include myofiber degeneration and regeneration, wide variation in myofiber size indicated by fiber splitting and hypertrophy, central nuclei, and hypercontracted muscle fibers (Figure 59-4). Mineralization within skeletal and cardiac muscle also is a prominent and characteristic abnormality.[37,38,40,41,46] This finding may be a result of repeated trauma and transient breaches and loss of integrity of the sarcolemma.[40] Gaschen demonstrated a selective loss of type 2A muscle fibers and fast twitch oxidative glycolytic fibers in dystrophin-deficient cats.[46] In human patients type 2B and fast twitch glycolytic fibers seem to be most sensitive to decreases in dystrophin.[38,40,46] Although atrophy, fibrosis, and adipose tissue proliferation are

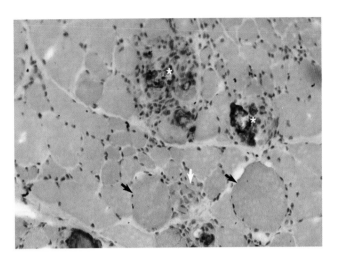

Figure 59-4 Transverse section of feline dystrophin-deficient skeletal muscle showing marked variability in myofiber size, hypertrophic myofibers *(black arrows)*, regions of degeneration/regeneration consisting of atrophic calcified myofibers and minimal mononuclear inflammatory response *(white asterisks)*, and a small area of regeneration consisting of small myofibers with larger nuclei *(white arrow)*. (H&E stain.) (Courtesy Dr. Frederic P. Gaschen. Copyright 2004 Elsevier B.V.)

common in Duchenne muscular dystrophy and canine muscular dystrophy, this is not the case in feline muscular dystrophy.[36,46] Muscle hypertrophy in cats associated with exercise seems to result from transient breaches in the sarcolemma and in efflux of CK accompanied by influx of proteins into the muscle cell, with the subsequent adaptive response of hypertrophy.[40] Transient breaches in the sarcolemma due to incompetency of the dystrophin-deficient membrane may simulate this effect. In dystrophin-deficient human beings and dogs, myofiber leakage may signal wound repair mechanisms leading to fibrosis, muscle wasting, and death.[40]

Feline dystrophin-deficient muscular dystrophy can lead to premature death from the physical effects of tongue and diaphragm hypertrophy. In addition, predisposition to fatal rhabdomyolysis and malignant hyperthermia associated with anesthesia and stress has been reported. Death associated with cardiac failure is uncommon. Still, dystrophin-deficient cats can live for many years, and some have survived the disease until 10 years of age.[46]

Cats with muscular dystrophy should be managed with supportive care. In order to reduce risk of malignant hyperthermia and rhabdomyolysis, it is important to avoid stress and excessive restraint, and limit excessive physical activity, inhalant anesthetic agents, and muscle relaxants.[35,42,44,46] Future therapeutic strategies may involve the use of the protein utrophin.[35] Utrophin is a structural and functional embryonic homolog of dystrophin, which is expressed at the sarcolemma before development of dystrophin and which is replaced gradually by dystrophin during late gestation. It has been shown to be spontaneously unregulated in Duchenne muscular dystrophy. Lin et al demonstrated upregulation of utrophin in feline muscular dystrophy during the regeneration phase of the muscle with associated restoration of dystrophin-associated proteins. Although spontaneous upregulation limited to the regeneration phase of muscle was not enough to overcome clinical disease, it was postulated that treatment strategies enabling maintenance of overexpression of the protein for longer periods at the sarcolemma may enhance efficacy.[35]

Laminin Alpha 2–Deficient Muscular Dystrophy

Laminin alpha 2–deficient muscular dystrophy has been documented in three female cats of different breeds: Siamese, domestic short hair, and Maine Coon.[43,47] Clinical signs of weakness were present by 6 months of age, and all three cats succumbed to the disease by 19 months of age. At time of death these cats were nonambulatory tetraparetic and in respiratory distress. The clinical features are quite different from the phenotypic expression of dystrophin-deficient feline muscular dystrophy. Marked muscle atrophy, weakness, contractures, and hypotonia and hyporeflexia suggestive of peripheral nerve involvement were consistent abnormalities. Serum CK elevations were moderate to marked, ranging from 4900 to 8000 IU/L. Electromyographic findings were normal or showed spontaneous activities. Motor nerve conduction velocities in all cases were reduced, consistent with myelinopathy. Histopathological findings were characteristic of the Duchenne muscular dystrophy phenotype, and included marked variation in myofiber size, atrophic and hypertrophic fibers, fibrosis, and accumulation of adipose tissue. Peripheral nerve and nerve roots were thinly myelinated. Immunohistochemistry examination revealed lack of laminin alpha 2 staining; however, dystrophin staining was normal. Laminin alpha 2 underlies the basement membrane surrounding each myofiber, and functions to anchor the sarcolemma to the basement membrane. Laminin alpha 2 also underlies the basement membrane of Schwann cells.

MYOTONIA CONGENITA

Myotonia is defined as sustained contraction of a muscle after cessation of volitional activity, and is characterized by muscle stiffness and spasm. Myotonia congenita has been reported in six kittens (three males and three females). Four kittens were related domestic shorthair cats,[48] and two were siblings, of which one was a domestic longhair and one a domestic shorthair.[49]

Onset of clinical signs ranged from 7 weeks to 5 months of age. Clinical signs included a stiff stilted gait in all limbs, being worse in the pelvic limbs. The pelvic limb gait was described as abduction secondary to reduced joint flexion. The stiffness was worse in cold temperatures and improved with exercise. When startled, the kittens would fall into lateral recumbency with hyperextension of the limbs due to extreme stiffness, and would remain in that position for several seconds. Flattening of the ears and prolonged blepharospasm also occurred in some cats. Dysphonia resulted from laryngeal spasm, and dysphagia was associated with difficulty in prehension of food.

Transient respiratory stridor and cyanosis was observed in one cat. Hypertrophy of proximal limb and tongue muscles was present in some affected cats.

Results of complete blood counts and serum chemistry profiles, including CK levels, were within the reference ranges in affected cats. Electromyographic studies showed classic myotonic discharges in all affected cases, and nerve conduction studies were normal. Percussion dimpling of the tongue was a prominent feature that was sustained for up to 30 seconds under anesthesia. Histopathological examination revealed mild to moderate diffuse muscle hypertrophy, occasional degeneration of individual muscle fibers, localized proliferation of nuclei, and few central nuclei. Immunohistochemical studies showed normal dystrophin staining. Electron microscopy of tissues was performed in one cat and showed mild dilation of the transverse tubules. All affected kittens managed relatively well without medication and were alive at the time of publication of their reports.

Congenital myotonia reported in kittens likely is genetic, and probably is reflective of a channelopathy, as is the case in human beings and dogs. Inherited channelopathies are ion channel disorders caused by genetic mutations that result in loss of normal transport of ions across the cell membrane, leading to abnormal cellular polarity and cellular dysfunction. Intriguingly, they seem to account for a vast array of neuromuscular disorders for which the underlying pathophysiology has been defined with advances in molecular biology. These diseases are known to include congenital myotonia, familial hemiplegic migraine, familial benign neonatal convulsions, episodic ataxia type 2, spinocerebellar episodic ataxia type 6, hyperkalemic periodic paralysis, hypokalemic periodic paralysis, and several other disorders.[50,51] The common clinical feature shared among these disorders is the paroxysmal onset of signs.

To date two conditions in cats that are thought to be channelopathies include hypokalemic paralysis, an abnormality of the calcium channel affecting Burmese kittens, and myotonia congenita, an abnormality in the chloride channel. Myotonia congenita in human beings and Chow Chow dogs is caused by alterations of the voltage-gated chloride channels. Chloride accounts for a majority of total resting ion conductance in normal muscle. After a change in the membrane potential, chloride ions act as a buffer and flow across the membrane to return it to resting membrane potential. In muscle with decreased chloride conductance, normally occurring potassium accumulation within T tubules is not buffered by chloride. The membrane fails to repolarize sufficiently prior to the next action potential. Subsequent action potentials can lead to depolarization of such magnitude that threshold is reached and spontaneous action potentials occur, resulting in clinical signs.[23]

Mutations causing channelopathies often affect a gene encoding one channel subunit. In affected human beings many different mutations have been demonstrated involving some region of the muscle chloride channel gene CLCN1, which contains 24 exons. Different mutations may result in different chloride channel abnormalities that may or may not result in different phenotypic expressions.[52,53] In people there are two major types of congenital myotonia involving mutation of the chloride channel: Thomsen's disease, an autosomal dominant inheritance, and Becker's disease, an autosomal recessive inheritance. Clinical myotonia is observed in both diseases, but Becker's disease also features transient weakness. Congenital myotonia in human beings also can be caused by a mutation of a highly conserved position in the sodium channel. This form of myotonia is responsive to acetazolamide, and is worsened by elevated serum potassium levels. Most channelopathies involving sodium channels, including hyperkalemic periodic paralysis and paramyotonia congenita, have episodic weakness as a clinical manifestation in addition to myotonia.[54] Understanding the molecular basis for myotonia congenita ultimately will determine the best therapies. For congenital myotonia in dogs and human beings associated with chloride channel abnormalities, the goal of treatment is to decrease repetitive activity in muscle by using antagonists to the voltage-gated sodium channel. Medications that have shown some effect are procainamide, mexiletine, phenytoin, and quinidine.[23]

HYPOKALEMIC PARALYSIS IN BURMESE KITTENS

A unique condition has been reported in young Burmese cats 2 to 12 months of age consisting of hypokalemia and associated episodic weakness.[23-25] Although the molecular basis has not been determined, most likely it is a channelopathy similar to hypokalemic periodic paralysis in human beings. Hypokalemic periodic paralysis is caused by mutations in voltage-sensitive calcium or sodium channels. Human patients with this condition experience episodic weakness or paralysis accompanied by mild decreases in serum potassium levels and increases in serum CK. Factors influencing potassium concentrations, such as insulin therapy, carbohydrate-rich meals, and rest after strenuous exercise, can precipitate episodes. Burmese cats show episodic weakness and affected cats are related. The weakness, although transient, can be severe and includes ventroflexion of the neck, head nodding, stiff stilted gait, exercise intolerance, and collapse. Serum potassium values during episodes typically are less than 3.2 mEq/L, similar to values associated with other causes of hypokalemic myopathy. However, the elevations in CK tend to be extreme, and are often higher than 50,000 IU/L.

Treatment includes potassium supplementation when acute episodes occur. Carbonic anhydrase inhibitors and dietary modification are used as preventative measures. Potassium supplementation appears to control the signs, with daily supplementation reported to be beneficial. Improvement may occur spontaneously in some affected cats.

NEMALINE ROD MYOPATHY

Congenital nemaline rod myopathy, likely having a genetic basis, has been reported in cats.[55,56] Ultrastructural

studies of congenital nemaline myopathy in human beings show nemaline rod inclusions composed of contractile cytoskeletal proteins, including thin filament proteins that normally make up the Z-band and Z-line. Mutations subsequently have been identified in five different thin-filament genes manifesting different phenotypes.

Clinical signs in affected cats were evident by 6 months to 1.5 years of age, and included progressive weakness and exercise intolerance. Five of the reported cats were born from the same queen. Males and females were affected. Euthanasia was chosen within 3 years because of extreme weakness and poor quality of life. Abnormal clinical findings included muscle atrophy more severe in the proximal limb muscles, thoracic limb weakness, again worse than the pelvic limbs, and fine tremors when walking. CK levels were normal or moderately elevated. Findings on EMG can be normal or may show abnormalities of spontaneous activity in muscle groups of the proximal thoracic limb muscles.

The predominant histopathological abnormality in all affected cats was the presence of abundant rodlike inclusions (Figure 59-5). Electron microscopy shows rods to be in structural continuity with, and arising from, Z-bands with smaller rods consisting of localized expansion of Z-bands (Figure 59-6). Areas of myofibrillar dissolution and haphazard arrangement of myofilaments were observed.[55,56]

The finding of nemaline rods in muscle biopsy is not specific for congenital nemaline rod myopathy. Nemaline rods can occur as a secondary pathophysiological process associated with other neuromuscular disease. In dogs, nemaline rods also have been observed in association with endocrine myopathies. Many other types of inclusion myopathies are described in human beings. Recently an inclusion myopathy has been described in

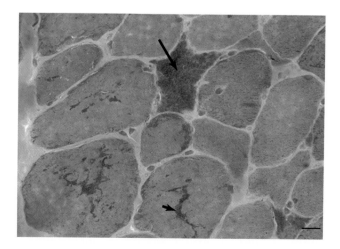

Figure 59-5 Feline nemaline rod myopathy. Fresh-frozen muscle biopsy sections from the triceps muscle prepared with modified Gomori trichome stain. Rod structures are readily visible. Focal central and diffuse staining is present *(arrows)*. Bar = 75 μm. (Courtesy Drs. Stephanie A. Kube and G. Diane Shelton. Copyright 2006 Elsevier B.V.)

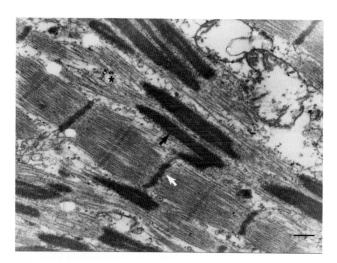

Figure 59-6 Nemaline rod myopathy. Electron micrographs showing rod bodies with the longitudinal axis parallel to that of the muscle fibers *(black arrow)*. The rods were in structural continuity with Z-discs *(white arrow)*, had the same electron density as Z-lines of adjacent sarcomeres, and had a similar lattice pattern. Areas of myofibrillar disarray also were apparent *(asterisk)*. Bar = 0.15 μm. (Courtesy Drs. Stephanie A. Kube and G. Diane Shelton. Copyright 2006 Elsevier B.V.)

two unrelated cats, in which the presence of tubulin-reactive inclusions was demonstrated.[57]

GLYCOGEN STORAGE DISEASES

Glycogen Storage Disease Type IV

Glycogen storage diseases result from defects in enzymes necessary for normal glycogen metabolism. As a consequence, accumulation of glycogen or polysaccharide storage material occurs within muscle and other tissues. A deficiency in the glycogen-branching enzyme alpha-1,4-D-glucan has been reported in an inbred family of Norwegian Forest cats.[58] In human beings this branching enzyme deficiency is known as glycogen storage disease type IV, and is a rare inherited defect that leads to the accumulation of an abnormal glycogen resembling amylopectin in skeletal, smooth, and cardiac muscles; central and peripheral nervous systems; and liver.

Clinically affected cats developed generalized muscle tremors, intermittent listlessness, and a bunny-hopping gait at 5 months of age. The muscle weakness was rapidly progressive, leading to tetraplegia by 7 months of age. One cat died of congestive heart failure. Serum alanine aminotransferase and CK levels were increased in all affected cats. Blood glucose levels and all other serum chemistries were normal. Electrodiagnostic studies were consistent with myopathic disease. Accumulations of abnormal glycogen were present in central nervous system, skeletal muscle, and heart. Although PAS-positive material was identified in hepatocytes, liver failure was not a clinical feature, as reported in human patients.

Although fasting hypoglycemia frequently is associated with glycogen storage disease, it was not a feature in these cats. Diagnosis of glycogen storage diseases typi-cally is made by identification of PAS-positive vacuoles within muscle biopsy sections. A polymerase chain reaction test is now available for the diagnosis of this disorder.

DEVON REX MYOPATHY

A myopathy has been reported in six closely related Devon Rex cats.[59] Onset of clinical signs ranged from 3 to 23 weeks of age. Abnormal findings on neurological examination included cervical spine ventroflexion, dorsal protrusion of the scapula, a hypermetric thoracic limb gait, head bobbing, megaesophagus, generalized weakness, and exercise intolerance. Abnormal prehension and swallowing of food presumably were due to pharyngeal weakness and laryngeal spasm. Death by choking on food is a hallmark feature of this myopathy. Four of the six cats died between 6 and 19 months of age due to laryngeal obstruction. One cat was euthanized at 2 years of age because of complications associated with megaesophagus. At the time of writing of the report, one cat was reported to be alive at 20 months of age, with only mild evidence of weakness.

CK activity and electrodiagnostic studies were within normal limits. Histopathological examination of muscle was consistent with a dystrophy. Abnormal findings include variation in myofiber size, internal nuclei, myofiber degeneration and regeneration, muscle atrophy and hypertrophy, and fibrosis. Although normal dystrophin staining was present in these cats, the myopathy may be associated with a form of muscular dystrophy as a result of deficiency of other proteins necessary for maintaining integrity and function of the muscle sarcolemma.

MISCELLANEOUS MYOPATHIES

MYOPATHY WITH TUBULIN-REACTIVE INCLUSIONS

This myopathy was described recently in two unrelated cats, a 6-year-old female spayed Devon Rex and a 6-year-old male neutered domestic shorthair, based on the presence of tubulin-reactive inclusions.[57] The inclusions consisted of crystalline structures that reacted positively with an antibody against tubulin, similar to that described in myopathy in human patients with tubulin-positive crystalline inclusions. Clinical signs in the two cats consisted of slowly progressive muscle weakness, and included prominent cervical ventroflexion, appendicular weakness, and moderate muscle atrophy. CK activity and electrodiagnostic testing were within normal limits.

MYOSITIS OSSIFICANS

Myositis ossificans is a rare idiopathic disorder that has been described in cats and dogs. The age of onset of signs in cats has been reported to range from 10 months to 2 years.[60,61] Disease progression is rapid and euthanasia usually occurs within 2 months of presentation. The underlying cause for this disease is unknown. Diagnosis is based on clinical signs, radiographic findings, and histopathological examination. Initial signs include mild thoracic or pelvic limb stiffness that progresses to involve severe stiffness and rigidity in all limbs and pain. Serum chemistry profiles are within normal limits. CK activity has been reported to be normal to increased. Radiography shows extensive mineralization of skeletal muscles. Histopathological findings include widespread fibrosis and ossification of skeletal muscles without evidence of inflammation. In one patient, the ectopic bone within the semimembranosus muscle had organized into a facsimile of a second femur, complete with a fatty marrow cavity.[60] Various treatments with corticosteroids, vitamin E, and diphosphonate disodium etidronate have been ineffective.[61]

FELINE HYPERESTHESIA SYNDROME

Feline hyperesthesia syndrome is a well-recognized clinical syndrome; however, the underlying etiology has remained enigmatic. Affected cats develop intermittent muscle spasms in the thoracolumbar epaxial muscles, and appear agitated and irritated with biting directed toward the back and flank regions, vocalization, frantic running, and exaggerated tail movements. An underlying myopathic disorder may be the cause in some cases.[62] Five cats between 5 and 8 years of age with a chronic history of signs consistent with feline hyperesthesia syndrome underwent electrodiagnostic testing. Electromyographic abnormalities were detected in the thoracic epaxial musculature of these five patients. Appendicular muscles were normal. On histopathological examination, vacuoles containing material staining positive with antibodies against β-amyloid and paired helical filaments were present within epaxial muscle sections, comparable to those found in inclusion body myositis in human beings.

SUMMARY

Hypokalemic and ischemic myopathy probably account for most feline myopathies encountered in clinical practice. Although reported sporadically, other myopathic disorders in cats include a vast array of inherited and acquired diseases, similar to those occurring in dogs, human beings, and other species. A thorough diagnostic evaluation will lead to recognition of the underlying disease process and appropriate therapeutic intervention.

REFERENCES

1. Maxwell LC, Barclay JK, Mohrman DE, et al: Physiological characteristics of skeletal muscle of dogs and cats, *Am J Physiol* 233:14, 1977.
2. Lappin MR, Greene CE, Winston S, et al: Clinical feline toxoplasmosis. Serologic diagnosis and therapeutic management of 15 cases, *J Vet Intern Med* 3:139, 1989.
3. Podell M: Inflammatory myopathies, *Vet Clin North Am Small Anim Pract* 32:147, 2002.
4. Edwards J, Ficken M, Luttgen P, et al: Disseminated sarcocystosis in a cat with lymphosarcoma, *J Am Vet Med Assoc* 193:831, 1988.
5. Dubey JP, Lindsay DS, Lipscomb TP: Neosporosis in cats, *Vet Pathol* 27:335, 1990.
6. Mansfield P, Wilt G, Powers R: Clostridial myositis associated with an intrathoracic abscess in a cat, *J Am Vet Med Assoc* 184:1150, 1984.
7. Poonacha K, Donahue J, Leonard W: Clostridial myositis in a cat, *Vet Pathol* 19:217, 1982.
8. Dewey CW: Myopathies: disorders of skeletal muscle. In Dewey CW, editor: *A practical guide to canine and feline neurology*, Iowa, 2003, Blackwell, p 413.
9. Podell M, Chen E, Shelton G: Feline immunodeficiency virus associated myopathy in the cat, *Muscle and Nerve* 21:1680, 1998.
10. Schunk KL: Feline polymyopathy. Proceedings of the 2nd Annual ACVIM Forum, 197, 1984.
11. Carpenter JL, Holzworth J: Thymoma in 11 cats, *J Am Vet Med Assoc* 181:248, 1982.
12. Braund KG: Endogenous causes of myopathies in dogs and cats, *Vet Med* 92:618, 1997.
13. Crickenberger GE: Polymyositis in the cat, *Pulse* 24:23, 1982.
14. Thomas WB: Use of corticosteroids in neurology. Proceedings of the Tufts Animal Expo, North Grafton, MA, 2002.
15. Sorjonen D, Braund KG, Hoff E: Paraplegia and subclinical neuromyopathy associated with primary lung tumor in a dog, *J Am Vet Med Assoc* 180:1209, 1982.
16. Griffiths IR: Neuromuscular disease in dogs: some aspects of its investigation and diagnosis, *J Small Anim Pract* 14:533, 1973.
17. Shelton GD: Rhabdomyolysis, myoglobinuria, and necrotizing myopathies, *Vet Clin North Am Small Anim Pract* 34:1469, 2004.
18. Dow SW, Fettman MJ, Curtis CR, et al: Hypokalemia in cats: 186 cases (1984-1987), *J Am Vet Med Assoc* 194:1604, 1989.
19. Eger C, Robinson W, Huxtable C: Primary aldosteronism (Conn's syndrome) in a cat: a case report and comparative aspects, *J Small Anim Pract* 24:293, 1983.
20. Fettman MJ: Feline kaliopenic polymyopathy/nephropathy syndrome, *Vet Clin North Am Small Anim Pract* 19:415, 1989.
21. Dow SW, LeCouteur RA, Fettman MJ, et al: Potassium depletion in cats: hypokalemic polymyopathy, *J Am Vet Med Assoc* 191:1563, 1987.
22. Knochel JP: Neuromuscular manifestations of electrolyte disorders, *Am J Med* 72:521, 1982.
23. Vite CH: Myotonia and disorders of altered muscle membrane excitability, *Vet Clin North Am Small Anim Pract* 32:169, 2002.
24. Mason K: A hereditary disease in Burmese cats manifested as an episodic weakness with head nodding and neck ventroflexion, *J Am Anim Hosp Assoc* 24:147, 1988.
25. Edwards CM, Belford CJ: Hypokalemic polymyopathy in Burmese cats, *Aust Vet Pract* 25:58, 1995.
26. Peterson ME: Hyperthyroidism. In Ettinger SJ, Feldman EC, editors: *Textbook of veterinary internal medicine*, ed 5, Philadelphia, 2000, Saunders, p 1400.
27. LeCouteur RA, Dow SW, Sisson AF: Metabolic and endocrine myopathies of dogs and cats, *Semin Vet Med Surg* 4:146, 1989.
28. Dow SW, Fettman MJ, LeCouteur RA, et al: Hypodypsic hypernatremia and associated myopathy in a hydrocephalic cat with transient hypopituitarism, *J Am Vet Med Assoc* 191:217, 1987.
29. Greco DS, Peterson ME: Feline hypoadrenocorticism. In Kirk RW, editor: *Current veterinary therapy X*, Philadelphia, 1989, Saunders, p 1042.

30. Platt SR: Neuromuscular complications in endocrine and metabolic disorders, *Vet Clin North Am Small Anim Pract* 32:125, 2002.

31. Luttgen PJ: Miscellaneous myopathies, *Semin Vet Med Surg* 4:168, 1989.

32. Lewis DD: Fibrotic myopathy of the semitendinosus muscle in a cat, *J Am Vet Med Assoc* 193:240, 1988.

33. Carberry CA, Flanders JA: Quadriceps contracture in a cat, *J Am Vet Med Assoc* 189:1329, 1986.

34. Dennis JM, Alexander RW: Nutritional myopathy in a cat, *Vet Rec* 111:195, 1982.

35. Lin S, Gaschen F, Burgunder JM: Utrophin is a regeneration-associated protein transiently present at the sarcolemma of regenerating skeletal muscle fibers in dystrophin-deficient hypertrophic feline muscular dystrophy, *J Neuropathol Exp Neurol* 57:780, 1998.

36. Gaschen L, Lang J, Lin S, et al: Cardiomyopathy in dystrophin-deficient hypertrophic feline muscular dystrophy, *J Vet Intern Med* 13:346, 1999.

37. Carpenter JL, Hoffman EP, Romanul FC, et al: Feline muscular dystrophy with dystrophin deficiency, *Am J Pathol* 135:909, 1989.

38. Kohn B, Guscetti F, Waxenberger M, et al: Muscular dystrophy in a cat, *Tierarztl Prax* 21:451, 1993.

39. Howard J, Jaggy A, Busato A, et al: Electrodiagnostic evaluation in feline hypertrophic muscular dystrophy, *Vet J* 168:87, 2004.

40. Gaschen FP, Hoffman EP, Goropse JR, et al: Dystrophin deficiency causes lethal muscle hypertrophy in cats, *J Neurol Sci* 110:149, 1992.

41. Vos JH, van der Linde-Sipman JS, Goedegeburre SA: Dystrophy like myopathy in the cat, *J Comp Path* 96:335, 1986.

42. Gaschen F, Gaschen L, Seiler G, et al: Lethal peracute rhabdomyolysis associated with stress and general anesthesia in three dystrophin-deficient cats, *Vet Pathol* 35:117, 1998.

43. O'Brien DP, Johnson GC, Liu LA, et al: Laminin alpha 2 (merosin)-deficient muscular dystrophy and demyelinating neuropathy in two cats, *J Neurol Sci* 189:37, 2001.

44. Winand NJ, Edwards M, Pradhan D, et al: Deletion of the muscle promoter in feline muscular dystrophy, *Neuromuscul Disord* 4:443, 1994.

45. Chetboul V, Blot S, Carlos Sampedrano C, et al: Tissue Doppler imaging for detection of radial and longitudinal myocardial dysfunction in a family of cats affected by dystrophin-deficient hypertrophic muscular dystrophy, *J Vet Intern Med* 20:640, 2006.

46. Gaschen F, Burgunder JM: Changes of skeletal muscle in young dystrophin-deficient cats: a morphological and morphometric study, *Acta Neuropathol* 101:591, 2001.

47. Poncelet A, Resibois A, Engvall E, et al: Laminin alpha 2 deficiency-associated muscular dystrophy in a Maine Coon cat, *J Small Anim Pract* 44:550, 2003.

48. Hickford FH, Jones BR, Gething MA, et al: Congenital myotonia in related kittens, *J Small Anim Pract* 39:281, 1998.

49. Toll J, Cooper B, Altschul M: Congenital myotonia in 2 domestic cats, *J Vet Intern Med* 12:116, 1998.

50. Surtees R: Inherited ion channel disorders, *Eur J Pediatr* 159:199, 2000.

51. Kullmann DM, Hanna MG: Neurological disorders caused by inherited ion-channel mutations, *Lancet Neurol* 1:157, 2002.

52. Sangiuolo F, Botta A, Mesoraca A, et al: Identification of five new mutations and three novel polymorphisms in the muscle chloride channel gene (CLCN 1) in 20 Italian patients with dominant and recessive myotonia congenita, *Hum Mutat* 11:331, 1998.

53. Brugnoni R, Galantini S, Confalonieri P, et al: Identification of three novel mutations in the major human skeletal muscle chloride channel gene (CLCN 1), causing myotonia congenita, *Hum Mutat* 14:447, 1999.

54. Ptacek LJ, Tawil R, Griggs RC, et al: Sodium channel mutations in acetazolamide-responsive myotonia congenita, paramyotonia congenita, and hyperkalemic periodic paralysis, *Neurology* 44:1500, 1994.

55. Kube SA, Vernau KM, LeCouteur RA, et al: Congenital myopathy with abundant nemaline rods in a cat, *Neuromuscul Disord* 16:188, 2006.

56. Cooper BJ, DeLahunta A, Gallagher EA, et al: Nemaline myopathy of cats, *Muscle Nerve* 9:618, 1986.

57. Shelton GD, Sturges BK, Lyons LA, et al: Myopathy with tubulin-reactive inclusions in two cats, *Acta Neuropathol* 114:537, 2007.

58. Fyfe JC, Giger U, Van Winkle TJ, et al: Glycogen storage disease type IV: inherited deficiency of branching enzyme activity in cats, *Pediatr Res* 32:719, 1992.

59. Malik R, Mepstead K, Yang F, et al: Hereditary myopathy of Devon Rex cats, *J Small Anim Pract* 34:539, 1993.

60. Norris AM, Pallett L, Wilcock B: Generalized myositis ossificans in a cat, *J Am Anim Hosp Assoc* 16:659, 1980.

61. Waldron D, Pettigrew V, Turk M, et al: Progressive ossifying myositis in a cat, *J Am Vet Med Assoc* 187:64, 1985.

62. March PA, Fischer JR, Potthoff A: Electromyographic and histologic abnormalities in epaxial muscles of cats with feline hyperesthesia syndrome (abstract), *J Vet Intern Med* 13:238, 1999.

SECTION
IX

Hematopoietic and Lymphatic Systems

Ann E. Hohenhaus, Section Editor

CHAPTER

60 Immune-Mediated Hemolytic Anemia

Barbara Kohn

ETIOLOGY AND PATHOGENESIS

PRIMARY AND SECONDARY IMMUNE-MEDIATED HEMOLYTIC ANEMIA

In immune-mediated hemolytic anemia (IMHA), the underlying pathogenesis involves destruction of red blood cells (RBCs) by a type II (antibody-dependent cytotoxicity) mechanism. Initiation of IMHA involves presentation of a self-antigen by major histocompatibility complex (MHC) molecules and interactions between autoreactive T- and B-lymphocytes resulting in synthesis of autoantibodies. Immunoglobulin (Ig) G or IgM antibody-coated RBCs may be removed after formation of the membrane attack complex of the terminal pathway of complement (intravascular lysis) or after opsonization by IgG and/or complement C3b and phagocytosis by macrophages in the spleen and liver (extravascular lysis).[1]

The antibody may attach to the surface of the RBCs by several different mechanisms. Antibodies may be directed against normal erythrocytes or against erythrocytes altered antigenically through interaction with secondary causes. If the stimulus responsible for antibody production can not be identified, the anemia is called *primary IMHA* (pIMHA) or *autoimmune hemolytic anemia* (AIHA). The "true" autoantibody binds to a structural component of the erythrocyte membrane (self-antigen) and may develop after primary immunological dysregulation. In dogs, major autoantigenic molecules, such as erythrocyte membrane glycoproteins (glycophorins), and compo-

nents of the erythrocyte anion exchange channel (band 3) have been identified.[2] However, there are no data available in cats to indicate the major autoantigen.

In many cases, there is a specific underlying cause for this antibody binding *(secondary IMHA [sIMHA])*. Mechanisms of antibody binding in sIMHA are (1) binding to a foreign epitope carried by an infectious agent (e.g., *Hemoplasma* spp.) or drug that is attached nonspecifically to the cell surface (innocent bystander destruction); (2) a drug (acting as a hapten) binds to a RBC surface molecule, creating a novel epitope recognized as foreign by the immune system (modified-self); (3) binding of a drug or microbe causes exposure of a previously cryptic determinant; and (4) alloantibody binding to a blood group antigen. Additionally, Ig or immune complexes may be absorbed nonspecifically onto the surface of the erythrocyte but will not necessarily mediate cell destruction (Figure 60-1).[1]

sIMHA in cats can be triggered by infectious agents, such as feline leukemia virus (FeLV), coronaviruses that induce feline infectious peritonitis (FIP), feline immunodeficiency virus (FIV), *Hemoplasma* spp., and *Hepatozoon* infection; inflammatory diseases (e.g., sterile and nonsterile abscesses, cholangiohepatitis, pyothorax, polyarthritis, nephritis, or lymphocytic enteritis), drugs (e.g., propylthiouracil, methimazole); or tumors (e.g., malignant lymphoma, erythroid leukemia, mast cell leukemia, or lymphoid leukemia). IMHA also has been described in cats suffering from amyloidosis and myelodysplasia.[3-12] Therefore an extensive search for an underlying disorder or trigger is always warranted, and IMHA only should be

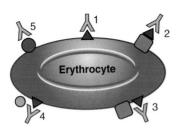

FIGURE 60-1 Possible mechanisms of antibody binding in pIMHA and sIMHA. *1,* Primary (autoimmune) IMHA; autoantibody binding to a structural component of the RBC membrane (self-antigen). *2-5,* Secondary IMHA: *2,* antibody binding to a foreign epitope carried by an infectious agent or drug; *3,* binding of a drug to a RBC membrane component creating a novel epitope; *4,* binding of a drug or microbe leads to exposure of a previously cryptic determinant; *5,* alloantibody binding to a blood group antigen. (Modified according to Day MJ, Mackin AJ: Immune-mediated haematological disease. In Day MJ, editor: *Clinical immunology of the dog and cat,* ed 2, London, 2008, Manson Publishing, p 94.)

defined as autoimmune in the absence of identifiable underlying factors.

Recent vaccination (within 1 month) has been implicated as a trigger for immune-mediated diseases such as IMHA[13] and polyarthritis[14] in dogs. Vaccination against calicivirus has resulted in polyarthritis in cats.[15] Therefore it appears likely that vaccines enhance a smoldering immune process. Three of 19 cats with pIMHA had been vaccinated in the 4 weeks before initial presentation.[11] However, it is difficult to define a vaccine reaction, and the mechanism underlying this association has not been ascertained.

IMHA and immune-mediated thrombocytopenia (IMTP) occur most commonly in isolation, but the two conditions may occur together (Evans' syndrome), which has been described in a small number of cats.[16,17] Moreover, IMHA can be part of the multisystemic autoimmune disease (e.g., systemic lupus erythematosus).[18,19]

IMHA often is associated with a strongly regenerative bone marrow erythroid response; however, a high percentage of cats do not have reticulocytosis at the time of diagnosis.[11] One possible reason for this may be peracute IMHA because 3 to 4 days are required for a substantial reticulocyte response to occur after the onset of anemia.[20] An absence of reticulocytosis in animals with anemia of greater than 5 days duration has been attributed to immune reactions directed against erythroid precursor cells. This can be due either to nonregenerative IMHA (associated with bone marrow erythroid hyperplasia or erythroid maturation arrest) or to pure red cell aplasia (PRCA) that is characterized by erythroid aplasia in the bone marrow.[21,22]

PRCA is an uncommon hematological syndrome characterized by severe anemia, reticulocytopenia, and leukocyte and platelet counts that are within reference ranges. PRCA can be primary (idiopathic) or secondary in origin, and secondary PRCA has been reported in cats infected with FeLV subtype C. Three of six cats in one study of

PRCA were Coombs' test–positive, supporting the theory of immune-mediated pathology in idiopathic cases of PRCA.[21]

Alloimmune hemolytic anemias, such as *hemolytic transfusion reactions* and *neonatal isoerythrolysis,* are caused by specific anti-erythrocytic alloantibodies. Unlike dogs, cats possess naturally occurring antibodies (alloantibodies) against the blood group they are lacking (see Chapter 61). These alloantibodies can lead to incompatibility reactions, such as hemolytic transfusion reactions, when incompatible transfusions are administered. Cats with blood type B who receive type A blood may develop a severe acute hemolytic transfusion reaction, with clinical signs such as lethargy, bradycardia, dyspnea, cardiac arrhythmia, salivation, vomition, defecation and urination, and neurological disorders. Death may occur during this phase. If the cats survive, they develop tachycardia, tachypnea, hemoglobinemia, and hemoglobinuria. If type A cats receive blood from type B cats, only mild incompatibility reactions, such as restlessness, tachycardia, and tachypnea, may be observed. However, the transfusion is not efficient because of the rapid destruction of erythrocytes.[23,24] These alloantibodies are the cause of neonatal isoerythrolysis, a very specific form of IMHA, Neonatal isoerythrolysis is an important disorder for breeders because type A kittens born to a type B queen are at risk. Besides the well-characterized AB blood grouping system, a newly recognized blood group, the *Mik* red cell antigen, with a corresponding clinically relevant, naturally occurring alloantibody, has been described in association with hemolysis.[25]

CATEGORIES OF IMMUNE-MEDIATED HEMOLYTIC ANEMIA

Classically, IMHA has been subdivided into five main categories based on the thermal reactivity of the anti-RBC antibodies and their major clinical effects at optimal temperature. This categorization system is derived by extrapolation from human beings; however, the five categories have been described in small animals. In cats, as well as in other species, IMHA typically is caused by warm reactive antibodies that exert their effects at body temperature. Three different categories have been described (Class I to III). Cold reactive antibodies are only reactive at cold temperatures; two categories (Class IV to V) have been described (Table 60-1).[26]

EPIDEMIOLOGY

IMHA was reported to be uncommon in cats. However, very few data are available regarding the occurrence of the different types of anemia in cats. One hundred cats who presented to the Small Animal Clinic, Freie Universität Berlin over a 2-year period with a hematocrit (Hct) <25 per cent were studied prospectively. Twenty-four cats suffered from hemolytic anemia: 12 of them from pIMHA, three from sIMHA, three cats had FIP, and one cat each with lymphoma, severe hypophosphatemia, and Heinz body anemia. The cause of hemolytic anemia remained

Table 60-1 Categories of Immune-Mediated Hemolytic Anemia

Category	Antibodies Involved	Pathomechanism
Class I	IgG, IgM; warm reactive	Autoantibodies agglutinate RBCs at body temperature; agglutination may be seen when a drop of blood is placed on a glass slide; RBCs are destroyed mainly by phagocytosis in the spleen (extravascular hemolysis).
Class II	IgM; warm reactive	Antibodies activate complement and destroy RBCs by intravascular hemolysis causing hemoglobinemia and hemoglobinuria.
Class III	IgG; warm reactive	Antibodies bind to RBCs at 37° C; they do not activate complement or agglutinate RBCs (affected cells are removed by splenic macrophages, extravascular hemolysis).
Class IV	IgM; cold reactive	Antibodies agglutinate RBCs at cold temperatures ("cold-agglutinins"); agglutination can occur within the vasculature of the extremities.
Class V	IgM, cold reactive	IgM antibodies will bind RBCs when chilled to 4° C but will not agglutinate them; these antibodies can activate complement leading to intravascular hemolysis.

Data from Tizard IR: *Veterinary immunology*, Philadelphia, 2004, Saunders.
IgG, Immunoglobulin G; *IgM,* immunoglobulin M; *RBCs,* red blood cells.

unknown in three cats. The following diagnoses were obtained in the other cats: anemia of inflammatory disease (29 per cent), acute blood loss anemia (22 per cent), chronic blood loss anemia (2 per cent), chronic kidney disease (9 per cent), nonregenerative anemia caused by retrovirus infection/bone marrow disease (9 per cent), and cause of anemia unknown (5 per cent).[9] In a retrospective study performed at the Utrecht University, all Coombs'-positive cats presented over an 11-year period were evaluated. Sixty-seven cats with underlying diseases were diagnosed with sIMHA and 29 cats were diagnosed with idiopathic IMHA. These two studies and other reports suggest that pIMHA and sIMHA occur more frequently in cats than recognized previously.[10,27]

SIGNALMENT

The age of 19 cats with pIMHA ranged from 6 months to 9 years (mean 3.2 years); 12 cats were younger than 3 years.[11] In other studies (involving five and 25 cats), the average age was 3 and 6.2 years, respectively.[27,28] Domestic Shorthair cats were affected primarily. A slightly higher incidence of pIMHA was reported in male cats.[3,11,27] The age of nine cats with idiopathic PRCA ranged from 8 months to 3 years.[21]

HISTORY

Most owners of the 19 cats with pIMHA sought veterinary care because of nonspecific clinical signs such as lethargy (n = 19) and inappetence (n = 13). Other clinical signs were pica (n = 5) and rarely vomiting (n = 2), pruritus, dyspnea, epistaxis, polydipsia, and obstipation (one cat each). Before initial evaluation, the cats had been sick between 1 and 56 days (median 8.5 days). Three of 19 cats with pIMHA had been vaccinated 3 to 4 weeks before initial presentation.[11] However, the association between vaccination and disease might have been coincidental.

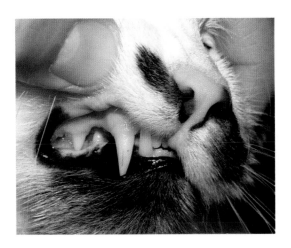

FIGURE 60–2 Pale mucous membranes in a cat with severe anemia caused by primary IMHA.

CLINICAL AND LABORATORY FINDINGS

Cats often are presented in a late stage of the disease because the major clinical signs of lethargy and inappetence are nonspecific. Moreover, cats appear to tolerate low Hct values better than dogs. Further findings often include pale mucous membranes (Figure 60-2), mild-to-moderate systolic heart murmurs (degree II-IV/VI), and rarely, hypothermia or hyperthermia. Heart murmurs may be due to changes in rheological properties of the blood because of severe anemia; however, it is possible that chronic anemia may lead to a secondary cardiomyopathy. Compared to dogs, icterus is rare in affected cats and was detected in only two of 19 patients, suggesting a slow, well-compensated hemolytic process in most cases.[11]

Cats reported in the literature suffered from extravascular hemolysis; intravascular hemolysis occurs less frequently in cats than in dogs, and a careful search for sIMHA (e.g., a result of hemoplasmosis) is warranted in these cases (Figure 60-3).

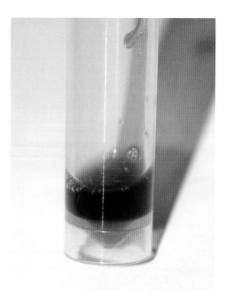

FIGURE 60-3 Hemolytic plasma in a rare case of intravascular IMHA in a cat.

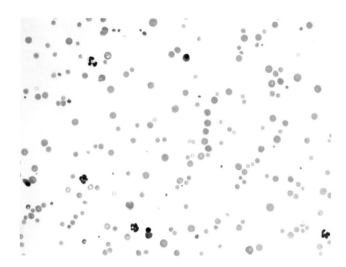

FIGURE 60-4 Blood smear of a cat with regenerative primary IMHA: polychromasia, anisocytosis, and nucleated RBCs. (May-Grünwald, ×1000.)

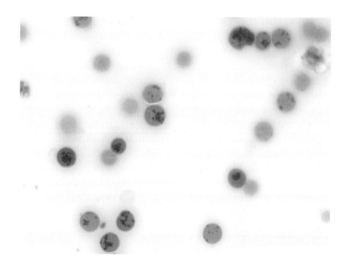

FIGURE 60-5 Blood smear of a cat with regenerative primary IMHA: numerous aggregated and few punctated reticulocytes. (brilliant cresyl blue, ×1000.)

A mean Hct of 12 per cent was reported in 30 cats with pIMHA at initial presentation.[27,28] In another study with 19 cats, the Hct ranged from 6 to 22 per cent (median 12 per cent); 79 per cent of the cats had a severe anemia with a Hct less than 15 per cent.[11] Twenty-nine cats with pIMHA had Hct values ranging from 6 to 23 per cent (median 9.5 per cent), which was significantly lower than the Hct values of a group of cats with sIMHA (n = 67; range 4 to 38 per cent, median 14 per cent).[10]

The median Hct of nine cats with idiopathic PRCA was 7 per cent (range 6 to 15 per cent).[21] In a study by Weiss (2008), the mean Hct of 29 cats with PRCA was 7 per cent (SD ± 2); twenty-four cats were diagnosed with nonregenerative IMHA with erythroid hyperplasia and four cats had nonregenerative IMHA with erythroid maturation arrest. The mean Hct in these cats was 13 and 14 per cent, respectively.[22]

Regeneration of RBCs in patients with hemolytic anemia is characterized by macrocytic and either hypochromic or normochromic erythrocytes. At initial evaluation, 13 of 19 cats with pIMHA had an increased mean corpuscular volume (MCV), but only eight of these patients had increased numbers of aggregated reticulocytes.[11] However, MCV also can be increased in patients with severe agglutination because it is difficult for cell counters to identify single RBCs resulting from agglutination.

Median absolute aggregate and punctate reticulocyte counts at initial presentation in two studies with 19 and 25 cats with pIMHA were 16,000 and 72,600/μL and 46,000 and 248,070/μL, respectively (Figures 60-4 and 60-5). In 11 of 19 cats (58 per cent) with pIMHA, the anemia was nonregenerative at initial evaluation, which makes a diagnosis of hemolytic anemia more challenging. The aggregated reticulocyte counts of these 11 cats ranged from 0 to 28,600/μL and increased in 10 cats after 7 to 33 days to greater than 40,000/μL.[11] Because bone marrow results of these cats were not available, some

patients might have suffered from nonregenerative IMHA or PRCA.[22]

Evaluation of blood smears revealed 1 to 20 nucleated RBCs/100 white blood cells (WBCs) (median 4) in 11 of 19 cats with pIMHA, only three of whom had a regenerative anemia with more than 40,000/μL aggregated reticulocytes. The number of Heinz bodies in these 19 cats was less than 5 per cent.[11]

In dogs, leukocytosis with a left shift is common in association with pIMHA. In cats, however, leukocytosis is rare. In two studies, neutrophilia was found in 10.5 per cent and 12 per cent of the cats, respectively, and a left shift was present in 5 per cent and 20 per cent.[11,27] Anemia-related hypoxia and thromboembolism causing tissue necrosis primarily in the liver, spleen, and lung are considered the main factors for leukocytosis in dogs with pIMHA.[29] No data are available concerning histopathological examinations of cats with pIMHA.

In two studies, lymphocytosis was present in 32 per cent and 52 per cent of cats with values from 4400 to 12,400/µL.[11,27] In approximately half of the cats, reactive lymphocytes were described that should not be mismatched with lymphoblasts. Lymphopenia was detected in 16 per cent of cats[11] and a monocytosis in 8 per cent and 31 per cent of cats with pIMHA.[11,27]

Thrombocytopenia was detected in 42 per cent and 33 per cent of cats in two different studies on pIMHA.[11,27] Low platelet counts may be caused by consumption caused by disseminated intravascular coagulation (DIC), sequestration in an enlarged spleen, or immune-mediated destruction. In dogs with pIMHA, approximately one-third also suffer from IMTP (Evans' syndrome). One of 19 cats with pIMHA suffered from both IMHA and thrombocytopenia. A direct platelet-bound antibody test was positive, supporting the diagnosis of Evans' syndrome.[11,27] DIC was present in 45 per cent of dogs suffering from IMHA[30] but only diagnosed in 8 per cent and 10 per cent of cats in two studies.[11,27] However, coagulation profiles were only performed in a small number of cats. Thrombocytopenia also may be due to bone marrow pathology described in 11 of 24 cats with nonregenerative IMHA.[22] Thromboembolic complications have been reported quite commonly in dogs with IMHA[29,30]; however, no reports about cats are in the literature. The author recently has seen thromboembolic events in a cat with severe intravascular pIMHA, leading to necrosis of several toes of both hind limbs. Liver enzyme activities, especially alanine aminotransferase (ALT), were increased in about 50 per cent of the cats with pIMHA.[11] Mild-to-moderate hyperbilirubinemia was present in 13 of 19 cats with pIMHA (plasma bilirubin concentration 0.4 to 1.9 mg/dL, median 0.7 mg/dL). In seven of the 13 cats with hyperbilirubinemia, the liver enzyme activities also were increased. The Hct of these cats was 6 to 13 per cent (median 9 per cent), suggesting liver damage as a result of hypoxia.[11] Liver necrosis caused by hypoxia was shown by histopathological examination in dogs with IMHA.[29] In six of 19 cats with pIMHA with Hct values ranging from 6 to 20 per cent, the plasma bilirubin concentrations were in the normal range, indicating a compensated chronic hemolysis.[11]

A majority of cats with pIMHA have hyperglobulinemia.[10,11] Lymphocytosis, hyperglobulinemia, and splenomegaly may indicate chronic antigenic stimulation of the immune system. This finding also has been described in other feline hemolytic anemias such as pyruvate kinase deficiency and increased erythrocytic osmotic fragility.[31,32]

COLD AGGLUTININ DISEASE

Obstruction of the blood supply to the peripheral vasculature as a result of agglutination can lead to ischemic necrosis of the tips of the ears or tail, the end of the nose, and the feet. This has been described in only one cat to date, who developed dry gangrene of both front paws, both ear tips, and the distal half of the tail. Abdominal palpation revealed mild splenomegaly. There was macroscopic agglutination present at 4° C but not at 37° C.

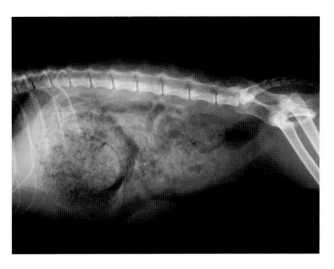

FIGURE 60-6 Lateral abdominal radiograph: splenomegaly in a 2-year-old British shorthair cat with primary IMHA.

Complete blood count revealed mild neutrophilia with a left shift, a drop of the Hct from 29 per cent to 18 per cent but no intravascular hemolysis.[33]

DIAGNOSTIC IMAGING

Radiographic and ultrasonographic examinations identified enlarged spleens with homogeneous parenchyma in 42 per cent of 19 cats with pIMHA (Figure 60-6).[11] In another study, three of five cats had splenomegaly.[28] Diffuse splenomegaly can be caused by inflammatory or infectious processes (e.g., splenitis as a result of FIP, *Mycoplasma haemofelis*, or toxoplasmosis), infiltration of abnormal cells (neoplastic or nonneoplastic, extramedullary hematopoiesis), congestion, or hyperplastic splenomegaly (e.g., associated with hemolysis). Cats suffering from other types of hemolytic anemia, such as increased erythrocyte osmotic fragility or pyruvate kinase deficiency, also had splenomegaly. The principal histopathological findings included lymphoreticular hyperplasia, extramedullary hematopoiesis, and hemosiderosis.[31] Results of pathological examinations of cats with pIMHA are not available.

DIFFERENTIAL DIAGNOSIS

In addition to pIMHA and sIMHA and A-B blood group incompatibilities, several other causes for hemolysis characterized by a shortening of the normal survival time of erythrocytes have been described in cats (Table 60-2).

DIAGNOSIS

The diagnosis of IMHA is based on persistent erythrocyte agglutination or detection of erythrocyte-bound IgG, IgM, or complement (direct differentiating Coombs' test). In dogs, numerous spherocytes are pathognomonic for IMHA. In cats, however, identification of spherocytes is

Table 60-2 Differential Diagnoses of Hemolytic Anemias in Cats

Immune-mediated	Primary IMHA Secondary IMHA Evans' syndrome Alloimmune hemolytic anemia (hemolytic transfusion reaction, neonatal isoerythrolysis)
Infectious diseases	Hemoplasmosis, FeLV infection, babesiosis, cytauxzoonosis, bacterial sepsis
Inherited erythrocytic defects	Pyruvate kinase deficiency (Abyssinians, Somalis, few domestic shorthair cats), "increased osmotic fragility of erythrocytes" (Abyssinians, Somalis), porphyria (Siamese)
Oxidant injury of erythrocytes	Chemicals and drugs (e.g., acetaminophen, phenacetin, vitamin K overdose, phenazopyridine, methylene blue, DL-methionine, zinc, benzocaine, lidocaine), food additives (e.g., onions, propylene glycol), certain diseases (e.g., diabetic ketoacidosis, hyperthyroidism, lymphoma, carcinoma), excessive Heinz body formation and/or methemoglobinemia, Heinz body anemia in severe cases
Microangiopathic hemolytic anemia	Associated with DIC, tumors (e.g., hemangiosarcoma) (often subclinical)
Hypophosphatemia (depletion of energy supply [adenosine triphosphate] to RBCs)	Associated with diabetes mellitus, hepatic lipidosis, refeeding syndrome, oral administration of phosphate- binding acids

IMHA, Immune-mediated hemolytic anemia; *FeLV,* feline leukemia virus; *DIC,* disseminated intravascular coagulation; *RBCs,* red blood cells.

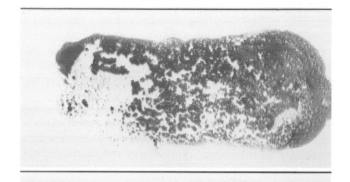

FIGURE 60-7 Macroscopic slide agglutination of erythrocytes in a cat with primary IMHA

present in all 19 cats with pIMHA. In most cats (15/19), however, agglutination did not persist after thorough washing of RBCs.[11] In another study, 40 per cent of the cats showed autoagglutination.[27] However, the method of testing was not described. Agglutination of RBCs, however, is not specific for IMHA because mild agglutination can be detected in cats without autoimmune diseases.[3,9]

A positive Coombs' test does not differentiate between pIMHA and sIMHA (i.e., a positive test result does not confirm if there are antiautologous antigens, antibodies against RBC-attached xenoantigens such as drugs or components of infectious agents, or immune-complexed antibodies bound nonspecifically to the surface of RBCs). Moreover, differences in test methods or use of reagents may have an effect on the test results.

The diagnostic importance of the Coombs' test has been questioned because of the occurrence of false-positive and false-negative results.[34] However, performing a Coombs' test in a qualified laboratory is strongly recommended in all cats with suspected IMHA, even if criteria, such as positive agglutination, already strongly suggest the diagnosis. A positive Coombs' test will support the diagnosis; if a differentiated Coombs' test is performed, the IMHA can be further characterized by determining the involvement of various immunoglobulin types (IgG and/or IgM) and complement.

The validity of a differentiated direct Coombs' test was tested by evaluating five healthy, 78 sick anemic, and nine sick nonanemic cats. None of the healthy or sick nonanemic cats had a positive Coombs' test result. In those cats suffering from blood loss anemia or nonregenerative anemia due to renal failure, retrovirus infection, or anemia of inflammatory disease, the Coombs' test results were negative, with the exception of one cat with cholangitis. Cats suffering from hemolysis not related to immunological processes, such as hypophosphatemia or Heinz body anemia, also tested negative. Eighteen of 76 cats had positive Coombs' test results. In 17 of the 18 cats who had positive Coombs' test results, hemolytic anemia was diagnosed by an increased osmotic fragility, hyperbilirubinemia, or increased numbers of reticulocytes. No other causes for anemia were detected in 15 cats who tested positive. Moreover, most of these cats experienced

difficult because feline RBCs are much smaller and do not have a central pallor. None of the tests, however, can differentiate between pIMHA and sIMHA, and the diagnosis of pIMHA therefore is one of exclusion.

Agglutination must be differentiated from rouleaux formation by adding a few drops of physiological saline; a rouleaux pattern will disperse. For confirmation of a persistent (auto) agglutination, RBCs are "washed" three times. Physiological saline is added to the tube containing the EDTA anticoagulated blood. After repeated mixing, the tube is centrifuged, and plasma and supernatant is removed. This process is repeated an additional two times. Agglutination will either "break up" or "persist" (Figure 60-7). True autoagglutination is indicative of an immune process and precludes the performance of Coombs' testing or blood typing. Varying degrees of agglutination, which remained after adding saline, were a favorable response to immunosuppressive therapy. Therefore the diagnosis of pIMHA was very likely. Three cats with positive Coombs' test results were diagnosed with sIMHA (associated with FeLV infection, lymphoma, or cholangitis).

Based on these results, the Coombs' test was considered very useful in diagnosing IMHA.[11] In the case of a negative result, cats should be reevaluated carefully for other causes of hemolysis. Negative results also may be due to technical reasons, insufficient quantities of bound antibodies, the presence of weakly bound antibodies, or the disease in remission. Person et al described five cats with pIMHA: all cats were Coombs' test positive for IgG antibodies.[28] The Coombs' test was positive in three cats at recurrence of disease after 10 months and in two cats after 5 and 6 months of immunosuppressive therapy. Therefore a Coombs' test can be of diagnostic value in both dogs and cats undergoing immunosuppressive therapy.

In two studies, a higher level of IgM antibodies was present in cats with IMHA as compared with dogs.[5,11] However, Person et al reported only IgG antibodies in five cats with pIMHA.[28] IgM antibodies that are active at 37° C can activate complement and cause intravascular hemolysis, which is described very rarely in cats.

Because spherocytes are not useful diagnostically in cats, the determination of the erythrocytic osmotic fragility (OF) can be an additional valuable diagnostic tool. The OF test measures the stability of erythrocytes in sodium chloride solutions ranging from 0.85 to 0 per cent. In IMHA, OF of RBCs is increased because of a reduced relationship of surface and volume.[35] Mean OF was moderately to severely increased in all 10 cats with pIMHA examined in one study (Figure 60-8).[11] Determination of mean OF can be an especially important diagnostic tool in cases of nonregenerative IMHA. However, an increased OF is not specific for IMHA. OF also can be increased in associations with infections with *Hemoplasma* spp.[4] or FeLV. Additional diseases

resulting in increased OF are lymphoma, hypophosphatemia, renal failure, or inflammatory disease (e.g., fat necrosis, FIP).[9]

Evaluation of the bone marrow may be indicated, especially if the patient's anemia is nonregenerative, a destruction process directed at RBC precursors is suspected, or another cytopenia is present. Results of bone marrow examinations of cats with nonregenerative IMHA and PRCA have been described in detail.[21,22]

Bone marrow findings in nine cats with idiopathic PRCA were the absence of erythroid precursors and numerous small mature lymphocytes comprising 12 to 45 per cent of the total marrow cells.[21] Besides erythroid aplasia, lymphoid hyperplasia also was the predominant finding in bone marrow aspirates and core biopsy specimens in 86 per cent of 29 cats with PRCA.[22] In the same study, bone marrow findings were described from 24 cats with nonregenerative IMHA and erythroid hyperplasia and from four cats with nonregenerative anemia associated with erythroid maturation arrest. Dysmyelopoiesis, myelonecrosis, myelofibrosis, interstitial edema, and acute inflammation were noted primarily in patients with evidence of erythroid hyperplasia compared to cats with PRCA or erythroid maturation arrest. These patients also were more often neutropenic and thrombocytopenic. The author concluded that the pathogenesis of the nonregenerative anemia in nonregenerative IMHA may involve both antibody-mediated destruction of bone marrow precursor cells and pathological events within the bone marrow, both resulting in ineffective erythropoiesis[22] (see Chapter 64).

TREATMENT

The severity of IMHA ranges from indolent to life-threatening disease. Therapy must be tailored for the unique needs of each cat and depends in part on whether the IMHA is primary or secondary. Removal of the

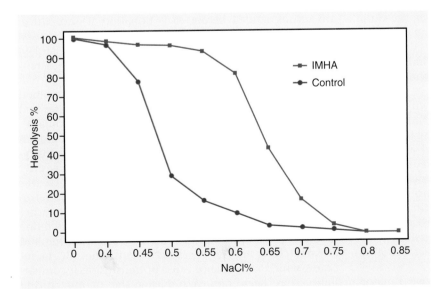

FIGURE 60-8 Increased osmotic fragility of erythrocytes in a cat with IMHA compared with a healthy control cat.

triggering agent or treatment of the underlying condition can bring the IMHA under control rapidly.

IMMUNOSUPPRESSIVE TREATMENTS

Immunosuppressive doses of prednisolone (initially 2 mg/kg PO q12h) or rarely, dexamethasone (0.15 mg/kg PO q12h) are administered in pIMHA or idiopathic PRCA.[11,21,27] After a response to therapy (stable Hct), prednisolone is reduced by approximately 20 to 25 per cent every 14 days. Tapering should be performed very slowly over a period of several months with constant monitoring of the Hct. In patients with insufficient response to prednisolone or with a relapse, an additional treatment with cyclosporine (initially 5 mg/kg PO q24h) or chlorambucil (0.1 to 0.2 mg/kg PO q24h) may be considered. In the study by Husbands et al, seven cats received cytotoxic drugs (cyclophosphamide, cyclosporine) in addition to prednisolone, as a result of lack of control or relapse.[27]

When PRCA is suspected, the author uses chlorambucil in addition to prednisolone from the beginning of therapy. Monitoring of WBC and platelet counts must be performed every 7 to 14 days because of the myelosuppressive effects of these cytostatic drugs. In a study involving 19 cats, complications of chronic prednisolone therapy were pancreatitis, diabetes mellitus, and cystic calculi.[27]

OTHER TREATMENTS

Administration of antibiotics (e.g., doxycycline, enrofloxacin) is indicated if hemoplasmosis is suspected and because of dysregulation or therapeutic suppression of the immune system. Administration of H_2-receptor antagonists is recommended because of the danger of gastrointestinal bleeding resulting from high doses of glucocorticoids and poor perfusion of the gastrointestinal tract. Restoration and maintenance of tissue perfusion with crystalloid fluids may be indicated even when it results in further lowering of the Hct. However, the clinician should administer fluids very carefully to cats with severe anemia, using infusion pumps for fluid administration. A further lowering of the Hct before administering RBC support might lead to decompensation and death of the patient.

Four of nine cats with PRCA were treated with human recombinant human erythropoietin (rHuEPO). However, this strategy can not be recommended because the therapeutic benefits are uncertain, and erythroid aplasia or hypoplasia has been induced in cats as a result of the drug's antigenicity. Measurement of EPO concentration in cats with PRCA is recommended; high concentrations would argue against the use of rHuEPO[21] (see Chapter 66).

One cat with suspected immune-mediated erythroid and megakaryocytic aplasia was treated successfully with human polyclonal immunoglobulins; however, proof of a beneficial effect requires further studies.[36]

Splenectomy, which is performed to remove a major site of erythrocyte destruction and antibody production, is controversial in the treatment of IMHA and only should be considered as a last resort in patients with life-threatening refractory anemia.[1] However, there are no detailed reports in the literature describing cats with IMHA who have been splenectomized.

TRANSFUSION THERAPY

When severe anemia and a dropping Hct result in signs of tissue hypoxia, RBC support is indicated and might be life-saving. The increased oxygen-carrying capacity provided by the transfused RBCs may be sufficient to maintain the cat's Hct for several days while other treatment modalities have time to become effective. A blood-type–compatible RBC transfusion is recommended for critically ill cats if the Hct falls below 10 to 15 per cent (see Chapter 61). However, even more important in making the decision to administer a blood transfusion is the overall condition of the patient.

In different studies, 53 to 64 per cent of the cats with pIMHA received packed RBCs, whole blood, or Oxyglobin.[10,11,27] Packed RBCs are the preferred blood product for patients with hemolytic anemia. However, the small blood volume collected and the difficulties in separation of blood elements often lead to transfusion of whole blood in feline patients.[37,38] In a study of 19 cats with pIMHA, 10 cats received transfusions with fresh or stored whole blood; the cats needed 1 to 4 transfusions over a period of 1 to 10 days. The Hct before transfusion was 5 to 17 per cent (median 11 per cent). After transfusion, an increase in the Hct of 1 to 11 per cent (median 3 per cent) was measured.[11] A lower than expected rise in Hct may be due to ongoing hemolysis. Moreover, any preexisting hypovolemia, the concomitant infusion of large volumes of crystalloids, or lysis of the transfused erythrocytes may cause a lower than expected rise in Hct.

In general, feline blood transfusions are safe and efficient; however, they are labor-intensive because blood typing of donor and recipient and possible crossmatching are needed.[25,37] Moreover, a clinical examination of the donor and a complete blood count and clinical chemistry are recommended before each donation. Donor infections with FeLV, FIV, *Hemoplasma* spp., and *Bartonella* spp. must be excluded, but absolute safety in regard to transmission of infectious diseases can never be guaranteed[39] (see Chapter 6).

The occurrence of autoagglutination may make blood typing and crossmatching impossible. In these cases and if blood-type–compatible (type B) blood is not available, the administration of an ultrapurified bovine hemoglobin solution in a modified Ringer's lactate solution (Oxyglobin, Biopure Corporation, Cambridge, MA) may offer an alternative in an emergency situation, although this solution is not yet approved for use in cats. In two retrospective studies, the reason for choosing Oxyglobin rather than feline blood products was a lack of available feline blood in the majority of the cases.[40,41] Blood typing and crossmatching are not necessary because the RBC membrane, which is the major cause of transfusion incompatibility, has been removed during the manufacturing process. A further advantage is that the transmission of

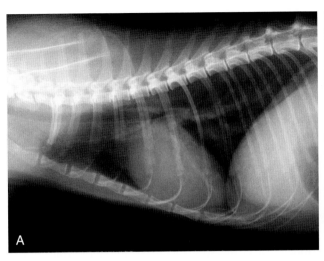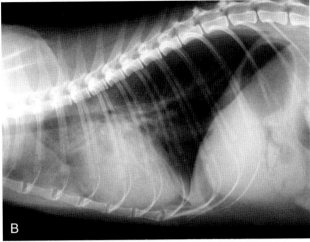

FIGURE 60-9 Lateral thoracic radiograph of a 6-year-old domestic shorthair cat with IMHA and cardiomyopathy before **(A)** and 36 hours after **(B)** receiving a bovine hemoglobin solution; the cat developed pleural effusion and pulmonary edema.

infectious diseases is believed to be minimal compared to blood products.[42] Oxyglobin has a storage life of 3 years at room temperature. However, once a bag has been opened, its contents must be used within 24 hours because of oxidation of hemoglobin to methemoglobin and possible bacterial growth.[43] In contrast to blood transfusions, special infusion sets are not needed for the administration of Oxyglobin. An advantage of the small molecular size is an even distribution within the vascular system.[44] In healthy dogs, the half-life of Oxyglobin is 24 hours after administration of 15 mL/kg. After 5 to 9 days, more than 95 per cent has been eliminated. Oxyglobin is metabolized by the reticuloendothelial system, except for the less than 5 per cent that exists as an unstable tetramer and is excreted by the kidney.[44] Comparable data are not available for cats.

Indications for administration of Oxyglobin are anemias, especially from hemolysis or blood loss, and hemorrhagic or hypovolemic shock. Treatment of an anemia caused by ineffective erythropoiesis (e.g., PRCA) is less effective because of the product's short half-life, but Oxyglobin can be life-saving until blood products are available.[44]

An increased risk for volume overload has been reported in patients suffering from cardiac and respiratory diseases or in patients with cerebral edema or oliguria/anuria as the result of acute renal failure.[40,41,43,44] Oxyglobin can cause vasoconstriction, which may result in increased systemic arterial pressure. The vasodilatory effect of nitric oxide, which is produced by endothelial cells, may be blocked by Oxyglobin.[42]

Pulmonary edema and/or thoracic effusion were described in 25 of 72 cats with different types of anemia who were treated with Oxyglobin. However, a pleural effusion and/or pulmonary edema was present in 10 cats before treatment. The median dose of Oxyglobin given to cats who developed circulatory overload was 21 mL/kg.[40] In a recently published study, life-threatening side effects, such as pulmonary edema, pleural effu-

sion, and respiratory distress, occurred in seven of 48 cats (15 per cent) with different types of anemia, and these seven cats had concurrent cardiac diseases (Figure 60-9). Four of these seven cats received additional blood transfusions on the same day, and six of them died. The dose of Oxyglobin given to these seven cats was 7 to 20 mL/kg in 24 hours (median 12 mL/kg in 24 hours). These results suggest that a significantly lower dose such as 5 to 7.5 mL/kg is recommended, especially in cats with preexisting cardiac disease. However, many cats with cardiomyopathy show no clinical signs. The administration of blood products and crystalloids in addition to Oxyglobin may be another risk factor for circulatory overload.

The rate of infusion of Oxyglobin ideally should be adjusted for each patient. The risk of volume overload might be decreased if a considerably lower infusion rate than 5 mL/kg/hr is administered by a perfusion pump (Figure 60-10). A careful examination, including respiratory and heart rates before, during, and after administration of Oxyglobin, is very important.

Other side effects of Oxyglobin administration include dose-related discoloration of mucous membranes and urine. Red discoloration of plasma interferes with colorimetric laboratory analyses (e.g., liver enzymes, bilirubin) (Figure 60-11).[40,45] Although the concentration of plasma hemoglobin increases, the Hct may be decreased by hemodilution after the infusion and can not be used as parameter to monitor the course of the anemia.

COURSE OF DISEASE AND PROGNOSIS

Median time to a normal Hct was 33 days (range 8 to 228 days) for 16 of 19 cats with pIMHA who responded to therapy. The mean oral prednisolone dose at discharge was 3.3 mg/kg/day. Three cats never achieved a normal Hct. Because of a lack of control or relapse, seven cats later received cyclophosphamide (n = 4), cyclosporine (n = 3), dexamethasone (n = 1) and/or were

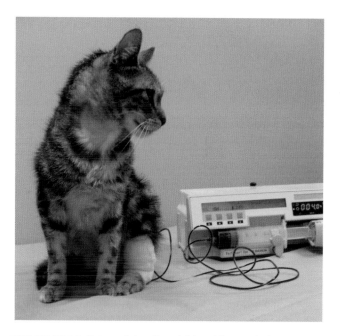

FIGURE 60-10 Cat receiving Oxyglobin with a perfusion pump.

Five of 16 cats (31 per cent) with pIMHA being monitored over a longer period of time (≥1 month) showed a recurrence of disease with a decrease in Hct. Four cats underwent a relapse after reducing the dosage of prednisolone; one cat relapsed 7 months after finishing the medication.[11]

In one study, 19 out of 25 cats with pIMHA survived to be discharged. Median survival time for these 19 cats was 1249 days.[27] In another study, the survival rate of 17 cats being monitored between 9 and 2400 days (median 345 days) was 76.5 per cent. Four of 17 cats were euthanized at their owners' request because of a relapse or because they failed to respond to therapy.[11] A calculated Kaplan-Meier 1-year survival of 29 cats with idiopathic IMHA was 69 per cent.[10] It would appear that the prognosis for cats with pIMHA is better than for dogs, with longer survival rates and fewer possible fatal complications such as DIC and thromboembolic events. The 60-day survival rate of 26 cats with PRCA was 88 per cent, which was higher compared than for 19 cats with nonregenerative anemia associated with erythroid maturation arrest (63 per cent).[22]

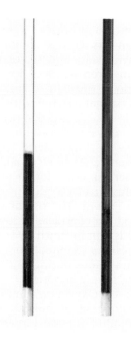

FIGURE 60-11 Feline serum sample before *(left)* and after *(right)* Oxyglobin infusion; red discoloration is visible.

splenectomized.[27] Fifteen of 17 cats with IMHA experienced an increase in Hct above 25 per cent within 8 to 42 days (median 20 days) after treatment with prednisolone.[11]

Six of 7 cats with primary PRCA responded (as indicated by an increase in the aggregate reticulocyte count or Hct) within 1.5 to 4 weeks of initiating immunosuppressive treatment with prednisolone or dexamethasone and cyclophosphamide. The Hct was within reference range within 3 to 5 weeks.[21]

REFERENCES

1. Day MJ, Mackin AJ: Immune-mediated haematological disease. In Day MJ, editor: *Clinical immunology of the dog and cat*, ed 2, London, 2008, Manson Publishing, p 94.
2. Day MJ: Antigen specificity in canine autoimmune haemolytic anaemia, *Vet Immunol Immunopathol* 69:215, 1999.
3. Scott DW, Schultz RD, Post JE, et al: Autoimmune hemolytic anemia in the cat, *J Am Anim Hosp Assoc* 9:530, 1973.
4. Maede Y, Hata R: Studies of feline haemobartonellosis. II. The mechanism of anemia produced by infection with *Haemobartonella felis*, *Jap J Vet Sci* 37:49, 1975.
5. Werner LL, Gorman NT: Immune-mediated disorders of cats, *Vet Clin North Am Small Anim Pract* 14:1039, 1984.
6. Peterson ME, Hurwitz AI, Leib MS, et al: Propylthiouracil-associated hemolytic anemia, thrombocytopenia, and antinuclear antibodies in cats with hyperthyroidism, *J Am Vet Med Assoc* 184:806, 1984.
7. Peterson ME, Kintzer PP, Hurvitz AI: Methimazole treatment of 262 cats with hyperthyroidism, *J Vet Intern Med* 2:150, 1988.
8. Gunn-Moore DA, Day MJ, Graham MEA, et al: Immune-mediated haemolytic anaemia in two sibling cats associated with multicentric lymphoblastic infiltration, *J Feline Med Surg* 1:209, 1999.
9. Kohn B: *Erythrozytenstudien bei gesunden und anämischen Katzen (Erythrocyte studies in healthy and anemic cats).* 2001, Habilitation thesis, Free University of Berlin.
10. Piek CJ, Dekker A, Junius G, et al: Idiopathic immune-mediated haemolytic anaemia (IMHA) in cats: differentiation from secondary IMHA and outcome of treatment. Proceedings of the 13th ECVIM-CA Forum, Uppsala: 162, 2003.
11. Kohn B, Weingart C, Ottenjann M, et al: Primary immune-mediated hemolytic anemia in 19 cats: diagnosis, therapy, and outcome (1998-2004), *J Vet Intern Med* 20:159, 2006.
12. Ottenjann M, Weingart C, Arndt G, et al: Characterization of the anemia of inflammatory disease in cats with abscesses, pyothorax or fat necroses, *J Vet Intern Med* 20:1143, 2006.
13. Duval D, Giger U: Vaccine-associated immune-mediated hemolytic anemia in the dog, *J Vet Intern Med* 10:290, 1996.

14. Kohn B, Garner M, Lübke S, et al: Polyarthritis following vaccination in four dogs, *Vet Comp Orthop Traumatol* 16:6, 2003.

15. Dawson S, McArdale F, Bennett D, et al: Investigation of vaccine reactions and breakdowns after feline calicivirus vaccination, *Vet Rec* 132:346, 1993.

16. Penhale WJ, Day MJ, Lines AD, et al: A review of cases submitted to Murdoch University for immunodiagnostic testing: 1978-1989, *Aust Vet J* 67:148, 1990.

17. Kohn B, Linden T, Leibold W: Platelet-bound antibodies detected by a flow cytometric assay in cats with thrombocytopenia, *J Feline Med Surg* 8:254, 2006.

18. Faircloth JC, Montgomery JK: Systemic lupus erythematosus in a cat presenting with autoimmune haemolytic anemia, *Fel Pract* 11:22, 1981.

19. Lusson D, Billiemaz B, Chabanne JL: Circulating lupus anticoagulant and probable systemic lupus erythematosus in a cat, *J Feline Med Surg* 3:193, 1999.

20. Meyer DJ, Harvey JW: *Veterinary laboratory medicine, interpretation and diagnosis*, ed 3, St Louis, 2004, Saunders.

21. Stokol T, Blue JT: Pure red cell aplasia in cats: 9 cases (1989-1997), *J Am Vet Med Assoc* 214:75, 1999.

22. Weiss DJ: Bone marrow pathology in dogs and cats with non-regenerative immune-mediated haemolytic anaemia and pure red cell aplasia, *J Comp Pathol* 138:46, 2008.

23. Griot-Wenk ME, Giger U: Feline transfusion medicine. Blood types and their clinical importance, *Vet Clin North Am Small Anim Pract* 25:1305, 1995.

24. Wardrop KJ: Transfusion medicine. In August JR, editor: *Consultations in feline internal medicine*, vol 4, Philadelphia, 2001, Saunders, p 461.

25. Weinstein NM, Blais MC, Harris K, et al: A newly recognized blood group in Domestic Shorthair cats: the Mik red cell antigen, *J Vet Intern Med* 21:287, 2007.

26. Tizard IR: *Veterinary immunology*. Philadelphia, 2004, Saunders.

27. Husbands BD, Smith SA, Weiss DJ: Idiopathic immune-mediated hemolytic anemia (IMHA) in 25 cats. Proceedings of the 20th ACVIM Forum, Dallas, 2002.

28. Person JM, Sicard M, Pellerin JL: Les anemies hemolytiques auto-immunes chez le chat: etude clinique et immunopathologique de cinq cas, *Revue Med Vet* 148:107, 1997.

29. McManus PM, Linden EC: Correlation between leukocytosis and necropsy findings in dogs with immune-mediated hemolytic anemia: 34 cases (1994-1999), *J Am Vet Med Assoc* 218:1308, 2001.

30. Scott-Moncrieff JC, Treadwell NG, McCullough SM, et al: Hemostatic abnormalities in dogs with primary immune-mediated hemolytic anemia, *J Am Anim Hosp Assoc* 37:220, 2001.

31. Kohn B, Goldschmidt HM, Hohenhaus AE, et al: Anemia, splenomegaly, and increased osmotic fragility of erythrocytes in Abyssinian and Somali cats, *J Am Vet Med Assoc* 217:1483, 2000.

32. Kohn B, Fumi C: Clinical course of pyruvate kinase deficiency in Abyssinian and Somali cats, *J Feline Med Surg* 10:145, 2008.

33. Schrader LA, Hurvitz AI: Cold agglutinin disease in a cat, *J Am Vet Med Assoc* 183:121, 1983.

34. Dunn JK, Searcy GP, Hirsch VM: The diagnostic significance of a positive direct antiglobulin test in anemic cats, *Can J Comp Med* 48:349, 1984.

35. Jain NC: Osmotic fragility of erythrocytes in dogs and cats in health and in certain hematologic disorders, *Cornell Vet* 63:411, 1973.

36. Zini E, Hauser B, Meli ML, et al: Immune-mediated erythroid and megakaryocytic aplasia in a cat, *J Am Vet Med Assoc* 230:1024, 2007.

37. Weingart C, Giger U, Kohn B: Whole blood transfusions in 91 cats: a clinical evaluation, *J Feline Med Surg* 6:139, 2004.

38. Klaser DA, Reine NJ, Hohenhaus AE: Red blood cell transfusions in cats: 126 cases (1999), *J Am Vet Med Assoc* 226:920, 2005.

39. Wardrop KJ, Reine N, Birkenheuer A, et al: Canine and feline blood donor screening for infectious disease, *J Vet Intern Med* 19:135, 2005.

40. Gibson GR, Callan MS, Hoffmann V, et al: Use of haemoglobin based oxygen carrying solutions in cats: 72 cases (1998-2000), *J Am Vet Med Assoc* 221:96, 2002.

41. Weingart C, Kohn B: Clinical use of a haemoglobin-based oxygen carrying solution (Oxyglobin) in 48 cats (2002-2006), *J Feline Med Surg* 10:431, 2008.

42. Muir WW, Wellmann ML: Hemoglobin solutions and tissue oxygenation, *J Vet Intern Med* 17:127, 2003.

43. Adamantos S, Boag A, Hughes D: Clinical use of a haemoglobin-based oxygen carrying solution in dogs and cats, *In Practice* 27:399, 2005.

44. Callan MS, Rentko VT: Clinical application of a haemoglobin-based oxygen carrying solution, *Vet Clin North Am Small Anim Pract* 33:1277, 2003.

45. Rentko VT, Sharpe TA: Red blood cell substitutes. In Feldman BF, Zinkl JG, Jain NC, editors: *Schalm's veterinary hematology*. Baltimore, 2000, Lippincott Williams & Wilkins, p 874.

Barbara Bighignoli, Sean D. Owens, Lutz Froenicke,
and Leslie A. Lyons

Progress in feline medicine, especially the increase in more complex surgeries such as renal transplantations, has raised the clinical importance of elucidating the feline blood group systems. Historically, blood groups of domestic cats have been considered to be fairly straightforward and not complex. However, such simplicity is an oddity for the animal world. Most species have a variety of blood group systems with a plethora of types, whereas the cat has had only one well-defined blood type system to date.

A review of the feline AB blood type system, describing the historical identification of the feline blood group and its importance for transfusion medicine, has been published previously in this series.[1,2] Since then, feline blood type research has seen several major advances. A new blood type system not correlated to the previously known AB system has been discovered. New data on the rare AB blood group, which had never been resolved clearly as either allelic caused by a second gene or by an epistatic mechanism, suggest that at least two or more AB variants exist. Further, the gene associated with the A and B blood groups has been identified. Additionally, extensive data on the frequencies of blood types for both domestic random-bred cats and fancy breeds have been published, and methods for serological typing have advanced. The recent advances of the feline blood group systems are reviewed in this chapter, from both the serological and genetic points of view.

BRIEF OVERVIEW

The long-recognized feline AB blood system displays two major blood types, A and B, as well as the rare type AB.

The A and the B types are alternate forms of the same gene, alleles; the allele *A*, for blood type A, is dominant to allele *b*, which controls blood type B. Although several studies have examined the rare AB type, which co-expresses both A and B antigens phenotypically, its heritability still needs to be elucidated.[3-6] The AB blood group has been found exclusively in breeds in which the B blood type occurs.[4]

Ontogenetically, erythrocyte antigens are developed in utero, whereas antibodies are developed postnatally. Both the cat anti-A and anti-B antibodies are naturally occurring antibodies. The anti-A antibodies are developed earlier than the anti-B antibodies, probably because epitopes similar to the A antigen are more common in the environment or are stronger immunological stimulants than the B antigens.[7]

The feline blood types are clinically important in two circumstances. The possession of a high titer of anti-A antibodies in a B-type cat leads to severe transfusion reactions if receiving blood from an A-type cat. Further, neonatal isoerythrolysis (NI) can occur, especially when a B-type queen nurses A-type kittens, because the antibodies pass through the colostrum.[1]

SEROLOGICAL TECHNIQUES FOR FELINE BLOOD TYPE DETECTION

Blood typing and cross-matching are critical components of pretransfusion testing in feline patients, and both techniques help to identify compatible blood donors correctly.[8] Blood typing identifies blood group antigens on the surface of erythrocytes, whereas cross-matching detects the presence of significant levels of antibodies directed against erythrocyte antigens. However, because blood typing is unable to detect blood group incompatibilities in the absence of naturally occurring alloantibodies, cross-matching remains the only method available to ensure that AB-system–compatible blood is transfused.[9]

Cross-matching refers to the testing that is performed to determine the compatibility of a donated unit of blood with its intended recipient. In short, erythrocytes from the donor unit are tested against the plasma of the patient in need of the blood transfusion. If the patient's plasma contains antibodies against the antigens present on the donor erythrocytes, agglutination will occur. Agglutination is considered a positive reaction, indicating that the donor unit is incompatible for that specific patient. If no agglutination occurs, the unit is deemed compatible and is safe to transfuse.

The principle of serological blood-typing reactions is based on the identification of macroscopically visible agglutination of erythrocytes following incubation with known antibodies or special agglutinin reagents.[10] Agglutination of erythrocytes signifies a positive reaction, whereas if no agglutination reaction occurs, the test is considered negative for the blood group antigen being examined.

Agglutination reactions were performed initially in test tubes or micro-well plates and were given a grade based on the degree of macroscopic erythrocyte agglutination observed. Grading of agglutination reactions gives an indication of the relative amount of antigen or antibody present. In grading agglutination reactions, a 4+ reaction yields a solid clump of erythrocytes and a 3+ reaction yields several small clumps. A 2+ reaction yields small- to medium-sized clumps with a clear background. A 1+ reaction yields several small clumps with a cloudy background, and a weak+ reaction reveals many tiny aggregates with a cloudy background.

Currently, all commercial serological blood typing tests for cats are based on agglutination reactions. Although the use of agglutination techniques for blood typing remains a simple, sensitive, and reliable test, agglutination techniques are only as sensitive as the antibodies or agglutinins used, so that new blood group antigens may be overlooked without the availability of specific antibodies and/or agglutinins.

Confirmation of blood typing results may be accomplished through the use of a back-typing test in which the plasma or serum of the cat being blood typed is evaluated for alloantibodies. Back-typing involves incubating known type-A and type-B erythrocytes with the patient's plasma. Plasma from type-A cats typically will agglutinate type-B erythrocytes weakly to moderately. Plasma from type-B cats will agglutinate type-A erythrocytes strongly. The back-typing test is similar to the cross-match test in circumstances in which the blood type of the blood donor is known and assists in confirming the patient's (transfusion recipient's) blood type.

The reagents used for feline blood typing are either polyclonal or monoclonal antibodies or lectins. The polyclonal anti-sera created from the serum of type-A and type-B positive cats has been used to blood type cats for decades; in particular, the anti-A serum from type-B cats has high erythrocyte agglutination activity.[9] The lectin

from *Triticum vulgaris* has replaced the feline anti-B serum because it agglutinates type-B positive erythrocytes preferentially, whereas it agglutinates type-A positive erythrocytes only at higher concentrations.[11]

Current serological methods used for feline blood typing include the Penn tube or slide agglutination assays (Transfusion Laboratory, Section of Medical Genetics, School of Veterinary Medicine, University of Pennsylvania, Philadelphia), blood typing card tests, and gel column tests. Both the Penn slide and tube assays use anti-A polyclonal serum and *T. vulgaris* lectin.[12] The Penn tube assay is reliable and has been considered the gold standard and has been utilized as the reference standard in several blood type frequency surveys.[10]

A tube assay using monoclonal antibodies to identify both A and B blood group antigens has been developed (Shigeta Animal Pharmaceuticals Inc, Komoridani, Oyabe City, Toyama Pref, Japan), thereby eliminating polyclonal antibodies and lectins entirely.[13] The Penn slide assay is a simplified version of the tube assays and allows typing of whole blood, thus lending itself to use in a practice setting. The tube methods have been confined mostly to diagnostic laboratories and research institutions, given their greater complexity and the technical expertise required to perform the assay. The card test (DMS Rapid-Vet-H [feline] blood typing card test, DMS Laboratories Inc, Flemington, NJ) uses a monoclonal anti-A antibody for the identification of type-A erythrocytes and the *T. vulgaris* lectin for identification of type-B erythrocytes. Use of a gel matrix column to fix the blood typing agglutination reaction has been developed for use in cats (DiaMed ID-Card Anti A+B [Cat], DiaMed AG, Cressier sur Morat, Switzerland). Like the other methods of determining blood type in cats, the gel matrix column uses an anti-A antibody and *T. vulgaris* lectin.

In a comparison of the previously mentioned blood typing assays, using the Penn tube test as a reference standard, Giger and colleagues found that the blood typing card tests allow identification of both type-A and type-B cats; however, weak reactions of type-AB blood with the monoclonal type-A antibody were a concern. Therefore type-AB and type-B results should be confirmed either by laboratory alloantibody testing or using another technique.[10] They further concluded that the gel test and the Japanese tube test appear to be reliable clinical laboratory methods for feline blood typing.

THE *Mik* ANTIGEN: A NEW BLOOD TYPE

The feline A, B, and AB blood group system is the only internationally recognized blood group system in cats. However, blood group antigen incompatibilities unrelated to the AB blood group system have been suspected after rare incompatible cross-match results from AB-type–compatible donors and recipients and because of very rare hemolytic transfusion reactions after AB-type–compatible blood transfusion.

In 2005, Weinstein and colleagues,[14] using standard tube and novel gel column cross-matching techniques, identified the presence of a clinically relevant alloantibody, formed against a newly discovered feline erythrocyte antigen, which was named *Mik*. The incidence of the *Mik* antigen in the feline population is not known at this time; however, the clinical significance of the *Mik* antigen was established after an acute hemolytic transfusion reaction from an inadvertent transfusion of *Mik*-positive blood to a *Mik*-negative renal transplant patient at the Veterinary Hospital of the University of Pennsylvania. Identification of previously unknown blood types typically follows the investigation of an unexpected acute hemolytic transfusion reaction.

Routine screening of potential blood donors and transfusion recipients for the *Mik* antigen may become necessary as part of pretransfusion blood typing pending the outcome of prevalence studies. Until such time, these transfusion reactions highlight the need to perform a cross-match before blood transfusion in the feline patient, even when there have not been any previous transfusions.

MOLECULAR STRUCTURES OF FELINE BLOOD TYPES

The earliest studies investigating glycoconjugates on feline erythrocyte membranes revealed the presence of seven different gangliosides. These first studies were carried out on cats of unknown blood types.[15,16] Later, the molecular structures of the antigens determining the blood type of the AB system were defined by Butler et al in 1991.[17]

Thin-layer chromatography suggested that the antigens are defined principally by the form of the neuraminic acid residues present on a ceramide dihexose backbone on the surface of the erythrocytes.[17] The major glycolipid and antigen of type-A cats is the disialoganglioside NeuGc-NeuGc-Galactose-Glucose-Ceramide ($[NeuGc]_2G_{D3}$), in which NeuGc represents *N*-glycolyl neuraminic acid. The major glycolipid of type-B cats is the disialoganglioside NeuAc-NeuAc-Galactose-Glucose-Ceramide ($[NeuAc]_2G_{D3}$), with NeuAc representing *N*-acetylneuraminic acid.[17]

Further studies on the composition of the erythrocyte antigens showed that the A-type cat also contains a minor amount of $(NeuAc)_2G_{D3}$ and two intermediate forms such as NeuAc-NeuGc-G_{D3} and NeuGc-NeuAc-G_{D3}.[12,18] Furthermore, minor amounts of monosialogangliosides such as $(NeuAc)G_{M3}$ and $(NeuGc)G_{M3}$, the latter not being found in type-B cats, were discovered (Table 61-1). Additionally, trisialoganglioside seems to be present in all of the three blood types.[12]

Cats of the rare AB type have both of the sialic acids, NeuGc and NeuAc, co-expressed on the erythrocyte membrane; even though they have the same composition as type-A cats, the relative amounts differ from those in type-A cats.[18] In contrast with previous findings that suggested a minor amount of B antigen in the AB-type than in the B-type,[4,12,18] a recent study demonstrated a higher expression in type-AB cats of $(NeuAc)G_{D3}$ as compared to $(NeuGc)G_{D3}$.[5] The amount of $(NeuAc)G_{D3}$ is reported to be similar to that in type-B cats, whereas the antigen

Table 61-1 Composition of the Gangliosides of Feline Erythrocyte Membrane Determining the Three Blood Types

Blood Type	Monosialogangliosides	Disialogangliosides
A type and AB type	$(NeuGc)G_{M3}$ $(NeuAc)G_{M3}$	$(NeuGc)_2G_{D3}$ $(NeuAc)_2G_{D3}$ NeuAc-NeuGc-G_{D3} NeuGc-NeuAc-G_{D3}
B type	$(NeuAc)G_{M3}$	$(NeuAc)_2G_{D3}$

$(NeuGc)G_{D3}$ was confirmed to be less expressed in type-AB than in type-A cats.[5]

Surprisingly, this study, which included four AB cats and used several types of monoclonal antibodies, showed differences between the A antigen of type-A and type-AB cats.[5] The authors concluded that at least two different phenotypes exist within the AB blood type, varying in amount and form of the A antigen. Therefore several slightly varying potential antigens may be present on the feline erythrocytes, suggesting that cats may have additional "subtypes." Extensive studies will be required to shed light on this hypothesis.

NeuAc and NeuGc are two of the most abundant forms of sialic acids in mammalian cells, with NeuGc being the predominant type. NeuGc is produced from NeuAc by a pathway involving the enzyme cytidine monophospho-*N*-acetylneuraminic acid hydroxylase (CMP-NeuAc).[19] CMP-NeuAc hydroxylase is an enzyme that converts NeuAc to NeuGc, which is expressed in all mammals except human beings. The absence of NeuGc in human beings is due to a partial deletion in the gene (*CMAH*) encoding the enzyme.[20,21] In human beings, NeuGc is an oncofetal antigen expressed in certain tumors but not in the normal adult tissue.[22] However, more recent studies found the presence of NeuGc not only in several human carcinomas but also in some healthy human tissues, raising the question as to whether other pathways could generate this molecule because the *CMAH* gene is nonfunctional. Bardor and colleagues found that exogenous free NeuGc can be incorporated via pinocytic/endocytic pathways, delivered to the lysosome, and then reach the cytosol by a sialic acid transporter.[23] Red meat and milk products can be dietary sources of free NeuGc.[23] Whether NeuGc is generated by alternate pathways in cats or if it is absorbed from dietary sources has not been studied to date.

GENETIC BASIS OF FELINE BLOOD TYPES

The lack of CMP-NeuAc hydroxylase had been suggested by several authors to be responsible for the absence of the NeuGc in the B-type cat.[5,12,17,18] Hence *CMAH* was the best candidate gene for defining the A and the B blood types in cats.[6]

The complete genetic sequence of *CMAH* was analyzed recently in cats of all blood types. Unlike human beings, no deletion that disrupts the coding sequence was identified, but several nucleotide differences were found between the type-A and type-B cats.

Five single nucleotide polymorphisms (SNPs), two in the control region of the gene and three mutations that cause amino acid changes in the coding parts of the gene, the exons, were found. In addition, an 18 nucleotide insertion/deletion (indel) in the 5′ untranslated region (UTR), before the translation of the protein begins, was found associated with the type-B cats. These associations were consistent in 107 type-A and 79 type-B cats. These mutations were found on the same strand of DNA and thus constitute a "haplotype" that is associated with the *b* allele, producing the B blood type when two *b* alleles are present. Therefore, at the genetic level, a cat with the B blood type was always homozygous for all these various mutations, having both inherited strands of DNA with the same mutations, and was designated as having a *bb* genotype. A type-A cat, because the *A* allele is dominant, can be either a homozygote (designated genotype *AA*) or heterozygote for the variants (designated genotype *Ab*).

The messenger ribonucleic acid (mRNA) produced by the *CMAH* gene was sequenced from four cats, one for each blood type (A, B, and AB) and one for an obligate *b* carrier. Unexpectedly, several different sequences of the *CMAH* mRNA, the so-called isoforms, were found (Figure 61-1). In some of these isoforms, the cat *CMAH* mRNA extended 121 nucleotides further than the known start site of protein translation in other species. An additional potential start site for protein translation was found within this 121bp extension, which could generate a longer *CMAH* protein than found in other species.

For type-B cats, the extended area contains an additional 18 nucleotides, altering the DNA sequence in a way that stops the translation of the CMAH protein. Therefore no CMAH enzyme would be produced from these transcripts, preventing the conversion of NeuAc to NeuGc. As a consequence, the stop mutation in these transcripts causes the presentation of the type-B antigen, NeuAc, on the erythrocytes. The extended mRNA isoforms, containing the alternative start codon, were not detected in the AB blood type cat but only in type-B cats and the obligate carrier (*Ab*) cat.

Other *CMAH* mRNA isoforms were found to be missing the exon 1 and having a part of intron 1 sequence spliced directly to exon 2.[6] For these isoforms, the G139A SNP detected in exon 2, associated to the *b* allele, generate an ATG start codon only in cats with the B blood type. Only more extensive genetic and serological studies in more cats will resolve the truly causative mutation.

The cat sampling for the *CMAH* study[6] consisted of 221 cats but was composed principally of the following three breeds: Birman, British Shorthair, and Devon Rex. All of these breeds have significant frequencies of the B blood type; therefore the breeders of these cats have concerns about neonatal isoerythrolysis. The *CMAH* study also included a few samples of other breeds, and the DNA mutation results proved to be consistent across all breeds. Altogether, 35 type-AB cats in this study displayed genotypes consistent with type-A cats, of both homozygous

and heterozygous status. No type-AB cats were found who had the homozygous DNA variants that are associated with a type-B cat. Therefore type-AB cats may be a result of a different genetic mechanism, or the DNA variants causing the AB allele have been missed and are very similar to the A allele.

Additional gene expression and protein level studies are needed to elucidate the translation of cat *CMAH*, as well as genetic sequence studies, to further define the mechanism of blood type determination and its exact causative mutations in cats.

The *CMAH* mutations have allowed the development of commercial tests to distinguish blood types genetically in cats. Commercial laboratories typically genotype both the 18-bp indel and one of the DNA variants that causes an amino acid change at the beginning of the protein (G139A SNP in exon 2) because these two mutations likely affect protein production. Three laboratories have continued to supply cat serology and genetic mutation screening data: the University of California Davis Veterinary Genetics Laboratory (VGL), Oy Triniini Company in Helsinki, Finland, and the University of Milan Vetogene Laboratory. The continued testing has revealed rare inconsistencies between serology and the genetic mutations in the Ragdoll breed, instigating a more thorough investigation of this breed. One hundred twenty-four Ragdoll blood samples were typed both serologically and genetically. The genetic test was conducted testing the 18-bp indel and the G139A SNP in exon 2 of *CMAH*. Serological and genetic results were concordant for 96.8 per cent of the cases. Four cats were serotype B, but three of these were *CMAH*-genotype homozygous (*AA*) and one cat was heterozygous (*Ab*). Among the tested Ragdoll cats, 15 AB-type cats were consistent with previous findings, being either heterozygous or homozygous for the type A DNA genotypes (unpublished data).

Based on these results, approximately 3.2 per cent of the tested Ragdoll cats are discordant for the blood group determined by genotyping versus serology. These data suggest that perhaps one of the identified SNPs in *CMAH* that are not genotyped routinely may be the causative mutation or that a secondary pathway may confer the serotype for these cats. These data support the need to examine all breeds closely to support the accuracy of genetic tests and suggest that the analysis of other SNPs should be considered in future studies. Similar discordances have not been detected in other cat breeds; however, few data are available for many of the other breeds, which are not blood typed routinely.

The entire dataset from the service laboratories (VGL and Vetogene), testing for both the 18bp indel and the G139A SNP, is reported in Table 61-2. Out of 1407 tested cats, 42.8 per cent were genotyped *AA*, 36 per cent were typed *A* carrying the *b* allele, and 20.3 per cent were *bb*. When interpreting these data, it should be noted that the genetic test can not discriminate between A and AB blood groups. In 13 cases, the results of the indel and the G139A SNP testing were not concordant. The discordant data represent 0.9 per cent of the overall sampling. Similar discordances were reported previously for two Sphynx cats who were typed AB.[6]

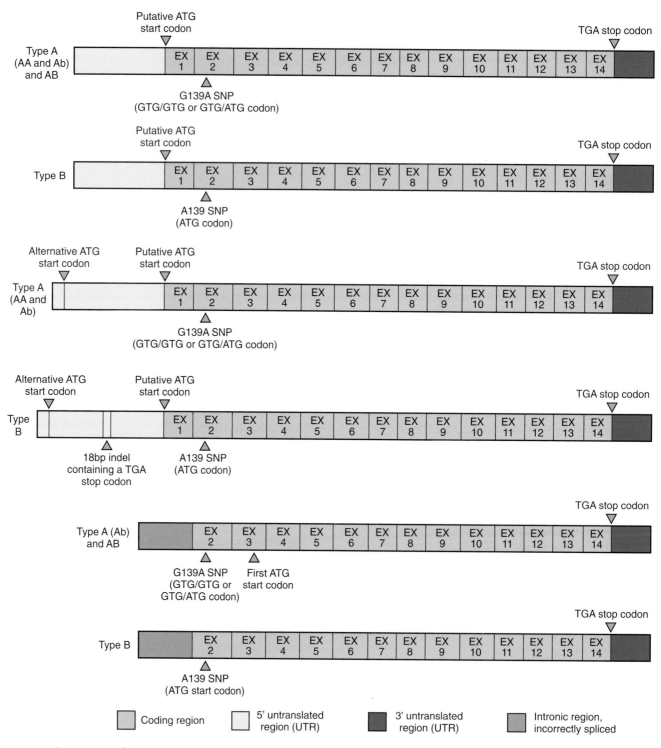

Figure 61-1 Schematic representation of the mRNA isoforms of the *CMAH* gene detected in A (*AA* and *Ab*), B, and AB blood types.

CLINICAL IMPLICATIONS OF GENETIC BLOOD TYPING

The small number of discrepancies between serological and genetic tests, as observed in the Ragdoll breed, has important implications for the practical transfusion medicine of the cat. To avoid hemolytic transfusion reactions,

it is vitally important to determine the cat's blood compatibility by blood typing and cross-matching.[2,8] Genetic testing is not sufficiently rapid for clinical applications and regardless of the genetic test, the determination of the overall serological interactions should remain the standard for transfusion medicine. The management of neonatal isoerythrolysis benefits from both genetic and

Table 61-2 Genotyping Results in Different Cat Breeds

Number of Cats	Breed	AA	Ab	bb
102	Abyssinian	49	35	18
3	Balinese	3	0	0
1	Bengal	1	0	0
172	Birman	71	77	24
546	British Shorthair (4)*	125	227	190
31	Cornish Rex	5	18	8
1	Chartreux	0	1	0
1	Domestic Mediumhair	0	1	0
71	Devon Rex (1)*	17	32	21
4	Domestic Shorthair	2	2	0
16	Exotic Shorthair	9	5	2
5	Himalayan	4	1	0
1	Japanese Bobtail	1	0	0
1	La-Perm	1	0	0
5	Maine Coon (1)*	2	1	1
7	Norwegian Forest Cat (1)*	6	0	0
48	Persian	35	9	4
235	Ragdoll (4)*	193	35	3
6	Siberian Cat	6	0	0
22	Scottish Fold	9	10	3
1	Siamese	1	0	0
29	Somali	18	11	0
32	Selkirk Rex	5	20	7
31	Sphynx	9	17	5
11	Turkish Angora (2)*	8	1	0
2	Turkish Van	2	0	0
23	Unknown and cross-breed	20	3	0
TOTAL 1407		602	506	286

*Number in parentheses indicates cats with discordant results between the indel and the G139A SNP genotyping.

serological testing. The genetic testing for blood groups allows breeders to determine blood type early and non-invasively, with a buccal swab, and also to detect type-B carriers, which can not be done with serology.

The detection of the type A cat carrying the b allele is possible solely with the genetic test; therefore breeders can avoid breeding two carriers, which could result in a type-A queen having type-B kittens. Two cats who are carriers, serologically type-A but genetically type-*Ab*, likely will produce 25 per cent kittens who are type A, genetically *AA*; 50 per cent kittens who are type A, genetically type *Ab*; and 25 per cent kittens who are type B, genetically type *bb*.

The *CMAH* genotype status is important information for breeders in the planning of the mating program. However, the 3 per cent discordance between the serological and DNA tests in the Ragdoll breed should be considered when advising cat breeders about genetic testing for blood types.

BLOOD TYPE FREQUENCIES OF THE AB SYSTEM

Several publications have reported the frequencies of A, B, and AB blood types in various regions all over the world, both in nonpedigreed and pure-bred cats. The earliest studies were conducted by Holmes in 1950 in Manchester, United Kingdom,[24] and by Eyquem in 1962 in Paris.[25] These studies, as well as the large survey of almost 2000 cats in Australia (Brisbane region) reported by Auer and Bell in 1980[26] and the first Japanese work by Ikemoto,[27] focused on the detection of the main blood type antigens and the determination of the mode of inheritance of the feline blood groups.

For these studies, the analyzed cats were reported simply as domestic cats, no information was provided as to the relatedness of the cats or if they were of particular breeds. A sampling of cats who are related will bias the interpretation of the frequency of the blood types in the populations.

Ejima and colleagues in 1986 determined the blood types of 238 Japanese cats, including a few representatives from the Siamese, Persian, Himalayan, and Abyssinian breeds. Similar to the previous studies, the primary goal was the investigation of the antibodies and antigens involved, and little information was provided regarding the relatedness of the cats. This study identified an unusually high prevalence of the AB blood type (9.2 per cent). On the other hand, only approximately 1 per cent of the "Japanese breed" was blood type B. This AB:B ratio is in contrast to the findings in other breeds and random-bred cats.[28] The only other region in which a higher prevalence of the AB blood type as compared to the B blood type has been reported is in the north of Portugal, where 6.8 per cent of cats were typed AB and 4.1 per cent were typed as B.[29] These authors commented that the unusual ratio may reflect random genetic drift or an interbreeding with purebred cats with a high AB-type frequency.[29]

The first studies focusing on feline blood type frequencies were conducted in the United States in the late 1980s. Kilrain and Giger sampled 100 cats from Philadelphia, 82 of whom were Domestic Shorthair (DSH) cats. The remaining cats represented several breeds. A single type-B cat, a Himalayan, was identified.[30] In a subsequent and more extensive study, just one other cat with the B blood type, a DSH from Florida, was identified.[31] Bird and colleagues sampled 100 cats (80 per cent of whom were DSHs), in New England and Virgin Gorda, one in the British Virgin Islands, and all cats were found to have the A blood type.[32] Over the years, more extensive studies have been conducted in the United States, Europe, Australia, and South America.[29,33-53]

The B blood type incidences have been found to vary significantly in nonpedigreed DSH and Domestic

Longhair (DLH) cats in different parts of the world (Table 61-3). As the map shows (Figure 61-2), the highest prevalence has been found in Turkey, and the type-B frequency decreases progressively towards the western Mediterranean area. However, variations in type B also may be due to the population of cats included in an individual study, and sampling biases may affect blood type frequencies.

Arikan et al suggested that the high frequencies of the type-B cats in the feral population from Turkey could be

Table 61-3 Worldwide Blood Type Frequencies of Type A, B, and AB in Domestic Shorthair/Domestic Longhair Cats

Region	Number of Cats	A%	B%	AB%
US (British Virgin Island)[32]	32	100	0	0
US (New England)[32]	69	100	0	0
Finland[36]	61	100	0	0
Hungary (Budapest area)[43]	73	100	0	0
US[31]	432	99.77	0.23	0
US (82% Philadelphia area)[33]	1072	99.72	0.28	0
Switzerland[38]	1014	99.6	0.4	0
Japan[28]	238	89.9	0.9	9.2
US (Northeast)[34]	1450	99.7	0.3	0
US (North Central)[34]	506	99.4	0.4	0.2
US (Southeast)[34]	812	98.5	1.5	0
US (Southwest)[34]	483	97.5	2.5	0
US (West Coast)[34]	812	94.8	4.7	0
Germany (Berlin and Brandenburg area)[50]	372	98.7	1.1	0.3
Denmark (Copenhagen area)[40]	105	98.1	1.9	0
Argentina (Buenos Aires area)[41]	76	96.1	2.6	1.3
Brazil (Rio de Janeiro area)[55]	172	94.8	2.9	2.3
Scotland[36]	70	97.1	2.9	0
Austria[39]	101	97	3	0
England (Manchester)[24]	477	97	3	0
Portugal (North)[29]	147	89.1	4.1	6.8
Netherlands[36]	95	94.8	4.2	0.1
Spain (Barcelona area)[46]	100	94	5	1
Germany (Gieben area)[37]	404	94.1	5.9	0
Gran Canaria[47]	97	88.7	7.2	4.1
Italy (Piedmont region)[51]	122	86.9	7.4	5.7
UK (Edinburgh area)[42]	139	87.1	7.9	5
Italy (Lombardy region)[53]	57	89.5	8.8	1.7
Japan (Tokyo)[27]	207	90	10	0
Italy (Tuscany region)[35]	363	87.1	12.9	0
France (Paris area)[25]	350	85	15	0
Greece[44]	207	78.3	20.3	1.4
Turkey[49]	301	73.1	24.6	2.3
Australia (Brisbane area)[26]	1895	73.3	26.3	0.4
England (Southeast)[52]	105	67.6	30.5	1.9
Australia (Sydney region)[48]	187	62	36	1.6

US, United States; *UK,* United Kingdom.

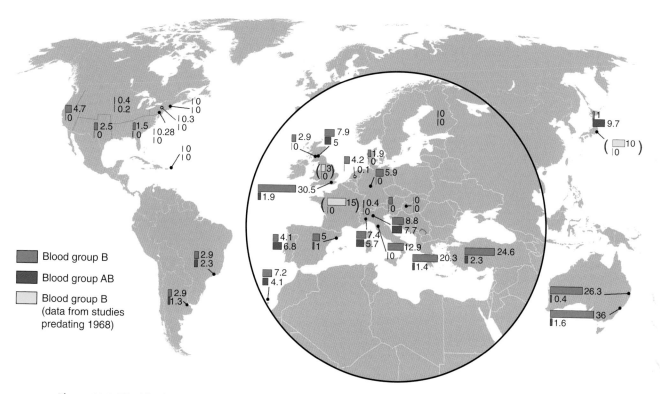

Figure 61-2 Worldwide distribution of blood types B and AB of Domestic Shorthair (DSH) and Domestic Longhair (DLH) cats.

the result of interbreeding with Turkish Angora and Turkish Van, which are the two breeds of cats originating from this country that also have the highest frequencies of B-type cats for any breed. This deduction supposedly is supported by the fact that the lowest frequency of type B has been recorded in the region of Turkey in which cats from these two breeds are less common and were introduced just recently.[49]

Minor regional variations in the B-type frequencies have been reported for neighboring regions in Italy, with 13 per cent type B in Tuscany, 8.8 per cent in Lombardy, and 7.4 per cent in Piedmont, even though these are bordering regions.[35,51,53] Conversely, significant differences were noted for nonjuxtaposed regions of the United Kingdom. Thirty-one per cent of the DSH/DLH cats in the south of England have B blood type,[52] whereas in Scotland the frequency is only 8 per cent.[42] Both datasets are similar because samples were collected from cats presented at the referral hospitals for other reasons.

A survey of more than 1000 cats from Switzerland revealed that the domestic random cats are 99.6 per cent type A. This dataset was collected mostly from veterinarians in private practice and from four different test laboratories.[38] The absence of the B blood type in Hungary could be explained by the relatively small sample size of 73 cats, all of whom were from Budapest.[43]

The Sydney region in Australia has been found recently to have the highest percentage (36 per cent) of B blood type in nonpedigreed cats among all of the countries in which such studies have been performed.[48] The authors suggested several explanations for the highest frequencies of the *b* allele in this region. First, the high type-B frequency could be the result of a founder effect, possibly

introduced early from England where the *b* allele has been found in a high frequency. Alternatively, a constant selection against the heterozygous A-type cats could exist; if the kittens are born from a B-type queen and NI occurs, the *A* allele could suffer a reduction in expression.[48]

In the United States, an extensive study throughout the country showed how the distribution of the B blood type increases from the East Coast to the West Coast. Giger et al suggested that the increase could be the result of more frequent cross-breeding with purebreds, an early introduction from Australia, and/or a random genetic drift effect.[33] Therefore regional variations of blood type frequencies do exist, likely the result of founder effects and different breed popularities.[33]

Contrary to the random-bred populations, the blood type frequencies in purebred cats from various regions of the world seem to be breed-specific and less variable geographically (Table 61-4). This could be caused by the international exchange and preferential mating of champion cats in the fancy breeds. However, some of this exchange is limited because of rabies-related import and export restrictions.

Some breeds, such as Siamese and related breeds, do not seem to possess the B blood type at all.[4] The only Asian breed that possesses the type-B antigens is the Birman. Even though this breed genetically appears to originate in Southeast Asia, according to folklore, the modern roots of this breed are located in France.[54] Furthermore, the color-pointed coat of the Birman resembles cats of the Siamese breed, but the coat is more like Persians. Therefore it is not unlikely that some Persian cats and with them the B blood type could have entered the stock of this breed.

Table 61-4 Worldwide Frequencies of Blood Types A, B, and AB in Different Breeds

Breed	Country/Reference	Number of Cats	A%	B%	AB%
Abyssinian	US[34]	230	86.5	13.5	0
Abyssinian	US[33]	194	79.9	20.1	0
Birman	US[33]	216	82.4	17.6	0
British Shorthair	UK[42]	121	39.7	58.7	1.6
British Shorthair	US[3]	85	41.2	58.8	0
British Shorthair	Germany[37]	33	54.5	45.5	0
British Shorthair	Germany[50]	35	71.4	28.6	0
British Shorthair	Denmark[40]	30	66.7	33.3	0
Burmese	Australia[48]	30	93	3	3
Burmese	US[33]	25	100	0	0
Chartreux (Kartäuser)	Germany[50]	27	77.8	18.5	3.7
Devon Rex	US[34]	288	50.3	49.7	0
Devon Rex	US[33]	100	57	43	0
Devon Rex*	Australia[48]	71	45	54	1.4
Himalayan	US[33]	35	80	20	0
Maine Coon	Germany[50]	25	96	4	0
Persian	US[34]	230	90.4	9.6	0
Persian	US[33]	170	75.9	24.1	0
Persian	Germany[37]	157	91.7	7.6	0.6
Persian	Denmark[40]	56	96.4	3.6	0
Persian	Italy[35]	38	97.4	2.6	0
Ragdoll	Italy[53]	36	72.2	8.3	19.4
Scottish Fold	US[33]	27	85.2	14.8	0
Siamese	US[33]	99	100	0	0
Siamese	Germany[37]	46	100	0	0
Siamese	Italy[35]	26	96.2	3.8	0
Somali	US[33]	27	77.8	22.2	0
Tonkinese	US[33]	31	100	0	0
Turkish Angora	Turkey[45]	28	53.6	46.4	0
Turkish Van	Turkey[45]	85	40	60	0

US, United States; *UK,* United Kingdom.
*Also includes hybrids.

Further and more extensive studies should be performed both in nonpedigreed and pure-bred cats to have a better worldwide picture of the frequencies of the different blood types. A good collection of the samples from mostly unrelated cats and the documentation of breed status and relatedness of the cats are essential in the accurate assignment of blood types and also could be helpful in biodiversity studies of cats.

In conclusion, the feline AB blood group system is the most significant system in cats. However, genetic and serological studies suggest that the feline blood group system is more complicated than considered previously. Several important questions remain unanswered. Genetic testing reveals discordances of about 3 per cent with serology in any given breed, suggesting alternative pathways and/or mutations controlling the B-type erythrocyte antigens in cats. Genetic tests need to be validated in all breeds and populations. The genetic base of the rare AB blood type still needs to be elucidated, including the mode of inheritance and genetic control. Moreover, recent serological testing has discovered that the AB type actually could be differentiated into at least two different types, further complicating the interpretation of the system. The discovery of the new *Mik* antigen raises the questions as to whether there are additional blood types still undetected and what role they might play in feline health. Additional investigation of *Mik* antigen frequency in feline populations and breeds should be performed, and its antigenic and genetic bases characterized.

The current recommendation is that veterinarians always should perform cross-matching in the clinical setting before proceeding with blood transfusions or organ transplantations in feline patients. The genetic test is an excellent tool for breeders for managing breeding programs, but the accuracies of blood typing, genetic testing methods, or other technologies should always be considered when selecting a blood typing method.

REFERENCES

1. Callan MB, Giger U: Transfusion medicine. In August JR, editor: *Consultations in feline internal medicine*, vol 2, Philadelphia, 1994, Saunders, p 525.
2. Wardrop KJ: Transfusion medicine. In August JR, editor: *Consultations in feline internal medicine*, vol 4, Philadelphia, 2001, Saunders, p 461.
3. Auer L, Bell K: The AB blood group system of cats, *Anim Blood Groups Biochem Genet* 12:287, 1981.
4. Griot-Wenk ME, Callan MB, Casal ML, et al: Blood type AB in the feline AB blood group system, *Am J Vet Res* 57:1438, 1996.
5. Green JL, Andrews GA, Wyatt CR: Phenotypic differences within the Ab blood type of the feline AB blood group system, *Comp Clin Pathol* 14:138, 2005.
6. Bighignoli B, Niini T, Grahn RA, et al: Cytidine monophospho-N-acetylneuraminic acid hydroxylase (CMAH) mutations associated with the domestic cat AB blood group, *BMC Genet* 8:27, 2007.
7. Knottenbelt CM: The feline AB blood group system and its importance in transfusion medicine, *J Feline Med Surg* 4:69, 2002.
8. Hohenhaus AE: Importance of blood groups and blood group antibodies in companion animals, *Transfus Med Rev* 18:117, 2004.
9. Giger U: Blood typing and crossmatching to ensure compatible transfusions. In Bonagura JD, editor: *Kirk's current veterinary therapy XIII*, Philadelphia, 2000, Saunders, p 396.
10. Stieger K, Palos H, Giger U: Comparison of various blood-typing methods for the feline AB blood group system, *Am J Vet Res* 66:1393, 2005.
11. Butler M, Andrews GA, Smith JE: Reactivity of lectins with feline erythrocytes, *Comp Haematol Int* 1:217, 1991.
12. Griot-Wenk M, Pahlsson P, Chisholm-Chait A, et al: Biochemical characterization of the feline AB blood group system, *Anim Genet* 24:401, 1993.
13. Kaoru A, Kyo K: Determination of canine and feline blood types using monoclonal antibodies, *Provet* 10:12, 2001.
14. Weinstein NM, Blais MC, Harris K, et al: A newly recognized blood group in domestic shorthair cats: the Mik red cell antigen, *J Vet Intern Med* 21:287, 2007.
15. Ando N, Yamakawa T: On the minor gangliosides of erythrocyte membranes of Japanese cats, *J Biochem* 91:873, 1982.
16. Furukawa K, Chait BT, Lloyd KO: Identification of N-glycolyl neuraminic acid-containing gangliosides of cat and sheep erythrocytes. 252Cf fission fragment ionization mass spectrometry in the analysis of glycosphingolipids, *J Biol Chem* 263:14939, 1988.
17. Butler M, Andrews GA, Smith JE, et al: Thin layer chromatography of erythrocyte membrane glycolipids from type A and type B cats, *Comp Haematol Int* 1:196, 1991.
18. Andrews GA, Chavey PS, Smith JE, et al: N-glycolylneuraminic acid and N-acetylneuraminic acid define feline blood group A and B antigens, *Blood* 79:2485, 1992.
19. Muchmore EA, Milewski M, Varki A, et al: Biosynthesis of N-glycolyneuraminic acid. The primary site of hydroxylation of N-acetylneuraminic acid is the cytosolic sugar nucleotide pool, *J Biol Chem* 264:20216, 1989.
20. Chou HH, Takematsu H, Diaz S, et al: A mutation in human CMP-sialic acid hydroxylase occurred after the Homo-Pan divergence, *Proc Natl Acad Sci USA* 95:11751, 1998.
21. Irie A, Suzuki A: CMP-N-Acetylneuraminic acid hydroxylase is exclusively inactive in humans, *Biochem Biophys Res Commun* 248:330, 1998.
22. Schauer R: Chemistry, metabolism, and biological functions of sialic acids, *Adv Carbohydr Chem Biochem* 40:131, 1982.
23. Bardor M, Nguyen DH, Diaz S, et al: Mechanism of uptake and incorporation of the non-human sialic acid N-glycolyneuraminic acid into human cells, *J Biol Chem* 280:4228, 2005.
24. Holmes R: Blood groups in cats, *J Physiol* 111:61p, 1950.
25. Eyquem A, Podliachouk L, Millot P: Blood groups in chimpanzees, horses, sheep, pigs, and other mammals, *Ann N Y Acad Sci* 97:320, 1962.
26. Auer L, Bell K: The A-B blood group system in the domestic cat, *Anim Blood Groups Biochem Genet* 11(suppl 1):63, 1980.
27. Ikemoto S, Sakurai Y, Fukui M: Individual difference within the cat blood group detected by isohemagglutinin, *Nippon Juigaku Zasshi* 43:433, 1981.
28. Ejima H, Kurokawa K, Ikemoto S: Feline red blood cell groups detected by naturally occurring isoantibody, *Nippon Juigaku Zasshi* 48:971, 1986.
29. Silvestre-Ferreira AC, Pastor J, Almeida O, et al: Frequencies of feline blood types in northern Portugal, *Vet Clin Pathol* 33:240, 2004.
30. Kilrain G, Giger U: Blood type frequencies in the Philadelphia population. Proceedings of the 5th ACVIM Forum, San Diego, CA: 891, 1987.
31. Giger U, Kilrain CG, Filippich LJ, et al: Frequencies of feline blood groups in the United States, *J Am Vet Med Assoc* 195:1230, 1989.
32. Bird MS, Cotter SM, Gibbons G, et al: Blood groups in cats, *Comp Anim Pract* 2:31, 1988.
33. Giger U, Bucheler J, Patterson DF: Frequency and inheritance of A and B blood types in feline breeds of the United States, *J Hered* 82:15, 1991.
34. Giger U, Griot-Wenk M, Bucheler J, et al: Geographical variation of the feline blood type frequencies in the United States, *Fel Pract* 19:21, 1991.
35. Continenza R, Lubas G, Gugliucci B: Indagini prelimisul sistema di gruppo sanguigno AB nel gatto allevato in Italia. Società Italiana delle Scienze Veterinarie, XLVI, (Conference Proceedings) XLVI:1493, 1992.
36. Giger U, Gorman NT, Hubler M, et al: Frequencies of feline A and B blood types in Europe. Proceedings of the 23rd International Society of Animal Genetics Conference, Interlaken, Switzerland, p 17, 1992.
37. Haarer M, Grunbaum EG: Blood group typing in the cat, *Tierarztl Prax* 21:339, 1993.
38. Hubler M, Arnold S, Casal M, et al: The blood group distribution in domestic cats in Switzerland, *Schweiz Arch Tierheilkd* 135:231, 1993.
39. Leidinger J, Leidinger E, Giger U: Distribution and importance of feline blood type-A and type-B in Austria, *Wiener Tierarztliche Monatsschrift* 80:10, 1993.
40. Jensen AL, Olesen AB, Arnbjerg J: Distribution of feline blood types detected in the Copenhagen area of Denmark, *Acta Vet Scand* 35:121, 1994.
41. Jacomet L, Montoro A, Rivero M, et al: Frecuencia de los distintos grupos sanguíneos en gatos de Buenos Aires, Argentina, *Revista de Medicina Veterinaria* 78:428, 1997.

42. Knottenbelt CM, Addie DD, Day MJ, et al: Determination of the prevalence of feline blood types in the UK, *J Small Anim Pract* 40:115, 1999.

43. Bagdi N, Magdus M, Leidinger E, et al: Frequencies of feline blood types in Hungary, *Acta Vet Hung* 49:369, 2001.

44. Mylonakis ME, Koutinas AF, Saridomichelakis M, et al: Determination of the prevalence of blood types in the non-pedigree feline population in Greece, *Vet Rec* 149:213, 2001.

45. Arikan S, Duru SY, Gurkan M, et al: Blood type A and B frequencies in Turkish Van and Angora cats in Turkey, *J Vet Med A Physiol Pathol Clin Med* 50:303, 2003.

46. Ruiz de Gopegui R, Velasquez M, Espada Y: Survey of feline blood types in the Barcelona area of Spain, *Vet Rec* 154:794, 2004.

47. Silvestre-Ferreira AC, Pastor J, Sousa AP, et al: Blood types in the non-pedigree cat population of Gran Canaria, *Vet Rec* 155:778, 2004.

48. Malik R, Griffin DL, White JD, et al: The prevalence of feline A/B blood types in the Sydney region, *Aust Vet J* 83:38, 2005.

49. Arikan S, Gurkan M, Ozaytekin E, et al: Frequencies of blood type A, B and AB in non-pedigree domestic cats in Turkey, *J Small Anim Pract* 47:10, 2006.

50. Weingart C, Arndt G, Kohn B: Prevalence of feline blood types A, B AB in non-pedigree and purebred cats in Berlin Brandenburg, *Kleintierpraxis* 51:189, 2006.

51. Cavana P, Picco S, Bellino C, et al: Distribuzione dei gruppi sanguigni nei gatti della regione Piemonte (Italia). 55th Congresso Nazionale di Medicina Felina, Milano (Conference Proceedings), p 267, 2007.

52. Forcada Y, Guitian J, Gibson G: Frequencies of feline blood types at a referral hospital in the south east of England, *J Small Anim Pract* 48:570, 2007.

53. Spada E, Proverbio D, Baggiani L, et al: Prevalenza dei gruppi sanguigni in una popolazione di gatti della regione Lombardia. Società Italiana delle Scienze Veterinarie, LXII San Benedetto del Tronto (Conference Proceedings), 2008.

54. The Cat Fanciers' Association, Inc: Breed Profile: Birman. [www.cfainc.org]. Retrieved September 19, 2008 from http://www.cfainc.org/breeds/profiles/birman.html.

55. Medeiros MA, Soares AM, Alviano DS, et al: Frequencies of feline blood types in the Rio de Janeiro area of Brazil, *Vet Clin Pathol* 37:272, 2008.

62 Disseminated Intravascular Coagulation

Michael A. Estrin and Elizabeth A. Spangler

Blood normally circulates throughout the body in a fluid state. The body's hemostatic system, composed of the coagulation cascade, platelets, vascular endothelium, and the fibrinolytic system, is responsible for maintaining the fluidity of blood while repairing vascular injuries. The coagulation cascade is activated during even minor states of disease or trauma. Normally, coagulation cascade activity is localized to the site of injury by natural anticoagulants and is in equilibrium with the fibrinolytic system. When there is sufficiently severe or prolonged activation, coagulation may occur unchecked and widespread microvascular thrombosis may occur, resulting in an often fatal condition known as disseminated intravascular coagulation (DIC). DIC has been defined as a disorder of systemic thrombosis and hemorrhage associated with underlying clinical situations and laboratory evidence of procoagulant activation, fibrinolytic activation, inhibitor consumption, and end-organ damage (Figure 62-1).[1]

ETIOLOGY

DIC is a disorder characterized in all species by the uncontrolled activation of the coagulation and fibrinolytic systems, resulting in widespread microvascular thrombosis and multiple organ dysfunction.[2] DIC always occurs in association with an underlying condition that triggers the coagulation cascade. The most common causes of DIC in human beings are sepsis or severe inflammation/infection, neoplasia including both hemic and solid tumors, trauma, burns, and organ destruction including pancreatitis.[1] In dogs, common underlying diseases include neoplasia (hemangiosarcoma, lymphoma, and other neoplasms), hepatic disease, sepsis, immune-mediated hemolytic anemia, renal disease, pancreatitis, trauma, immune-mediated thrombocytopenia, heat stroke, nonseptic peritonitis, gastric dilatation-volvulus, and benign splenic disease.[3,4]

A retrospective study published in 1995 evaluating hemostatic disorders in cats identified 21 patients fulfilling diagnostic criteria for DIC. The most common associated disorders were neoplasia, hepatic disease, and feline infectious peritonitis.[5] Thomas et al identified 10 cats meeting criteria for DIC, with systemic infection, hepatic disease, and neoplasia as the most common underlying disorders.[6] In a recent retrospective study of DIC in cats, the most common associated underlying disorders were neoplasia, pancreatitis, sepsis, and other infectious diseases (Table 62-1).[7]

Figure 62-1 Pathogenesis of DIC. An underlying disorder causes activation of coagulation primarily by tissue factor expression on endothelial cells and activated mononuclear cells. Fibrinolysis also is activated. When activation is severe or prolonged, inhibitors of coagulation and fibrinolysis are consumed or downregulated. Microvascular thrombosis leads to end-organ damage.

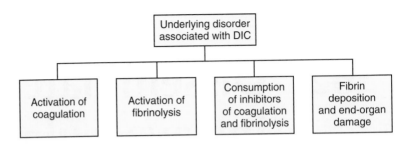

Table 62-1 Final Diagnoses in Cats with Disseminated Intravascular Coagulation

System or Category	Number Affected	Disorder (Number of Cats)
Neoplasia	19	Lymphoma (8), biliary adenocarcinoma (2), hepatocellular carcinoma (1), mastocytosis in spleen and bone marrow (1), metastatic pulmonary adenocarcinoma (1), multiple myeloma (1), metastatic carcinoma (1), pancreatic adenocarcinoma (1), myeloproliferative disease (not further characterized) with secondary IMHA (1), intrascapular fibrosarcoma (1), metastatic anaplastic neoplasia—not further characterized (1)
Pancreatic disease	12	Pancreatitis (12)
Sepsis	9	Cutaneous abscess/cellulitis (4), bacterial peritonitis (3), peritonitis secondary to intraabdominal neoplasia (2)
Infectious disease	6	Toxoplasmosis (2), yeast septicemia (1), feline panleukopenia virus (1), feline infectious peritonitis (1), feline leukemia virus (1)
Urinary system	4	Pyelonephritis (2), glomerular and renal medullary amyloidosis (1), uroabdomen (1)
Trauma/tissue necrosis	2	Trauma—fell four stories (1), tissue necrosis secondary to biliary cystadenoma (1)
Other	3	Immune-mediated hemolytic anemia (2), vaccine reaction (1)

From Estrin MA, Wehausen CE, Jessen CR, et al: Disseminated intravascular coagulation in cats, *J Vet Intern Med* 20:1334, 2006.

EPIDEMIOLOGY

Because DIC is always secondary to a variety of underlying disease processes, all ages and breeds of cats are susceptible to developing the problem. From a veterinary teaching hospital population of 86 cats who fulfilled laboratory criteria for DIC (microscopic evidence of intravascular fibrin deposition or thrombosis in more than one organ on necropsy evaluation and/or three or more of the following: prolonged prothrombin time [PT], prolonged activated partial thromboplastin time [aPTT], thrombocytopenia, hypofibrinogenemia, and elevated fibrin/fibrinogen degradation products [FDPs]), the median age was 9 years with a range of 7 weeks to 23 years. Forty-four (51.1 per cent) of the cats were neutered males, one (1.1 per cent) cat was an intact male, 40 (46.5 per cent) cats were spayed females, and one cat (1.1 per cent) was an intact female. The median body weight was 4.5 kg (n = 84, range 0.76 to 9 kg). Sixty (69.8 per cent) of the cats were Domestic Shorthairs, while the remaining consisted of 15 Domestic Longhairs, two Siamese, and one of each of the following breeds: Persian, Himalayan, Abyssinian, Devon Rex, Birman, Ragdoll, British Blue, Norwegian Forest Cat, and a Domestic Mediumhair cat. Of those cats for whom data were available, 50 (58.1 per cent) cats lived indoors exclusively and 23 (26.7 per cent) cats lived both indoors and outdoors; none of the cats lived outdoors exclusively.[8] The actual prevalence of DIC in the feline population is unknown.

COAGULATION IN THE NORMAL STATE

PHYSIOLOGY OF COAGULATION AND FIBRINOLYSIS

The process of hemostasis is a result of a complex series of interactions among the endothelium, platelets, and the coagulation cascade. In health, hemostasis is limited to the site of vascular injury by natural inhibitors of coagulation and the fibrinolytic system. The endothelium normally is resistant to thrombus formation, and the endothelial surface contains several modulators of coagulation, including a negative surface charge, thrombomodulin, heparan sulfate, and a protein C receptor.[9] In states of vascular injury, circulating platelets are exposed to subendothelial connective tissue and von Willebrand factor (vWF). Platelets then bind to collagen and vWF via surface glycoprotein receptors and become activated, secreting molecules including thromboxane A_2 and adenosine diphosphate (ADP) that activate locally circulating platelets. The activated platelets that cover the disrupted endothelium adhere via glycoprotein IIb/IIIa receptor binding to fibrinogen, which serves as a bridge to other activated platelets and leads to formation of a platelet aggregate.[9] Receptors for activated coagulation factors are exposed on the platelet surface in states of activation (Figure 62-2).

The coagulation cascade was described previously as two separate pathways, intrinsic and extrinsic, both of which activated a common pathway. It is now considered as a series of interdependent enzymatic reactions involving coagulation factors, anticoagulant factors, and fibrinolytic factors (Figure 62-3). Coagulation factors circulate as inactive enzymes (prozymogens).

Tissue factor (TF) is an intrinsic membrane protein present on fibroblasts, neoplastic cells, and most other cell types not normally in contact with blood. Certain stimuli, such as cytokines interleukin-1 (IL-1) and tumor necrosis factor (TNF), can induce monocytes and endothelial cells to synthesize TF.[9] Factor VII is capable of autoactivation, with activated factor VII (factor VIIa) normally present as 1 per cent of factor VII concentration. Factor VII and factor VIIa bind readily to TF, forming a complex on the cell surface. The TF-VIIa complex is

capable of activating additional factor VII bound to TF. The TF-VIIa complex also activates factor IX and factor X, resulting in membrane-bound factor IXa and factor Xa. Factor IX also is activated by factor XIa, a protein in the contact system that is activated by thrombin and by factor XIIa. Factor XII is part of the contact system, which plays a role in fibrinolysis, inflammation, complement activation, and kinin formation but not in the initiation of coagulation.[9] Activation of factor IX by factor XIa is thought to be less important in vivo than TF-VIIa activation because deficiency of factor XI results in a clinically mild hemostatic disorder in affected individuals.[10] Similarly, a deficiency of factor XII and its cofactor, high-molecular-weight kininogen, does not result in a hemorrhagic tendency. Factor VIII, which circulates in plasma bound to vWF, can be activated by factor Xa or thrombin. Factor VIIIa serves as a cofactor for factor IXa and the resultant "Xase" complex is the most potent activator of factor X. Factor Xa converts prothrombin to thrombin in a slow reaction. The presence of factor Va helps form a prothrombinase complex on the cell surface and accelerates the formation of thrombin markedly. Factor V can be activated by both factor Xa and thrombin. Thrombin cleaves fibrinogen, forming a fibrin monomer. Fibrin monomers polymerize spontaneously and then are cross-linked covalently to form a stable fibrin clot by factor XIIIa, which is activated by thrombin.

Procoagulant activity of the coagulation factors is balanced by inhibitors of coagulation (Figure 62-4). Several physiological mechanisms inhibit coagulation. TF pathway inhibitor regulates the activation of factors IX and X by the TF-VIIa complex. Antithrombin (AT) inhibits thrombin, factor Xa, and factor IXa.[11] The activity of AT is enhanced greatly by heparin. Factor Xa also is inhibited by Z protease inhibitor and protein Z.[9] Thrombin bound to thrombomodulin on the endothelial surface is not capable of activating factors V and VIII but does activate protein C. Activated protein C (APC), along with its cofactor protein S, inactivates factors Va and VIIIa.[11] This serves as an important regulatory pathway because the inactivated factors V and VIII are no longer able to participate in the coagulation cascade.

The fibrinolytic system solubilizes fibrin clots, maintaining the balance between fibrin clot formation and

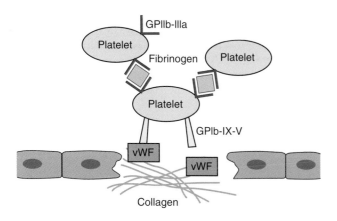

Figure 62-2 Endothelial damage exposes vWF, which is a target for platelet binding via the glycoprotein Ib-IX-V receptor complex. Platelet adhesion results in activation and degranulation. Activated platelets aggregate via binding of fibrinogen and vWF to the glycoprotein IIb-IIIa receptor complex. Activation leads to exposure of anionic phospholipid on the platelet membrane, which provides a procoagulant surface to support thrombin generation. Fibrinogen = purple; vWF = green; vascular endothelial cells = brown.

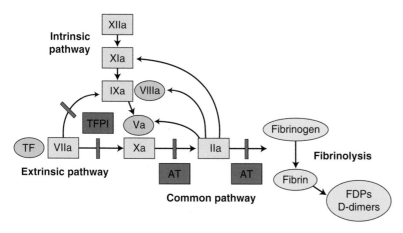

Figure 62-3 The coagulation cascade. Coagulation is initiated primarily by tissue factor. Tissue factor is inactivated rapidly by TFPI, but the thrombin produced activates factors XIa, VIIIa, and Va, which perpetuate and accelerate coagulation. *AT,* Antithrombin; *TFPI,* tissue factor pathway inhibitor. Red bars indicate sites of inhibition by TFPI and AT. Blue = coagulation enzymes; green = TF and enzyme cofactors; red = inhibitors of coagulation.

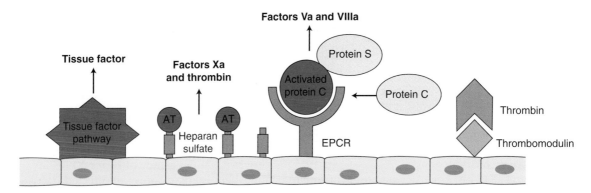

Figure 62-4 Physiological mechanisms that downregulate coagulation. Tissue factor pathway inhibitor limits activation of coagulation by tissue factor, AT directly inhibits factors Xa and thrombin, while the protein C pathway inactivates factors Va and VIIIa, which are cofactors in the activation of factors Xa and thrombin. *AT,* Antithrombin; *EPCR,* endothelial protein C receptor. Red = inhibitory factors; beige = vascular endothelium.

dissolution. Thrombin stimulates endothelial cells to release tissue-type plasminogen activator (tPA).[11] Plasminogen is activated to plasmin by tPA when both are bound to fibrin. Plasmin splits fibrinogen and fibrin to produce fibrin degradation products (FDPs). These products are themselves anticoagulants, inhibiting thrombin and fibrin polymerization.[11] Cross-linked fibrin is relatively more resistant to plasmin degradation. Urokinase plasminogen activator acts similarly to tPA and is formed by activation of prourokinase. Prourokinase bound to its receptor on activated endothelial cells is activated by plasmin, by autoactivation, and by kallikrein, a component of the contact system.[11] Urokinase then cleaves plasminogen to form plasmin. The fibrinolytic system is regulated by α-2 antiplasmin, plasminogen activator inhibitor-1 (PAI-1), and thrombin-activated fibrinolysis inhibitor.

DISRUPTION OF NORMAL PROCOAGULANT, ANTICOAGULANT, AND FIBRINOLYTIC BALANCE

DIC results from excess systemic generation of thrombin, which leads to a disruption of balance between coagulation and fibrinolysis. Major causes of marked activation of coagulation sufficient to lead to DIC include endothelial injury, tissue injury, and monocyte activation. TF is the key event in most cases of initiation of DIC, and studies in animal models of *Escherichia coli* endotoxemia showed that inhibition of the TF pathway eliminated thrombin production.[12] Systemic generation of thrombin has been demonstrated to be mediated by the extrinsic pathway of coagulation via TF and factor VIIa.[12] TF is expressed on activated mononuclear cells, endothelial cells, and neoplastic cells.[2] Endotoxin, IL-1, and TNF induce TF synthesis and expression on endothelial cells.[13] TNFα transcription is stimulated by the TF-VIIa complex, leading to increased TF synthesis and resulting in a positive feedback loop.[13] TNFα stimulates the release of other cytokines, including IL-1 and IL-6.[13] IL-6 contributes to systemic thrombin generation by causing TF expression on mononuclear cells.

PLATELET DYSFUNCTION AND CONSUMPTION

FDPs D and E have a tendency to bind to platelet membranes, leading to platelet dysfunction. Platelet consumption and incorporation into thrombi lead to thrombocytopenia, which may range from mild to severe in patients with DIC. Persistent activation of the coagulation cascade may result in consumption of coagulation factors, prolongation of coagulation times, and hemorrhage.

ABNORMALITIES OF THE FIBRINOLYTIC SYSTEM

As a result of widespread thrombin production and subsequent release of tPA, plasminogen is converted to plasmin and increased levels of plasmin circulate systemically during DIC, acting on fibrin and fibrinogen to produce FDPs X, Y, D, and E.[4] Plasmin also splits cross-linked fibrin, creating the D-dimer fragment. Other enzymes degraded by plasmin include factors V, VIII, IX, and XI, which results in decreased concentrations of these clotting factors.[1] The FDPs in circulation interfere with fibrin polymerization, leading to hemorrhage. FDPs sometimes are referred to as fibrin split products (FSPs) or fibrin-related antigens.[14] FDPs activate macrophages and monocytes to release IL-1, IL-6, and PAI-1, a potent inhibitor of fibrinolysis.[1] During peak activation of coagulation, endotoxin, IL-1, and TNF increase PAI-1 synthesis and reduce thrombomodulin expression, thus inhibiting fibrinolysis and favoring coagulation.[2]

INHIBITOR CONSUMPTION

AT and protein C concentrations decrease in patients with DIC. AT levels are reduced in DIC because of consumption, reduced synthesis, and degradation by neutrophil elastase.[2] Protein C activity is compromised as a result of reduced synthesis, reduced thrombomodulin expression on endothelial cells, and binding of cofactor protein S to C4b-binding protein.[2] TF pathway inhibitor function also is insufficient in states of DIC.[2]

END-ORGAN DAMAGE

Systemic circulation of thrombin results in the splitting of fibrinogen to form fibrinopeptides A and B and the fibrin monomer.[1] Fibrin monomers polymerize spontaneously and factor XIII, activated by thrombin, stabilizes the cross-linked fibrin, forming a clot that contributes to tissue ischemia. IL-1 and IL-6 cause vascular endothelial disruption and thus contribute to end-organ damage.[15] Thrombin-induced release of endothelin from endothelial cells leads to vasoconstriction and vasospasm, predisposing to thrombus formation and vascular occlusion.[1]

CLINICAL FEATURES

The clinical signs in cats with DIC are nonspecific and often reflect the particular underlying disorder. A review of 86 hospitalized cats with DIC revealed that depression and lethargy were the primary complaint, followed by anorexia, weakness, vomiting, dyspnea, and diarrhea. Common physical examination abnormalities included hypothermia, weak femoral pulses, tachycardia, hyperthermia, a palpable abdominal mass, cardiac murmur, bradycardia, and presence of a gallop rhythm.[8]

Physical examination findings compatible with a coagulation disorder are uncommon despite frequent alterations in laboratory tests of coagulation. Lack of spontaneous hemorrhage is common in cats with abnormal laboratory tests of coagulation. Peterson et al found evidence of spontaneous bleeding in only one of 21 cats with DIC.[5] In a study by Estrin et al,[7] hemorrhage was noted in only 14 of 86 (16.3 per cent) cats. Petechiae or ecchymoses were noted in six of 86 (seven per cent) cats. Other sources of hemorrhage consisted of hemoabdomen (5), rectal bleeding (2), epistaxis (3), hemothorax (3), and hematuria (1) (Figure 62-5). One cat had both rectal bleeding and epistaxis, while another cat had both a hemothorax and hemoabdomen. The three cats with the lowest platelet counts (1,000 to 13,000/μL) exhibited hemorrhage. One cat had epistaxis and petechiae, one had rectal bleeding and petechiae, and one developed hemoabdomen. Hemorrhage was noted in five of 12 cats

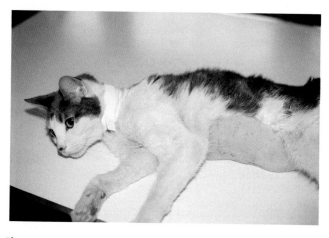

Figure 62-5 Petechiae on the abdomen of a cat with DIC secondary to feline leukemia virus–associated disease.

with a prothrombin time (PT) of 120 seconds or higher (reference range 7.4 to 12.8 seconds) and in six of 14 cats with an activated partial thromboplastin time (aPTT) of 120 seconds or higher (reference range 11.1 to 16.4 seconds).[7]

Hemorrhage is more common in dogs with DIC than in cats. Spontaneous bleeding was noted in 26 per cent of dogs with DIC in a retrospective study.[4] Severe hemorrhage is uncommon in human beings with DIC, occurring in only 5 to 12 per cent of patients with severe sepsis and DIC, but severe hemorrhage occurs four to five times more often when platelet counts fall below 50,000/μL.[2] While hemorrhage may be a more commonly recognized sign of DIC, microvascular and large vessel thrombosis causing tissue hypoxia and irreversible organ damage are more important consequences of DIC.

DIFFERENTIAL DIAGNOSIS

Conditions that may be mistaken for DIC include inherited disorders such as hemophilia A or B (factor VIII and factor IX deficiency, respectively), as well as anticoagulant rodenticide toxicosis. Thrombocytopenia may be present as a result of platelet consumption during excessive hemorrhage. The patient's clinical history, coagulation factor analysis, toxicological assays, or rapid correction of hemorrhage with appropriate component therapy allow the clinician to distinguish hemophilia readily from DIC. Cats with liver disease may develop prolonged coagulation times, especially PT and aPTT, because of decreased factor synthesis.[16] Fibrinogen may be low as a result of decreased hepatic synthesis. In addition, FDPs may be elevated in hepatic disease because of decreased clearance. Therefore differentiating cats with hepatic disease, DIC, and hepatic disease with concurrent DIC may be difficult.

PATHOLOGICAL FINDINGS

Necropsy findings will vary, depending on the underlying disorder that triggers DIC.

DIC-specific findings include evidence of intravascular fibrin deposition or thrombosis in more than one organ on histopathological evaluation (Figure 62-6, *A* and *B*), but this may not be evident because of postmortem fibrinolysis. Paradoxical hemorrhage also may be found (Figure 62-6, *C*). Necrosis of tissue affected with fibrin or thrombi is another common finding. DIC was identified in 19 of 24 (79.2 per cent) cats based on histopathological examination.[7] Thrombi were identified most commonly within the hepatic and pulmonary vasculature.

DIAGNOSIS

LABORATORY EVALUATION OF COAGULATION STATUS

Diagnostic tests that are available most commonly for evaluation of coagulation status in cats include tests for

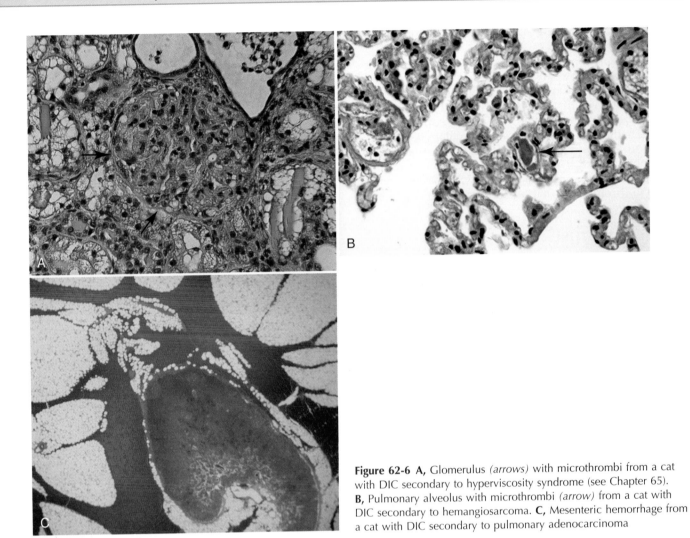

Figure 62-6 A, Glomerulus *(arrows)* with microthrombi from a cat with DIC secondary to hyperviscosity syndrome (see Chapter 65). **B,** Pulmonary alveolus with microthrombi *(arrow)* from a cat with DIC secondary to hemangiosarcoma. **C,** Mesenteric hemorrhage from a cat with DIC secondary to pulmonary adenocarcinoma

PT, aPTT, AT, fibrinogen, FDPs, D-dimer, and platelet count. As indicated, the diagnosis of DIC requires the presence of a predisposing condition, together with a combination of laboratory abnormalities that may include thrombocytopenia, activation of coagulation with production of thrombin, depletion of coagulation inhibitors, and activation of fibrinolysis. No single test is sufficient to identify a patient with DIC.

An algorithm for the diagnosis of DIC in human beings that makes use of routine tests such as those listed was proposed in 2001 by the International Society of Thrombosis and Haemostasis.[17] As outlined in Box 62-1, the DIC score is based on assessment of the PT, platelet count, and the concentration of fibrinogen and fibrin-related markers (FDPs or D-dimer). In human beings, a score greater than or equal to 5 is compatible with overt DIC. In this proposal, the working definition for DIC is further divided into two phases: nonovert DIC is characterized by subtle abnormalities of hemostasis, and overt DIC is a severe, decompensated state. A DIC score less than 5 in a patient with an underlying condition known to be associated with DIC is suggestive of nonovert DIC. It

Box 62-1 Diagnostic Algorithm for Disseminated Intravascular Coagulation in Human Patients

1. Does the patient have a predisposing condition that has been associated with DIC?
If yes, proceed; if no, do not use this algorithm.
2. Order coagulation tests (platelet count, prothrombin time [PT], fibrinogen, fibrin/fibrinogen degradation product [FDP], or D-dimer)
3. Score coagulation test results
   - Platelet count (>100,000/μL = 0; <100,000/μL = 1; <50,000/μL = 2)
   - FDP or D-dimer (no increase: 0; moderate increase: 2; strong increase: 3)
   - PT (<3 sec = 0; >3 sec but <6 sec = 1; >6 sec = 2)
   - Fibrinogen concentration (>1 g/L = 0; <1 g/L = 1)
4. Calculate score
5. If ≥5, compatible with overt DIC; if <5, suggestive (not affirmative) for nonovert DIC

Modified from Levi M, de Jonge E, Meijers J: The diagnosis of disseminated intravascular coagulation. *Blood Reviews* 16:217, 2002.

Box 62-2 Guidelines for Diagnosis of DIC in Cats

1. Does the patient have a predisposing condition that has been associated with DIC?
   If yes, DIC is a consideration; if no, DIC is not present.
2. Order coagulation tests. Test that are commonly available include measurement of the prothrombin time (PT), activated partial thromboplastin time (aPTT), antithrombin (AT) activity, fibrinogen concentration, fibrin/fibrinogen degradation product (FDP) or D-dimer levels, platelet count, and evaluation of red blood cell (RBC) morphology.
3. If three or more of these parameters are abnormal, then DIC is likely.

seems likely that evaluation of abnormal trends in the coagulation parameters will be useful for more conclusive identification of nonovert DIC.[18]

Strategies that have been applied to the identification of DIC in veterinary species are similar, but the coagulation tests that are available vary between different institutions and no standardized algorithm for determination of a DIC score has been accepted. Diagnosis of DIC in veterinary patients often is based on the presence of a predisposing condition, accompanied by at least three of the following abnormalities: (1) prolonged PT or aPTT, (2) low plasma AT activity, (3) low plasma fibrinogen concentration, (4) high plasma concentration of FDPs or D-dimer, (5) low platelet count, and (6) presence of schistocytes on a blood smear (Box 62-2). Only a few studies have been published that assess the utility of these parameters for diagnosis of DIC in dogs.[14,19] One retrospective analysis of hemostasis in 46 cats with DIC included evaluation of the PT, aPTT, fibrinogen, FDPs, and platelet count.[7] In that study, prolongation of the aPTT was seen most often, but abnormalities of the other parameters were present in 50 per cent or more of cats. Another study included assessment of AT activity, as well as the PT, aPTT, fibrinogen, FDPs, platelet count, and red blood cell (RBC) morphology, for a total of 73 cats, including seven who were diagnosed with DIC.[20] This study also found the aPTT to be abnormal most often in cats with DIC and concluded that AT was not useful for the diagnosis of DIC in cats. These results suggest that a diagnostic scheme similar to that used for human beings will be applicable to cats; however, additional studies will be necessary to determine which coagulation tests are most informative. An algorithm that can differentiate between overt and nonovert DIC in cats has not been established.

SAMPLE COLLECTION AND ANALYSIS

Most of the commercially available kits for coagulation tests are developed for human plasma and may not perform optimally when applied to plasma samples from cats; therefore it is important to verify that each test has been validated for this species. In addition, the absolute numbers obtained in different laboratories or on different instruments can not be compared directly because the methodology used will affect the results. Biological variation of the measured coagulation parameters also may be significant. A recent study in dogs emphasizes the need for caution when interpreting subtle changes in tests of coagulation because normal dogs sometimes show values that are slightly abnormal relative to the accepted standard or show variation from day to day that is not truly significant.[21] No studies have been completed to assess the significance of biological variation in cats.

Blood sample collection and handling can have a significant impact on tests that evaluate coagulation status. Platelet clumping is a common problem in cats and may cause an artifactual decrease in the measured platelet count. Excitement during the blood draw and/or repeated attempts to hit the vessel can lead to platelet activation and release of TF, both of which will result in artifactual changes in the measured coagulation times. If collection of a blood sample from one site is difficult in a cat, the best strategy is to move to another vessel. Most standard coagulation tests are performed on plasma collected from blood that has been anticoagulated with 3.2 or 3.8 per cent trisodium citrate (anticoagulant choice determined by the laboratory), at a ratio of one part citrate to nine parts blood. In-house analyzers that use citrated whole blood are available for some assays. The ratio of anticoagulant to blood in the sample is important because a precise amount of calcium must be added back to the sample to allow controlled initiation of coagulation for testing. Deviation from this ratio, as in a "short sample," will limit calcium availability in the assay because there will be an excess amount of anticoagulant available. Ethylenediaminetetraacetic acid (EDTA) is the optimal anticoagulant for assessment of the platelet count but is not an acceptable anticoagulant for other coagulation tests because it binds calcium much more avidly than citrate, impairing the controlled initiation of coagulation.

Blood drawn for coagulation testing should flow freely from the vessel. The blood can be drawn directly into a syringe or vacuum tube containing citrate or may be collected into a syringe and transferred directly to the citrate tube. The preferred strategy for blood sample collection should be the one recommended by your clinical pathology laboratory. If several different blood sample tubes are to be filled after collection of a sample, the citrate-containing tube should be filled before those containing any other anticoagulant to avoid contamination of the sample. If blood is taken from an intravenous catheter, the first 5 mL drawn from the catheter should be set aside before collection of the sample for coagulation testing. Ideally, blood samples for coagulation testing should not be collected from a heparinized catheter.

The blood sample should be mixed promptly but gently with the anticoagulant by repeated inversion of the tube. The sample should be centrifuged, and the plasma removed within 30 minutes of the blood draw. If coagulation tests can not be performed immediately, the plasma may be stored at 4° C for several hours without a loss of enzyme activity. If a plasma sample must be frozen (i.e., for shipping to an outside laboratory), it should be frozen rapidly and transported at –20° C or lower. The sample should be packed in dry ice for shipping to ensure that it remains frozen.

PLATELETS

Platelets initiate and promote the process of blood coagulation. Platelets adhere to any site of damage to the vascular endothelium and aggregate subsequently at that site. They release factors that promote transient vasoconstriction and hemostasis, and the platelet membrane provides a negatively charged lipid surface for assembly of coagulation complexes. Thrombocytopenia is often present in cats with DIC, although some cats maintain a normal platelet count despite having other coagulation abnormalities consistent with DIC.[7,20] Feline platelets may not be counted accurately by automated hematology analyzers because of clumping and because they are often large enough to exceed the size limit for detection established for the instrument. A blood smear always should be evaluated to confirm a low platelet count in cats. An estimate of the platelet count can be based on evaluation of a blood smear by multiplying the average number of platelets per 100× field (based on evaluation of at least 10 fields) by 15,000 to 20,000/μL.

In the past, coagulation was viewed as a cascade of events involving two separate pathways (intrinsic and extrinsic) that converge to activate the common pathway leading to thrombin production. Although this model does not characterize the process of coagulation accurately or completely, it is useful to describe some basic laboratory tests that are available for assessment of coagulation status (Figure 62-7).

ACTIVATED CLOTTING TIME

Activated clotting time (ACT) is a point-of-care coagulation test that uses whole blood to screen for abnormalities of the intrinsic (surface-activated) and common

pathways. The ACT test is not very sensitive, and depletion of factors to less than 90 per cent of normal may be necessary for a prolonged result. To perform this test, blood is drawn into a prewarmed (37° C) tube, which contains diatomaceous earth that provides a surface to activate the intrinsic pathway of coagulation. The blood is mixed by inverting the tube several times, and the tube then is incubated at 37° C for 60 seconds. After this, the tube is checked by gentle inversion every 5 to 10 seconds to detect the first evidence of clot formation. The time from addition of blood to the tube to clot formation is the ACT. Using this method, the ACT was determined to be less than 165 seconds in clinically normal cats and was not affected significantly by sedation with acepromazine and ketamine or by moderately traumatic venipuncture.[22] Automated point-of-care instruments are available for measurement of the ACT (SCA2000 Veterinary Coagulation Analyzer, Synbiotics, Kansas City, MO; i-STAT, Heska Corporation, Loveland, CO), and the use of such instruments may help minimize the variability that results from differences in sample handling.

ACTIVATED PARTIAL THROMBOPLASTIN TIME

The activated partial thromboplastin time (aPTT) is measured using citrated plasma and evaluates the intrinsic (surface-activated) and common pathways of coagulation. The aPTT is more sensitive than the ACT and is prolonged when there is roughly a 70 per cent decrease in factor activity. The test plasma is combined first with particulate material (e.g., kaolin, silicates, or ellagic acid) to activate the contact factors, together with an excess amount of procoagulant phospholipid to provide a surface for assembly of coagulation complexes. Because TF is not present in the phospholipid, the reagent does not activate the extrinsic (TF) pathway. Subsequent addition of calcium chloride allows progression of the coagulation cascade to produce an insoluble fibrin clot that can be detected optically or electromechanically, depending on the instrument. The reaction is carried out at 37° C. The time from addition of calcium chloride to the reaction to detection of a clot is the aPTT.

PROTHROMBIN TIME

The prothrombin time (PT) is measured using citrated plasma and evaluates the extrinsic (TF) and common pathways. The test plasma is combined with a reagent that contains calcium, phospholipid, and excess TF at 37° C. Factor activation leads to formation of an insoluble fibrin clot that can be detected either optically or electromechanically, depending on the instrument. The time from mixing of the test plasma with the reagent to detection of clot formation is the PT.

For both the PT and aPTT, assay results will vary, depending on the source of phospholipid and/or TF in the reagent kit. Kits that are valid for human beings may not give accurate results in cats. In addition, feline reference intervals may differ significantly from those established for human plasma. The assay method to be used

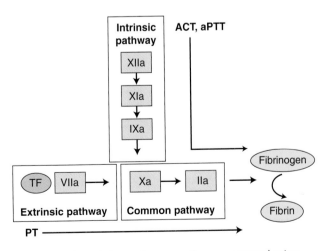

Figure 62-7 Coagulation pathways as they are assessed using the ACT, PT, and aPTT. *ACT*, Activated clotting time; *PT*, prothrombin time; *aPTT*, activated partial thromboplastin time. Green = TF; blue = coagulation enzymes.

must be validated for the species under investigation, and species-specific reference intervals must be established for the methodology in use. Characteristics of the sample, such as hemolysis, bilirubinemia, or lipemia, may interfere with optical detection of clot formation. Several point-of-care analyzers have been developed for use in veterinary species that make use of either citrated plasma or citrated whole blood for analysis of the PT and aPTT (SCA2000 Veterinary Coagulation Analyzer, Synbiotics, Kansas City, MO; i-STAT, Heska Corporation, Loveland, CO; IDEXX Coag Dx Analyzer, IDEXX, Westbrook, MA).

ANTITHROMBIN

Antithrombin (AT) is a protease inhibitor and is the major physiological anticoagulant in blood. AT is a small protein (molecular weight 62,000 daltons) that is synthesized by the liver. It is active against thrombin and factor Xa, as well as several other factors. AT forms a complex with the protease that is removed from the circulation by binding to receptors on hepatocytes. AT is consumed in this reaction and as a result may become depleted in patients with DIC. AT also may be decreased because of a lack of hepatic production or as a result of protein-losing diseases such as protein-losing enteropathy or protein-losing nephropathy. In human beings, AT activity less than 70 per cent of normal is an independent risk factor for thrombosis.[23]

AT activity is measured using a functional assay in which the test plasma is combined with heparin, an excess amount of a protease (thrombin or factor Xa), and a chromogen-labeled substrate. Protease activity will result in cleavage of the substrate, producing a color change that is detected by a spectrophotometer. AT inhibits the activity of the protease, resulting in less of a color change. AT activity is reported as the per cent activity in the test plasma relative to a pool of normal human plasma or species-specific control plasma.

One study showed that AT activity often is decreased in cats who fulfill other diagnostic criteria for DIC[6]; however, more recent work suggests that AT is not useful for the diagnosis of DIC in cats.[20] AT activity is not included in the recommended scoring system for identification of overt DIC in human patients.[18] Further work is needed to determine whether assessment of this parameter adds significantly to the information provided by other tests in cats with particular disease states.

FIBRINOGEN

Fibrinogen is a plasma protein that is synthesized by the liver. Activation of thrombin leads to cleavage of fibrinogen to fibrin, which is cross-linked subsequently to form a fibrin clot. Fibrinogen concentration can be assessed using several strategies, but fibrinogen that is capable of forming a clot is measured most commonly using an assay based on the time to clot formation when excess thrombin is added to a sample of plasma (thrombin time [TT]). The plasma sample is diluted so that fibrinogen is the rate-limiting factor in the reaction. As a result, the TT

is inversely proportional to the fibrinogen concentration, which is read from a standard curve and reported as mg/dL or μmol/L.[24] In theory, depletion of fibrinogen will result when activation of thrombin is increased. However, fibrinogen concentration is not a straightforward indicator of DIC because it is influenced by many factors that are not related directly to coagulation. Fibrinogen is an acute phase reactant, and as a result, plasma levels can increase or remain within the reference interval despite ongoing consumption.[12] Likewise, fibrinogen production may decrease as a result of decreased hepatic function, although the demand for clot formation is not increased.

FIBRINOGEN/FIBRIN DEGRADATION PRODUCTS

Plasmin cleaves both fibrinogen and fibrin at specific sites to produce a variety of fragments called fibrin and fibrinogen degradation products (FDPs), collectively. D-dimers are formed specifically through the breakdown of cross-linked fibrin and as such, their formation indicates that both coagulation and fibrinolysis have occurred. Plasma FDPs can be measured using a latex agglutination method in which latex beads are coated with antibody to human FDPs (FDP Plasma, Diagnostica Stago, Parsippany, NJ). Serial dilutions of the plasma sample are assayed and visual detection of agglutination of the beads is used to provide a semiquantitative assessment of FDP concentration. Validation of this assay method for cats has not been published, and its use is based on anecdotal reports.

Several kits are available for measurement of D-dimer concentration in plasma. All make use of latex agglutination methodology to produce a semi-quantitative or quantitative assessment of D-dimer concentration. Strategies for detection of agglutination include visual inspection of the reaction on a plate, or automated assessment of light transmittance through the sample. As for the FDP measurement, detection of D-dimer in plasma samples requires recognition of feline D-dimer by the antibody in the kit. A few kits have been shown to perform adequately in feline patients (Minutex D-dimer, Trinity Biotech, Ireland; IL Test D-Dimer, Instrumentation Laboratory Company, Lexington, MA).[25] There are two publications using another kit for measurement of feline D-dimer (STA-Liatest D-DI, Diagnostica Stago, Parsippany, NJ) that yield inconsistent results, suggesting that antibody recognition of feline D-dimer is not optimal with this reagent kit.[20,26]

SUMMARY

The diagnostic tests that are discussed here are generally available, and several have been shown to provide useful information regarding the diagnosis of DIC in cats. The ideal combination of tests to make that diagnosis is still uncertain. Monitoring of trends in these parameters over time is likely to be more powerful than a single measurement and may be useful in the diagnosis of nonovert DIC, as well as providing a measure of response to treatment.

Table 62-2 Strategies for Treatment of DIC in Cats

Therapeutic Strategy	Desired Outcome	Limitations
Unfractionated heparin	Limit microvascular thrombosis to prevent end-organ damage	Unpredictable pharmacokinetics. Contraindicated when active hemorrhage is present.
Low-molecular-weight heparin (LMWH)	Limit microvascular thrombosis to prevent end-organ damage	More predictable pharmacokinetics in human beings; however, the optimal dose and frequency of administration have not been determined for cats.
Plasma transfusion	Provide coagulation factors and antithrombin	No proven benefit. Indicated in cats who are bleeding actively and/or require invasive procedures.
Activated protein C (APC)	Inhibition of coagulation and antiinflammatory effects	Species specificity prevents use of the human product in small animals—feline APC is not available at the present time.

Treat the underlying disorder and provide supportive care.

TREATMENT

To the authors' knowledge, no clinical trials evaluating treatment modalities and their influence on survival in small animal patients with DIC have been published. The optimal strategy for management of cats with DIC remains unknown, but the most important component of a treatment plan for any patient with DIC, including cats, is to treat the underlying disorder aggressively. A rational treatment approach should be tailored to the individual patient and differs according to the underlying pathophysiology of the inciting disorder. Available therapy in small animal patients includes treatment of the underlying cause of DIC, supportive care, blood component therapy, and heparin (Table 62-2).

ADDRESS UNDERLYING DISEASE AND INCITING CAUSE

The hallmark of treatment of the patient with DIC is specific therapy for the inciting disorder. If the underlying disease can be eliminated, the nidus for the consumptive coagulopathy no longer exists. This is evident in cases of abruptio placentae in human beings, in which DIC resolves with delivery of the fetus and evacuation of the uterus.[13] Unfortunately, rapid successful treatment of the common diseases underlying feline DIC (sepsis, neoplasia, or pancreatitis) often is difficult or impossible.

SUPPORTIVE CARE

Supportive care for the patient with DIC should be coupled with treatment for the underlying disorder. Patient monitoring is critical to determining appropriate supportive measures. Such measures include monitoring oxygen saturation, blood pressure, body temperature, and fluid and electrolyte balance. Nutritional support is necessary to prevent concurrent hepatic lipidosis and to maintain gastrointestinal mucosal integrity. Other treatments that may be indicated are oxygen supplementation in hypoxemic cats and pressor therapy if hypotension persists despite adequate volume resuscitation.

HEPARIN THERAPY

Heparin is a commonly used anticoagulant therapy in human patients with DIC. The goal of heparin therapy is to reduce end-organ damage by decreasing activation of coagulation and limiting thrombus formation. The efficacy, dose, and preferred route of administration of heparin therapy in human patients with DIC are controversial. Conflicting data exist in the human literature regarding the benefit of heparin in human patients with DIC, with some clinical trials supporting a beneficial role of heparin and others showing either no benefit or increased risk of hemorrhagic complications.[13,27-29] Two major forms of heparin (unfractionated heparin and low-molecular-weight heparin [LMWH]) are available for therapeutic use. Unfractionated heparin is inexpensive and used more widely in veterinary patients; however, concerns of unpredictable pharmacokinetics, the need for aPTT monitoring, and risk of hemorrhage have led to increased use of LMWH in human beings. LMWHs have more predictable bioavailability, require less frequent dosing, do not typically require monitoring, and are associated with a reduced bleeding tendency in human patients.[30] A recent retrospective study evaluating the use of a LMWH (dalteparin, median dose 99 U/kg SQ q24h or q12h) in 57 feline patients, with the intent of reducing the risk of thromboembolic disease, found that it was well tolerated with bleeding events that may or may not have been attributable to dalteparin noted in 9 per cent of cats.[31] However, the optimal dose and frequency of administration for LMWH in cats is not known. A prospective study evaluating commonly used doses of LMWH in five healthy cats found rapid absorption and elimination kinetics and failure to achieve therapeutic anti-Xa activity.[32] In that study, unfractionated heparin at a dose of 250 IU/kg SQ q6h resulted in sustained therapeutic anti-Xa activity in all cats.[32] Because of these limitations, the authors do not recommend the use of LMWH in the treatment of feline DIC.

Heparin is contraindicated in cats with excessive hemorrhage or any active hemorrhage into vital areas such as the brain, spinal cord, pericardium, or respiratory tract. The optimal dose and frequency of administration of heparin is not known, and various low-dose and high-dose protocols exist. Based on available evidence, the authors recommend the use of unfractionated heparin at a starting dose of 200 to 250 IU/kg SQ q6h to q8h in cats with DIC. A full coagulation panel, including aPTT, PT, platelet count, fibrinogen, FDP/D-dimer, and AT (if available), should be performed on cats receiving heparin initially on a daily basis to monitor both the effect of heparin on aPTT prolongation, as well as the status of the coagulopathy. The heparin dose should be reduced if aPTT prolongation greater than 1.5 to 2 times normal occurs and if the elevation can be attributed to heparin therapy. Because the effect of heparin on coagulation depends on AT, adequate AT activity is necessary for a maximum beneficial effect. For this reason, fresh frozen plasma transfusions (containing AT) may be needed concurrently with heparin therapy in cats with low AT activity.

TRANSFUSION THERAPY

Replacement of platelets or coagulation factors may be indicated in some patients with DIC. The presence of abnormal coagulation tests does not necessitate blood component therapy. RBC transfusion therapy should be performed in cats with anemia severe enough to result in inadequate oxygen-carrying capacity (see Chapter 60). Plasma should be administered to cats who are actively bleeding and in hypocoagulable cats who require surgery or other invasive procedures. Blood typing and/or cross-matching should be performed before administration of both plasma and RBCs (see Chapter 61). If available, fresh frozen plasma is the preferred therapy for cats with active hemorrhage or before invasive procedures because it contains all of the coagulation factors, as well as AT, and is less likely to produce volume overload compared to whole blood. Multiple transfusions may be necessary to raise coagulation factor levels adequately and minimize hemorrhage. Frozen platelets and platelet-rich plasma are not readily available and probably are of limited benefit because of ongoing platelet consumption in cats with severe thrombocytopenia. A recent retrospective study of DIC in cats found no survival benefit from transfusion therapy of any type.[7] However, the number of surviving cats was very low, and transfusion therapy remains a rational treatment option for patients with active and clinically significant hemorrhage. The possibility of exacerbating thrombosis and tissue ischemia or "adding fuel to the fire" by transfusing clotting factors to patients with DIC is a theoretical concern that has not been proved in veterinary patients and is only encountered rarely in human beings.[13]

ACTIVATED PROTEIN C

Protein C levels are reduced in human patients with DIC, and treatment with APC has been shown to result in a statistically significant survival benefit in a large randomized controlled trial in human beings with severe sepsis.[33] The mortality rate for those patients receiving APC was 24.7 per cent compared to 30.8 per cent in the placebo group, resulting in a 19.4 per cent relative-risk reduction.[33] Patients in this study with DIC received the most benefit from APC therapy.[34] In another randomized, double-blind trial comparing APC and unfractionated heparin in 132 human patients with DIC, the 28-day all-cause mortality rate was significantly lower in the APC group compared to the heparin group (20.4 per cent vs. 40 per cent, $p < 0.05$).[30] In addition to its effects on coagulation, the survival benefit from protein C therapy may be a result of its antiinflammatory effects, including reduced IL-6 levels, TNF release, and reduced leukocyte adhesion.[35] APC therapy for DIC has not been studied in cats, and the human recombinant APC product is not recommended in small animals because of rapid elimination, high species specificity necessitating a fifteenfold to twentyfold dose to achieve an equivalent effect, and as a result of its antigenic properties and potential for anaphylactic hypersensitivity reactions with repeated administration in nonhuman species.[35]

ANTITHROMBIN AND OTHER THERAPIES

Activation of thrombin is one of the key events leading to DIC. Inhibition of TF or factor VIIa has been demonstrated in laboratory animal models of sepsis to eliminate endotoxin-induced thrombin generation.[2] However, treatment with TF pathway inhibitor in human patients with severe sepsis in a phase III randomized controlled clinical trial failed to result in increased survival.[36] By restoring a deficient natural anticoagulant pathway, AT replacement therapy is another theoretically beneficial treatment modality. Unfortunately, a large-scale phase III randomized controlled clinical trial evaluating AT concentrate therapy in human patients with severe sepsis showed no significant increase in 28-day survival.[37]

PROGNOSIS

The prognosis for cats with DIC likely is poor because of its association with serious underlying diseases. In a recent study, only three of 46 cats (6.5 per cent) with DIC survived beyond 2 weeks after discharge from the hospital.[7] Each surviving cat had a different underlying disorder: one cat had hepatic lipidosis and lymphoma, one cat had immune-mediated hemolytic anemia, and one cat had pancreatitis. No prognostic factors or differences in therapy between survivors and nonsurvivors were identified in this study. However, this study was biased toward nonsurvivors because cases for inclusion were selected in part based on necropsy findings. Survival has been evaluated in a large number of dogs with DIC in an abstract presented in 2002. In that study, survival at discharge was

49 per cent and 90-day survival was 28 per cent.[3] Dogs with trauma and benign splenic disease had the highest survival rate.[3]

SUMMARY

Feline DIC remains a challenging clinical problem and carries a poor prognosis despite our advancing understanding of the physiology of hemostasis. Optimal diagnostic tests and treatments remain to be elucidated. Moreover, the process of feline hemostasis may differ subtly from that which occurs in human beings or dogs, so future studies involving species-specific assessment of diagnosis and treatment will be essential. Efforts to identify patients in early, compensated stages of DIC may be helpful in identifying and developing interventional therapies to halt the progression of this disorder. Although treatment directed at restoring normal hemostasis, including replacement of deficient coagulation factors and inactivation of excessive thrombin, has a role in the management of affected patients, aggressive treatment of the underlying cause for DIC, as well as comprehensive supportive care, remain the most important components of therapy.

REFERENCES

1. Bick RL: Disseminated intravascular coagulation: current concepts of etiology, pathophysiology, diagnosis, and treatment, *Hematol Oncol Clin North Am* 17:149, 2003.
2. Levi M: Disseminated intravascular coagulation, *Crit Care Med* 35:2191, 2007.
3. Ross SJ, Smith SA, Lekcharoensuk C: Disseminated intravascular coagulation (DIC) in dogs: 252 cases (1999-2000) Abstract, *J Vet Intern Med* 16:350, 2002.
4. Couto CG: Disseminated intravascular coagulation in dogs and cats, *Vet Med* 94:547, 1999.
5. Peterson JL, Couto CG, Wellman ML: Hemostatic disorders in cats: a retrospective study and review of the literature, *J Vet Intern Med* 9:298, 1995.
6. Thomas JS, Green RA: Clotting times and antithrombin III activity in cats with naturally developing diseases: 85 cases (1984-1994), *J Am Vet Med Assoc* 213:1290, 1998.
7. Estrin MA, Wehausen CE, Jessen CR, et al: Disseminated intravascular coagulation in cats, *J Vet Intern Med* 20:1334, 2006.
8. Estrin MA: Unpublished data, 2005.
9. Colman RW, Clowes AW, George JN, et al: Overview of hemostasis. In Colman RW, Marder VJ, Clowers JN, et al, editors: *Hemostasis and thrombosis: basic principles and clinical practice*, ed 5, Philadelphia, 2006, Lippincott Williams & Wilkins, p 3.
10. Roberts HR, Ma AD: Overview of inherited hemorrhagic disorders. In Colman RW, Marder VJ, Clowers JN, et al, editors: *Hemostasis and thrombosis: basic principles and clinical practice*, ed 5, Philadelphia, 2006, Lippincott Williams & Wilkins, p 877.
11. Colman RW, Marder VJ, Clowes AW: Overview of coagulation, fibrinolysis, and their regulation. In Colman RW, Marder VJ, Clowers JN, et al, editors: *Hemostasis and thrombosis: basic principles and clinical practice*, ed 5, Philadelphia, 2006, Lippincott Williams & Wilkins, p 17.
12. Levi M, Ten Cate H: Disseminated intravascular coagulation, *N Engl J Med* 341:586, 1999.
13. Marder VJ, Feinstein DI, Colman RW, et al: Consumptive thrombohemorrhagic disorders. In Colman RW, Marder VJ, Clowers JN, et al, editors: *Hemostasis and thrombosis: basic principles and clinical practice*, ed 5, Philadelphia, 2006, Lippincott Williams & Wilkins, p 1571.
14. Bateman SW, Mathews KA, Abrams-Ogg AC, et al: Diagnosis of disseminated intravascular coagulation in dogs admitted to an intensive care unit, *J Am Vet Med Assoc* 215:798, 1999.
15. Bick RL: Disseminated intravascular coagulation: pathophysiological mechanisms and manifestations, *Semin Thromb Hemost* 24:3, 1998.
16. Liscandro SC, Hohenhaus AE, Brooks MB: Coagulation abnormalities in 22 cats with naturally occurring liver disease, *J Vet Intern Med* 12:71, 1998.
17. Taylor FB Jr, Toh CH, Hoots WK, et al: Towards definition, clinical and laboratory criteria, and a scoring system for disseminated intravascular coagulation, *Thromb Haemost* 86:1327, 2001.
18. Toh CH, Hoots WK: The scoring system of the Scientific and Standardization Committee on Disseminated Intravascular Coagulation of the International Society on Thrombosis and Haemostasis: a 5-year overview, *J Thromb Haemost* 5:604, 2007.
19. Bateman SW, Mathews KA, Abrams-Ogg ACG: Disseminated intravascular coagulation in dogs: review of the literature, *J Vet Emerg Crit Care* 8:29, 1998.
20. Brazzell JL, Borjesson DL: Evaluation of plasma antithrombin activity and D-dimer concentration in populations of healthy cats, clinically ill cats, and cats with cardiomyopathy, *Vet Clin Pathol* 36:79, 2007.
21. Wiinberg B, Jensen AL, Kjelgaard-Hansen M, et al: Study on biological variation of haemostatic parameters in clinically healthy dogs, *Vet J* 174:62, 2007.
22. Bay JD, Scott MA, Hans JE: Reference values for activated coagulation time in cats, *Am J Vet Res* 61:750, 2000.
23. Dahlback B: Advances in understanding pathogenic mechanisms of thrombophilic disorders, *Blood* 112:19, 2008.
24. Stockham SL, Scott MA: *Fundamentals of veterinary clinical pathology*, ed 2, Ames, 2008, Blackwell.
25. Spangler EA: Personal communication, 2008.
26. Bedard C, Lanevschi-Pietersma A, Dunn M: Evaluation of coagulation markers in the plasma of healthy cats and cats with asymptomatic hypertrophic cardiomyopathy, *Vet Clin Pathol* 36:167, 2007.
27. Pernerstorfer T, Hollenstein U, Hansen J, et al: Heparin blunts endotoxin-induced coagulation activation, *Circulation* 100:2485, 1999.
28. Hoffmann JN, Wiedermann CJ, Juers M, et al: Benefit/risk profile of high-dose antithrombin in patients with severe sepsis treated with and without concomitant heparin, *Thromb Haemost* 95:850, 2006.
29. Chojnowski K, Trelinski J, Wawrzyniak E, et al: The influence of low molecular weight heparin on the intravascular activation of the coagulation system in patients with acute leukemia during induction chemotherapy–report of a prospective randomized study, *Leuk Lymphoma* 43:1021, 2002.
30. Aoki N, Matsuda T, Saito H, et al: A comparative double-blind randomized trial of activated protein C and unfractionated heparin in the treatment of disseminated intravascular coagulation, *Int J Hematol* 75:540, 2002.
31. Smith CE, Rozanski EA, Freeman LM, et al: Use of low molecular weight heparin in cats: 57 cases (1999-2003), *J Am Vet Med Assoc* 225:1237, 2004.
32. Alwood AJ, Downend AB, Brooks MB, et al: Anticoagulant effects of low-molecular-weight heparins in healthy cats, *J Vet Intern Med* 21:378, 2007.

33. Bernard GR, Vincent JL, Laterre PF, et al: Efficacy and safety of recombinant human activated protein C for severe sepsis, *N Engl J Med* 344:699, 2001.

34. Dhainaut JF, Yan SB, Joyce DE, et al: Treatment effects of drotrecogin alfa (activated) in patients with severe sepsis with or without overt disseminated intravascular coagulation, *J Thromb Haemost* 2:1924, 2004.

35. Hopper K, Bateman SW: An updated view of hemostasis: mechanisms of hemostatic dysfunction associated with sepsis, *J Vet Emerg Crit Care* 15:83, 2005.

36. Abraham E, Reinhart K, Opal S, et al: Efficacy and safety of tifacogin (recombinant tissue factor pathway inhibitor) in severe sepsis: a randomized controlled trial, *JAMA* 290:238, 2003.

37. Warren BL, Eid A, Singer P, et al: Caring for the critically ill patient. High-dose antithrombin III in severe sepsis: a randomized controlled trial, *JAMA* 286:1869, 2001.

63 Selection of Treatment Protocols for Lymphoma

Ann E. Hohenhaus

Lymphoma is the most important tumor of the domestic cat, and veterinarians have been treating the disease since the late 1960s.[1] Initially, selection of a treatment protocol was simple because prednisone was the only treatment administered to these cats. The current state-of-the-art treatment may include surgical resection, multi-agent chemotherapy, adjuvant radiation therapy, and increasingly, investigational therapies. The variety of extremely similar treatment protocols may be confusing to veterinarians and may make protocol selection complicated.

The purpose of this chapter is to review commonly recommended treatment protocols used as first-line treatment and those used in "rescue" or relapse situations. This chapter also will discuss the various factors that impact the selection of a lymphoma treatment protocol. These factors include issues affecting the owner of the cat with lymphoma, the veterinarian prescribing cancer treatment, and the cat diagnosed with lymphoma.

REVIEW OF PROTOCOLS

Chemotherapy protocols for the treatment of feline lymphoma can be classified in several different ways (Table 63-1). They may be classified by the number of drugs used: single-agent and multi-agent protocols. Primary protocols are those used as first-line therapy for lymphoma, and rescue protocols are those used when the disease relapses. Finally, protocols may be classified as those with or without doxorubicin. Multi-agent protocols containing doxorubicin are referred to commonly as CHOP-based protocols. The acronym CHOP refers to the drugs included in the protocol representing cyclophos-

phamide, doxorubicin (hydroxydaunomycin), Oncovin (vincristine), and prednisone. In general, most oncologists believe multi-agent protocols that include doxorubicin result in a longer survival time than those without doxorubicin; however, multi-agent protocols likely require more patient visits to the veterinarian, which incur a greater cost for the owners and require a larger drug inventory for the veterinarian.[2-5] Single-agent doxorubicin, which is a very successful protocol in dogs, is not recommended because it is much less successful in cats with lymphoma.[2,5-8]

FACTORS INFLUENCING PROTOCOL SELECTION FOR INITIAL TREATMENT

A variety of chemotherapy treatment protocols have been developed for the treatment of cats with lymphoma. When reviewing potential treatment protocols for use in their practices, veterinarians should familiarize themselves with the anticipated remission rate and duration, survival time, and the frequency of toxicity. This information will be essential in communicating with the cat owner during the decision-making process about lymphoma treatment. Table 63-1 contains some of this information for commonly used chemotherapy protocols.

If a single-agent treatment protocol was optimal for the treatment of all cats with lymphoma, veterinary oncologists would not continue investigations to identify better treatments. Most studies of treatment protocols for feline lymphoma are retrospective, making comparisons between published data difficult because of the variations in the cat population studied. For example, the COP

Table 63-1 Common Protocols for the Treatment of Feline Lymphoma

Protocol	Reference	Drugs Included	Frequency of Visits	Common Toxicity
SINGLE-AGENT PROTOCOLS				
Prednisone	1	Prednisone	Monthly	None
Doxorubicin	7, 8	Doxorubicin	Every 3 weeks	Anorexia common Myelosuppression less common
MULTI-AGENT PROTOCOLS WITHOUT DOXORUBICIN				
Cyclic combination chemotherapy	27	L-Asparaginase, vincristine, cyclophosphamide, methotrexate, prednisone	Weekly for 8 weeks, then every 10 days for 8 treatments, then every 14 days	Few side effects
COP	4, 9, 10	Cyclophosphamide, vincristine (Oncovin), prednisone	Weekly for 4 weeks, then every 3 weeks	Few side effects
CHOP-BASED PROTOCOLS (CYCLOPHOSPHAMIDE, DOXORUBICIN, VINCRISTINE, PREDNISONE)				
University of Wisconsin, Madison	24	L-Asparaginase, vincristine, cyclophosphamide, doxorubicin, prednisone	Weekly for 9 weeks with 1-week breaks, then every other week	34% of cats had neutropenia resulting in treatment delay
Current Veterinary Therapy X	3, 25, 53	L-Asparaginase, vincristine, cyclophosphamide, doxorubicin, methotrexate, prednisone	Weekly for 6 weeks, then every 10 days for 6 treatments, then every 14 days	Mild anorexia, low-grade neutropenia, especially with vincristine Low-grade gastrointestinal toxicity, especially with vincristine and L-asparaginase
VELCAP-C	26	L-Asparaginase, vincristine, cyclophosphamide, doxorubicin, prednisone	Weekly with 1- to 2-week breaks	49% of cats had dose reductions due to toxicity
RESCUE OR RELAPSE PROTOCOLS				
CCNU (Lomustine)	11	CCNU	Every 6 weeks	Neutropenia dose-limiting
MOPP	12	Nitrogen mustard, Oncovin, procarbazine, prednisone	Treat 2 consecutive weeks, then no treatment for 2 weeks	Well-tolerated

(cyclophosphamide, Oncovin, prednisone) protocol was used to treat cats in the United States and The Netherlands.[9,10] In these studies, the median remission duration was 8 months in the Dutch study and 5 months in the American study. These data suggest that the COP protocol works better in 2002 than it did in 1983; however, a critical review of the publications suggests that the study populations were very different between the two countries. The feline leukemia virus (FeLV) status differed tenfold between the two countries, with 7 per cent of Dutch cats and 70 per cent of the American cats testing positive for the virus. Both studies reported approximately 30 per cent of cats with the mediastinal form of lymphoma; however, the Dutch study had a large proportion of young, FeLV-negative Siamese cats with mediastinal lymphoma. These cats had among the highest percentages of remission and longest survival rates ever reported for cats with lymphoma. No young, FeLV-negative Siamese cats were reported in the American study. Veterinarians should avoid comparing the success of retrospectively evaluated treatment protocols without considering the differences in cat population included in the studies. These examples highlight the critical need for

veterinarians to review the reported data carefully and to determine how the data apply to the cats in their practices before selecting a treatment protocol for feline lymphoma.

FACTORS INFLUENCING PROTOCOL SELECTION WHEN LYMPHOMA PROGRESSES OR RELAPSES

Progression of the tumor during treatment or relapse of the tumor after discontinuation of therapy are poor prognostic indicators. Suggested guidelines for selection of a rescue protocol are included in Table 63-2. Little has been written on the success of additional chemotherapy treatment for feline lymphoma once progression or relapse occurs. Response to treatment was reported in 10 cats who relapsed after receiving a multi-agent chemotherapy protocol that did not contain doxorubicin.[3] In nine of these cats, the original treatment protocol was continued at more frequent, weekly intervals and achieved a response rate of 66 per cent. The tenth cat received doxorubicin followed by mitoxantrone for a second complete response of 40 weeks. A phase I clinical trial of CCNU (Lomustine)

Table 63-2 Guidelines for Selection of a Rescue Protocol

Initial Protocol	Rescue Protocol
Single-agent	Multi-agent
No doxorubicin	Single-agent doxorubicin or CHOP-based
Chemotherapy discontinued >2 months	Restart previous protocol
Progression while on chemotherapy or chemotherapy discontinued <2 months	Select protocol with different drug(s)
CHOP-based protocol	Change class of drugs used Consider platinum drug or antimetabolite
Prednisone	Switch to different corticosteroids (i.e., dexamethasone or methylprednisolone)
L-Asparaginase used in protocol	Repeat L-asparaginase if only 1 previous administration

CHOP, Cyclophosphamide, doxorubicin (hydroxydaunomycin), Oncovin (vincristine), prednisone.

in cats with a variety of refractory tumors reported the response of 13 cats with lymphoma.[11] Five of 13 cats had a partial response to treatment with CCNU. The use of Mustargen (nitrogen mustard), Oncovin, procarbazine, and prednisone (MOPP) has been reported for the treatment of cats with relapsed lymphoma.[12] Fifty-six per cent of cats treated with MOPP had a measurable response and a median MOPP survival time of 65 days. The median survival time in cats after relapse of lymphoma is similar to that in dogs, approximately 2 months, regardless of the protocol chosen.[13,14]

FACTORS IMPACTING THE CAT OWNER'S DECISION ABOUT LYMPHOMA TREATMENT

CAT OWNER AND VETERINARIAN COMMUNICATION

The diagnosis of lymphoma is devastating to cat owners. Because of cats' innate ability to hide the seriousness of their illnesses, owners may not be expecting a terminal diagnosis. Veterinarians need to anticipate the cat owner's need for sympathy, crying, and some handholding. Each cat owner will react somewhat differently to the news, and the veterinarian will need to respond a little differently in each situation. The cat owner also may need some time to digest the information and will need to schedule time in the future to discuss the implications of the diagnosis of lymphoma. Others will have many questions immediately about treatment and prognosis.

Client expectations of their relationship with their veterinarian have been studied, and several points are

Box 63-1 Questions for Owners Considering Chemotherapy Treatments for Their Cat

- What are the owner's goals for performing chemotherapy?
  - To provide the cat with a good quality of life and alleviate clinical signs of the tumor?
  - To have a chance for the longest survival possible?
  - To keep their cat alive until a particular time such as a holiday or for the visit of a family member?
- How much money is the owner prepared to spend?
- How much time is the owner prepared to expend?
- How much toxicity is the owner willing to accept?
- How does the cat's personality impact chronic, recurring visits to the veterinarian for treatment?

applicable to the owner of a cat with lymphoma[15] (Box 63-1). Cat owners take their cats to the veterinarian less frequently than dog owners take their dogs to the veterinarian; however, pet owners seeking high-level medical care have a stronger bond with their pet and take their pet to the veterinarian 40 per cent more often.[16] Strongly bonded cat owners are those who typically pursue chemotherapy for lymphoma.

Communication regarding expectations for cats on chemotherapy is critical because there is a perception by the pet-owning public that treatment with chemotherapy causes pain and suffering in companion animals.[17] In a survey of cat owners who treated their cats for lymphoma, 78 per cent expressed apprehension about embarking on a course of chemotherapy for their cat.[18] Cat owners are more highly educated than dog owners and should be excellent candidates to understand the medical needs of their cat with lymphoma, if the veterinarian allows adequate time to discuss treatment.[16] Adequate time may require one long session with the owners to answer their questions or multiple short phone calls and e-mails to answer short questions.

From the owner's viewpoint, an important factor in their compliance with veterinarian-recommended protocols is the level of communication from the veterinarian about the importance of the recommended treatment.[16,19] Communication skills play a critical role in the veterinarian's ability to develop a strong relationship with the pet owner. Pet owners who feel their veterinarian provides them with adequate information on pet care, communicates well, and recommends only what their pet needs have favorable opinions about their veterinarian, resulting in a strong client-veterinarian bond. Eighty-four per cent of clients with a strong bond to their veterinarian follow their veterinarian's recommendations, whereas only 48 per cent of those with a weak relationship follow their veterinarian's recommendations.[16] Finally, an important determinant in compliance with the administration of recommended drugs is if the owner feels the veterinarian spent adequate time during the examination explaining the need for drug administration.[20]

Pet owners expect informational material on diagnosis and treatment to be available in various forms. This is because adults vary significantly in their optimal learning style. Some learn by hearing or asking questions and others by visual means. Veterinarians need to provide information about lymphoma treatment in formats other than a conversation such as handouts, fact sheets, websites, or pamphlets.[19] Repetition of the message to the client by a veterinary practice team member other than the primary veterinarian improves compliance with recommended treatment.[19] Some cat owners may require time to consider the information and ask more questions, whereas others will make a decision immediately.

Pet owners expect treatment options to be discussed at the time of diagnosis.[15] Options for treatment of a cat with lymphoma include no treatment, euthanasia, or treatment. For some cat owners, treatment of any sort is not an option because of time, finances, or personal preference. A variety of options exist for owners electing treatment. Prednisone alone, a chemotherapy protocol administered by the family veterinarian, or referral to a veterinary oncologist for discussion of chemotherapy protocols, adjuvant radiation therapy, or investigational therapy all should be presented as options for the cat with lymphoma.

Pet owners have varying degrees of health care literacy. When receiving information about potential treatments for lymphoma, the owner expects the veterinarian to tailor the discussion to their individual ability to understand medical information. Veterinarians should never use medical terms or jargon when discussing treatment with owners. The veterinarian should attempt to understand the owner's goals for chemotherapy in their cat and help them to set realistic expectations regarding their cat's cancer therapy (Box 63-2). Open-ended questions (How do you feel about treating your cat with chemotherapy? What will be the problems you anticipate with the treatment protocol I have described?) should be asked to determine if the owner comprehends the discussion.[21] By asking questions frequently (Have I given you enough information about the potential chemotherapy side effects?) the veterinarian can clarify the client's level of understanding.

Sixty-eight per cent of people making decisions about their own health care prefer the decision making to be a shared process between themselves and their physician.[21]

Box 63-2 Pet Owner Expectations Regarding Veterinarian-Client Communication

- Expect information to be explained
- Expect information to be presented up-front
- Expect information to be available in various forms
- Expect to be presented with a range of options
- Expect veterinarians to be respectful of their decisions
- Expect a partnership in the care of their pets
- Expect veterinarians to use language that clients understand
- Expect veterinarians to listen
- Expect veterinarians to ask the right questions

From Coe JB, Adams CL, Bonnett BN: A focus group study of veterinarians' and pet owners' perceptions of veterinarian-client communication in companion animal practice, *J Am Vet Med Assoc* 233:1072, 2008.

Similar studies in veterinary medicine have not been performed; however, owners have expressed a strong preference for the care of their pet to be a partnership between themselves and the veterinarian and for having multiple treatment options discussed, irrespective of the cost.[15,19] Pet owners can be confused by the presentation of multiple options when the "best" option is not identified.[15,19] There is no "best" option for the treatment of lymphoma because the disease is controllable but not curable by any currently available treatment. The benefits and risks of the available treatment options for each individual cat should be discussed, and the owner should be helped to choose the best treatment protocol for their cat and their family. Once a treatment decision is made, pet owners expect veterinarians to respect their decision.[15]

The various chemotherapy treatment protocols utilize different treatment schedules. A survey of Australian cat owners whose cats were undergoing therapy for lymphoma considered chemotherapy a substantial time commitment.[18] As part of the decision-making process, veterinarians must outline the anticipated frequency of visits to allow the client to determine if they can comply with the recommended schedule.

Most cats treated for lymphoma will receive medications administered by their owners. Owner noncompliance with the recommended treatment schedule is a barrier to therapeutic success. Market research suggests that veterinarians are considered by pet owners to be the main source for information on oral medication administration.[22] Despite this, veterinarians typically wait until the client expresses difficulty in administering oral medications to discuss interventions to make it more successful. Therefore, during selection of a lymphoma treatment protocol, a veterinarian or technician should enlist the owner as a partner in the treatment of their cat and discuss the importance and techniques of oral medication administration. In addition to spending time with the owner explaining the importance of the prescribed medication, there are other interventions to facilitate drug administration. These include the use of "pill pockets," compounded formulations of medication with flavorings to improve palatability, or transdermal administration. Because of the risk of human exposure to chemotherapy drugs, there are limited options for compounded formulations of these drugs. (See Chapter 18 in the fifth volume of this series for a discussion on the use of transdermal medications.)

FACTORS INFLUENCING THE VETERINARIAN'S SELECTION OF LYMPHOMA TREATMENT PROTOCOL

The decision to offer chemotherapy for feline lymphoma is an individual choice for each veterinary practice. Points to consider when making this decision include the veterinary staff's training and experience in treating a cat for lymphoma, the proximity to a veterinary oncologist, and the willingness and ability of the veterinary practice to comply with federal, state, and local guidelines for safe handling of chemotherapy drugs as workplace hazards[23] (see Chapter 73). Chemotherapy protocols containing multiple chemotherapy agents require significant investment in maintaining an adequate drug inventory. Given the small amount of drug administered to a cat, chemotherapy drugs often expire before the contents of the bottle can be utilized completely, if the practice does not treat many cats with lymphoma. This must be taken into account when developing the fees associated with chemotherapy administration. Alternatively, chemotherapy drugs can be ordered from some pharmacies that deliver premeasured, individual doses conveniently. Veterinary practices may decide to limit their usage of chemotherapy protocols to one or two commonly used protocols. This decision will allow the staff to become familiar with the treatment protocol and the anticipated toxicities and also will limit the required drug inventory. Owners desiring other treatment options can be referred to a veterinary oncologist.

Veterinarians should set expectations for the owner regarding the anticipated complete remission rate, survival time, and quality of life for each cat undergoing treatment for lymphoma (see Table 63-1). Slightly more than 50 per cent of pet owners expected the visible tumor to shrink when their cat was treated with chemotherapy.[17] Remission rate varies based on the protocol used, the cat population studied, and the predominant anatomical form of the disease. In general, owners should be informed that the complete remission rate for lymphoma is 38 to 75 per cent.[3,10,24-27]

In a 2003 pet owner survey, 87 per cent of owners expected that their pet would live longer, and in a separate cat-owner survey, 85 per cent were completely satisfied with their decision to pursue chemotherapy.[17,18] The high rate of satisfaction was in part because 70 per cent of the cats had a marked clinical improvement. This information was corroborated in a separate study in which the owners of eight of 10 cats treated for lymphoma reported that their cat's well-being had improved on chemotherapy.[17] Nearly 90 per cent of pet owners who treated their pets for cancer would do so again. The outcome of cancer treatment impacted the data only slightly. If the pet had died before the time the owners were surveyed, only 75 per cent reported that they still would treat their pet again.

The decision-making process regarding treatment of a cat with lymphoma can be complicated by factors that the veterinarian can control[19] (see Box 63-2). Every veterinarian has experienced an owner who is preoccupied by a nervous pet or an owner who keeps answering cell phone calls during the discussion of a serious medical condition. When discussing the diagnosis and treatment of lymphoma, there is a large amount of information to present. Scheduling time when the cat owner and the veterinarian can talk without interruption, without the presence of the cat or cell phones, will improve the veterinarian's ability to communicate the diagnostic and therapeutic recommendations effectively to the cat owner.

Median survival time has been reported for many different chemotherapy protocols and ranges widely (Table 63-3). Most protocols utilize similar combinations of drugs; therefore some attribute the variation in survival

Table 63-3 Median Survival of Cats Treated for Lymphoma Based on Selected Prognostic Factors

	Reported Median Survival	Reference
Nasal lymphoma	456 days	2
Alimentary lymphoma	40 weeks	3
Mediastinal lymphoma, young Siamese or Oriental Shorthair cat	"Very prolonged survival"	10
Mediastinal lymphoma	69 days 262 days	2, 10
FeLV-positive cat	21 days 37 days	2, 8
Complete remission	654 days 253 days	2, 24
Doxorubicin in protocol	281 days 225 days	2, 5

FeLV, Feline leukemia virus.

time to factors other than the treatment protocol. Response to treatment possibly is the strongest predictor of survival time in cats diagnosed with lymphoma, and cats achieving a complete remission have a longer median survival than those who fail to do so.[10,24,25,27] Survival time varies with the anatomical form of the disease being treated; for example, nasal lymphoma has been reported to have a survival in excess of 1 year.[2,28] Infection with feline immunodeficiency virus (FIV) has not been shown to affect survival time; however, FeLV infection does decrease survival time.[2,18,27] Communicating the expected survival time to the owner is an important feature of any discussion with a cat owner about lymphoma. In addition to a discussion of survival time, a conversation about the unpredictable nature of lymphoma is equally important.

Accurately communicating the anticipated level of toxicity from a treatment protocol is critical in setting expectations for the owner. Overstating the risk of toxicity may prevent clients from even attempting lymphoma treatment, whereas understating the risk may result in owner dissatisfaction with the chemotherapy experience. Toxicity is different in cats than in dogs, with certain chemotherapy toxicities seen in dogs being rare in cats. These include cyclophosphamide-induced sterile hemorrhagic cystitis and doxorubicin-induced cardiotoxicity.[9,29] Cat owners may have had experience with family or friends receiving chemotherapy. It is critical to explain to them the differences between human and feline patients. Cats do not lose all their hair from chemotherapy as do people, and the gastrointestinal side effects are minimal because of the dosing strategies used in cats. Despite these differences, 95 per cent of owners expected side effects in their cats undergoing chemotherapy for lymphoma.[17] Given the high expectation clients have for chemotherapy-related toxicity, it is important for owners to understand that there are interventions designed to mitigate toxicity. Those interventions include treatment delay in the face of an inadequate neutrophil count, administration of medications to prevent nausea and vomiting, dosage reductions when toxicity is repeatable, and discontinuation of the drug or even discontinuation of treatment if toxicity is unmanageable. Owners want decision making to be a partnership between themselves and their veterinarians.[15] When the veterinarian provides alternatives to lessen chemotherapy toxicity to an owner who thought they had none, the owner's expectation of a partnership is met.

Several studies have reported the occurrence of toxicity in cats receiving chemotherapy for lymphoma. When reviewing this information, it is essential to assess not only the rate of occurrence of toxicity but also the severity of toxicity. The Veterinary Co-operative Oncology Group has developed common terminology criteria for reporting adverse events after chemotherapy.[30] These criteria grade the severity of toxicity according to a scale from 0 to 5 with 0 representing no toxicity, grade 4 representing life-threatening toxicity, and grade 5 equal to death.

Veterinarians are conflicted when discussing the cost of veterinary care because of the fee-for-service nature of veterinary medicine[31] (Box 63-3). Compounding the veterinarian's internal conflict is the pet-owning public, who desire a veterinarian who loves animals and cares for them without regard to monetary gain. Pet owners also would like a veterinarian who offers payment plans or other financial alternatives when the cost of care exceeds the owner's financial resources.[31]

Veterinarians fear a client's primary objection to accepting recommended treatment will be the associated costs.[19] However, the cost of care does not prevent most clients from following treatment recommendations for feline lymphoma. Fifty-five per cent of owners surveyed reported cost alone was not a major factor in the decision to proceed with chemotherapy.[18] Confusion, uncertainty, and misunderstanding of the need for and the goals of the recommended treatment are the likely barriers.[16] Some pet owners are experienced consumers of veterinary care and are aware of the costs associated with routine care.[31] Most cat owners are not aware of the costs associated with diagnosis, chemotherapy administration, and

---

Box 63-3   Barriers the Veterinarian Faces When Communicating with Clients

- Discussions of cost
- Client misinformation
- Involvement of more than one client
- Lack of available time
- Client disability
- Language barriers
- Level of "health care literacy"
- Client cell phone usage

From Coe JB, Adams CL, Bonnett BN: A focus group study of veterinarians' and pet owners' perceptions of veterinarian-client communication in companion animal practice, *J Am Vet Med Assoc* 233:1072, 2008.

---

management of toxicity associated with the treatment of lymphoma. Pet owners expect the veterinarian to initiate a discussion of cost before initiating a treatment plan, but these discussions do not always occur.[31] Furthermore, pet owners expect the cost of care to be given in the context of the anticipated prognosis. Veterinarians recommending and administering chemotherapy should be prepared to give the cat owner an estimate of the cost of each individual chemotherapy visit and an estimate of the total cost if the cat were to survive the median time expected for that anatomical form of lymphoma. Factors included in this estimate of total cost should include the visits, safety testing, drugs and administration, and medications administered at home by the owner. Owners need to be aware that the cost of management of treatment-related toxicity can not be predicted, although most toxicity can be managed on an outpatient basis. Toxicity requiring hospitalization typically is uncommon; however, it can be very expensive. Providing this level of detail regarding the cost of treatment will help meet the owner's expectations concerning communication and will assist them in making an informed decision.

The team composed of the family veterinarian, the cat owner, and the cat with lymphoma may benefit from additional members such as a veterinary oncologist, veterinary radiation oncologist, or a veterinary surgeon. A consultation with an oncology specialist will help the cat owner understand the issues related to treatment of lymphoma and, as mentioned previously, when the owner hears the treatment recommendation from a team member other than the primary veterinarian, owner compliance improves.[19] Oncology specialists will have access to new or investigational treatments and clinical trials not available to the family veterinarian. The oncologist and family veterinarian may be able to share treatment of the cat, which is often more convenient for the cat owner. Finally, the family veterinarian will have the knowledge and support of the oncologist should uncommon adverse events occur. The surgeon may be added to the team if a surgical procedure such as a biopsy or resection of an intestinal mass is required.

The team also may benefit from the addition of a social worker, grief counselor, or veterinary practice member with excellent client communication skills (see Chapter 72). In large referral centers, these professionals can help the cat owner overcome the impersonal feeling of a large facility and the feeling of being alone when they receive devastating information about their cat. The training and skills of professionals allow them to assist the cat owner in decision making about treatment, to translate the "doctor speak" into understandable terms, and to reiterate the treatment recommendations of the veterinarian. The client embarking on a treatment protocol also will need support for their decision to treat their cat for cancer. Friends and family members are not always supportive or understanding of the decision to treat a cat with chemotherapy, and the cat owner will need affirmation of their decision. Ultimately, the social worker, grief counselor, or veterinary practice member will become a resource for the cat owner when the cat dies or a decision about euthanasia must be made.

FACTORS INFLUENCING THE SELECTION OF A LYMPHOMA TREATMENT PROTOCOL

ANATOMICAL FORM OF LYMPHOMA

Feline lymphoma has been categorized into four anatomical forms: alimentary, multicentric, thymic, and an atypical (extranodal) form; although not all studies use an identical classification scheme[2,32,33] (Table 63-4). Certain features of the various anatomical forms of lymphoma impact the selection of the treatment protocol and are outlined in Table 63-3.

In the 1980s, mediastinal lymphoma was seen most commonly in young FeLV-positive cats and carried a poor prognosis.[33] Over the past 30 years, there has been a marked decrease in the incidence of FeLV infection and an increase in gastrointestinal lymphoma (see Chapter 17). Recently, reports from around the world have described mediastinal lymphoma in young, FeLV-negative Siamese and Oriental Shorthair cats.[7,10,33,34] These cats have a longer median survival compared to the median survival of cats with gastrointestinal lymphoma, 262 days versus 191 days, respectively, suggesting the disease is very chemotherapy-responsive regardless of the treatment protocol selected.[10,18]

Lymphoma of the nasal cavity presents typically with nasal discharge, ocular discharge, facial deformity, or respiratory stertor. This anatomical form of lymphoma often is localized to the nasal cavity but occurs as a component of disseminated lymphoma in approximately 20 per cent of patients with nasal lymphoma.[28,35] Nasal lymphoma appears to confer a better prognosis than some other forms of lymphoma, and the median survival has been reported to approach two years.[2,10,28] Adjuvant radiation therapy often is used in the treatment of nasal lymphoma. Some oncologists have reported radiation therapy as a successful treatment for nasal lymphoma when it is used as the sole treatment modality.[36] Most veterinary oncologists recommend that chemotherapy and radiation therapy should be used concurrently because of the risk of systemic lymphoma.[28]

Lymphoma can occur primarily in the brain and spinal cord, and it can occur secondary to the spread of lymphoma from another anatomical site. Lymphoma in the brain often causes ataxia, altered consciousness, and aggression[37] (see Chapter 55). Spinal cord lymphoma occurs at the thoracolumbar location, has a predilection for male cats, and often occurs as a result of FeLV infection.[38,39] Reported characteristics of renal lymphoma in cats include renomegaly, clinical and laboratory abnormalities associated with renal failure, and cytological or histological confirmation of malignant lymphocytes in the kidney (see Chapter 51).[40] At least two studies have reported a high frequency of central nervous system (CNS) metastasis, and in one study, 40 per cent of cats with renal lymphoma died from CNS lymphoma.[27,41]

Treatment of primary and secondary CNS lymphoma is complicated by the blood-brain barrier, which prevents most chemotherapy agents from entering the brain and spinal cord in therapeutic levels. One exception to this situation is cytosine arabinoside, an antimetabolite chemotherapy agent. After subcutaneous administration, cytosine arabinoside crosses the blood-brain barrier and penetrates into the CNS.[42] The use of cytosine arabinoside has been recommended in cats with renal lymphoma because of the frequent concurrence of CNS involvement.[41] In cats with lymphoma of either the brain or spinal cord, the addition of cytosine arabinoside to the chemotherapy protocol should be strongly considered. Radiation therapy is another mode of treatment that can cross the blood-brain barrier.

Radiation therapy typically is utilized in specific situations as an adjunct to chemotherapy for the treatment of lymphoma. It is rarely used as the sole therapy for lymphoma because lymphoma typically is a systemic disease and radiation therapy treats only the tumor within the radiation field. Because of its ability to penetrate all tissue, radiation is a useful adjunctive treatment in cases of lymphoma in the brain or spinal cord, in which the blood-brain barrier prevents therapeutic concentrations of most chemotherapy drugs. A life-threatening condition caused by lymphoma is another indication for use of radiation therapy, for example, dyspnea from a cranial mediastinal mass or tracheal mass.[43,44] Radiation therapy as an adjunct to the treatment of nasal lymphoma has been discussed in a previous section.

The available information on lymphoma immunophenotype in cats is not as well-defined as in dogs, in whom

Table 63-4 Classification Scheme of Lymphoma Based on Anatomical Form

Anatomical Category				Reference
Thymic	**Multicentric**	**Alimentary**	**Extranodal (Atypical)**	32

Mediastinal	Mixed	Abdominal
		• Alimentary
		  ○ Renal
		  ○ Other
		• Combination of above categories
			Atypical nonlymphoid tissue	33, 46

Mediastinal	Multicentric	Alimentary	Extranodal • Nasal • Renal • Hepatic • Other	2, 25

the immunophenotype is a strong predictor of median survival time.[45] Dogs with B-cell lymphoma have a longer median survival time than those with T-cell lymphoma. The two largest and most recent studies of immunophenotype in feline lymphoma report that approximately 25 per cent of cats have T-cell lymphoma.[2,46] These studies contradict earlier studies that report higher percentages of T-cell lymphoma but included more FeLV-positive cats and studied smaller populations. A correlation between immunophenotype and histological findings or response to therapy could not be made in these studies. The gastrointestinal form of lymphoma may be a T-cell disorder predominantly, although only a small number of cats have been studied.[3,47]

Low-grade lymphoma may represent a subset of lymphoma that is very responsive to therapy and that has a long median survival time. Approximately 10 per cent of lymphomas in cats overall are classified as low grade and occur most commonly in the gastrointestinal tract[46,48] (see Chapter 17). Some authors recommend that treatment of cats diagnosed with low-grade lymphoma should be limited to chlorambucil and prednisone; however, not all cats with low-grade lymphoma will respond to this treatment.[48,49] Furthermore, superior efficacy of chlorambucil/prednisone has not been proved in a randomized, controlled clinical trial, comparing response to treatment and median survival time in cats with low-grade lymphoma to a multi-agent chemotherapy protocol.

CONCURRENT FELINE LEUKEMIA VIRUS INFECTION

Cats with lymphoma and concurrent FeLV infection have shorter median remission duration and median survival time than cats not infected with FeLV.[2,8,27] In one study, median remission duration in FeLV-positive cats with lymphoma was 27 days compared to 146 days in FeLV-negative cats with lymphoma.[2] Median survival time in these two groups of cats was 37 days and 170 days, respectively.

THE PERSONALITY OF THE PATIENT

Most cats are very cooperative during phlebotomy for blood sampling and during chemotherapy. Those cats who resist these procedures require special handling. When handling cats for venipuncture or catheter placement, less restraint often results in a more relaxed, cooperative cat (see Chapter 73). Wrapping the cat in a towel may protect the people involved in the process from injuries. If the cat is still unmanageable, sedation may be required to safely obtain a blood sample for a complete blood count and to administer chemotherapy. If sedation is required for every treatment, a vascular access port (VAP) should be considered.

A VAP is a surgically implanted device that allows ready vascular access for administering a sedative, obtaining blood samples, or administering chemotherapy. Use of the VAP requires fewer personnel to draw a blood sample than traditional venipuncture methods and will facilitate the procedure in a fractious cat.[50] The blood samples obtained from VAPs have been shown to be suitable for monitoring cats receiving chemotherapy.[51] As with any surgical procedure, there are potential complications, including seroma, infection, dermatitis, breaking the port-catheter junction, port occlusion, and port migration.[50-52] The occurrence of port complications is uncommon, and most owners of pets with cancer with implanted ports are satisfied with the use of a VAP.[52]

REFERENCES

1. Brick JO, Roenigk WJ, Wilson GP: Chemotherapy of malignant lymphoma in dogs and cats, *J Am Vet Med Assoc* 153:47, 1968.
2. Vail DM, Moore AS, Ogilvie GK, et al: Feline lymphoma (145 cases): proliferation indices, cluster of differentiation 3 immunoreactivity and their association with prognosis in 90 cats, *J Vet Intern Med* 12:349, 1998.
3. Zwahlen CH, Lucroy MD, Kraegel SA, et al: Results of chemotherapy for cats with alimentary malignant lymphoma, *J Am Vet Med Assoc* 213:1144, 1998.
4. Mahony OM, Moore AS, Cotter CM, et al: Alimentary lymphoma in cats: 28 cases (1988-1993), *J Am Vet Med Assoc* 207:593, 1995.
5. Moore AS, Cotter SM, Frimberger AE, et al: A comparison of doxorubicin and COP for maintenance of remission in cats with lymphoma, *J Vet Intern Med* 10:372, 1996.
6. Carter RF, Harris CK, Withrow SJ, et al: Chemotherapy of canine lymphoma with histopathological correlation: doxorubicin alone compared to COP as first treatment regimen, *J Am Anim Hosp Assoc* 23:587, 1987.
7. Peaston AE, Maddison JE: Efficacy of doxorubicin as an induction agent for cats with lymphosarcoma, *Aust Vet J* 77:442, 1999.
8. Kristal O, Lana SF, Ogilvie GK, et al: Single agent chemotherapy with doxorubicin for feline lymphoma: a retrospective study of 19 cases (1994-1997), *J Vet Intern Med* 15:125, 2001.
9. Cotter SM: Treatment of lymphoma and leukemia with cyclophosphamide, vincristine and prednisone: II. Treatment of cats, *J Am Anim Hosp Assoc* 19:166, 1983.
10. Teske E, van Straten G, van Noort R, et al: Chemotherapy with cyclophosphamide, vincristine and prednisolone (COP) in cats with malignant lymphoma: new results with an old protocol, *J Vet Intern Med* 16:179, 2002.
11. Rassnick KM, Gieger TL, Williams LE, et al: Phase I evaluation of CCNU (Lomustine) in tumor bearing cats, *J Vet Intern Med* 15:196, 2001.
12. Mauldin GE, Mooney SC, Mauldin GN: MOPP chemotherapy as rescue for cat with refractory lymphoma. Proceedings of the Veterinary Cancer Society, Chicago, Illinois, 1997, p 98.
13. Van Vechten M, Helfand SC, Jeglum KA: Treatment of relapsed canine lymphoma with doxorubicin and dacarbazine, *J Vet Intern Med* 4:187, 1990.
14. Lucroy MD, Phillips BS, Kraegel SA, et al: Evaluation of single-agent mitoxantrone as chemotherapy of relapsing canine lymphoma, *J Vet Intern Med* 12:325, 1998.
15. Coe JB, Adams CL, Bonnett BN: A focus group study of veterinarians' and pet owners' perceptions of veterinarian-client communication in companion animal practice, *J Am Vet Med Assoc* 233:1072, 2008.
16. Lue TW, Patenburg DP, Crawford PM: Impact of the owner-pet and client-veterinarian bond on the care that pets receive, *J Am Vet Med Assoc* 232:531, 2008.

17. Bronden LB, Rutteman G, Flagstad A, et al: Study of dog and cat owners' perceptions of medical treatment for cancer, *Vet Rec* 152:77, 2003.

18. Malik R, Gabor LJ, Foster SF, et al: Therapy for Australian cats with lymphosarcoma, *Aust Vet J* 70:808, 2001.

19. *Executive Summary of Compliance in Companion Animal Practices*, Lakewood, CO, 2003, American Animal Hospital Association.

20. Grave K, Tanem H: Compliance with short-term oral antibacterial drug treatment in dogs, *J Small Anim Pract* 40:158, 1999.

21. Timmins R: Getting the message across. DVM Newsmagazine. May 2008, p 44.

22. Tyrone Research Proprietary Studies with veterinary and pet owner panels, February 2008.

23. National Institute for Occupational Safety and Health Alert, Department of Health and Human Services, Centers for Disease Control and Prevention: Preventing occupational exposures to antineoplastic and other hazardous drugs in health care settings, 2004. NIOSH Publication, 2004: 165. http://www.cdc.gov/niosh/docs/2004-165/. Accessed November 17, 2008.

24. Milner RJ, Peyton J, Cooke K, et al: Response rates and survival times for cats with lymphoma treated with the University of Wisconsin-Madison chemotherapy protocol: 38 cases (1996-2003), *J Am Vet Med Assoc* 227:1118, 2005.

25. Simon D, Eberle N, Laacke-Singer L, et al: Combination chemotherapy in feline lymphoma: treatment outcome, tolerability and duration in 23 cats, *J Vet Intern Med* 22:394, 2008.

26. Hadden AG, Cotter SW, Rand W, et al: Efficacy and toxicosis of VELCAP-C treatment of lymphoma in cats, *J Vet Intern Med* 22:153, 2008.

27. Mooney SC, Hayes AA, MacEwen EG, et al: Treatment and prognostic factors in lymphoma in cats: 103 cases (1977-1981), *J Am Vet Med Assoc* 194:696, 1989.

28. Sfiligoi G, Theon AP, Kent M: Response of nineteen cats with nasal lymphoma to radiation therapy and chemotherapy, *Vet Radiol Ultrasound* 48:388, 2007.

29. O'Keefe D, Sisson D, Gelberg H, et al: Systemic toxicity associated with doxorubicin administration in cats, *J Vet Intern Med* 7:309, 1993.

30. Veterinary Co-operative Oncology Group: Veterinary Co-Operative Oncology Group-Common terminology criteria for adverse events (VCOG-CTCAE) following chemotherapy or biological antineoplastic therapy in dogs and cats v1.0, *Vet Comp Oncol* 2:194, 2004.

31. Coe JB, Adams CL, Bonnett BN: A focus group study of veterinarians' and pet owners' perceptions of the monetary aspects of veterinary care, *J Am Vet Med Assoc* 231:1510, 2007.

32. Theilen GH, Madewell BR: Hematopoietic neoplasms, sarcomas and related conditions, Part II feline. In Theilen GH, Madewell BR, editors: *Veterinary cancer medicine*, Philadelphia, 1987, Lea & Febiger, p 354.

33. Louwerens M, London CA, Pedersen NC, et al: Feline lymphoma in the post feline leukemia virus era, *J Vet Intern Med* 19:329, 2005.

34. Gabor LJ, Malik R, Canfield PJ: Clinical and anatomical features of lymphosarcoma in 118 cats, *Aust Vet J* 76:725, 1998.

35. Day MJ, Henderson SM, Belshaw Z, et al: An immunohistochemical investigation of 18 cases of feline nasal lymphoma, *J Comp Pathol* 130:152, 2004.

36. Elmslie RE, Ogilvie GK, Gillette EL, et al: Radiotherapy with and without chemotherapy for localized lymphoma in 10 cats, *Vet Radiol Ultrasound* 32:277, 1991.

37. Troxel MT, Vite CH, van Winkle TJ, et al: Feline intracranial neoplasia: retrospective review of 160 cases (1985-2001), *J Vet Intern Med* 17:850, 2003.

38. Lane SB, Kornegay JN, Duncan JR, et al: Feline spinal lymphosarcoma: a retrospective evaluation of 23 cats, *J Vet Intern Med* 8:99, 1994.

39. Spodnick GJ, Berg J, Moore FM, et al: Spinal lymphoma in cats: 21 cases (1967-1989), *J Am Vet Med Assoc* 200:373, 1992.

40. Weller RE, Stann SE: Renal lymphosarcoma in the cat, *J Am Anim Hosp Assoc* 19:363, 1983.

41. Mooney SC, Hayes AA, Matus RE, et al: Renal lymphoma in cats: 28 cases (1977-1984), *J Am Vet Med Assoc* 191:1473, 1987.

42. Scott-Moncrieff JC, Chan TCK, Samuels ML, et al: Plasma and cerebrospinal fluid pharmacokinetics of cytosine arabinoside in dogs, *Cancer Chemother Pharmacol* 29:13, 1991.

43. Calia CM, Hohenhaus AE, Fox PR, et al: Acute tumor lysis syndrome in a cat with lymphoma, *J Vet Intern Med* 10:409, 1996.

44. Brown MR, Rogers KS, Mansell KJ, et al: Primary intratracheal lymphosarcoma in four cats, *J Am Anim Hosp Assoc* 39:468, 2003.

45. Greenlee PG, Filippa DA, Quimby FW, et al: Lymphomas in dogs: a morphologic, immunologic and clinical study, *Cancer* 60:199, 1990.

46. Gabor LJ, Canfield PJ, Malik R: Immunophenotypic and histological characterization of 109 cases of feline lymphosarcoma, *Aust Vet J* 77:436, 1999.

47. Carreras JK, Goldschmidt M, Lamb M, et al: Feline epitheliotropic intestinal malignant lymphoma: 10 cases (1997-2000), *J Vet Intern Med* 17:326, 2003.

48. Kiselow MA, Rassnick KM, McDonough SP, et al: Outcome of cats with low-grade lymphocytic lymphoma: 41 cases (1995-2005), *J Am Vet Med Assoc* 232:405, 2008.

49. Fondacaro JV, Richter KP, Carpenter JL, et al: Feline gastrointestinal lymphoma: 67 cases (1988-1996), *Eur J Comp Gastroenterol* 4:5, 1999.

50. Morrison J, Lauer SK, Baldwin CJ, et al: Evaluation of the use of subcutaneous implantable vascular access ports in feline blood donors, *J Am Vet Med Assoc* 230:855, 2007.

51. Henry CJ, Russell LE, Tyler JW, et al: Comparison of hematologic and biochemical values for blood samples obtained via jugular venipuncture and via vascular access port in cats, *J Am Vet Med Assoc* 220:482, 2002.

52. Cahalane AK, Rassnick RM, Flanders JA: Use of vascular access ports in femoral veins of dogs and cats with cancer, *J Am Vet Med Assoc* 231:1354, 2007.

53. Matus RM: Chemotherapy of lymphoma and leukemia. In Kirk RW, editor: *Current veterinary therapy X*, Philadelphia, 1989, Saunders, p 482.

CHAPTER

64 Feline Bone Marrow Disorders

Douglas J. Weiss

Bone marrow disorders have been categorized as primary bone marrow disorders and those occurring secondary to diseases of other organs or systems.[1,2] Several primary bone marrow disorders of cats, including acute myelogenous leukemias, acute lymphocytic leukemia, chronic lymphocytic leukemias, multiple myeloma, and pure red cell aplasia (PRCA), are diagnosed routinely.[3-5] However, bone marrow disorders occurring secondary to other diseases frequently are confusing both to clinicians and pathologists. Routine methods of evaluating these disorders, including single or repeated complete blood counts, serum chemistry profiles, feline leukemia virus (FeLV) and feline immunodeficiency virus (FIV) testing, and bone marrow aspiration, often provide only a description of the pathological condition and a list of differential diagnoses.[1] When the diagnostic information is fragmented—as can occur when different people interpret the blood smear, bone marrow aspirate, and bone marrow core biopsy specimen or when the clinician and pathologist(s) fail to communicate—the problem is compounded. However, with a careful evaluation of the case history and a coordinated evaluation of the blood smear, bone marrow aspiration smear, and bone marrow core biopsy specimen, the clinician frequently can make an etiopathological diagnosis.

In this chapter, I will begin with a discussion of general lesions in bone marrow that need to be understood both by the pathologist interpreting bone marrow specimens and the clinician applying the results to a particular case.

Thereafter, I will discuss specific bone marrow disorders occurring in cats, including the clinical, hematological, and bone marrow features needed to achieve an etiopathological diagnosis. An overall diagnostic approach for evaluation of hematological disorders in cats has been presented elsewhere.[1] The diagnostic plan for evaluation of hematological disorders should be conducted in several phases. The initial phase should include results of a complete history (including exposure to drugs and toxins), physical examination, complete blood count, and blood smear examination. Thereafter, infectious diseases (FeLV, FIV, *Mycoplasma* spp., parvovirus) and immune-mediated diseases should be evaluated with appropriate diagnostic tests. Because mild to moderate nonregenerative anemias frequently occur secondary to inflammatory, renal, hepatic, neoplastic, or certain endocrine disorders, a serum chemistry profile and other appropriate diagnostic tests to detect these conditions are indicated. If the initial phase of testing does not achieve an etiological diagnosis, a bone marrow aspiration and core biopsy are indicated. Both the aspirate and core are essential for complete evaluation of bone marrow disorders. Although bone marrow differential cell counts are performed infrequently, they can be useful, and determining the percentage of myeloblasts in the aspiration smear is recommended. In selected cases, additional testing may be needed. These tests include immunophenotyping of leukemias, determination of clonality, and FeLV testing on the bone marrow aspirate.

HISTOPATHOLOGICAL ALTERATIONS IN BONE MARROW

Several histopathological changes are seen frequently in feline bone marrow and contribute to bone marrow failure.[6-9] Although these changes can be associated with several disease conditions, they can be used to identify the general type of marrow injury and to focus the search for an etiological diagnosis. A core biopsy specimen is needed to identify these lesions. These pathological changes generally are subclassified as acute or chronic bone marrow injury.[6,10] Lesions associated with acute marrow injury include myelonecrosis and acute inflammation, and lesions associated with chronic marrow injury include chronic inflammation, myelofibrosis, and osteosclerosis. These conditions may occur concurrently and usually are described and defined by which process is the most prominent. All of these conditions occur secondary to other disease processes. Therefore the goal should be to identify and treat the underlying condition. If the primary condition is treated successfully, the bone marrow failure usually resolves.

ACUTE MARROW INJURY

Myelonecrosis

Myelonecrosis is thought to result from ischemic injury to marrow.[11] Necrosis can be associated with toxic injury to marrow sinusoids associated with sepsis or with immune-mediated injury or ischemia associated with thrombosis such as in disseminated intravascular coagulation or marrow neoplasia.[8,11] Myelonecrosis can appear as multifocal areas of coagulation-type necrosis or as individual cell necrosis.[8,11,12] Coagulation-type necrosis is rare in cats.[11] Individual cell necrosis, a frequent finding in cat bone marrow, is characterized by large numbers of degenerating, frequently anuclear cells and increased pink amorphous background material (Figure 64-1).[11] The most frequent causes of bone marrow necrosis are immune-mediated hemolytic anemia (IMHA) (see Chapter 60) and sepsis.[11,13] Other causes include myelodysplastic syndromes, myeloproliferative diseases, and chronic kidney disease. Therefore identifying significant necrosis in the absence of evidence of a myelodysplastic syndrome or myeloproliferative disease in marrow should prompt a search for IMHA or sepsis. IMHA frequently is accompanied by lymphocytosis in bone marrow, further helping to identify an immune etiology.

ACUTE INFLAMMATORY INJURY

Acute marrow inflammation results from injury to bone marrow sinusoids resulting in altered permeability.[9,13,14] Histopathological changes associated with altered vascular permeability include sinusoidal dilation or congestion, interstitial edema, or hemorrhage.[9,13] Interstitial edema is seen as amorphous pink homogeneous material between hematopoietic cells (Figure 64-2).[13] Vascular injury also can result in exudation characterized by mul-

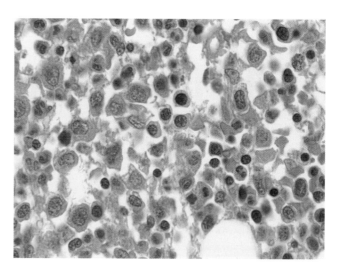

Figure 64-1 Individual cell necrosis in a core biopsy section from a cat with nonregenerative immune-mediated hemolytic anemia. Note the presence of many anuclear cells and cellular debris. (Hematoxylin & eosin stain, original magnification 1000×.)

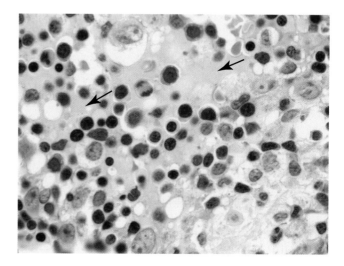

Figure 64-2 Interstitial edema *(arrows)* in a bone marrow core biopsy section from a cat with nonregenerative immune-mediated hemolytic anemia. Edema is seen as amorphous pink material between cells. (Hematoxylin & eosin stain, original magnification 1000×.)

tifocal fibrin deposits or multifocal infiltrates of neutrophils.[13,14] Fibrin appears as pink fibrillar material that can be identified on hematoxylin-eosin–stained sections, but it stains selectively with Frazier-Lundrum stain (Figure 64-3).[9] These fibrin deposits frequently contain variable numbers of segmented neutrophils.[13,15] Causes of acute inflammation in feline bone marrow include IMHA and infectious diseases including bacterial sepsis, parvovirus infection, and feline infectious peritonitis (FIP).[8,9,13,16,17] Fibrin is particularly prominent in cats with FIP.[8] Therefore identifying acute inflammation in marrow should prompt a search for these conditions.

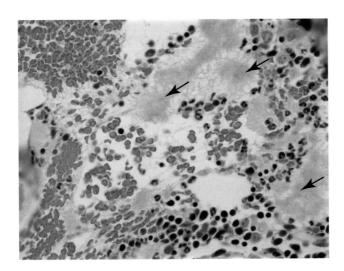

Figure 64-3 Fibrinous inflammation in a bone marrow core biopsy section from a cat with bacterial sepsis. Note the presence of pink, fibrous strands of fibrin *(arrows)*, hemorrhage, and an infiltrate of neutrophils. (Hematoxylin & eosin stain, original magnification 500×.)

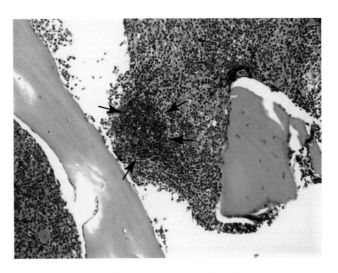

Figure 64-4 Lymphoid aggregate *(arrows)* in a bone marrow core biopsy section from a cat with nonregenerative immune-mediated hemolytic anemia. (Hematoxylin & eosin stain, original magnification 100×.)

CHRONIC BONE MARROW INJURY

Chronic bone marrow injury can occur as a chronic manifestation of acute marrow injury or arise independently.[8,13] Bone marrow cellularity is variable but typically is decreased. Chronic injury frequently is accompanied by myelofibrosis.[13]

Chronic Inflammation

Types of chronic inflammation observed in cats include lymphocytosis and plasma cell hyperplasia.[3,13,18] Lymphocytosis is the most frequent type of chronic inflammation.[13,18] In a retrospective study of 203 clinical bone marrow reports from cats, lymphocytosis (i.e., lymphocytes >15 per cent of all nucleated cells) was observed in 15.6 per cent of the specimens.[6] In some cats, lymphocyte numbers exceeded 50 per cent of all nucleated cells in the bone marrow.[6,13,18] More than 80 per cent of cats with lymphocytosis have a diagnosis of nonregenerative IMHA.[18] Other, less frequent, causes of bone marrow lymphocytosis include cholangiohepatitis and idiopathic reactive lymphadenopathy.[13,18] Differentiating benign lymphocytosis from chronic lymphocytic leukemia can be problematic. The age of the affected cat should be considered. Whereas many conditions that induce benign lymphocytosis, including IMHA (see Chapter 60), PRCA, and idiopathic reactive lymphadenopathy, are conditions of young cats, chronic lymphocytic leukemia is a disease of old cats.[18] Lymphocyte morphology and distribution also provide some clues. In chronic lymphocytic leukemia, lymphocytes frequently are mildly pleomorphic and have cleaved or lobulated nuclei.[18] Benign lymphocytes frequently are arranged in small, multifocal aggregates in bone marrow, whereas they are distributed diffusely in chronic lymphocytic leukemia (Figure 64-4).[18] Furthermore, the number of lymphocytes in blood helps differentiate benign lymphocytosis from chronic lymphocytic leukemia.[18,19] More than 25,000 lymphocytes/μL in blood

is suggestive of chronic lymphocytic leukemia, while more than 50,000 lymphocytes/μL usually is diagnostic for chronic lymphocytic leukemia.[19,20] Additionally, immunophenotyping of lymphocytes in bone marrow may be useful. Benign lymphocytes in bone marrow are mostly B cells, whereas malignant lymphocytes in chronic lymphocytic leukemia usually are T cells.[18,19]

Because plasma cells are distributed unevenly in bone marrow, plasmacytosis usually is evaluated subjectively in bone marrow aspirates or core biopsy specimens.[12] Plasmacytosis has been observed in 6 per cent of feline bone marrow specimens.[6] Plasmacytosis in cats has been associated with IMHA, PRCA, immune-mediated thrombocytopenia, and FIP.

Myelofibrosis and Osteosclerosis

Myelofibrosis is a frequent finding in feline bone marrow and is characterized by the presence of fibroblasts or by deposition of collagen or reticulin fibers (Figure 64-5).[6,21] Special stains are needed to detect reticulin fibrosis (e.g., Gomori's stain).[15] Reticulin fibrosis is present in the majority of cats with acute myelogenous leukemia.[21] Extensive reticulin fibrosis may interfere with obtaining a bone marrow aspirate, resulting in a "dry tap" even when the marrow is hypercellular.[21] Other conditions associated with myelofibrosis include nonspecific myelonecrosis, nonregenerative IMHA, myelodysplastic syndromes, chronic kidney disease, hypertrophic cardiomyopathy, and FIP.[8] Rare cases of idiopathic myelofibrosis, a rare form of chronic myeloproliferative disease, have been reported in cats.[22]

Cats with myelofibrosis typically have a severe nonregenerative anemia.[8] Leukopenia and thrombocytopenia are less frequent findings. Ovalocytes and other erythrocyte shape changes are seen rarely in cats. The prognosis for secondary myelofibrosis varies with the primary condition.[8] Cats with myelofibrosis secondary to IMHA or idiopathic myelonecrosis frequently recover, and the

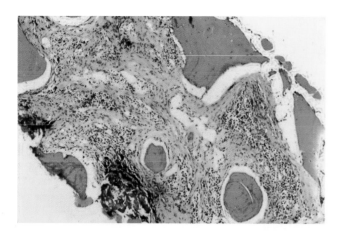

Figure 64-5 Myelofibrosis in a bone marrow core biopsy section from a cat. (Hematoxylin & eosin stain, original magnification 50×.)

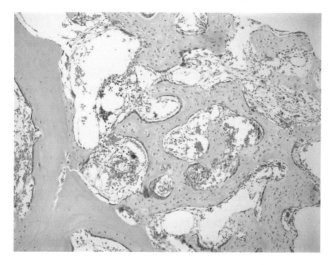

Figure 64-6 Osteosclerosis in a bone marrow core biopsy section from a feline leukemia virus–infected cat. Note the presence of new bone proliferation decreasing the size of the marrow cavity. (Hematoxylin & eosin stain, original magnification 100×.)

fibrosis resolves with successful treatment of the primary condition.[8] Alternatively, myelofibrosis associated with myeloproliferative disease, myelodysplastic syndromes, FIP, and chronic kidney disease tends to be progressive presumably because the initiating factors persist. Therefore the prognosis for myelofibrosis should be based on the primary disease condition, the severity of the anemia present, and the degree of hypocellularity of the bone marrow.[8]

Osteosclerosis (also termed *myelosclerosis*) is a condition in which the marrow cavity is reduced in size or obliterated as a result of bony proliferation (Figure 64-6). When severe, the associated thickening of bone is visible radiographically.[22] This type of severe osteosclerosis has been associated with FeLV infection.[23,24] Mild osteosclerosis frequently is associated with cases of severe myelofibrosis. These changes are seen in core biopsy sections as thickened trabeculae with irregular edges that contain increased numbers of osteoblasts.

SPECIFIC BONE MARROW DISORDERS

HEMATOLOGICAL DISORDERS ASSOCIATED WITH INFLAMMATION AND NEOPLASIA

Inflammatory diseases are accompanied consistently by a mild to moderate normocytic normochromic nonregenerative anemia.[25,26] This appears to be the most frequent cause of anemia in cats.[25] The hematocrit drops within the first few days after onset of inflammation and then stabilizes.[25,26] The pathogenesis is complex. At least three factors have been implicated, including impaired bone marrow response to anemia, iron sequestration in macrophages making it unavailable for erythrocyte production, and shortened erythrocyte lifespan.[25] Proinflammatory cytokines, including tumor necrosis factor-α and interleukin-1, play a prominent role in the anemia. Tumor necrosis factor-α and interleukin-1 induce ferritin synthesis (the major protein involved in iron sequestration), inhibit proliferation and differentiation of erythroid progenitor cells in bone marrow, reduce formation of erythropoietin, and reduce responsiveness of erythroid precursor cells to erythropoietin. More recent studies incriminate hepcidin, an acute phase protein that regulates iron metabolism, as a mediator of the anemia of inflammatory disease (AID).[27] Diagnosis of AID is based on identifying a mild to moderate normocytic normochromic nonregenerative anemia and detecting an underlying inflammatory disease process. Bone marrow usually is essentially normal. However, marrow may be hypercellular with an increased myeloid-to-erythroid ratio due to myeloid hyperplasia in response to chronic inflammation. Differentiating AID from iron deficiency can be problematic. Both conditions are characterized by low serum iron; however, cats with AID typically have high serum ferritin levels, whereas cats with iron deficiency have low serum ferritin levels.[26,28] Other differentiating characteristics frequently associated with iron deficiency include microcytosis or hypochromasia and increased platelet count.[29] In dogs, absence of hemosiderin in bone marrow is a reliable indicator of iron deficiency; however, healthy cats lack stainable iron in bone marrow.[29] Unlike AID, iron deficiency appears to be a rare condition in adult cats, occurring mostly in kittens as a result of blood loss.[29]

Hematological alterations accompany large or metastatic malignancy consistently. Disseminated malignancy is accompanied almost invariably by AID, resulting in a mild to moderate normocytic normochromic nonregenerative anemia.[30,31] Acute or chronic blood loss also accompanies disseminated or metastatic malignancy frequently. Chronic external blood loss can cause iron deficiency, which impairs erythropoiesis and results in a microcytic or hypochromic anemia. However, as mentioned previously, iron deficiency occurs rarely in adult cats.[29]

Increased numbers of normal or atypical nucleated erythroid cells or leukocytes have been observed in the blood or bone marrow of cats with neoplastic processes.[30,31] This condition has been termed *leukoerythroblastic anemia* or *megaloblastic anemia*.[30,31] However, the author prefers to use the general term *secondary dysmyelopoiesis* for this condition. Secondary dysmyelopoiesis is defined as nonclonal dysplastic changes in blood or bone marrow that occur secondary to other disease processes, drug treatments, or toxin exposure.[32]

Microangiopathic hemolytic anemia also can contribute to anemia associated with neoplasia.[30,31] Microangiopathic hemolytic anemia results from direct traumatic damage to erythrocyte membranes. It can result from damage to vascular endothelium or from fibrin deposition within blood vessels. Fibrin deposits within blood vessels are common in disseminated intravascular coagulation (see Chapter 62). The hallmark of this process is the presence of schistocytes and keratocytes in the blood of affected cats. Other, less frequent, causes of hematological disorders associated with neoplasia include secondary immune-mediated hemolytic anemia and hemophagocytic syndrome.[30,31]

HEMATOLOGICAL DISORDERS ASSOCIATED WITH RENAL DISEASE

The major hematological problem for cats with chronic kidney disease is mild to severe normocytic normochromic nonregenerative anemia.[33-35] Whereas 32 per cent of uremic cats and 65 per cent of cats with end-stage kidney disease were anemic, only 4 per cent of cats with chronic kidney disease were leukopenic. The anemia results primarily from decreased erythropoietin production and is responsive to erythropoietin replacement therapy (see Chapter 66).[34] Bone marrow evaluation usually reveals variable degrees of erythroid hypoplasia.

A small percentage of cats with chronic kidney disease develop pancytopenia.[36] Evaluation of bone marrow indicates that the marrow is extremely hypocellular consistent with a diagnosis of aplastic anemia. Despite the pancytopenia and aplastic bone marrow, three of five cats in one study lived more than 1 year after diagnosis.[36]

INFECTIOUS DISEASES INVOLVING THE HEMATOPOIETIC SYSTEM

Several organisms infect hematopoietic cells and induce hematological dyscrasias. These include FeLV, FIV, feline parvovirus, and *Ehrlichia* spp.

Feline Leukemia Virus

FeLV infection can result in a broad spectrum of hematological alterations. Nonregenerative anemia with erythroid hypoplasia in the bone marrow is the most frequent hematological alteration.[37] Clinically, the anemia typically is macrocytic and nonregenerative. Granulocytopenia also may occur. Both thrombocytosis with increased mean platelet volume and thrombocytopenia can occur. Bone marrow in infected cats is characterized by granulocyte hypoplasia or by a maturation arrest at the myelocyte or metamyelocyte stage. Other hematological dyscrasias that have been documented include PRCA, myelodysplastic syndromes, aplastic anemia, myelofibrosis, hemolytic anemia, and a panleukopenia-like syndrome.[38] These syndromes are seen most frequently in cats infected with FeLV subgroup C. In vitro, FeLV-Sarma subgroup V infects up to 90 per cent of bone marrow mononuclear cells and causes depletion of early erythroid progenitor cells.[39]

Feline Immunodeficiency Virus Infection

FIV-infected cats are lymphopenic and neutropenic. Both transient neutropenia and persistent lymphopenia are seen.[37,40,41] As clinical illness develops, a mild, nonregenerative anemia is a frequent finding and thrombocytopenia occurs occasionally. Bone marrow alterations in symptomatic cats include granulocytic and erythroid hyperplasia and dysplastic changes in erythroid and megakaryocytic cell lineages.

Parvovirus Infection

Parvovirus invades and destroys rapidly proliferating intestinal epithelial and bone marrow precursor cells in cats.[16] Infection is characterized by acute onset of diarrhea and panleukopenia. The bone marrow is characterized by hypocellularity, sinusoidal congestion, edema, degenerative changes in hematopoietic precursor cells, and the presence of many phagocytic macrophages.[17] The sinusoidal congestion and edema most likely result from microvascular injury secondary to septicemia or endotoxemia. Bone marrow pathology and leukopenia resolve rapidly if affected cats survive the secondary bacterial infection.[16]

Ehrlichiosis

Granulocytic ehrlichiosis has been reported in one cat and monocytic ehrlichiosis has been reported in several cats.[42,43] In monocytic ehrlichiosis, nonregenerative anemia is a consistent finding, and neutropenia and thrombocytopenia are present in some cats. In one study, all three affected cats tested positive for antinuclear antibodies.[42] This suggests that ehrlichiosis can be confused with primary immune-mediated diseases. Because intracellular morulae are detected infrequently in the blood of infected cats, polymerase chain reaction (PCR) testing is recommended for detection of ehrlichiosis.[42]

MYELODYSPLASTIC SYNDROMES

Myelodysplastic syndromes (MDSs) are a heterogeneous group of acquired clonal hematological disorders that originate from acquired genetic mutations in hematopoietic stem cells.[32,44-46] Myelodysplastic syndromes are characterized by cytopenias in the blood and prominent dysplastic changes in one or more cell lineages in blood or bone marrow (Figure 64-7).[32] Bone marrow is frequently normocellular or hypercellular. Cytopenias result from a combination of defects in growth and differentiation and increased apoptosis of hematopoietic cells. Both FeLV-positive and FeLV-negative MDS has been described in cats.[32,46]

MDSs have been classified by the French-American-British cooperative group and the World Health Organization (WHO) and have been modified for dogs and cats.[32,46,47] Although the modified dog/cat classification

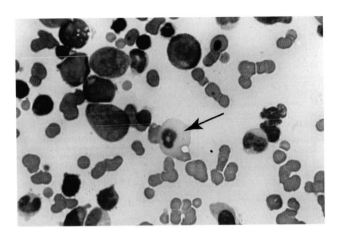

Figure 64-7 Myelodysplastic syndrome with excess blasts in a bone marrow aspirate from a cat. Note the presence of increased numbers of myeloblasts and a large rubricyte with asynchronous maturation of the nucleus and cytoplasm (arrow). (Wright-Giemsa stain, original magnification 1000×.)

system has been recommended for use, the WHO classification will be used here to maintain uniform terminology within the medical literature. The WHO system categorizes MDS into seven categories, four of which have been identified in cats.[32,46,47] The WHO categories include refractory anemia (RA), RA with ringed sideroblasts (RARS), refractory cytopenias with multilineage dysplasia (RCMD), RA with excess blasts–1 (RAEB-1), and RAEB-2. RA is characterized by a nonregenerative anemia and dysplastic features in the erythroid lineage. RARS is characterized by a nonregenerative anemia with large numbers of siderocytes (i.e., erythrocytes containing iron particles) and ringed sideroblasts (nucleated erythroid precursor cells that contain a ring of iron surrounding the nucleus). RCMD is characterized by dysplastic changes in all hematopoietic cell lineages but no increase in the percentage of myeloblasts in bone marrow. RAEB-1 is defined by dysplastic features in all cell lineages and 5 to 10 per cent myeloblasts in bone marrow; RAEB-2 is defined by dysplastic features in all cell lineages and 10 to 20 per cent myeloblasts in bone marrow. Acute leukemia is defined as greater than 20 per cent myeloblasts in bone marrow. Chronic myelomonocytic leukemia is not included within the definition of MDS.

In general, the higher the percentage of myeloblasts, the greater the likelihood for progression of MDS to acute myelogenous leukemia and the poorer the prognosis.[32] Therefore pathologists should report a myeloblast count as a percentage of the total nucleated cells in the bone marrow. It is important to keep in mind that myeloblasts can be increased in certain benign conditions. Toxic injury to marrow from a variety of causes can result in suppression of hematopoiesis. Subsequent recovery will result in the appearance of many blast cells and very few mature precursor cells in the marrow. Low numbers of these immature cells also may be seen in the peripheral blood. In general, it takes about 3 days for these primitive precursor cells to mature. Additionally, in cases of sepsis, mature granulocytes are mobilized rapidly from the bone

marrow, and bacterial toxins may destroy granulocyte precursors or alter their maturation, resulting in a transient increase in the percentage of myeloblasts in bone marrow.

In a retrospective study of clinical bone marrow reports at a veterinary teaching hospital, 11.6 per cent had a diagnosis of MDS.[32] Of these, 4.8 per cent had a diagnosis of RCMD, and 6.8 per cent had a diagnosis of RAEB.

Refractory Anemia

Cats categorized previously as RA or MDS with refractory cytopenia have multiple cytopenias in the blood and dysplastic features in two or more cell lineages in blood or bone marrow. Therefore they are best categorized as RCMD.[32,46]

Refractory Anemia with Ringed Sideroblasts

A small number of cases of RARS have been described.[32,46] Unlike dogs, cats with RARS have a macrocytic normochromic anemia. Bone marrow is characterized by dyserythropoiesis, less than 5 per cent myeloblasts, the presence of siderocytes, and variable numbers of ringed sideroblasts. Normal cats do not have siderocytes in bone marrow.

Refractory Cytopenia with Multilineage Dysplasia

Cats with previous diagnoses of RA and MDS with refractory cytopenia and some cats with a diagnosis of RARS fit into the RCMD category because of the presence of multiple cytopenias in the blood and multilineage dysplasia in bone marrow.[32,46] However, cytogenetic analysis used for classification of the condition in human beings is not available for cats. A small number of cats have been reported with macrocytic normochromic anemia, siderocytes, ringed sideroblasts, and multilineage dysplasia.[32] Most cats with RCMD did not have sideroblastic changes. The age and FeLV status of these cats varied between studies. In studies in which most of the cats were FeLV-positive, the median age was approximately 3 years, whereas in studies in which few cats were FeLV-positive, the median age was 8.7 years.[32,46] In general, these cats were less severely ill than cats with RAEB. Frequently encountered clinical signs include anorexia, depression, weakness, and weight loss. Affected cats have a moderate to severe macrocytic normochromic nonregenerative anemia and frequently have metarubricytosis and autoagglutination. Most cats are thrombocytopenic and some are leukopenic. Bone marrow is normocellular or hypercellular. Although myeloblasts are less than 5 per cent of all nucleated cells, rubriblasts frequently are increased. Dysplastic features are present in the erythroid line of all cats and frequently are present in the granulocyte and megakaryocyte lineages. Myelonecrosis and myelofibrosis are present in approximately one third of cats with RCMD.[32]

Although the prognosis is guarded, some cats with RCMD respond partially or completely to symptomatic therapy and have prolonged survival.[32] Survival is considerably longer than for cats with RAEB, with some cats living for several years after diagnosis.[32] RCMD progresses infrequently to acute myeloid leukemia. Therapy has consisted of prednisolone, prednisolone and cytarabine, cyclosporine A, or combination chemotherapy consisting of daunorubicin, cytarabine, vincristine, and prednisolone.[46]

Refractory Anemia with Excess Blasts

Cats with RAEB are characterized by multiple cytopenias, multilineage dysplasia, and 5 to 20 per cent myeloblasts in bone marrow.[32] In studies in which most affected cats were FeLV-positive, the median age was approximately 3 years, whereas in studies in which the majority of affected cats were FeLV-negative, the median age was approximately 9 years.[30,43] Cats with RAEB tend to be severely ill with clinical signs including anorexia, weakness, depression, weight loss, fever, vomiting, diarrhea, and platelet-related bleeding. Affected cats have a moderate to severe nonregenerative anemia and may have metarubricytosis or autoagglutination. Most cats are thrombocytopenic and some are leukopenic. Bone marrow usually is normocellular or hypercellular, but it can be hypocellular, particularly in FeLV-positive cats. Dysplastic features typically are present in all cell lines. Myelonecrosis or myelofibrosis is present in bone marrow of some affected cats.[32] Presently, survival for cats with RAEB varies from days to a few months with frequent progression to acute myeloid leukemia.[32,46]

Secondary Dysmyelopoiesis

Detection of secondary dysmyelopoiesis is important because it is a frequent cause of marrow failure and it can be confused easily with myelodysplastic syndromes. In a retrospective study of clinical bone marrow reports in cats, 6.3 per cent were categorized as secondary dysmyelopoiesis.[6] Disease conditions associated with secondary dysmyelopoiesis include IMHA, PRCA, immune-mediated thrombocytopenia, lymphosarcoma, glomerulonephritis, and FIP.[32] Bone marrow has normal or increased cellularity, and dysplastic features are most prominent in the erythroid lineage but can be found in the granulocyte and megakaryocyte lineages. In general, these changes are similar to those seen in MDS except that myeloblasts and rubriblasts are not increased, the percentage of dysplastic changes usually is not as high, and megaloblastic changes are seen infrequently. Secondary dysmyelopoiesis resolves frequently with successful treatment of the primary condition.

Secondary dysmyelopoiesis associated with IMHA is difficult to differentiate from myelodysplastic syndromes. Both syndromes are characterized by severe nonregenerative anemia and metarubricytosis.[32] Additionally, both syndromes can be accompanied by autoagglutination. Several factors are useful in differentiating these conditions. Marked macrocytosis (i.e., MCV >65 fl) is a useful indicator of RCMD. Dysplastic changes in bone marrow also are helpful. The percentage of dysplastic changes is higher in MDS than in secondary dysmyelopoiesis. Additionally, megaloblastic changes typically are prominent in MDS but are seen rarely in IMHA. Also, myeloblasts and rubriblasts are less than 5 per cent of all nucleated cells in cats with IMHA. Alternatively, all cats with RAEB have increased myeloblasts, and most cats with RCMD have increased rubriblasts. An increased number of small lymphocytes in bone marrow is a con-

sistent finding in IMHA and PRCA.[32] Lymphoid aggregates may be present.

APLASTIC ANEMIA

Aplastic anemia is a relatively frequent diagnosis in cats, accounting for 10.2 per cent of bone marrow diagnoses in one study.[6] Aplastic anemia is defined as the presence of a bicytopenia or pancytopenia in the blood, and an acellular bone marrow that is replaced by adipose tissue.[36] Conditions associated with aplastic anemia include chronic kidney disease, FeLV infection, and adverse drug reactions, including griseofulvin, chemotherapeutic agents, and methimazole.[36,39,48-50] Idiopathic causes also have been described.[16] Chronic kidney disease typically is associated with nonregenerative anemia, and aplastic anemia is an infrequent complication.[34] Most affected cats have a history of prolonged anorexia before developing aplastic anemia, and adipose tissue in marrow of some cats has a pink, granular appearance consistent with serous atrophy of fat.[36] This suggests that a nutritional deficiency secondary to starvation may be involved in the pathogenesis of the marrow failure.

FeLV infection has been associated with a variety of bone marrow disorders, including aplastic anemia.[39] These syndromes are seen most frequently in cats infected with FeLV subgroup C.[37,39] Survival time of these cats usually is short.

Many cats with a diagnosis of idiopathic aplastic anemia have a history of prolonged partial or complete anorexia with associated cachexia.[36] For example, cats may have a history of chronic oral or gastric ulcers or other conditions that induce inanition. One of five reported cases had evidence of serous atrophy of fat in bone marrow, providing further evidence of emaciation. Therefore starvation may play a role in the development of idiopathic aplastic anemia.

IMMUNE-MEDIATED ANEMIAS

Immune-mediated hemolytic anemia occurs in cats as a primary (i.e., idiopathic) condition or secondary to other disease processes (see Chapter 60).[13,48-52] Reported associated conditions include infectious agents (e.g., FeLV, FIP virus, *Mycoplasma haemofelis,* Candidatus *Mycoplasma haemominutum,* Candidate *Mycoplasma turicensis,* Ehrlichia spp.), drug treatments (e.g., propylthiouracil, methimazole, griseofulvin), and malignant lymphoma.[13,48-52] More than 50 per cent of cats with IMHA have a nonregenerative anemia when first evaluated.[48] Changes in bone marrow in cats with nonregenerative IMHA are quite variable. Most cats have either erythroid hyperplasia or PRCA.[13,51] A few cats have a maturation arrest in the erythroid series.[13] Unlike cats with PRCA and maturation arrest, cats with erythroid hyperplasia have a variety of histopathological changes in the marrow that may contribute to their nonregenerative anemia.[13] These histopathological changes include myelonecrosis, myelofibrosis, acute inflammation, and dysmyelopoiesis.[13] Dyserythropoiesis is a frequent finding in cats with nonregenerative IMHA.[13] Dyserythropoiesis is known to result in increased ineffective erythropoiesis due to decreased maturation and accelerated apoptosis of erythroid precursor cells. Many cats with nonregenerative IMHA also have prominent individual cell necrosis.[13] These cats also have pancytopenia in the blood in spite of normal or hypercellular bone marrows. Other cats with erythroid hyperplasia have evidence of acute inflammation in bone marrow.[13]

Bone marrow lymphocytosis (i.e., >15 per cent small lymphocytes) is present in more than 80 per cent of cats with IMHA.[13,18] Lymphocytes are virtually all small lymphocytes and can exceed 50 per cent of all nucleated marrow cells. Lymphoid aggregates are present in biopsy specimens from some cats. Because of this frequent occurrence, lymphocytosis in bone marrow can be used as a test to support the diagnosis of IMHA.[13] Alternatively, marked lymphocytosis can be confused with well-differentiated acute lymphocytic leukemia or chronic lymphocytic leukemia.

Diagnosis of IMHA is based on the presence of moderate to severe anemia, autoagglutination or positive direct Coombs' test, and exclusion of other causes of anemia.[48] It is particularly important to exclude oxidant-induced hemolysis, characterized by detecting the presence of Heinz bodies in erythrocytes, and microangiopathic hemolytic anemia by detecting the presence of keratocytes and schistocytes in the blood. *Mycoplasma* spp. infection should be excluded by use of repeated blood smear examinations for organisms or by PCR testing.[48] Autoagglutination can be confused with rouleaux formation. True autoagglutination can be distinguished from rouleaux formation by adding one or two drops of saline to one drop of blood.[48] Rouleaux disperses but agglutination persists. Autoagglutination can be seen in cats with MDSs. Peripheral blood lymphocyte counts in the high-normal to slightly increased range are common in IMHA.[48]

Pure red cell aplasia is a frequent cause of nonregenerative IMHA.[6,13] Pure red cell aplasia can be caused by antibody-mediated destruction of erythroid progenitor cells in bone marrow or by FeLV subgroup C infection.[38] Affected cats usually are young and are severely anemic (median hematocrit ≈ 7 per cent), with total leukocyte and platelet counts within or above reference intervals. The bone marrow contains few or no erythroid cells; however, rare rubriblasts and prorubricytes are present in some cats. The percentage of small lymphocytes is increased in more than 90 per cent of cases and can exceed 50 per cent of all nucleated cells in bone marrow.[13,18] Lymphoid aggregates are seen frequently in bone marrow core biopsy sections.[13,18] This benign lymphocytosis can be confused easily with a lymphoid malignancy.

DRUG-INDUCED HEMATOLOGICAL DISORDERS

Several drug-associated hematological dyscrasias have been documented in cats. Chemotherapeutic agents are toxic for bone marrow at or near the therapeutic dose; however, the myelosuppressive potential of chemotherapeutic agents varies.[53] Because of their high mitotic rate, progenitor and proliferative cells in bone marrow are predisposed to injury. Bone marrow suppression by chemotherapeutic agents is dose-dependent and follows a predictable course. Neutropenia typically occurs 5 to 7 days after initiation of treatment, and thrombocytopenia occurs at 7 to 10 days.[53] Because stem cells are spared, hematopoietic recovery usually is rapid once chemotherapy is discontinued.

Griseofulvin is used for treatment of mycotic diseases. Hematological dyscrasias occur as an idiosyncratic reaction.[54] In most cases, neutropenia or panleukopenia occurs several weeks after initiation of treatment. The bone marrow is hypoplastic, but the majority of cats recover after discontinuation of the drug.

A high incidence of immune-mediated drug reactions have been reported in hyperthyroid cats treated with propylthiouracil or methimazole.[55,56] These reactions vary from mild leukopenia to severe agranulocytosis and thrombocytopenia. These changes usually occur within the first 2 months of treatment. An immune-mediated mechanism is indicated by positive direct Coombs' and antinuclear antibody test results in many affected cats. However, some affected cats have an aplastic bone marrow.[36] The cytopenias usually resolve within 2 weeks after discontinuing treatment.

HEMATOLOGICAL DISORDERS ASSOCIATED WITH NONLEUKEMIC NEOPLASTIC INFILTRATION OF BONE MARROW

Multiple Myeloma

Multiple myeloma (see Chapter 65) is a relatively common tumor of older cats, being diagnosed in approximately 4 per cent of clinical bone marrow specimens.[6] Myeloma also occurs frequently at extramedullary sites in cats.[57] The diagnosis of multiple myeloma is dependent on the presence of a combination of increased numbers of plasma cells and atypical plasma cells in bone marrow. Features typical of malignant plasma cells include large size, anisocytosis, anisokaryosis, and frequent binucleation. These anaplastic features are important in differentiating multiple myeloma from plasma cell hyperplasia associated with immune-mediated diseases and FIP. Hematological alterations are associated frequently with multiple myeloma. These include nonregenerative anemia (69 per cent), thrombocytopenia (50 per cent), and hyperglobulinemia (88 per cent).[58] Cats with multiple myeloma frequently have extramedullary tumor involvement including spleen, liver, and lymph nodes.[58] Lytic bone lesions are present in approximately 50 per cent of cats with multiple myeloma.[58]

Malignant Histiocytosis

Malignant histiocytosis (also termed *disseminated histiocytic sarcoma*) has been reported infrequently in cats, but was diagnosed in 1 per cent of clinical bone marrow specimens in a retrospective study.[6] Malignant histiocytosis is a malignancy of dendritic cells and is characterized by infiltration of multiple organs with large histiocytic cells with variable degrees of cytophagia. Spleen, liver, lymph nodes, and bone marrow are the tissues involved most frequently. Most affected cats have a nonregenerative anemia and some are thrombocytopenic.[6,59] The diagnosis of malignant histiocytosis frequently is based on cell number or morphology; however, cytochemical staining or immunophenotyping may be useful in differentiating malignant histiocytosis from other round cell malignancies. Malignant histiocytosis also should be differentiated from benign macrophage proliferations in bone marrow, liver, or spleen. In bone marrow, macrophage proliferation is associated most frequently with myelonecrosis. In general, cells in malignant histiocytosis tend to be larger and have atypical features. Some cells are multinucleate.

SUMMARY

A few primary bone marrow disorders are well defined in cats. These include acute and chronic leukemias, multiple myeloma, PRCA, and FeLV-associated myelosuppression. On the other hand, many bone marrow disorders are associated with a group of histopathological alterations that occur secondary to a variety of disease conditions or drug treatments. Detection of unique features in bone marrow can provide important clues that point toward a diagnosis. For example, the presence of a mature lymphocytosis frequently is associated with IMHA. Because the diagnosis of IMHA in cats frequently is difficult and the majority of cases have a nonregenerative anemia when first examined, lymphocytosis is an important diagnostic clue. Likewise, the presence of myelonecrosis, interstitial edema, or fibrin deposits is associated with IMHA and infectious diseases. Extensive fibrin deposits, particularly when accompanied by plasma cell hyperplasia, should make one suspicious of FIP. If dysmyelopoiesis is identified, it is essential to determine if it is the result of a myelodysplastic syndrome or is occurring secondary to another disease process such as IMHA or lymphoma. Although aplastic anemia is a pathological diagnosis, it has been associated with a limited number of conditions in cats, including chronic kidney disease, FeLV infection, adverse drug reactions, and starvation. Therefore, although an etiopathological diagnosis frequently is not possible solely by examination of blood and bone marrow samples, the combination of careful evaluation of blood and bone marrow combined with a knowledge of the case history and additional diagnostic testing often can establish an etiological diagnosis.

REFERENCES

1. Rentko VT, Cotter SM: Feline anemia: the classifications, causes, and diagnostic procedures, *Vet Med* 85:584, 1990.
2. Weiser MG: Correlative approach to anemia in dogs and cats, *J Am Anim Hosp Assoc* 17:286, 1981.
3. Jain NC: Classification of myeloproliferative disorders in cats using criteria proposed by the animal leukemia study group: a retrospective study of 181 cases (1969-1992), *Comp Haematol Int* 3:125, 1993.
4. Kociba GJ: Hematologic consequences of feline leukemia virus infection. In Kirk R, editor: *Current veterinary therapy IX*, Philadelphia, 1986, WB Saunders, p 488.
5. Shelton GH, Linenberger ML: Hematologic abnormalities associated with retroviral infections in the cat, *Semin Vet Med Surg (Small Anim)* 10:220, 1995.
6. Weiss DJ: A retrospective study of the incidence and classification of bone marrow disorders of cats (1996-2004). *Compar Clin Pathol* 14:179, 2006.
7. Weiss DJ: Bone marrow pathology in dogs and cats with non-regenerative immune-mediated hemolytic anaemia and pure red cell aplasia, *J Compar Pathol* 138:46, 2008.
8. Weiss DJ: Feline myelonecrosis and myelofibrosis: 22 cases 1996-2006, *Compar Clin Pathol* 16:18, 2007.
9. Weiss DJ, Greig B, Aird B, et al: Inflammatory disorders of bone marrow, *Vet Clin Pathol* 21:79, 1992.
10. Weiss DJ, Evanson OA: A retrospective study of feline pancytopenia, *Compar Clin Pathol* 10:50, 2000.
11. Weiss DJ: Bone marrow necrosis in dogs: 34 cases (1996-2004), *J Am Vet Med Assoc* 227:263, 2005.
12. Shimoda T, Shiranaga N, Mashita T, et al: Bone marrow necrosis in a cat infected with feline leukemia virus, *J Vet Med Sci* 62:113, 2000.
13. Weiss DJ: Bone marrow pathology in dogs and cats with nonregenerative immune-mediated hemolytic anemias, *J Compar Pathol* 138:46, 2008.
14. Weiss DJ: Acute stromal disorders of bone marrow in the dogs, *Compar Clin Pathol* 16:223, 2007.
15. Weiss DJ: A review of the techniques for preparation of histopathologic sections of bone marrow, *Vet Clin Pathol* 16:90, 1987.
16. Bentinck-Smith J: Feline panleukopenia (feline infectious enteritis). A review of 574 cases, *North Amer Vet* 30:379, 1949.
17. Langheinrich KA, Neilsen SW: Histopathology of feline panleukopenia: a report of 65 cases, *J Am Vet Med Assoc* 158:863, 1971.
18. Weiss DJ: Differentiating benign and malignant causes of lymphocytosis in feline bone marrow, *J Vet Intern Med* 19:855, 2005.
19. Workman HC, Vernau W: Chronic lymphocytic leukemia in dogs and cats: the veterinary perspective, *Vet Clin North Am Small Anim Pract* 33:1379, 2003.
20. Kohn B, Goldschmidt MH, Hohenhaus AE: Anemia, splenomegaly and increased osmotic fragility of erythrocytes in Abyssinian and Somali cats, *J Am Vet Med Assoc* 217:1483, 2000.
21. Blue JT: Myelofibrosis in cats with myelodysplastic syndrome and acute myelogenous leukemia, *Vet Pathol* 24:154, 1988.
22. Bruer W, Darbes J, Hermanns W, et al: Idiopathic myelofibrosis in a cat and in three dogs, *Compar Haematol Inter* 9:17, 1999.
23. Flecknell PA, Gibbs C, Kelly DF: Myelosclerosis in a cat, *J Compar Pathol* 88:627, 1978.
24. Hoover EA, Kociba GJ: Bone lesions in cats with anemia induced by feline leukemia virus, *J Natl Cancer Inst* 53:1277, 1974.
25. Weiss DJ, Krehbiel JD, Lund JE: Studies of the pathogenesis of anemia of inflammation: mechanisms of impaired erythropoiesis, *Am J Vet Res* 44:1832, 1983.
26. Ottenjann M, Weingart C, Arndt G, et al: Characterization of the anemia of inflammatory disease in cats with abscesses, pyothorax or fat necrosis, *J Vet Intern Med* 20:1143, 2006.
27. Fry MM, Liggett JL, Baek SJ: Molecular cloning and expression of canine hepcidin, *Vet Clin Pathol* 33:223, 2004.
28. Stone MS, Freden GO: Differentiation of anemia of inflammatory disease from anemia of iron deficiency, *Compend Contin Educ Pract Vet* 12:963, 1990.
29. Harvey JW: Microcytic anemias. In Feldman BF, Zinkl JG, Jain NC, editors: *Schalm's veterinary hematology*, Philadelphia, 2000, Lippincott Williams & Wilkins, p 200.

30. Madewell BR, Feldman BF: Characterization of anemias associated with neoplasia in small animals, *J Am Vet Med Assoc* 176:419, 1980.

31. Couto CG: Hematologic abnormalities in small animal cancer patients. Part I. Red cell abnormalities, *Compend Contin Educ Pract Vet* 6:1059, 1984.

32. Weiss DJ: Evaluation of dysmyelopoiesis in cats: 34 cases (1996-2005), *J Am Vet Med Assoc* 228:893, 2006.

33. DiBartola SP, Rutgers HC, Zack PM, et al: Clinicopathologic findings associated with chronic renal disease in cats: 74 cases (1973-1984), *J Am Vet Med Assoc* 190:1196, 1987.

34. Cowgill LD: Pathophysiology and management of anemia of chronic progressive renal failure, *Semin Vet Med Surg (Small Anim)* 7:175, 1992.

35. Elliott J, Barber PJ: Feline chronic renal failure: clinical findings in 80 cases diagnosed between 1992 and 1995, *J Small Anim Pract* 39:78, 1998.

36. Weiss DJ: Aplastic anemia in cats—clinicopathological features and associated disease conditions 1996-2004, *J Feline Med Surg* 8:203, 2006.

37. Jordan H: Feline leukemia virus and feline immunodeficiency virus. In Feldman BF, Zinkl JG, Jain NC, editors: *Schalm's veterinary hematology*, ed 5, Philadelphia, 2000, Lippincott Williams & Wilkins, p 727.

38. Abkowitz JL: Retrovirus-induced feline pure red cell aplasia: pathogenesis and response to suramin, *Blood* 77:1442, 1991.

39. Dornsife RE, Gasper PW, Mullins JI, et al: In vitro erythrocytopathic activity of an aplastic anemia-inducing feline retrovirus, *Exp Hematol* 17:138, 1989.

40. Shelton GH, Linenberger ML, Grant CK, et al: Hematologic manifestations of feline immunodeficiency virus infections, *Blood* 76:1104, 1990.

41. Walker C, Canfield P: Haematological findings in cats naturally infected with feline immunodeficiency virus, *Compar Clin Pathol* 6:77, 1996.

42. Breitschwerdt EB, Abrams-Ogg ACG, Lappin MR, et al: Molecular evidence supporting *Ehrlichia canis*-like infection in cats, *J Vet Intern Med* 16:642, 2002.

43. Bjoersdorff A, Svendenius L, Owens JH, et al: Feline granulocytic ehrlichiosis—a report of a new clinical entity and characterization of the infectious agent, *J Small Anim Pract* 40:20, 1999.

44. Shimoda T, Shiranaga N, Mashita T, et al: A hematologic study on thirteen cats with myelodysplastic syndrome, *J Vet Med Sci* 62:59, 1999.

45. Hisasue M, Nishigaki K, Katae H, et al: Clonality analysis of various hematopoietic disorders in cats naturally infected with feline leukemia virus, *J Vet Med Sci* 62:1059, 2000.

46. Hisasue M, Okayama H, Okayama T, et al: Hematologic abnormalities and outcome of 16 cats with myelodysplastic syndromes, *J Vet Intern Med* 15:471, 2001.

47. Germing U, Strupp C, Kuendgen A, et al: Prospective validation of the WHO proposals for the classification of myelodysplastic syndromes, *Haematologica* 91:1596, 2006.

48. Kohn B, Weingart C, Eckmann V, et al: Primary immune-mediated hemolytic anemia in 19 cats: diagnosis, therapy, and outcome (1998-2004), *J Vet Intern Med* 20:159, 2006.

49. Werner LL, Gorman NT: Immune-mediated disorders of cats, *Vet Clin North Am Small Anim Pract* 14:1039, 1984.

50. Scott DW, Schultz RD, Post JE, et al: Autoimmune hemolytic anemia in the cat, *J Am Anim Hosp Assoc* 9:530, 1973.

51. Stokol T, Blue JT: Pure red cell aplasia in cats: 9 cases (1987-1997), *J Am Vet Med Assoc* 214:75, 1999.

52. Sykes JE, Terry JC, Lindsay LL, et al: Prevalences of various hemoplasma species among cats in the United States with possible hemoplasmosis, *J Am Vet Med Assoc* 232:373, 2008.

53. Couto CG: Toxicity of anticancer chemotherapy. In Campfield WW, editor: *Kal Kan Symposium for the treatment of small animal diseases*, Vernon, Calif, 1986, Kal Kan Pet Foods, p 37.

54. Helton KA, Nesbitt GH, Cariolo PL: Griseofulvin toxicity in cats: literature review and report of seven cases, *J Am Anim Hosp Assoc* 22:453, 1986.

55. Peterson ME, Hurvitz AI, Leib MS: Propylthiouracil-associated hemolytic anemia, thrombocytopenia, and antinuclear antibody in cats with hyperthyroidism, *J Am Vet Med Assoc* 184:806, 1984.

56. Peterson ME, Kintzer PP, Hurvitz AI: Methimazole treatment of 262 cats with hyperthyroidism, *J Vet Intern Med* 2:150, 1988.

57. Mellor PJ, Haugland S, Murphy S, et al: Myeloma-related disorders in cats commonly present as extramedullary neoplasms in contrast to myeloma in human patients; 24 cases with clinical follow-up, *J Vet Intern Med* 20:1376, 2006.

58. Patek RT, Caceres A, French AF, et al: Multiple myeloma in 16 cats: a retrospective study, *Vet Clin Pathol* 34:341, 2005.

59. Fitz D, Georges C, Hopfner CL: Malignant histiocytosis in a cat, *Feline Pract* 27:6, 1999.

65 Plasma Cell Disorders

Virginia L. Gill and Nicole F. Leibman

Plasma cell disorders represent a spectrum of neoplasms derived from a clonal proliferation of plasma cells. This leads to an accumulation of immunoglobulin (IgA, IgG, IgM, IgE, IgD)–producing B lymphocytes within hematopoietic or medullary (multiple myeloma) and extrahematopoietic or extramedullary (plasmacytoma) sites. Because these disorders are considered to arise from a single B lymphocyte, the resultant gammopathy is characteristically monoclonal; however, biclonal and polyclonal plasma cell disorders exist. The most commonly reported plasma cell diseases in cats are multiple myeloma and extramedullary plasmacytoma (EMP), respectively. Other diseases in the spectrum include monoclonal gammopathy of unknown significance (MGUS), a clinically benign condition, Waldenström macroglobulinemia, plasma cell leukemia, and solitary osseous plasmacytoma (SOP) (Tables 65-1 and 65-2).

MULTIPLE MYELOMA AND RELATED PLASMA CELL DISORDERS

INCIDENCE AND ETIOLOGY

Multiple myeloma (MM) is an uncommon disease in cats, accounting for less than 1 per cent of all malignant neoplasms in two large compilations of feline neoplasms.[1,2] Similarly, in one recent report of feline MM, the disease represented less than 1 per cent of all feline neoplasms diagnosed at the Veterinary Hospital of the University of Pennsylvania from 1996 to 2004.[3] Related plasma cell disorders, such as MGUS, Waldenström macroglobulinemia, and plasma cell leukemia, are rare, with only a few case reports existing in the feline literature. MM is a disease of older cats (median age ≈12 years), with no breed or gender predilection. A slight increase in incidence in male cats has been suggested; however, the total number of cases reported is low, making this predilection difficult to verify.[3,4]

The etiology of the disease is unknown. Although the development of B lymphoid neoplasms has been associated with the prevalence of retroviruses in several domestic species, there is no association with FeLV or FIV in cats with MM.[4,5] There also is no association with feline coronavirus.[4] In human beings, exposure to ionizing radiation (including occupational exposure), as well as exposure to metals, benzenes, petroleum products, and silicon, have been considered potential risk factors. Familial associations have been reported in human patients and inbred mice, supporting the role of hereditary and genetic factors.[6] A potential familial association was suggested in one report of a pair of sibling cats with MM.[7] Chronic immune stimulation has been suggested as a predisposing factor in human beings and mice. In a case series of 24 cats with "myeloma-related disorders," Mellor et al examined medical records for antecedent inflammatory disease. One cat had a history of severe, recurrent dental disease, and one cat had unilateral uveitis of unknown origin. No other evidence of chronic antigenic stimulation or inflammation preceding the development of the disease was found.[8] In a case report of a cat with an intraocular plasmacytoma, previous trauma had occurred to the involved eye, and the authors hypothesized that chronic inflammation played a role in the development of the plasmacytoma.[9] Although it is uncommon, solitary extramedullary plasmacytomas can precede MM in several species, and a cutaneous EMP has been reported to precede MM in a cat.[10] This also has been reported occasionally in dogs and human beings.[11,12]

Table 65-1 Definitions of Plasma Cell Disorders*

Disorder	Definition
Multiple myeloma (MM) (see Boxes 65-1 and 65-2)	
Light chain myeloma	MM characterized by light chain proteinuria without monoclonal gammopathy
Nonsecretory myeloma	MM characterized by bone marrow plasmacytosis of >20% and skeletal lytic lesions without monoclonal gammopathy or light chain proteinuria
Extramedullary plasmacytoma (EMP)	One plasma cell tumor originating in soft tissues, with no skeletal lytic lesions, monoclonal gammopathy, or light chain proteinuria
Solitary osseous plasmacytoma (SOP); also referred to as solitary plasmacytoma of bone (SPB)	One plasma cell tumor originating in bone, with no other skeletal lytic lesions, monoclonal gammopathy, or light chain proteinuria
Waldenström macroglobulinemia (WM)	IgM monoclonal gammopathy, often with concurrent hyperviscosity syndrome, and infiltration of the liver and spleen
Monoclonal gammopathy of unknown significance (MGUS)	Monoclonal gammopathy with bone marrow plasmacytosis of <10%, with no skeletal lytic lesions, monoclonal gammopathy or light chain proteinuria, and no clinical, hematological, or biochemical abnormalities
Plasma cell leukemia (PCL)	>20% bone marrow plasmacytosis and >2000 plasma cells/μL in peripheral blood
Heavy chain disease (HCD)	Elevated M protein with an incomplete heavy chain, lacking a light chain

*References 3, 4, 6, 10, 14-19.

Table 65-2 Commonly Used Terms*

Term	Definition	Synonym
Monoclonal gammopathy	Elevation in a single type or component of immunoglobulin	M protein, M component, paraprotein
Light chain (L chain)	Lighter molecular weight polypeptide chain of antibody/immunoglobulin molecule. There are two light chains per immunoglobulin unit	κ or λ chains
Heavy chain (H chain)	Heavier molecular weight polypeptide chain of antibody/immunoglobulin molecule. There are two heavy chains per immunoglobulin unit	IgA, IgG, IgM, IgE, IgD
Fab	Fragment of antibody containing the antigen binding portion	
Light chain proteinuria	Excess of monoclonal light chains in urine	Bence Jones proteinuria
Hyperviscosity syndrome (HVS)	Sequela of increased serum viscosity secondary to increased circulating serum immunoglobulins in MM or WM. This also can be secondary to increases in RBCs or WBCs in other diseases	
Cryoglobulin	Proteins, often immunoglobulins, that precipitate as serum is cooled to temperatures less than body temperature and dissolve on rewarming	
Extramedullary	Outside of the bone marrow, in cats commonly the spleen and liver	
Amyloidosis	Tissue deposition of protein aggregates systemically or locally in bundles of β-sheets	AA amyloidosis—reactive AL amyloidosis—light chain

*References 4, 6, 19-21, 28, 44.

PATHOLOGY AND PATHOGENESIS

MM is derived from a clonal proliferation of malignant plasma cells (immunoglobulin-secreting B lymphocytes). It is a systemic disease arising typically from the bone marrow. The malignant plasma cells range from well differentiated to atypical on cytological and histological preparations. In a recent retrospective study, atypical cytological changes were noted in plasma cells in the majority of cats with MM. These changes included increased size, multiple nuclei, clefted nuclei, anisocytosis, anisokaryosis, variable N:C ratios, decreased chromatin density, and variably sized nucleoli.[3] Flame cells, characterized by peripheral eosinophilic cytoplasmic projections, or Mott cells, characterized by Russell bodies representing globules of immunoglobulin, may be present (Figure 65-1).

MM is characterized by the presence of a monoclonal gammopathy (M protein, M component, paraprotein) signifying the production of a single immunoglobulin from the neoplastic cells (Figure 65-2). In cats, this is represented most commonly by IgG gammopathy. The second most common M protein is IgA.[3,13] Biclonal spikes also occur in cats, and this may be due to two independent secretory tumor cell lines each secreting a unique M protein, one tumor cell line producing two separate M proteins, or a spurious biclonal spike secondary to an increase in the dimeric protein IgA. A monoclonal increase in the pentamer IgM (Waldenström macroglobulinemia) has been reported in one cat.[14] Waldenström macroglobulinemia in human beings is characterized by the absence of skeletal lytic lesions and the involvement of liver, spleen, and/or lymph nodes; more recently, it has been classified as a lymphoplasmacytic lymphoma in human beings.[6] Production of the entire immunoglobulin is most common in cats; however, light chain myeloma has been reported in two cats, as well as in a dog.[15-17]

Light chain myeloma is characterized by the presence of light chains (L chains) in urine without a concurrent monoclonal gammopathy. Nonsecretory disease, characterized by marrow plasmacytosis and skeletal lytic lesions, occurs in dogs and human beings,[18] although it has not been reported in cats. This manifestation typically carries a poor prognosis in human beings.[6] In heavy chain disease, which is rare in human patients and has been reported in one dog, the M protein is characterized by an incomplete heavy chain, lacking a light chain.[19] Cryoglobulinemia has been reported in one cat.[20] This is characterized by the oversecretion of an M protein that is insoluble at low temperatures. Clinical signs associated with cryoglobulinemia result from precipitation of the cryoglobulin in small-diameter blood vessels and include purpura, cold intolerance, and ulceration and necrosis of the skin of distal extremities. To evaluate for cryoglobu-

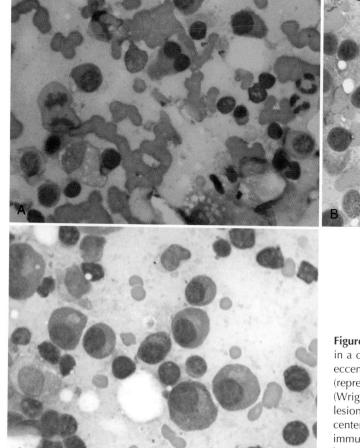

Figure 65-1 A, A cytological sample from a hepatic plasmacytoma in a cat with multiple myeloma. Note the pleomorphic cells with eccentrically placed nuclei and a perinuclear clear zone (representing the Golgi body). A mitotic figure also is present. (Wright-Giemsa, 100×.) **B,** A cytological sample of a skeletal lytic lesion in a cat with multiple myeloma. Note the Mott cell in the center (cell containing Russell bodies representing globules of immunoglobulin within a plasma cell). (Wright-Giemsa, 100×.) **C,** A bone marrow aspirate of a cat with multiple myeloma. (Wright-Giemsa, 100×.)

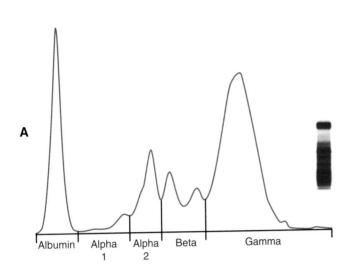

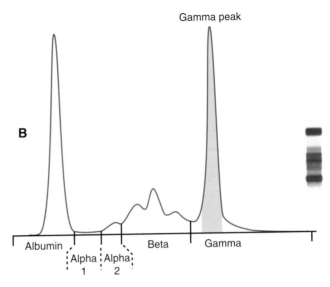

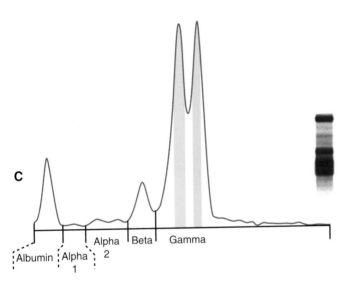

Figure 65-2 A, Serum protein electrophoresis from a cat with a nonspecific polyclonal gammopathy (stained cellulose acetate electrophoretic strip with accompanying densitogram). **B,** Serum protein electrophoresis from a cat with multiple myeloma. Note the large M component spike in the gamma region (interpreted as a monoclonal gammopathy). **C,** Serum protein electrophoresis representing a biclonal gammopathy.

lins, blood must be collected and serum separated at 37° C to avoid precipitation of the protein in the clot. Plasma cell leukemia can be diagnosed as either primary, without a previous diagnosis of MM, or secondary, with concurrent myeloma or plasmacytoma. This is a rare disease that has been reported in one cat with a cutaneous extramedullary plasmacytoma that progressed to MM with secondary plasma cell leukemia.[3,10]

CLINICAL SIGNS AND MANIFESTATIONS

In the three most recent compilations of feline MM cases, the most common presenting clinical signs are nonspecific and consist of lethargy, decreased appetite, and weight loss.[3,7,8] Other clinical signs and physical examination abnormalities include polyuria/polydipsia, vomiting, diarrhea, lameness or paresis/paralysis, central nervous system signs, fundic changes (retinal hemorrhages, retinal detachment), palpable hepatosplenomegaly, other evidence of bleeding (epistaxis, oral bleeding), and concurrent skin masses.

The clinical manifestations associated with MM include bony involvement, extramedullary involvement, hyperviscosity syndrome, cardiac disease, bleeding diathesis, chronic kidney disease, hypercalcemia, and possible increased susceptibility to infections. The resulting manifestations often occur due to high levels of circulating M protein or organ/bone infiltration by neoplastic plasma cells.

Bone lesions are characterized by lysis and are classically described as "punched-out" lesions (Figure 65-3). They can be single or multiple or represented by diffuse osteopenia or pathological fractures. Reported sites of skeletal lytic lesions are the pelvis, ribs, vertebrae, and long bones. Reports of the frequency of bone lesions in cats with MM are conflicting, ranging from 8 to 60 per cent.[3,7,8]

Extramedullary infiltration by neoplastic plasma cells is a common finding in feline MM. By contrast, extramedullary involvement is uncommon in human beings and dogs with MM.[4,6] A recent report examining cats diagnosed with MM reported that approximately 40 per cent had cytologically or histologically confirmed plasma

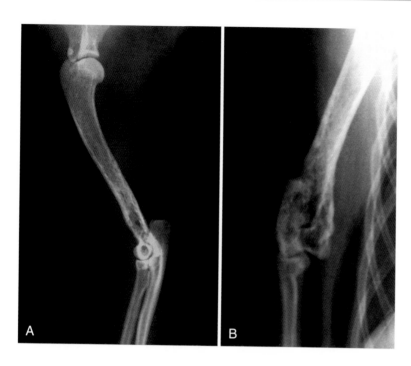

Figure 65-3 Lateral **(A)** and anteroposterior **(B)** radiographic views of the elbow of a cat with multiple myeloma. This cat had concurrent cutaneous plasma cell tumors, in conjunction with systemic evidence of multiple myeloma.

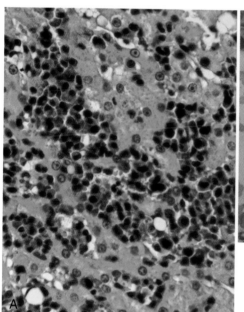
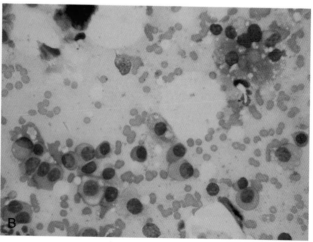

Figure 65-4 A, A liver biopsy from a cat with multiple myeloma. The biopsy consists of hepatocytes with intermixed plasma cells arranged in sheets. The neoplastic cells are round to oval with eccentrically placed nuclei. (H&E, 40×.) **B,** Fine-needle aspirate cytological sample of the liver of the same cat. Note the binucleate plasma cells and the cluster of hepatocytes in right upper corner.

cell neoplasia in the spleen, liver, and abdominal lymph nodes, with splenic infiltration being the most common (Figure 65-4).[3] Additionally, in a report evaluating the spectrum of myeloma-related disorders in cats, 50 per cent of cats with plasma cell infiltration in the bone marrow had concurrent involvement of abdominal organs. Several cats in this report had abdominal organ involvement without concurrent bone marrow infiltration. However, all of these cats had concurrent monoclonal gammopathy.[8]

Hyperviscosity syndrome (HVS) results from elevations in circulating M protein leading to increased serum viscosity. Incidence is highest with IgM due to the high molecular weight of IgM, a pentamer, followed by IgA, a dimer that can polymerize, and IgG. HVS also may be more common with cryoglobulinemia. High serum viscosity can lead to central nervous system abnormalities, such as mentation changes and seizures. It also can lead to increased cardiac workload and cardiac failure, retinal hemorrhages, and coagulation abnormalities. These complications are thought to occur secondary to sludging of blood in small vessels and ineffective delivery of oxygen to tissues.[21,22] HVS was present in 40 per cent (four of nine) of cats in one study; however, serum viscosity is not measured routinely at most institutions.[7]

Bleeding diathesis or coagulation defects can result from several mechanisms, including M protein interfering with clotting factors and platelets, the Fab fragment of the M protein binding to fibrin preventing its aggregation, or adsorption of minor clotting proteins. Additionally, bone marrow infiltration (myelophthisis) may lead to thrombocytopenia.[4,6] Evidence of bleeding diathesis or bleeding abnormalities was noted in approximately 30 per cent of cats in recent reports.[3,7,8]

Chronic kidney disease may be present for a variety of reasons in cats with MM. In three recent reports of MM in cats, 25 to 40 per cent of cats were azotemic.[3,7,8] Light chain proteinuria occurs due to an unbalanced production of kappa (κ) or lambda (λ) light chains. These excessive light chains are filtered freely by the glomerulus leading to their presence in urine. Filtered light chains can form protein precipitates that lead to tubular damage and resulting azotemia. Other possible mechanisms of kidney disease include hypercalcemia, amyloidosis, renal infiltration by neoplastic plasma cells, decreased renal perfusion secondary to HVS, or pyelonephritis.[4,6] Light chain proteinuria was reported in 40 to 50 per cent of cats with MM in recent reports.[3,7] Amyloidosis, the systemic deposition of light-chain (AL) amyloid in organs (including the kidney), is rare in cats with MM.

Hypercalcemia may result from direct tumor lysis of infiltrated bone or osteoclast activation. Osteoblast inhibition also is cited as a mechanism of hypercalcemia in affected human beings. In human patients, osteoclast activation occurs secondary to aberrant production of interleukin (IL)-1β (previously called osteoclast activating factor), tumor necrosis factor (TNF)-β, and IL-6. Receptor activator of nuclear factor-κB ligand (RANKL) also is elicited by parathyroid hormone (PTH), PTHrp, and IL-1β, and likely plays a role in hypercalcemia associated with MM. RANK (the receptor for RANKL) is located on osteoclasts and becomes activated with the binding of RANKL on stromal cells, osteoblasts, and possibly tumor cells (Figure 65-5).[6,23] Hypercalcemia is reported to occur in 20 to 40 per cent of cats in recent reports.[3,7]

A number of factors contribute to the increased risk of infection in MM patients. In human beings with MM, there are documented decreases in the levels of uninvolved immunoglobulins, which increases patients' risk for bacterial infections. Additionally, B-cell and T-cell function may be dysregulated secondary to immunosuppressive cytokines (e.g., TGF-β), and neutropenia may result from myelophthisis.[6] One recent report includes three cats (approximately 20 per cent of the study group) with concurrent infectious processes, including upper respiratory infection, severe dental disease, and terminal bacteremia[3]; however, overwhelming infection is not reported commonly in feline MM patients.

Cytopenias were relatively common in recent reports, with approximately 55 to 75 per cent of cats being anemic, 30 per cent being neutropenic, and 50 per cent being thrombocytopenic. Anemia in cats with MM typically is nonregenerative, normochromic, and normocytic.[3,6]

Clinical signs and clinicopathological abnormalities in cats with MM reported since 2000 are summarized in Tables 65-3 and 65-4.

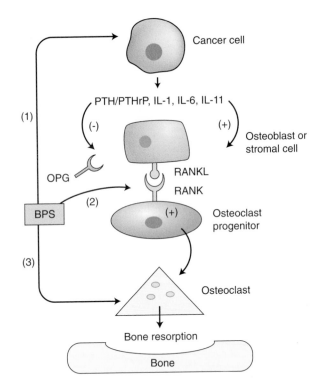

Figure 65-5 Graphic depiction of neoplastic mechanisms of hypercalcemia. Receptor activator of nuclear factor-κB ligand (RANKL) is located on osteoblasts or stromal cells while RANK is located on osteoclasts or osteoclast progenitors. The numbers indicate hypothesized mechanisms of bisphosphonates (BPS) on cancer cells. (From Milner RJ, Farese J, Henry CJ, et al: Bisphosphonates and cancer, *J Vet Intern Med* 18:597, 2004.)

Table 65-3 Clinical Signs in Cats with Multiple Myeloma*

Clinical Sign or Finding	Approximate Percentage
Anorexia	70
Lethargy	65
Bleeding abnormalities/evidence of bleeding diathesis	30
Lameness/hindlimb ataxia/weakness	30
Palpable abdominal organomegaly/mass	25
Vomiting/diarrhea	25
Polydipsia/polyuria	20
Neurological disease	15
Skin masses[†]	10

N = 52.

*References 3, 7, 8, 10, 13, 19, 23.

[†]Mellor et al included cats with "myeloma-related disorders." Five cats with solitary cutaneous plasma cell tumors with no systemic involvement were excluded from this summary.

Table 65-4 Clinicopathological Abnormalities in Cats with Multiple Myeloma*

Abnormality	Approximate Percentage
M-protein	100
Monoclonal	80
Biclonal/polyclonal	20
Anemia	60
Bence Jones proteinuria	40
Azotemia	40
Thrombocytopenia	40
Neutropenia	30
Hypercalcemia	25
FeLV/FIV seropositive	0

N = 28.
*References 3, 7, 10, 13, 19, 23.

DIAGNOSIS

The diagnostic criteria for MM are relatively straightforward in human beings and dogs,. Major criteria in human patients consist of (1) plasmacytoma on tissue biopsy, (2) bone marrow plasmacytosis with more than 30 per cent plasma cells, and (3) monoclonal gammopathy (>3.5 g/dL for IgG or >2 g/dL for IgA) or light chain proteinuria (κ- or λ-light chain excretion >1.0 g/dL when measured by protein electrophoresis performed on a sample of urine collected over 24 hours) with amyloidosis. Amyloidosis is determined in human medicine by biopsy of abdominal fat or rectum. These biopsy methods are reflective of amyloid deposit within multiple organs, including the heart and kidneys. Minor criteria consist of (a) bone marrow plasmacytosis of 10 to 30 per cent, (b) monoclonal gammopathy less than the level defined in the major criteria, (c) lytic bone lesions, and (d) suppressed uninvolved immunoglobulins. The presence of two major criteria; the combination of major criterion 1 plus minor criteria b, c, or d or of major criterion 3 plus minor criteria a or c; or the combination of minor criteria a and b with c or d are diagnostic of MM in human patients. MGUS is diagnosed in the presence of a monoclonal gammopathy, bone marrow plasmacytosis of less than 10 per cent, and in the absence of bone lesions, light chain proteinuria and clinical symptoms. Plasma cell leukemia is diagnosed if there is more than 20 per cent marrow plasmacytosis and greater than 2000 plasma cells/μL in peripheral blood.[6,10]

In dogs, the above criteria from the human literature have been modified to include bone marrow plasmacytosis greater than 20 per cent, monoclonal gammopathy, lytic bone lesions, and light chain proteinuria. Two of the four criteria are required (Box 65-1).[25-27] Variations of these diagnostic criteria include marrow plasmacytosis of greater than 5 to 10 per cent in earlier reports[25-27] and the requirement of three of four criteria. In cats, the inclusion of extramedullary involvement has been suggested as an additional diagnostic criterion. Extramedullary infiltra-

Box 65-1 **Diagnostic Criteria* for Multiple Myeloma in Dogs**[24-26]

- Bone marrow plasmacytosis (>20%)
- Monoclonal gammopathy
- Skeletal lytic lesions
- Bence Jones proteinuria/light chain proteinuria

*Most sources indicate 2 of 4 for diagnosis of MM; however, some clinicians prefer to use 3 of 4.

Box 65-2 **Proposed Criteria* for Diagnosis of Multiple Myeloma in Cats**[3]

MAJOR CRITERIA
1. Bone marrow plasmacytosis (>20%)
2. Monoclonal gammopathy or Bence Jones/light chain proteinuria
3. Skeletal lytic lesions

MINOR CRITERIA
a. Bone marrow plasmacytosis (5% to 20% with atypia)
b. Splenic/hepatic plasmacytoma

*Diagnosis of MM if two major criteria or one major criterion and one minor criterion are met.

tion was a common finding in recent reports of cats with MM and "myeloma-related disorders," and the use of this finding as a diagnostic criterion may aid in making a diagnosis in cats who do not have skeletal lytic lesions or in cats in whom bone marrow aspirates can not be acquired.[3,4] Additionally, Patel and colleagues have suggested including atypical plasma cell morphology, especially in cases with marrow plasmacytosis of less than 20 per cent.[3] A proposed set of diagnostic criteria is listed in Box 65-2.

In contrast to human beings, systemic amyloidosis is a rare occurrence in feline patients with MM. Amyloidosis is described as insoluble protein aggregates deposited systemically or locally, typically in bundles of β-pleated sheets. Amyloid protein can be either reactive amyloid (AA amyloid) with the amyloid protein synthesized in the liver, or light chain amyloid (AL amyloid), the more common form associated with MM.[28] Only two cases of systemic AL amyloidosis associated with plasma cell disorders have been reported in veterinary medicine, a cat with an EMP of the tarsus and a horse with MM.[28,29]

Because the typical cat with MM has vague clinical signs, a complete blood count and serum biochemical profile often is performed as part of a medical evaluation. Identification of hyperglobulinemia, hypercalcemia, azotemia, or cytopenias will increase the index of suspicion for MM and should provoke additional tests. These laboratory evaluations should include urinalysis and urine culture to characterize azotemia (if present) and to assess for proteinuria and concurrent secondary infection. Hyperglobulinemia often is the first abnormality noted in cats with MM. If hyperglobulinemia is confirmed, a serum protein electrophoresis should be performed to identify a monoclonal spike. Immunoelectrophoresis or immunofixation can be performed to categorize the immunoglobulin involved; however, the prognostic value of identifying the class of immunoglobulin being produced is unknown in feline medicine. In human beings, IgA-secreting disease is associated with a worse prognosis.[6] Immunoelectrophoresis or immunofixation may be a more sensitive method than serum protein electrophoresis for detecting monoclonal immunoglobulins in cats.[17] Hypocholesterolemia, also identified frequently in cats with MM, is believed to occur secondary to decreased hepatic production in the face of hyperglobulinemia.[3]

Heat precipitation to detect urine light chain proteins or urine protein electrophoresis should be performed in cases with an index of suspicion for plasma cell disease. Urine dipsticks are not reliable for detecting light chain proteinuria, but sulfosalicylic acid (SSA) may be an adequately sensitive determinant. The SSA technique detects albumin, globulins, light chain proteins, polypeptides, and proteases, while urine dipsticks detect albumin primarily. False-positive results can occur in human beings when heat precipitation is used to detect urine light chain proteins, due to excess polyclonal light chains in conditions such as chronic kidney disease, nonmyeloma malignancies, and connective tissue disorders. Therefore urine electrophoresis for a monoclonal increase in κ- or λ-light chains may be a more specific test for detecting true monoclonal light chain proteinuria.[3] Retinal fundic examination, coagulation profile, and serum viscosity determination are additional recommendations in cats with suspected plasma cell diseases. Retinal fundic examination to assess for retinal changes, such as dilated or tortuous retinal vessels or retinal hemorrhages, should be performed in all cats with suspected plasma cell diseases. Coagulation profiles and serum viscosity measurements should be performed in all cats with clinical evidence of bleeding or hyperviscosity syndrome, such as altered mentation, seizures, or retinal fundic abnormalities.

Imaging recommendations include routine three-view thoracic radiographs, abdominal ultrasound, and survey skeletal films. Abdominal ultrasound is recommended in all cats with suspected plasma cell disorders due to the high proportion of cats with MM who have extramedullary involvement.[3,8] In a recent retrospective study, ultrasonographic abnormalities were reported most frequently in the spleen and liver of cats with MM. Splenic changes included splenomegaly with diffuse mottling, diffuse or nodular hypoechogenicity, and nodular hyperechogenicity. Hepatic changes included hepatomegaly and diffuse or nodular hyperechogenicity. Abdominal lymphadenopathy and renomegaly also may be present in cats with MM.[3] MM or visceral plasmacytoma should be included in the list of differential diagnoses for cats with hepatosplenomegaly. Survey skeletal films are preferred to bone scans using nuclear scintigraphy, because bone scans detect areas of osteoblastic activity predominantly and MM is characterized by osteolytic activity with osteoblastic inactivity.[4,6] In human oncology, bone mineral density measured by dual-energy X-ray absorptiometry (DEXA) is recommended because of the frequent occurrence of bone demineralization (osteoporosis) in MM. Magnetic resonance imaging of the bone marrow is used to detect occult bone marrow involvement in patients

with solitary plasmacytomas in bone.[6] Neither of these techniques has been evaluated routinely in cats.

Bone marrow aspirate and occasionally biopsy, as well as aspirate or biopsy of visceral organs, are required for definitive diagnosis of MM (see Chapter 64). Normal marrow plasmacytosis is less than 5 per cent, and the current recommendations in dogs for diagnosis of MM is a value of greater than 20 per cent. As mentioned above, inclusion of plasma cell atypia may be useful in cases with marrow plasmacytosis of less than 20 per cent. Occasionally, bone marrow aspirates need to be performed at multiple sites. Additionally, it has been recommended that bone marrow aspirates or bone biopsies be performed at the areas of radiographic bony lysis in order to increase the likelihood of obtaining a diagnosis.[3,4] Patel and colleagues note in their case series that plasma cell infiltrates were found in abdominal organs of normal size, suggesting that routine aspiration of the spleen and liver might be performed in any cat with a suspected plasma cell disorder.[3]

A clinical staging system for MM exists for human beings and has been suggested for dogs; however, neither of these systems has been evaluated for prognostic significance in cats.[4,6]

DIFFERENTIAL DIAGNOSIS

Differential diagnoses for monoclonal gammopathy include infectious diseases, such as leishmaniasis, ehrlichiosis, and feline infectious peritonitis; other B-cell neoplasms, such as lymphoma, acute and chronic leukemias; Waldenström macroglobulinemia, and MGUS.[4] One cat has been reported with MGUS that progressed to MM 9 years later.[3] Monoclonal gammopathy of unknown significance progresses to MM or other lymphoproliferative diseases in 25 per cent of human patients affected with the syndrome.[30]

TREATMENT

Due to the disseminated nature of MM, chemotherapy is the treatment of choice. The standard treatment in dogs is melphalan, an oral alkylating agent, and prednisone. The standard or best chemotherapy protocol in cats remains controversial. Melphalan and prednisone can be used in cats; however, some clinicians report the protocol to be more myelosuppressive in cats than in dogs. This observation may be related to the reported increased toxicity of melphalan in smaller patients when dosed using body surface area. Due to this potential increased toxicity, the use of body weight (mg/kg) to dose smaller patients has been recommended.[31] A suggested dosing schedule, similar to the protocol reported for dogs, is 0.1 mg/kg PO q24h for 10 to 14 days, followed by 0.1 mg/kg PO q48h until there is clinical improvement or leukopenia develops.[4,7] Hanna et al define clinical improvement as reduction in clinical signs, laboratory evidence of response to therapy as measured by a decrease in serum total protein, and radiographic evidence of reduction or resolution of skeletal lytic lesions.[7] Due to tablet size

(2 mg), this dosing regimen equates to approximately one tablet every 4 days for a 5-kg cat. The melphalan tablet should not be split because it is covered by a protective coating and dividing it will result in human exposure to the drug. A continuous maintenance protocol for cats of 0.1 mg/kg PO q7d has been reported,[7] although this would be difficult to administer due to tablet size. The recommended maintenance protocol in dogs is 0.05 mg/kg PO q24h continuously until clinical relapse or myelosuppression occurs.[4] This equates to approximately one 2-mg tablet q7d for a 5-kg cat. Prednisolone is given concurrently at a dose of 0.5 mg/kg PO q24h.[7] In dogs, prednisone is reduced to 0.5 mg/kg PO q48h after 10 days and then discontinued after 60 days of therapy.[4] The duration of corticosteroid administration has not been reported in cats. Complete blood counts must be monitored regularly, because cytopenias such as neutropenia and thrombocytopenia are the most common toxicity associated with melphalan in veterinary medicine and myelosuppression may be more severe in cats. A complete blood count and platelet count should be performed every 7 to 14 days for the first 1 to 2 months and then monthly thereafter. If myelosuppression occurs, the drug can be discontinued and restarted at a decreased dose or frequency once bone marrow recovery has occurred.

Some clinicians advocate the use of faster acting alkylating agents to alleviate clinical signs more quickly. There is no evidence that these agents are more effective, however. Cyclophosphamide, combination protocols such as cyclophosphamide-vincristine-prednisone (COP), and lomustine (CCNU) have been reported for the treatment of MM in a small number of cats.[8,32] Chlorambucil, another slow alkylator similar to melphalan, also has been used to treat cats with MM.

Radiation therapy can be used as an adjuvant or for palliation in cats with MM with bony lesions resulting in pathological fractures or in spinal cord compression. Treatment with radiation therapy has been reported in dogs with vertebral plasma cell tumors, using doses of 36 and 48 Gy.[33] Treatment of one cat with a vertebral plasmacytoma using radiation therapy has been reported. This cat was treated with a total of 12 Gy. The patient had a solitary vertebral lesion, with no systemic evidence of MM.[34]

MANAGEMENT

Evaluation of Response

The goal of chemotherapy is to relieve clinical signs and decrease tumor burden. Evaluation of response to therapy is measured by subjective improvement in clinical signs, such as lameness/bone pain, lethargy, anorexia, and objective improvement in clinicopathological parameters and radiographic appearance of skeletal lesions. Clinicopathological parameters are measured as decreases in serum globulin level or improvement in the complete blood count. A serum protein electrophoresis and heat precipitation for urine light chain proteins or urine protein electrophoresis can be performed monthly to help define response, then less frequently if there is a good response. In a recent report by Hanna et al, cats who responded to treatment with melphalan and prednisone showed clinical improvement within 4 weeks of initiation of therapy, with radiographic improvement of skeletal lesions within 8 weeks.[7] Objective improvement in clinicopathological parameters (serum immunoglobulin level and urine light chain protein level) occurs within 3 to 4 weeks in dogs.[4] If cytopenias persist or develop during treatment, another bone marrow aspiration may be required to differentiate between myelosuppression secondary to chemotherapy or disease relapse.

Supportive Care

Management of cats with MM may involve the treatment of hypercalcemia, chronic kidney disease, hyperviscosity syndrome, and bleeding diathesis. These problems should resolve with response to chemotherapy; however, in the short term they may need to be addressed symptomatically.

Hypercalcemia can be managed with standard therapies, including fluid diuresis with 0.9 per cent sodium chloride or furosemide, once the patient has been rehydrated. For refractory hypercalcemia, medications such as pamidronate, salmon calcitonin, and prednisone (once diagnostic samples have been obtained) can be used. Fluid diuresis also will assist in the management of chronic kidney disease while the patient is in the hospital. If azotemia results in ongoing clinical signs, subcutaneous fluids can be continued when the cat is discharged from the hospital.

Hyperviscosity syndrome is uncommon in cats with MM; however, those patients with severe clinical signs associated with HVS can be managed with plasmapheresis. To perform intermittent plasmapheresis, whole blood (10 to 15 mL/kg) is removed from the patient and collected in transfer packs with anticoagulant. The blood then is centrifuged to separate plasma from packed red blood cells; plasma is removed and discarded. The red blood cells are resuspended in 0.9 per cent sodium chloride to restore the blood to its original volume and, finally, readministered to the patient with the use of a filter set.[22] Continuous plasmapheresis via plasma filtration also can be performed with the use of hemodialysis equipment. Bleeding diatheses typically resolve with the resolution of HVS; however, some patients may require whole blood or plasma transfusions.

Careful monitoring for infections is important in human patients with MM. This is due to a concurrent decrease in uninvolved immunoglobulins, as well as dysregulation of immune effector cells.[5] This has been recognized infrequently in feline patients; however, prophylactic antibiotics in MM patients are recommended by some clinicians.[25] Periodic urine cultures may be indicated because cats with MM frequently are azotemic and are being treated concurrently with corticosteroids.

PROGNOSIS

Information regarding survival times in cats with MM is limited. In three recent compilations of cases, approximately 60 per cent of cats treated with chemotherapy responded to therapy (melphalan and prednisone and cyclophosphamide-based protocols). Survival times were short in most cats (1 to 4 months); however, there was a subset of long-term responders (up to 24 months). Untreated cats or cats who did not respond to therapy had rapidly progressive disease.[3,7,8] Mellor et al describe a case series of cats with "myeloma-related disorders." Cats with extramedullary involvement, bone marrow involvement, or both who were treated with chemotherapy (n = 7) had a median survival time of 284 days, with responders (clinical improvement/reduced globulinemia) having a median survival of 373 days.[8] Prognostic factors have not been identified in cats; however, Hanna et al divided cases into two categories—*aggressive* (hypercalcemia, bony lesions with pathological fracture, anemia, light chain proteinuria, azotemia, no or little change in globulin level after treatment, no or little clinical improvement) and *less aggressive* (normocalcemia, bony lesions without pathological fractures, absence of azotemia, absence of anemia, absence of light chain proteinuria, return of serum protein level to normal following 8 weeks of treatment). Cats in the aggressive group had a median survival time of 5 days, and patients in the less aggressive group had a median survival time of 387 days. Due to the small numbers of cats in each group, no statistical analysis was performed.[7] Negative prognostic factors identified in dogs include hypercalcemia, light chain proteinuria, and extensive bony lysis.[26]

INVESTIGATIONAL/NOVEL THERAPIES

In human oncology, patients often are treated initially with melphalan and prednisone or melphalan-based myeloablative chemotherapy, followed by bone marrow or peripheral blood stem cell transplant. Additional therapies include thalidomide, thalidomide analogs, arsenic trioxide, and bortezomib.[6,35,36] Thalidomide exerts its activity through antiangiogenic mechanisms. Its use is restricted in feline medicine due to concerns regarding teratogenic effects in human beings handling the drug. Arsenic trioxide works through several mechanisms including induction of apoptosis of myeloma cells and decreased binding of myeloma cells to bone marrow stromal cells. Bortezomib is a proteosome inhibitor. Its use is approved in human beings with MM who have failed other therapies. The use of arsenic trioxide or bortezomib has not been reported in feline medicine.

Bisphosphonates, such as pamidronate and zoledronate, decrease the number of skeletal complications and bone pain in human patients with MM.[37] The use of pamidronate and zoledronate has been reported in cats with hypercalcemia and oral squamous cell carcinoma, respectively, and these agents may be useful for palliation in cats with skeletal lesions or hypercalcemia. Pamidronate is given at a dose of 1.5 to 2 mg/kg IV diluted in 0.9 per cent sodium chloride over 2 hours.[38,39] Zoledronate is used at a dose of 0.2 mg/kg IV diluted in 25 mL of 0.9 per cent saline, given as an infusion over 15 minutes every 28 days.[40] Because bisphosphonates can cause renal tubular damage, monitoring of renal function is critical when using bisphosphonates to treat cats with MM. The risk of renal failure is associated with the length of infusion and total dose, with rapid infusions of large quantities carrying the highest risk.[23,39,40] A serum chemistry profile and a urine specific gravity should be performed prior to each infusion to assess renal function.

SOLITARY OSSEOUS AND EXTRAMEDULLARY PLASMACYTOMAS

Solitary extramedullary plasmacytomas (EMP) are diagnosed less often than MM in cats.[4] As discussed above, however, cats with MM frequently have extramedullary involvement.[3,8] Additionally, cats with plasmacytomas of the spleen and/or liver have been reported without marrow plasmacytosis and both with and without monoclonal gammopathy, reinforcing that plasma cell diseases are a spectrum of syndromes.[8,41] Solitary EMP are diagnosed most frequently in the skin; other sites include the oral cavity, gastrointestinal tract, abdominal organs, retroperitoneum, subcutaneous tissues, and orbit[9,41-45] (see Chapter 70). An intracerebral plasma cell tumor also has been reported; however, serum protein electrophoresis and examination of the urine for light chains was not performed, and the cat did not undergo a full necropsy examination.[46] Solitary osseous plasmacytoma (SOP) has been reported in two cats in the lumbar and sacral vertebrae.[34]

In dogs, plasmacytomas of the skin and oral cavity typically are benign, with gastrointestinal plasmacytomas often exhibiting more aggressive behavior, metastasizing most commonly to local lymph nodes. SOP is thought to progress eventually to MM in most dogs. Solitary osseous plasmacytoma in dogs may behave similarly to the disease in human beings, in which more than 50 per cent of patients develop MM in a median time of 2 to 4 years.[47] The behavior of solitary plasmacytomas in cats is not as predictable.[4]

CLINICAL SIGNS

Cutaneous plasmacytomas typically are solitary, smooth, and nodular. Cutaneous and oral forms of EMP frequently have no related clinical signs. Solitary osseous plasmacytomas often occur in the spine in dogs,[4,33] and the two reported cases in cats also had a vertebral location. Clinical signs in these cats were pain on palpation of the region and neurological deficits. A bony mass at the sacrum also was palpable in one cat.[34] Signs related to an elevated M protein, such as HVS, may be associated rarely with secretory EMP or SOP. Monoclonal and biclonal gammopathies have been reported in cats with cutaneous, orbital, retroperitoneal, hepatic, and splenic plasmacytomas, without bone marrow involvement.[8-9,41,44]

DIAGNOSIS AND PATHOLOGY

Extramedullary plasmacytomas and SOP are solid tumors comprised of monoclonal proliferations of terminally differentiated B lymphocytes. Fine-needle aspirate or biopsy

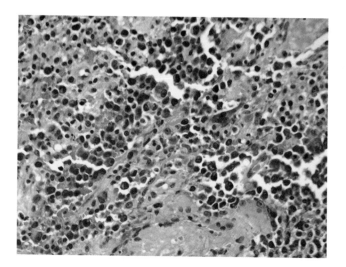

Figure 65-6 A solitary cutaneous extramedullary plasmacytoma in a cat. The biopsy consists of cutaneous extramedullary plasmacytomas with homogeneous eosinophilic amyloid deposits. (H&E, 40×.)

is required for diagnosis. Tumor cells are round with pleomorphic, often eccentric nuclei. The cells may be binucleated or multinucleated with a perinuclear clear zone representing the Golgi body. Cytological examination of EMP or SOP may reveal two variants of plasma cells. Flame cells, characterized by eosinophilic cytoplasmic projections, or Mott cells, characterized by Russell bodies representing globules of immunoglobulin, may be identified. Tumor cells of EMP are located in the dermis and subcutis of the skin and lamina submucosa of the oral cavity. Tumors typically are expansile and rarely infiltrative. On histopathological examination, tumor cells are arranged in sheets. A histopathological classification scheme of EMP has been modified from human beings, with mature, hyaline, cleaved, asynchronous, and polymorphous-blastic types described; however, the prognostic significance of this scheme is unknown in cats.[42]

Amyloid is found frequently in human EMP and has been identified in feline EMP (Figure 65-6). The proteinaceous extracellular deposits in various tissues and organs, which are characteristic of amyloidosis, have common morphological, structural, and staining properties but variable protein composition. Two types of amyloidosis are described: amyloid A (AA) amyloidosis and amyloid L (AL) amyloidosis. AA amyloidosis is reactive amyloidosis, in which amino terminal portions of acute-phase protein serum amyloid A are deposited. AL amyloidosis, on the other hand, consists of amino terminal fragments and complete immunoglobulin light chains. These are derived from B-cell tumors that synthesize and secrete a monoclonal protein that forms amyloid deposits.[48] This localized production of monoclonal protein is too low to be reflected as a serum or urine monoclonal gammopathy. Amyloid L lambda (λ)-amyloid was identified in nine of 21 reported cases of feline EMP.[42] Amyloid deposits stain positively with Congo red and display light-green birefringence when examined under polarized light.

Immunohistochemical stains that are useful in identifying plasma cell tumors include those for light chains (λ, κ) and heavy chains (IgG, IgA, IgM). The majority (>90 per cent) of plasma cell tumors in cats are positive for λ light chains.[42]

Staging tests (serum protein electrophoresis, heat precipitation for urine light chain proteins or urine protein electrophoresis, bone marrow aspirate, skeletal survey radiographs) should be performed in cats with EMP or SOP. In a report by Mellor et al, 5 of 7 cats with cutaneous plasmacytomas were not systemically ill or hyperglobulinemic, while cats with abdominal organ plasmacytomas typically were systemically ill and hyperglobulinemic, with six of 12 cats having concurrent bone marrow plasmacytosis.[8]

TREATMENT

Surgery is the treatment of choice for cats with solitary EMP. Thorough staging should be performed prior to surgery because cats with EMP seem to have a higher incidence of systemic involvement than affected dogs. If systemic involvement is not identified with staging tests, the question of whether to recommend adjuvant chemotherapy is debatable (see Prognosis below). In human oncology, noncutaneous EMP and SOP have a high likelihood of local lymph node metastasis or progression to MM, respectively. It has been shown that there is no benefit to treating human patients with solitary EMP or SOP with chemotherapy prior to the documentation of systemic disease.[4,47] In cats with tumors in areas other than the skin, adjuvant chemotherapy may be a reasonable consideration due to the possible progression to systemic disease; however, the need for adjuvant chemotherapy is unknown due to the small numbers of cases reported. Chemotherapy (melphalan, cyclophosphamide) may be used as an adjuvant to local therapy (surgery, radiation therapy) or as the primary therapy in cats with systemic involvement.

Plasma cell tumors are radiosensitive, and radiation therapy can be used in sites not amenable to surgical excision. In one recent case report of a cat with SOP of the lumbar vertebrae, the patient was treated with a total of 12 Gray (Gy), delivered in three weekly fractions of 4 Gy.[34] Doses of 40 to 50 Gy are recommended in human beings with EMP or SOP.[6,47]

PROGNOSIS

The rarity of the disease and the small number of reported cases make determination of prognosis difficult for cats with EMP and SOP. In one recent study of cats with a variety of plasma cell disorders, patients with cutaneous plasmacytomas who received either no treatment or treatment with corticosteroids alone (n = 3) had a median survival of 93 days, compared to a median survival of 663 days for cats who underwent surgical excision of the cutaneous mass (n = 4). However, two of the cats in this study had a monoclonal gammopathy and evidence of abdominal involvement, and it is difficult to determine if these cats were not treated or received corticosteroids alone.[8] It is likely that the cats who were not treated or received corticosteroids alone had evidence of systemic involvement, resulting in the shorter survival time. Although cutaneous plasma cell tumors are largely benign in dogs, systemic involvement, most commonly a monoclonal gammopathy, and progression to MM have been reported in cats.[8,10] In a report of two cats with SOP, the patients were treated with either melphalan and prednisone chemotherapy or radiation therapy alone. The cats had survival times of 6 years and greater than 4 years, respectively. One cat had no evidence of progression to MM over 4 years; the other cat had possible evidence of a monoclonal gammopathy at the time of euthanasia, 6 years after initial diagnosis.[34] Due to the unpredictable nature of this disease, close monitoring is recommended for any cat with an extramedullary or solitary osseous plasmacytoma.

REFERENCES

1. Engle GC, Brodey RS: A retrospective study of 395 feline neoplasms, *J Am Anim Hosp Assoc* 5:21, 1969.
2. Carpenter JL, Andrews LK, Holzworth J: Tumors and tumor like lesions. In Holzworth J, editor: *Diseases of the cat: medicine and surgery*, Philadelphia, 1987, WB Saunders, p 406.
3. Patel RT, Caceres A, French AF, et al: Multiple myeloma in 16 cats: a retrospective study, *Vet Clin Pathol* 34:341, 2005.
4. Vail DM: Plasma cell neoplasms. In Withrow SJ, Vail DM, editors: *Withrow & MacEwens's small animal clinical oncology*, ed 4, St Louis, 2007, Saunders Elsevier, p 769.
5. Sydney SE, Cassady JR: Plasma cell neoplasms. In DeVita VT, Hellman S, Rosenberg SA, editors: *Cancer: principles and practice of oncology*, ed 5, Philadelphia, 1997, Lippincott-Raven, p 2347.
6. Munshi, NC, Anderson KC: Plasma cell neoplasms. In DeVita VT, Hellman S, Rosenberg SA, editors: *Cancer: principles and practice of oncology*, ed 7, Philadelphia, 2000, Lippincott Williams & Wilkins, p 2155.
7. Hanna F: Multiple myeloma in cats, *J Feline Med Surg* 7:275, 2005.
8. Mellor PJ, Haughland S, Murphy S, et al: Myeloma-related disorders in cats commonly present as extramedullary neoplasms in contrast to myeloma in human patients: 24 cases with clinical follow-up, *J Vet Intern Med* 20:1376, 2006.
9. Michau TM, Proulx DR, Rushton SD, et al: Intraocular extramedullary plasmacytoma in a cat, *Vet Ophthalmol* 6:177, 2003.
10. Radhakrishnan A, Risbon RE, Patel RT, et al: Progression of a solitary, malignant cutaneous plasma cell tumor to multiple myeloma in a cat, *Vet Comp Oncol* 2:36, 2004.
11. Lester AE, Carpenter JL: A solitary plasmacytoma in a dog with progression to disseminated myeloma, *Can Vet J* 21:284, 1980.
12. Hauschild A, Haferlach T, Löffler H, et al: Multiple myeloma first presenting as cutaneous plasmacytoma, *J Am Acad Dermatol* 34:146, 1996.
13. Bienzle D, Silverstein DC, Chaffin K: Multiple myeloma in cats: variable presentation with different immunoglobulin isotypes in two cats, *Vet Pathol* 37:370, 2000.
14. Yamada T, Ogura A, Inoue J, et al: A case of feline macroglobulinemia, *Nippon Juigaku Zasshi* 45:395, 1983.
15. Yamada O, Tamura K, Yagihara H, et al: Light-chain myeloma in a cat, *J Vet Diagn Invest* 19:443, 2007.
16. Cowgill ES, Neel JA, Ruslander D: Light-chain myeloma in a dog, *J Vet Intern Med* 18:119, 2004.
17. Appel AL, Moens NMM, Abrams-Ogg ACG, et al: Multiple myeloma with central nervous system involvement in a cat, *J Am Vet Med Assoc* 233:743, 2008.
18. MacEwan EG, Patnaik AK, Hurvitz AI, et al: Nonsecretory multiple myeloma in two dogs, *J Am Vet Med Assoc* 170:511, 1977.
19. Hoenig M: Multiple myeloma associated with the heavy chains of immunoglobulin A in a dog, *J Am Vet Med Assoc* 190:1191, 1987.
20. Hickford FH, Stokol T, vanGessel YA, et al: Monoclonal immunoglobulin G cryoglobulinemia and multiple myeloma in a domestic shorthair cat, *J Am Vet Med Assoc* 217:1029, 2000.
21. Forrester SD, Greco DS, Relford RL: Serum hyperviscosity syndrome associated with multiple myeloma in two cats, *J Am Vet Med Assoc* 200:79, 1992.
22. Forrester SD, Relford RL: Serum hyperviscosity syndrome: its diagnosis and treatment, *Vet Med* 87:48, 1992.
23. Milner RJ, Farese J, Henry CJ, et al: Bisphosphonates and cancer, *J Vet Intern Med* 18:597, 2004.
24. King AJ, Davies DR, Irwin PJ: Feline multiple myeloma: literature review and four case reports, *Aust Vet Pract* 32:146, 2002.
25. MacEwen EG, Hurvitz AI: Diagnosis and management of monoclonal gammopathies, *Vet Clin North Am Small Anim Pract* 7:119, 1977.
26. Matus RE, Leifer C, MacEwen EG, et al: Prognostic factors for multiple myeloma in the dog, *J Am Vet Med Assoc* 188:1288, 1986.
27. Ogilvie GK, Moore AS: Plasma cell tumors. In Ogilvie GK, Moore AS, editors: *Managing the veterinary cancer patient*, Trenton, NJ, 1995, Veterinary Learning Systems, p 280.
28. Carothers MA, Johnson GC, DiBartola SP, et al: Extramedullary plasmacytoma and immunoglobulin-associated amyloidosis in a cat, *J Am Vet Med Assoc* 195:1593, 1989.
29. Kim DY, Taylor W, Eades SC, et al: Systemic AL amyloidosis associated with multiple myeloma in a horse, *Vet Pathol* 42:81, 2005.
30. Kyle RA, Therneau TM, Rajkaumar SV, et al: A long-term study of prognosis in monoclonal gammopathy of undetermined significance [comment], *N Engl J Med* 346:564, 2002.
31. Page RL, Macy DW, Thrall DE, et al: Unexpected toxicity associated with use of body surface area dosing melphalan in the dog, *Cancer Res* 48:288, 1998.
32. Fan TM, Kitchell BE, Dhaliwal RS, et al: Hematological toxicity and therapeutic efficacy of lomustine in 20 tumor-bearing cats: critical assessment of a practical dosing regimen, *J Am Anim Hosp Assoc* 38:357, 2002.
33. Rusbridge C, Wheeler SJ, Lamb CR, et al: Vertebral plasma cell tumors in 8 dogs, *J Vet Intern Med* 13:126, 1999.
34. Mellor PJ, Polton GA, Brearley M, et al: Solitary plasmacytoma of bone in two successfully treated cats, *J Feline Med Surg* 9:72, 2007.
35. Barlogie B, Shaughnessy J, Tricot G, et al: Treatment of multiple myeloma, *Blood* 103:20, 2004.
36. Bruno B, Giaccone L, Rotta M, et al: Novel targeted drugs for the treatment of multiple myeloma: from bench to bedside, *Leuk* 19:1729, 2005.
37. Berenson JR, Lichtenstein A, Porter L, et al: Efficacy of pamidronate in reducing skeletal events in patients with advanced multiple myeloma. Myeloma Aredia study group, *N Engl J Med* 334:488, 1996.
38. Hostutler RA, Chew DJ, Jaeger JQ, et al: Uses and effectiveness of pamidronate disodium for treatment of dogs and cats with hypercalcemia, *J Vet Intern Med* 19:19, 2005.
39. Fan TM: The role of bisphosphonates in the management of patients that have cancer, *Vet Clin North Am Small Anim Pract* 37:1091, 2007.

40. Wypij JM, Fan TM, Fredrickson RL, et al: In vivo and in vitro effects of zoledronate for treating oral squamous cell carcinoma in cats, *J Vet Intern Med* 22:151, 2008.

41. Larsen AE, Carpenter JL: Hepatic plasmacytoma and biclonal gammopathy in a cat, *J Am Vet Med Assoc* 205:708, 1994.

42. Majzoub M, Breuer W, Platz SJ, et al: Histopathologic and immunophenotypic characterization of extramedullary plasmacytomas in nine cats, *Vet Pathol* 40:249, 2003.

43. Zikes CD, Spielman B, Shapiro W, et al: Gastric extramedullary plasmacytoma in a cat, *J Vet Intern Med* 12:381, 1998.

44. Mandel NS, Esplin DG: A retroperitoneal extramedullary plasmacytoma in a cat with a monoclonal gammopathy, *J Am Anim Hosp Assoc* 30:603, 1994.

45. Ward DA, McEntee MF, Weddle DL: Orbital plasmacytoma in a cat, *J Small Anim Pract* 38:576, 1997.

46. Greenberg MJ, Schatzberg SJ, deLahunta A, et al: Intracerebral plasma cell tumor in a cat: a case report and literature review, *J Vet Intern Med* 18:581, 2004.

47. Soutar R, Lucraft H, Jackson G, et al: Guidelines on the diagnosis and management of solitary plasmacytoma of bone and solitary extramedullary plasmacytoma, *Br J Haematol* 124:717, 2004.

48. Platz SJ, Breuer W, Geisel O, et al: Identification of λ light chain amyloid in eight canine and two feline extramedullary plasmacytomas, *J Comp Pathol* 116:45, 1997.

CHAPTER

66 Clinical Use of Erythropoietin in Feline Medicine

Cathy E. Langston

Erythropoietin (EPO) is the hematopoietic growth factor responsible for stimulating erythrogenesis in response to anemia. EPO is a 30.4 kilodalton glycoprotein characterized by a 165–amino acid protein backbone with 4 carbohydrate chains, each containing two to four sialic acid residues.[1] The majority of EPO is produced in the peritubular interstitial cells of the inner renal cortex and outer renal medulla; however, the liver produces 10 to 15 per cent of the total EPO.[2] EPO has a circulating half-life of 6 to 10 hours. The main trigger for the synthesis of EPO is renal hypoxemia, which increases production of hypoxia-inducible factor (HIF). HIF stimulates transcription of the EPO gene and is inactivated by HIF-alpha prolyl and asparaginyl hydroxylases. HIF-alpha hydroxylases require oxygen and iron to function (Figure 66-1).[3]

EPO stimulates proliferation and maturation of erythrocytes in the bone marrow directly by binding specific growth factor receptors on the red blood cell precursors. EPO has the greatest effect on the colony-forming unit erythroid cell (CFU-E), although it has some effect also on the differentiation of the burst-forming unit erythroid cell (BFU-E) and erythroblasts (Figure 66-2).[4] In the absence of EPO, these progenitor cells undergo apoptosis, whereas they differentiate and proliferate in the presence of EPO.[5] It takes approximately 5 days from stimulation by EPO for the release of reticulocytes into the circulation.[6]

In addition to its effects on red blood cell differentiation, EPO induces synthesis of hemoglobin and red blood cell membrane proteins. It facilitates release of reticulocytes into the blood by lowering the barrier between the marrow and the blood.[7]

ERYTHROPOIESIS-STIMULATING AGENTS (ESA)

The gene sequence for EPO was determined in 1983, and recombinant human EPO (rHuEPO) became available in 1985.[8] Epoetin alfa varies from epoetin beta in the glycosylation, but there is no difference in clinical efficacy.[9] These products have a half-life of 4 to 9 hours after IV injection and 24 hours after SQ injection (Table 66-1).[5] Darbepoetin was licensed for use in human beings in 2001. Darbepoetin has a 165–amino acid protein backbone that varies from the human EPO sequence by 5 amino acids and is more highly glycosylated than epoetin alfa and beta. The glycosylation slows clearance of this product, allowing a reduction in frequency of administration while maintaining efficacy.[10-12]

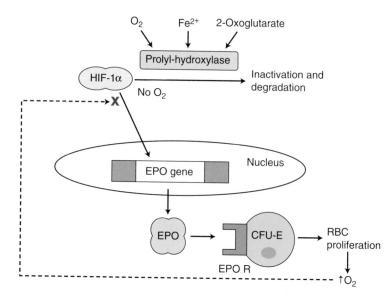

Figure 66-1 Stimulation of erythropoietin production. Hypoxia-inducible factor 1a (HIF-1a) is produced continually. In normoxic conditions, the enzyme prolylhydroxylase, with iron and 2-oxoglutarate, causes HIF-1a to be inactivated and degraded rapidly. In hypoxic conditions, HIF-1a migrates to the nucleus and increases transcription of the EPO gene, increasing circulating EPO levels. EPO binds receptors on CFU-E, decreasing apoptosis and thus allowing proliferation. The increase in red blood cells increases oxygen carrying capacity, which feeds back negatively on HIF-1a. *HIF-1a,* Hypoxia inducible factor; *EPO,* erythropoietin; *EPO R,* EPO receptor.

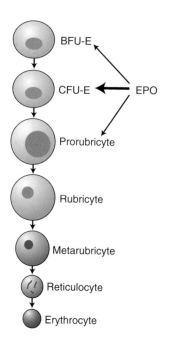

Figure 66-2 Red blood cell maturation. Erythropoietin binds to receptors found predominantly on the colony-forming unit erythron. The blast-forming unit erythron and prorubricytes have smaller numbers of receptors. Erythropoietin inhibits apoptosis (programmed cell death) and stimulates these cells to proliferate. Over approximately 7 days, they pass through various stages to become mature erythrocytes.

Feline EPO has a greater amino acid sequence homology with human EPO (83.3 per cent) than the canine amino acid sequence (81.3 per cent).[13,14] Although the gene sequence is adequately conserved for human products to have a clinical effect in cats and dogs, the absence of complete homology results in the possibility of antibody formation that leads to development of pure red cell aplasia (PRCA) in both species.

Recombinant feline EPO (rFeEPO) and recombinant canine EPO have been produced but are not available commercially.[13] In a small number of cats with anemia of chronic kidney disease (CKD) treated with rFeEPO, hematocrit increased in the majority of patients. Unfortunately, a small number of treated cats, both those who had never received rHuEPO and those receiving rFeEPO as a salvage treatment after development of PRCA from rHuEPO, developed PRCA in response to rFeEPO. The reasons for this adverse complication are under investigation, but proposed theories include gene polymorphism in the population or use of an aberrant gene in the initial gene sequencing.[15] Recombinant canine EPO has been shown to stimulate erythrocyte production successfully in clinically normal dogs and dogs with CKD without causing PRCA, a complication that was encountered in rHuEPO-treated dogs.[16,17] Canine EPO was not uniformly effective in increasing hematocrit in dogs with PRCA induced by rHuEPO.[17]

The gene for feline EPO has been transfected into an adenovirus vector and introduced into healthy cats via IM injection. Gene transcription with attendant increase in hematocrit was present in the high-dose group. Some cats developed polycythemia, and surgical excision of the injected muscle controlled polycythemia in some of the affected animals. However, some cats continued to produce excessive EPO, and virus particles could be found in surrounding tissue. One cat developed PRCA, which resolved after excision of the injected muscle.[18,19] In order to control gene expression, a doxycycline response gene has been inserted and may make this technology feasible in the future.[20]

Continuous EPO receptor activator (CERA) has the same protein sequence as EPO and has a large carbohydrate chain attached to the protein backbone, doubling its molecular weight compared to EPO.[3] Because of its long half-life, the sustained effect on stimulating the EPO receptor increases erythropoiesis[21] (see Table 66-1). Initial reports projected that it would need to be administered monthly. Although CERA was approved by the FDA for use in human patients in 2007, it is not yet available commercially, and there is no information about its use in cats or dogs.

Table 66-1 Erythropoiesis-Stimulating Agents

Compound	Brand	Company	Aa	Kdal	Half-Life	Initial Dose	Route	Availability
rHuEPO-α	Epogen, Procrit, Eprex	Amgen, Ortho Biotech	165	30.4	4-9 hr IV, 24 hr SQ	100 U/kg 3 times a week	SQ, IV	Worldwide
rHuEPO-β	NeoRecormon	Roche	165	30	*	*	*	Europe
Darbepoetin-α	Aranesp	Amgen	165	37	70-105 hr SQ	0.45-1 µg/kg/wk	SQ, IV	Worldwide
CERA	Mircera	Roche	165	60	130-140 hr IV or SQ	NA (every 2-4 wk)	SQ, IV	Europe
Pegylated dimeric peptidic ESA	Hematide	Affymax	20		30-90 hr	NA (monthly)	SQ, IV	In Phase III trials

*Same as rHuEPO-α.

A small peptide of 20 amino acids (Hematide) unrelated in sequence to EPO that can stimulate the EPO receptor is in Phase III clinical trials in people (see Table 66-1). Once-monthly IV or SQ injections are effective in treating anemia in human patients.[3] This drug is dissimilar to epoetin or native EPO, and therefore it holds promise as a rescue agent for patients with PRCA because it is not inactivated by anti-EPO antibodies. This concept has been shown in mice, and this drug has been used for this purpose in human beings.[3,22] When this drug becomes available, its use could be considered for treatment of PRCA in cats.

BENEFITS OF TREATMENT OF ANEMIA

Treating anemia has many benefits, including improving tissue oxygenation, which enhances exercise capacity, central nervous system function, and endocrine and cardiac function.[23] In people, control of anemia decreases the number of hospital admissions and reduces cardiovascular morbidity.[24] Treatment of anemia improves cognitive function, decreasing depression and increasing quality of life.[25] Although these factors are difficult to quantify in animals, owners volunteer comments frequently about the improvement in attitude and social behaviors of their companion animals. Interestingly, this improvement may happen at initiation of rHuEPO treatment, prior to any substantial increase in hematocrit.[17,26]

Treatment of anemia may slow the progression of renal disease in human beings.[28] Hypoxia increases extracellular matrix formation and interstitial fibrosis, and treatment of anemia decreases renal cellular hypoxia. In a randomized clinical trial in human patients, early treatment of anemia (hemoglobin 9 to 11.5 g/dL) decreased the risk of doubling of creatinine, starting dialysis, or death by 60 per cent, compared to delayed treatment of anemia (hemoglobin < 9 g/dL).[29] It is interesting to speculate on the effect of early treatment of anemia in veterinary renal patients. Unfortunately, the currently available treatments (mainly rHuEPO) carry the risk of substantial adverse effects, making a clinical trial of early treatment (prior to onset of clinical signs of anemia) difficult to design ethically. New ESAs with lower risk may obviate this dilemma.

INDICATIONS FOR ERYTHROPOIESIS-STIMULATING AGENTS

Human recombinant EPO is approved for use in human beings to treat anemia associated with hemodialysis or chronic kidney disease, cancer patients on chemotherapy, human immunodeficiency virus (HIV) patients on zidovudine (AZT) therapy, and for anemic patients preparing for major surgery who wish to minimize allogeneic blood transfusions. rHuEPO and darbepoetin are used primarily to treat anemia of CKD in cats and dogs but also have been used to treat feline leukemia virus (FeLV) and feline immunodeficiency virus (FIV) infections, idiopathic PRCA in cats, myelodysplastic and myelofibrotic disorders, and for autologous transfusions in dogs.[30-38]

ANEMIA OF CHRONIC KIDNEY DISEASE

Anemia is a common abnormality noted in patients with CKD, affecting 32 to 65 per cent of cats with CKD.[39-41] The mechanism of development of anemia of CKD is multifactorial. Reasons for increased loss of erythrocytes include bleeding from gastrointestinal ulceration and uremic platelet dysfunction and decreased survival in the uremic environment.[42-44] Decreased production may result from uremic toxins that inhibit erythropoiesis,[1,42,44-47] nutritional deficiencies (e.g., B vitamins),[45,48,49] bone marrow fibrosis,[43,45,50-52] and concurrent inflammation.

The most significant reason for development of anemia associated with CKD is a relative EPO deficiency. Several studies have demonstrated that EPO levels in uremic anemic patients are within the normal range or mildly elevated, in contrast to nonuremic anemic patients, who have markedly elevated EPO levels.[43,46,53,54] As the kidneys fail, EPO production decreases, the bone marrow becomes less proliferative, and a slowly developing nonregenerative anemia develops. This relative EPO deficiency can be reversed by treatment with rHuEPO.

Many therapies have been suggested for treatment of anemia of CKD, including minimizing blood loss from gastric ulcers, controlling blood sampling, and administering blood transfusions. Supplementation of the water-soluble B vitamins may be beneficial in CKD patients.[55] Anabolic steroids have been utilized for the treatment of the anemia of CKD. Results have been variable and generally disappointing, with a long delay to effect and the effect being minor. Their use can not be recommended due to the lack of efficacy and the potential for hepatotoxicity.[48,55,56]

Epoetin and darbepoetin have been used successfully for treatment of anemia of CKD in human beings, cats, and dogs. rHuEPO increases the hematocrit effectively in a dose-dependent manner and has been used to treat naturally occurring CKD in cats and dogs.[16,27,57,58] In addition to resolving anemia, the majority of patients treated with rHuEPO have improved appetite, weight gain, increased energy, alertness, playfulness, and physical strength, greater affection, and improved grooming.*

CANCER PATIENTS ON CHEMOTHERAPY

Anemia in cancer patients often is multifactorial. The most common mechanisms include anemia of chronic disease, blood loss, decreased production from bone marrow infiltration, and suppression secondary to chemotherapy. Cancer patients may have an inadequate EPO response to an anemia (relative EPO deficiency).[61] Erythropoiesis-stimulating agents have been used in human cancer patients in an effort to minimize the need for blood transfusions. Although the improvement in quality of life from resolution of anemia is unquestioned, concern exists about the effect of ESAs on tumor progression and patient survival times.[62] EPO may improve sensitivity to radiation therapy and chemotherapy by increasing tumor oxygenation, but it also promotes angiogenesis, which may support tumor growth.[5,63] There are no reports of the use of rHuEPO in veterinary cancer patients.

MYELODYSPLASTIC DISORDERS

Myelodysplastic syndrome (MDS) refers to myeloproliferative disorders associated with anemia, neutropenia, and/or thrombocytopenia with the presence of less than 30 per cent dysplastic hematopoietic precursor (blast) cells in the bone marrow (see Chapter 64). rHuEPO has been used successfully to treat human beings, cats, and dogs with MDS. Approximately 25 per cent of human patients with MDS respond to rHuEPO treatment.[64] Response to rHuEPO in four cats with PRCA not induced by rHuEPO administration was difficult to determine due to concurrent immunosuppressive therapy but appeared to be of no benefit in two cats.[33] There have been reports of successful treatment of myelodysplasia in dogs with rHuEPO in combination with immunosuppressive

therapy.[34,35] rHuEPO also has been used (in combination with immunosuppressive therapy) for the treatment of myelofibrosis in dogs.[37,65]

INTENSIVE CARE UNIT PATIENTS

Relative EPO deficiency has been well documented in critically ill patients.[66] Impaired iron availability may play a significant role in anemia associated with critical illness.[67] rHuEPO treatment appears to be most useful in critically ill patients who have a protracted ICU stay, which corresponds to a limited population in veterinary medicine.

VIRAL IMMUNOSUPPRESSIVE DISEASES

rHuEPO is indicated for treatment of anemic HIV-infected people receiving the antiviral agent zidovudine (AZT) who have low endogenous serum EPO levels. Of the 60 to 80 per cent of HIV patients on zidovudine who had low EPO levels, rHuEPO treatment reduced transfusion requirements by 43 per cent, and 17 per cent were transfusion-independent.[68,69] Transfusion requirements did not change in patients with endogenous EPO levels greater than 500 mU/mL. rHuEPO has been suggested as a treatment for anemic cats with FeLV infection, although many patients do not respond.[70] Serum EPO levels are elevated in anemic cats infected with FeLV,[30,31] so exogenous EPO would not be predicted to be helpful. A short course (2 weeks) of rHuEPO was effective at raising hematocrit in nonanemic FIV-infected cats and did not result in anti-rHuEPO antibody formation.[71]

PREOPERATIVE AUTOLOGOUS TRANSFUSIONS

rHuEPO is approved for use in anemic human patients preoperatively, and it has been used as an adjunct to preoperative autologous blood donation in people and dogs.[72,73] Preoperative autologous transfusions have been used successfully in cats with meningiomas, but rHuEPO was not administered as part of the transfusion protocol.[74]

OTHER POTENTIAL USES

EPO has been used to treat myelotoxicity from adverse drug events. Although there are no reports of its use in cats for this indication, simultaneous treatment with rHuEPO and granulocyte colony-stimulating factor was used successfully in a dog with pancytopenia secondary to myelotoxicity from captopril, although it is unclear whether the bone marrow would have recovered without therapy.[36]

---

*References 4, 27, 48, 55, 57, 59, 60.

GUIDELINES FOR USE OF ERYTHROPOIESIS-STIMULATING AGENTS

The decision to treat anemia is based on a variety of factors. Cats can adapt to slowly developing anemia and may exhibit minimal clinical signs. The risks associated with the available treatment options always must be weighed against the benefit of diminishing the anemia. Because 50 to 70 per cent of cats treated with rHuEPO develop adverse events (unpublished data, Langston and Kittrell, 2006), treatment is recommended only if clinical signs are present.[27] Clinical signs include exercise intolerance, tachypnea, tachycardia, development of a new heart murmur or worsening of a preexisting murmur, anorexia, or lethargy.[75] Therapy is reserved for patients with moderate to severe anemia that is not attributable to transient causes of anemia (e.g., bleeding from gastric ulceration). Changes to this recommendation are not warranted until information about the risk of newer ESAs in cats and evidence of benefit of earlier treatment are available. rHuEPO and darbepoetin are not licensed for use in cats, and owners should provide informed consent prior to administration.

Hematocrit generally starts to increase within 1 to 2 weeks of starting ESA therapy and usually takes several weeks to achieve the target hematocrit. For immediately life-threatening anemia, or in cases in which relatively rapid control of anemia is desired, transfusion of blood-type and crossmatch-compatible red blood cells is the recommended treatment (see Chapter 61). Hemoglobin products (Oxyglobin) can be used in an emergency, but the duration of effect (1 to 2 days) renders it a temporary solution (see Chapter 60).

EPOETIN

The recommended starting dose is 100 U/kg SQ three times a week until the hematocrit is at the low end of the target range (25 to 30 per cent for cats), which usually takes 4 to 12 weeks. The dose then is reduced to twice-weekly administration until the hematocrit is in the middle of the target range. The maintenance dose usually is 50 to 100 U/kg once to twice weekly and is titrated to maintain the hematocrit in the middle of the target range. Higher doses have been advocated in human patients in ICU or for preoperative autologous blood transfusions.

DARBEPOETIN

The recommended starting dose for darbepoetin for people is 0.45 μg/kg SQ or IV once weekly. The frequency of administration can be decreased to every second week once the hematocrit has reached the low end of the target range. Few patients are able to maintain the target hematocrit with administration every three weeks. In the author's experience, most cats started at 0.45 μg/kg required a dose increase, and now I routinely start at 1 μg/kg. For patients being converted from rHuEPO

Table 66-2 Conversion of Epoetin to Darbepoetin Dosing Chart

Epoetin (IU/wk)	Darbepoetin (μg/wk)
<2500	6.25
2500-4999	12.5
5000-10,999	25
11,000-17,999	40
18,000-33,999	60
34,000-90,000	100
>90,000	200

Box 66-1 Key Points About Erythropoiesis-Stimulating Agent Use in Cats

KEY POINTS
rHuEPO
    Administer 100 U/kg three times a week
    Decrease to 50-100 U/kg once or twice weekly
    Monitor for PRCA, develops in 25 per cent of patients
Darbepoetin
    Administer 0.45-1 μg/kg once weekly, decreasing to every 2nd or 3rd week
    Monitor for PRCA, risk of PRCA unknown
Routine monitoring
    Perform physical examination, hematocrit, reticulocyte count, blood pressure
        Weekly during loading period (until target hematocrit reached)
        Every other week when maintenance dose is stable
        Eventually monthly
Administer iron at start of therapy; monitor and supplement as needed

therapy, 200 U of rHuEPO is equivalent to 1 μg of darbepoetin, or a conversion chart (Table 66-2) can be used. Some clinicians have adopted a set dose of 6.25 μg per cat once weekly, regardless of body weight.

MONITORING

Regular monitoring of response to therapy is required for optimal results (Box 66-1). The hematocrit and reticulocyte count should be checked weekly until the hematocrit has been stable for 4 weeks. Monthly monitoring usually is sufficient once the hematocrit has been stabilized. A complete blood count should be checked monthly to bimonthly for the duration of therapy. Blood pressure should be evaluated prior to therapy and at each visit after starting therapy.

ADJUVANT THERAPY: IRON

Iron administration in conjunction with ESA therapy is necessary for maximal response.[16,27,76] Human patients

...ments					
...on Product	Route of Administration	How Supplied	Elemental Iron	Daily Dose*
	IM	100 mg/mL	100 mg/mL	50 mg/mo
...Pet-Tinic	PO	2.82 mg/mL		3.5-7 mL
Ferrous fumarate	Favor	PO	5 mg		2-4 tabs
Ferrous sulfate	Feosol	PO	44 mg/mL	8.8 mg/mL	1-2 mL
Ferrous sulfate	Slow FE	PO	160 mg	50 mg	$\frac{1}{4}$-$\frac{1}{2}$ tab
Ferrous sulfate		PO	325 mg	65 mg	$\frac{1}{8}$-$\frac{1}{4}$ tab
Ferrous gluconate		PO	325 mg	35 mg	$\frac{1}{4}$ tab

*Recommended daily dose (except where noted otherwise) for a 5-kg cat.
mo, Monthly dose.

treated with iron had higher hemoglobin levels and required a lower dose of rHuEPO to maintain the target hemoglobin level.[77] Despite iron administration, iron indices in people do not rise during initial rHuEPO therapy, indicating that large amounts of iron are being utilized.[17] In dogs, iron indices actually decreased, despite oral iron supplementation.[17] Although oral iron is inexpensive, it is poorly absorbed and gastrointestinal side effects limit compliance in people. Intramuscular iron dextran injections (50 mg/cat IM monthly or based on iron parameters) may be a practical therapy. Various oral iron supplements are available (Table 66-3).

Monitoring iron parameters is recommended in human patients prior to and 1 month after starting EPO therapy and then monthly to bimonthly thereafter. A serum iron panel consisting of serum iron (a measure of mobile iron), total iron-binding capacity (an indirect measure of transferrin, the carrier molecule for iron in the serum), and ferritin (a storage form of iron) is preferred. Hemosiderin is a storage form present in the bone marrow that can be estimated by evaluating a bone marrow aspirate when necessary. The transferrin saturation can be calculated from the equation:

% saturation = serum iron ÷ total iron-binding capacity

and represents the amount of transferrin that is bound to iron. Transferrin saturation normally is about 33 per cent.[78,79] The mean hemoglobin content of reticulocytes (CHr) is a measure of iron status in human beings that is more sensitive than other methods. It may prove to be a reliable early indicator in veterinary medicine, but limited data are available as yet.[80,81]

Diagnosing iron deficiency is not always a straightforward matter. Serum iron can be decreased by infection or inflammation in addition to iron deficiency, whereas ferritin is an acute-phase protein that can be increased by infection or inflammation.

COMPLICATIONS OF THE USE OF ERYTHROPOIETIN

Adverse events reported in cats and dogs receiving rHuEPO include refractory anemia, systemic hypertension, polycythemia, seizures, vomiting, iron deficiency,

injection discomfort, skin reactions, cellulitis, cutaneous or mucocutaneous reactions, fever, arthralgia, and PRCA.[55] The adverse effects of darbepoetin in human trials are similar to those of epoetin. One would expect the same to hold true in veterinary patients.

Hypertension has been associated with EPO therapy in both people and animals. EPO causes vascular vasoconstriction from increased cytoplasmic calcium concentrations, which leads to resistance to the vasodilatory action of nitric oxide.[5] Increases in blood pressure developed in 40 to 50 per cent of cats and dogs treated with EPO, and the author's clinical experience corroborates this observation.[27] Therapy for hypertension may need to be started or intensified.

Seizures have been reported in association with EPO administration. Two of 11 cats and one of six dogs in one series developed seizures,[27] as did an additional cat in a case report.[57] Of 53 cats and 11 dogs treated with rHuEPO at the Animal Medical Center in New York City, one cat and one dog developed seizures terminally. In most animals, seizures were associated with moderate to severe azotemia, and hypertension was documented in the three patients in whom blood pressure was measured. The etiology of seizures is uncertain, but it is thought to be related to compensatory adaptations to increases in red blood cell mass and not to rHuEPO directly.[27] However, uremia and hypertension (independent of rHuEPO use) are associated with seizures.[82,83]

Injection discomfort or skin reactions are reported in human beings, but are not recognized commonly in animal patients. In one study of 11 cats and six dogs, one cat and one dog developed hypersensitivity-like reactions.[27] The manifestations resolved within days of discontinuing the drug and did not recur when administration was reinstituted. rHuEPO preparations contain human serum albumin, which may be antigenic to animals.

Polycythemia can occur with an excessive dose of EPO.[27] Adequate monitoring with appropriate dose adjustment will prevent its occurrence. It will resolve with decreasing the dose.

Refractory anemia in patients on rHuEPO therapy has many potential causes. A careful review of the patient and the clinical pathology results may indicate iron deficiency, ongoing blood loss, or anemia of chronic inflammatory disease. More than 75 per cent of human patients who fail to respond to rHuEPO have underlying infection or inflammation.[84] In a retrospective study of cats, 25 per cent of patients did not reach the target hematocrit and were suspected of having infection or inflammation (unpublished data, Langston and Kittrell, 2006). Higher doses of rHuEPO do not overcome the resistance; control of the infection or inflammatory state is necessary. Refractory anemia may represent formation of anti-rHuEPO antibodies causing PRCA.

PURE RED CELL APLASIA

Antibodies to native EPO have been described rarely in people with PRCA.[85,86] Prior to 1998, there were only three reports of this condition in human beings; however, to date more than 400 people have been identified with this complication.[87-91] Although all types of EPO (including epoetin alfa, epoetin beta, and darbepoetin) have been involved, the majority of cases involved a particular brand supplied in prefilled syringes. Identification and removal of the risk factors (replacement of human serum albumin with glycine and polysorbate 80, SQ administration, and leachates from the rubber stoppers of the syringes) caused the incidence of this condition to wane after 2003.[91]

Antibodies directed against rHuEPO can develop because rHuEPO is dissimilar antigenically to both canine and feline EPO. These antibodies appear to cross-react with native EPO. Antibodies to rHuEPO developed in 63 to 100 per cent of healthy dogs receiving rHuEPO, and 22 to 100 per cent developed a concurrent anemia.[16,92] In cats and dogs with naturally occurring CKD treated with rHuEPO, five of seven cats treated for more than 180 days, and two of three dogs treated for more than 90 days, developed refractory anemia attributed to anti-rHuEPO antibodies.[27] Similarly, eight of 37 cats and two of seven dogs treated more than 21 days at the Animal Medical Center in New York City developed refractory anemia. Therefore 20 to 70 per cent of patients will develop a clinically significant immunological reaction to rHuEPO. Antibodies usually develop within the first few months of administration, although a later onset could occur.

Pure red cell aplasia seems less common in cats treated with darbepoetin compared to rHuEPO. Of 18 cats treated for 30 days or longer by the author, none were known to have developed PRCA, although two cats had progressive anemia with low reticulocyte counts immediately prior to death. At least one dog has been documented by bone marrow cytological examination to have PRCA following darbepoetin administration. More experience is needed to estimate the real risk of PRCA with darbepoetin therapy in cats.

The primary sign of anti-rHuEPO antibodies is a precipitously declining hematocrit. Reticulocyte counts will decrease to zero prior to the reduction in hematocrit. There currently is no commercially available test for the presence of antibodies. Bone marrow aspiration cytology may show a very high myeloid-to-erythroid ratio (typically M:E >8:1), ranging from 2.5:1 to 299:1 (Figure 66-3).[16,27]

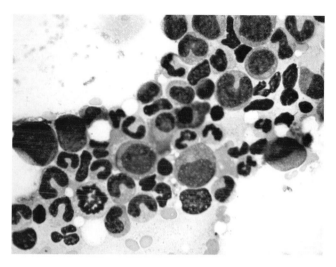

Figure 66-3 Micrograph of bone marrow aspiration cytological specimen showing pure red cell aplasia secondary to rHuEPO administration in a cat. The myeloid precursors seen here are present in normal numbers and are maturing normally. No erythroid precursors are present. The megakaryocytic cell line was normal. (1000×.) (Courtesy Dr. Andrew S. Loar, Animal Medical Center, New York.)

If anti-rHuEPO antibodies are suspected, administration of rHuEPO is discontinued, and blood transfusions will be required. The antibody concentration can decline to a subclinical level over 2 to 12 months and the hematocrit can return to the pretreatment level. Although anti-rHuEPO antibodies can be a reversible problem, blood cross-match compatibility problems with repeated transfusions, the cost of repeated transfusions, and the persistence of the pretreatment level of anemia frequently lead to the death or euthanasia of the affected cat.

Approximately 66 per cent of human patients with PRCA were treated with immunosuppressive drugs. The condition resolved in about one third of the patients, with the majority in the group receiving immunosuppressive therapy (57 per cent vs. 2 per cent).[93] A variety of immunosuppressive strategies were used. Although successful reintroduction of a different ESA in human patients after resolution of PRCA has been reported, this is not recommended because of the high degree of homology between most ESAs. Hematide, a small-protein ESA with a structure unrelated to other ESAs, has been used to "rescue" rats with rHuEPO-induced PRCA and may play a role in treatment of cats with PRCA if it becomes available commercially.[22]

SUMMARY

EPO is a hematopoietic growth factor that is decreased in feline chronic kidney disease. Administration of EPO treats hypoproliferative anemia associated with feline chronic kidney disease effectively and thereby improves the quality of life of these cats. Other uses of EPO are poorly characterized in feline medicine. Careful monitoring of therapy is necessary for optimal results. Several complications are associated with the use of rHuEPO in feline patients. The production of anti-rHuEPO antibodies is the most significant and can be a life-threatening event. Darbepoetin appears to pose a lower risk of this complication compared to rHuEPO. Alternatives to human EPO are being sought for cats to provide the beneficial effects while avoiding antibody formation.

REFERENCES

1. Eschbach JW: The anemia of chronic renal failure: pathophysiology and the effects of recombinant erythropoietin, *Kidney Int* 35:134, 1989.
2. Car B: Erythropoiesis and erythrokinetics. In Feldman BF, Zinkl JG, Jain NC, editors: *Schalm's veterinary hematology*, ed 5, Philadelphia, 2000, Lippincott Williams & Wilkins, p 105.
3. Macdougall IC: Novel erythropoiesis-stimulating agents: a new era in anemia management, *Clin J Am Soc Nephrol* 3:200, 2008.
4. Giger U: Erythropoietin and its clinical use, *Compend Contin Educ Pract Vet* 14:25, 1992.
5. Fisher JW: Erythropoietin: physiology and pharmacology update, *Exp Biol Med* 228:1, 2003.
6. Duncan R, Prasse K: Erythrocytes. In Duncan R, Prasse K, editors: *Veterinary laboratory medicine*, ed 2, Ames, 1986, Iowa State University Press, p 4.
7. Bunn H: Erythropoietin: current status, *Yale J Biol Med* 63:381, 1990.
8. Egrie JC, Strickland TW, Lane J, et al: Characterization and biological effects of recombinant human erythropoietin, *Immunobiology* 172:213, 1986.
9. Storring PL, Tiplady RJ, Gaines Das RE, et al: Epoetin alfa and beta differ in their erythropoietin isoform compositions and biological properties, *Br J Haematol* 100:79, 1998.
10. Locatelli F, Del Vecchio L, Marai P: Clinical experience with darbepoetin-alfa (Aranesp), *Contrib Nephrol* 137:403, 2002.
11. Macdougall IC: Darbepoetin alfa: a new therapeutic agent for renal anemia, *Kidney Int* 61:S55, 2002.
12. Macdougall IC, Padhi D, Jang G: Pharmacology of darbepoetin alfa, *Nephrol Dial Transplant* 22:iv2, 2007.
13. MacLeod JN, Tetreault JW, Lorschy KAS, et al: Expression and bioactivity of recombinant canine erythropoietin, *Am J Vet Res* 59:1144, 1998.
14. MacLeod JN: Species-specific recombinant erythropoietin preparations for companion animals. Proceedings of the 19th ACVIM Forum, Denver, CO: 578, 2001.
15. Randolph JF, Scarlett JM, Stokol T, et al: Expression, bioactivity, and clinical assessment of recombinant feline erythropoietin, *Am J Vet Res* 65:1355, 2004.
16. Randolph JF, Stokol T, Scarlett JM, et al: Comparison of biological activity and safety of recombinant canine erythropoietin with that of recombinant human erythropoietin in clinically normal dogs, *Am J Vet Res* 60:636, 1999.
17. Randolph JF, Scarlett JM, Stokol T, et al: Clinical efficacy and safety of recombinant canine erythropoietin in dogs with anemia of chronic renal failure and dogs with recombinant human erythropoietin-induced red cell aplasia, *J Vet Intern Med* 18:81, 2004.
18. Beall CJ, Phipps AJ, Mathes LE, et al: Transfer of the feline erythropoietin gene to cats using a recombinant adeno-associated virus vector, *Gene Ther* 7:534, 2000.
19. Walker MC, Mandell TC, Crawford C, et al: Expression of erythropoietin in cats treated with a recombinant adeno-associated viral vector, *Am J Vet Res* 66:450, 2005.
20. Levy JK, Walker M, Byrne B: Gene therapy in companion animals: lessons from feline erythropoietin. Proceedings of the 19th ACVIM Forum, Denver, CO: 580, 2001.
21. Macdougall IC, Robson R, Opatrna S, et al: Pharmacokinetics and pharmacodynamics of intravenous and subcutaneous continuous erythropoietin receptor activator (C.E.R.A.) in patients with chronic kidney disease, *Clin J Am Soc Nephrol* 1:1211, 2006.
22. Woodburn KW, Fan Q, Winslow S, et al: Hematide is immunologically distinct from erythropoietin and corrects anemia induced by antierythropoietin antibodies in a rat pure red cell aplasia model, *Exp Hematol* 35:1201, 2007.
23. Fishbane S, Masani N: Anemia in chronic kidney disease. In Pereira BJG, Sayegh MH, Blake P, editors: *Chronic kidney disease, dialysis, and transplantation*, ed 2, Philadelphia, 2005, Elsevier Saunders, p 122.
24. Xia H, Ebben J, Ma JZ, et al: Hematocrit levels and hospitalization risks in hemodialysis patients, *J Am Soc Nephrol* 10:1309, 1999.
25. Moreno F, Sanz-Guajardo D, Lopez-Gomez JM, et al: Increasing the hematocrit has a beneficial effect on quality of life and is safe in selected hemodialysis patients, *J Am Soc Nephrol* 11:335, 2000.
26. Langston CE: New concepts in anemia management. Advanced Renal Therapies Symposium, 2006.
27. Cowgill LD, James KM, Levy JK, et al: Use of recombinant human erythropoietin for management of anemia in dogs and cats with renal failure, *J Am Vet Med Assoc* 212:521, 1998.
28. Rossert J, Froissart M, Jacquot C: Anemia management and chronic renal failure progression, *Kidney Int* 68:S76, 2005.
29. Gouva C, Nikolopoulos P, Ioannidis JPA, et al: Treating anemia early in renal failure slows the decline of renal function: A randomized controlled trial, *Kidney Int* 66:753, 2004.
30. Wardrop KJ, Kramer JW, Abkowitz JL, et al: Quantitative studies of erythropoiesis in the clinically normal, phlebotomized, and feline leukemia virus-infected cats, *Am J Vet Res* 47:2274, 1986.
31. Kociba GJ, Lange RD, Dunn CDR, et al: Serum erythropoietin changes in cats with feline leukemia virus-induced erythroid aplasia, *Vet Pathol* 20:548, 1983.
32. Arai M, Darmen J, Lewis A, et al: The use of human hematopoietic growth factors (rhGM-CSF and rhEPO) as a supportive therapy for FIV-infected cats, *Vet Immunol Immunopathol* 77:71, 2000.
33. Stokol T, Blue J: Pure red cell aplasia in cats: 9 cases (1989-1997), *J Am Vet Med Assoc* 214:75, 1999.
34. Boone L, Knauer K, Rapp S, et al: Use of human recombinant erythropoietin and prednisone for treatment of myelodysplastic syndrome with erythroid predominance in a dog, *J Am Vet Med Assoc* 213:999, 1998.
35. Weiss D, Smith S: Primary myelodysplastic syndromes of dogs: a report of 12 cases, *J Vet Intern Med* 14:491, 2000.
36. Holland M, Stobie D, Shapiro W: Pancytopenia associated with administration of captopril to a dog, *J Am Vet Med Assoc* 208:1683, 1996.
37. Weiss D, Smith S: A retrospective study of 19 cases of canine myelofibrosis, *J Vet Intern Med* 16:174, 2002.
38. Suzuki K: Use of recombinant human erythropoietin as adjuvant therapy for blood banking for autotransfusion in dogs, *Vet J* 155:239, 1998.
39. Elliott J, Barber PJ: Feline chronic renal failure: clinical findings in 80 cases diagnosed between 1992 and 1995, *J Small Anim Pract* 39:78, 1998.
40. Lulich JP, Osborne CA, O'Brien TD, et al: Feline renal failure: questions, answers, questions, *Compend Contin Educ Pract Vet* 14:127, 1992.
41. DiBartola SP, Rutgers HC, Zack PM, et al: Clinicopathologic findings associated with chronic renal disease in cats: 74 cases (1973-1984), *J Am Vet Med Assoc* 190:1196, 1987.

42. Remuzzi G, Rossi EC: Hematologic consequences of renal failure. In Brenner BM, editor: *Brenner and Rector's the kidney*, ed 5, Philadelphia, 1996, WB Saunders, p 2170.

43. King LG, Giger U, Diserens D, et al: Anemia of chronic renal failure in dogs, *J Vet Intern Med* 6:264, 1992.

44. Himmelfarb J: Hematologic manifestations of renal failure. In Greenberg A, editor: *Primer on kidney diseases*, ed 2, New York, 1998, Academic Press, p 465.

45. Eschbach JW, Adamson JW: Anemia of end-stage renal disease (ESRD), *Kidney Int* 28:1, 1985.

46. McGonigle RJS, Wallin JD, Shadduck RK, et al: Erythropoietin deficiency and inhibition of erythropoiesis in renal insufficiency, *Kidney Int* 25:437, 1984.

47. Petrites-Murphy MB, Pierce KR, Fisher JW: Effect of incorporation of serum from dogs with renal impairment on canine erythroid bone marrow cultures, *Am J Vet Res* 50:1537, 1989.

48. Polzin DJ, Osborne CA, Jacob F, et al: Chronic renal failure. In Ettinger SJ, Feldman EC, editors: *Textbook of veterinary internal medicine*, ed 5, Philadelphia, 2000, WB Saunders, p 1634.

49. Watson ADJ, Canfield PJ: Nutritional deficiency anemias. In Feldman BF, Zinkl JG, Jain NC, editors: *Schalm's veterinary hematology*, ed 5, Philadelphia, 2000, Lippincott Williams & Wilkins, p 190.

50. Boxer M, Ellman L, Geller R, et al: Anemia in primary hyperparathyroidism, *Arch Intern Med* 137:588, 1977.

51. Zingraff J, Drueke T, Marie P, et al: Anemia and secondary hyperparathyroidism, *Arch Intern Med* 138:1650, 1978.

52. Barbour GL: Effect of parathyroidectomy on anemia in chronic renal failure, *Arch Intern Med* 139:889, 1979.

53. Cook SM, Lothrop CDJ: Serum erythropoietin concentrations measured by radioimmunoassay in normal, polycythemic, and anemic dogs and cats, *J Vet Intern Med* 8:18, 1994.

54. Pechereau D, Martel P, Braun JP: Plasma erythropoietin concentrations in dogs and cats: reference values and changes with anaemia and/or chronic renal failure, *Res Vet Sci* 62:185, 1997.

55. Cowgill LD: Pathophysiology and management of anemia in chronic progressive renal failure, *Semin Vet Med Surg (Small Anim)* 7:175, 1992.

56. Harkin KR, Cowan LA, Andrews GA, et al: Hepatotoxicity of stanozolol in cats, *J Am Vet Med Assoc* 217:681, 2000.

57. Bloomberg RM, Pook HA, Jacobs RM, et al: Human recombinant erythropoietin therapy in a cat with chronic renal failure, *Can Vet J* 33:612, 1992.

58. Henry P: Human recombinant erythropoietin used to treat a cat with anemia caused by chronic renal failure, *Can Vet J* 35:375, 1994.

59. Cowgill LD: Application of recombinant human erythropoietin in dogs and cats. In Kirk RW, Bonagura JD, editors: *Current veterinary therapy XI*, Philadelphia, 1992, WB Saunders, p 484.

60. Cowgill LD: CVT update: use of recombinant human erythropoietin. In Bonagura JD, editor: *Current veterinary therapy XII*, Philadelphia, 1995, WB Saunders, p 961.

61. Beguin Y: Prediction of response and other improvements on the limitations of recombinant human erythropoietin therapy in anemic cancer patients, *Haematologica* 87:1209, 2002.

62. Glaspy JA: Erythropoiesis-stimulating agents in oncology, *J Natl Compr Canc Netw* 6:565, 2008.

63. Ludwig H: rHuEPO and treatment outcomes: the preclinical experience, *Oncologist* 9(suppl5):48, 2004.

64. Langston CE, Reine NJ, Kittrell D: The use of erythropoietin, *Vet Clin North Am Small Anim Pract* 33:1245, 2003.

65. Manire C, Rhinehart H: Use of human recombinant erythropoietin for the treatment of nonregenerative anemia in a rough-toothed dolphin (Steno bredanensis), *J Zoo Wildl Med* 31:157, 2000.

66. Rogiers P, Zhang H, Leeman M, et al: Erythropoietin response is blunted in critically ill patients, *Intensive Care Med* 23:159, 1997.

67. van Iperen CE, Gaillard C, Kraaijenhagen R, et al: Response of erythropoiesis and iron metabolism to recombinant human erythropoietin in intensive care unit patients, *Crit Care Med* 28:2773, 2000.

68. *Epogen (Epoetin alfa) for Injection*, Thousand Oaks, Calif, 1999, Amgen.

69. Fischl M, Galpin JE, Levine JD, et al: Recombinant human erythropoietin for patients with AIDS treated with zidovudine, *N Engl J Med* 322:1488, 1990.

70. Levy JK: FeLV and non-neoplastic FeLV-related disease. In Ettinger SJ, Feldman EC, editors: *Textbook of veterinary internal medicine*, ed 5, Philadelphia, 2000, WB Saunders, p 424.

71. Arai M, Darman J, Lewis A, et al: The use of human hematopoietic growth factors (rhGM-CSF and rhEPO) as a supportive therapy for FIV-infected cats, *Vet Immunol Immunopathol* 78:217, 2001.

72. Goodnough LT, Rudnick S, Price TH, et al: Increased preoperative collection of autologous blood with recombinant human erythropoietin therapy, *N Engl J Med* 321:1163, 1989.

73. Goodnough LT, Price TH, Friedman KD, et al: A phase III trial of recombinant human erythropoietin therapy in nonanemic orthopedic patients subjected to aggressive removal of blood for autologous use: dose, response, toxicity, and efficacy, *Transfusion* 34:66, 1994.

74. Fusco JV, Hohenhaus AE, Aiken SW, et al: Autologous blood collection and transfusion in cats undergoing partial craniectomy, *J Am Vet Med Assoc* 216:1584, 2000.

75. Kerl ME, Langston CE: Treatment of anemia of chronic kidney disease. In Bonagura JD, Twedt DC, editors: *Current veterinary therapy XIV*, Philadelphia, 2009, Elsevier Saunders, p 913.

76. Eschbach JW, Abdulhadi MH, Browne JK, et al: Recombinant human erythropoietin in anemic patients with end-stage renal disease: results of a phase III multicenter clinical trial, *Ann Intern Med* 111:992, 1989.

77. Schiesser D, Binet I, Tsinalis D, et al: Weekly low-dose treatment with intravenous iron sucrose maintains iron status and decreases epoetin requirement in iron-replete haemodialysis patients, *Nephrol Dial Transplant* 21:2841, 2006.

78. Smith JE: Iron metabolism in dogs and cats, *Compend Contin Educ Pract Vet* 14:39, 1992.

79. Stone MS, Freden GO: Differentiation of anemia of inflammatory disease from anemia of iron deficiency, *Compend Contin Educ Pract Vet* 12:963, 1990.

80. Steinberg JD, Olver CS: Hematologic and biochemical abnormalities indicating iron deficiency are associated with decreased reticulocyte hemoglobin content (CHr) and reticulocyte volume (rMCV) in dogs, *Vet Clin Pathol* 34:23, 2005.

81. Fry MM, Kirk CA: Reticulocyte indices in a canine model of nutritional iron deficiency, *Vet Clin Pathol* 35:172, 2006.

82. Wolf AM: Canine uremic encephalopathy, *J Am Anim Hosp Assoc* 16:735, 1980.

83. Jacob F, Polzin DJ, Osborne CA, et al: Association between initial systolic blood pressure and risk of developing a uremic crisis or of dying in dogs with chronic renal failure, *J Am Vet Med Assoc* 222:322, 2003.

84. Macdougall IC: Role of uremic toxins in exacerbating anemia in renal failure, *Kidney Int* 59:S67, 2001.

85. Casadevall N, Dupuy E, Molho-Sabatier P, et al: Brief report: autoantibodies against erythropoietin in a patient with pure red-cell aplasia, *N Engl J Med* 334:630, 1996.

86. Peschle C, Marmont AM, Marone G, et al: Pure red cell aplasia: studies on an IgG serum inhibitor neutralizing erythropoietin, *Br J Haematol* 30:411, 1975.

87. Prabhakar SS, Muhlfelder T: Antibodies to recombinant human erythropoietin causing pure red cell aplasia, *Clin Nephrol* 47:331, 1977.

88. Casadevall N, Nataf J, Viron B, et al: Pure red-cell aplasia and antierythropoietin antibodies in patients treated with recombinant erythropoietin, *N Engl J Med* 346:469, 2002.

89. Gershon SK, Luksenburg H, Cote TR, et al: Pure red-cell aplasia and recombinant erythropoietin (letter), *N Engl J Med* 346:1584, 2002.

90. Casadevall N, Mayeux P: Pure red-cell aplasia and recombinant erythropoietin (author reply), *N Engl J Med* 346:1585, 2002.

91. Pollock C, Johnson DW, Horl WH, et al: Pure red cell aplasia induced by erythropoiesis-stimulating agents, *Clin J Am Soc Nephrol* 3:193, 2008.

92. Cowgill LD, Neal L, Egrie JC, et al: Antigenicity of recombinant human erythropoietin (r-HuEPO) in normal dogs (abstract), *J Vet Intern Med* 8:167, 1994.

93. Bennett CL, Cournoyer D, Carson KR, et al: Long-term outcome of individuals with pure red cell aplasia and antierythropoietin antibodies in patients treated with recombinant epoetin: a follow-up report from the Research on Adverse Drug Events and Reports (RADAR) Project, *Blood* 106:3343, 2005.

Oncology

Kenita S. Rogers, Section Editor

67 Mast Cell Tumors

Corey F. Saba

Mast cells are normal inflammatory cells that play a critical role in type I hypersensitivity reactions. They are produced in the bone marrow, enter the blood, and mature in connective tissues. They are found normally in a variety of organs including skin, lymph nodes, bone marrow, gastrointestinal tract, and respiratory tract. Mast cells are large (20 to 30 microns in diameter) round cells, with eccentric nuclei. They often are easily identified by their associated metachromatic granules, best seen with toluidine blue, Giemsa, and Romanowsky stains (Figure 67-1). These granules contain biologically active amines, including, but not limited to, histamine and heparin. As a result, significant mast cell degranulation can lead to complications including gastrointestinal ulceration, hypersensitivity reactions, coagulation disorders, and/or decreased wound healing.[1,2]

Neoplastic proliferation of mast cells results in the formation of a mast cell tumor (MCT). In cats MCTs typically present in one of three forms: cutaneous, visceral-splenic, and visceral-intestinal. Cats present occasionally with concomitant forms, but the relationship between these tumors remains unclear.[2-4]

ETIOLOGY OF MAST CELL TUMORS

The etiology of feline MCT is unknown and possibly multifactorial. A genetic predisposition seems plausible because of the high incidence of cutaneous MCTs in Siamese cats.[5,6] Association with feline leukemia virus (FeLV) and feline immunodeficiency virus (FIV) has not been reported.[3] Studies of canine MCTs have demonstrated mutations in the protooncogene c-kit. Most commonly these mutations consist of internal tandem duplications in exons 11 and 12. It is believed that such mutations result in dysregulation of the tyrosine kinase receptor Kit, leading to progression of mast cell disease.[7-9] The role of c-kit mutations in feline MCT is controversial. In a study of 10 formalin-fixed feline splenic MCTs, no such mutations were identified by means of polymerase chain reaction (PCR). Based on these results, the authors concluded that Kit dysregulation was an unlikely cause of splenic MCT in cats.[10] In a separate study, mast cells were aspirated from the tumor of a cat with systemic mastocytosis. An internal tandem duplication was identified in exon 8 within the c-kit cDNA of this patient. The cat subsequently was treated with imatinib mesylate (Gleevec), a protein tyrosine kinase inhibitor with selectivity for c-kit in human beings (as well as Bcr-Abl and platelet-derived growth factor),[11] and had a favorable response.[12]

FELINE MAST CELL TUMORS: CUTANEOUS

EPIDEMIOLOGY

Cutaneous MCTs are the second most common skin tumor in cats, accounting for up to 21 per cent of all reported skin tumors. Historically this was thought to be a much less common disease. However, more recent analysis has suggested that the lesions were misdiagnosed previously as eosinophilic granuloma.[5] Cutaneous MCTs generally are categorized into one of three distinct histological forms—compact mastocytic, diffuse mastocytic, or histiocytic. Mastocytic forms of MCTs occur most commonly and are similar histologically to MCTs in dogs. The compact or well-differentiated mastocytic form is most

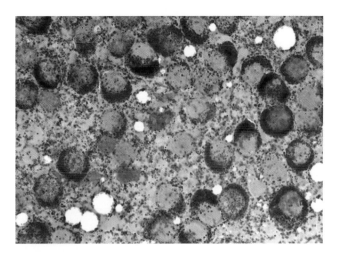

Figure 67-1 Intact feline mast cells with free granules in the background from an imprint of a splenic MCT. (Wright's stain. 1000×.) (Courtesy Dr. Bruce LeRoy.)

common, comprising 50 to 90 per cent of cutaneous MCTs in cats. These tumors are well circumscribed and superficial. Neoplastic mast cells appear well differentiated and are accompanied by few eosinophils. Mitotic figures are infrequent, and this form is associated with a more benign behavior.[13-15] The diffuse or anaplastic mastocytic form is far less common. Neoplastic mast cells are poorly differentiated with marked anisocytosis, and they often are accompanied by many eosinophils. Diffuse mastocytic MCTs are very infiltrative and generally have a more malignant behavior.[13-15] The histiocytic form is rare and usually is seen on the heads of young Siamese cats. Clinically they occur as deep dermal or subcutaneous papulonodular lesions. Histologically there is a mixed population of well-differentiated mast cells, histiocytes, eosinophils, and lymphocytes. These tumors often regress spontaneously.[5,6,14,15] The remainder of this section will focus on the compact mastocytic MCT.

Cutaneous MCTs occur typically in middle-age to older cats. However, they can affect cats of any age, and as mentioned, the histiocytic form of the disease occurs most commonly in young cats less than 4 years of age.[4,5,15-17] Studies have suggested that Siamese cats are predisposed to both mastocytic and histiocytic MCTs, but no definitive gender predilection has been identified.[5,6]

CLINICAL SIGNS

Cutaneous MCTs are often solitary, raised, well-circumscribed hairless nodules (Figure 67-2), but they occur also as flat, plaquelike, and sometimes ulcerated lesions. They typically involve the dermis, but in some cases may extend into the subcutis.[14,15,18] They are located most commonly on the head and neck, especially at the base of the pinna, but also may be seen on the trunk and limbs.[2,4,5,16,19] They generally are small in size but range from 0.2 to 5 cm.[2,13] Up to 43 per cent of cases present with multiple MCTs.[16]

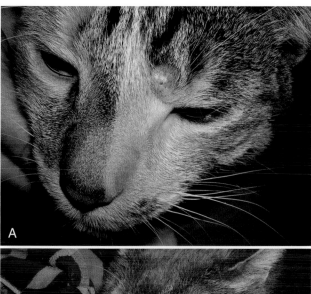

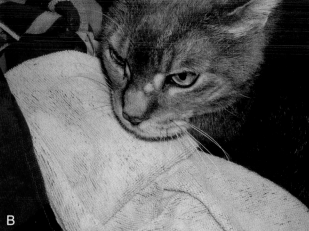

Figure 67-2 A, Solitary cutaneous mastocytic mast cell tumor on the head of a cat. **B,** Solitary cutaneous mastocytic mast cell tumor on the head of a cat. (Courtesy Dr. Carrie Kosarek.)

DIAGNOSTIC EVALUATION

Metastasis to local lymph nodes and/or visceral organs is uncommon, occurring in 0 to 22 per cent of cases.[4,14,16,19] For this reason the utility of staging cats with solitary cutaneous MCTs is debatable. At a minimum, tumor measurements, fine-needle aspiration and cytological examination of the mass and regional lymph node, and thorough abdominal palpation with close attention to splenic size should be performed. Because cells within these tumors exfoliate well, MCTs often are diagnosed easily with cytological evaluation.[5] Photographs of the tumor also provide valuable information for the medical record. Other testing, including complete blood count, biochemical profile, FeLV antigen and FIV antibody tests, serum thyroxine (T$_4$), urinalysis, thoracic and abdominal imaging, bone marrow aspiration, and buffy coat smear, provides a more thorough clinical picture of the cat's overall health but rarely identifies disseminated disease. Staging cats with multiple cutaneous MCTs is recommended, because it has been proposed that the skin may be a metastatic site for visceral MCT.[4,20] Histopathological examination is useful in confirming the diagnosis of cuta-

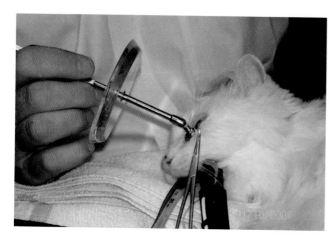

Figure 67-3 Strontium-90 irradiation.

neous MCT. However, it is important to note that tumor grade does not correlate with biological behavior or prognosis in cats, as it does in dogs.[16,18] Additionally, a study by Johnson failed to correlate cellular pleomorphism with outcome in cats with cutaneous MCT.[21]

TREATMENT

Surgical excision is a commonly used treatment for cutaneous MCTs, and in many cases, narrow margins are acceptable. The incidence of local recurrence is low (0 to 36 per cent), even in patients in whom the tumor is excised incompletely.[4,14,16,19] The role of postoperative radiation therapy in cats with incompletely excised MCTs has not been reported.

For small, superficial tumors, strontium 90β (Sr-90) radiation therapy may be considered when surgery is not feasible (Figure 67-3). Most commonly this treatment modality is used for tumors on the face, nasal planum, and eyelids. In a study investigating this treatment modality, 54 primary cutaneous MCTs in 35 cats were treated with a median dose of 135 Gy of Sr-90 irradiation. Local tumor control was achieved in 98 per cent of affected cats with a median follow-up of 783 days and a median survival of 1075 days. Adverse effects of the treatment, including alopecia, crusting, pruritus, leukotrichia, and thinning and depigmentation of skin, were mild and self-limiting.[22]

Chemotherapy is rarely indicated in the treatment of cutaneous MCTs, except in cases of metastatic and/or nonresectable disease. The role of chemotherapy is largely unknown, and treatment protocols frequently are extrapolated from those recommended for dogs.

PROGNOSIS

Overall, the prognosis for cats with cutaneous MCTs is good because the incidence of local recurrence and/or metastasis is low. However, multiple cutaneous tumors, recurrent tumors, and/or evidence of systemic disease all carry a more guarded prognosis.[4]

FELINE MAST CELL TUMORS: VISCERAL-SPLENIC

EPIDEMIOLOGY

Visceral MCT occurs more commonly in cats than in dogs. MCT is the most common tumor of the feline spleen, accounting for 15 per cent of all splenic diseases.[23] Affected cats typically are older, and no breed or sex predilections have been reported.[4,24,25]

CLINICAL SIGNS

Presenting complaints in cats with splenic MCTs are variable and nonspecific. Clinical signs may include decreased appetite, lethargy, weight loss, vomiting, and/or abdominal distension; however, some affected cats are asymptomatic. Physical examination usually reveals a massive, diffusely enlarged spleen. Abdominal effusion also may be noted.[16,24,26]

DIAGNOSTIC EVALUATION

Metastasis to organs including liver, lymph nodes, bone marrow, and lungs is far more common in cats with splenic MCT than in those patients with cutaneous MCT.[17,24,26] Therefore cats with suspected splenic MCT should be staged completely. Diagnosis often is obtained via fine-needle aspirate and cytological examination of the spleen, as well as affected lymph nodes and effusions if present. Anemia is noted in up to one third of cats with visceral MCT, and peripheral mastocytosis is noted in some cases.[17,24] Biochemical profile and urinalysis often are normal or reveal unrelated abnormalities; however, both provide insight into the overall health status of the cat. Thoracic radiographs are useful for evaluation of metastasis to lungs (occurring in approximately 20 per cent of cases) and in detection of neoplastic pleural effusions.[17] Abdominal imaging, both radiographs and ultrasound, also provides valuable information. Although not specific for splenic MCT, diffuse splenomegaly of varying severity is the most consistent finding, but discrete masses or nodules also may be seen. More commonly the spleen appears hypoechoic, but hyperechoic splenic changes have been reported.[26,27] In fact, it has been suggested that although uncommon, small hyperechoic nodules or diffuse hyperechogenicity may be specific findings for splenic MCT in cats. In addition to the splenic changes, neoplastic abdominal effusion is identified in up to one third of cases.[26] Other abdominal organs including lymph nodes and liver also should be evaluated thoroughly for metastatic disease.[17,24,26,27] Approximately 50 per cent of cats with splenic MCT have evidence of bone marrow and/or buffy coat involvement.[24] Bone marrow invasion without peripheral mastocytosis may occur, making bone marrow evaluation a more sensitive test than a buffy coat smear. However, buffy coat examination is a less invasive test to perform, and may have substantial diagnostic utility. In contrast to dogs, in whom buffy coat examinations are relatively insensitive and nonspecific for mast cell disease,[28] healthy cats and cats sick from non–mast-cell disease have negative buffy coat smears, possibly suggesting that a positive buffy coat is more likely to be specific for feline MCT.[29] Furthermore, if positive at diagnosis, the number of mast cells in the buffy coat smear may decline postoperatively, suggesting clinical remission of disease. In such cases, the buffy coat examination is a simple monitoring tool for disease remission and subsequent progression.[3] Coagulation profiles also are indicated; in one report, up to 90 per cent of cats with splenic MCT had coagulation abnormalities.[24]

TREATMENT

Splenectomy, even in cases with confirmed metastasis, is integral to the treatment of splenic MCT, and resolution of clinical signs reportedly often occurs after surgery.[30] The reported median survival times in cats treated with splenectomy alone is up to 19 months.[24,25] Prognostic factors associated with a worse outcome include anorexia, significant weight loss, and male gender.[24]

The role of chemotherapy in the treatment of feline MCT is largely unknown, and many oncologists use the same chemotherapy agents utilized in dogs. These include vinblastine, lomustine, cyclophosphamide, and prednisone, alone or in a variety of combinations.[31-34] In one report Rassnick and colleagues treated 38 cats with measurable MCT with lomustine at a target dose of 50 mg/m[2]. The reported overall response rate was 50 per cent, with a median duration of response of 168 days. In general the treatment was well tolerated, and neutropenia and thrombocytopenia were the most common toxicoses. Although the majority of the cats in the study had cutaneous MCTs, the results suggest that lomustine has antitumor activity against feline MCTs and may be considered a viable adjuvant treatment option for cats with more aggressive forms of the disease.[20] There are no reports on the role of prednisone in the treatment of feline MCT. When used in canine MCT, response rates of 20 to 70 per cent have been reported,[35,36] and anecdotally, similar responses have been seen in cats.

Because of the risk of complications associated with mast cell degranulation, including gastrointestinal ulceration and hypotensive shock, histamine blockers are indicated in cats with high disease burdens. H_1 blockers (famotidine, cimetidine, or ranitidine) and H_2 blockers (diphenhydramine) are believed to ameliorate these effects at least partially.[3] There is some evidence to suggest that serotonin is found in feline mast cells located within the respiratory tract[37]; therefore it has been proposed that cyproheptadine, a serotonin antagonist, may aid in symptomatic relief.[17,38] Other investigators have suggested that mast cells are not homogeneous, and that there may be morphological and histochemical differences between mast cells of varying anatomical sites within the same species.[39] Based on this argument, the exact content of granules from MCTs from various sites is unknown. Although future studies may help to clarify this issue, for now it is best to provide symptomatic care on a case-by-case basis.

PROGNOSIS

Overall the prognosis for cats with splenic MCT is guarded, because the incidence of metastasis is high. However, cats with disseminated disease have experienced return to good qualities of life and long survival times following splenectomy. Additionally, future studies evaluating chemotherapy may help to improve the prognosis for this disease.

FELINE MAST CELL TUMORS: VISCERAL-INTESTINAL

EPIDEMIOLOGY

Of the three common forms, intestinal MCT is the least common. MCT is the third most common intestinal tumor in cats, with lymphoma and adenocarcinoma occurring more frequently.[17] As with splenic MCTs, intestinal MCTs usually affect older cats, and no breed or gender predilections have been reported.[17,39,40]

CLINICAL SIGNS

Presenting complaints in cats with intestinal MCTs are variable and nonspecific; clinical signs may include lethargy, inappetence, weight loss, vomiting, and/or diarrhea. Intraabdominal mass(es) and/or diffusely thickened intestines may be palpated on physical examination. Masses are located most commonly in the small intestine. Abdominal effusion also may be noted.[17,39-41]

DIAGNOSTIC EVALUATION

Widespread metastasis is extremely common in cats with intestinal MCT.[17,40] Therefore these patients should be staged completely as described for splenic MCT. Diagnosis often is obtained via fine-needle aspiration and cytological examination of the intestinal mass, affected regional lymph nodes, and/or effusions if present. In contrast to cats with splenic MCT, circulating mastocytosis is seen uncommonly,[17,41] but eosinophilia has been reported.[41] Metastasis of MCT to lungs is rare; however, neoplastic pleural effusion has been detected. Abdominal imaging, both radiographs and ultrasound, likely provide the most diagnostic information. Solitary masses are common, but diffuse infiltrative disease also occurs. Loss of layering of the intestinal wall is noted commonly on ultrasound examination[27] (see Figure 16-33, C). As mentioned with splenic MCT staging, other abdominal organs including lymph nodes and liver should be evaluated thoroughly for metastatic disease.[17,27,40,41]

TREATMENT

Intestinal resection and anastomosis are often attempted in cases of intestinal MCT; however, it is important to note that wide resection of 5 to 10 cm of normal bowel on either side of the mass is recommended. Additionally, dehiscence is a concern because of the diffuse nature of this disease and the difficulty in achieving complete resection.[17] Unfortunately, the prognosis for cats with intestinal MCT treated with surgery alone is poor because of high rates of local recurrence and metastasis.[3]

The role of chemotherapy is, for the most part, unknown. Lomustine has shown some activity in the therapy of feline MCT, and should be considered in the treatment of intestinal MCT because of its aggressive biological behavior.[20] Haney and colleagues reported on the treatment response of 18 cats with intestinal MCT. Although various chemotherapy drugs and protocols were used, a favorable response rate of 61 per cent was noted. The median survival time was 240 days, and cats with weight loss had significantly shorter survival times compared with those without weight loss.[40]

Also in contrast to splenic MCTs, intestinal MCTs typically are not associated with gastric ulceration. In one study, evaluation of intestinal MCTs failed to demonstrate the typical metachromatic granules seen with cutaneous and splenic MCTs. Authors of this study concluded that intestinal MCTs may lack or be deficient in histamine, thereby explaining the absence of gastric ulceration in their series of affected cats.[39]

PROGNOSIS

Overall the prognosis for cats with intestinal MCT is poor. The incidences of recurrence and metastasis are high, and survival times are short. Future studies evaluating chemotherapy may help to improve the prognosis for this disease.

SUMMARY

Feline MCTs present and behave differently from similar tumors in dogs, and tumor location is a major predictor of behavior and prognosis in cats. In most cases, surgery is a cornerstone of treatment. Hopefully, future studies will help determine the usefulness of chemotherapy in treatment of the more aggressive forms of this disease.

REFERENCES

1. Scott MA, Stockham SL: Basophils and mast cells. In Feldman BF, Zinkl JG, Jain NC, editors: *Schalm's veterinary hematology*, ed 5, Philadelphia, 2000, Lippincott Williams & Wilkins, p 313.
2. Macy DW, Reynolds HA: The incidence, characteristics, and clinical management of skin tumors in cats, *J Am Anim Hosp Assoc* 17:1026, 1981.
3. Thamm DH, Vail DM: Mast cell tumors. In Withrow SJ, Vail DM, editors: *Withrow and MacEwen's small animal clinical oncology*, ed 4, St. Louis, 2007, Saunders, p 402.
4. Litster AL, Sorenmo KU: Characteristics of the signalment, clinical and survival characteristics of 41 cats with mast cell neoplasia, *J Feline Med Surg* 8:177, 2006.
5. Miller MA, Nelson SL, Turk JR, et al: Cutaneous neoplasia in 340 cats, *Vet Pathol* 28:389, 1991.
6. Chastain CB, Turk MAM, O'Brien D: Benign cutaneous mastocytomas in two litters of Siamese kittens, *J Am Vet Med Assoc* 193:959, 1988.
7. London CA, Galli SJ, Yuuki T, et al: Spontaneous canine mast cell tumors express tandem duplications in the proto-oncogene c-kit, *Exp Hematol* 27:689, 1999.
8. Ma Y, Longley BJ, Wang X, et al: Clustering of activating mutations in c-KIT's juxtamembrane coding region of canine mast cell neoplasms, *J Invest Dermatol* 112:165, 1999.
9. Dank G, Chien MB, London CA: Activating mutations in the catalytic or juxtamembrane domain of c-kit in splenic mast cell tumors in cats, *Am J Vet Res* 63:1129, 2002.
10. Downing S, Chien MB, Kass PH, et al: Prevalence and importance of internal tandem duplications in exons 11 and 12 of c-kit in mast cell tumors in dogs, *Am J Vet Res* 63:1718, 2002.
11. Cohen MH, Williams G, Johnson JR, et al: Approved summary for imatinib mesylate capsules in the treatment of chronic myelogenous leukemia, *Clin Cancer Res* 8:935, 2002.
12. Isotani M, Tamura K, Yagihara H, et al: Identification of a c-kit exon 8 internal tandem duplication in a feline mast cell tumor case and its favorable response to the tyrosine kinase inhibitor imatinib mesylate, *Vet Immunol Immunopathol* 114:168, 2006.
13. Holzinger EA: Feline cutaneous mastocytomas, *Cornell Vet* 63:87, 1973.
14. Wilcock BP, Yager JA, Zink MC: The morphology and behavior of feline cutaneous mastocytomas, *Vet Pathol* 23:320, 1986.
15. Goldschmidt MH, Hendrick MJ: Mast cell tumor. In Meuten DJ, editor: *Tumors in domestic animals*, Ames, 2002, Iowa State Press, p 107.
16. Buerger RG, Scott DW: Cutaneous mast cell neoplasia in cats: 14 cases (1975-1985), *J Am Vet Med Assoc* 190:1440, 1987.
17. Carpenter JL, Andrews LK, Holzworth J: Tumors and tumor-like lesions. In Holzworth J, editor: *Diseases of the cat: medicine and surgery*, Philadelphia, 1987, Saunders, p 569.
18. Molander-McCrary H, Henry CJ, Potter K, et al: Cutaneous mast cell tumors in cats: 32 cases (1991-1994), *J Am Anim Hosp Assoc* 34:281, 1998.
19. Lepri E, Ricci G, Leonardi L, et al: Diagnostic and prognostic features of cutaneous mast cell tumours: a retrospective analysis of 40 cases, *Vet Res Commun* 27:707, 2003.
20. Rassnick KM, Williams LE, Kristal O, et al: Lomustine for treatment of mast cell tumors in cats: 38 cases (1999-2005), *J Am Vet Med Assoc* 232:1200, 2008.
21. Johnson TO, Schulman FY, Lipscomb TP, et al: Histopathology and biological behavior of pleomorphic mast cell tumors in fifteen cats, *Vet Pathol* 39:452, 2002.
22. Turrel JM, Farrelly J, Page RL, et al: Evaluation of strontium 90 irradiation in treatment of cutaneous mast cell tumors in cats: 35 cases (1992-2002), *J Am Vet Med Assoc* 228:898, 2006.
23. Spangler WL, Culbertson MR: Prevalence and type of splenic diseases in cats: 455 cases (1985-1991), *J Am Vet Med Assoc* 201:773, 1992.
24. Feinmehl R, Matus R, Mauldin GN, et al: Splenic mast cell tumors in 43 cats (1975-1992), *Proc Annu Conf Vet Cancer Soc* 12:50, 1992.
25. Liska WD, MacEwen EG, Zaki FA, et al: Feline systemic mastocytosis: a review and results of splenectomy in seven cases, *J Am Anim Hosp Assoc* 15:589, 1979.
26. Hanson JA, Papageorges M, Girard E, et al: Ultrasonographic appearance of splenic disease in 101 cats, *Vet Radiol Ultrasound* 42:441, 2001.
27. Sato AF, Solano M: Ultrasonographic findings in abdominal mast cell disease: a retrospective study of 19 patients, *Vet Radiol Ultrasound* 45:51, 2004.

28. McManus PM: Frequency and severity of mastocytemia in dogs with and without mast cell tumors: 120 cases (1995-1997), *J Am Vet Med Assoc* 215:335, 1999.

29. Garrett LD, Craig CL, Szladovits B, et al: Evaluation of buffy coat smears for circulating mast cells in healthy cats and ill cats without mast cell tumor-related disease, *J Am Vet Med Assoc* 231:1685, 2007.

30. Guerre R, Millet P, Groulade P: Systemic mastocytosis in a cat: remission after splenectomy, *J Small Anim Pract* 20:769, 1979.

31. Thamm DH, Turek MM, Vail DM: Outcome and prognostic factors following adjuvant prednisone/vinblastine chemotherapy for high-risk canine mast cell tumour: 61 cases, *J Vet Med Sci* 68:581, 2006.

32. Thamm DH, Mauldin EA, Vail DM: Prednisone and vinblastine chemotherapy for canine mast cell tumor—41 cases (1992-1997), *J Vet Intern Med* 13:491, 1999.

33. Rassnick KM, Moore AS, Williams LE: Treatment of canine mast cell tumors with CCNU (lomustine). *J Vet Intern Med* 13:601, 1999.

34. Camps-Palau MA, Leibman NF, Elmslie R, et al: Treatment of canine mast cell tumours with vinblastine, cyclophosphamide, and prednisone: 35 cases (1997-2004), *Vet Comparat Oncol* 5:156, 2007.

35. Stanclift RM, Gilson SD: Evaluation of neoadjuvant prednisone administration and surgical excision in treatment of cutaneous mast cell tumors in dogs, *J Am Vet Med Assoc* 232:53, 2008.

36. McCaw DL, Miller MA, Ogilvie GK, et al: Response of canine mast cell tumors to treatment with oral prednisone, *J Vet Intern Med* 8:406, 1994.

37. Padrid PA, Mitchell RW, Ndukwu IM, et al: Cyproheptadine-induced attenuation of type I-hypersensitivity reactions of airway smooth muscle for immune-sensitized cats, *Am J Vet Res* 56:109, 1995.

38. Moore AS, Ogilvie GK: Splenic, hepatic, and pancreatic tumors. In Moore AS, Ogilvie GK, editors: *Feline oncology: a comprehensive guide to compassionate care*, Trenton, 2001, Veterinary Learning Systems, p 295.

39. Alroy J, Leav I, DeLellis RA, et al: Distinctive intestinal mast cell neoplasms of domestic cats, *Lab Invest* 33:159, 1992.

40. Haney SM, Clifford CA, de Lorimier LP, et al: Feline intestinal mast cell tumors: biologic behavior and response to treatment in 18 cats, *Proc Annu Conf Vet Cancer Soc* 25:8, 2005.

41. Bortnowski HB, Rosenthal RC: Gastrointestinal mast cell tumors and eosinophilia in two cats, *J Am Anim Hosp Assoc* 28:271, 1992.

CHAPTER
68 Cardiac Neoplasia

Ashley B. Saunders

Tumors of the heart and pericardium are unusual in feline medicine, with an incidence of less than 0.3 per cent of the population in one report.[1] Primary cardiac and pericardial tumors occur with lower frequency than metastasis to the heart and pericardium. The most commonly reported primary heart tumors in cats include lymphoma and chemodectoma, followed by myxoma, hemangiosarcoma, sarcoma, and rhabdomyosarcoma.[2-7] Metastasis to the heart has been documented with lymphoma, hemangiosarcoma, pulmonary carcinoma, mammary gland carcinoma, tonsillar carcinoma, salivary gland adenocarcinoma, oral melanoma, and carcinomatosis.[8-12]

Primary pericardial tumors are reported rarely, having been identified at necropsy as mesothelioma and hemangiosarcoma.[9,13] Metastasis to the pericardium has been demonstrated with lymphoma, bronchoalveolar carcinoma, mammary gland adenocarcinoma, pulmonary adenocarcinoma, and melanoma.[8,10] Metastasis to the heart and pericardium is identified predominately at postmortem examination with the exception of lymphoma, and the most common locations for metastasis are the left ventricular free wall and interventricular septum.[9]

No breed, age, or gender predilections have been reported with feline cardiac neoplasms.[1] In a review of the literature, the most commonly reported signalment was Domestic Shorthair breed 5 years of age or older. The clinical effects of cardiac tumors are related principally to compression or obstruction of cardiac structures, infiltration of the myocardium, and fluid production. Effusions result from obstruction of venous return and pericardial pathology. Small masses may not cause clinical signs of disease and remain undetected.

CLINICAL SIGNS

Clinical signs in most feline patients with cardiac neoplasia are nonspecific and include lethargy, anorexia, and weight loss. Tachypnea and dyspnea are common complaints in the presence of pleural effusion and pulmonary edema. Other clinical signs may be unique and are related specifically to tumor location. Neoplastic cells may infiltrate the myocardium and affect the conduction system resulting in arrhythmias, conduction abnormalities, and syncope.[14] Cough was reported in one cat with an aortic body tumor that had penetrated the trachea and occluded the right pulmonary bronchus completely.[15]

Physical examination findings may include tachypnea, dyspnea, and muffled heart and lung sounds in the presence of pleural or pericardial effusion. Auscultatory abnormalities including murmur and gallop rhythm may be detected in association with myocardial disease or anemia.[10] An abnormal heart rate or rhythm often is attributed to neoplastic myocardial infiltration affecting the conduction system. Signs of right heart failure or increased right heart pressures include jugular venous distension and hepatomegaly, which occur infrequently in cats. Pale mucous membranes and decreased femoral pulse quality may occur with hemodynamic instability.

DIAGNOSIS

In general comprehensive laboratory evaluation including complete blood count, biochemical analysis, urinalysis, and retroviral testing (feline leukemia virus [FeLV] antigen and feline immunodeficiency virus [FIV] antibody) is recommended. Careful examination for primary tumors should focus on lymph nodes, the gastrointestinal tract, kidneys, mammary glands, and oral cavity.

Cardiac tumors typically are detected with echocardiography or discovered at necropsy evaluation. Echocardiography provides a noninvasive means of imaging the heart and surrounding structures, and is superior to conventional radiography for identifying masses, myocardial infiltrative lesions, and pericardial effusion.[10] Tumors most often are located at the heart base or within the ventricular myocardium, and assessment of both the right and left imaging windows may be required for successful localization. Pericardial effusion appears as a hypoechoic space surrounding the heart and is helpful for visualizing tumors. In addition to identifying pericardial effusion, echocardiography can provide evidence of cardiac tamponade by documenting diastolic collapse of the right atrium and ventricle when intrapericardial pressures exceed right atrial or ventricular end-diastolic pressures.[16]

Cardiac tumors are not identified routinely with thoracic radiographs. Dorsal deviation of the trachea and visualization of a heart base mass has been reported rarely with chemodectoma and carcinomatosis.[13,15,17] A globoid cardiac silhouette suggests pericardial effusion, whereas small volume pericardial effusions may go undetected. Cardiomegaly can occur with neoplastic infiltrative lesions. Pericardial calcification has been reported in a cat with pulmonary carcinoma metastasized to the pericardium.[8] Radiographic evidence of pulmonary metastasis has been reported in a cat with chemodectoma.[18] Thoracic radiographic findings in dyspneic patients may include pleural effusion or pulmonary edema with pulmonary venous distension.

Arrhythmias and conduction abnormalities most often are related to neoplastic myocardial infiltration. Electrocardiographic evaluation is recommended for cats with abnormally slow or rapid heart rates, irregular heart rhythm, or a history of syncope (see Chapter 42). Reported abnormalities in cats with cardiac neoplasia consist of electrical alternans, changes in the ST segment, atrial tachycardia, ventricular premature beats, atrioventricular block, bundle branch block, and sinus arrest.[8,14] Although low voltage QRS complexes may be associated with pericardial effusion in cats, it is important to recognize that QRS complexes typically are small in cats, making this an insensitive indicator of effusion.

The most common causes of pericardial effusion in cats are congestive heart failure secondary to myocardial disease, neoplasia, and infectious diseases.[10] Most cardiac tumors do not exfoliate well, and for this reason pericardial fluid analysis and cytological examination often are unrewarding for identifying feline cardiac tumors. Careful cytological evaluation is required so that reactive mesothelial cells are not mistaken for neoplastic cells. Lymphoma is the only tumor that may be diagnosed from pericardial fluid analysis, and lymphoblasts and atypical lymphocytes were identified in some but not all cases.[19,20] Chylous effusion has been documented in a cat with chemodectoma.[21]

Feline cardiac tumors are located principally near important vascular structures, making definitive diagnosis challenging and obtained most often at postmortem examination. Ultrasound-guided fine-needle aspirates of heart base tumors and surgical excisional biopsy have been performed occasionally to identify chemodectoma.[15,22] Multiple tumor types have been identified using immunohistochemistry including a chemodectoma positive for chromogranin A (CgA), neuron-specific enolase (NSE), and synaptophysin (SY) characteristic of neuroendocrine tumors.[23] Immunopositivity for CD3 consistent with T lymphocytes has been documented in a cat with chemodectoma.[17] Immunohistochemistry

demonstrated positive staining for alpha-actin and desmin that aided in identifying a primary rhabdomyosarcoma.[7] Diagnosis of right atrial hemangiosarcoma was confirmed with positive immunohistochemical staining for factor VIII–related antigen.[5]

TREATMENT

Critically ill cats with cardiac neoplasia require immediate stabilization. Cats with pleural effusion or pericardial effusion require thoracocentesis or pericardiocentesis to relieve clinical signs of dyspnea or hemodynamic collapse. Small volume pleural or pericardial effusions typically do not require immediate removal. Dyspneic patients benefit from oxygen therapy. Diuretic therapy is indicated in the rare instance of pulmonary edema, but does not remove free fluid reliably from the chest or pericardium and can contribute to further hemodynamic collapse. Intravenous fluid therapy is recommended for cats with pericardial effusion and evidence of hemodynamic compromise.

Palliative or definitive cancer therapy rarely is successful in cats with cardiac neoplasia. Complete surgical excision of chemodectoma was considered in several cases but deemed too difficult intraoperatively because of tumor proximity to vital structures. Radiation therapy for cardiac tumors has not been reported in cats. The prognosis generally is poor for cats with cardiac neoplasia unless in the rare instance there is a positive response to chemotherapy for lymphoma.

LYMPHOMA

Lymphoma is the most common neoplasia diagnosed in cats; however, cardiac involvement is not common.[2] Primary cardiac tumors and metastasis to the heart have both been documented (Figures 68-1 to 68-3). There is an increased risk of lymphoma in FeLV-positive cats. Ten to 15 per cent of cats with lymphoma have been reported to have myocardial infiltrates, whereas a slightly higher percentage (20 per cent) of myocardial infiltrates are reported in FeLV-positive cats.[2] Resolution of lymphoma infiltrating the myocardium has been reported with the administration of combination chemotherapy that included prednisone, cyclophosphamide, and vincristine.[24]

CHEMODECTOMA

Chemodectomas may be referred to as nonchromaffin paragangliomas and typically affect the aortic body in cats. Chemoreceptor cells are found in groups at the ventrolateral surface of the aorta and the bifurcation of the carotid artery near the base of the heart.[25] The chemoreceptor system responds to changes in pH and the partial pressure of arterial oxygen and carbon dioxide in the blood. The tumors tend to be slow growing and locally invasive, causing compression or infiltration of structures in the area. Invasion of the pericardium and

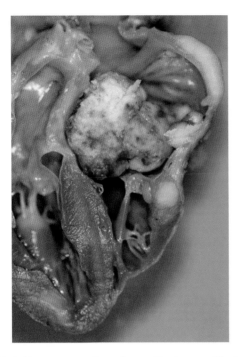

Figure 68-1 Necropsy specimen from a Persian cat. The heart has been transected longitudinally to display a prominent mass arising from and invading the right atrial wall and also present in the right ventricular free wall. (Courtesy Drs. Kelly Nitsche and Matthew Miller.)

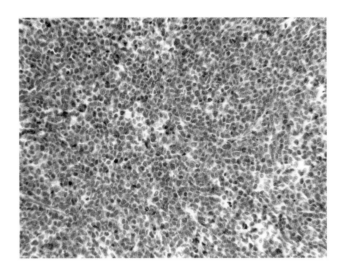

Figure 68-3 The round cells exhibited positive immunohistochemical staining for CD3 confirming a T cell lymphoma. (20×.) (Courtesy Drs. Kelly Nitsche and Matthew Miller.)

HEMANGIOSARCOMA

Right atrial and auricular involvement is very uncommon and has only been reported in a single cat with a primary tumor, whereas metastasis to the heart was reported with 22 per cent of hemangiosarcomas in cats.[5,26]

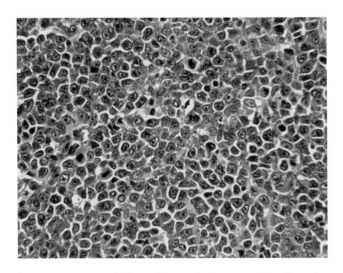

Figure 68-2 Histopathology of a neoplastic mass arising from the right atrial wall in the cat from Figure 68-1. The densely cellular mass is composed of sheets of round cells with prominent nucleoli and minimal cytoplasm indicative of lymphocytes. (H&E 40×.) (Courtesy Drs. Kelly Nitsche and Matthew Miller.)

right atrium has been reported and metastasis can occur.[8] Chemodectomas are intimately associated with vascular structures, making complete surgical excision and radiation therapy problematic. The use of chemotherapy for this tumor type has not been reported in cats.

REFERENCES

1. Ware WA: Cardiac neoplasia. In Bonagura JD, editor: *Current veterinary therapy XII*, Philadelphia, 1995, Saunders, p 873.
2. Fox PR: Feline myocardial disease. In Fox PR, editor: *Feline and canine cardiology*, New York, 1988, Churchill Livingstone, p 435.
3. Yates WDG, Lester SJ, Mills JHL: Chemoreceptor tumors diagnosed at the Western College of Veterinary Medicine 1967-1979, *Can Vet J* 21:124, 1980.
4. Campbell MD, Gleberg HB: Endocardial ossifying myxoma of the right atrium in a cat, *Vet Pathol* 37:460, 2000.
5. Merlo M, Bo S, Ratto A: Primary right atrium haemangiosarcoma in a cat, *J Feline Med Surg* 4:61, 2002.
6. Pessier AP, Flom JO: Primary sarcoma of the heart in cat, *Feline Practice* 18:25, 1990.
7. Venco L, Kramer L, Sola LB, et al: Primary cardiac rhabdomyosarcoma in a cat, *J Am Anim Hosp Assoc* 37:159, 2001.
8. Tilley LP, Bond B, Patnaik AK, et al: Cardiovascular tumors in the cat, *J Am Vet Med Assoc* 17:1009, 1981.
9. Aupperle H, Marz I, Ellenberger C, et al: Primary and secondary heart tumours in dogs and cats, *J Comp Pathol* 136:18, 2007.
10. Rush JE, Keene BW, Fox PR: Pericardial disease in the cat: a retrospective evaluation of 66 cases, *J Am Anim Hosp Assoc* 26:39, 1990.
11. Kraje AC, Mears EA, Hahn KA, et al: Unusual metastatic behavior and clinicopathologic findings in eight cats with cutaneous or visceral hemangiosarcoma, *J Am Vet Med Assoc* 214:670, 1999.
12. Lusk RH, Ettinger SJ, Barr EA: Ultrasound diagnosis of a feline heart tumor, cardiac carcinomatosis in a cat, *Calif Vet* 41:9, 1987.

13. Tilley LP, Owens JM, Wilkins RJ, et al: Pericardial mesothelioma with effusion in a cat, *J Am Anim Hosp Assoc* 11:60, 1975.

14. Meurs KM, Miller MW, Mackie JR, et al: Syncope associated with cardiac lymphoma in a cat, *J Am Anim Hosp Assoc* 30:583, 1994.

15. Tillson DM, Fingland RB, Andrews GA: Chemodectoma in a cat, *J Am Anim Hosp Assoc* 30:586, 1994.

16. Gidlewski J, Petrie JP: Pericardiocentesis and principles of echocardiographic imaging in the patient with cardiac neoplasia, *Clin Tech Small Anim Pract* 18:131, 2003.

17. Willis R, Williams AE, Schwarz T, et al: Aortic body chemodectoma causing pulmonary edema in a cat, *J Small Anim Pract* 42:20, 2001.

18. George C, Steinberg H: An aortic body carcinoma with multifocal thoracic metastases in a cat, *J Comp Pathol* 101:467, 1989.

19. Shinohara N, MacGregor JM, Calo A, et al: Presumptive primary cardiac lymphoma in a cat causing pericardial effusion, *J Vet Cardiol* 7:65, 2005.

20. Zoia A, Hughes D, Connolly DJ: Pericardial effusion and cardiac tamponade in a cat with extranodal lymphoma, *J Small Anim Pract* 45:467, 2004.

21. Fossum TW, Miller MW, Rogers KS, et al: Chylothorax associated with right-sided heart failure in five cats, *J Am Vet Med Assoc* 204:84, 1994.

22. Paola JP, Hammer AS, Smeak DD, et al: Aortic body tumor causing pleural effusion in a cat, *J Am Anim Hosp Assoc* 30:281, 1994.

23. Paltrinieri S, Riccaboni P, Rondena M, et al: Pathologic and immunohistochemical findings in a feline aortic body tumor, *Vet Pathol* 41:195, 2004.

24. Brummer DG, Moise NS: Infiltrative cardiomyopathy responsive to combination chemotherapy in a cat with lymphoma, *J Am Vet Med Assoc* 195:1116, 1989.

25. Buergelt CD, Das KM: Aortic body tumor in a cat, *Path Vet* 5:84, 1968.

26. Patnaik AK, Liu SK: Angiosarcoma in cats, *J Small Anim Pract* 18:191, 1977.

69 Tumors of the Ear

Heather M. Wilson

Neoplasia of the ear represents a very small portion of the otic disorders of cats. Tumors can arise from any of the normal structures of the ear. The pinna and the external ear canal are affected more commonly than the middle and inner ear. Neoplasms spanning all three tumor types are found in the feline ear. Tumors of epithelial and adnexal origin include squamous cell carcinoma (SCC), basal cell tumors, ceruminous gland tumors, and sebaceous gland tumors. Tumors of round-cell origin include mast cell tumors, lymphoma, and cutaneous plasma cell tumors. Finally, tumors of mesenchymal origin include fibroma/fibrosarcoma, chondroma/chondrosarcoma, rhabdomyoma/rhabdomyosarcoma, and hemangioma/hemangiosarcoma.

Benign tumors occur less often than malignant tumors in the ears of cats; however, benign masses including inflammatory polyps, basal cell tumors, papillomas/fibropapillomas (feline sarcoids), and ceruminous or apocrine gland adenomas are diagnosed with some frequency. In descending order, the ear tumors diagnosed most commonly in cats are inflammatory polyps, SCC of the pinna, and ceruminous gland adenocarcinomas.[1]

INCIDENCE AND ETIOLOGY

There are many possible etiologies for the various ear tumors diagnosed in cats. Chronic inflammation has been associated with malignant transformation of normal cells of the ear.[2] Ear tumors typically are diagnosed in older cats, although mast cell tumors and inflammatory polyps are seen commonly in younger cats. No gender predilection has been associated with any type of feline ear tumor.

TUMORS OF THE PINNA

SCC is the most commonly diagnosed neoplasm of the feline pinna. These tumors often are actinically induced as a result of DNA damage secondary to solar radiation. Thin-haired and light-color coated cats are at an increased risk for developing cutaneous SCC. White cats are 13.4 times more likely to develop SCC than cats with other coat colors.[1] These tumors occur frequently on the face where the hair is thin and exposure to sunlight is common. Lesions are found commonly on the inner ear pinna, at the ear base, preaurally, periocularly, and on the nasal planum (Figure 69-1). Indoor cats also are at risk. Any cat who sunbathes (whether on the patio or in the skylight) is exposed to solar radiation. The incidence of cutaneous SCC is highest in areas of the country receiving the highest levels of solar radiation annually (up to 26.9 cats out of 10,000).[3]

Mutations of the tumor suppressor gene *p53* have been identified in nine of 11 cats in one study and in two of four cats in another study who were diagnosed with SCC of the ear pinna.[4,5] This mimics the same pathway of malignant transformation as seen in human beings. It is often associated with head and neck cancer in people. Retroviral status plays no known role in this disease process; however, the two may represent dual risk factors

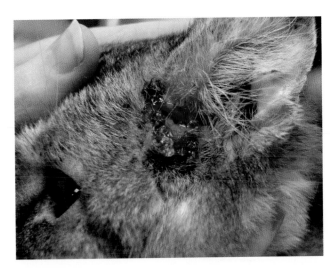

Figure 69-1 Invasive periaural squamous cell carcinoma with ulceration, hemorrhage, and scabbing.

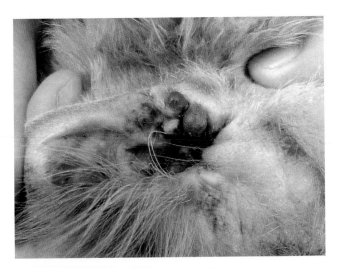

Figure 69-2 Multiple ceruminous gland adenomas in the ear of a cat. These tumors have been slowly progressive over several years. (Courtesy Dr. John August, Texas A&M University.)

because outdoor cats have a higher risk of exposure to both sunlight and retroviruses.

Other tumors of the ear pinna in cats also have been associated with sunlight exposure. Basal cell tumors, hemangiomas, and hemangiosarcomas have been associated with UVB exposure in cats. Additionally, specific breeds, such as Siamese, Persians, and Himalayans, may be predisposed to developing basal cell tumors.[6]

PAPILLOMAS AND FIBROPAPILLOMAS (FELINE SARCOIDS)

Papillomas are rare tumors that occur most commonly on the face (typically on the nose, lip, and pinna) of cats. They also can be found within the external ear canal and on the digits.[7] These tumors frequently are pedunculated and rarely ulcerated. Although the causative factor has not been described definitively, a viral etiology most certainly is the culprit. In a study of 19 feline sarcoids, a papilloma virus most similar to bovine papilloma virus I was identified positively in 17 of the lesions.[8] The prevalence of feline sarcoids increases in cats with exposure to cattle.

TUMORS OF THE EXTERNAL EAR CANAL

External ear canal tumors are more aggressive in cats than in dogs. More than 85 per cent of these tumors are malignant in cats.[9] They arise from the epithelial and adnexal structures of the auditory meatus. Ceruminous gland adenocarcinomas (CGA) are the most common malignant tumors; however, SCC, sebaceous gland adenocarcinomas (SGA), and carcinomas of unknown origin have been described. These tumors may be associated with chronic inflammation of the external ear canal. Benign tumors such as ceruminous gland adenomas and sebaceous gland adenomas also occur. These tumors may be pigmented or nonpigmented (Figures 69-2 and 69-3).

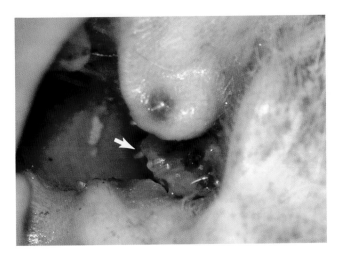

Figure 69-3 Inflammation and ulceration associated with a nonpigmented ceruminous gland adenoma in a cat *(arrow)*. There is also a small basal cell tumor located on the auricular fold of this cat's ear.

INFLAMMATORY POLYPS

Inflammatory polyps do not represent a neoplastic process; however, they are one of the most commonly identified benign ear masses of cats. These polyps arise from the mucosal lining of the middle ear, Eustachian tubes, or pharynx. They can extend into the external ear canal where they may be visualized with an otoscope, or they may protrude into the nasopharynx. A definitive etiology has not been elucidated, but several causes are suspected to play a role in the development of this disease. Chronic inflammation of the upper respiratory tract or chronic otitis media are commonly accepted factors. Polyps may be congenital in origin or may be secondary to a chronic ascending infection from the nasopharynx. Viruses such as feline herpesvirus-1 (FHV-1) and feline calicivirus (FCV) also have been incriminated, but this possible etiology is controversial. One study of 41 polyps found no virus particles in any of the lesions, whereas other studies have found FHV-1 or FCV in some of the polyps studied.[10-13] Although these viruses probably are not necessary for tumor formation, a possible role in development can not be excluded.

MIDDLE EAR TUMORS

Middle ear tumors are quite rare in cats, and very little information exists on their true incidence and possible etiologies. The few reports of middle ear tumors in cats include two carcinomas, three lymphomas (LSA), small numbers of SCC, and one fibrosarcoma. Of the cats with LSA, only one was tested and it was found to be negative for retrovirus infection. Retroviral status of the other cats was not reported.[1,14,15]

BIOLOGICAL BEHAVIOR AND PATHOGENESIS

Ear tumors in cats tend to be aggressive. Their behavior often is characterized by rapid local invasion, and lymphatic or vascular spread. Distant metastasis is uncommon. Five of 56 cats with various carcinomas of the ear canal had evidence of metastasis to local lymph nodes; none had evidence of lung metastasis during the study, although lung metastases were found in one cat during a postmortem examination.[9] Benign tumors are less likely to be ulcerated and tend to have a narrow base of attachment. Additionally, they are more likely to be lobulated and typically do not invade into the cartilage like their malignant counterparts.[9]

TUMORS OF THE PINNA

SCCs of the pinna tend to start as hyperemic lesions, and progress to erythematous crusts and ulcerated lesions. Premalignant lesions often are described as actinic keratosis on histopathological examination. These neoplasms tend to be locally invasive with a low metastatic rate. If these tumors metastasize, they usually spread first to the local lymph nodes, then to the lungs. Approximately 15 per cent of affected cats will have multicentric actinically induced lesions involving the pinna, nasal planum, and/or the periorbital region.[1]

Basal cell tumors arise from the uncommitted basal reserve cells of the skin. These tumors usually are benign basal epitheliomas and are referred to collectively as basal cell tumors. These tumors often are pigmented and can be mistaken for melanomas. Basal cell carcinomas do occur but are rare. When they occur, they often are aggressive lesions invading into local structures as well as into vascular and lymphatic vessels.

Mesenchymal tumors of the pinna are rare. Rhabdomyomas are benign striated skeletal muscle tumors that have been reported in four cats.[16] No association with sun exposure or other etiological factors has been identified. Fibrosarcomas of the pinna are non–vaccine-related soft-tissue sarcomas that are locally invasive with a low

metastatic rate of approximately 15 per cent.[2] Non–vaccine-associated fibrosarcomas tend to occur on the head and extremities and usually are less aggressive than their vaccine-induced counterparts. Vascular tumors tend to occur in the inguinal region and on the ears of white cats. An association with UVB radiation has been proposed.[17]

Hemangiosarcomas tend to be locally invasive, although metastasis is rare. However, full staging is still recommended for cats with malignant vascular tumors.[6,17]

Melanomas (MSA) are rare in cats. They occur most commonly as ocular tumors (see Chapter 70); however, dermal MSAs have been diagnosed on the pinnae of cats. One study of 23 cats with dermal MSA included four cats with MSA of the pinna. Three of these cats were cured with surgery alone, whereas one cat experienced recurrence with evidence of distant metastasis.[18] These tumors can be considered to have a benign behavior, although a subset exists with a more aggressive phenotype.

Cutaneous mast cell tumors are uncommon in cats; however, when they occur, they are commonly located on or near the ear (see Chapter 67). These tumors have a benign behavior and often are cured with surgery alone. These tumors rarely recur even with incomplete surgical margins.

Papillomas/fibropapillomas (feline sarcoids) do not metastasize and generally have a benign behavior. However, they are likely to recur after surgery. This behavior is consistent with the proposed viral etiology, because these tumors behave similarly to virally-induced papillomas of other species.[7]

TUMORS OF THE EXTERNAL EAR CANAL

Tumors of the external ear canal are often slow to metastasize and are locally invasive. Occasionally cats present with a very aggressive phenotype with early spread to local lymph nodes and lungs. The degree of invasion is prognostic for these tumors.[9] Ceruminous gland carcinomas often destroy the adjacent soft tissues and are capable of distant metastasis. They have the longest median survival time of the malignant external ear canal tumors when treated aggressively.[9]

SCC of the external ear canal is a very aggressive tumor. These tumors often are ulcerated, painful, and highly invasive into the local structures. The lesions are difficult to excise completely, and they respond poorly to adjunct therapies such as radiation or chemotherapy (see Figure 69-4). Carcinomas of unknown origin have a similar prognosis to SCC of the external ear canal.[9]

Two cats reportedly have been diagnosed with meningeal carcinomatosis secondary to SCC of the ear. Both patients had been diagnosed previously with SCC of the pinna and had recurrence within the external ear canal or along the previous pinnectomy site. Both cats presented with neurological signs, with one patient being slowly progressive over several months whereas the other presented with an acute onset of neurological abnormalities.[19]

Inflammatory polyps are benign masses that can either extend through the eustachian tube to the pharynx or

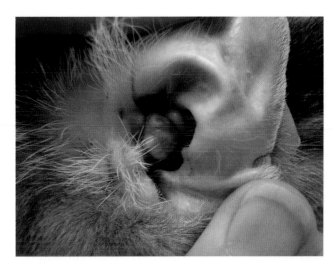

Figure 69-4 Ulcerated ceruminous gland adenoma of the external ear canal in an 11-year-old spayed female cat.

through the tympanic membrane into the external ear canal. They are not neoplastic and do not metastasize. They are irritating to the cat because they act as a space-occupying lesion.

MIDDLE EAR TUMORS

Middle ear tumors also are locally invasive with rare reports of distant metastasis. Metastases tend to occur to the local lymph nodes. LSA of the middle ear tends to present as a solitary extranodal site, but thorough staging is recommended.

CLINICAL SIGNS ASSOCIATED WITH EAR TUMORS

The clinical signs associated with various ear tumors often depend on the location of the tumor, the degree of invasion into the normal structures, and whether metastases are present. The severity of signs often depends on the size of the tumor and the chronicity of the lesion.

TUMORS OF THE PINNA

SCCs often start as small hyperemic lesions that progress to erythema. Eventually crusting is seen when the lesion progresses to ulceration and then to an invasive lesion that is highly destructive, painful, and often open and draining. These tumors can invade deep into the ear canal and even affect the facial nerves, causing hearing loss, Horner's syndrome, or facial nerve paralysis. Eventually these tumors can invade the brain stem or the brain itself.[1]

Basal cell tumors are dermal, well-circumscribed, pigmented masses that may be filled with a brown fluid. They may be nonpigmented or hyperpigmented. They

are nonpainful, but occasionally can ulcerate. They have been reported to range from 0.5 to 3 cm in size and are slow growing.[1] These tumors almost always are benign but rare carcinomas do occur. Invasiveness is prognostic, and a mass that appears to invade into underlying structures should be treated more aggressively.

Rhabdomyomas are often well-circumscribed smooth firm masses under the skin of the pinna. If allowed to grow large enough, they may eventually ulcerate the skin. Fibromas have a similar clinical appearance to rhabdomyomas and may require histopathological examination to be differentiated. Fibrosarcomas are more invasive and less well circumscribed than rhabdomyomas and fibromas.

Vascular tumors, such as hemangioma and hemangiosarcoma (HSA), often are dermal and dark purple to dark red in color. They may be well circumscribed (hemangioma) or more diffuse in nature (HSA). These tumors tend to bleed easily and can involve deeper tissues. The masses can be soft or firm depending on the degree of cavitation.

MSAs are round, well-circumscribed dark masses within the dermis and epidermis. These tumors metastasize rarely to local lymph nodes or distant sites such as the lungs, but thorough staging still should be performed.

Mast cell tumors typically are well circumscribed. They are dermal in location with intact overlying skin. They may be erythematous and edematous, but rarely are ulcerated. These masses tend to be slow growing with little impact on the cat's quality of life. Young Siamese cats are at an increased risk for developing multiple mast cell tumors of the head. These tumors may resolve on their own with time.[4]

TUMORS OF THE EXTERNAL EAR CANAL

SCC in this location is more likely to invade deep into normal structures and cause neurological signs, when compared with other tumors of the external ear canal (Figure 69-4). All external ear canal tumors can cause otorrhea with dark, bloody, and often foul smelling discharge. Secondary infections due to the breakdown of the natural protective barriers also are common. Most cats demonstrate pain and often will guard the affected ear. Sedation may be needed for a thorough otoscopic examination.

INFLAMMATORY POLYPS

These ear masses typically affect cats less than 3 years of age (Figure 69-5). Upper respiratory signs commonly accompany a polyp. Nasal discharge, sneezing, stertor, voice change, dyspnea, otitis media, otitis interna, head tilt, loss of balance, nystagmus, and Horner's syndrome all are possible signs of an inflammatory polyp. Occasionally a mass will be visible within the external ear canal along with otorrhea and head shaking. Inflammatory polyps usually are unilateral, and Abyssinian cats may be overrepresented.[10-12,20]

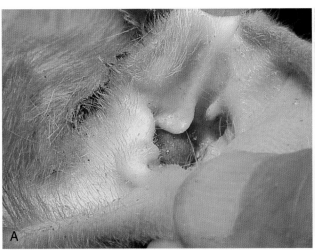

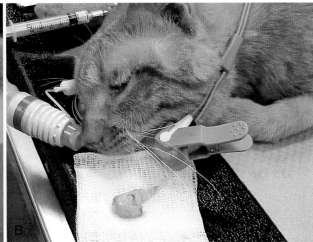

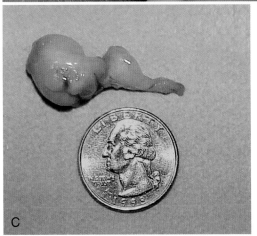

Figure 69-5 A, External ear canal polyp in a 1-year-old neutered male Domestic Shorthair cat. The polyp arose in the middle-ear cavity and had ruptured through the tympanic membrane, leading to bacterial otitis media. The patient recovered satisfactorily following a right lateral bulla osteotomy and appropriate antimicrobial therapy. **B,** The same patient minutes after traction avulsion of the middle-ear polyp through the external ear canal. **C,** Middle-ear polyp removed from the patient in **A** and **B**. (Courtesy Dr. John R. August, Texas A&M University.)

MIDDLE EAR TUMORS

Cats with middle ear tumors commonly present with chronic signs such as therapy-resistant otitis media. Vestibular signs such as head tilt, loss of balance, nystagmus, and Horner's syndrome may occur. Additionally, these patients may present with signs of otitis externa, head shaking, pain upon opening the mouth, otorrhea, and facial nerve paralysis. Rarely these tumors extend to involve the pharynx.

DIAGNOSIS AND STAGING OF EAR TUMORS

A definitive diagnosis, along with full staging, is necessary in order to determine treatment options and prognosis for ear tumors (Table 69-1). Imaging plays a very important role in the diagnosis and staging of ear tumors, and several imaging modalities are helpful.

Radiographs are useful for examining the osseous structures of the ear. They also may reveal soft-tissue opacity in the bulla, mineralization of the tissues, and stenosis of the canal. Care must be taken to use good technique and positioning in order to achieve diagnostic films. Skull radiographs typically require general anesthesia in order to achieve proper positioning. Specific views

Table 69-1 Clinical Stages of Feline Tumors of Epidermal Origin, According to the World Health Organization

Site	Stage	Description
Primary tumor	T_{is}	Carcinoma in situ (precancerous)
	T_0	No evidence of tumor
	T_1	Tumor <2 cm maximum diameter, superficial or exophytic
	T_2	Tumor 2-5 cm maximum diameter, or with minimal invasion regardless of size
	T_3	Tumor >5 cm maximum diameter, or with invasion of the subcutis regardless of size
	T_4	Tumor invading other structures such as fascia, muscle, bone, or cartilage
Regional lymph node involvement	N_0	No evidence of regional lymph node involvement
	N_1	Regional lymph node involvement
Distant metastasis	M_0	No evidence of distant metastasis
	M_1	Evidence of distant metastasis

From Owen LN: *TNM classification of tumours in domestic animals,* Geneva, 1980, World Health Organization.

that should be acquired include a lateral, dorsoventral or ventrodorsal, 20-degree lateral, ventrolaterodorsal oblique, rostro-30 degree angle, and a ventral caudodorsal open mouth oblique.[21] Three-view thoracic radiographs also are needed for identifying distant lung metastasis, thoracic lymph node enlargement, as well as possible lung or cardiovascular pathology that may increase the patient's anesthetic risk. Although radiographs are relatively easy to perform and inexpensive compared with other imaging modalities, this imaging technique is not as sensitive as computed tomography (CT) or magnetic resonance imaging (MRI) for identifying the lesion or determining the extent of tumor invasion preoperatively.[9] Radiographs typically are unable to determine mild to moderate lymph node enlargement within the head and neck region.

Computed tomographic scanning is used to determine the presence and extent of the mass or polyp within the normal tissues. This modality is more sensitive than radiographs, but also requires general anesthesia and careful positioning. CT can be used to evaluate both the soft tissues and bony structures in good detail. Unlike radiographs, it can differentiate between fluid and soft tissues. Additionally, contrast agents can be used to determine the extent of blood flow to a suspicious lesion. CT often is only available at private specialty hospitals and university teaching hospitals.

MRI is not used as often as CT for ear tumors, but has better soft-tissue contrast than the other two modalities and often is helpful for differentiating central versus peripheral causes of vestibular disease.[21] MRI also requires general anesthesia and precise positioning. It is not as capable of evaluating the bony structures as CT, but may be better at diagnosing otitis interna than the other two modalities. Contrast agents also may be used to identify blood flow to a suspicious lesion. MRI is the most expensive of the three imaging modalities and often is only available at private specialty hospitals and universities. (The reader is directed to Chapter 31 for a complete discussion of diagnostic imaging of the ear.)

Imaging is quite helpful for narrowing down the list of differential diagnoses; however, a tissue sample is still required for definitive diagnosis (Table 69-2). There are several methods available for procuring a tissue sample and the best method depends on the tumor type suspected.

TUMORS OF THE PINNA

SCCs can be difficult to diagnose in the early stages. Often, the crusting and scaling is overlooked by owners until more advanced disease is present. Additionally, these lesions are associated with inflammation secondary to keratin release into the tissues causing a foreign body reaction. It can be quite challenging to differentiate inflammation from neoplasia, especially when epithelial cells are involved.[2,22]

For small superficial lesions, excisional biopsy is the most appropriate diagnostic tool. These lesions often are too small or thin for fine-needle aspiration (FNA) or needle core biopsy techniques. Biopsy also will clarify the

Table 69-2 Differential Diagnoses Associated with Various Ear Tumors

Location of Tumor	Differential Diagnoses
Pinna	
Squamous cell carcinoma	Immune-mediated diseases (pemphigus, lupus), inflammation (dermatitis), vasculitis, deep mycosis, foreign body, other carcinomas
Pigmented pinnal mass	Basal cell tumor, ceruminous gland cyst, apocrine gland cyst, hemangioma, hemangiosarcoma, melanoma
Mast cell tumors	Eosinophilic plaques, feline sarcoids, granulomas
External ear canal	
Squamous cell carcinoma	CGA, other carcinoma, deep mycosis, foreign body
Ceruminous gland adenocarcinoma	SCC, other carcinomas, deep mycosis, foreign body
Carcinoma of unknown origin	CGA, SCC, other carcinomas, deep mycosis, foreign body
Inflammatory polyps	Deep mycosis, tumors of the external ear canal and pharynx
Middle ear	Idiopathic vestibular disease, deep mycosis, therapy-resistant otitis media

invasive nature of the lesion and whether the margins are completely free of tumor.

Larger lesions may allow for a FNA or needle core biopsy with cytological evaluation. The inflammation associated with many SCCs interferes with the diagnosis, necessitating a biopsy. Biopsies of larger lesions can either be incisional (only a small portion of the mass is removed) or excisional (an attempt is made to remove the entire mass while procuring the biopsy sample). The size of the mass and its location will help to determine whether an incisional or excisional biopsy technique is more appropriate.

Once a diagnosis of SCC has been made, staging is performed. Baseline laboratory testing, including a complete blood count (CBC), biochemistry panel, urinalysis, and retroviral testing, helps to determine if the cat has any systemic disease that may limit treatment options. Positive retroviral status has not been associated with this disease, but testing is important for determining the overall prognosis. Three-view thoracic films are necessary to rule out distant metastasis to the lungs, and to determine if there is lung or cardiovascular pathology that may limit therapeutic options. Aspirates of the regional draining lymph node should be performed, if possible, to exclude nodal involvement.

Basal cell tumors often can be diagnosed with a FNA of the mass. A brown fluid often is obtained from the aspirate, and the mass may decrease in size significantly after aspiration. It can be difficult to differentiate between benign and malignant basal cell tumors cytologically. Basal cell carcinomas are very rare and typically are more invasive than their benign counterparts. If there is any suspicion that a mass may be malignant, a biopsy should be performed. Staging is only necessary for malignant tumors. The staging plan for a basal cell carcinoma is identical to that of a SCC.

Rhabdomyomas and fibrosarcomas often do not exfoliate well with FNAs. It may be possible to get a diagnosis using this technique; however, biopsy of the mass often is required for definitive diagnosis. Biopsies can be either excisional or incisional depending on the size of the tumor. Staging for malignant tumors includes baseline laboratory evaluation (defined above) and three-view thoracic radiographs. Soft-tissue sarcomas rarely metastasize to lymph nodes; nevertheless, any enlarged lymph node should be aspirated.

Vascular tumors often appear as small purple to red lesions on the ear. Cytological evaluation of these tumors often only reveals blood. They bleed regularly after an aspiration procedure. A biopsy is required for a definitive diagnosis. Although hemangiomas tend to be less invasive and well circumscribed in comparison to HSA, a biopsy is necessary to differentiate between the two definitively. For malignant tumors, staging includes baseline laboratory evaluation as well as three-view thoracic films. It is unlikely for this disease to involve the spleen; however, abdominal ultrasound can be included for thorough staging. Like other soft-tissue sarcomas, HSA rarely metastasizes to the lymph nodes, but any enlarged lymph node should be aspirated.

MSAs are often diagnosed easily using a FNA or needle core technique. These tumors exfoliate well and tend to be heavily pigmented when located on the ear of cats. The tumor cells may appear as round cells with a fine dusting of small gray cytoplasmic granules, mesenchymal cells with indistinct cell borders and wispy cytoplasm, or a mixed population of round and mesenchymal cells. Amelanotic MSAs may require special stains for confirmation. Pinnal MSAs in cats typically have a benign behavior. Occasionally an aggressive phenotype exists that necessitates full staging.[18] Tumors with a more aggressive behavior likely will be more locally invasive, may not be well circumscribed, have decreased pigmentation, and a higher mitotic index than more benign lesions. Full staging includes baseline laboratory evaluation, three-view thoracic radiographs, and aspirates of the draining lymph nodes (when accessible).

Mast cell tumors are easily identified with a FNA or needle core technique. These round cell tumors often exfoliate well and have characteristic metachromatic granules within the cytoplasm. They may be accompanied by varying numbers of eosinophils. Occasionally the granules will fail to take up Diff-quick stain, requiring a Wright-Giemsa stain to be visualized. These tumors normally have a benign behavior in the cat and often do not require full staging. Conversely, if a cat is systemically ill (weight loss, vomiting, anorexia), or has splenomegaly or other signs suggestive of systemic disease, full staging is recommended.[4] Full staging would include baseline laboratory testing, abdominal ultrasound, two-view thoracic

radiographs, and aspirates of abnormal organs (see Figure 67-1) and regional lymph nodes (see Figure 71-28).

TUMORS OF THE EXTERNAL EAR CANAL

The diagnosis of an external ear canal tumor starts with a good otoscopic examination (see Chapter 30). Sedation may be required in order to fully evaluate the ear canal in which a mass or ulcerated lesion is detected. Radiographs may be helpful for detecting stenosis of the ear canal, mineralization of the soft tissues, osteolysis, or fluid/soft tissue in the bulla. Ultimately CT or MRI is needed to determine the extent of the mass lesion within the normal structures (Figure 69-6). Aggressive lesions may have obliterated the ear canal and can even cause lysis of the calvarium.

A FNA is able to diagnose a CGA 86 per cent of the time and a benign tumor 80 per cent of the time; however, a biopsy remains the gold standard for diagnosing external ear canal tumors.[23]

Staging for malignant external ear canal tumors typically is the same regardless of the tumor type. Baseline laboratory evaluation, three-view thoracic radiographs, and aspirates of the draining lymph nodes should be performed to complete staging.

The clinician may have a strong suspicion of an inflammatory polyp based on history, clinical signs, and signalment. Additional imaging often can support the diagnosis and determine the location and extent of the polyp. A soft-tissue mass may be detectable on skull radiographs; however, the mass may be difficult to identify in some cats due to summation with surrounding normal structures. A 20-degree oblique lateral view or a ventral-laterodorsal oblique view may be the best way to identify a polyp using radiographs. A 30-degree rostroventral cau-

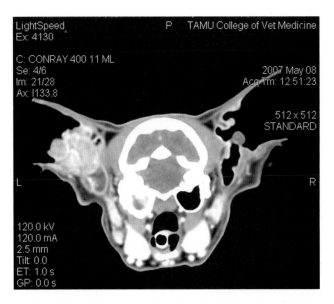

Figure 69-6 Contrast-enhanced image of a cat with a ceruminous gland adenocarcinoma located in the left external ear canal. This mass is obstructing the vertical ear canal and secondary otitis externa and otitis media are present.

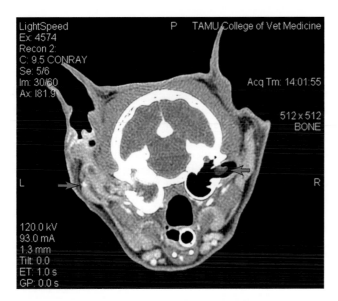

Figure 69-7 Contrast-enhanced image of a cat with a large inflammatory polyp of the left ear canal and a small early polyp of the right ear canal (indicated by the *red arrows*).

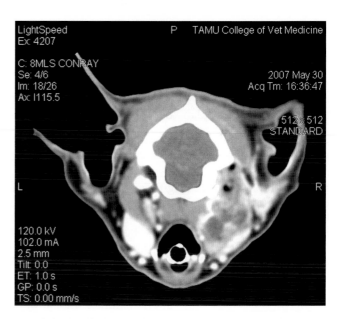

Figure 69-8 Contrast-enhanced image of a cat with a large ceruminous gland adenocarcinoma of the right middle ear. The tumor has invaded the local structures.

dodorsal open-mouth oblique view also is valuable for identifying polyps.[14] Bilateral or unilateral soft tissue opacities may be seen within the tympanic bulla, and sclerosis of the osseous bulla also may be present (see Chapter 31). In some cases, otitis externa with soft-tissue opacity within the horizontal ear canal may be seen. In other cases soft-tissue opacity may be seen within the nasopharyngeal region. Radiographs do not provide enough detail in most patients to delineate the mass from adjacent structures and can only support a presumptive diagnosis of an inflammatory polyp.

CT and MRI are the best modalities for locating these masses and determining their size. Computed tomographic views that provide the most information include sagittal, transverse, and parasagittal views[21] (see Chapter 31). CT can identify which bulla is involved and the extent of involvement. The mass may be outlined as extending from the tympanic membrane into either the external ear canal or the nasopharyngeal region (Figure 69-7). Thickening of the tympanic membrane also may be seen. There are only two reported cases of MRI imaging of inflammatory polyps. These polyps had strong contrast enhancement on T1-weighted images. One of the cats also had contrast enhancement on T2-weighted images.[24]

Although advanced imaging, signalment, and clinical signs can make a strong case for the diagnosis of an inflammatory polyp, all polyps should be submitted for histopathological evaluation to ensure that appropriate therapy is initiated. Microbial culture and sensitivity testing of the mass should be performed to allow for the selection of appropriate antibiotic therapy.

MIDDLE EAR TUMORS

The diagnosis of a middle ear tumor begins with a thorough physical examination. Occasionally it may be possible to visualize a mass through a ruptured or irregular tympanic membrane with an otoscope (see Chapter 30). A FNA may even be attempted, with sedation if the mass is visible. Full staging includes baseline laboratory evaluation, thoracic radiographs, aspirates of any enlarged lymph nodes, retroviral testing, and advanced imaging.

High-quality skull films may reveal bony destruction of the bulla and adjacent structures. Soft-tissue opacity also may be visible within the tympanic bulla, with or without sclerosis of the bulla. A CT scan or MRI of the head often is necessary for therapeutic planning. Lysis of the tympanic bulla, petrous temporal bone, and adjacent calvarium may be seen in addition to a soft-tissue mass within (and possibly extending through) the tympanic bulla.[21] It is important to note that osteolysis may not be seen with all tumors. Contrast enhancement may help to delineate the tumor and determine the degree of blood flow to the tumor (Figure 69-8). A biopsy may be taken through a myringotomy while the cat is under general anesthesia, but after the imaging procedure. Most often, the surgical biopsy is obtained at the time of excision.

For cats with LSA of the middle ear, a diagnosis often is achieved with a FNA if the mass can be aspirated.[15] Full staging for lymphoma patients is required before the appropriate course of therapy may be selected. Full staging includes baseline laboratory evaluation (including retroviral testing), two-view thoracic radiographs, abdominal ultrasound, and possibly a bone-marrow aspirate.

TREATMENT FOR EAR TUMORS

TUMORS OF THE PINNA

SCC of the ear pinna often can be cured if diagnosed early and treated aggressively. Surgery remains the mainstay of therapy for this disease. Pinnectomy with wide surgical margins often is easy to perform, cosmetically satisfactory, and the best option for long term control (Figure

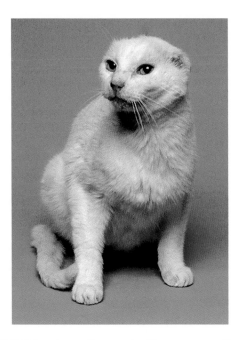

Figure 69-9 This cat was diagnosed with squamous cell carcinomas of both pinnas as a result of UV-induced tumor formation. Bilateral pinnectomies have been performed and are often considered cosmetically satisfactory by owners. (Courtesy Dr. Kenita Rogers, Texas A&M University.)

69-9). In one study 18 cats treated with surgical resection had no local recurrence and a median survival time (MST) of 799 days.[25]

Cryosurgery is a reasonable option if pinnectomy is not possible, or if the owners would be dissatisfied with the cosmetic outcome of surgery. Cryosurgery involves minimal equipment costs and is available to general practitioners and specialty clinics. The drawbacks to this procedure include the fact that no surgical margins can be assessed, and only small, superficial lesions (<5 mm) amenable to thorough freezing can be treated. However, if used early in the disease process for carefully selected cases, it can be a very successful therapy. In one study all 12 cats with SCC of the ear pinna and eyelid were treated successfully and had a complete response to cryotherapy. Unfortunately, cats with SCC on the nasal planum did not respond as well.[26]

Photodynamic therapy (PDT) involves the administration of a photosensitizing agent that is retained preferentially by neoplastic tissue. The agent then is activated by applying a light source (typically a specific diode) to the tissue of interest that is of a specific wavelength of light generating cytotoxic free radicals. The agents used most commonly include 5-aminolevulinic acid and aluminum phthalocyanine tetrasulfonate. The success of PDT depends on the tumor type, the photosensitizing agent used, and the energy dose. The light source does not penetrate deeply into the tissues; therefore only superficial lesions may be treated. Tumor responses have been variable and the disease free interval (DFI) associated with this treatment has been generally disappointing compared with other therapies.[27-29] After treatment cats should be kept out of direct sunlight to avoid generalized photosensitivity. Other side effects include depression, facial edema, and blistering or ulceration of nonpigmented skin.[27-29]

Local current field radiofrequency hyperthermia is used for large nonresectable tumors in human beings and enhances the effects of chemotherapy and radiation therapy (RT). Temperatures exceeding 42° C are used to kill cells within minutes. This modality has been used in cats and dogs with pinnal and nasal planum SCC with an overall response rate (ORR) of 68 per cent.[30]

RT typically is not necessary for pinnal SCC because the response to surgery is so positive. However, megavoltage radiation (cobalt 60) and brachytherapy (strontium applicators) have been used (see Figure 67-3). Megavoltage RT to the ear pinna may result in significant side effects to the pinna itself as well as the ear canal, with ulceration and fibrosis likely to occur. Additionally, responses and MST with this therapy are not particularly good.[2] Conversely, brachytherapy can be very successful for the right patient. It is particularly effective for superficial lesions and is relatively inexpensive. Proton beam RT has been used for nasal lesions in cats with a 93 per cent ORR and a MST of 946 days.[31] This therapy has not been applied to pinnal SCC in cats.

Intralesional chemotherapy is another option for pinnal SCC. There is less systemic absorption and therefore less toxicity associated with this route of administration. Chemotherapy agents that have been used intralesionally in cats include cisplatin, 5-fluorouracil (5-FU), and carboplatin. The lack of systemic absorption allows the use of drugs that typically would be fatal if given to a cat systemically (i.e., cisplatin and 5-FU).[32,33]

There are limited data regarding therapy for mesenchymal tumors of the ear pinna such as rhabdomyomas and fibrosarcomas. The limited information available suggests that excellent long-term control can be achieved with complete surgical excision.[16] This typically requires an aggressive surgical procedure because these tumors have long finger-like projections extending away from the primary mass into the surrounding tissues.

Hemangiosarcomas and hemangiomas of the ear pinna in cats also are often treated with surgery alone. Surgery typically is curative for hemangiomas; however, hemangiosarcomas often recur even after aggressive surgery. In one study, four cats with pinnal HSA had recurrence within 9.5 months.[17] A combination of surgery and electron beam RT may provide longer DFI and MSTs.

MSAs of the ear pinna in cats often are cured with surgery alone; however, there is a subset of more aggressive MSAs in cats that recur and/or metastasize. Adjunct therapy may be needed for those cats with a more aggressive phenotype. Carboplatin chemotherapy and treatment with other agents have been attempted with minimal success in dogs. There are no reports of successful chemotherapy protocols for cats with MSA of the ear pinna. RT has been effective for lymph node metastases and local recurrences in dogs and also may be appropriate therapy for cats. Immunotherapy, such as the Merial Melanoma Vaccine, is largely untested in cats. The vaccine has been given to a small number of cats with MSA (none of whom had pinnal MSA) safely; however, no responses have been documented thus far.[34]

Basal cell tumors and mast cell tumors have been treated successfully with surgery alone. A small basal cell tumor may be removed with minimal margins because most of these tumors are benign. A histopathological diagnosis of a basal cell carcinoma would potentially require an additional, more aggressive surgery.

Mast cell tumors in cats also tend to have a benign behavior requiring less aggressive surgery than is necessary in dogs. Premedication with antihistamines and corticosteroids can counter the release of vasoactive substances during surgery.

TUMORS OF THE EXTERNAL EAR CANAL

Surgery is the mainstay of therapy for all external ear canal tumors. These tumors are challenging and often impossible to remove completely. Conservative approaches, such as a lateral ear canal resection (LECR), tend to result in incomplete surgical margins and early recurrence.[35] More aggressive approaches, such as a total ear canal ablation (TECA), are more likely to result in clean surgical margins but result in deafness. In addition to surgery, adjuvant RT may be helpful when the margins are incomplete. Chemotherapy also may be used for tumors with a high metastatic potential.

CGA is the most common external ear canal tumor seen in cats. A study of 22 cats included 16 patients who underwent a TECA and six cats who underwent a LECR. The median disease free interval (MDFI) for cats treated with a TECA was 42 months with a recurrence rate of 25 per cent, compared with a MDFI of 10 months and a 66.7 per cent recurrence rate for those cats treated with a LECR.[35,36] There is limited information regarding RT for CGA in cats. In a study evaluating six cats with both microscopic and macroscopic disease treated with megavoltage radiation to 48 Gy total dose, a few cats achieved a complete response, but most eventually developed recurrence or metastases.[37]

Therapy for inflammatory polyps typically involves simple traction avulsion for pharyngeal polyps and polyps not associated with the middle ear. Corticosteroid use after surgery is controversial, but may decrease recurrence.[11] Appropriate antibiotic therapy should be initiated, based on microbial culture and sensitivity testing. For cats with tympanic cavity involvement or recurrence, a ventral bulla osteotomy, with or without a TECA, may be necessary; however, there is a higher complication rate with this surgery compared with other less invasive methods of polyp removal. The most common postoperative complication seen is temporary Horner's syndrome. Occasionally, vestibular signs and transient facial nerve paralysis are seen.[20,38] The recurrence rate for traction avulsion alone is approximately 30 per cent, and less than 8 per cent for those cats undergoing a ventral bulla osteotomy.[11,20,38]

THERAPY FOR MIDDLE EAR TUMORS

Surgery provides the greatest chance for long-term disease control. A TECA typically is required in order to achieve the appropriate margins, but complete margins are not possible for all tumors. Adjunct RT for incompletely excised carcinomas of the middle ear may provide longer DFIs and MSTs than surgery alone. Cats diagnosed with LSA of the middle ear should be staged completely. If the disease is confined to the ear canal, RT is likely to be very successful. If the disease has spread beyond the ear canal, or RT is not a good option for the cat, then chemotherapy may be another good option. These therapies are not likely to be curative, but may result in an improved quality and quantity of life.

Tumors of the middle ear often are diagnosed at an advanced stage, which leads to a poor or guarded prognosis for malignant tumors. Benign tumors still carry a good prognosis, as local and regional control is crucial for long-term survival.

PREVENTION OF EAR TUMORS

Many tumors of the pinna are actinically induced (SCC, HSA, hemangioma, possibly basal cell tumor), especially in cats with light-colored coats. Decreasing the cats' lifetime exposure to UV light may prevent tumor formation. Cats with light coat colors should be kept indoors to avoid excess sun exposure. Additionally, UV shields can be used on windows to limit the exposure of frequent sunbathers. It also is possible to apply infant-safe sunscreen to the ears and nose of light-colored cats who have frequent or prolonged exposure to sunlight.

Chronic inflammation associated with ear infections increases the risk of developing an ear tumor.[2] A thorough evaluation for ear infections followed by appropriate therapy and regular recheck examinations may help to limit inflammation and decrease the likelihood of malignant transformation later in life (see Chapter 32).

SUMMARY

Ear tumors are relatively rare in cats, but tend to be more aggressive than similar tumors in dogs. They occur most commonly on the pinna or in the external ear canal, and many tumor types can be caused by chronic sun exposure. As with most tumors, early intervention increases the likelihood for long-term success. Thorough physical examination including an otoscopic examination may help to detect some ear tumors earlier in the disease process and to increase the probability for therapeutic success.

REFERENCES

1. Fan TM, de Lorimier LP: Inflammatory polyps and aural neoplasia, *Vet Clin North Am Small Anim Pract* 34:489, 2004.
2. Vail DM, Withrow SJ: Ear canal tumors in dogs and cats. In Vail DM, Withrow SJ, editors: *Small animal clinical oncology*, ed 4, Philadelphia, 2007, Saunders, p 393.
3. Dorn CR, Taylor DO, Schneider R: Sunlight exposure and risk of developing cutaneous and oral squamous cell carcinoma in white cats, *J Natl Cancer Inst* 199:1357, 1971.
4. Teifke JP, Lohr CV: Immunohistochemical detection of p53 overexpression in paraffin wax-embedded squamous cell carcinomas of cattle, horses, cats and dogs, *J Comp Pathol* 114:205, 1996.

5. Nasir L, Krasner H, Argyle DJ, et al: Immunocytochemical analysis of tumour suppressor protein (p53) in feline neoplasia, *Cancer Lett* 155:1, 2000.

6. Matousek JL: Diseases of the ear pinna, *Vet Clin North Am Small Anim Pract* 34:511, 2004.

7. Hanna PE, Dunn D: Cutaneous fibropapilloma in a cat (feline sarcoid), *Can Vet J* 44:601, 2003.

8. Schulman FY, Krafft AE, Janczewski T: Feline cutaneous fibropapillomas: clinicopathologic findings and association with papillomavirus infection, *Vet Pathol* 38:291, 2001.

9. London CA, Dubilzeig RR, Vail DM, et al: Evaluation of dogs and cats with tumors of the ear canal: 145 cases (1978-1992), *J Am Vet Med Assoc* 208:1413, 1996.

10. Muilenburg RK, Fry TR: Feline nasopharyngeal polyps, *Vet Clin North Am Small Anim Pract* 32:839, 2002.

11. Anderson DM, Robinson RK, White RAS: Management of inflammatory polyps in 37 cats, *Vet Rec* 147:684, 2000.

12. Kudnig ST: Nasopharyngeal polyps in cats, *Clin Tech Small Anim Pract* 17:174, 2002.

13. Veir JK, Lappin MR, Foley JE: Feline inflammatory polyps: historical, clinical and PCR findings for feline calici virus and feline herpes virus-1 in 28 cases, *J Feline Med Surg* 4:195, 2002.

14. Trevor PB, Martin RA: Tympanic bulla osteotomy for treatment of middle-ear disease in cats: 19 cases (1984-1991), *J Am Vet Med Assoc* 37:99, 1993.

15. De Lorimier LP, Alexander SD, Fan TM: T-cell lymphoma of the tympanic bulla in a feline leukemia virus-negative cat, *Can Vet J* 44:987, 2003.

16. Roth L: Rhabdomyoma of the ear pinna in four cats, *J Comp Pathol* 103:237, 1990.

17. Miller MA, Ramos JA, Kreeger JM: Cutaneous vascular neoplasia in 15 cats: clinical, morphologic and immunohistochemical studies, *Vet Pathol* 29:173, 1992.

18. Luna LD, Higginbotham ML, Henry CJ, et al: Feline nonocular melanoma: a retrospective study of 23 cases (1991-1999), *J Feline Med Surg* 1:173, 2000.

19. Salvadori C, Cantile C, Arispici M: Meningeal carcinomatosis in two cats, *J Comp Path* 131:246, 2004.

20. Little CJ: Nasopharyngeal polyps. In August JR, editor: *Consultations in feline internal medicine*, vol 3, Philadelphia, 1997, Saunders, p 310.

21. Bischoff MG, Kneller SK: Diagnostic imaging of the canine and feline ear, *Vet Clin North Am Small Anim Pract* 34:734, 2004.

22. Venker-van Haagen AJ, van der Gaag I: Tumors of the external ear, *Vet Quart* 20:S7, 1998.

23. Lorenzi DD, Bonfanti U, Masserdotti C, et al: Fine needle biopsy of external ear canal masses in the cat: cytologic results and histologic correlations in 27 cases, *Vet Clin Pathol* 34:100, 2005.

24. Allgoewer I, Lucas S, Schimtz SA: Magnetic resonance imaging of the normal and diseased feline middle ear, *Vet Radiol Ultrasound* 41:413, 2000.

25. Lana SE, Olgilvie GK, Withrow SJ, et al: Feline cutaneous squamous cell carcinoma of the nasal planum and pinnae: 61 cases, *J Am Anim Hosp Assoc* 33:329, 1997.

26. Clarke RE: Cryosurgical treatment of cutaneous squamous cell carcinoma, *Aust Vet Pract* 21:148, 1991.

27. Peaston AE, Leach MW, Higgins RJ: Photodynamic therapy for nasal and aural squamous cell carcinoma in cats, *J Am Vet Med Assoc* 202:1261, 1993.

28. Hahn KA, Panjehpour M, Legendre AM: Photodynamic therapy response in cats with cutaneous squamous cell carcinoma as a measure of fluence, *Vet Dermatol* 9:3, 1998.

29. Stell AJ, Dobson JM, Langmack K: Photodynamic therapy of feline superficial squamous cell carcinoma using topical 5-aminolaevulinic acid, *J Small Anim Pract* 42:164, 2001.

30. Grier RL, Brewer WG Jr, Theilen GH: Hyperthermic treatment of superficial tumors in cats and dogs, *J Am Vet Med Assoc* 177:227, 1980.

31. Fidel JL, Egger E, Blattman H, et al: Proton irradiation of feline nasal planum squamous cell carcinomas using an accelerated protocol, *Vet Radiol Ultrasound* 43:501, 2002.

32. Theon AP, Van Vechten MK, Madewell BR: Intratumoral administration of carboplatin for treatment of squamous cell carcinomas of the nasal plane in cats, *Am J Vet Res* 57:205, 1996.

33. Orenberg EK, Luck EE, Brown DM: Implant delivery system: intralesional delivery of chemotherapeutic agents for treatment of spontaneous skin tumors in veterinary patients, *Clin Dermatol* 9:561, 1991.

34. Personal communication: Dr. Andrea Flory, Animal Medical Center, New York, NY, 4/11/2008.

35. Marino DJ, MacDonald JM, Matthiesen DT: Results of surgery in cats with ceruminous gland adenocarcinoma, *J Am Anim Hosp Assoc* 30:54, 1994.

36. Moisan PG, Watson GL: Ceruminous gland tumors in dogs and cats: a review of 124 cases, *J Am Anim Hosp Assoc* 32:449, 1996.

37. Theon AP, Barthez PY, Madewell BR, et al: Radiation therapy of ceruminous gland carcinomas in dogs and cats, *J Am Vet Med Assoc* 205:566, 1994.

38. Lanz OI, Wood BC: Surgery of the ear and pinna, *Vet Clin North Am Small Anim Pract* 34:567, 2004.

70 Ocular Tumors

*Carolina Naranjo, Joan Dziezyc, and
Nicholas J. Millichamp*

Ocular, orbital, and adnexal tumors are rare in cats, affecting 0.34 per cent of all feline patients presented for veterinary consultation.[1] These tumors are classified as *primary*, if they arise in the eye, or *secondary*, if they involve the eye as a direct extension from a tumor in an adjacent structure (e.g., nasal cavity, brain, or sinuses) or if the tumors are metastatic from another part of the body. In the latter situation, the first clinical evidence of these tumors may be detected in the eye. Ocular tumors can involve the globe, the orbit, or the ocular adnexa (eyelids, conjunctiva, and third eyelid).

PRIMARY TUMORS

EYELID TUMORS

Eyelid tumors are uncommon in cats compared with dogs, occurring in 0.13 per cent of feline patients presented for treatment at veterinary hospitals, and their relative risk increases with age.[2] Eyelid tumors in cats are more likely to be malignant than those occurring in dogs; therefore complete surgical resection may require aggressive surgery with or without adjunctive therapy. If the globe is to be preserved, special skin and mucosal flaps are essential to restore the eyelid functionality and maintain the health of the ocular surface. More extensive tumors may require enucleation with skin grafting procedures to obtain adequate margins.[3]

The most common eyelid tumor in cats is squamous cell carcinoma, accounting for up to two-thirds of the tumors in this location.[2] This tumor can be found in the eyelids, conjunctiva, nictitating membrane, and orbit, and in advanced cases, it may be difficult to establish the primary site. There is a predilection for the lower eyelid and medial canthus of white cats,[1] which suggests that exposure to ultraviolet (UV) radiation and lack of pigmentation may play a role (Figure 70-1). Metastasis usually occurs late in the course of the disease, most often to the regional lymph nodes and lungs[4]; however, because of the invasiveness of this tumor, local recurrence is common if excised incompletely. As mentioned previously, multiple cutaneous and mucosal flaps may be necessary for restoration of eyelid function.[5,6] Other modalities of treatment, in combination with surgery or alone, have been described for squamous cell carcinomas, including intralesional chemotherapy, radiation therapy, photodynamic therapy, and brachytherapy.[7-10]

Apocrine hydrocystomas or cystadenomas arise from the apocrine sweat glands in the skin of the eyelids or eyelid margin (from the glands of Moll). Results from two recent case reports suggest that these are adenomatous proliferative tumors and not mere retention cysts.[11,12] They usually appear in middle-aged to old cats, with a possible predilection for Persian cats because six of the seven cases reported are from this breed.[11-13] They usually appear as multiple, well-circumscribed, firm to fluctuant, smooth, pigmented nodules that are 2 to 10 mm in diameter and located in the superior and inferior eyelid, although more typically they arise on the face, neck, and extremities of cats.[13] Fine-needle aspirate of these masses usually reveals a dark brown translucent fluid with variably admixed neutrophils or macrophages, and biopsy is needed for definitive diagnosis.[11] These proliferations usually are benign, but recurrence and development of new masses may arise at other sites in the eyelids.[11,13] Some authors recommend observation without treatment because of the benign nature of the tumor; however, drainage and/or surgical excision are recommended if the lesion is causing discomfort to the ocular structures or resulting in corneal disease.[11,13] Chemical ablation with trichloroacetic acid has been suggested as a

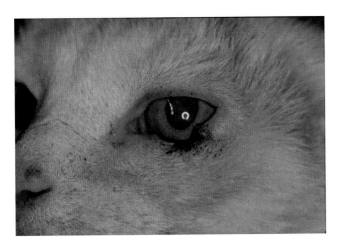

Figure 70-1 Squamous cell carcinoma of the lower eyelid in a white cat.

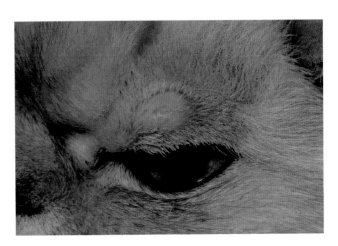

Figure 70-2 Mast cell tumor of the upper eyelid.

complement to surgical excision and in the one case report, resulted in no recurrences of the masses 12 months postoperatively.[12]

Peripheral nerve sheath tumors, also known as schwannomas, neurilemomas, neurogenic sarcomas, neurofibromas, or neurofibrosarcomas, are seen infrequently in the periocular skin of middle-aged to old cats, with a tendency to occur in the superior eyelid.[14] These tumors arise as firm nodular masses and, although they usually do not metastasize, local aggressive recurrence after surgical excision is common even when ancillary procedures, such as cryoablation and laser ablation, are used. Radical surgical procedures often are necessary, including enucleation or exenteration of a visual eye.[14]

Cutaneous hemangiosarcomas involving the eyelid have been described infrequently and in both reported cases involved the lower eyelid.[15,16] One case occurred in a white cat, and an association with actinic changes was proposed.[16] When compared to its visceral counterparts, cutaneous hemangiosarcomas in cats are associated with a more favorable prognosis[17] and have a tendency to recur locally. Metastatic behavior has been reported rarely[18]; therefore this neoplasm carries a good prognosis when complete surgical resection is achieved.[15]

Sebaceous and meibomian gland tumors (adenoma, adenocarcinoma, and epithelioma), so prevalent in dogs, occur rarely in cats.[19] Mast cell tumors and melanocytic tumors can occur in the dermal side of the eyelid (Figure 70-2). No specific behavior has been attributed to either of these neoplasms when affecting the eyelids[19,20] (see Chapter 67).

CONJUNCTIVAL AND THIRD EYELID TUMORS

Neoplasms of the conjunctiva or third eyelid in the cat are uncommon.[19] Conjunctival melanoma has been reported rarely in cats.[21,22] Although the number of reported cases of conjunctival melanoma is small, three of the four affected cats were euthanized because of systemic spread of the neoplasm. Local excision was attempted in these patients; however, recurrence of the tumor prompted enucleation. No criteria have been established to predict malignant behavior, and it is unclear if there is any difference if the melanoma arises from the bulbar or palpebral conjunctiva; however, the tumor arose from the bulbar conjunctiva in all three cases in one report.[22] These findings suggest that this tumor manifests malignant behavior, necessitating early surgical intervention. A malignant melanoma arising from the nictitating membrane also has been reported,[23] with metastases to the brain and lungs. The conjunctiva and orbit were involved extensively, so primary conjunctival or orbital involvement could not be excluded.

Primary hemangioma and hemangiosarcoma of the conjunctiva (bulbar, palpebral, or in the conjunctiva lining the third eyelid) have been reported rarely in cats,[24,25] and little is known about their risk factors and prognosis. Distinction between these two tumors is based on histological degree of differentiation and local invasive behavior.[20,25] A retrospective study including six hemangiomas and two hemangiosarcomas revealed that six of seven cats in whom gender was reported were neutered males,[25] similar to findings for feline cutaneous hemangiomas and hemangiosarcomas.[17] Most of the affected patients were middle-aged to old cats. The tumors tended to occur in cats of variably or poorly pigmented hair coats, and the patients lived in states with higher UV radiation levels.[25] The most common site of involvement was the leading edge of the nictitating membrane, usually in locations where the conjunctiva was not pigmented. The tumors presented as red-to-brown, smooth-to-multilobulated exophytic nodules. Metastasis appears to be rare, and surgical excision alone was curative in most of the tumors in the series; however, local recurrence may occur when hemangiosarcomas are resected incompletely, necessitating more aggressive procedures such as excision of the entire third eyelid or enucleation. Ancillary therapies, such as laser (neodymium-yttrium-aluminum-garnet [ND:YAG]) and cryotherapy, have been used at the time of excision, but the number of patients in whom these modalities have been used is too low to draw conclusions.[24,25]

Lymphoma has been reported to occur in the conjunctiva without systemic involvement.[26] Another report described a Hodgkin's-like lymphoma in the conjunctiva of a cat, with various enlarged peripheral lymph nodes; however, histopathological examination was not performed on lymph node tissue to determine if neoplastic tissue was present.[27] The cat was reported to be alive 3 years after the diagnosis, after undergoing chemotherapy and radiation therapy.

Adenocarcinoma of the gland of the third eyelid has been reported in one cat.[28] The case report described a mass present in the bulbar aspect of the nictitating membrane, causing its protrusion, indentation of the adjacent cornea, and eventually exophthalmos. On histopathological examination, there was a pleomorphic population of anaplastic polygonal cells, with some cells showing intracytoplasmic secretory material and occasional acinar and tubular formations. The cat was euthanized 4 weeks after presentation, with extensive metastatic disease found on necropsy examination. Based on this single case report in the literature, it appears that this tumor has metastatic potential, and radical surgery, such as excision of the nictitating membrane, is recommended at early stages of the disease.[28]

Mast cell tumors of the third eyelid have been reported in a cat with concurrent eosinophilic conjunctivitis and herpesvirus infection, with no recurrence reported 1 year after local excision.[29] Feline cutaneous mast cell tumors usually have a benign course, but it has not been determined if the behavior of conjunctival or third eyelid mast cell tumors in cats differs from their dermal counterparts[30] (see Chapter 67).

Squamous cell carcinomas can invade the conjunctiva and third eyelid. The tumors have not been reported as a primary conjunctival neoplasm in cats but rather occur as an extension of eyelid tumors.[19]

TUMORS OF THE ORBIT

Orbital neoplasms are reported to be rare in cats,[31,32] accounting for 4 per cent of feline neoplasms.[33] Approximately 90 per cent are malignant,[1,31,33] with the average survival time after diagnosis being 1 to 2 months.[31,33] The tumors may be primary within the orbit, secondary by extension from adjacent structures (nasal cavity, sinuses), or secondary by metastatic spread,[31,32,34] with an estimated percentage of 14, 71, and 14 for each of these categories, respectively.[33] These neoplasms tend to occur in older cats, with no breed or gender predilections. The most common clinical sign is exophthalmos, but enophthalmos, protrusion of the third eyelid, epiphora, and strabismus also have been described.[31,33] Fine-needle aspirates of these tumors can be useful diagnostically. Advanced imaging techniques (computed tomography [CT] and magnetic resonance imaging [MRI]) have proved to be very useful in the diagnosis of orbital tumors, especially when trying to differentiate these tumors from nonneoplastic diseases.[35-37] MRI is less specific for bony structures than CT, but it offers more detailed imaging of the soft tissues of the orbit.[38]

Epithelial tumors, particularly squamous cell carcinoma, are the orbital tumors reported most commonly in cats, accounting for two-thirds of the tumors in one study.[33] In this study, orbital squamous cell carcinoma always occurred secondary by extension from the nasal or oral cavities, conjunctiva, eyelids, or maxillary bone. A variety of other tumors have been reported in the feline orbit, including zygomatic gland tumors,[31] adenocarcinoma from the frontal sinuses or nasal cavity,[33] lymphoma (associated with systemic involvement or by extension from the nasal cavity),[31,33,36] zygomatic osteoma,[39] osteosarcoma,[31,38,40] fibrosarcoma,[31,33,36] melanoma,[33] and plasmacytoma[41]; however, any tissue present in the orbit (including extraocular muscles, adipose tissue, lacrimal gland, and orbital vessels and nerves) can give rise to a primary orbital tumor.

Melanomas have been reported to occur in the orbit by extension from uveal melanomas,[33] but only a few cases of primary orbital melanoma without intraocular involvement have been reported.[35,42] In both cases, the neoplasms were very advanced at the time of presentation and the possibility of a conjunctival tumor extending into the orbit could not be excluded. Orbital meningiomas, reported commonly in dogs, are extremely rare in cats.[31,35]

Most orbital neoplasms are malignant. Treatment frequently is unsuccessful because the majority of tumors are secondary to extension from adjacent structures or metastatic from distant sites. Multiple treatment modalities have been described, including surgical excision (usually exenteration of the orbit), radiation therapy, and chemotherapy. Unfortunately, even with the use of multiple treatment modalities, survival time averages 4.3 months.[33]

Deserving special mention is orbital pseudotumor (retrobulbar pseudotumor, idiopathic sclerosing orbital pseudotumor), a term borrowed from the human literature, which is used to identify any idiopathic mass lesion with accompanying inflammation. It is discussed here because its clinical presentation, behavior, and prognosis are similar to those of a neoplasm.[43] This rare condition has been described in the feline orbital area,[44,45] occurring primarily in old cats and is characterized by an insidious and progressive course that frequently involves both eyes. The clinical signs usually are related to the orbital disease and include exophthalmos, lagophthalmos, varying degrees of keratitis with possible ulceration and perforation, resistance to manual retropulsion of the globe, and reduced ocular mobility. Histopathologically, the lesion is characterized by an extensive infiltration of the orbit, eyelids, and third eyelid by a variably dense, poorly delineated population of spindle cells (fibroblasts) encircling the eye and dissecting between the orbital adipose and connective tissue, extraocular muscles, and dermal collagen of the eyelids, with variable deposition of collagen and multifocal inflammatory foci. These foci are composed mainly of lymphoplasmacytic infiltrates; however, eosinophilic infiltrates also have been described. Response to treatment (systemic corticosteroids with topical treatment for the secondary corneal disease) in the cases reported is poor, and enucleation is a final outcome in all of the cases reported. Because of the

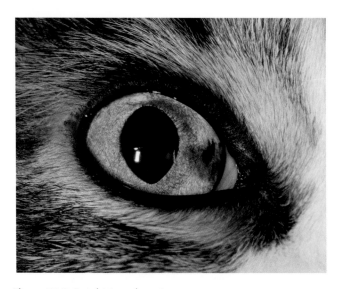

Figure 70-3 Focal iris melanosis.

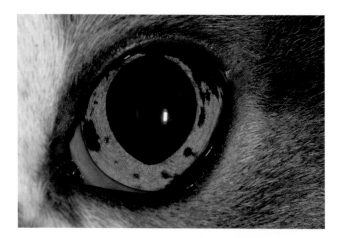

Figure 70-4 Diffuse iris melanoma (early stages) in which the iris has multiple areas of flat pigmentation with no discomfort or visual disturbance.

involvement of the contralateral orbit, euthanasia was elected in seven of the eight cases described in the literature.[44,45]

TUMORS OF THE GLOBE

Melanocytic Tumors

Tumors of melanocytic origin are the most common primary intraocular tumor in cats,[20,46-48] and in turn, the eye is the most common site for melanocytic neoplasms to occur in this species.[22] The most common melanocytic tumor involving the ocular structures is the diffuse iris melanoma, which is characterized by a diffuse, slowly progressive pigmentation of the iris without the presence of a mass lesion, often over a period of years. There are no known breed or gender predilections, but the incidence increases in older cats. In the first stage (Figure 70-3), called *iridal melanosis,* single or multiple localized nonneoplastic pigmented foci are noted, which can expand and coalesce over several years, progressing to a diffuse pigmentation of the iris and malignant transformation (Figures 70-4 and 70-5). Clinically, a diffusely pigmented iris should be differentiated from chronic uveitis, which also can lead to a change in pigmentation of the uvea.[1] In more advanced cases, affected eyes often develop glaucoma, which presumably is associated with proliferation of neoplastic cells in the iridocorneal (drainage) angle (Figure 70-6).

Histopathologically, iridal melanosis is characterized by one to a few layers of angular pigmented cells that have a small round bland nucleus and are carpeting the anterior iris surface, without invading the iris stroma (Figure 70-7, *A*). These lesions can remain static or progress slowly for years before the development of neoplasia. The diagnosis of feline diffuse iris melanoma is made when the pigmented cells invade the iris stroma (Figure 70-7, *B*), expand and distort the iris profile, and eventually extend and invade other ocular structures such as the iridocorneal angle, ciliary body, and sclera (Figure 70-8).

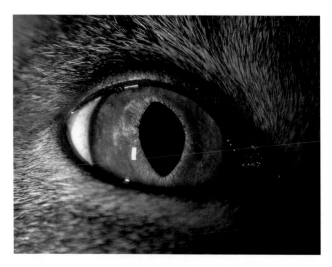

Figure 70-5 Diffuse iris melanoma. The pigmented areas are slightly raised, and the pupil did not constrict as well as the pupil in the unaffected eye.

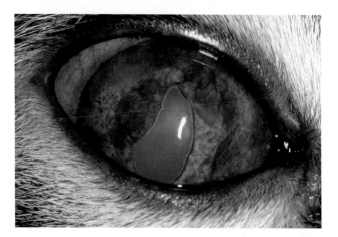

Figure 70-6 More advanced diffuse iris melanoma with iris swelling, pupil distortion (dyscoria), and secondary glaucoma.

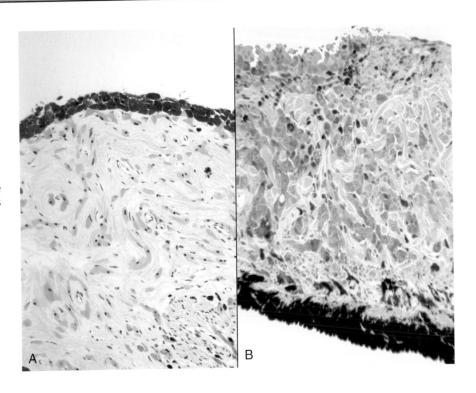

Figure 70-7 A, In iris melanosis, the anterior surface of the iris is carpeted by a few layers of bland, angular pigmented cells without cellular atypia. **B,** Early feline diffuse iris melanoma. The pigmented cells have invaded the iris stroma and show moderate anisokaryosis, with prominent nucleoli. (Hematoxylin & eosin, 200×.) (Courtesy Dr. Richard R. Dubielzig.)

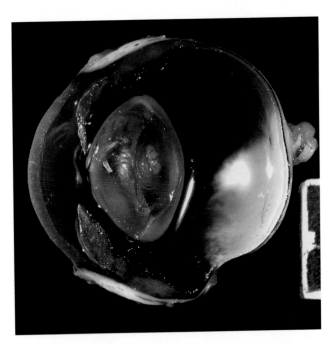

Figure 70-8 Feline diffuse iris melanoma, extensive: The iris and ciliary body are diffusely and homogeneously expanded by a neoplastic population of pigmented cells. Bar = 1 cm. (Courtesy Dr. Richard R. Dubielzig.)

This usually is accompanied by a change in cellular morphology, with increased anaplastic features and cellular atypia that are not appreciated clinically.[47,49] Multiple histological forms are found; the most common is composed of pleomorphic round plump cells, followed by spindle cells and finally balloon cells, with mixtures of all types seen frequently; however, no prognostic significance has been attributed to the different morphological types.[22,46] Amelanotic forms also are noted, which are more difficult to diagnose clinically because of the lack of a mass lesion and can be confused with changes associated with uveitis. Multiple morphological criteria may influence the outcome and metastatic potential of these tumors, but most of the criteria do not predict the outcome clearly in any individual cat. The only histopathological features that have been suggested to influence the prognosis are the extent of ocular involvement, with decreasing survival times when the tumor infiltrates the ciliary body and sclera,[46,47] and with mitotic rate.[46] Although the rate of metastasis has been reported to vary from 20 to 66 per cent or higher,[22,32,46,47] few documented cases with confirmed metastasis are found in the literature. When these tumors metastasize, they do so primarily to the regional lymph nodes, liver, and lungs; therefore survey abdominal ultrasound and thoracic radiographs are recommended.[22,46]

Because of the long time between initial change in pigmentation and development of overt neoplasia with metastatic potential, controversy exists as to when to enucleate the affected eye. On the one hand, this tumor has metastatic potential. Conversely, enucleating an eye that can be comfortable and visual for many years before metastasis occurs has ethical implications. Ideally, the eye should be enucleated immediately before the development of glaucoma, which implies invasion into the iridocorneal angle and a possible route for the neoplastic cells to exit the eye and metastasize.[49] Obviously, it is impossible to determine this precise timing clinically, so periodic evaluation of the lesion for change in size usually is recommended.[1] Other clinical criteria mentioned in the literature include exfoliation of pigmented cells into the anterior chamber, gonioscopic evidence of infiltration of the iridocorneal angle, and changes in pupillary shape and mobility.[1,19] Ablation of small focal hyperpigmented foci on the iris with a diode laser has been attempted, but the success rate and side effects of this procedure are unknown.[1]

Atypical forms have been described in which the tumor originates from any portion of the uvea (ciliary body and choroid, as opposed to the iris) and forms nodular, frequently multifocal masses that subsequently may coalesce and distort the globe.[34,49,50] The fact that they originate posteriorly may explain the delay in clinical diagnosis, thereby explaining the extensive involvement of the ocular structures and increased risk of metastasis in these cats.[47,50] Histopathologically, the neoplastic cells of these atypical forms are uniformly round, plump, and heavily pigmented with absence of nuclear atypia, as opposed to the morphological features described for the neoplastic cells of diffuse iris melanomas.[34,50] In a small series of cats with these atypical tumors,[50] two of the six patients were thought to have metastatic disease, although no histopathological examination was performed to confirm it.

Limbal melanoma or melanocytoma, although reported sporadically in cats,[51-54] is considered the most common primary tumor of the cornea and sclera in this species,[19] with similar clinical presentation and behavior as in dogs.[51] The cases described occurred in middle-aged to old cats, with no breed or gender predilections. All of the tumors occurred in the dorsolateral limbus, appearing as slow-growing, minimally invasive, and slightly raised, darkly pigmented masses. The lesion should be differentiated from conjunctival melanoma, and the involvement of the iridocorneal angle should be assessed by gonioscopy. The tumors are composed histopathologically of two populations of pigmented cells: round plump and spindle.[51] Multiple treatment modalities have been described, from surgical excision alone (lamellar or full-thickness keratectomy and sclerectomy), with an autogenous graft of nictitans cartilage,[54] to surgical excision with adjuvant therapies such as cryotherapy[51] or laser photocoagulation.[55] Many authors consider the tumor to be benign[51]; however, metastases presumed to be from primary limbal melanomas have been reported in two cases.[52,53]

Feline Posttraumatic Sarcoma

Feline posttraumatic sarcoma, also named primary ocular sarcoma or feline ocular sarcoma, is a unique, highly malignant neoplasm occurring in this species and is the second most common primary ocular tumor.[19,56] This malignant neoplasm has been associated repeatedly with a previous traumatizing insult to the eye, including blunt and penetrating trauma, intraocular surgery (such as evisceration or lens extraction), or intraocular gentamicin injection.[19,20,57] These neoplasms are associated with previous longstanding ocular inflammatory disease, and owners often report that the cat was found as a stray and that the eye already looked abnormal. Even when there is no historical evidence of trauma, which occurs in approximately one-half of the reported cases, these tumors have a typical histopathological pattern that helps in their recognition. This tumor does not appear to be associated with infection with feline leukemia virus (FeLV) or feline sarcoma virus.[57] No breed or gender is

overrepresented, and old cats are affected most commonly. The latency period after the traumatizing event is approximately 5 years but ranges from months to 10 years.[58]

The most common clinical sign is a color change of the eye to white or pink and an alteration in shape or consistency,[1,56] with the tumor precluding evaluation of intraocular structures. In the earlier stages, the tumor may be masked by uveitis, glaucoma, or intraocular hemorrhage.[19] The uniqueness of this tumor is related to the fact that at least one-third to one-half of the lesions arise from malignant transformation of released lens epithelial cells.[58,59]

Typically, the globe is filled with a solid tan neoplasm, and lens material may not be visible grossly (Figure 70-9). Histopathologically, the typical features of this tumor are rupture of the lens capsule, organization of neoplastic cells circumferentially around the globe that differentiates the tumor from rare metastatic sarcomas, and the tendency to infiltrate optic nerve and peripheral nerves within the sclera and orbit.[49,56,58] Three histopathological variants of this tumor have been described.[58,59] The most common by far is the spindle cell variant, which is reported to arise from lens epithelial cells. An abundant deposition of collagen (usually type IV) is encountered in the lens capsule,[59] and variably thick basement membranes are present between the neoplastic cells. The neoplastic cells are positive for vimentin and crystallin alpha A, demonstrating lens epithelial origin.[59] The second most common variant is the round cell type, which may be a form of lymphoma.[60] This variant is characterized by a typical pattern of solid sheets of round cells, with survival of tumor cells around blood vessels and extensive

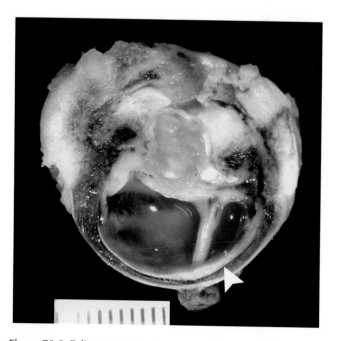

Figure 70-9 Feline posttraumatic sarcoma. The neoplastic infiltrate is surrounding the ruptured lens, filling the anterior chamber and carpeting the inner aspect of the choroid *(arrowhead)*. The retina is detached and also infiltrated by the neoplasm. Bar = 1 cm. (Courtesy Dr. Richard R. Dubielzig.)

necrosis away from the vessels. Finally, the least common type is an osteosarcoma/chondrosarcoma variant, which is very rare. It is unclear if this latter form derives from the spindle cell variant.[61,62]

Because of its malignant behavior, enucleation is the recommended treatment for this tumor. As described previously for feline diffuse iris melanoma, the exact time at which to enucleate is controversial. Few clinicians advocate for early prophylactic enucleation of blind globes, although it is known that a traumatized feline globe is at risk for developing a neoplasm and that invasion of the optic nerve occurs soon after the tumor appears.[63,64] Some ophthalmologists would observe that because the tumor is uncommon, enucleation of a nonpainful phthisical feline eye is not recommended unless there is a change in appearance. Periodic monitoring of blind phthisical eyes or eyes with chronic uveitis is advised[19] because the prognosis is best when enucleation is performed before the tumor invades the optic nerve or sclera.[49] Chemotherapy or radiation protocols have not been described.[1,49]

Because of the tendency of this tumor to infiltrate the optic nerve and scleral and peripheral nerves, a frequent outcome is the development of contralateral blindness and neurological signs, caused by the ascendant infiltration of the tumor toward the brain.[58,65] Recurrence in the orbit and distant metastases also have been reported.[58,64] Death or euthanasia related to the tumor occurs in up to 60 per cent of the cases, with a survival time from enucleation to euthanasia ranging from 0 days to months.[58,63]

Iridociliary Tumors

Tumors of the epithelium of the ciliary body and iris are rare in cats.[66] These neoplasms arise from the pigmented or nonpigmented epithelium of the iris or ciliary body, which is of neuroectodermal origin. There are no breed or gender predilections, affected cats are middle-aged to old, and the tumor usually presents as a solitary, slow-growing, smooth, solid or cystic, nonpigmented mass visible through the pupil. The tumor can displace the iris and lens and if large enough, can lead to a localized nonpigmented mass that is visible in the anterior chamber (Figures 70-10 to 70-12). These neoplasms rarely infiltrate the sclera, which is the criterion proposed to differentiate adenomas from carcinomas.[66] Metastatic disease from this tumor has not been recognized, but enucleation is recommended.[19]

Other Tumors of the Globe

Scattered reports of other types of primary ocular neoplasia in cats are found in the literature. These include an astrocytoma of the retina[67] and an intraocular extramedullary plasmacytoma.[68]

SECONDARY (METASTATIC) TUMORS

A variety of metastatic tumors have been reported to occur in the feline eye, with a tendency for the metastatic lesions to infiltrate the choroid, alone or in conjunction with the anterior uvea.[69] These metastatic lesions do not always cause a mass lesion, which frequently poses a diagnostic challenge. Additionally, these tumors often are

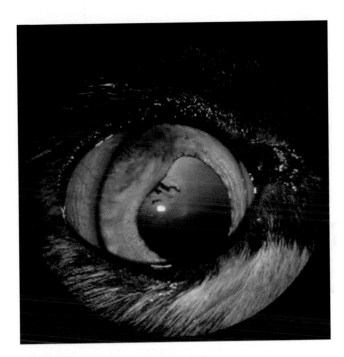

Figure 70-10 Iridociliary adenoma: Ciliary processes are seen displaced into the pupil.

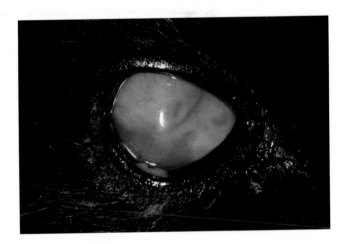

Figure 70-11 Iridociliary carcinoma with uveitis.

accompanied by hemorrhage, exudation, inflammation, retinal detachment, and secondary glaucoma, which can obscure the neoplastic changes.[1,69]

Lymphoma is the most common metastatic tumor to the feline eye[19,32,34] (Figures 70-13 and 70-14). The lesion frequently involves the iris and may appear as a solitary mass, or as a diffuse infiltrate throughout the uvea,[70] making the iris appear thickened and velvety, as is often seen with uveitis. These diffuse neoplastic changes make differentiation between inflammation and neoplasia very difficult clinically. In one study, 17 of 49 cats with ocular lymphoma had been diagnosed initially with uveitis.[70] The retina, cornea, and sclera also can become involved by infiltration with neoplastic cells. Cytological examination of the aqueous humor frequently confirms the diagnosis.[19]

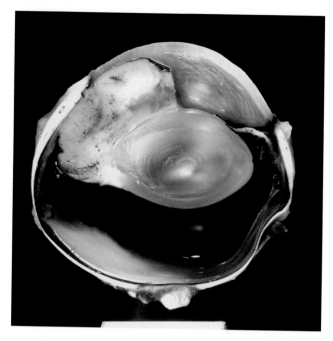

Figure 70-12 Feline iridociliary adenoma. There is a well-delineated, nonencapsulated white mass arising from the ciliary body and cradling the lens, pushing the iris leaflet forward. Bar = 1 cm. (Courtesy Dr. Richard R. Dubielzig.)

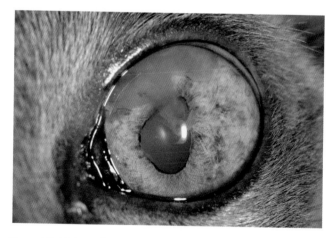

Figure 70-13 Lymphosarcoma at pupil base, extending into the anterior chamber, and iritis.

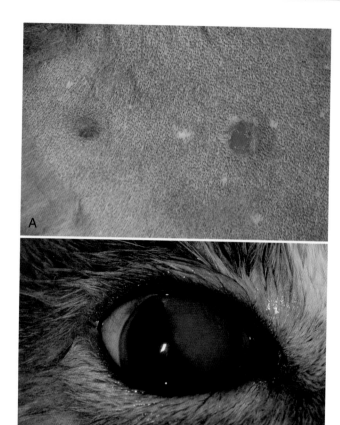

Figure 70-14 Cutaneous (**A**) and ocular (**B**) (anterior uveal) lymphosarcoma (mycosis fungoides).

Other neoplasms that metastasize to the feline eye are carcinomas,[34] which include squamous cell carcinoma of pulmonary or aural origin, and adenocarcinoma of pulmonary,[71,72] mammary, sweat gland, and uterine origin. Hemangiosarcoma and fibrosarcoma metastasizing to the eye also have been reported rarely in cats.

Of special interest are pulmonary carcinomas, which tend to metastasize to the eye in cats,[71,72] similar to the metastatic behavior found in lung-digit syndrome.[69] These ocular tumors also can go unnoticed clinically because they do not form mass lesions and usually appear as angular areas of choroidal and retinal degeneration and necrosis from infarction caused by neoplastic infiltration of choroidal blood vessels.[72] The primary pulmonary tumor can range from a large mass to small foci within the lung lobes.[69]

SUMMARY

In summary, a variety of tumors can affect the feline eye and adnexal structures. Many of them are malignant, making an accurate diagnosis key to assessing the extent of the disease in other organs and to determining the most appropriate treatment modalities.

REFERENCES

1. Miller PE, Dubielzig RR: Ocular tumors. In Withrow SJ, Vail DM, editors: *Withrow & MacEwen's small animal clinical oncology*, ed 4, St. Louis, 2007, Saunders, p 686.
2. McLaughlin SA, Whitley RD, Gilger BC, et al: Eyelid neoplasms in cats: a review of demographic data (1979 to 1989), *J Am Anim Hosp Assoc* 29:63, 1993.
3. Aquino SM: Management of eyelid neoplasms in the dog and cat, *Clin Tech Small Anim Pract* 22:46, 2007.
4. Riis RC, Vitali CM, Simons JB: Eyelid tumors. In Peiffer RL, Simons KB, editors: *Ocular tumors in animals and humans*, Ames, 2002, Iowa State Press, p 25.
5. Stiles J, Townsend W, Willis M, et al: Use of a caudal auricular axial pattern flap in three cats and one dog following orbital exenteration, *Vet Ophthalmol* 6:121, 2003.

6. Schmidt K, Bertani C, Martano M, et al: Reconstruction of the lower eyelid by third eyelid lateral advancement and local transposition cutaneous flap after "en bloc" resection of squamous cell carcinoma in 5 cats, *Vet Surg* 34:78, 2005.

7. Théon AP, VanVechten MK, Madewell BR: Intratumoral administration of carboplatin for treatment of squamous cell carcinomas of the nasal plane in cats, *Am J Vet Res* 57:205, 1996.

8. Magne ML, Rodriguez CO, Autry SA, et al: Photodynamic therapy of facial squamous cell carcinoma in cats using a new photosensitizer, *Lasers Surg Med* 20:202, 1997.

9. Hardman C, Stanley R: Radioactive gold-198 seeds for the treatment of squamous cell carcinoma in the eyelid of a cat, *Aust Vet J* 79:604, 2001.

10. Melzer K, Guscetti F, Rohrer Bley C, et al: Ki67 reactivity in nasal and periocular squamous cell carcinomas in cats treated with electron beam radiation therapy, *J Vet Intern Med* 20:676, 2006.

11. Cantaloube B, Raymond-Letron I, Regnier A: Multiple eyelid apocrine hidrocystomas in two Persian cats, *Vet Ophthalmol* 7:121, 2004.

12. Yang SH, Liu CH, Hsu CD, et al: Use of chemical ablation with trichloroacetic acid to treat eyelid apocrine hidrocystomas in a cat, *J Am Vet Med Assoc* 230:1170, 2007.

13. Chaitman J, van der Woerdt A, Bartick TE: Multiple eyelid cysts resembling apocrine hidrocystomas in three Persian cats and one Himalayan cat, *Vet Pathol* 36:474, 1999.

14. Hoffman A, Blocker T, Dubielzig R, et al: Feline periocular peripheral nerve sheath tumor: a case series, *Vet Ophthalmol* 8:153, 2005.

15. McAbee KP, Ludwig LL, Bergman PJ, et al: Feline cutaneous hemangiosarcoma: a retrospective study of 18 cases (1998-2003), *J Am Anim Hosp Assoc* 41:110, 2005.

16. Hartley C, Ladlow J, Smith KC: Cutaneous haemangiosarcoma of the lower eyelid in an elderly white cat, *J Feline Med Surg* 9:78, 2007.

17. Miller MA, Ramos JA, Kreeger JM: Cutaneous vascular neoplasia in 15 cats: clinical, morphologic and immunohistochemical studies, *Vet Pathol* 29:329, 1992.

18. Kraje AC, Mears EA, Hahn KA, et al: Unusual metastatic behavior and clinicopathologic findings in eight cats with cutaneous or visceral hemangiosarcoma, *J Am Vet Med Assoc* 214:670, 1999.

19. Stiles J, Townsend WM: Feline ophthalmology. In Gelatt KN, editor: *Veterinary ophthalmology*, ed 4, Ames, 2007, Blackwell Publishing, p 1095.

20. Wilcock B, Dubielzig RR, Render JA: Intraocular tumors. In WHO histological classification of ocular and otic tumors of domestic animals, Series 2, Vol. IX. Washington, DC, 2002, Armed Forces Institute of Pathology, p 58.

21. Cook CS, Rosenkrantz W, Peiffer RL, et al: Malignant melanoma of the conjunctiva in a cat, *J Am Vet Med Assoc* 186:505, 1985.

22. Patnaik AK, Mooney S: Feline melanoma: a comparative study of ocular, oral, and dermal neoplasms, *Vet Pathol* 25:105, 1988.

23. Roels S, Ducatelle R: Malignant melanoma of the nictitating membrane in a cat *(Felis vulgaris)*, *J Comp Pathol* 119:189, 1998.

24. Multari D, Vascellari M, Mutinelli F: Hemangiosarcoma of the third eyelid in a cat, *Vet Ophthalmol* 5:273, 2002.

25. Pirie CG, Dubielzig RR: Feline conjunctival hemangioma and hemangiosarcoma: a retrospective evaluation of eight cases (1993-2004), *Vet Ophthalmol* 9:227, 2006.

26. Radi ZA, Miller DL, Hines ME II: B-cell conjunctival lymphoma in a cat, *Vet Ophthalmol* 7:413, 2004.

27. Holt E, Goldschmidt MH, Skorupski K: Extranodal conjunctival Hodgkin's-like lymphoma in a cat, *Vet Ophthalmol* 9:141, 2006.

28. Komaromy AM, Ramsey DT, Render JA, et al: Primary adenocarcinoma of the gland of the nictitating membrane in a cat, *J Am Anim Hosp Assoc* 33:333, 1997.

29. Larocca RD: Eosinophilic conjunctivitis, herpes virus and mast cell tumor of the third eyelid in a cat, *Vet Ophthalmol* 3:221, 2000.

30. Gross TL, Ihrke PJ, Walder EJ, et al: *Skin diseases of the dog and cat: clinical and histopathological diagnosis*, ed 2, Ames, 2005, Blackwell Science Ltd.

31. Attali-Soussay K, Jegou JP, Clerc B: Retrobulbar tumors in dogs and cats: 25 cases, *Vet Ophthalmol* 4:19, 2001.

32. Grahn BH, Peiffer RL: Fundamentals of veterinary ophthalmic pathology. In Gelatt KN, editor: *Veterinary ophthalmology*, ed 4, Ames, 2007, Blackwell Publishing, p 155.

33. Gilger BC, McLaughlin SA, Whitley RD, et al: Orbital neoplasms in cats: 21 cases (1974-1990), *J Am Vet Med Assoc* 201:1083, 1992.

34. Wilcock BP: Eye and ear. In Maxie MG, editor: *Jubb, Kennedy and Palmer's pathology of domestic animals*, ed 5, Philadelphia, 2007, Saunders, p 459.

35. Grahn BH, Stewart WA, Towner RA, et al: Magnetic resonance imaging of the canine and feline eye, orbit, and optic nerves and its clinical application, *Can Vet J* 34:418, 1993.

36. Calia CM, Kirschner SE, Baer KE, et al: The use of computed tomography scan for the evaluation of orbital disease in cats and dogs, *Vet Comp Ophthalmol* 4:24, 1994.

37. Källberg ME: Ophthalmic examination and diagnostics. Part 2: Ocular imaging. In Gelatt KN, editor: *Veterinary ophthalmology*, ed 4, Ames, 2007, Blackwell Publishing, p 484.

38. Ramsey DT, Gerding PA, Losonsky JM, et al: Comparative value of diagnostic imaging techniques in a cat with exophthalmos, *Vet Comp Ophthalmol* 4:198, 1994.

39. Foley RH: Zygomatic osteoma in a cat, *Feline Pract* 21:26, 1993.

40. Heldmann E, Anderson MA, Wagner-Mann C: Feline osteosarcoma: 145 cases (1990-1995), *J Am Anim Hosp Assoc* 36:518, 2000.

41. Ward DA, McEntee MF, Weddle DL: Orbital plasmacytoma in a cat, *J Small Anim Pract* 38:576, 1997. Erratum in: *J Small Anim Pract* 39:230, 1998.

42. De Lorimier LP: Primary orbital melanoma without ocular involvement in a Balinese cat, *Can Vet J* 47:225, 2006.

43. Dubielzig RR: Personal communication, May 16, 2008.

44. Miller SA, van der Woerdt A, Bartick TE: Retrobulbar pseudotumor of the orbit in a cat, *J Am Vet Med Assoc* 216:356, 2000.

45. Billson FM, Miller-Michau T, Mould JR, et al: Idiopathic sclerosing orbital pseudotumor in seven cats, *Vet Ophthalmol* 9:45, 2006.

46. Duncan DE: Morphology and prognostic indicators of anterior uveal melanomas in cats, *Prog Vet Comp Ophthalmol* 1:25, 1991.

47. Kalishman JB, Chappell R, Flood LA, et al: A matched observational study of survival in cats with enucleation due to diffuse iris melanoma, *Vet Ophthalmol* 1:25, 1998.

48. Colitz CM: Feline uveitis: diagnosis and treatment, *Clin Tech Small Anim Pract* 20:117, 2005.

49. Dubielzig RR: Tumors of the eye. In Meuten DJ, editor: *Tumors in domestic animals*, ed 4, Ames, 2002, Iowa State Press, p 739.

50. Harris BP, Dubielzig RR: Atypical primary ocular melanoma in cats, *Vet Ophthalmol* 2:121, 1999.

51. Harling DE, Peiffer RL, Cook CS: Feline limbal melanoma: four cases, *J Am Anim Hosp Assoc* 22:795, 1986.

52. Day MJ, Lucke VM: Melanocytic neoplasia in the cat, *J Small Anim Pract* 36:207, 1995.

53. Betton A, Healy LN, English RV, et al: Atypical limbal melanoma in a cat, *J Vet Intern Med* 13:379, 1999.

54. Kanai K, Kanemaki N, Matsuo S, et al: Excision of a feline limbal melanoma and use of nictitans cartilage to repair the resulting corneoscleral defect, *Vet Ophthalmol* 9:255, 2006.

55. Sullivan TC, Nasisse MP, Davidson MG, et al: Photocoagulation of limbal melanoma in dogs and cats: 15 cases (1989-1993), *J Am Vet Med Assoc* 208:891, 1996.

56. Dubielzig RR: Feline ocular sarcomas. In Peiffer RL, Simons KB, editors: *Ocular tumors in animals and humans*, Ames, 2002, Iowa State Press, p 283.

57. Cullen CL, Haines DM, Jackson ML, et al: The use of immunohistochemistry and the polymerase chain reaction for detection of feline leukemia virus and feline sarcoma virus in six cases of feline ocular sarcoma, *Vet Ophthalmol* 1:189, 1998.

58. Dubielzig RR, Everitt J, Shadduck JA, et al: Clinical and morphologic features of post-traumatic ocular sarcomas in cats, *Vet Pathol* 27:62, 1990.

59. Zeiss CJ, Johnson EM, Dubielzig RR: Feline intraocular tumors may arise from transformation of lens epithelium, *Vet Pathol* 40:355, 2003.

60. Naranjo C, Dubielzig RR: Round cell variant of feline post-traumatic sarcoma: 7 cases, *Invest Ophthalmol Vis Sci* 48:E-Abstract 3596, 2007.

61. Woog J, Albert DM, Gonder JR, et al: Osteosarcoma in a phthisical feline eye, *Vet Pathol* 20:209, 1983.

62. Miller WW, Boosinger TR: Intraocular osteosarcoma in a cat, *J Am Anim Hosp Assoc* 23:317, 1987.

63. Peiffer RL, Monticello T, Bouldin TW: Primary ocular sarcomas in the cat, *J Small Anim Pract* 29:105, 1988.

64. Hakanson N, Shively JN, Reed RE, et al: Intraocular spindle cell sarcoma following ocular trauma in a cat: case reports and literature review, *J Am Anim Hosp Assoc* 26:63, 1990.

65. Barrett PM, Merideth RE, Alarcon FL: Central amaurosis induced by an intraocular, posttraumatic fibrosarcoma in a cat, *J Am Anim Hosp Assoc* 31:242, 1995.

66. Dubielzig RR, Steinberg H, Garvin H, et al: Iridociliary epithelial tumors in 100 dogs and 17 cats: a morphological study, *Vet Ophthalmol* 1:223, 1998.

67. Gross SL, Dubielzig RR: Ocular astrocytomas in a dog and cat, *Trans Ann Proc Am Coll Vet Ophthalmol* 15:243, 1984.

68. Michau TM, Proulx DR, Rushton SD, et al: Intraocular extramedullary plasmacytoma in a cat, *Vet Ophthalmol* 6:177, 2003.

69. Dubielzig RR, Grendahl RL, Orcutt JC, et al: Metastases. In Peiffer RL, Simons KB, editors: *Ocular tumors in animals and humans*, Ames, 2002, Iowa State Press, p 337.

70. Corcoran KA, Peiffer RL, Koch SA: Histopathologic features of feline ocular lymphosarcoma: 49 cases (1978-1992), *Vet Comp Ophthalmol* 5:35, 1995.

71. Gionfriddo JR, Fix AS, Niyo Y, et al: Ocular manifestations of a metastatic pulmonary adenocarcinoma in a cat, *J Am Vet Med Assoc* 197:372, 1990.

72. Cassotis NJ, Dubielzig RR, Gilger BC, et al: Angioinvasive pulmonary carcinoma with posterior segment metastasis in four cats, *Vet Ophthalmol* 2:125, 1999.

71 The Dilemmas of Cytological Evaluation of the Feline Lymph Node

Mark C. Johnson

Cytological examination of tissues is an integral part of the veterinary diagnostic repertoire in cats. Practically any tissue of the body, including peripheral and internal lymph nodes, is amenable to direct or ultrasound-guided fine-needle aspiration. Studies in dogs and cats have evaluated the sensitivity and specificity of cytological evaluation of various tissues compared with histopathology, and for the assessment of metastasis to lymph nodes.[1-3] Remarkably, these studies have shown that in lymph nodes, cytopathology correlates well to histopathology about 50 per cent of the time, and is highly sensitive (100 per cent) and specific (96 per cent) for detecting metastasis.[1,2] The most important challenge associated with cytological evaluation of feline lymph nodes is to differentiate the normal changes from the various abnormal processes involving these tissues, and to identify specific diseases. This chapter will illustrate a systematic approach for resolving the cytological dilemmas of lymph node evaluation in cats.

SAMPLE ACQUISITION AND SMEAR PREPARATION OF LYMPH NODES

Veterinarians can perform fine-needle aspiration of enlarged lymph nodes routinely in cats, similar to dogs. Proper sample acquisition and smear preparation are just as important to the overall cytological interpretation of lymph node samples as the microscopic evaluation, because inferior collection and preparation techniques often lead to poor cellular preservation of the notoriously fragile lymphocyte.[4-6] Fine-needle core or "stab" tech-

nique samples often are superior to fine-needle "aspiration" techniques in terms of cellular integrity during the collection process.[6] Gentle vertical pull-apart "squash smears" (Figure 71-1) or "blood smear" methods provide the best morphological preservation of lymphocytes.[6] Horizontal pull-apart smears (Figure 71-2) should be avoided, because they often induce lysis of lymphocytes (Figure 71-3).[6]

Samples typically are stained with rapid Romanowsky-type cytological stains, such as Diff-Quick, Wright's, or a modified Wright's stain.[6,7] Unstained samples that are shipped to a diagnostic laboratory should be submitted separately from any formalin-fixed tissues, because exposure to either formalin or the formalin fumes causes an excessively blue-staining, nondiagnostic sample.[6,8] A good practice for veterinarians to employ, even if they are skilled cytologists, is to send similar slides to a pathologist to verify the cytological diagnosis. Likewise, histological examination of tissues remains the gold standard for definitive diagnosis.

NORMAL LYMPH NODE CYTOLOGY

The initial challenge in lymph node cytology is to determine if the sample is normal or abnormal. In reality this can be a challenging task, particularly with feline lymph nodes because what constitutes normal lymph node cytology is somewhat dependent on the location of the node. For example, normal mesenteric lymph nodes may have a higher percentage of immature lymphocytes and plasma cells compared with their normal peripheral

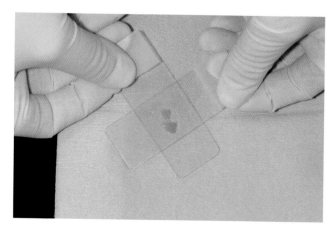

Figure 71-1 Vertical pull-apart technique for lymph node aspirate. One of the preferred methods for preservation of lymphocyte morphology.

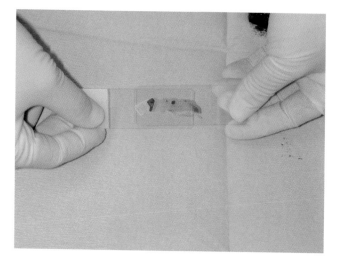

Figure 71-2 Horizontal pull-apart technique for lymph node aspirate. Avoid this method, because lysis of lymphocytes is common.

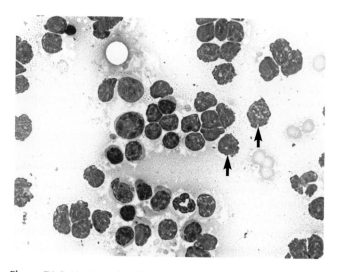

Figure 71-3 Horizontal pull-apart smear. Note the numerous lysed lymphocytes at the tip of the *arrows*. (Diff-Quick stain—100× oil immersion objective.)

counterparts.[7,8] This difference is hypothesized to occur because mesenteric lymph nodes are exposed to larger numbers of antigens derived from the intestinal tract compared with peripheral lymph nodes.[7,8]

Small lymphocytes in most normal peripheral lymph node cytology samples represent approximately 85 to 90 per cent of the entire lymphocyte population.[6-9] Likewise, immature lymphocytes typically compose the remaining 10 to 15 per cent of the population. Immature lymphocytes are large or medium-sized cells, or a combination of both. Small numbers of plasma cells, macrophages, neutrophils, eosinophils, and mast cells also are seen in cytology samples from normal lymph nodes, but each should represent less than 1 per cent of the entire nucleated cell population.[6-8,10,11]

ABNORMAL LYMPH NODE CYTOLOGY: THE INITIAL DILEMMA

Lymphadenopathy is defined as an enlargement of one or more lymph nodes. When multiple lymph nodes are enlarged throughout the body, the designation of generalized lymphadenopathy is used. Generalized lymphadenopathy is recognized in cats, but this finding is certainly more common in dogs.[7] Causes of generalized lymphadenopathy in cats include infectious diseases such as feline immunodeficiency virus (FIV) and feline leukemia virus (FeLV), systemic bacterial or fungal infections, lymphoma, and dermatopathic conditions.[12-19] Three references are reported documenting unusual generalized lymphadenopathy in cats: one detailing a distinctive peripheral lymphadenopathy resembling lymphoma in six cats, five of whom subsequently resolved; one describing peripheral lymph node hyperplasia in young cats; and one attributing lymphadenopathy to methimazole treatment for hyperthyroidism.[20-22] Latter portions of this chapter will discuss changes in lymph nodes associated with some of these diseases. Enlargement of solitary lymph nodes is a relatively common occurrence in cats, as is mesenteric lymphadenopathy, which is more difficult to detect clinically. Accordingly, it is extremely important for clinicians to be able to palpate enlarged peripheral lymph nodes for collection of quality cytological samples. Ultrasound-guided aspiration of lymph nodes generally is recommended for mesenteric or mediastinal lymphadenopathy.

Feline lymph nodes typically are quite small, so palpable lymphadenopathy should be considered an abnormal clinical finding. However, it is important for the clinician to remember that palpable changes in lymph node size are not sufficient for a definitive diagnosis; cytological or histopathological examinations are required. Additionally, minimal enlargement of a lymph node does not exclude the potential for disease within the node. One study in dogs and cats evaluated the predictability of determining metastatic disease based on palpable lymph node enlargement compared with histopathological and cytopathological examinations.[2] The results of this study showed there is relatively good sensitivity (93 per cent) but poor specificity (14 per cent) using lymph node palpation alone when the lymph nodes are significantly enlarged.[2] However, when lymph nodes are only mildly increased in size, the sensitivity for metastasis based on palpation alone decreased substantially (60 per cent).[2] In contrast, cytopathology compares relatively well to histopathology, and cytological evaluation of lymph nodes is recommended for assessing lymph nodes for metastatic disease.[2]

The initial cytological dilemma is classifying the cause of lymphadenopathy. In the most simplistic approach to this classification strategy, causes of lymphadenopathy are divided into three separate categories: (1) reactive hyperplasia, (2) inflammatory, and (3) neoplastic. The inflammatory and neoplastic categories are subdivided further into groups based on the type of inflammatory cells present, and whether the neoplasia is primary or secondary. Each of these three categories has unique cytological features that aid in their classification. What makes evaluation of many cytological samples extremely challenging is that these categories often overlap. In the following sections, these three categories will be discussed based on their cellular features and which specific feline disorders may elicit such cytological changes.

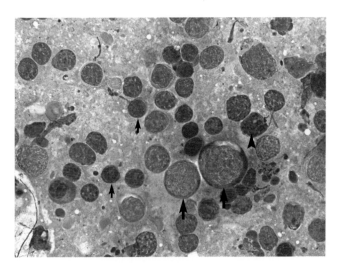

Figure 71-4 Hyperplastic lymph node in a cat. Note the predominance of small lymphocytes *(small arrows)* and the two large lymphocytes *(large arrows)*. (Diff-Quick stain—100× oil immersion objective.)

THE REACTIVE HYPERPLASTIC LYMPH NODE DILEMMA

By definition, hyperplastic lymph nodes have increased numbers of lymphocytes, generally reflecting an increased number of immature lymphocytes within the tissue.[6,8] Although some veterinarians use this term synonymously with "reactive" lymph nodes, reactive lymph nodes typically imply increased numbers of plasma cells within the node. These two processes often are commingled within the same lymph node, leading some clinicians to use the two terms interchangeably. The percentage of immature lymphocytes in a hyperplastic lymph node is increased compared with normal lymph nodes, varying from 15 to 20 per cent to approximately 35 to 40 per cent (Figure 71-4) in marked hyperplasia.[6,8] Higher percentages of immature lymphocytes raise a strong suspicion for lymphoma. Plasma cell numbers also are usually increased, often representing greater than 5 per cent of the total nucleated cell population within the lymph node (Figure 71-5). Extremely high percentages of plasma cells (>50 per cent) in a lymph node cytological sample may represent an extramedullary plasma cell neoplasm.[23-25]

A variety of nonspecific disorders are capable of inducing these lymph node changes. Antigenic stimulation, although a vague and nonspecific term, is thought to stimulate these changes in the lymph nodes. Lymph nodes filter and process antigens, so exposure to new or excessive amounts of these antigens can lead to proliferation of lymphocytes and production of antibodies by plasma cells.[6-8] Many infectious, inflammatory, allergic, and neoplastic disorders are capable of eliciting this type of response. This response is nonspecific and an etiology often is not identified in the cytological sample. However, thorough microscopic examination for potential causes of reactive hyperplasia, such as metastatic neoplasia and inflammation from infectious diseases, is recommended when reactive hyperplasia is evident cytologically. Spe-

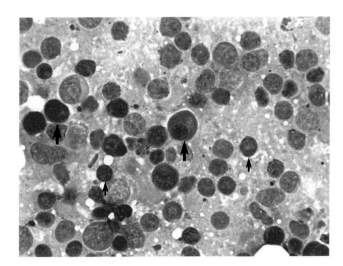

Figure 71-5 Reactive lymph node in a cat. Note the numerous plasma cells *(large arrows)* and predominance of small lymphocytes *(small arrows)*. (Diff-Quick stain—100× oil immersion objective.)

cific types of neoplasia and infectious diseases common to cats will be discussed in later sections of this chapter.

THE INFLAMMATORY LYMPH NODE DILEMMA

Increased numbers of inflammatory cells in a lymph node cytological sample are abnormal, but it is often difficult to differentiate a true lymphadenitis from the presence of inflammatory cells resulting from drainage of a regional inflammatory site. Reactive hyperplasia frequently is present in addition to the inflammatory infiltrate. The inflammatory cells are neutrophils most commonly, but macrophages, multinucleated giant cells, eosinophils, or a combination of these cells often are present. Mast cells

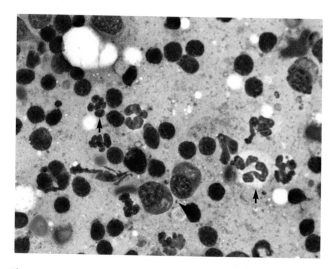

Figure 71-6 Suppurative lymphadenitis and reactive lymph node in a cat. Note the numerous neutrophils *(small arrows)* and plasma cells *(large arrow)*. (Diff-Quick stain—100× oil immersion objective.)

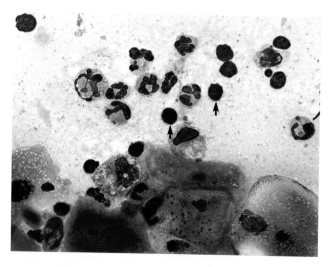

Figure 71-7 Metastatic squamous cell carcinoma in the submandibular lymph node of a cat. Note the large superficial squamous epithelial cells in the lower half of the image and numerous neutrophils in the upper half. Only occasional residual small lymphocytes are present from the lymph node *(small arrows)*. (Diff-Quick stain—100× oil immersion objective.)

also are present occasionally as a component of inflammation, but if these cells are present in larger numbers, they may represent disseminated mast cell disease.[26,27] Basophils are seen rarely in peripheral tissues and lymph nodes.

Increased neutrophils in a lymph node cytological sample indicates suppurative lymphadenitis, or as mentioned previously, drainage of suppurative inflammation distal to the node. If neutrophil numbers are increased considerably and multiple lymph nodes are involved, infectious etiologies are most likely (Figure 71-6). *Bartonella henselae* (bartonellosis, cat scratch disease), *Francisella tularensis* (tularemia), and *Yersinia pestis* (*Pasteurella pestis*, plague) are known causes of suppurative inflammation within multiple lymph nodes in cats.[17,28-31] Microscopic identification of any of these specific bacteria in the lymph node cytological sample is rare. Therefore culture and sensitivity testing and molecular-based tests such as polymerase chain reaction (PCR) for specific microorganisms often are required for identification of the causative agent. Early in the disease course of systemic or local fungal diseases, neutrophilic infiltration into lymph nodes also may occur. However, with time, the inflammatory component will change from suppurative to a mixed population of inflammatory cells. Neutrophilic infiltrates in feline lymph nodes also is seen with metastatic neoplasia, especially squamous cell carcinoma (Figure 71-7). The inflammation often is confined to regional draining lymph nodes, so generalized lymphadenopathy usually is not present.

Pyogranulomatous lymphadenitis is a relative uncommon finding in feline lymph node cytological samples. Neutrophils, macrophages, and occasional multinucleated giant cells typically comprise this type of inflammation. Eosinophils also are seen occasionally with pyogranulomatous inflammation. Some clinical pathologists choose to use the term mixed-cell inflammation interchangeably with pyogranulomatous inflammation, and if a neutrophilic component is absent, the designa-

tion of granulomatous inflammation is appropriate. The main components of this type of inflammation are macrophages and giant cells, which suggest a more insidious type of inflammatory process within the lymph node. In cats, fungal and certain bacterial diseases are the primary causes for this type of inflammation, but feline infectious peritonitis (FIP) is known to cause a similar inflammatory infiltrate in lymph nodes.[32,33]

One of the most common systemic fungal diseases responsible for lymphadenopathy in cats is histoplasmosis.[19] *Histoplasma capsulatum* infection often presents with systemic disease, including lymphadenopathy, so the clinical history, physical examination findings, and other diagnostic evidence of disseminated disease also are paramount for the diagnosis.[19] Although peripheral lymph nodes are easier to sample if enlarged, mesenteric lymph nodes often are a good source for detecting histoplasmosis, especially if gastrointestinal signs are present. Cytological examination of lymph nodes from cats with histoplasmosis often reveals reactive hyperplasia, but increased numbers of macrophages, occasional multinucleated giant cells, and neutrophils often are present.[19,34] Careful microscopic examination for the yeast of *H. capsulatum* is indicated if these inflammatory cells are noted and histoplasmosis is on the list of differential diagnoses. The yeast are approximately 2 to 4 μm in diameter, have a round to oval shape and a thin nonstaining capsule with a round to comma-shaped blue-staining nucleus (Figure 71-8).[19] Budding yeasts are identified occasionally (Figure 71-9). The organisms often are found both within inflammatory cells and free in the background of the smears. In a related finding, *H. capsulatum* also is identified occasionally in leukocytes found in peripheral blood smears (Figure 71-10).[19,34-36] Additionally, several diagnostic tests, including a specific test for *H. capsulatum* cell-wall polysaccharide antigen (performed preferably

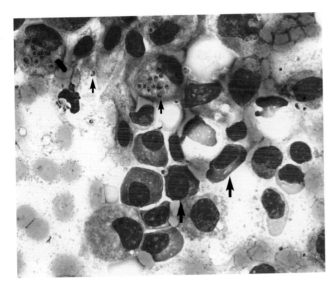

Figure 71-8 Granulomatous lymphadenitis from *Histoplasma capsulatum* infection in a cat. Note the large numbers of yeasts *(small arrows)* within macrophages and some free in the background of the smear. Many plasma cells *(large arrows)* with fewer small lymphocytes also are present. (Diff-Quick stain—100× oil immersion objective.)

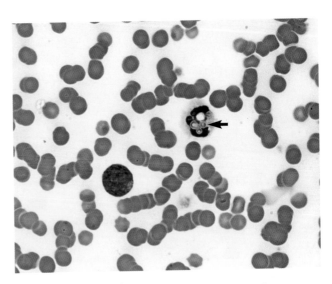

Figure 71-10 Peripheral blood smear of a cat. Note the numerous yeasts *(small arrow)* of *Histoplasma capsulatum* within a neutrophil. A reactive lymphocyte is present in the lower left portion of the image. (Diff-Quick stain—100× oil immersion objective.)

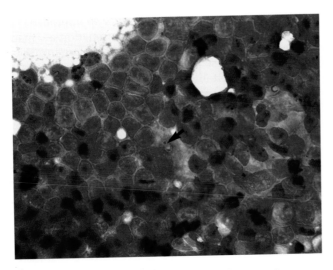

Figure 71-9 Granulomatous lymphadenitis from *Histoplasma capsulatum* infection in a cat. Note the small budding yeast *(small arrow)* within a macrophage admixed with numerous small lymphocytes. (Diff-Quick stain—100× oil immersion objective.)

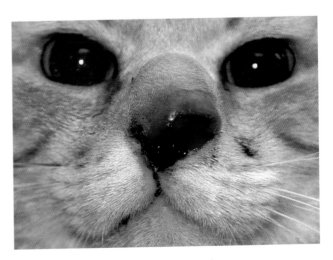

Figure 71-11 Granulomatous deforming rhinitis caused by *Cryptococcus neoformans* infection in a cat. Submandibular lymphadenopathy also was present.

with urine), are available to aid in the diagnosis of histoplasmosis.[37-39]

Cryptococcus neoformans is another fungal organism capable of inducing lymphadenopathy in cats.[36,40] The lymphadenopathy generally is confined to the head and neck because the primary disease usually is located in the nasal cavity and sinuses (Figure 71-11). While organisms may be identified in nasal discharge, lymph nodes also are a readily available source for possible identification of this fungus. Like histoplasmosis, the inflammatory component within the lymph node often is pyogranulomatous, but eosinophils also may be present. Similarly, the node often is reactive and hyperplastic. The yeast of *C.*

neoformans is more variable in size compared with *H. capsulatum*, ranging from 5 to 30 µm in diameter including the polysaccharide capsule.[40] It usually has a large nonstaining capsule, although acapsular forms are reported, and is characterized by narrow-based budding (Figure 71-12).[37,41] The cryptococcal antigen latex agglutination test also is available for aiding in the diagnosis of this fungal disease.[37,40-42]

Sporothrix schenckii, the cause of cutaneous sporotrichosis, is another fungal organism that is involved occasionally in regional lymphadenopathy in cats.[36,43] Initial cutaneous lesions often are similar in appearance to cat-bite abscesses, and are characterized by draining tracts that do not respond to antibiotic therapy. Cytological evaluation of these lesions varies from suppurative to

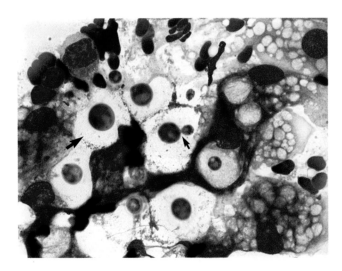

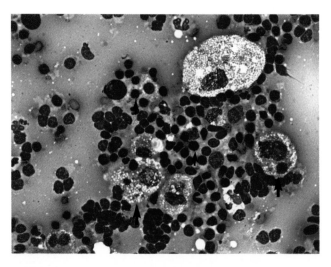

Figure 71-12 Impression smear from a nasal lesion in a cat. Note the numerous large yeasts with a nonstaining clear capsule *(large arrow)* surrounding a round purple nucleus from *Cryptococcus neoformans*. The yeasts are surrounded by many macrophages and other inflammatory cells. The yeast in the center of the image *(small arrow)* is exhibiting narrow-based budding. (Diff-Quick stain—100× oil immersion objective.)

Figure 71-14 Pyogranulomatous lymphadenitis in the mesenteric lymph node of a cat. Note the large foamy macrophages *(large arrows)* admixed with many small lymphocytes *(small arrows)* and occasional neutrophils. (Diff-Quick stain—100× oil immersion objective.)

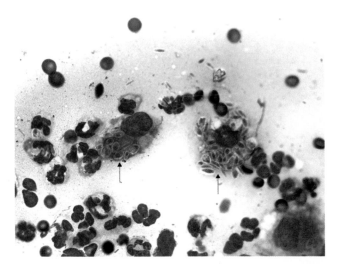

Figure 71-13 Impression smear of a draining subcutaneous lesion in a cat. Note the numerous round to cigar-shaped extracellular yeasts of *Sporothrix schenckii (small arrows)*. (Diff-Quick stain—100× oil immersion objective.)

pyogranulomatous inflammation, with affected draining lymph nodes sharing similar cytological features in addition to reactive hyperplasia. The yeasts are somewhat similar in appearance to *H. capsulatum*, but are slightly larger in size, and have round but also elongated or "cigar-shape" nuclei in addition to the nonstaining thin capsule (Figure 71-13).[38] Other fungal diseases, such as blastomycosis and coccidioidomycosis, are reported in cats, but are less common.[36]

A reemerging disease that is often associated with lymphadenopathy in cats is mycobacteriosis. There are several distinct types of mycobacterial diseases in cats:

feline leprosy, cutaneous tuberculosis, rapidly growing mycobacteriosis, and disseminated mycobacteriosis.[44-49] Discussing the clinical features and the specific genus and species of *Mycobacteria* associated with these manifestations is beyond the scope of this chapter; however, most of these infections can be associated with local, peripheral, or generalized lymphadenopathy. Rapidly or fast-growing mycobacteriosis, formerly known as atypical mycobacteriosis, often is associated with draining subcutaneous tracts involving fatty tissues, especially near mammary glands on the lower inguinal region, but widespread dissemination to lymph nodes is unusual.[47] Cytological examination of enlarged lymph nodes in cats with suspected mycobacterial disease may elucidate the microorganisms. Similar to the fungal diseases, the lymph nodes often exhibit reactive hyperplasia and have pyogranulomatous to granulomatous inflammation. Macrophages and multinucleated giant cells often are heavily vacuolated or "foamy" in appearance (Figure 71-14). Careful observation of these cells occasionally reveals nonstaining (negative staining) small linear structures compatible with bacteria (Figure 71-15), because the bacteria do not normally stain with routine cytological stains.[45,48] Acid-fast stains (Figure 71-16) and specialized culture techniques of these lymph nodes are recommended, as is PCR for speciation of the bacteria.[44-49] Infections of *Actinomyces* spp. and *Nocardia* spp. usually do not cause a generalized lymphadenopathy, although local or regional lymph node involvement is reported (Figure 71-17).[50,51]

Eosinophils occasionally are seen in increased numbers in cytological samples from feline lymph nodes, often as a result of drainage of eosinophilic inflammation distal to the node. These cells typically are observed in conjunction with other inflammatory cells, and in addition to fungal infections, are associated commonly with allergic conditions, parasites, certain tumors (e.g., mast cell

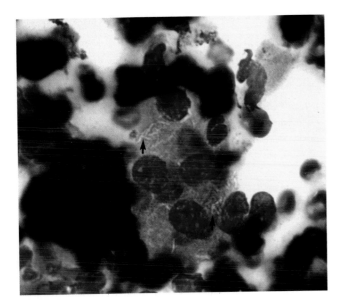

Figure 71-15 Pyogranulomatous inflammation from a subcutaneous lesion in the inguinal region of a cat. Note the three macrophages in the center of the image contain numerous clear, cylindrical nonstaining bacteria *(small arrows)* of *Mycobacterium* spp. (Diff-Quick stain—100× oil immersion objective.)

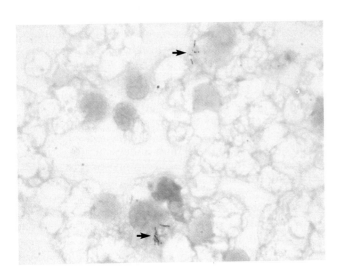

Figure 71-16 Acid-fast stain on the pyogranulomatous lesion from Figure 71-15. Note the positive red-staining *Mycobacterium* spp. *(small arrows)*. (Kinyoun acid-fast stain—100× oil immersion lens.)

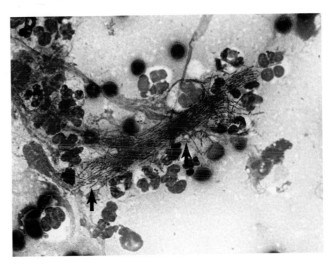

Figure 71-17 Impression smears from a draining subcutaneous lesion in a cat. Note the numerous bacteria with a beaded filamentous shape *(arrows)* within neutrophils and free in the background. These bacteria are consistent with *Actinomycetes* spp. or *Nocardia* spp. (Diff-Quick stain—100× oil immersion objective.)

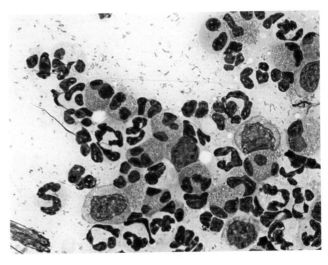

Figure 71-18 Suppurative and eosinophilic inflammation from a raised plaque-like skin lesion on the upper rear leg in a cat with a presumptive diagnosis of eosinophilic plaque. This type of inflammation also can be seen in lymph node cytology samples. (Diff-Quick stain—100× oil immersion objective.)

tumors, T cell lymphoma), and idiopathic causes such as eosinophilic plaques (Figure 71-18).[52-63] One reference is reported documenting eosinophilic infiltration into tissues, including lymph nodes, associated with methicillin-resistant *Staphylococcus*.[64] The combination of eosinophilic infiltrates in organs, including lymph nodes, and a substantial peripheral eosinophilia is very suggestive of a primary eosinophilic disorder such as hypereosinophilia syndrome (HES) or chronic eosinophilic leukemia (Figure 71-19).[58,65-67]

THE NEOPLASTIC LYMPH NODE DILEMMA

Neoplasia is a noted cause for lymphadenopathy in cats, albeit less common than other disorders. Depending on whether the neoplasia is primary, such as lymphoma, or secondary in the case of metastatic disease, the anatomical location and number of lymph nodes affected may be quite variable. Lymphoma is the most common primary neoplasia affecting lymph nodes in cats and is associated with both retroviral infections and nonretroviral causes.[14,15] Prior to the 1980s up to 70 per cent of cases of lymphoma in cats were associated with FeLV infec-

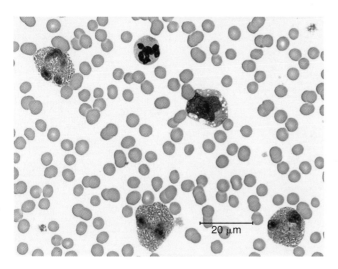

Figure 71-19 Blood smear from a cat with hypereosinophilia syndrome (HES). (Wright's stain—100× oil immersion objective.)

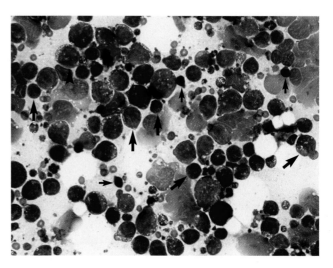

Figure 71-20 Medium to large cell lymphoma from a mesenteric lymph node in a cat. Note the heterogeneous appearance to the medium *(medium arrows)* and large lymphocytes *(large arrows)*. Small lymphocytes are rare *(small arrow)*. (Diff-Quick stain—60× oil immersion objective.)

tion.[14,15,68,69] Although FeLV-associated lymphoma still occurs in cats, the incidence of FeLV-associated lymphoma has diminished significantly.[14,15,68,69] FeLV-associated lymphoma often is multicentric (generalized), so a generalized lymphadenopathy often is present.[14-15,68] FIV infection also is known to increase the risk of lymphoma significantly, up to fivefold to sixfold, but the prevalence of FIV-associated lymphoma has not changed significantly over the years.[15,70]

As a result of this trend for FeLV, lymphoma in cats now is non–retroviral associated most frequently, and often is confined to specific anatomical sites such as the organs or lymph nodes in the abdominal cavity.[14,15,68] This creates a dilemma in itself because the lymphadenopathy often is difficult to detect with conventional palpation techniques, so cytological examination of these lymph nodes often requires the aid of ultrasound[71] (see Chapter 16). Equally challenging with cats is the difficulty of differentiating mesenteric lymphadenopathy caused by inflammatory bowel disease from enlarged lymph nodes caused by lymphoma[71-74] (see Chapter 17). Likewise, secondary neoplasia in lymph nodes also is confined frequently to anatomical locations (e.g., gastrointestinal tract) that are not amenable to routine palpation and cytological evaluation. However, the cytological principles for detecting primary or secondary neoplasia in cats are similar regardless of the anatomical nodal location.

Based on the revised European-American and World Health Organization (REAL-WHO) classification of lymphoid neoplasms in human beings and the National Cancer Institute working formulation (NCI WF), there are numerous separate categories for non-Hodgkin's lymphoma in people.[75-78] Interestingly, a Hodgkin's-like lymphoma has been characterized in cats.[79] These categories often are applied to lymphoid neoplasms in veterinary medicine, including cats, but a combination of histopathological examination, cytological features, immunophenotyping characteristics, and anatomical location are needed to place lymphomas in these groups.[78,80-83] This approach is not feasible with many cases of feline lymphoma, especially if the diagnosis is made only with cytological examination. Traditionally, the more practical approach with cytological examination is to diagnose lymphoma based on size and percentages of lymphocytes within the samples. Accordingly, based on the previous discussion of what constitutes the normal cellular population of a lymph node, small cell lymphoma is not a diagnosis made readily with cytological examination unless a marked small cell lymphocytosis also is present in the peripheral blood.[6] Medium cell, mixed medium and large cell, and large cell lymphoma generally are the descriptive size categories that are used with lymphoma based on cytological examination.[6]

It is important to not only recognize the size of lymphocytes but also the percentages of the different sizes. Generally if 50 per cent or more of the lymphocytes in a lymph node cytological sample are of medium to large size, a cytological diagnosis of lymphoma is made.[6-8] Cytological samples that contain a heterogeneous population of lymphocytes, to include plasma cells, are more compatible with reactive hyperplasia. However, mixed medium and large cell lymphomas, especially if a residual population of small lymphocytes and plasma cells also are present, often appear heterogeneous (Figure 71-20). In these samples it is important to distinguish this heterogeneity from reactive hyperplasia.

The key to the cytological diagnosis of lymphoma in cats is to recognize the size of the lymphocyte that corresponds to the majority of the lymphocytes present. Because most microscopes are not equipped with micrometers, cytologists must use other indicators to aid them in determining the size of the lymphocytes correctly. Feline red blood cells are approximately 5 to 6 μm in diameter and neutrophils are roughly 15 μm in diameter. Small lymphocytes are slightly larger than red blood cells, but smaller than neutrophils, and have a round nucleus with condensed dark blue clumped chromatin and scant amount of clear to light blue cytoplasm (Figure 71-21).

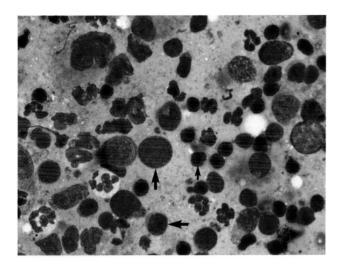

Figure 71-21 Suppurative lymphadenitis and reactive lymph node in a cat. Note the size of lymphocytes compared with the neutrophils: small lymphocytes *(small arrow),* large lymphocytes *(large arrow),* medium lymphocyte *(medium arrow).* (Diff-Quick stain—100× oil immersion objective.)

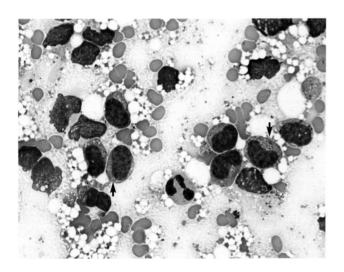

Figure 71-22 Large granular lymphocyte lymphoma from a mesenteric lymph node of a cat. Note the many fine magenta granules *(small arrows)* within the lymphocytes. (Wright's stain—100× oil immersion objective.)

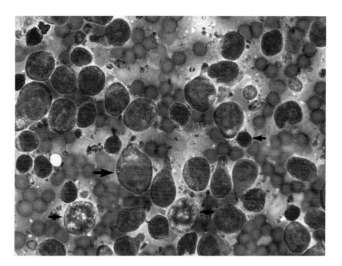

Figure 71-23 Large cell lymphoma from a mesenteric lymph node of a cat. Note the size of the large lymphocyte *(large arrow)* compared with the few small lymphocytes *(small arrow)* and many erythrocytes present. The large lymphocytes occasionally contain faint nucleoli and have a deep blue cytoplasm with a small "Golgi zone" clearing adjacent to the nucleus. Two large lymphocytes undergoing mitosis also are present *(medium arrows).* (Diff-Quick stain—100× oil immersion objective.)

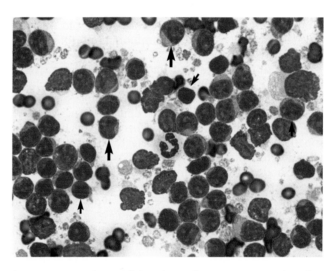

Figure 71-24 Medium cell lymphoma from a mesenteric lymph node of a cat. Note the predominance of medium-sized lymphocytes *(large arrows)* with only rare small lymphocytes *(small arrows)* and a neutrophil present for size comparison. (Diff-Quick stain—100× oil immersion objective.)

Medium lymphocytes are roughly the size of a neutrophil or approximately 1.5 times the size of a red blood cell (see Figure 71-21).[6,8,78,80] These cells have a round to cleaved to irregularly shaped nucleus with a slightly increased amount of cytoplasm that can vary from clear to dark blue. One to two inconspicuous to prominent nucleoli are seen occasionally within the nuclei, which have light pink to purple, smooth chromatin. The morphology of these cells and large lymphocytes is influenced greatly by whether they are T, B, or large granular lymphocytes (LGL) (Figure 71-22).[6,8,78,80,84] Large lymphocytes are greater in size than neutrophils, or approximately two to three times the size of a red blood cell (see Figure 71-21).[6,8,78,80] Nuclei are round to pleomorphic and are placed centrally to eccentrically within a moderate

amount of light to deep blue cytoplasm that occasionally contains a prominent Golgi zone. Nuclear chromatin is smooth to clumped and light pink to purple, with one to several notable nucleoli (Figure 71-23). Cytological examples of medium, mixed medium and large, and large lymphomas are depicted in Figures 71-24, 71-20, and 71-23 respectively.

Metastatic neoplasia in cats, as in other species, generally implies a guarded to poor prognosis. Cytological evaluation of lymph nodes for metastatic neoplasia is not only beneficial, but is fairly reliable in terms of identifying metastatic disease and generally correlates well with histopathological examination.[2,85] The dilemma for most cytopathologists is to recognize metastatic cells in the presence of the large population of lymphocytes. A distinguishing criterion that may aid in this determination is to compare potential metastatic cells in lymph nodes to neoplastic cells within the primary tumor, and to evaluate these cells for cytological criteria of malignancy (Figures 71-25 and 71-26). Additionally, the mere presence of nonresident cells in a lymph node suggests metas-

tasis, even if cellular atypia is not identified. However, in the case of small numbers of mast cells seen in lymph node cytological samples, it is not always possible to discern if the presence of nonresident cells truly represents metastatic disease or a concurrent inflammatory infiltrate.[11] The goal then for evaluating lymph nodes for metastatic disease in cats is to (1) identify the presence of the nonresident cells, (2) compare these cells to neoplastic cells in a primary tumor if possible, and (3) determine if the number of these cells indicates metastatic disease unequivocally.

Although many types of primary tumors can metastasize to lymph nodes in cats, carcinomas and mast cell tumors perhaps are identified most commonly.[26,27,85-92] Metastasis to mediastinal lymph nodes and mesenteric lymph nodes are common with pulmonary and gastrointestinal neoplasms respectively, but these lymph nodes may be difficult to sample routinely without the aid of ultrasound.[27,87-92] However, the presence of epithelial cells within a cytological sample from one of these lymph nodes is strongly supportive of metastatic carcinoma (Figure 71-27).

Facial and oral cutaneous squamous cell carcinoma (SCC) is common in cats, but neither is associated frequently with lymph node metastasis.[93-95] Regardless of the primary location, cytological samples from lymph nodes with suspected SCC often are reactive and hyperplastic owing to either the presence of metastatic cells or the generalized antigenic stimulation that occurs in response to the primary neoplasm. Additionally, neutrophils may be increased within these samples indirectly, as a result of drainage of suppurative inflammation associated with the primary tumor, or directly by the presence of the carcinoma (see Figure 71-7). While it is unclear

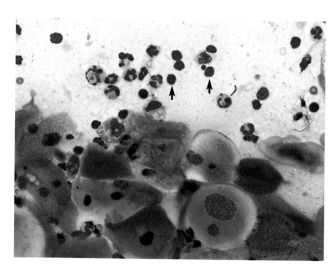

Figure 71-25 Metastatic squamous cell carcinoma in the submandibular lymph node of a cat. Note the large atypical-appearing squamous epithelial cells in the lower portion of the image, one notably with a retained large nucleus. Many neutrophils also are present and only occasional small lymphocytes *(small arrows)* are present suggesting total infiltration of the lymph node by the neoplasm. (Diff-Quick stain—60× oil immersion objective.)

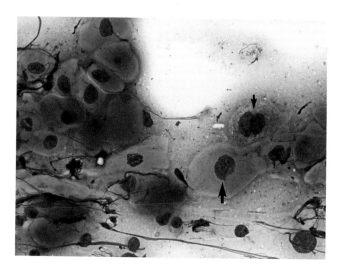

Figure 71-26 Primary oral squamous cell carcinoma from the cat in Figure 71-25. Compare the squamous epithelial cells in this sample to the ones in Figure 71-25. The retained large nucleus *(large arrow)* and binucleation *(small arrow)* are cytological features of malignancy for squamous epithelial cells. (Diff-Quick stain—100× oil immersion objective.)

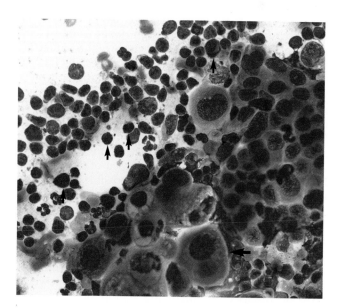

Figure 71-27 Metastatic carcinoma of unknown origin in the prescapular lymph node of a cat. Note the large numbers of cohesive and bizarre-appearing epithelial cells *(large arrow)* admixed with numerous small lymphocytes *(small arrow)* and plasma cells *(medium arrow)*. (Diff-Quick stain—100× oil immersion objective.)

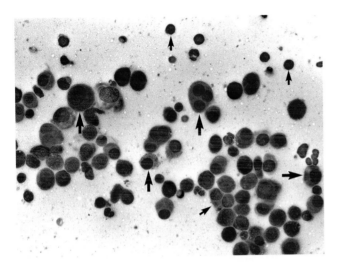

Figure 71-28 Metastatic mast cell tumor in a mesenteric lymph node of a cat. Note the numerous mast cells *(large arrows)* containing very fine red granules with only rare small lymphocytes *(small arrows)* and plasma cells *(medium arrows)* present. Many of the mast cells are exhibiting cytological criteria of malignancy to include multinucleation and macrokaryosis. (Diff-Quick stain—100× oil immersion objective.)

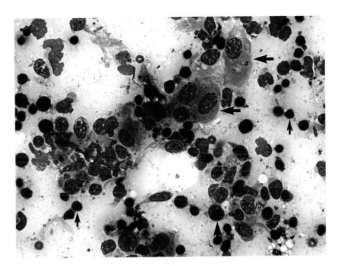

Figure 71-29 Locally invasive vaccine-associated sarcoma in the popliteal lymph node of a cat. Note the large spindle shape cells *(large arrow)* with bright pink material (presumably adjuvant) within the cytoplasm, as well as fewer fibroblastic type cells. Numerous small lymphocytes *(small arrows)* and rare plasma cells *(medium arrow)* are present as the residual lymphocyte population. (Diff-Quick stain—100× oil immersion objective.)

what increases neutrophils directly in SCC and multiple factors are likely to be involved, several references have documented an association with increased neutrophils in SCC and metastatic SCC to altered expression of interleukin-8 (IL-8), interleukin-1 (IL-1), nuclear factor-κB (NF-κB), and granulocyte colony-stimulating factor (G-CSF).[96-99] One human study correlated higher levels of IL-8 and inflammation with metastatic esophageal SCC.[98]

The challenge associated with establishing a cytological diagnosis of metastatic SCC is recognizing the epithelial cells. Rare superficial squamous epithelial cells are seen occasionally in normal lymph nodes from cats and likely originate from the skin during the collection process. Larger numbers of these cells, especially if atypical features are present, are strongly supportive of metastatic SCC (see Figure 71-25). In some cases the SCC metastatic infiltration of the lymph node displaces the lymphocyte resident population completely, and in those instances it often is a challenge to verify that the sample originated from a lymph node (see Figure 71-25). Likewise, if the metastatic SCC is composed of smaller basaloid or parabasaloid cells, it is still possible to diagnose metastatic carcinoma, but it is difficult to conclude definitively that the carcinoma is SCC.

Other tumors are capable of metastasizing to lymph nodes in cats, including mast cell tumors and soft tissue sarcomas.[26,27,100-102] Cutaneous mast cell tumors are common in cats, but unlike dogs, generally exhibit a benign biological behavior[26] (see Chapter 67). However, systemic mastocytosis involving lymph nodes, spleen, liver, and gastrointestinal tissue is reported in cats.[26,27] In these instances mast cells seen in high numbers in lymph node cytological aspirates indicate metastasis (Figure 71-28). Conversely, solitary mast cells in low numbers in lymph node cytological samples generally are a nonspecific finding.[11] Although rare, atypical appearing spindle

cells in lymph node cytological preparations are highly suspicious for a sarcoma, either by local extension into the lymph node or via metastasis (Figure 71-29). The quandary in these samples is to differentiate reactive fibroblasts, commonly associated with fibrosis, from neoplastic fibroblasts. In many instances it is not possible to make this distinction, but reactive fibroblasts often accompany chronic inflammatory processes, so the presence of inflammation is more likely to indicate a reactive population of cells.

SUMMARY

There are many challenges associated with cytological evaluation of lymph node samples in cats. Equally challenging is the fact that lymphadenopathy in cats often is difficult to detect when the affected lymph nodes are located within body cavities such as the mediastinum or mesentery. The goal for cytological examination of enlarged lymph nodes is to determine if the samples are reactive and hyperplastic, inflammatory, neoplastic, or a combination of all three. A systematic approach is best employed when evaluating for these changes and involves recognizing (1) normal lymphocyte sizes and percentages, (2) increased numbers and types of inflammatory cells and potential etiologic agents, and (3) the presence of nonresident cells and what significance they represent.

REFERENCES

1. Cohen M, Bohling MW, Wright JC, et al: Evaluation of sensitivity and specificity of cytologic examination: 269 cases (1999-2000), *J Am Vet Med Assoc* 222:964, 2003.

2. Langenbach A, McManus PM, Hendrick MJ, et al: Sensitivity and specificity of methods of assessing the regional lymph nodes for evidence of metastasis in dogs and cats with solid tumors, *J Am Vet Med Assoc* 218:1424, 2001.

3. Ménard M, Fontaine M, Morin M: Fine needle aspiration biopsy of malignant tumors in dogs and cats: a report of 102 cases, *Can Vet J* 27:504, 1986.

4. Sandhaus LM: Fine-needle aspiration cytology in the diagnosis of lymphoma. The next step, *Am J Clin Pathol* 113:623, 2000.

5. De Delorenzi D, Bertoncello D, Bottero E: Squash-preparation cytology from nasopharyngeal masses in the cat: cytological results and histological correlations in 30 cases, *J Feline Med Surg* 10:55, 2008.

6. Cowell RK, Tyler RD, Meinkoth JH, et al: *Diagnostic cytology and hematology of the dog and cat*, ed 3, St. Louis, 2008, Mosby.

7. Baker R, Lumsden JH: *Color atlas of cytology of the dog and cat*, St. Louis, 2000, Mosby.

8. Raskin RE, Meyer DJ: *Atlas of canine and feline cytology*, Philadelphia, 2001, Saunders.

9. Lucas PF: Lymph node smears in the diagnosis of lymphadenopathy, *Blood* 10:1030, 1955.

10. Gossett KA, Root CR, Cleghorn B, et al: Effects of heartworm and intestinal parasitic infections on hematology and peripheral lymph node cytology in Louisiana dogs, *Vet Clin Pathol* 16:97, 1987.

11. Bookbinder PF, Butt MT, Harvey HJ: Determination of the number of mast cells in lymph node, bone marrow, and buffy coat cytologic specimens from dogs, *J Am Vet Med Assoc* 200:1648, 1992.

12. Pedersen NC, Ho EW, Brown ML, et al: Isolation of a T-lymphotropic virus from domestic cats with an immunodeficiency-like syndrome, *Science* 235:790, 1987.

13. Hoover EA, Perryman LE, Kociba GJ: Early lesions in cats inoculated with feline leukemia virus, *Cancer Res* 33:145, 1973.

14. Couto CG: What is new on feline lymphoma? *J Feline Med Surg* 3:171, 2001.

15. Louwerens M, London CA, Pedersen NC, et al: Feline lymphoma in the post-feline leukemia virus era, *J Vet Intern Med* 19:329, 2005.

16. Gunn-Moore DA, Jenkins PA, Lucke VM: Feline tuberculosis: a literature review and discussion of 19 cases caused by an unusual mycobacterial variant, *Vet Rec* 138:53, 1996.

17. Breitschwerdt EB: Feline bartonellosis and cat scratch disease, *Vet Immunol Immunopathol* 123:167, 2008.

18. Meinkoth KR, Morton RJ, Meinkoth JH: Naturally occurring tularemia in a dog, *J Am Vet Med Assoc* 225:545, 2004.

19. Brömel C, Sykes JE: Histoplasmosis in dogs and cats, *Clin Tech Small Anim Pract* 20:227, 2005.

20. Mooney SC, Patnaik AK, Hays AA, et al: Generalized lymphadenopathy resembling lymphoma in cats: six cases (1972-1976), *J Am Vet Med Assoc* 190:897, 1987.

21. Moore FM, Emerson WE, Cotter SM, et al: Distinctive peripheral lymph node hyperplasia of young cats, *Vet Pathol* 23:386, 1986.

22. Niessen SJ, Voyce MJ, De Villiers L, et al: Generalised lymphadenomegaly associated with methimazole treatment in a hyperthyroid cat, *J Small Anim Pract* 48:165, 2007.

23. Majzoub M, Breuer W, Platz SJ, et al: Histopathologic and immunophenotypic characterization of extramedullary plasmacytomas in nine cats, *Vet Pathol* 40:249, 2003.

24. Patel RT, Caceres A, French AF, et al: Multiple myeloma in 16 cats: a retrospective study, *Vet Clin Pathol* 34:341, 2005.

25. Carothers MA, Johnson GC, DiBartola SP, et al: Extramedullary plasmacytoma and immunoglobulin-associated amyloidosis in a cat, *J Am Vet Med Assoc* 195:1593, 1989.

26. Litster AL, Sorenmo KU: Characterisation of the signalment, clinical and survival characteristics of 41 cats with mast cell neoplasia, *J Feline Med Surg* 8:177, 2006.

27. Sato AF, Solano M: Ultrasonographic findings in abdominal mast cell disease: a retrospective study of 19 patients, *Vet Radiol Ultrasound* 45:51, 2004.

28. Baldwin CJ, Panciera RJ, Morton RJ, et al: Acute tularemia in three domestic cats, *J Am Vet Med Assoc* 199:160, 1991.

29. Woods JP, Panciera RJ, Morton RJ, et al: Feline tularemia, *Compend Contin Educ Pract Vet* 20:442, 1998.

30. Watson RP, Blanchard TW, Mense MG, et al: Histopathology of experimental plague in cats. *Vet Pathol* 38:165, 2001.

31. Eidson M, Thilsted JP, Rollag OJ: Clinical, clinicopathologic, and pathologic features of plague in cats: 119 cases (1977-1988), *J Am Vet Med Assoc* 199:1191, 1991.

32. Kipar A, Köhler K, Leukert W, et al: A comparison of lymphatic tissues from cats with spontaneous feline infectious peritonitis (FIP), cats with FIP virus infection but no FIP, and cats with no infection, *J Comp Pathol* 125:182, 2001.

33. Kipar A, Bellman S, Kremendahl J, et al: Cellular composition, coronavirus antigen expression and production of specific antibodies in lesions in feline infectious peritonitis, *Vet Immunol Immunopathol* 65:243, 1998.

34. Clinkenbeard KD, Cowell RL, Tyler RD: Disseminated histoplasmosis in cats: 12 cases (1981-1986), *J Am Vet Med Assoc* 190:1445, 1987.

35. Wolf AM, Belden MN: Feline histoplasmosis: a literature review and retrospective study of 20 new cases, *J Am Anim Hosp Assoc* 20:995, 1984.

36. Davies C, Troy GC: Deep mycotic infections in cats, *J Am Anim Hosp Assoc* 32:380, 1996.

37. Dial SM: Fungal diagnostics: current techniques and future trends, *Vet Clin North Am Small Anim Pract* 37:373, 2007.

38. Kauffman CA: Endemic mycoses: blastomycosis, histoplasmosis, and sporotrichosis, *Infect Dis Clin North Am* 20:645, 2006.

39. Wheat LJ, Garringer T, Brizendine E, et al: Diagnosis of histoplasmosis by antigen detection based upon experience at the histoplasmosis reference laboratory, *Diagn Microbiol Infect Dis* 43:29, 2002.

40. Gionfriddo JR: Feline systemic fungal infections, *Vet Clin North Am Small Anim Pract* 30:1029, 2000.

41. Laurenson IF, Ross JD, Milne LJ: Microscopy and latex antigen negative cryptococcal meningitis, *J Infect* 36:329, 1998.

42. Medleau L, Marks MA, Brown J, et al: Clinical evaluation of a cryptococcal antigen latex agglutination test for diagnosis of cryptococcus in cats, *J Am Vet Med Assoc* 196:1470, 1990.

43. Schubach TM, Schubach A, Okamoto T, et al: Evaluation of an epidemic of sporotrichosis in cats: 347 cases (1998-2001), *J Am Vet Med Assoc* 224:1623, 2004.

44. Fyfe JA, McCowan C, O'Brien CR, et al: Molecular characterization of a novel fastidious mycobacterium causing lepromatous lesions of the skin, subcutis, cornea, and conjunctiva of cats living in Victoria, Australia, *J Clin Microbiol* 46:618, 2008.

45. Baral RM, Metcalfe SS, Krockenberger MB, et al: Disseminated *Mycobacterium avium* infection in young cats: over-representation of Abyssinian cats, *J Feline Med Surg* 8:23, 2006.

46. Davies JL, Sibley JA, Myers S, et al: Histological and genotypical characterization of feline cutaneous mycobacteriosis: a retrospective study of formalin-fixed paraffin-embedded tissues, *Vet Dermatol* 17:155, 2006.

47. Malik R, Wigney DI, Dawson D, et al: Infection of the sub-cutis and skin of cats with rapidly growing mycobacteria: a review of microbiological and clinical findings, *J Feline Med Surg* 2:35, 2000.

48. Jang SS, Hirsh DC: Rapidly growing members of the genus mycobacterium affecting dogs and cats, *J Am Anim Hosp Assoc* 38:217, 2002.

49. Couto SS, Artachio CA: *Mycobacterium fortuitum* pneumonia in a cat and the role of lipid in the pathogenesis of atypical mycobacterial infections, *Vet Pathol* 44:543, 2007.

50. Murakami S, Yamanishi MW, Azuma R: Lymph node abscess due to *Actinomyces viscosus* in a cat, *J Vet Med Sci* 59:1079, 1997.

51. Malik R, Krockenberger MB, O'Brien CR, et al: Nocardia infections in cats: a retrospective multi-institutional study of 17 cases, *Aust Vet J* 84:235, 2006.

52. Rakich PM, Grooter AM, Tang KN: Gastrointestinal pythiosis in two cats, *J Vet Diagn Invest* 17:262, 2005.

53. Roosje PJ, Koeman JP, Thepen T, et al: Mast cells and eosinophils in feline allergic dermatitis: a qualitative and quantitative analysis, *J Comp Pathol* 131:61, 2004.

54. Taglinger K, Day MJ, Foster AP: Characterization of inflammatory cell infiltration in feline allergic skin disease, *J Comp Pathol* 137:211, 2007.

55. Reinero CR, Cohn LA, Delgado C, et al: Adjuvanted rush immunotherapy using CpG oligodeoxynucleotides in experimental feline allergic asthma, *Vet Immunol Immunopathol* 121:241, 2008.

56. McConnell JF, Sparkes AH, Blunden AS, et al: Eosinophilic fibrosing gastritis and toxoplasmosis in a cat, *J Feline Med Surg* 9:82, 2007.

57. Hoover EA, Dubey JP: Pathogenesis of experimental pulmonary paragonimiasis in cats, *Am J Vet Res* 39:1827, 1978.

58. Lilliehöök I, Tvedten H: Investigation of hypereosinophilia and potential treatments, *Vet Clin North Am Small Anim Pract* 33:1359, 2003.

59. Howl JH, Petersen MG: Intestinal mast cell tumor in a cat: presentation as eosinophilic enteritis, *J Am Anim Hosp Assoc* 31:457, 1995.

60. Molander-McCrary H, Potter K, Tyler JW, et al: Cutaneous mast cell tumors in cats: 32 cases (1991-1994), *J Am Anim Hosp Assoc* 34:281, 1998.

61. Johnson TO, Schulman FY, Lipscomb TP, et al: Histopathology and biologic behavior of pleomorphic cutaneous mast cell tumors in fifteen cats. *Vet Pathol* 39:452, 2002.

62. Barrs VR, Beatty JA, McCandlish IA, et al: Hypereosinophilic paraneoplastic syndrome in a cat with intestinal T cell lymphosarcoma, *J Small Anim Pract* 43:401, 2002.

63. Maeda S, Okayama T, Ohmori K, et al: Molecular cloning of the feline thymus and activation-regulated chemokine cDNA and its expression in lesional skin of cats with eosinophilic plaque, *J Vet Med Sci* 65:275, 2003.

64. Ozaki K, Yamagami T, Nomura K, et al: Abscess-forming inflammatory granulation tissue with gram-positive cocci and prominent eosinophil infiltration in cats: possible infection of methicillin-resistant staphylococcus, *Vet Pathol* 40:283, 2003.

65. Gelain ME, Antoniazzi E, Bertazzolo W, et al: Chronic eosinophilic leukemia in a cat: cytochemical and immunophenotypical features, *Vet Clin Pathol* 35:454, 2006.

66. Sharifi H, Nassiri SM, Esmaelli H, et al: Eosinophilic leukaemia in a cat, *J Feline Med Surg* 9:514, 2007.

67. Huibregtse BA, Turner JL: Hypereosinophilic syndrome and eosinophilic leukemia: a comparison of 22 hypereosinophilic cats, *J Am Anim Hosp Assoc* 30:591, 1994.

68. Ettinger SN: Principles of treatment for feline lymphoma, *Clin Tech Small Anim Pract* 18:98, 2003.

69. Shelton GH, Grant CK, Cotter SM, et al: Feline immunodeficiency virus and feline leukemia virus infections and their relationships to lymphoid malignancies in cats: a retrospective study (1968-1988), *J Acquir Immune Defic Syndr* 3:623, 1990.

70. Beatty J, Terry A, MacDonald J, et al: Feline immunodeficiency virus integration in B-cell lymphoma identifies a candidate tumor suppressor gene on human chromosome 15q15, *Cancer Res* 62:7175, 2002.

71. Grooters AM, Biller DS, Ward H, et al: Ultrasonographic appearance of feline alimentary lymphoma, *Vet Radiol Ultrasound* 35:468, 1994.

72. Willard MD: Feline inflammatory bowel disease: a review, *J Feline Med Surg* 1:155, 1999.

73. Richter KP: Feline gastrointestinal lymphoma, *Vet Clin North Am Small Anim Pract* 33:108, 2003.

74. Evans SE, Bonczynski JJ, Broussard JD, et al: Comparison of endoscopic and full-thickness biopsy specimens for diagnosis of inflammatory bowel disease and alimentary tract lymphoma in cats, *J Am Vet Med Assoc* 229:1447, 2006.

75. Harris NL, Ferry JA: Classification of non-Hodgkins lymphoma. In Knowles DM, Thompson DD, editors: *Neoplastic hematopathology*, ed 2, Philadelphia, 2000, Lippincott Williams & Wilkins, p 691.

76. Harris NL, Jaffe ES, Stein H, et al: A revised European-American classification of lymphoid neoplasms: a proposal from the International Lymphoma Study Group, *Blood* 84:1361, 1994.

77. National Cancer Institute sponsored study of classifications of non-Hodgkin's lymphomas: summary and description of a working formulation for clinical usage. The non-Hodgkin's lymphoma pathologic classification project, *Cancer* 49:2112, 1982.

78. Valli VE: *Veterinary comparative hematopathology*, Ames, 2007, Blackwell.

79. Walton RM, Hendrick MJ: Feline Hodgkin's-like lymphoma: 20 cases (1992-1999), *Vet Pathol* 38:504, 2001.

80. Valli VE, Jacobs RM, Norris A, et al: The histologic classification of 602 cases of feline lymphoproliferative disease using the National Cancer Institute working formulation, *J Vet Diagn Invest* 12:295, 2000.

81. Carter RF, Valli VE, Lumsden JH: The cytology, histology and prevalence of cell types in canine lymphoma classified according to the National Cancer Institute working formulation, *Can J Vet Res* 50:154, 1986.

82. Teske E, van Heerde P, Rutteman GR, et al: Prognostic factors for treatment of malignant lymphoma in dogs, *J Am Vet Med Assoc* 205:1722, 1994.

83. Vernau W, Valli VE, Dukes TW, et al: Classification of 1,198 cases of bovine lymphoma using the National Cancer Institute working formulation for human non-Hodgkin's lymphomas, *Vet Pathol* 29:183, 1992.

84. Roccabianca P, Vernau W, Caniatti M, et al: Feline large granular lymphocyte (LGL) lymphoma with secondary leukemia: primary intestinal origin with predominance of a CD3/CD8 (alpha)(alpha) phenotype, *Vet Pathol* 43:15, 2006.

85. Herring ES, Smith MM, Robertson JL: Lymph node staging of oral and maxillofacial neoplasms in 31 dogs and cats, *J Vet Dent* 19:122, 2002.

86. Monteiro CB, O'Brien RT: A retrospective study on the sonographic findings of abdominal carcinomatosis in 14 cats, *Vet Radiol Ultrasound* 45:559, 2004.

87. Cribb AE: Feline gastrointestinal adenocarcinoma: a review and retrospective study, *Can Vet J* 29:709, 1988.

88. Amorim FV, Souza HJ, Ferreira AM, et al: Clinical, cytological and histopathological evaluation of mammary masses

in cats from Rio de Janeiro, Brazil, *J Feline Med Surg* 8:379, 2006.

89. Wilson HM, Chun R, Larson VS, et al: Clinical signs, treatments, and outcome in cats with transitional cell carcinoma of the urinary bladder: 20 cases (1990-2004), *J Am Vet Med Assoc* 231:101, 2007.

90. Hahn KA, McEntee MF: Primary lung tumors in cats: 86 cases (1979-1994), *J Am Vet Med Assoc* 211:1257, 1997.

91. Turk MA, Gallina AM, Russell TS: Nonhematopoietic gastrointestinal neoplasia in cats: a retrospective study of 44 cases, *Vet Pathol* 18:614, 1981.

92. Birchard SJ, Couto CG, Johnson S: Nonlymphoid intestinal neoplasia in 32 dogs and 14 cats, *J Am Anim Hosp Assoc* 22:533, 1986.

93. Lana SE, Ogilvie GK, Withrow SJ, et al: Feline cutaneous squamous cell carcinoma of the nasal planum and the pinnae: 61 cases, *J Am Anim Hosp Assoc* 33:329, 1997.

94. Rogers KS: Feline cutaneous squamous cell carcinoma, *Feline Pract* 22:7, 1994.

95. Hayes AM, Adams VJ, Scase TJ, et al: Survival of 54 cats with oral squamous cell carcinoma in United Kingdom general practice, *J Small Anim Pract* 48:394, 2007.

96. Dole RS, MacPhail CM, Lappin MR: Paraneoplastic leukocytosis with mature neutrophilia in a cat with pulmonary squamous cell carcinoma, *J Feline Med Surg* 6:391, 2004.

97. Lind MH, Rozell B, Wallin RP, et al: Tumor necrosis factor receptor 1-mediated signaling is required for skin cancer development induced by NF-kappaB inhibition, *Proc Natl Acad Sci USA* 101:4972, 2004.

98. Krzystek-Korpacka M, Matusiewicz M, Diakowska D, et al: Elevation of circulating interleukin-8 is related to lymph node and distant metastases in esophageal squamous cell carcinomas—implication for clinical evaluation of cancer patient, *Cytokine* 41:232, 2008.

99. Sato K, Fujii Y, Kakiuchi T, et al: Paraneoplastic syndrome of hypercalcemia and leukocytosis caused by squamous carcinoma cells (T3M-1) producing parathyroid hormone-related protein, interleukin 1α, and granulocyte colony-stimulating factor, *Cancer Res* 49:4740, 1989.

100. Pinard J, Wagg CR, Girard C, et al: Histiocytic sarcoma in the tarsus of a cat, *Vet Pathol* 43:1014, 2006.

101. Culp WT, Drobatz KJ, Glassman MM, et al: Feline visceral hemangiosarcoma, *J Vet Intern Med* 22:148, 2008.

102. Cook JL, Turk JR, Tomlinson JL, et al: Fibrosarcoma in the distal radius and carpus of a four-year-old Persian, *J Am Anim Hosp Assoc* 34:31, 1998.

72 Facilitating Client Grief

Zachary M. Wright and Kenita S. Rogers

As family pets have transitioned to the role of friends and confidants, many owners now believe that their cats provide a more stable and unconditional love than most human relationships.[1] Consequently the loss of that emotional companion can be very damaging psychologically. Simplistically, grief is viewed as the emotional response to a personal loss, and in today's society this loss often includes the death of a family pet. Of equal importance is the fact that grief also can present itself as physical, emotional, or behavioral changes.[2] Thirty per cent of pet owners in a recent survey admitted to experiencing some level of grief after the death of their pet.[2] Aiding clients through the grief process after the loss of a pet is now of fundamental importance to veterinarians treating companion animals.

RELAYING DIFFICULT NEWS

The first indication of how a client will handle the grieving process may be exhibited during the initial discussion of the pet's condition. Indeed, it is exceptionally important that the veterinarian understand the subtleties of relaying "difficult news," because veterinarians who are better trained and prepared for delivering this type of information have less anxiety toward the event and deliver the news in a more acceptable and compassionate manner to their clients.[1]

A working definition of difficult news would include situations in which there is a feeling of no hope, a threat to a person's mental or physical well-being, a risk of upsetting an established lifestyle, or when a message is given that conveys to an individual fewer choices in his or her life.[3] In reality difficult news is a relative term because all clients interpret and respond to information differently. In any case the veterinarian should relay the distressing information to the client in a consistent,

caring manner, and should be prepared to take the time necessary to allow the client to have a full understanding of the pet's condition.

The first step in relaying unfortunate news to the client is to select an ideal time.[1] Whenever possible, bad news should be reported in person and by the veterinarian, rather than by a member of the support staff. Although particular emergency situations may not allow for a scheduled discussion, a diagnosis of cancer or other life-threatening illness usually can be discussed at the convenience of both the client and the veterinarian. Furthermore, the client's support group of family and friends should be given the opportunity to attend the meeting.[1,4]

The location of the conversation also can influence a client's response to the news substantially. The very busy waiting room or lobby offers obvious limitations, notably noise and lack of privacy. Ideally the room should be away from the busy flow of a normal practice, and should be arranged in a friendly, accommodating manner with comfortable seating and tissue paper available. Personnel who are not involved directly in this patient's care should excuse themselves, because the lack of privacy can hinder the client's need to express her or his grief and may invoke a stronger response.[4]

The veterinarian's initial body language and attitude often set the tone for the entire conversation. A few deep breaths and a conscious decision to relax prior to entering the room can help to reassure the client. An anxious and unfocused veterinarian brings added stress to an already anticipatory situation.[4] When conveying the news, the veterinarian should not have any furniture, including an exam table, or person between herself or himself and the client.[4,5] Sitting or standing at or below the level of the owners reduces the intimidation associated with conversations with the veterinarian. Interacting with the cat while talking to owners helps to confirm your compassion toward the situation. Body language such as folded arms, or a short interpersonal distance, represents a forceful demeanor.[5] Numerous studies have found that empathy from the veterinarian or physician influences the situation positively.[1,4] Touching the client during difficult news is often viewed favorably by the client, but is not appropriate in all settings.[4]

Most veterinarians are able to gauge their clients' ability accurately to comprehend medical explanations. Their ability to understand may be further diminished in this stressful setting and more simplistic verbiage may be required when bad news is presented.[1] Should they desire it, owners usually will ask for a more scientifically complex explanation. Beginning with a statement that sets the tone for the conversation such as "Unfortunately, we have some bad news," helps minimize the shocking effect of a declarative statement such as "We found cancer," midway through the discussion.[1,4]

Inexperienced veterinarians often struggle with relaying a guarded prognosis for fear of being associated with the bad news, a well-documented phenomenon for many physicians.[1] Although it is acceptable to always offer some level of hope, unrealistic expectations, even if beneficial in the early stages, eventually will lead to a more devastating reality and grieving process when death of the pet occurs. Phrases such as, "We expect the cancer to behave in a particular way, but every disease has unique behavior in each pet" can be used to convey the small chance of hope without undermining the justifiably poor prognosis. Most clients are grateful for an honest answer or disease description at the beginning of the discussion.

Many clients are overwhelmed by the gravity of the news and the extent of the information. Whenever possible, allow for questions throughout the conversation.[4] This is not a lecture at a podium; it is a very delicate discussion about their pet. Set the pace of the conversation to meet the needs of the client.[4] Sending follow-up discharge instructions allows the owner to further process the information in the privacy of their home. Discharge instructions also may provide a more scientific explanation that allows the owner the opportunity for further research.[1,4] Finally, visual aids can be excellent tools for relaying the gravity of a medical condition. Visualizing the size and extent of a tumor on a radiograph, ultrasound, computed tomographic image, or magnetic resonance image certainly can facilitate your explanation of the severity of a disease process. Even showing normal laboratory parameters compared with their cat's values can be a very helpful visual exercise to increase understanding of the scale of the illness.

EUTHANASIA

DECIDING WHEN IT IS TIME FOR EUTHANASIA

For many chronic diseases, including cancer, the decision for euthanasia typically is a process requiring numerous conversations; only rarely does the owner need to make a decision immediately. It is helpful to introduce the owner of patients with terminal cancer to the concept of euthanasia very early in the disease process.[6] At the time of diagnosis, trigger phrases such as "terminal disease" and "noncurable" are repeated so that owners have a true understanding of the expected disease progression. Furthermore, detailed explanation of the predicted decline of the pet will forewarn clients of the changes anticipated in the future.

Many owners are fearful that they will be unable to recognize when the time for euthanasia is appropriate. For these situations, the authors routinely recommend the "Rule of Three."[7] The owners are encouraged to remember their pet at its healthiest time (which may or may not be the time of diagnosis). During that period of the pet's life, a list of the pet's three favorite activities should be made. When a pet can not accomplish two of the three activities on that list, quality of life is reasonably compromised and euthanasia should be considered. The owners are encouraged to write down the "Rule of Three" because writing down the activities serves two purposes. First, the list is easier to remember and less likely to be forgotten conveniently during emotional distress. Second, a written list serves psychologically as a contract for the owners that should not be broken, even in times of severe grief and confusion. The authors have found great success in helping owners recognize significant decline in patient quality of life before true patient suffering occurs when the "Rule of Three" is implemented early in the disease process. Other options include discussing a list of eventual clinical signs of disease and a hospital-designed brochure on planning for death and euthanasia that may be given to owners at the onset of their pet's diagnosis.[6,8]

It is exceptionally important to provide a support network when owners elect euthanasia for their pets.[9] It should be noted that 16 per cent of owners in a recent euthanasia survey felt that the decision to euthanize their pet was equivalent to murder and views of euthanasia are wide ranging among owners (Table 72-1).[2] The ethical dilemma of euthanasia for healthy or adoptable pets will not be discussed here. Instead, the focus will be on euthanasia decisions for those pets with terminal disease or severe injury. Owners elect euthanasia for a variety of reasons. Financial limitations should not invoke a judgmental reaction from the veterinarian or her/his staff. Even the slightest hint of judgment could influence these owners to delay euthanasia for a future pet because of unnecessarily held guilt, because up to 50 per cent of owners admit to some level of guilt after euthanizing their pets.[2] Additionally, casual use of certain words such as "stop" or "quit" should be avoided because they imply that the owner has abandoned her or his pet. This belief in abandonment can extend and increase the severity of the grieving process. Empathy from the veterinary staff concerning the difficulty in their decision is imperative to the owners' future mental health.[9,10]

THE PROCEDURE

Once the decision of euthanasia has been made, a checklist of steps should be used to ensure that the emotional event occurs as smoothly as possible. Legal authorization

Table 72-1 Responses in a Client Survey to Items Associated with Attitude Toward Euthanasia

Attitudes Toward Euthanasia	No.	Agree (%)	Disagree (%)	Neutral (%)	Missing Value (%)
I believe that euthanasia is a good option to humanely end my pet's life.	154	84	2	2	13
It bothered me to have my pet euthanatized.	152	64	18	4	14
One of the hardest things about the death of my pet was leaving the veterinary clinic without my pet.	138	61	12	5	22
My experience following pet death can be characterized as questioning whether I made the right decision.	153	46	33	7	14
After the death of my pet I felt guilty because I made the decision to euthanatize.	152	45	32	9	14
I felt like a murderer having my pet euthanatized.	153	16	61	10	14
I felt like I was rushed into making a decision to euthanatize.	154	6	79	2	13

From Adams CL, Bonnett BN, Meek AH: Predictors of owner response to companion animal death in 177 clients from 14 practices in Ontario, *J Am Vet Med Assoc* 217:1303, 2000, with permission.

should be obtained as quickly as possible. The initial euthanasia discussion should focus on whether or not the owners, specifically children, would like to be present for the procedure.[6] Although it is an added stress to the veterinarian, it is important for some owners to witness the process, because many clients need to make sure the procedure was not traumatic to their pet.[11] Decisions regarding the pet's remains (cremation, burial, or routine disposal) also should be discussed because owners often feel angry or suspicious if this information is not offered.[9]

All veterinary hospitals should have an established hospital policy on billing for euthanasia. The authors' hospital provides a mailed bill to clients in good standing. If payment is required, it may be best to collect the fees prior to the procedure so that an emotional client can avoid a crowded waiting room after the loss of their pet. Finally, as with all end-of-life discussions, clients appreciate an explanation of the euthanasia process.[9] Medical jargon is not required, but a brief explanation of the mechanisms of action of the drug used in euthanasia helps to eliminate the owners' fears of pet suffering during the procedure.

A veterinary hospital should develop routine procedures for euthanasia to ensure that mistakes are minimized. The trauma of a poorly placed catheter and subsequent slow death can haunt an owner for years. Provide medical proof that the animal has died, either via auscultation or palpation of a pulse. Confirm that the patient is dead or passed away; avoid terms such as sleeping or gone, as use of these phrases may be particularly confusing to children who are present.[10] Based on client surveys, owners should be allowed to spend time with their pet both before and after the euthanasia is performed; most owners take no more than 15 to 20 minutes to say goodbye.[9,11,12] As stated previously, allowing owners to leave from an exit other than the waiting room may help them feel more comfortable in their distressed emotional state.[6,9]

POSTEUTHANASIA AND THE GRIEVING PROCESS

Owners may experience some level of grief during the delivery of the diagnosis or during discussions of euthanasia. However, a compassionate veterinarian who is skilled in handling the grief process is especially valuable to clients after the loss of their pets.[6,9,12]

One half of all clients feel that grief and sadness toward the loss of a pet is socially unacceptable.[2,10] In a survey conducted by Adams et al, grief caused by the loss of a pet was defined as a search to determine how to feel and behave within a society that does not recognize the nature of the human-animal relationship or sanction the emotions that may result from a pet dying.[9] Consequently it is imperative that the first step in handling clients who have lost a pet is to provide confirmation that their relationship with their pet and their subsequent feelings toward the loss are normal and acceptable.[2,6,9,13] When not influenced by the perceived societal pressure (that grieving for companion animals is unnecessary), the owner then can experience a more natural and psychologically beneficial grieving process.

The second step in handling client grief is to care for certain details surrounding the process. After euthanasia, the pet's medical records should be updated immediately, and reminder mailings should be removed from data bases. A personal phone call or personalized mailed sympathy card signed by the staff is often gratefully received.[6,9,12] The authors' hospital offers a decorated clay impression of the deceased pet's paw print. Table 72-2 describes the results of a detailed survey regarding clients' needs and wishes regarding euthanasia.

Perhaps the most important step for the veterinary staff is recognizing which clients are the most likely to have difficulty in dealing with the loss of their pet. In a recent client survey study on grief following the death of a pet, dog owners were three times more likely to grieve

Table 72-2 Responses in a Client Survey to Items Related to Professional Support

Veterinarian Should Provide or Respondents Would Have Appreciated	No.	Agree (%)	Disagree (%)	Neutral (%)	Missing Value (%)
Emotional support following pet death	174	87	5	7	2
Time with the veterinarian to discuss whether euthanasia is the best option	152	67	12	7	14
The option to stay during euthanasia	151	67	16	4	15
An opportunity to discuss options available for the aftercare of pet	173	66	25	7	2
An explanation of what happens to the pet's body after it dies	173	66	25	7	2
A condolence card	174	54	33	11	2
An opportunity to discuss the medical aspect of euthanasia with the veterinarian	151	54	23	8	15
Bill payment on a day other than the day of euthanasia	149	51	24	10	16
A telephone call following the pet's death	173	38	50	9	2
Time alone with the pet following euthanasia	149	34	45	7	16
Information regarding grief associated with pet death	175	22	70	13	2
Bill payment for euthanasia somewhere other than the reception area	157	32	36	21	11

From Adams CL, Bonnett BN, Meek AH: Predictors of owner response to companion animal death in 177 clients from 14 practices in Ontario, *J Am Vet Med Assoc* 217:1303, 2000, with permission.

than cat owners.[2] First-time pet owners were more likely to experience grief compared with those who have had multiple pets.[2] Women were more likely to experience grief from pet loss compared with men, and age was inversely correlated with the level of grief.[2,12,14] Those owners whose pets were euthanized were more likely to experience some level of grief compared with pets who died of natural causes.[2] Finally, clients who had a strong support system, including their veterinarian and hospital support staff, were better able to cope with grief.[2]

THE FIVE STAGES OF GRIEF

Rarely is the grieving process of a client straightforward. Instead, it is often a waxing and waning progression through the five stages of grief.[6] These five stages are denial, anger, bargaining, depression, and resolution. Although progression through these stages is often orderly, it is not unusual for a client to skip a step or even take a step backward as they experience grief.[6] The complexity of grief can result in a variety of behaviors toward the veterinarian and staff, making it imperative for professional personnel to understand the stages of grief and the emotional spectrum of behavior associated with each stage.

Denial often is witnessed during the initial discussion of bad news. With a cancer diagnosis, clients often say that their pet is "not sick enough to have cancer." Repetition often is required to convince owners of the reality of the situation. As mentioned previously, visual aids (such as imaging modalities) and the same message delivered by multiple staff members (if not multiple veterinarians) may move the owner into acceptance of the situation. Often the denial may simply be a façade or first reaction while in the exam room, and after a night at home, the owner returns much more accepting of the situation.

Anger is the stage of grief that affects the veterinary hospital most directly.[10,15] Verbal, and less often physical, assaults often are directed at the staff instead of the veterinarian. Whether this behavior is a subconscious decision to respect the position of authority (veterinarian) or a display of power and control (against the staff) is not understood completely. In times of severe grief-induced anger, it is important to take a level-headed approach. Reacknowledgment of the loss of their pet and subsequent understanding of the clients' behavior often is enough to enlighten them regarding their aggressive behavior. However, although the grief process should be allowed, every veterinary hospital should limit the extent to which anger is acceptable.

In veterinary medicine, bargaining seems to be the step skipped most often and is usually a fairly short phase. Bargaining most often is expressed as the clients' desire to make sure that the diagnosis could not be a more benign disease. Wealthy owners may offer unlimited funding for superfluous tests and treatments. Although on the surface this appears to be a dedicated owner, subconsciously it is bargaining behavior.

The longest phase of grief usually is depression and on average can last for 6 weeks.[13] Depression can be expressed in a variety of ways. Studies have documented that over 90 per cent of owners who had a significantly ill pet or experienced the death of a pet reported an alteration in their general behavior ranging from insomnia and nightmares to diet change to social anxiety.[2,9,15,16] Symptoms of depression can be so severe that it is the primary reason listed for attendance in a bereavement support group organized by a veterinary teaching hospital.[15]

Resolution of grief often is missed by the veterinarian as the client reenters a more stable period of her or his life. However, it is during the period of resolution that the client may return to discuss the details of the pet's death. At this stage in the process, clients are most amenable to detailed discussions of laboratory findings, biopsy, or necropsy results, and their previous decision-making process. It is important to remember that in-depth discussion may trigger any of the previous phases of grief. Once acceptance is reached, clients also may seek guidance on obtaining a new pet.[10]

SPECIAL NEEDS CLIENTS

The majority of families with children own pets. Consequently children are regular visitors to the veterinary clinic and may be forced to deal with the mortality of their pet. During the death of a pet, many owners are more concerned with their children's emotional needs than their own—25 per cent of one pet-loss hotline survey concerned child grief.[17]

When the bad news is delivered to both parents and children, different strategies are needed depending on the age group of the child. Always give the parents the opportunity to remove their child from the conversation. Many owners may not realize that difficult news will be delivered and, in hindsight, would have preferred their child not be present. Deliver the information as discussed previously but do not discredit the children's actions or questions. Offer an explanation to a child's question at a level appropriate with their knowledge and emotional base. Children may begin to behave poorly or pout in the examination room as a way to express their concern. Although they may not fully understand details of the adult discussion, they may realize that the situation is sad or difficult. Offer to speak directly to the child and begin by dropping down to eye level with them.[5]

Euthanasia requires a more complicated approach to the family client dynamic. Again, ensure that the parents want their children to be present. The veterinarian's role is to explain the details of euthanasia to the parent, but it is not to decide what is or is not an appropriate experience for a child. As with all euthanasia, it is important to confirm that the pet is dead by using definitive statements. Saying the pet is "asleep" may lead to a terrified child afraid to go to bed at night. If children are crying, reassure them that it is okay to be upset and give them every opportunity to ask questions. Even sadness may not completely remove a child's inherent intuitiveness.

Parents may seek advice on how to console their children. Brandt and colleagues believe that dishonesty regarding death of a pet leads a child to create their own, often more detrimental, answer.[17] Injury and death are natural occurrences in life, and sheltering a child only delays their understanding of the inevitable reality of

death.[17] The reader is directed to Box 72-1 for more detailed recommendations on pet loss literature for children.

As the Baby Boomer population ages, veterinarians will be faced with a growing population of elderly pet owners. Interaction with the elderly regarding the mortality of their pets may present many challenges. Many elderly people have pets as their primary source of companionship, substituting for lost human relationships.[6,18] Pets can provide an avenue for communication, daily structure, a feeling of being needed, and tactile stimulation that an elderly person otherwise may not have available.[18] Often an elderly client's pet is the last link to a dead spouse. Because single pet owners are more likely to experience significant grief, the loss of a pet can be even more psychologically damaging to an elderly client.[2,6,10,18]

Box 72-1 Recommended Books on Grieving and Pet Loss

GENERAL PET LOSS

When Your Pet Dies: How to Cope with Your Feelings. Quakenbach & Graveline, 1985.
On Death and Dying. Elisabeth Kubler-Ross, 1969.
Ten Tips on How to Cope with the Loss of Your Pet. Anderson, 1989.
Grieving the Death of a Pet. Betty J. Carmack, 2003.
Goodbye My Friend. Herb and Mary Montgomery, 2001.
A Final Act of Caring. Herb and Mary Montgomery, 1993.
Journey Through Pet Loss. Deborah Antinori, 2000.
Pets Living with Cancer: A Pet Owner's Resource. Robin Downing, 2000.
Surviving the Heartbreak of Choosing Death for Your Pet: Your Personal Guide for Dealing with Pet Euthanasia. Linda Mary Peterson, 1997.
Goodbye, Friend: Healing Wisdom for Anyone Who Has Ever Lost a Pet. Gary Kowalski, 1997.

FOR CHILDREN

When a Pet Dies. Fred Rogers, 1988, Ages 4-8.
Remembering My Pet. Nechama Liss-Levinson and Molly Phinney Baskette, 2007, Ages 7-13.
Goodbye Mousie. Robie Harris, Simon and Schuster Children's, 2001, Ages 5-8.
Healing Your Grieving Heart for Kids. Alan Wolfelt, 2001.
The Tenth Good Thing About Barney. Judith Viorst, 1975, Ages 4-8.
A Special Place for Charlee: A Child's Companion Through Pet Loss. Debra Morehead, 1996, Ages 4-12.
Cat Heaven. Cynthia Rylant, 1997, Ages 4-8.
Dog Heaven. Cynthia Rylant, 1995, Ages 4-8.

FOR PARENTS

Talking About Death: A Dialogue Between Parent and Child. Earl Grollman, Beacon Press, 1991.
When Your Pet Dies: Dealing With Your Grief and Helping Your Children Cope. Christine Adamec, 2000.
When Children Grieve. John W. James, 2002.
Healing the Bereaved Child. Alan Wolfelt, 1996.
A Child's View of Grief. Alan Wolfelt, 1999.

Furthermore, studies have shown that elderly people tend to have a lesser understanding of basic medical concepts.[17] This means that the veterinarian should be diligent and should dedicate more time to careful explanation of the pet's condition to ensure the owner has an accurate understanding of the disease. Degenerative aging changes such as hearing loss and cognitive dysfunction should be recognized early and the dialogue altered appropriately and compassionately.[17] Many elderly people have companions who provide transportation and/or who provide a trusted voice in the conversation. It is important not to discredit these individuals because their influence on their elderly companions may be significant.[17] Finally, the loss of a companion animal may trigger thoughts about an elderly owner's own mortality. Although the veterinarian is not a psychologist or part of the client's medical team, simple acknowledgement of these feelings can influence the client positively.[17]

Some clients may be dealing with their own terminal disease, such as cancer, that is similar to their pet's medical condition. Again, truthful discussion about the treatment options and prognosis are imperative. The authors' have not found an obvious correlation with behavior when clients with cancer have pets with cancer. It is our experience that the owners obviously are more knowledgeable about the disease process and treatment options. However, their treatment decisions and propensity for grief can not be predicted accurately. When an owner and pet share a diagnosis of malignancy, the veterinarian should observe the owners closely for signs of transposition, because the owner may view the outcome of the pet's illness as an indicator of their own future prognosis.[6] In cases of euthanasia of the pet, this can lead to severe client grief and stress. In these situations it is important to offer all treatment options carefully (regardless of the likelihood for success), because the strong empathy for their pet may force a terminally ill owner to pursue even the rarest and most unlikely of treatment options.[6]

For many clients, regardless of age or maturity, the loss of a pet truly can be overwhelming and debilitating. For severely grief-stricken clients, more aggressive involvement with their mental health may be required. Social workers should be recommended for cases of long-term grief, clients who exhibit suicidal tendencies, or those who obviously are predisposed to severe grief and depression. First, the veterinarian is encouraged to direct the client to literature on the subject of pet loss (see Box 72-1). Many veterinary practices also establish a relationship with a local social worker or therapist who has experience with pet loss or general grief counseling. Referring clients to a therapist can be intimidating for many veterinarians because they do not wish to suggest that a client's grieving is beyond the realm of normal. Human psychologists suggest that veterinarians have discussions with a local therapist to address the most appropriate ways to make such a referral.[10] Larger practices, or a group of hospitals, may research the possibility of establishing a support group that is led by a certified counselor. The benefit of these support groups is that they validate the feelings associated with pet loss by showing the client that other people share similar feelings.[15,18] Support

groups also may serve to help with the euthanasia decision.[15] Finally, many universities offer telephone help lines for grieving pet owners (Box 72-2), and some are under the direction of staff social workers who are experts in the pet-loss field.

Box 72-2 Grief Telephone Hotlines and Web Sites

GRIEF HOTLINES
Most hotlines are staffed by volunteers, veterinarians, and/or veterinary students.
Veterinary Schools
University of California, Davis: 530-752-3602, or toll free 800-565-1526
University of Florida: 352-392-4700; then dial 1 and 4080
Michigan State University: 517-432-2696
Virginia-Maryland Regional College of Veterinary Medicine: 540-231-8038
The Ohio State University: 614-292-1823
Tufts University: 508-839-7966
Iowa State University: 888-478-7574
Cornell University: 607-253-3932
University of Illinois: 217-244-2273 or toll-free 877-394-2273
Colorado State University: 970-491-4143
Washington State University: 509-335-5704
Others
The Iams Company's Pet Loss Support Center: 888-332-7738
Chicago Veterinary Medical Association: 630-325-1600

WEB SITES
Veterinary Schools
University of California, Davis: http://www.vetmed.ucdavis.edu/petloss/index.htm
Tufts University: http://www.tufts.edu/vet/petloss/
University of Florida: http://www.vetmed.ufl.edu/patientcare/petlosssupport/
Michigan State University: http://cvm.msu.edu/petloss/index.htm
Iowa State University: http://www.vetmed.iastate.edu/animals/petloss/
Cornell University: http://www.vet.cornell.edu/Org/PetLoss/
University of Illinois: http://vetmed.illinois.edu/CARE
Washington State University: http://www.vetmed.wsu.edu/plhl/index.htm
Colorado State University Argus Institute: http://www.argusinstitute.colostate.edu/grief.htm
Associations
American Veterinary Medical Association: http://www.avma.org/careforanimals/animatedjourneys/goodbyefriend/plhotlines.asp
Association for Pet Loss and Bereavement: http://www.aplb.org
Additional Web Sites
http://www.griefhealing.com/pet-loss-links.htm
http://www.chancesspot.org
http://www.petloss.com

SUMMARY

An important part of veterinary medicine is the care of patients with terminal diseases. It is in our clients' best interest for the veterinarian to be knowledgeable about the emotional and psychological toll that the loss of a family pet may take on a client's overall well-being. The more prepared and experienced veterinarians are with these situations, the more support they can offer clients as they progress through the natural grieving process. As a result, this support will strengthen the future veterinarian-client relationship.

REFERENCES

1. Ptacek JT, Leonard K, McKee TL: "I've got some bad news …": veterinarians' recollections of communicating bad news to clients, *J Appl Soc Psychol* 34:366, 2004.
2. Adams CL, Bonnett BN, Meek AH: Predictors of owner response to companion animal death in 177 clients from 14 practices in Ontario, *J Am Vet Med Assoc* 217:1303, 2000.
3. Bor R, Miller R, Goldman E, et al: The meaning of bad news in HIV disease: counselling about dreaded issues revisited, *Counselling Psychol Quarterly* 6:69, 1993.
4. Ptacek JT, Eberhardt TL: Breaking bad news. A review of the literature, *JAMA* 276:496, 1996.
5. Carson CA: Nonverbal communication in veterinary practice, *Vet Clin North Am Small Anim Pract* 37:49, 2007.
6. Hancock G, Yates J: Client services for geriatric pets, *Vet Clin North Am Small Anim Pract* 19:187, 1989.
7. Barton C: *The rule of three*, 2008, College Station, TX (personal communication).
8. Frid MH, Perea AT: Euthanasia & thanatology in small animals, *J Vet Behav Clin Applic Res* 2:35, 2007.
9. Adams CL, Bonnett BN, Meek AH: Owner response to companion animal death: development of a theory and practical implications, *Can Vet J* 40:33, 1999.
10. Sharkin BS, Knox D: Pet loss: issues and implications for the psychologist, *Professional Psychology: Research and Practice* 34:414, 2003.
11. Sanders CR: Killing with kindness: veterinary euthanasia and the social construction of personhood, *Sociological Forum* 10:195, 1995.
12. Stutts JC: Veterinarians and their human clients, *J Am Vet Med Assoc* 210:1742, 1997.
13. Clements PT, Benasutti KM, Carmone A: Support for bereaved owners of pets, *Perspect Psychiatr Care* 39:49, 2003.
14. Gage MG, Holcomb R: Couples perception of stressfulness of death of the family pet, *Family Relations* 40:103, 1991.
15. Dunn KL, Mehler SJ, Greenberg HS: Social work with a pet loss support group in a university veterinary hospital, *Soc Work Health Care* 41:59, 2005.
16. Quackenbush JE, Glickman L: Helping people adjust to the death of a pet, *Health Soc Work* 9:42, 1984.
17. Brandt JC, Grabill CM: Communicating with special populations: children and older adults, *Vet Clin North Am Small Anim Pract* 37:181, 2007.
18. Carmack BJ: Pet loss and the elderly, *Holist Nurs Pract* 5:80, 1991.

73 Chemotherapy Administration

Krystal G. Schneider and Heather M. Wilson

Administration of chemotherapy has become a common procedure in many general veterinary practices, necessitated by the incidence of neoplasia in our feline patients. Thirty per cent of all cats over the age of 10 will be diagnosed with some type of cancer.[1] Many small animal and feline practices now are quite comfortable administering chemotherapy on-site rather than referring these patients to specialty hospitals. The increasing demand for veterinarians and their nursing staff to administer these drugs highlights the need for improved guidelines and more accurate information regarding chemotherapy administration for our feline patients. This chapter will cover basic chemotherapy safety and administration, as well as provide helpful charts, client handouts, and sedation protocols.

CHEMOTHERAPY SAFETY

Maintaining safe working conditions remains the highest priority for all veterinarians and nursing staff when administering chemotherapy. Many issues must be considered before the first dose of chemotherapy is administered. First, those individuals who are administering the chemotherapy are at the greatest risk for exposure. Women of childbearing age must use special caution when handling chemotherapy drugs, and women who are pregnant should be strongly discouraged from handling any chemotherapy drugs.[2] Second, veterinary hospitals should have a standard operating procedure (SOP) in place for chemotherapy administration; all staff members should be familiar and comfortable with this document and should be able to locate it easily. In accor-

dance with Occupational Safety and Health Administration (OSHA) guidelines, all nursing staff involved in the administration of hazardous drugs should wear the following protective gear:

Gloves: Veterinary hospitals can purchase specially made chemotherapy administration gloves. These gloves are thicker than the average latex glove and come in specific sizes for a better fit to enhance manual dexterity. If chemotherapy administration gloves are not available, latex gloves with minimal or no powder are preferred, because the powder can absorb contamination.[3,4] Double-gloving is recommended to minimize the risk of exposure to hazardous drugs, when using latex gloves.[3] Gloves always should be removed immediately if they are punctured, torn, or contaminated from a spill. Nursing staff always should wash their hands prior to putting the gloves on and again after they are removed.

Gowns: Disposable gowns should be worn that are made of lint-free, low-permeability fabric, with a closed front, long sleeves, and elastic or knit cuffs. Gloves should be placed over the cuff of the gown, and if two pairs of latex gloves are worn, the inner pair should be inserted under the gown cuff and the outer pair should be worn over the gown cuff. If gowns are not available, a buttoned-up lab coat with long sleeves may be worn in the same fashion. A plastic-backed absorbable pad may be placed over the administrator's lap to prevent any contamination of clothing underneath. The lab coat should be removed and washed after drug administration.

Masks: OSHA guidelines state that a Biologic Safety Cabinet (BSC) or vertical airflow fume hood should be used for the preparation of all hazardous drugs. Recognizing that few veterinary hospitals have access to such a hood, a National Institute for Occupational Safety and Health (NIOSH)–approved respirator may be worn during drug preparation. A surgical mask is not appropriate because it does not prevent the inhalation of aerosolized drugs. If hazardous drugs are not being prepared in your hospital, a surgical mask may be appropriate to protect your face from any splash or chemotherapy spill during administration.

Goggles: Goggles with a fitted nosepiece and side shields are appropriate to protect the administrator's eyes from any splash or spill from chemotherapy drugs. A full-face shield and a respirator always should be worn for preparation of hazardous drugs. It also is recommended that a functional eye-washing station be available in all hospitals.

In addition to the use of protective clothing, many other safety measures should be observed in hospitals in which chemotherapy is administered. These measures are recommended to help minimize spills, and to protect the nursing staff and patient from unnecessary exposure to hazardous chemicals.

The room in which chemotherapy is administered should be a low-traffic, quiet area with good ventilation and lighting. There should be no eating, drinking, smoking, chewing gum, applying cosmetics, or food storage where chemotherapy is prepared or administered. The preparation and administration of all chemotherapy drugs should be performed over a plastic-backed absorbable pad. A designated sharps container should be available for chemotherapy use only and labeled as such. The storage of chemotherapy drugs should be kept separate from other drugs and human food products. Areas housing chemotherapy drugs should be labeled clearly, and the drugs should be stored in bins with barrier fronts. If refrigeration is required, a separate unit should be used.[5]

It is always preferable to use Luer-Lok syringes to minimize the chances of aerosolization and chemotherapy spills. Never fill a syringe to more than 75 per cent of its capacity volume. This will minimize the chances of accidentally pulling the plunger out of the syringe resulting in a spill. If removing a needle and syringe from a bottle of chemotherapy drug is required, and a fume hood is not available, wrap a 70 per cent alcohol-soaked gauze around the chemotherapy bottle and needle. The alcohol-soaked gauze will serve as an absorptive barrier for any chemotherapy that may aerosolize from the bottle (Figure 73-1). As with any medication, accurate labeling of all syringes is crucial. When preparing a flushing syringe, it is best to use saline rather than a heparinized saline mixture because heparin precipitates with some chemotherapy agents. A chemotherapy dispensing pin can be used if mixing or reconstituting drugs is required (B. Braun Medical Inc, Bethlehem, PA). This "chemo-pin" has hydrophobic filters that help to equalize the pressure inside the bottle that is being mixed, further reducing the risk of exposure during mixing (Figure 73-2).

Most chemotherapy pills can not be broken and capsules should never be opened. However, chlorambucil, a commonly used chemotherapy drug for feline small cell gastrointestinal lymphoma, can be broken in half if necessary. Chlorambucil is available in 2-mg tablets. These

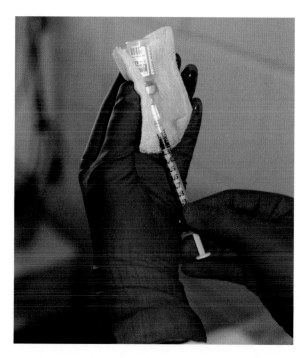

Figure 73-1 Wrapping a 70 per cent alcohol-soaked gauze square around the chemotherapy bottle while removing the needle and syringe minimizes the aerosolization of chemotherapy drug.

tablets are coated and may be broken carefully for 1-mg dose increments. When prescribing more than one tablet per dose, it often is easiest to place the tablet (or tablet halves) in an empty clear gelatin capsule so that the entire dose may be administered at one time. All clients and staff members should wear gloves when handling or administering this medication, regardless of whether it is in a gelatin capsule. If tablets need to be cut in half, this ideally should be done under a hood. If no hood is available, this can be performed over an absorbent pad. The person handling the medication should wear a mask if pills are being broken into halves, and the area subsequently should be cleaned with diluted bleach. The absorbent pad should be discarded as chemotherapy waste along with the gloves and mask.[6]

Wherever chemotherapy drugs are being mixed or administered, a clearly labeled hazardous chemical spill kit should be easily accessible. All staff members should be aware of its contents, how to use the components, and how to clean up a spill properly. The American Society of Hospital Pharmacists (ASHP) recommends that kits contain the following items: one to two pairs of chemical splash goggles, two pairs of gloves, two pairs of utility gloves, a low-permeability gown, two (12″ × 12″) absorbent pads, a sharps container, a small scoop to collect glass fragments, and two hazardous drug disposal bags (Figure 73-3).[3]

RECORD KEEPING

When dose calculation and administration of chemotherapy drugs are performed, it is vital to have a calcula-

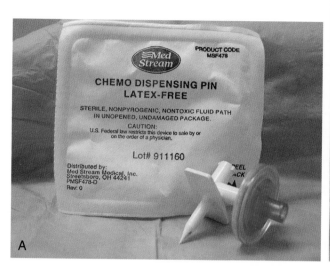
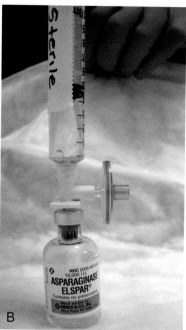

Figure 73-2 A, Chemotherapy dispensing pins should be used when mixing or reconstituting drugs without a fume hood. **B,** Chemotherapy dispensing pins have hydrophobic filters that equalize the pressure in the bottle while reconstituting the contents. These filters allow the drug to be reconstituted and then drawn back into the syringe without pressure build-up in the bottle. The pins further reduce the risk of exposure during mixing and decrease the possibility of aerosolization of chemotherapy drugs.

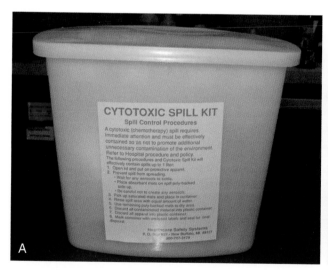
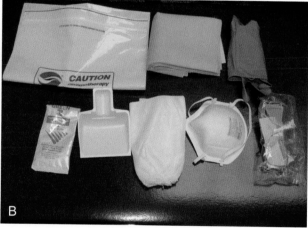

Figure 73-3 A, A chemotherapy spill kit always should be easily accessible wherever chemotherapy is being administered. All staff members should be aware of its location, contents, and how to clean up a spill properly. **B,** A chemotherapy spill kit, in accordance with The American Society of Hospital Pharmacists (ASHP), should contain: one to two pairs of chemical splash goggles, two pairs of gloves, two pairs of utility gloves, a low-permeability gown, two (12″ by 12″) absorbent pads, a "sharps" container, a small scoop to collect glass fragments, and two hazardous drug disposal bags.

tion sheet and log sheet as part of the cat's medical record. It not only helps to minimize errors, but also enhances communication between veterinarians and nursing staff.

The chemotherapy administration form (Figure 73-4) is designed to have all the pertinent information on one

sheet. The patient is identified (square shaded box located in the upper right corner of Figure 73-4), complete blood count and other pertinent test results can be recorded, and the patient's weight in pounds (lb), kilograms (kg), and meter squared (m²) body surface area is recorded for each dose of chemotherapy. One should always refer to

CHEMOTHERAPY ADMINISTRATION

CBC: Date_____ RDVM   TAMU

WBC/Neutrophils: _____ / _____

PCV: _____

Platelets: _____

BUN/Crea: _____

Urine SG: _____

ECG [ ] _____ Echo _____

Wt: _____ lbs _____ kg _____ M^2

ADMINISTRATION DATE: _____ **DIAGNOSIS:** _____

PREMEDICATIONS

Benadryl: _____ mg   IV   IM   SQ   _____ AM   PM _____ minutes pre-chemo

_____ mg   IV   IM   SQ   _____ AM   PM _____ minutes pre-chemo

CHEMOTHERAPY   Drug used: _____

Butterfly catheter [ ]   Indwelling catheter [ ]   Cath size _____ SQ [ ]   Oral [ ]

Dose: _____ mg per M^2 kg = _____ mg   Dose given _____

Diluted in _____ ml NaCl   SQ injection given: R   L _____

Catheter placed in R   L _____ Vein   Flushed with _____ ml NaCl before administration of chemotherapy.

Drug infused over _____ minutes.

Catheter was flushed with _____ ml NaCl post-administration. It was then pulled, and a light pressure bandage was applied.

MARKER LESION MEASUREMENTS   _____

_____

_____

_____

COMMENTS _____

_____

Dose verified by: _____ _____ _____ _____
                         DVM   Tech   RPh   Student

Created by Diane Green, RVT

Figure 73-4 The chemotherapy administration sheet is designed to have all the pertinent information on one sheet. This is where the patient's current weight is documented, premedications are recorded, chemotherapy is calculated, and all administration information is noted.

the kg to m^2 conversion chart each time when calculating chemotherapy drugs that are administered based on body surface area (Table 73-1). If a patient's weight in kg does not match precisely with the numbers on the chart, it is advisable to extrapolate between numbers and round the numbers down. There also is a section designated for recording any premedications, sedatives, or antihistamines that are administered. This form provides a place for listing the chemotherapy drug being administered, the route by which it was given, catheter placement information including location, and notes about marker lesion assessment. It also provides a site for the person(s) calculating the chemotherapy dose to initial or sign. Ideally more than one person should calculate and check the chemotherapy dose before administration. This form should be incorporated into the medical record at each visit, so that any comments or important information can be accessed conveniently.

Chemotherapy log sheets are important for all patients receiving chemotherapy. Some patients may receive several weeks or months of chemotherapy and the log sheet allows staff members to transfer the information from the administration sheet (see Figure 73-4) to the log sheet so that each visit involving chemotherapy can be found easily. The log sheet can be the first page of a patient's record, but at the very least should be near the front of the record so that it is accessible (Figure 73-5). The information on a log sheet should include the date, the cat's weight, chemotherapy drug administered, the calculated and administered dose (occasionally these are different), and any toxicities noted after the patient's last therapy, including the grade of toxicity noted (Table 73-2).[7] It also is prudent to record whether sedation was required for the treatment and if a previous sedation protocol was adequate or should be adjusted for future use. This log sheet should be updated each time the cat receives chemotherapy. It also is important to record any delays in the chemotherapy administration protocol, and their reasons (e.g., grade 3 neutropenia), on the log sheet.

CHEMOTHERAPY ADMINISTRATION

Before administering chemotherapy, it is important to assess the cat's attitude and stress level to determine if physical restraint will be adequate, or if chemical restraint will be required. When restraining cats, less restraint often is more effective than a more aggressive approach. It is essential to be prepared and to have an effective plan of action. An Elizabethan collar (e-collar) (Figure 73-6) is an excellent option when considering physical restraint of a cat for chemotherapy administration. These plastic e-collars facilitate the positioning of patients without scruffing or stretching them, minimizing stress and the risk of a staff member receiving a bite wound. Gentle physical restraint often is adequate to allow a short infusion or a bolus chemotherapy administration; however, chemical restraint may be required for a long infusion or for a fractious patient. When choosing a sedation protocol for the cat, select a protocol that can be administered subcutaneously (SQ), or intramuscularly (IM) (Table 73-3). This obviates the need for venipuncture prior to intravenous (IV) chemotherapy. Many drugs that are administered IV are tissue vesicants, requiring a perfect venipuncture to a vein that has not been used for several days.

Table 73-1 Feline Kilogram (kg) to Meter Squared (m^2) Conversion Chart*

kg	m^2	kg	m^2
0.5	0.06	26.0	0.88
1.0	0.10	27.0	0.90
2.0	0.15	28.0	0.92
3.0	0.20	29.0	0.94
4.0	0.25	30.0	0.96
5.0	0.29	31.0	0.99
6.0	0.33	32.0	1.01
7.0	0.36	33.0	1.03
8.0	0.40	34.0	1.05
9.0	0.43	35.0	1.07
10.0	0.46	36.0	1.09
11.0	0.49	37.0	1.11
12.0	0.52	38.0	1.13
13.0	0.55	39.0	1.15
14.0	0.58	40.0	1.17
15.0	0.60	41.0	1.19
16.0	0.63	42.0	1.21
17.0	0.66	43.0	1.23
18.0	0.69	44.0	1.25
19.0	0.71	45.0	1.26
20.0	0.74	46.0	1.28
21.0	0.76	47.0	1.30
22.0	0.78	48.0	1.32
23.0	0.81	49.0	1.34
24.0	0.83	50.0	1.36
25.0	0.85		

*Conversion of body weight in kilograms to body surface area in meters.

ORAL ADMINISTRATION

Most oral chemotherapy pills or capsules should not be split or crushed for administration or dosing, with the exception of chlorambucil. It is best to contact a veterinary pharmacy and request that the drugs be recompounded into exact doses. Chemotherapy gloves (or two pairs of latex gloves) must be worn when administering oral chemotherapy. When the patient allows, administer the pill in a treat (pill pocket or baby food) or by placing the pill/capsule in the back of the mouth and

**CHEMOTHERAPY
ADMINISTRATION LOG**

Date/ wt	Chemotherapy agent	Calc dose	Admin dose	Toxicities	Comments	Sedation agent/dose

Figure 73-5 The chemotherapy log sheet should be placed at the very beginning of the patient's medical record. It should contain the date, patient's weight, chemotherapy drug administered, the calculated and administered doses (occasionally these are different), and any toxicities noted after the patient's last therapy including the grade of toxicity. The effectiveness of sedation protocols also is a useful piece of information to be documented on this sheet.

Table 73-2 National Cancer Institute Guidelines for Grading Chemotherapy-Associated Toxicities

Adverse Event	Grade				
	0	**1**	**2**	**3**	**4**
Anorexia	None	Partial inappetence	Appetite significantly decreased	Requirement for IV fluids	Requirement for feeding tube or parenteral nutrition
Vomiting	None	1 episode in 24 hours over pretreatment	2-5 episodes in 24 hours over pretreatment	≥6 episodes in 24 hours over pretreatment, or need for IV fluids	Requirement for parenteral nutrition, or physiologic consequences necessitating intensive care, or hemodynamic collapse
Diarrhea	None	Increase of <4 stools/day over pretreatment	Increase of 4-6 stools/ day or nocturnal stools	Increase of ≥7 stools/ day or incontinence or need for parenteral support for dehydration	Physiologic consequences requiring intensive care, or hemodynamic collapse
Neutropenia	None	≥1500 to <2000 neutrophils/μL	≥1000 to <1500 neutrophils/μL	≥500 to <1000 neutrophils/μL	<500 neutrophils/μL
Thrombocytopenia	None	≥75,000 to <180,000 platelets/μL	≥50,000 to <75,000 platelets/μL	≥10,000 to <50,000 platelets/μL	<10,000 platelets/μL

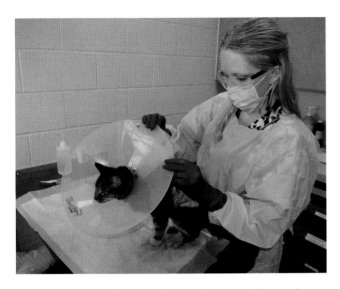

Figure 73-6 An Elizabethan collar (e-collar) should be used whenever physical restraint is required. E-collars help to minimize the amount of restraint necessary and also reduce patient stress.

Table 73-3 Drugs Used Commonly for Sedation During Chemotherapy Administration

Drug	Dose	Route of Administration
Butorphanol	0.2-0.4 mg/kg	SQ or IM
Acepromazine	0.01 mg/kg	SQ or IM
Midazolam	0.1-0.2 mg/kg	SQ or IM
Hydromorphone	0.1-0.2 mg/kg	SQ or IM
Buprenorphine	0.01-0.02 mg/kg	SQ, IM, sublingual

encouraging the cat to swallow. A pill gun or pill popper should be used if patient compliance is poor and if there is concern that the patient may bite the pill or the administrator. It is important to ensure that the patient has swallowed the pill. This may be facilitated by following the pill administration with a syringe of water. If an owner is administering oral chemotherapy at home, they should be provided with latex gloves, and should be advised to wash their hands before and after administration of the drugs.

SUBCUTANEOUS ADMINISTRATION

Subcutaneous chemotherapy can be given quickly with minimal stress and restraint to the patient; however, the same safety protocols need to be followed. An absorbent diaper should be placed under the patient during drug administration. Subcutaneous chemotherapy injections can be administered like other injections by this route, with the needle pointed down and away from any member of the nursing staff who is holding the cat. Check for negative pressure and be sure that the needle

has not been inserted into any small blood vessels before injecting the chemotherapy agent. After the injection has been completed, place all needles and syringes into the chemotherapy sharps container. Use a chemotherapy dispensing pin if the chemotherapy drug is formulated as a powder and requires the addition of a diluent. This will minimize the risk of aerosolization when the chemotherapy drug is prepared and the dose is drawn into the syringe (see Figure 73-2).

INTRAVENOUS ADMINISTRATION

Many chemotherapy drugs are administered intravenously (IV); most are irritants or vesicants, requiring perfect venipuncture. Before placing an IV catheter or a butterfly catheter, a small amount of fur over the vein should be shaved to the skin and prepared with an alcohol and antiseptic cleaning. Never scrub the cat's skin because this may lead to small abrasions. Catheter placement must be in a peripheral vein that has not been used for venipuncture within 48 hours.

Butterfly Catheter

The assistant restraining the cat occludes the vein while the administrator placing the catheter holds the patient's foot firmly. A flushed butterfly catheter (primed with saline) is placed into the vein. The needle must go directly into the vein and not through it. If the catheter goes through the vein, the nursing team should stop and redirect efforts to another vein. The administrator must not "back into" the vein; only forward motion (with no redirecting) ensures proper needle placement. Placing the entire butterfly needle in the vein is ideal, because this minimizes the chances of the needle backing itself out during administration and allowing extravasation. Once the catheter is in place, a three-way stopcock with a syringe containing 10 to 12 mL of sterile saline and a syringe with the chemotherapy dose is attached to the end of the butterfly line (Figure 73-7). The three-way stopcock always should be turned to the off position for the syringe containing the chemotherapy drug when it is attached to the butterfly catheter. The assistant then should stop occluding the vein, allowing for normal blood flow while maintaining a firm hold on the cat's leg. The chemotherapy administrator should begin by flushing two to three mL of saline into the patient's vein, to allow assessment of vascular integrity. If saline extravasates (creating a fluid-filled bubble under the skin) or if the saline does not flush easily, the catheter should be removed and puncture of another vein should be attempted. The assistant should be able to feel the pulsing of the flushed saline proximal to the butterfly needle. A small amount of blood should be aspirated back into the butterfly line, and two to three mL of saline flushed again. This process can be repeated several times until the administrator and the assistant are comfortable with the catheter placement. The stopcock is positioned to the off position for the saline syringe and to the on position for the syringe containing the chemotherapy agent, and the chemotherapy is bolused into the line. It is important not to aspirate back once the chemotherapy has been given,

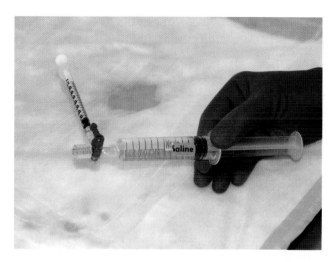

Figure 73-7 A three-way stopcock is used when administering IV bolus chemotherapy. The three-way stopcock has a syringe with chemotherapy drug and a syringe with saline flush attached to it (all using Luer-Lok syringes). Once the catheter is placed, the stopcock is attached to the end of the butterfly line. The purpose of this device is to minimize movement and exposure of the administrator to chemotherapy. This is considered a "closed system."

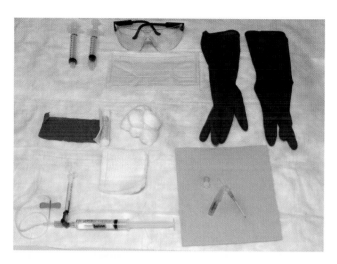

Figure 73-8 The equipment necessary for IV infusion administration is shown. A short catheter is placed, and a butterfly catheter then is placed into the PRN adaptor. The butterfly line is attached to the 3-way stopcock.

because this increases the possibility of extravasation or spill of chemotherapy agent and phlebitis.

Once the chemotherapy drug has been administered, the stopcock should be turned to the off position for the chemotherapy drug, and to the on position for the saline flush. The remainder of the saline then is flushed into the vein. The butterfly catheter is removed, with the three-way stopcock still attached, and is discarded into the chemotherapy sharps container as one piece. Finally, a pressure bandage is applied over the venipuncture site.

Intravenous Catheter Administration

Short-term catheters can be placed when a longer infusion of chemotherapy is required or when a butterfly catheter is not indicated (Figure 73-8). Extreme caution must be used when placing these catheters and when administering these chemotherapy agents, because several infusion chemotherapy drugs are severe vesicants. Because catheter placement must be perfect, the patient should be very relaxed and still, making sedation an attractive method for restraint. The catheter must be placed directly into the vein and fed easily with no resistance or redirection. Once the catheter is placed, a valved adaptor (i.e., a PRN adaptor) is attached to the Luer-Lok system on the end of the catheter and the catheter is taped to the cat's leg. The tape should be applied firmly, and the external tip of the catheter should be palpable and visible. The catheter should be flushed with a generous amount of sterile saline to ensure the accuracy of placement; 10 to 15 mL usually is adequate. Aspirating blood back into the syringe is discouraged.

Drug administration begins when the nursing staff members are comfortable with the catheter placement. Cats typically weigh less than their canine counterparts and require a smaller volume of chemotherapy drug. Therefore the chemotherapy drug should be diluted with sterile saline in a syringe, rather than diluting the agent in a partial bag of fluids, for better control over the amount the patient is receiving in the allotted time. Using the same setup with the three-way stopcock as described previously, place the needle of the butterfly catheter into the PRN adaptor, attach the butterfly line to the three-way stopcock, and begin administering the calculated volume slowly over 10 to 15 minutes. A gauze square should be placed between the butterfly catheter and the cat's leg at the point where the needle enters the PRN adaptor, creating a barrier between the patient's skin and the chemotherapy agent in case of leaks (Figure 73-9). When all of the chemotherapy dose has been administered, the stopcock should be turned to the off position for the chemotherapy drug and to the on position for the saline flush. Flush in the remainder of the saline, or at the very least, enough saline to flush the chemotherapy drug out of the butterfly line and into the cat. Remove the butterfly catheter, with the three-way stopcock still attached, and discard the whole apparatus into the chemotherapy sharps container. Flush an additional 5 to 10 mL of saline through the catheter before it is removed to ensure that no residual chemotherapy drug is present. It is important to note that heparinized saline should not be used as a flush for chemotherapy administration because it may precipitate some drugs, such as doxorubicin. Once removed, the combined catheter and chemotherapy administration apparatus should be discarded into the chemotherapy sharps container, and a pressure bandage applied over the venipuncture site.

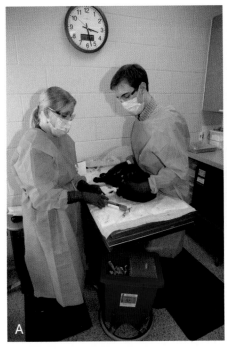
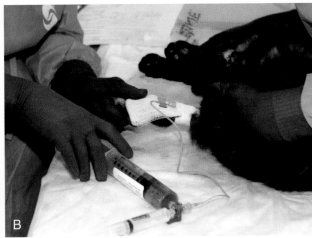

Figure 73-9 A, Oncology nursing staff are administering chemotherapy. All necessary safety equipment and clothing are being worn, the patient is lying on top of a plastic backed absorbable pad, and a chemotherapy sharps bucket is readily accessible. **B,** Chemotherapy is being administered to a patient using a short intravenous catheter. A butterfly line with a three-way stopcock has been placed in the PRN adaptor. A gauze square is placed between the patient's skin and the chemotherapy line.

POSTCHEMOTHERAPY CLEAN-UP

All "sharps" or materials that come in direct contact with chemotherapy should be discarded in a designated chemotherapy sharps container. All other protective clothing and equipment (gloves, masks, and plastic-backed absorbable pads) should be discarded in a designated thick plastic biohazard bag. Patients should be placed in a quiet comfortable area after chemotherapy administration, with access to a litter box and fresh water. Latex gloves and a disposable gown should be worn when cleaning up excrement from a patient who has received chemotherapy within the past 48 hours. Eye protection should be worn if splashing may occur. When cleaning a cage in which a chemotherapy patient has been housed, it is important to avoid spraying disinfectant cleaner directly into the cage. Rather spray a towel with the disinfectant and use the moist towel to clean the area, thereby minimizing the aerosolization of chemotherapy-contaminated feces or urine.

Linens soiled after chemotherapy administration should be handled in accordance with the Bloodborne Pathogens Standard.[8] They should be placed in a marked laundry bag and then in a labeled impervious bag. The laundry bag and the linen should be prewashed separately before they can be washed again with other laundry. Plastic-backed absorbable diapers are a better choice for lining cages than nondisposable linens, and are safer for the nursing staff responsible for cleaning up after these patients. Cages should be labeled clearly so that all staff members are aware that these patients have received chemotherapy and that there is a risk of drug exposure. Larger hospitals may require these cages to be labeled

with the drug's name, dose, and the date and time of administration.

CLIENT COMMUNICATION

Client communication is an essential component of the care of all patients receiving chemotherapy. Clients need to understand all the risks, complications, and potential side effects associated with chemotherapy and its administration. If they have more than one pet, they may need to take extra precautions with the treated pet's excrement and medications. Clients should be able to call with questions or concerns. Ideally a take-home standard written discharge instruction sheet should be provided after every visit. A simple, client take-home sheet on hazardous medications (Figure 73-10) should be provided, so that the clients have a quick resource for many of their questions.

SUMMARY

Properly trained staff who are well versed in standard operating procedures, safe chemotherapy administration, and thorough client communication, are essential for the provision of excellent care for our feline oncology patients. Having staff who are prepared, experienced, and knowledgeable is crucial when handling chemotherapy.

Although the safety precautions, record keeping, and basic care may be the same regardless of the medication, each chemotherapy drug comes with its own risks and possible complications.

Client Take-Home Sheet

Texas A&M Veterinary Medical Teaching Hospital

Hazardous medication (chemotherapy) safety instructions

Feline Patients

- Pregnant individuals, those trying to become pregnant, or nursing mothers should not handle hazardous medications (chemotherapy drugs) or excrement (urine, feces, vomit) of a pet who has received these medications until 48 hours after the last dose. Inform your physician of your pet's chemotherapy treatment for further precautions and recommendations.

- Wear gloves when administering chemotherapy medication to your pet, and wash your hands with soap and water after removing the gloves.

- Wear gloves when cleaning urine, feces, and vomit until 48 hours after the last dose of chemotherapy has been given.

- Place all contaminated items (gloves, paper towels, urine and feces from the litter box) in a sealable plastic bag and seal the top before discarding in outside trash. Wash hands thoroughly with soap and water.

- Use low-dust litter and clean the box frequently, wear gloves and dust mask if needed until 48 hours after the last dose of chemotherapy has been given.

- If your pet is allowed to go outside and defecate where other animals may ingest feces, pick up feces and place them in a sealable bag and discard.

- When medicating your pet with oral chemotherapy, if he/she bites the pill in half or crushes the pill or capsule, discard it in a sealable bag and contact your veterinarian for further advice.

- If linens or clothes are contaminated, wash them as soon as possible. Wash them separately from other laundry to prevent cross-contamination.

- If skin exposure to the medications or contaminated products occurs accidentally, wash immediately with soap and water.

- If eye exposure to medication or contaminated products occurs accidentally, flush with copious amounts of water. Seek medical advice for any large exposure or continued symptoms after flushing.

Figure 73-10 The client take-home sheet provides information on how to manage and care for a pet after chemotherapy administration.

REFERENCES

1. Reisen JS: Epidemiology and incidence of cancer. In Withrow S, Vail D, editors: *Small animal clinical oncology*, Philadelphia, 2007, Saunders, p 68.
2. Ogilvie GK, Moore AS: Drug handling and administration. In Ogilvie GK, Moore AS, editors: *Feline oncology. a comprehensive guide to compassionate care*, Trenton, 2001, Veterinary Learning Systems, p 53.
3. American Society of Hospital Pharmacists: ASHP Technical Assistance Bulletin on Handling Cytotoxic and Hazardous Drugs, *Am J Hosp Pharm* 47:1033, 1990.
4. U.S. Department of Health and Human Services: Guidelines for Protecting the Safety and Health of Health Care Workers. Public Health Service, Centers for Disease Control, National Institute for Occupational Safety and Health. DHHS (NIOSH) Publication No. 88-119, 1988.
5. U.S. Department of Labor: OSHA Technical Manual. Chemical Protective Clothing. Section VIII: Chapter 2, 1991. Available at http://www.osha.gov/dts/osta/otm/otm_viii/otm_viii_2.html
6. Wilson HM: Feline alimentary lymphoma: demystifying the enigma, *Top Companion Anim Med* 23:177, 2008.
7. Rogers KS, Green D: Medical record keeping for the oncology patient. In August JR, editor: *Consultations in feline internal medicine*, vol 5, St. Louis, 2006, Elsevier Saunders, p 627.
8. U.S. Department of Labor, Occupational Safety and Health Administration: Occupational Exposure to Bloodborne Pathogens Standard. Section VI: Chapter 2, 1991. Available at http://www.osha.gov/dts/osta/otm/otm_vi/otm_vi_2.html

Population Medicine

Margaret R. Slater, Section Editor

74 Shelter Population Health Management

Claudia J. Baldwin

Companion animal shelters continue to be a necessity for housing of free-roaming and relinquished cats. The number of cats in shelters in the United States is unknown, but it is estimated that six to eight million cats and dogs enter shelters each year.[1] It also is known that in some areas of the United States, cats represent greater than 75 per cent of companion animals entering shelters, but only 2 to 5 per cent of cats entering shelters are reclaimed. A large free-roaming cat population exists in the United States and its relationship with owned and sheltered populations is unknown.[2] The roles of animal shelters vary from animal control units to adoption or rehoming facilities to sanctuaries to a combination of these. Shelters may have open, limited, or closed access policies for admission depending on the shelter's role, mission, and funding. Successful shelter population health management is dependent on the design of the facility, and the staff's ability to minimize pathogen load and transmission; segregate populations based on health and life stage; minimize stress; afford strong preventative health care interventions; and recognize disease and provide treatment of individual animals without jeopardizing the population. Prevention of overcrowding is extremely important to maintain population health, and this can be accomplished by limiting intake when possible, utilizing strong fostering and adoption programs, and managing population density.

FACILITY AS IT RELATES TO POPULATION HEALTH

FACILITY DESIGN

The first consideration for the layout of the facility should be focused on limiting disease transmission. Many facilities being used to house populations of animals were not intended for that use. Rather, facilities are secured and modified for sheltering. These, and newly constructed facilities, should have clearly defined zones. Box 74-1 lists components of zones within shelters, identified as public and restricted.

Some larger shelters will have many of the rooms that are listed whereas others will not, but care should be taken to organize the zones and delineate between them with appropriate signage to the extent possible. Minimizing public traffic into the restricted zone will help to reduce spread of disease. Another vital concept for all traffic is to move from the healthy young animal areas to the healthy adult, to those potentially incubating disease, to those recovering from or with clinical signs of disease. Use of personal protective equipment (PPE), including lab coat or uniform, gloves, and in some instances of potential zoonotic disease, masks and goggles, is needed when staff work in restricted areas and must move back to

Box 74-1 Zones Within the Shelter Facility

PUBLIC ZONE
Entry
Adoption rooms
Get-acquainted room
Education and public activity rooms

RESTRICTED ZONE
Staff office area
Receiving room for incoming cats
Holding room for incoming healthy cats
Examination room for health assessments and treatment
Isolation room(s) for incoming and resident cats with
    signs of disease
Quarantine room for observation of cats for rabies/bites
Surgical facilities
Kitchen and laundry area
Secure storage area

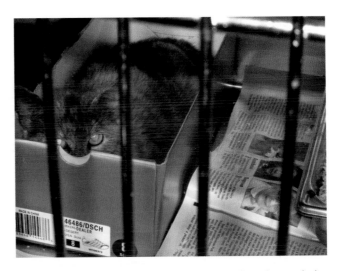

Figure 74-1 Cat housed in a box style cage with a place to hide as it acclimates to the shelter.

healthy areas in the shelter. Shelter access to owners looking for lost pets must be afforded. Escorting the individual so as not to move from restricted to public zones is recommended. Likewise, volunteers should be assigned to specific areas with understanding of strict traffic patterns. Separate areas to perform intake and preventative care on healthy animals and examination areas to treat cats with illness should be designated carefully. Within the facility, all floor and wall surfaces should be impervious to avoid harboring of pathogens and standing water.

SECURE STORAGE

Secure storage areas are needed in the restricted zone to hold foods, litter, equipment, cleaning agents and disinfectants, and other supplies. Ideally a separate area to clean and disinfect water and food dishes and litter pans, outside of animal housing rooms, should be available. Some of these areas also store food and serve as a kitchen, although some shelters utilize a mobile cart stocked with food, water, and bowls to be used during feeding times. An area to perform laundry is needed. Pest control is essential and can be achieved through securing food and eliminating waste. Intervention with traps and baits may be necessary, but caution when using chemical baits is necessary to prevent inadvertent consumption by animals in the shelter. As veterinary professionals working with shelters, we certainly can advise directors on zones, traffic control, signage, PPE, storage, and pest control. Prior to renovation or building of a shelter, professionals with experience in shelter design definitely should be consulted.[3]

HOUSING

Cages in the cat areas, benches, resting places, perches, and other equipment in communal areas should be nonporous so they can be cleaned and disinfected. Food bowls, litter pans, toys, and bedding should be washed

and disinfected, or disposable and discarded, after use. Housing of cats in cages is essential for incoming housing, isolation, and quarantine. Segregation of cats based on life stage (e.g., nursing kittens and queens, weaning/post weaning, adolescent, and adult) is ideal because the housing and animal care needs are different as well as their immune status and function. Adoption rooms in many facilities continue to use cages. Box style cages, similar to those used in veterinary hospitals, are easy to clean and disinfect but do not meet the behavioral needs of the cats. Cages should be large enough to accommodate litter boxes and bowls with adequate distance between them, and the size of the cage should meet minimum requirements.[4] Use of a vertical platform is helpful, as is a place to rest or hide, which can be as simple as a disposable shoe box or paper bag (Figure 74-1). Double-sided cages afford more space and facilitate cleaning. Cleaning with cat "in residence" or using other methods of minimizing cage moves is important to prevent stress, to prevent compromising the immune system and stimulating the recrudescence of viral pathogens. When cleaning "in residence," the process should be restricted to cleaning of debris, and cleaning or replacement of litter boxes and feed bowls. When more thorough cleaning is needed, the use of a carrier designated for each individual cat is one method to minimize cage moves (Figure 74-2). Cleaning and disinfection of cages to prevent spread of disease should be performed between occupants.

Communal housing is being utilized more frequently in shelters to reduce stress and improve welfare.[5] Animals entering communal housing, however, should be fully vaccinated, treated for endoparasites and ectoparasites, tested for feline leukemia virus (FeLV) and feline immunodeficiency virus (FIV), and free from infectious disease. Observation and removal of cats with aggressive behavior should be done routinely. Size of colonies should be limited to a maximum of 10 cats and age matching is important. Structures that can not be cleaned and disinfected easily, such as wood, should be avoided except in closed colony situations (Figure 74-3).

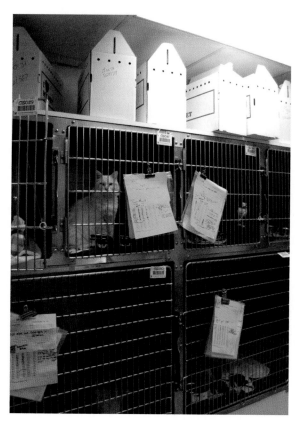

Figure 74-2 Designated holding carriers (here stored above the cages) for each individual cat can be helpful when more thorough cage cleaning is needed.

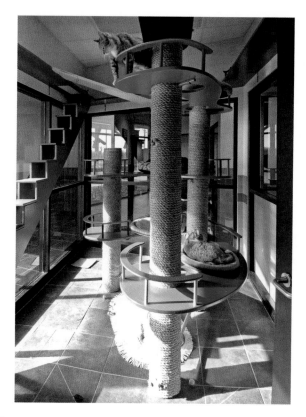

Figure 74-4 Natural light is provided by windows in this open housing area. (Courtesy Mr. Brent Isenberger.)

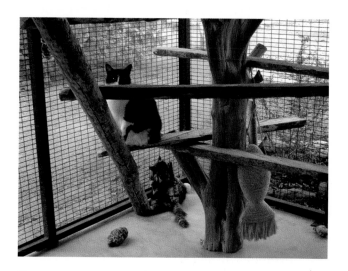

Figure 74-3 Structures such as wood that can not be cleaned and disinfected easily should be avoided except in closed colony situations.

LIGHT AND VENTILATION

Good lighting is essential. The addition of natural light is recommended and can be provided by windows and skylights (Figure 74-4). Use of low-emission glass can protect from heat loss and gain to the building. Light fixtures should be waterproofed to protect them during cleaning. Good light quality is needed to allow for adequate cleaning. Cats require light and dark periods daily, and lights should be turned on during the day and off at night. Sound should be minimized to reduce stress on the cats and personnel.

Ventilation systems should move air effectively and be kept in good working condition with fresh air also available whenever possible (Figure 74-5). Separate ventilation systems for individual rooms, or zones, is highly recommended. Air exchange recommendations range from 8 to 15 per hour, but the energy requirements may not be affordable for many shelters. Acceptable temperature and humidity ranges are 10° to 29° C (50° to 85° F) and 10 to 50 per cent, respectively. High humidity and poor air quality caused by urine odor and chemical fumes, hair, and dust from litter, along with inadequate ventilation, may contribute to respiratory tract irritation and perhaps disease by disruption of natural mucosal barriers.

ENVIRONMENTAL INFECTION CONTROL

MINIMIZE PATHOGEN LOAD

Environmental infection control is aimed at minimizing pathogen load within the confines of the shelter. For most animal shelters, a transient environment exists with a constant influx of animals from the community. An important concept to recognize is that cats will carry with them pathogens from the environment in which they

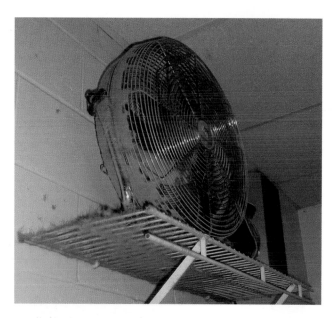

Figure 74-5 Fan covered in hair and dust can not perform the function of moving air.

originated. In dense and overcrowded populations, these pathogens can become concentrated and put the entire population at risk. Stress and other potential factors contributing to decreased immunity can lead to limiting a cat's ability to fight infection. It also can lead to recrudescence of latent infections, creating shedding and/or clinical disease. Initial evaluation of incoming cats is essential, as is isolation and preventative health care to minimize pathogen load and expression and transmission of disease. Sanitation or cleaning of the environment followed by disinfection can be a powerful way to minimize pathogens and infection. Good infection control measures should maintain optimal cat health, influence vaccination decisions, guide cleaning and disinfection decisions, take facility design and management into consideration, and serve as an opportunity to educate staff and volunteers.

KNOWLEDGE OF TRANSMISSION OF PATHOGENS

Transmission of disease can occur via aerosolized droplets (airborne), oral or ingestion, direct contact, fomites, vectors, the environment, reproductive transmission, or by multiple routes. Respiratory pathogens (e.g., feline herpesvirus-1 [FHV], feline calicivirus [FCV], and *Bordetella bronchiseptica*) can be transmitted via aerosolized droplets in cats housed within four feet, but can be spread easily through direct contact, the environment, and most frequently, fomites. Oral ingestion of pathogens can occur through contaminated food, water, or objects such as food and water bowls, litter pans, or toys. Rodents also can play a role in direct transmission of pathogens to food or objects. Feline panleukopenia virus (FPV) often is transmitted by the oral route. Direct contact occurs when an infected animal transmits a pathogen directly to a

susceptible animal. This may include rubbing, licking, or biting. Dermatophytosis is a very significant shelter pathogen that can be transmitted by direct contact.

Vector-borne transmission of disease to cats may occur commonly, as in the case of *Dipylidium caninum* transmitted by fleas. In one recent study of community-source blood donors, DNA from hemoplasma or *Bartonella henselae* was detected in 21.3 per cent and 22.7 per cent of the cats allowed outdoors or those with known flea exposure, respectively.[6] Additionally, fleas have been proposed as a possible means of transmission of FeLV, based on detection of FeLV RNA in fleas and their feces.[7] Environmental transmission occurs with pathogens that survive for extended periods of time in the environment. Route of infection may be through ingestion, direct contact, and airborne. Reproductive transmission in the shelter environment should be limited to vertical transmission during gestation or nursing. Of emerging pathogens, Group G *Streptococcus canis* can be transmitted to kittens born vaginally.[8] Transmission of zoonoses may occur via transmission from animals to human beings or from human beings to animals. Dermatophytosis is an example of such transmission. Use of PPE helps to minimize spread to human beings as does effective treatment or control of zoonotic disease in shelters.[9-10]

HYGIENE PRACTICES

Contaminated hands and clothes, acting as fomites, can be a significant means of spread of disease in a shelter. Shelter staff, volunteers, and the public all may contribute. Hand washing can be one of the most effective strategies available to us in animal shelters in preventing spread of disease. Hand washing, however, does take time when done between handling of all animals and can be hard to reinforce with staff and the public. Availability of washing stations in all areas of the shelter is ideal. Signage, posted by each station, will serve as a reminder.[11] When hand-washing stations are not available, use of alcohol-based hand sanitizers between handling of individual animals can be substituted if hands are not visibly dirty. Stationary units facilitate use. Not all hand sanitizers contain the same percentage or type of alcohol, making careful selection necessary. The unenveloped viruses (FPV and FCV) and dermatophytes may not be inactivated by some products.[12] Efficacy studies continue to conclude that sanitizers with less than 60 per cent alcohol, although available commercially, are inferior.[13] Using signs in the shelter environment, and asking the public to not touch cats without assistance from staff, may be of benefit in minimizing spread of disease. For staff, use of disposable gloves changed after handling of each cat is another consideration.

Pathogens may be spread from clothing as well, making utilization of lab coats, scrub tops, disposable gowns, or aprons that can be sanitized, a useful tool. These items always should be used if staff must move from the restricted zone to the public zone. Policies are needed for storage of the clean items and transport of potentially infected items to an area for cleaning and disinfection, or disposal.

Box 74-2 Cleaning and Disinfection Protocol

1. Clean/scrub off all visible debris
2. Wash the area with soap or detergent and water
3. Completely rinse the area of all residue because some detergents will inactivate disinfectants
4. Dry the area manually or allow it to air-dry
5. Apply disinfectant
6. Allow contact time as recommended by manufacturer. Most disinfectants should stand for a minimum of 10 minutes
7. Rinse the disinfectant thoroughly from the area, and manually dry or allow the area to air-dry

CLEANING AND DISINFECTION

Cleaning and disinfection of the shelter is necessary to maintain population health. Box 74-2 outlines a proper cleaning and disinfection protocol. Protocols should be selected, reviewed frequently, and posted to remind staff and volunteers of the protocol and its importance. Cleaning to remove dirt and organic material should be done initially. Cleaning agents then should be used on all surfaces to remove residual dirt and organic material. Following cleaning, the area should be rinsed to remove all cleaner residues and allowed to dry.

An appropriate disinfectant then can be applied at the recommended concentration, with contact time as recommended by the manufacturer. Quaternary ammonium compounds are general good spectrum disinfectants and are the primary type used in many shelters. Other disinfectants that are effective against unenveloped viruses (FCV and FPV) include sodium hypochlorite and potassium peroxymonosulfate. Potassium peroxymonosulfate, although more costly, may be chosen as the standard because of efficacy against unenveloped viruses. Care should be taken to use appropriate concentrations. Dermatophytes can be inactivated by sodium hypochlorite at a higher concentration with repeated applications. Selection of a disinfectant should be based on the known or suspected pathogen population in the shelter (Tables 74-1 and 74-2). Of importance, phenolic compounds are toxic to cats and should not be available in the shelter. Following application of the chosen disinfectant and required period of time, the area should be rinsed with water and allowed to dry. On large areas, such as floors, standing water can increase humidity beyond a comfortable level for the cats and people. A squeegee can be used to facilitate removal of standing water. Rotation of disinfectants is done commonly in shelters and may be of benefit.

Cleaning and disinfection of public areas to which animals have access, in addition to restricted areas where animals are housed or examined, is extremely important to minimize accumulation of pathogens and present a clean and odor-free shelter that is inviting to the public. Other areas, such as the kitchen and laundry, should not be overlooked when cleaning.[12,14] The best way this author has found to assess cleaning and disinfection in the shelter environment is to observe and shadow the animal caretakers. Feedback to the shelter is in the form of what they are doing well, where they need to make improvements, and how to accomplish this.

INFECTIOUS DISEASE POLICIES AND PROTOCOLS

Infectious disease policies and protocols are highly beneficial for animal shelters. Development of policies should be based on shelter philosophy (e.g., not accepting animals with obvious infectious disease if a limited admission shelter) and human and financial resources. Policies should be in place for specific diseases or conditions regarding treatment, adoption, or rescue with or without treatment, and euthanasia. General protocols in reference to body system involvement (e.g., respiratory, dermatological, gastrointestinal), and potential diseases or conditions also are beneficial. Brief policies and protocols can be posted for easy reference for the staff. Specific protocols should include information regarding clinical signs of the disease or condition, diagnostic tests available, incubation time, transmission routes, cleaning and disinfection as it relates to the pathogen, treatment, posttreatment shedding, prognosis, and zoonotic potential. Care should be taken to address impact on the population, as well as the adopter, if the cat is released while ill or shedding posttreatment. Many shelter personnel have little training in this area and will benefit from general and specific written policies and protocols.[15] Profiles for common infectious diseases are readily available on line.[16]

PREVENTATIVE HEALTH CARE

Protocols for intake should include an initial assessment of health as well as a history, including type of admission (e.g., animal control, owner unknown, surrender). For animal control and owner unknown cases, location and any history should be recorded. If the cat is surrendered, dates of vaccination, surgical procedures, and health concerns should be recorded, as should reason for surrender. Cats who appear healthy should be taken to the healthy intake examination area, and those who appear to be ill from infectious disease should be examined in a separate area designated for infectious disease, if available. A general examination with attention to presence of ectoparasites, haircoat or skin disease, any suggestion of upper respiratory disease (URD), and/or diarrhea should be conducted. Body weight should be recorded on entry. Scanning and recording for the presence of a microchip is essential in an attempt to reunite an owner with a lost pet. Record keeping may be hand written in smaller shelters, but computer programs developed for animal shelters are available that allow data to be collected, tabulated, and searched. These data can be used for individual cat care, such as reminders for vaccination or deworming or end of holding period, and also to determine daily census or count and many other parameters of great value for the health of the population.[17]

Table 74-1 The Antimicrobial Spectrum of Disinfectants

Chemical Disinfectants

Note: Removal of organic material must always precede the use of any disinfectant.

susceptibility of microorganisms to chemical disinfectants	Acids (hydrochloric acid, acetic acid, citric acid)	Alcohols (ethyl alcohol, isopropyl alcohol)	Aldehydes (formaldehyde, paraformaldehyde, gluteraldehyde)	Alkalis (sodium or ammonium hydroxide, sodium carbonate)	Biguanides (chlorhexidine*, Nolvasan*, Chlorhex*, Virosan*, Hibistat*)	Halogens hypochlorite	Halogens iodine	Oxidizing Agents (hydrogen peroxide, peroxyacetic acid, Trifectant*, Virkon-S*, Oxy-Sept 333*)	Phenolic Compounds (Lysol*, Osyl*, Amphyl*, TekTrol*, Pheno-Tek II*)	Quaternary Ammonium Compounds (Roccal*, Zepharin*, DiQuat*, Parvosol*, D-256*)
most susceptible										
mycoplasmas	++	++	++	++	++	++	++	++	++	+
gram-positive bacteria	+	++	++	+	++	+	+	+	++	++
gram-negative bacteria	+	++	++	+	+	+	+	+	+	+
pseudomonads	+	+	++	+	+I	+	+	+	+	I
rickettsiae	+I	+	+I	+	+I	+	+	+	+[a]	+I
enveloped viruses	+I	+I	++	+	+	+	+	+I	+I	+I
chlamydiae	I	I	+	+I	+	+I	+I	+I	+I	+I
non-enveloped viruses	+I	+I	+	+	I	+	+	+I	I	I
fungal spores	+	N	+	+	+I	+	+	+	+	I
picornaviruses (i.e. FMD)	N	N	+	N	N	N	N	N	N	N
parvoviruses	I	+	+	+	N	N	N	+I	N	I
acid-fast bacteria	+I	I	+	+I	I	+	+	+I	+I	N
bacterial spores	I	I	+	+[c]	I	I	I	+[b]	I	I
coccidia	I	I	I	+	I	I	I	I	+[d]	I
prions	I	I	I	I	I	I	I	I	I	I
most resistant										

LEGEND

++ highly effective	I no activity	
+ effective	N information not available	
+I limited activity		

a – varies with composition
b – peracetic acid is sporicidal
c – ammonium hydroxide
d – some have activity against coccidia

DISCLAIMER: The use of trade names does not in any way signify endorsement of a particular product. For additional product names, please consult the most recent Compendium of Veterinary Products.

ADAPTED FROM: Linton AH, Hugo WB, Russel AD. Disinfection in Veterinary and Farm Practice. 1987. Blackwell Scientific Publications; Oxford, England; Quinn PJ, Markey BK. Disinfection and Disease Prevention in Veterinary Medicine, In: Block SS, ed., Disinfection, Sterilization and Preservation. 5th edition. 2001. Lippincott, Williams and Wilkins: Philadelphia.

Table 74-2 Characteristics of Selected Disinfectants

Disinfectant Category	Alcohols	Aldehydes	Biguanides	Halogens: Hypochlorites	Halogens: Iodine Compounds	Oxidizing Agents	Phenols	Quaternary Ammonium Compounds (QAC)
Sample Trade Names	Ethyl alcohol Isopropyl alcohol	Formaldehyde Glutaraldehyde	Chlorhexidine Nolvasan® Virosan®	Bleach	Betadyne® Providone®	Hydrogen peroxide Peracetic acid Virkon S® Oxy-Sept 333®	One-Stroke Environ® Pheno-Tek II® Tek-Trol®	Roccal® DiQuat® D-256®
Mechanism of Action	• Precipitates proteins • Denatures lipids	• Denatures proteins • Alkylates nucleic acids	• Alters membrane permeability	• Denatures proteins	• Denatures proteins	• Denature proteins and lipids	• Denatures proteins • Alters cell wall permeability	• Denatures proteins • Binds phospholipids of cell membrane
Advantages	• Fast acting • Leaves no residue	• Broad spectrum	• Broad spectrum	• Broad spectrum • Short contact time • Inexpensive	• Stable in storage • Relatively safe	• Broad spectrum	• Good efficacy with organic material • Non-corrosive • Stable in storage	• Stable in storage • Non-irritating to skin • Effective at high temperatures and high pH (9-10)
Disadvantages	• Rapid evaporation • Flammable	• Carcinogenic • Mucous membranes and tissue irritation • Only use in well ventilated areas	• Only functions in limited pH range (5–7) • Toxic to fish (environmental concern)	• Inactivated by sunlight • Requires frequent application • Corrodes metals • Mucous membrane and tissue irritation	• Inactivated by QACs • Requires frequent application • Corrosive • Stains clothes and treated surfaces	• Damaging to some metals	• Can cause skin and eye irritation	
Precautions	Flammable	Carcinogenic		Never mix with acids; toxic chlorine gas will be released			May be toxic to animals, especially cats and pigs	
Vegetative Bacteria	Effective	Effective	Effective	Effective	Effective	Effective	Effective	YES—Gram Positive Limited—Gram Negative
Mycobacteria	Effective	Effective	Variable	Effective	Limited	Effective	Variable	Variable
Enveloped Viruses	Effective	Effective	Limited	Effective	Effective	Effective	Effective	Variable
Non-enveloped Viruses	Variable	Effective	Limited	Effective	Limited	Effective	Variable	Not Effective
Spores	Not Effective	Effective	Not Effective	Variable	Limited	Variable	Not Effective	Not Effective
Fungi	Effective	Effective	Limited	Effective	Effective	Variable	Variable	Variable
Efficacy with Organic Matter	Reduced	Reduced	?	Rapidly reduced	Rapidly reduced	Variable	Effective	Inactivated
Efficacy with Hard Water	?	Reduced	?	Effective	?	?	Effective	Inactivated
Efficacy with Soap/Detergents	?	Reduced	Inactivated	Inactivated	Effective	?	Effective	Inactivated

? Information not found

DISCLAIMER: The use of trade names does not in any way signify endorsement of a particular product. For additional product names, please consult the most recent Compendium of Veterinary Products.

ADAPTED FROM: Linton AH, Hugo WB, Russel AD. Disinfection in Veterinary and Farm Practice. 1987. Blackwell Scientific Publications; Oxford, England; Quinn PJ, Markey BK. Disinfection and Disease Prevention in Veterinary Medicine, In: Block SS, ed, Disinfection, Sterilization and Preservation. 5th edition. 2001. Lippincott, Williams and Wilkins: Philadelphia.

COSD_Z0606

the Center for
Food Security
& Public Health
IOWA STATE UNIVERSITY®
www.cfsph.iastate.edu

Preventative health care minimally should include vaccination, deworming, and treatment for ectoparasites. Vaccination upon arrival, unless vaccination within the last year can be documented, is essential to afford immunity as soon as possible. In a recent study of 61 adult feral cats not thought to have been vaccinated previously, protective antibody titers for FPV, FHV, FCV, and rabies were present in 33 per cent, 21 per cent, 64 per cent, and 3 per cent respectively. Based on the results of this study and others, a substantial proportion of this population was susceptible to infection.[18] Unowned and unvaccinated cats entering shelters may be equally vulnerable to infection in the face of a high pathogen load, stress, and crowding.

The 2006 American Association of Feline Practitioners Feline Vaccine Advisory Board Panel Report includes guidelines for cats housed in multi-cat environments and shelters.[19] The panel recognizes that shelters with low admission rate and turnover, essentially sanctuaries, may not hold more risk of infectious disease than cats living in multiple-cat households. Cats housed in transient populations fall into a higher risk category of likelihood of exposure to infectious pathogens. To avoid consequences of infection in these populations, a more intense vaccination program is needed to prevent or minimize disease. Furthermore, they recommend only administration of vaccines when a clear benefit against common and serious shelter diseases can be afforded. Core vaccines in a shelter environment include FPV, FHV, and FCV.

Modified live virus (MLV) vaccines are recommended because of the rapid onset of protection, and their ability to better overcome maternal-derived antibodies in kittens. One drawback of MLV vaccines is their ability to create mild clinical signs of URD. Similarly, intranasal (IN) vaccines can create mild clinical signs; however, onset of immunity is faster, making this a desirable choice in some shelters. Vaccination of kittens as young as 4 to 6 weeks of age, and then at 2- to 4-week intervals up until 16 weeks of age is recommended for FPV, FHV, and FCV. For adult cats and kittens greater than 4 months of age, two vaccines 3 to 4 weeks apart are recommended. It also is recommended that vaccines be given upon intake in transient environments regardless of general health. Additionally, vaccination guidelines should be changed in environments challenged with high viral load and disease.

Inclusion of IN *B. bronchiseptica* vaccine should be based on documentation of the pathogen within the shelter, especially when kittens are becoming extremely ill and developing bronchopneumonia. Feline leukemia virus vaccine should be considered in group housing situations. Rabies vaccine is not considered to be essential, but is recommended in some situations. The reader is referred to the complete Advisory Panel Report for further information.[19]

Parasite control is important for the feline population, as well as for the individual cat, and also is important to prevent transmission to human beings. Deworming with pyrantel pamoate should be performed in all kittens 3 weeks of age or older and repeated three to four times at 2-week intervals, along with nursing queens. Older kittens and adults should be treated and transitioned to a broader spectrum topical preparation monthly, which also may protect against fleas, ear mites, and heartworm infection. Broader spectrum and more expensive anthelmintics, such as pyrantel pamoate/praziquantel are desirable if tapeworms are detected.

Testing feces for parasites has the value of identifying specific pathogens and determining the complexity and load of parasite infection within the shelter. In a recent study of five shelters, the prevalence of common gastrointestinal parasites was 37 per cent and included *Ancyclostoma*, *Trichuris*, *Giardia*, cestodes, coccidia, and ascarid spp.[20] In one shelter in this study, 41 per cent of the cats in the adoption area tested positive for ascarid ova. Recommendations for all shelters are to administer pyrantel pamoate to all cats on intake, and to repeat treatment as described previously to prevent environmental contamination and reduce the risk of zoonotic transmission. Parasitism is well documented as a cause of diarrhea in kittens and cats, resulting from coccidia, *Giardia* spp., *Tritrichomonas foetus*, and *Cryptosporidium* spp. (see Chapter 18). Diagnosis can be difficult and treatment can be costly.[21] Dosing all kittens and cats with the antiprotozoal drug ponazuril is becoming more common in animal shelters for empirical treatment for coccidia. The use is off-label, but use testimonials suggest that it has high efficacy and dosing occurs q24h from 1 to 3 days, in comparison with other drugs that may need to be used for up to 20 days.[22]

Ectoparasite examination should occur at intake, with fleas and ear mites being troublesome in populations. Topical antiparasitic drugs, such as ivermectin and synthetic avermectins, are effective against a variety of parasites. Selamectin, as one example, is approved for prevention of heartworms and control of fleas, mites, ascarids, and hookworms in cats. It can be given to kittens as young as 8 weeks of age. Nitenpyram, an oral antiparasitic drug, can kill over 90 per cent of fleas within 6 hours on cats. It can be used in conjunction with avermectins, is desirable when live fleas are present, and can be administered to kittens older than 4 weeks of age (see Chapter 37).

FeLV AND FIV TESTING

Testing for retroviruses using an in-house combination test may be part of the preventative health care plan for cats in many shelters, but the cost may preclude this as standard practice. With the relatively small percentage of healthy cats testing positive, an alternative plan may be to target those cats who are more likely to be infected. This includes older males, sexually intact cats, and cats with bite wounds and cutaneous abscesses. In a recent study of seroprevalence of retroviruses in cats with bite wounds or abscesses, combined seropositivity rate was 19.3 per cent.[23] In addition, it is recommended that cats with clinical illness be tested. However, the limitation of testing only once in a shelter environment must be considered. Negative results may occur for both of these viruses following infection; therefore retesting at 28 and 60 days, for FeLV and FIV respectively, is recommended. Positive test results for FeLV antigen can occur following exposure, although many cats will clear the infection effectively. With FIV, seropositivity for antibody may persist for up to 1 year following vaccination.[24] Kittens born to vaccinated queens may not be seronegative until 12 weeks of age.[25] (See Chapter 6 for additional information about testing for retroviral infections.)

NUTRITION

Nutrition is extremely important in a shelter situation. In addition to representation of all life stages of cats, cats may come through the intake area with body conditions ranging from emaciated because of lack of food or illness to grossly obese. Careful evaluation on intake of body condition and measurement of body weight, and recording of these data, are important. Body condition or scoring systems are available from several sources. Utilization of only one system for each facility is beneficial. Posters are available to hang on the wall to help with consistency in evaluation. Feeding of individual cats must take life stage and body condition into account. Veterinarians can provide nutritional information (e.g., feeding requirement during gestation, lactation, feeding of kittens and for growth, and maintenance) including calories required. Monitoring of body weight is essential in the shelter population.

Feeding diets approved by the National Research Council is important and foods that are tested in live animals to support various life cycles are ideal. Unfortunately, because of financial constraints, shelters may need to accept and feed donations of foods that are not optimal, designed to be fed as prescription diets, or outdated. For perspective, a shelter with an annual intake of 19,000 animals may spend $250/day to feed them. As veterinarians, we can guide the shelters to let the public know what types of food they would like to receive, give them prescription diet information so they can learn about donated foods before feeding, and recommend foods that are balanced and suitable for life stages.

In the shelter environment, optimal weight performance (e.g., gaining when undernourished, or maintaining weight) can be challenging because of strange foods, stress, competition when housed with other cats, illness, or underfeeding. Weight loss in the obese cat may be a result of these conditions or anorexia. Fresh food and water should be made available daily, and because cats eat frequently, should be available throughout the day. Offering canned foods may stimulate appetite; however, some cats simply will not eat canned food. Feeding the same food consistently will help to avoid gastrointestinal upsets. Cats failing to eat should be brought to the attention of the staff or contract veterinarian for evaluation. Off-label use of appetite stimulants may be beneficial. Mirtazapine currently is being investigated and used in cats for antinausea, antiemetic, and appetite stimulating properties.

Failure to maintain body weight can compromise the immune system and lead to onset of infectious disease. In a recent investigation of 142 cats from two shelters followed for 4 weeks, cats losing weight during the first week of sheltering were 7.1 times more likely to develop URD.[26] In another study of 61 cats aimed at assessing body weight change, behavioral stress score, and develop-

ment of URD, weight loss occurred in 59 per cent of cats during the first 2 weeks of sheltering and those who lost weight during the first week of sheltering were at greater risk for URD.[27] Careful attention to adequate nutrition, consumption of food by individual cats, and measurement of body weights should help to identify cats at risk. Changes in husbandry directed at maintenance of body weight may result in a lower incidence of URD.

DISEASE SURVEILLANCE

Disease surveillance is essential to maintenance of a healthy shelter population. Animal caretakers can be trained to walk through the housing units on a daily basis, before feeding and cleaning, moving from adoption to holding, to inspect each cat visually. During these daily rounds, attitude, appetite, water consumption, stool character, presence of urination, evidence of vomition, changes in haircoat or skin, and clinical signs of URD should be noted. Animals who are not completely healthy should be identified and brought to the attention of a veterinarian on staff or the designated shelter health representative. Posting of a clinical signs sheet in each room can be helpful to record clinical signs in cats throughout the day, as well as engaging all shelter workers in the surveillance team. The power of daily surveillance allows animals who are not eating to receive extra attention to avoid weight loss, and those with clinical signs to be removed from the healthy population. This is an extremely important process for maintenance of health. Animals in isolation should be assessed daily for response to treatment.

POPULATION HEALTH CHALLENGES

DERMATOLOGICAL DISEASE

Skin disorders of cats in animal shelters are not uncommon, with some diseases putting the entire population at risk. Many cats in shelters come with no history, thus all changes in haircoat or skin should be noted on initial presentation and during the shelter stay. Odors may be localized to the skin/haircoat or other areas (e.g., mouth, perineal area). Crusting, scaling, erythema or oily skin, alopecia, broken hairs and salivary staining, ulceration, and masses should be noted. Fleas, ticks, ear mites, and matted hair coats can be managed easily, and wounds, apparent bite wounds, or cutaneous abscesses can be addressed. Some disorders, such as dermatophytosis, mites, lice, and other parasites must be detected very early to avoid spread to the environment and population. In addition, treatment can be successful in those shelters with the resources to address these disorders. As an example, dermatophytosis can be treated effectively with use of specific protocols.[28] Once allowed in the general population, however, dermatophytosis can be challenging to control and the facility can be difficult to disinfect. A triage strategy for common skin diseases in animal shelters has been published recently.[29] See Chapter 37 for further information on treatment of ectoparasites.

GASTROINTESTINAL DISEASE

Gastrointestinal disease may derive from metabolic, neoplastic, nutritional, iatrogenic, inflammatory, infectious, toxic, or parasitic causes. In the shelter population, iatrogenic, nutritional, infectious, and parasitic causes predominate. Sometimes the cause can not be identified. Nutritional causes of poor stool character may be a result of poor quality food or frequent changes in the diet. When diarrhea occurs at unusual rates in otherwise healthy cats, investigation of current feeding protocols, including treats, should occur to exclude an iatrogenic cause. Of great concern to shelters is FPV. Feline panleukopenia virus infection may occur in unvaccinated cats, especially the young, although adult cats also are at risk for this disease. Cats exposed within 7 days of vaccination are most susceptible. The best prevention is vaccination with an MLV vaccine upon entry into a shelter (see the Preventative Health Care section), combined with disease surveillance, thorough cleaning and disinfection, and avoidance of crowding. Sudden death of cats in the population should lead the attending veterinarian to consider FPV first. Clinical signs other than sudden death include depression, vomiting, diarrhea that may be bloody, and dehydration. Suspects should be isolated and postmortem examinations should be performed. Diagnostic testing of feces for parvovirus antigen can be done using tests developed for parvovirus in dogs, but tests also may be weakly positive following vaccination.[30] Once FPV infection occurs in the shelter, careful attention must be paid to cleaning and disinfection, and limiting admission is necessary. Parasitism is well documented as a cause of diarrhea in cats, resulting from coccidia, *Giardia* spp., *Tritrichomonas foetus*, and *Cryptosporidium* spp. Diagnosis and treatment, however, can be tedious and costly. In addition, bacterial causes of diarrhea are recognized in cats (see Chapter 5 in the fifth volume of this series).[21,31] Management of diarrhea is dependent on whether a cause is identified, and whether it is occurring in a single cat, a litter, or throughout the population. Probiotics are recent additions to therapeutic options for affected cats. In one published trial of probiotics in kittens 2 to 12 months of age, both the control and treated groups experienced an outbreak of diarrhea.[32] Sixty per cent of the kittens fed the control diet developed diarrhea severe enough to require treatment, whereas only 9.5 per cent of the group also given probiotics had clinical signs severe enough to need treatment. Additionally, resolution of the diarrhea in untreated kittens occurred in 45 days, compared with 18 days in the treated group.[32] (See Chapter 11 for a further discussion on the use of probiotics.) Bathing of cats and having a sleeping area away from the litter box is highly recommended to reduce pathogen load (Figure 74-6). (See Chapters 8, 18, and 22 for additional information on the management of diarrhea.)

UPPER RESPIRATORY DISEASE

Upper respiratory disease (URD) complex is a significant challenge in cat populations and may be enzootic or epizootic in shelters. Previous studies evaluating infec-

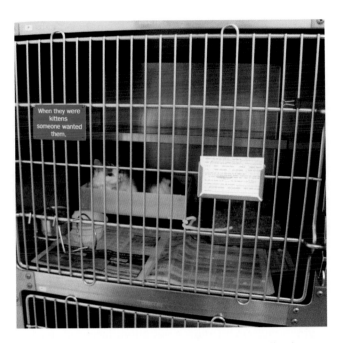

Figure 74-6 Use of a box for resting is not only visually pleasing to the public, but also offers a place to rest outside of the litter box.

tious disease transmission confirm that transmission of disease in populations is rapid and efficient. Viral pathogens of primary importance in feline populations are FHV and FCV. Other pathogens include *B. bronchiseptica*, *Chlamydophila felis*, and *Mycoplasma* spp. A comprehensive recent review of these pathogens, their involvement in URD, and control measures is available.[33] Clinical scoring of signs of disease at the time of detection and continued daily for the individual cat is valuable to assess progression of disease and time to recovery objectively. Combining the scoring process with recommended treatment in a format that can be posted will help to standardize individual care. Staff should be trained to recognize the clinical signs. Serous ocular or oculonasal discharge is characteristic of viral pathogens, whereas discharge or sneezing that is mucopurulent is characteristic of bacterial involvement requiring antibiotic treatment (Figures 74-7 and 74-8). Failure to maintain body weight has been shown to be a factor in development of disease.[26,27] In the investigation of 147 cats, those who were sheltered for more than 28 days were approximately 40 per cent more likely to develop URD than cats in residence for less than 28 days.[26] In addition, an investigation looking for environmental and group health risk factors for URD in shelters showed a correlation of decreased disease incidence in the shelter that minimized cage moves and cleaned with cats in residence, management practices that are thought to decrease stress.[34] During this same study period, the shelter with the higher incidence of URD appeared to pay close attention to disease surveillance, thorough cleaning of hands between handling of animals, and cleaning and disinfection. Infection rate in that shelter dropped from 40 per cent on day 1 to 6 per cent on day 28 of the study.[15]

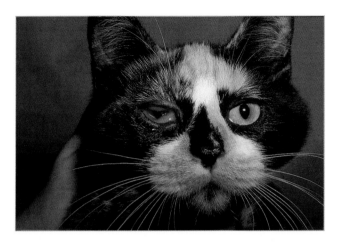

Figure 74-7 Ocular disease in a cat with FHV infection without evidence of mucopurulent discharge.

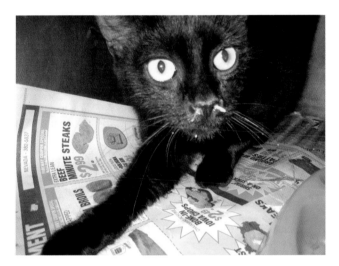

Figure 74-8 Mucopurulent nasal discharge in a cat with *B. bronchiseptica* infection signifying a bacterial component to the disease.

A standardized treatment protocol should be developed for the individual shelter. This author's preference is to use antibiotics that can be dosed q24h (e.g., doxycycline and fluoroquinolones). When character or magnitude of URD in the population changes, review of management practices, cleaning and disinfection protocols, and antibiotic choice should occur. Diagnostic testing, inclusive of necropsy is invaluable. Use of a data entry system that can calculate total incidents of URD, repeat incidents, mean severity score, and mean duration of illness in a population is desirable and has been made available to cooperating shelters.[35] When a data system and diagnostic test results are used, decisions can be made that are data driven and much more powerful. Diagnostic polymerase chain reaction (PCR) panels are available commercially for shelters, and samples can be pooled to determine the complexity and depth of pathogens within individual housing areas in the shelter. Bacterial culturing of individual cats and the environment

also can be done. Sampling of 15 to 20 per cent of the population is recommended. Pathogen complexity and load varies among shelters. A recent investigation evaluating prevalence of respiratory pathogens and comparison of anatomical sampling sites (nasal and pharyngeal) in shelter cats with URD revealed a high prevalence of FHV and *Mycoplasma* spp., with only one cat testing positive for FCV.[36] Recovery rates from pharynx and nasal swabs were similar. Of interest, *B. bronchiseptica* was isolated from only 3 of 59 cats sampled and was cultured only from nasal swabs.[36] This same group of investigators studied the efficacy of amoxicillin and azithromycin as empirical treatments in shelter cats with signs of bacterial URD. No significant differences in response to either therapy were found.[37] Studies such as these help to build evidence in the shelter environment for the practice of high quality medicine.

STREPTOCOCCUS CANIS INFECTION

Streptococcus canis is an emerging shelter pathogen that is noteworthy. It belongs to the Group G *Streptococcus* organisms and can be transmitted to kittens born vaginally.[8] It also is a common constituent of feline skin and upper respiratory tracts. Although this commensal and opportunistic pathogen is known to cause problems in catteries, it is now being reported to do so in shelters. Fatal *S. canis* infections were detected in intensively housed shelter cats in three independent shelters over a 3-year period.[38] It was estimated that more than 150 cats were affected, with a mortality rate of up to 30 per cent. Two distinct pathological presentations were described. The first included ulceration of the skin and URD that progressed in some cats to necrotizing sinusitis and meningitis. The second presentation was necrotizing fasciitis with skin ulceration that progressed to toxic shock–like syndrome, sepsis, and finally death. In most instances, *S. canis* was the only pathogen detected.[38] An additional presentation, in the form of subcutaneous abscessation, was investigated in a newly constructed spacious shelter that was at half capacity.[39] At least 14 cases of abscessation had occurred over the previous 8 months. There was no correlation with age, area of the shelter in which the affected cats were housed, contact with other cats, prior history of URD and treatment, or surgical sterilization. Most affected cats were treated with antibiotics and recovered. On investigation, a new cat who had been neutered recently was identified with axillary and scrotal abscesses and oronasal ulceration. Bacterial culture revealed *S. canis* infection, treatment with penicillin was recommended, and the cat recovered. The use of a 1:15 dilution of household bleach, which was irritating to the investigators upon entry to the shelter, was discontinued in favor of a 1:32 dilution, which is effective against many pathogens and much less irritating to the mucous membranes of cats and human beings. No further cases have been identified.[39] *S. canis* infection is a concern for cats housed in shelters, and more information is needed on occurrence rate, clinical presentations, cat density, potential means of transmission, and treatment outcome.

SUMMARY

Overcrowding can be a serious health threat in any shelter population. Overcrowding increases the pathogen load, diminishes our ability to segregate cats, increases stress, decreases our ability to recognize and treat disease, and impairs our ability to clean and disinfect the environment effectively. It also can compromise staff time and financial resources, such that appropriate preventative health care is not administered on admission or at all. Prevention of disease is a much more effective use of resources than treating disease in the population, is much more humane, and should result in placing more cats in homes. A problem-detection system model is available to define capacity, determine needed adoption capacity, manage staff time, and calculate animal care days or length of stay as it relates to shelter capacity.[35] In addition to limiting admission and the use of foster care to manage population density, reducing the turnover time of cats by maintaining a healthy population can lead to increased adoptions.[13,17,29]

As veterinarians, we can contribute to the sheltering of homeless companion animal populations by working with our shelters to educate them on minimization of pathogen load and disease transmission, segregation of populations, stress reduction, strong preventative health care, disease recognition and treatment, and prevention of overcrowding. Education and participation with development of policies and standard procedures are powerful and can be life saving.

REFERENCES

1. Humane Society of the United States. HSUS Pet Overpopulation Estimates. Available at http://www.hsus.org/pets/issues_affecting_our_pets/pet_overpopulation_and_owner ship_statistics/hsus_pet_overpopulation_estimates.html
2. Scarlett J: Pet populations dynamics and animal shelter issues. In Miller L, Zawistowski S, editors: *Shelter medicine for veterinarians and staff*, Ames, 2004, Blackwell, p 11.
3. Johnson T: The animal shelter building: design and maintenance of a healthy and efficient facility. In Miller L, Zawistowski S, editors: *Shelter medicine for veterinarians and staff*, Ames, 2004, Blackwell, p 55.
4. Miller L: Dog and cat care in the animal shelter. In Miller L, Zawistowski S, editors: *Shelter medicine for veterinarians and staff*, Ames, 2004, Blackwell, p 95.
5. Griffin B, Hume KR: Recognition and management of stress in housed cats. In August JR, editor: *Consultations in feline internal medicine*, vol 5, St. Louis, 2006, Saunders, p 717.
6. Hackett TB, Jensen WA, Lehman TL, et al: Prevalence of DNA of *Mycoplasma haemofelis*, 'Candidatus *Mycoplasma haemominutum*,' *Anaplasma phagocytophilum*, and species of *Bartonella*, *Neorickettsia*, and *Ehrlichia* in cats used as blood donors in the United States, *J Am Vet Med Assoc* 229:700, 2006.
7. Hartmann K: Feline leukemia virus infection. In Greene CE, editor: *Infectious diseases of the dog and cat*, ed 3, St. Louis, 2006, Saunders, p 105.
8. Greene CR, Prescott JF: Streptococcal and other Gram-positive bacterial infections. In Greene CE, editor: *Infectious diseases of the dog and cat*, ed 3, St. Louis, 2006, Saunders, p 302.
9. Petersen CA, Dvorak G, Steneroden K, et al: Introduction to infection control for animal shelters. In Petersen CA, Dvorak G, Spickler AR, editors: *Maddie's infection control manual for animal shelters for veterinary personnel*, Ames, 2008, Center for Food Security and Public Health, p 2.
10. Center for Food Security and Public Health, Iowa State University. Feline transmission of disease information sheets, 2005. Available at http://www.cfsph.iastate.edu/brm/resources/stationary/DiseaseBRMFelineMarch2005.pdf
11. Center for Food Security and Public Health, Iowa State University. Hand washing sign, 2005. Available at http://www.cfsph.iastate.edu/brm/resources/stationary/WashHands SignSmallMarch2005.pdf
12. Steneroden K, Spickler AR, Dvorak G, et al: Principles of infection control for animal shelters. In Petersen CA, Dvorak G, Spickler AR, editors: *Maddie's infection control manual for animal shelters for veterinary personnel*, Ames, IA, 2008, Center for Food Security and Public Health, p 18.
13. Hurley KF: Feline infectious disease control in shelters, *Vet Clin North Am Small Anim Pract* 35:21, 2005.
14. Reynolds SA, Levy F, Walker ES: Hand sanitizer alert [letter]. *Emerg Infect Dis [serial on the internet] Mar* 2006. Available at http://www.cdc.gov/ncidod/EID/vol12no03/05-0955.htm
15. Hurley KF, Baldwin CJ: Developing infectious disease policies and protocols in an animal shelter. In Petersen CA, Dvorak G, Spickler AR, editors: *Maddie's infection control manual for animal shelters for veterinary personnel*, Ames, IA, 2008, Center for Food Security and Public Health, p 66.
16. UC Davis Koret Shelter Medicine Program information sheets on common infectious diseases. Click on shelter medicine at http://www.sheltermedicine.com
17. Hurley KF: Implementing a population health plan in an animal shelter. In Miller L, Zawistowski S, editors: *Shelter medicine for veterinarians and staff*, Ames, 2004, Blackwell, p 211.
18. Fischer SM, Quest CM, Dubovi EJ, et al: Response of feral cats to vaccination at the time of neutering, *J Am Vet Med Assoc* 230:52, 2007.
19. Richards JR, Elston TH, Ford RB, et al: The 2006 American Association of Feline Practitioners Feline Vaccine Advisory Panel Report, *J Am Vet Med Assoc* 229:1405, 2006.
20. Meythaler-Mullins L, Brown S, Jarvinen AC, et al: Prevalence of *Tritrichomonas foetus* and common gastrointestinal parasites in Iowa shelter cats. 2005. Located under Veterinary Student Education, Summer Scholars at http://www.maddiesfundisu.org
21. Marks SL, Willard MD: Diarrhea in kittens. In August JR, editor: *Consultations in feline internal medicine*, vol 5, St. Louis, 2006, Elsevier Saunders, p 133.
22. Companion Animal Parasite Control. Available at http://www.capcvet.org/index.html
23. Goldkamp CE, Levy JK, Edinboro CH: Seroprevalence of feline leukemia virus and feline immunodeficiency virus in cats with abscesses or bite wounds and rate of veterinarian compliance with current guidelines for retrovirus testing, *J Am Vet Med Assoc* 232:1152, 2008.
24. Levy JK, Crawford PC, Slater MR: Effect of vaccination against feline immunodeficiency virus on results of serologic testing in cats, *J Am Vet Med Assoc* 225:1558, 2004.
25. MacDonald K, Levy JK, Tucker SJ, et al: Effects of passive transfer of immunity on results of diagnostic tests for antibodies against feline immunodeficiency virus in kittens born to vaccinated queens, *J Am Vet Med Assoc* 225:1554, 2004.
26. Polak K, Byers S, Baldwin CJ, et al: Risk factors for feline upper respiratory disease complex in animal shelters and correlation with body weight performance. 2008. Located under "Veterinary Student Education, Summer Scholars" at http://www.maddiesfundisu.org

27. Hurley KF: Personal communication, February 12, 2009.

28. Moriello KA, DeBoer DJ: Recent research on dermatophytosis. In August JR, editor: *Consultations in feline internal medicine*, vol 5, St. Louis, 2006, Elsevier Saunders, p 291.

29. Newbury S, Moriello KA: Skin diseases of animals in shelters: triage strategy and treatment recommendations for common diseases, *Vet Clin North Am Small Anim Pract* 38:59, 2006.

30. Patterson EV, Reese MJ, Tucker SJ, et al: Effect of vaccination on parvovirus antigen testing in kittens, *J Am Vet Med Assoc* 230:359, 2007.

31. Willard MD, Marks SL: Bacterial causes of diarrhea. In August JR, editor: *Consultations in feline internal medicine*, vol 5, St. Louis, 2006, Elsevier Saunders, p 39.

32. Czarnecki-Maulden GL, Cavadini C, Lawler D: *E. faecium* SF68 helps minimize naturally occurring diarrhea in kittens. In Kelly M, editor: *The role of probiotics in GI tract health*, St. Louis, 2006, Ralston Purina Co, p 14.

33. Scarlett JM: Controlling feline respiratory disease in animal shelters. In August JR, editor: *Consultations in feline internal medicine*, vol 5, St. Louis, 2006, Elsevier Saunders, p 735.

34. Jenkins C, Byers S, Baldwin CJ: Environmental and group health risk factors for feline upper respiratory disease complex in animal shelters, 2007. Located under Veterinary Student Education, Summer Scholars/Research Program, Summer Scholars Research Posters at http://www.maddiesfundisu.org

35. UC Davis Koret Shelter Medicine Program. Available at http://www.sheltermedicine.com/portal/uri_project.shtml

36. Veir JK, Ruch-Gallie R, Spindel ME, et al: Prevalence of selected infectious organisms and comparison of two anatomic sampling sites in shelter cats with upper respiratory tract disease, *J Feline Med Surg* 10:551, 2008.

37. Ruch-Gallie RA, Veir JK, Spindel ME, et al: Efficacy of amoxicillin and azithromycin for the empirical treatment of shelter cats with suspected bacterial upper respiratory infections, *J Feline Med Surg* 10:542, 2008.

38. Pesavento PA, Bannasch MJ, Bachmann R, et al: Fatal *Streptococcus canis* infections in intensively housed shelter cats, *Vet Pathol* 44:218, 2007.

39. Dvorak G, Petersen CA, Spickler AR, et al: Disinfection 101. In Petersen CA, Dvorak G, Spickler AR, editors: *Maddie's infection control manual for animal shelters for veterinary personnel*, Ames, IA, 2008, Center for Food Security and Public Health, p 42.

CHAPTER
75 A Review of Neutering Cats

Brenda Griffin, Brian A. DiGangi, and Mark W. Bohling

"One cat leads to another..."

—Ernest Hemingway

Neutering is widely accepted as an essential component of preventive healthcare for cats and represents the best method of birth control for the species. In this chapter the authors review the importance of these procedures, describe recommended veterinary medical guidelines and techniques for neutering cats, and present various models of targeted large-scale spay-neuter programs.

IMPLICATIONS FOR FELINE WELFARE

FELINE OVERPOPULATION AND STRATEGIES FOR CONTROL

Although exact estimates do not exist, it is believed that between three and four million cats enter animal shelters in the United States each year and nearly 75 per cent of them are euthanized.[1] Indeed, cat impoundments and euthanasias significantly outnumber those of dogs. Of cats entering shelters with an unknown ownership status, less than 2 per cent are reunited with their owners compared with as many as 15 to 19 per cent of lost dogs.[2-4] Many cats are relinquished by their owners, with "too

many in house" being cited as the leading reason.[5] Millions of other cats survive as free-roaming strays with their reproduction resulting in generations of unsocialized feral cats.[6] In fact, as much as 50 per cent of the total cat population in a given community may be feral.[7] These cats represent both an effect of feline overpopulation and a significant source of it. Free-roaming and feral queens may produce up to 80 per cent of the kittens born annually in the United States.[7] The reader is referred to Chapter 71 in the fourth volume of this series for a discussion of the control of feral cat populations.

Four nonlethal strategies for reducing feline overpopulation have been described: increasing sterilization of cats, increasing owner retention of cats, increasing adoption of cats from animal shelters, and increasing educational efforts and laws designed to help owners be more responsible.[8] Certainly efforts should emphasize preventing cats from entering animal shelters through proactive strategies to decrease their birthrates and keep them in their homes. Neutering cats not only prevents reproduction and decreases the number of unwanted, unowned cats, but also improves the odds that owned cats will be retained in their homes because being sexually intact has

776

been identified as the leading risk factor for owner relinquishment of cats.[9-11] Thus neutering cats represents the core strategy to reduce feline overpopulation humanely. In order to maximize their impact, sterilization efforts should target recognized sources of surplus cats in communities. Box 75-1 contains recommended target groups of cats for sterilization.[8]

These groups consist of those cats who otherwise would not likely be neutered, including both unowned free-roaming and feral cats and pet cats from low-income households. Ensuring the availability of affordable services for all cats regardless of ownership status is critical to success. Given that relinquished cats are likely to originate from low-income households,[5] sterilization programs should strive to provide opportunities for affordable surgery for this population. Successful marketing of services is required to ensure owner acceptance and compliance with neutering of their cats. Sustainable programs that ensure a large majority of cats are neutered in a timely fashion are required for population control.

Neutering all cats prior to adoption represents another important target or goal for spay-neuter programs. Approximately 18 per cent of owned cats are acquired from animal shelters.[12] These organizations generally require cats to be neutered; however, neutering is not always performed prior to adoption. Adoption agencies employ a variety of programs to encourage sterilization of pets after adoption including monetary incentives, contracts, and vouchers; however, national compliance rates for neutering after adoption average only 50 to 60 per cent.[13] This is clearly an unacceptable outcome and has the potential to contribute to pet overpopulation rather than to reduce it. In its policy statement on dog and cat population control, the American Veterinary Medical Association (AVMA) concludes that "Public policies should prohibit the sale or adoption of intact dogs and cats by humane organizations and animal control agencies."[14] Published veterinary medical guidelines for spay-neuter programs state that neutering is best performed prior to adoption.[15] Neutering all cats prior to adoption, including kittens as young as 6 weeks of age, ensures control of reproduction and sets an example of responsible ownership for the community.

To prevent pregnancy and to avoid contributing to overpopulation, neutering must be performed before puberty. Pediatric, early-age, or prepubertal sterilization refers to the neutering of patients between the ages of 6 and 16 weeks of age and is supported by the AVMA.[16] Given that queens may experience estrus as early as 4 to 5 months of age,[17] delaying spaying of juvenile cats is

likely to result in a significant number of unintentional litters. In fact, many queens are neutered after sexual maturity and are allowed to have one or more litters prior to being spayed.[18-20] Educating pet owners about the appropriate timing of surgery is a crucial task, because they are seldom aware of the precocious nature of cats and often believe that their pets are too young for surgery. One survey of pet owners indicated that 20 per cent of owned cats were allowed to have one or more litters prior to neutering,[20] and another survey showed that a majority of cat owners believed that it was better to allow cats to have a litter prior to neutering.[9]

Most owned pet cats are neutered in private veterinary practices in the United States. Currently most practices recommend 6 to 9 months of age as the appropriate timing for surgery.[21] This recommendation is not based on a scientifically defined optimal age for neutering, but on a historical clinical sentiment that this is the appropriate age for these procedures. It probably was chosen originally because anesthetic and surgical techniques were less advanced at the time and surgical success was more likely in a larger patient. Despite considerable advances in anesthetic and surgical techniques and published data that illustrate shorter surgical times and lower complication rates for younger patients,[22] these recommendations have persisted. Many practitioners routinely see kittens for a series of vaccinations and preventive healthcare between 6 and 16 weeks of age, then advise owners to return a few months later for neutering. This gap in care contributes to many cats being spayed after puberty and the birth of many unintentional litters. In the authors' opinion, owned pet cats with private veterinarians are best served by neutering at 4 to 5 months of age after standard vaccinations. This allows time for cats to develop immunity through vaccination while ensuring they are neutered prior to sexual maturity. Because there is no gap in veterinary care between the vaccine series and the surgical appointment, owner compliance may be improved because the owner establishes a routine of veterinary appointments for their cat during kittenhood visits. In 2008 the "Spay Before Five" campaign (http://www.fivesaveslives.org) was launched, and serves as a spay-neuter public awareness campaign to encourage owners and veterinarians to spay cats before 5 months of age in order to ensure that they do not reproduce and that they reap the health benefits associated with being spayed prior to puberty.

BENEFITS OF NEUTERING ON HEALTH

PHYSICAL HEALTH

Whereas there are numerous indications for neutering as a treatment option for a variety of disease states, its value as a preventive healthcare measure also deserves emphasis. Most notably, when complete ovariohysterectomy or orchiectomy is performed, diseases of the uterus, ovaries, and testes are eliminated.[23] These include cystic endometrial hyperplasia, pyometra, prostatitis, and various cancers of the gonads themselves. Additionally, there are reports of significant reduction in the risk of mammary carcinoma in spayed versus intact female cats—as high as 91 per cent in cats spayed before 6 months of age.[24,25] Feline mammary carcinomas typically occur in middle-age to older cats and are characterized by both aggressive local invasion and metastasis. Even with treatment, median survival times usually are less than 1 year.[24] Given that mammary tumors are the third most common tumor in cats and that as many as 96 per cent of them are malignant, this is a significant benefit.

BEHAVIORAL HEALTH

Perhaps the greatest benefit of sterilization for feline welfare is that of a reduction in behaviors that are objectionable to human beings. Indeed, behavioral problems are leading reasons for relinquishment of companion animals and their subsequent euthanasia.[5,9,11,26-28] Among the most commonly cited behavioral reasons for relinquishment of pet cats are inappropriate elimination and various forms of aggression. Urine spraying, one form of inappropriate elimination, is very common in sexually mature tomcats. In addition, queens may spray urine occasionally during estrus. Neutering frequently results in the disappearance of this highly objectionable behavior.[29] It also reduces urine odor, fighting, and roaming significantly in tomcats. In addition, both male and female cats are reportedly less aggressive and more affectionate after neutering.[30] These behavioral effects serve to enhance the human-animal bond and increase the odds that cats will be retained in their homes. It is important to recognize that only sexually dimorphic behaviors can be expected to be influenced by sterilization and the degree to which they may be altered varies among individuals.[31]

PEDIATRIC NEUTERING

More than 30 years ago humane organizations began sterilizing young puppies and kittens. Understandably, many veterinarians expressed concerns and questions regarding the short- and long-term safety of sterilizing pediatric patients. In response to these concerns, numerous controlled prospective studies and retrospective cohort studies have been performed to verify the safety of early age sterilization.[21,22,30,32-40] Data from these studies suggest that early age sterilization is not associated with serious health problems and is surgically and medically sound. In addition, early age sterilization offers many advantages including safe anesthetic and surgical techniques, shorter surgical and recovery times, and avoidance of the stresses and costs associated with spaying while in estrus, pregnant, or with pyometra.

Perhaps the single greatest concern expressed by veterinary practitioners regarding early age neutering of cats involves the influence of early neutering on urinary tract development and health of male kittens. Anecdotally, veterinarians have expressed concern that neutering young kittens may result in decreased urethral size increasing the risk of feline lower urinary tract disease

and urethral obstruction. Numerous studies have evaluated urethral size, function, and health in neutered cats.[30,32,33,35-37] Based on contrast retrograde urethrograms and urethral pressure profiles, neither urethral diameters nor dynamic urethral function differ significantly between intact tomcats and neutered cats regardless of age of neuter (7 weeks versus 7 months).[30,35-37] In addition, the incidence of urethral obstruction and lower urinary tract disease has not been shown to be different regardless of age of neuter.[32,33]

More recently concerns have been raised regarding the relationship between prepubertal sterilization and spontaneous femoral capital physeal fractures in cats.[41,42] Overweight male cats who were neutered prior to puberty and physeal closure have been shown to be at greatest risk for these fractures. Timing of physeal closure of the long bones is controlled in part by gonadal hormones; thus gonadectomy prior to physeal closure may delay the process. Studies of physeal closure in cats have not demonstrated significant differences in time to closure between cats neutered at 7 weeks of age compared with those neutered at 7 months of age.[30,43]

Physeal closure in normal intact cats begins at 4 to 7 months of age and is complete by 14 to 20 months of age.[43] The risks associated with performing sterilization prior to puberty and physeal closure must be weighed against any theoretical orthopedic benefit of delaying surgery. Keeping in mind that many tomcats begin to exhibit urine spraying after attaining puberty at 8 to 10 months of age, delaying surgery until after physeal closure may not be feasible for most clients.

VETERINARY MEDICAL GUIDELINES FOR SPAY-NEUTER PROGRAMS

It is a common misperception that veterinarians who perform a high volume of surgical sterilizations per day or who perform surgical procedures at a reduced cost are not providing quality care for their patients.[44,45] Although exceptions may exist, this is not the case in the majority of situations. Increasing the volume of procedures or lowering costs is not obtained by reducing quality. To the contrary, concentrating on a single practice area has already been used very successfully in human surgery both in the United States and abroad to improve outcomes and reduce complications while reducing costs simultaneously. The goals of dedicated spay-neuter surgeons are achieved by efficient use of support staff, equipment, and protocols to provide safe, high-quality surgical sterilization at low cost to large numbers of companion and feral cats and dogs. In fact, the mortality rates reported by high volume spay-neuter programs are lower than those published for elective surgeries in small animal private practice and teaching hospitals.[46-48]

State practice acts and professional organizations provide recommended guidelines for the practice of veterinary medicine.[49-51] Guidelines that specifically address spay-neuter practice also have been published and serve as a valuable adjunct to state and local practice acts.[15] Guidelines for medical and surgical care must take into consideration the population being served. For example, a standard recommendation is that a physical examination should be performed on every patient prior to an anesthetic event. In the case of feral cats, however, physical examination can not be performed safely or humanely prior to anesthesia. Despite this difference, it is still possible to provide quality veterinary care.

Although specific protocols and procedures necessarily will differ among programs, certain aspects should remain consistent.[15] Attentive care to preoperative procedures is necessary in order to ensure patient safety and minimize client, patient, and staff stress. A veterinarian (or veterinary student under their supervision) should examine every patient, and medical records should be prepared in compliance with state practice acts. Medical records should include informed owner consent for surgery, medical history (if available), physical examination findings, body weight, dosages of all drugs administered or prescribed and routes of administration, the surgical procedure performed, any abnormalities that are identified, and any other pertinent information regarding the animal's condition. Standardized operative reports may be used, but should allow for additions when necessary. Systems for infectious disease control should be in place to prevent or minimize transmission among patients. Vaccination is recommended prior to surgery; however, perioperative vaccination is acceptable when necessary and has been demonstrated to induce immunity effectively in cats and kittens.[52,53]

Balanced anesthetic protocols are required, including the provision of adequate analgesia for all patients. Protocols for general use, as well as those for high-risk patients, should be available. Care should be taken to ensure thermoregulation throughout the perioperative period, and cats should be monitored continuously by vigilant, trained hands-on observers. In addition, emergency readiness plans always should be in place.[15]

Regarding surgery, aseptic technique must never be compromised and separate instruments that have been sterilized via steam, gas, or plasma should be used for all patients. Veterinarians (or veterinary students under their direct supervision) must perform all surgical procedures. For female patients, ventral midline, flank, and laparoscopic approaches are acceptable for ovariohysterectomy or ovariectomy. The general surgical principles of gentle tissue-handling, meticulous hemostasis, and aseptic technique are required, and hemostasis must be ensured and verified prior to completion of any procedure. Either an interrupted or continuous suture pattern is acceptable for abdominal closure. Perioperative antibiotics should not be used routinely.[15]

In the postoperative period care should be taken to provide patients with a smooth transition from the anesthetized state to wakeful comfort for return to their home environments. Patients should be evaluated immediately prior to release. Cat owners, caregivers, or their agents should be provided with clear instructions (written and verbal) for postoperative care. Finally, regular policies for managing complications and emergencies that occur within the 48-hour period after surgery must be in place.[15]

SPECIAL CONCERNS FOR FELINE PATIENTS IN THE SPAY-NEUTER CLINIC

STRESS REDUCTION

Naturally possessing heightened fight or flight responses, feline patients are particularly prone to experiencing acute stress and fear in novel environments. Both acute stress and fear are accompanied by catecholamine release, which can induce tachycardia and increase the risk of serious cardiac arrhythmias during anesthetic induction.[54] Behaviorally, fearful cats may be overtly aggressive or may be "teetering on the edge" of defensive aggression. Such responses can not only compromise cat welfare, but staff safety as well. For these reasons spay-neuter programs should have protocols in place to minimize stress for feline patients beginning prior to their arrival at the clinic and continuing until their discharge. Caregivers should be required to present cats for surgery in individual carriers or traps. From the time they arrive at the clinic, care should be taken not to place cats within spatial, visual, or auditory range of other species, especially dogs. Tractable juvenile and adult cats should be housed individually throughout their stays in the facility. Pediatric littermates or house mates generally benefit from being housed together to prevent stress induced by separation. Cats instinctively feel more secure when they can perch at a high point and studies indicate that feline stress responses are significantly reduced when cats are housed in elevated cages compared with floor-level cages.[55] For these reasons, carriers containing cats should never be placed on the floor, and cats preferentially should be transferred to the highest available holding cage. When possible, and in a manner that does not interfere with perianesthetic monitoring, the provision of a hiding box or towel to cover the cage can reduce the stress of a feline patient substantially. Indeed, the ability to control aversive stimuli through hiding decreases stress hormones profoundly in cats.[56] If cats are to be held for more than 12 hours, a litterbox should be provided once the patient is ambulatory.

Intractable or feral cats should be housed in traps or other enclosures that allow for administration of anesthetics without extensive handling in order to minimize stress and safety for both cats and personnel. They should only be removed from their trap or enclosure after heavy sedation and should be returned to the holding enclosure when adequately recovered. During holding, traps should be elevated to allow urine and feces to fall through the wire bottoms away from the patient. Feral cats should be returned to their environments as soon as they are fully recovered from anesthesia (e.g., when their mental status and motor coordination have returned to normal).[15]

In the context of spay-neuter programs, handling and restraint of cats of varying ages, personality types, social experiences, and stress levels require skill, knowledge of normal feline behavior and signaling, finesse, and proper equipment. Minimal, gentle restraint should be used to handle tractable cats, because research indicates that gentle human contact can attenuate the adverse effects of unpleasant stimuli, eliminate fear responses, and alleviate signs of pain in animals.[57] Providing time for cats to acclimate to new surroundings prior to handling, avoiding escapes and the need to recapture, and using transport carriers also are helpful methods of reducing stress when handling cats in the spay-neuter clinic. In some cases, chemical restraint should be administered with the use of humane restraint equipment such as nets or squeeze devices. Control poles should never be used to restrain cats. Finally, the use of commercially available diffusers containing synthetic analogues of naturally occurring feline facial pheromones (Feliway, Veterinary Product Laboratories, Phoenix, AZ) also may aid in reducing patient stress.[58]

ANESTHETIC PROTOCOLS

The induction of a balanced state of anesthesia is required for all patients undergoing any surgical sterilization procedure. The specific protocol used may vary, but it must provide rapid, reversible loss of consciousness, immobility with muscle relaxation, anxiolysis, and analgesia. By definition, surgical sterilization induces tissue damage, which can result in pain; therefore administration of analgesics is not optional.[59,60] Anesthetic protocols that combine multiple analgesic agents in a single protocol (multimodal analgesia) are preferred.[15,61] Numerous balanced anesthetic protocols have been utilized successfully for neutering cats.[62-68] Sample protocols are presented in Table 75-1 and Box 75-2. When selecting an anesthetic protocol for a spay-neuter program, consideration should be given to a number of factors, including the type and number of patients, an individual animal's physical

examination findings and risk assessment, the procedure to be performed, the duration of anesthesia and analgesia desired, whether or not a reversible protocol is desired, the organization's physical and economic resources, the technical skill of clinic staff, and the efficiency of the surgeon.[15]

Historically, proper intubation with an endotracheal tube has represented the gold standard for maintaining a patent, protected airway in surgical patients. Typically tomcats are not intubated routinely because of the brief duration of surgery for the male patient, whereas female cats may be intubated depending on the anesthetic protocol selected for general use. When considering whether or not cats undergoing ovariohysterectomy should be intubated routinely, the pros and cons of this procedure should be considered carefully in the context of the individual spay-neuter program.[15] Intubation requires technical proficiency, time, and the proper depth of anesthesia. In some cases it may complicate, delay, or even compromise effective delivery of care in the setting of a spay-neuter program. In addition, endotracheal tubes are associated with tracheal irritation and can serve as fomites for transmission of respiratory pathogens that are common in cats, particularly those housed in animal shelters. Of particular concern is feline calicivirus as it is a nonenveloped virus that is not easily destroyed and many cats are asymptomatic carriers, shedding the virus for months or even years after natural infection.[69] Thorough cleaning of endotracheal tubes, including the inflated cuff, followed by the application of freshly prepared 1:32 bleach solution or properly diluted potassium peroxymonosulfate (Trifectant, Vetoquinol, Buena, NJ) is required for deactivation of this common viral pathogen of cats. Thus intubation may increase the risk of

Table 75-1 Balanced Anesthetic Protocols Utilizing Inhalant Gas Anesthetics for Feline Surgery[66]

Premedication	Induction	Maintenance*	Analgesia
Acepromazine 0.04 mg/kg IM + butorphanol 0.2 mg/kg IM	Ketamine 5 mg/kg IV + diazepam 0.25 mg/kg IV OR Propofol 6 mg/kg IV	Isoflurane OR sevoflurane	Buprenorphine 0.01 mg/kg SQ AND/OR meloxicam 0.2 mg/kg SQ
Acepromazine 0.05 mg/kg IM + buprenorphine 0.005 mg/kg IM	Tiletamine-zolazepam 5 mg/kg IM or IV	Isoflurane OR sevoflurane	Meloxicam 0.1 mg/kg SQ

IM, Intramuscularly; *IV*, intravenously; *SQ*, subcutaneously.
*For queens, inhalant gas anesthesia via endotracheal tube is required. In the majority of cases, intubation and inhalant gas anesthesia will not be required for tomcats.
Note: splash blocks containing local anesthetics may be used to enhance postoperative analgesia.[67]
Mix 2 parts 0.5% bupivacaine, 1 part 2% lidocaine, and 1 part 0.9% NaCl and splash 0.22 mL per kilogram of body weight onto the incision after closure of the linea but before closure of the subcutaneous tissue and skin.

Box 75-2 Balanced Injectable Anesthetic Protocols for Feline Surgery

Mix together and administer intramuscularly[62-65]:

Tiletamine-zolazepam
(8 mg/kg)
+
butorphanol
(0.2 mg/kg)

Tiletamine-zolazepam
(3 mg/kg)
+
butorphanol
(0.15 mg/kg)
+
dexmedetomidine*
(7.5 µg/kg)

Morphine
(0.2 mg/kg)
+
dexmedetomidine*
(30 µg/kg)
+
ketamine
(5 mg/kg)

Dexmedetomidine*
(20 µg/kg)
+
ketamine
(15 mg/kg)
+
buprenorphine
(0.01 mg/kg)

IM, Intramuscularly; *IV,* intravenously; *SQ,* subcutaneously.
*Dexmedetomidine may be reversed with atipamezole given IM at an equal volume to the amount of dexmedetomidine given.
For feral patients or when accurate body weight can not be obtained prior to administration, mix together[62-65] tiletamine-zolazepam (500 mg), ketamine (400 mg), and xylazine (100 mg). (Xylazine may be reversed with yohimbine given IV at a dose of 0.1 mg/kg.) Administer 0.25 mL IM for adult cats or 0.15 mL for kittens.
Buprenorphine (0.01 mg/kg) is administered SQ or transmucosally for analgesia.[67]
Note: splash blocks containing local anesthetics may be used to enhance postoperative analgesia.

respiratory infection in cats, particularly in high-risk populations.

Whereas intubation is not a requirement, it must be available for all feline patients in the case of an emergency situation.[15] In addition, intubation usually is indicated for obese and brachycephalic cats, as well as for those cats with preexisting respiratory tract compromise, especially of the upper airway. The use of anesthetic facemasks for delivery of inhalant anesthetics during neutering should be minimized in order to reduce environmental contamination of waste gases, bronchial irritation, and the risk of aspiration of gastric contents. In spay-neuter programs, occasional mask supplementation may be required; however, if its use becomes frequent, other options should be considered to ensure patient and staff safety by utilizing injectable protocols that employ better combinations of analgesics and sedatives or delivery of inhalant anesthesia via an endotracheal tube.[15]

SURGICAL TECHNIQUES

The "conventional" surgical techniques for ovariohysterectomy and orchiectomy have been described thoroughly in the literature.[23,70] The basic techniques, with many minor variations, are taught to all veterinary students and practiced by the vast majority of small animal practitioners. Less well-known are several modifications that have been developed to improve efficiency in surgery. These techniques have been utilized for decades and are becoming increasingly popular among veterinarians engaged in high volume spay-neuter practice. In the authors' experience, these techniques have objective benefits of decreasing anesthetic and surgical time and of decreasing the amount of suture material implanted. Subjectively, a decrease in postoperative pain also may be seen. It also is important to note that no additional risks for intraoperative or postoperative complications have been noted in comparison to so-called *conventional* techniques.

LATERAL FLANK OVARIOHYSTERECTOMY

The flank approach has been described as an alternative to the ventral midline approach for feline ovariohysterectomy.[66,71-74] Indications for this approach may include lactation, mammary gland hyperplasia, and severe ventral abdominal dermatitis. The flank approach also has been recommended for ovariohysterectomy of feral cats because it offers the opportunity for convenient postoperative observation of the surgical site from a distance. Other purported advantages include shorter surgical and anesthetic time when performed by an experienced surgeon, and reduced risk of evisceration in the event of incisional dehiscence. The flank approach, however, is not without disadvantages. The small size and dorsal location of the incision render thorough abdominal exploration impossible; therefore the flank approach is not recommended for those patients suspected of having uterine pathology or abnormal reproductive anatomy. Increasing the exposure necessitates a large incision in the muscles of the lateral abdominal wall, with its attendant morbidity; therefore the ventral midline approach is a better choice in pregnant cats or those with pyometra. If pregnancy or pyometra is discovered on entering the abdominal cavity, closing the incision and utilizing a ventral midline approach may be advisable. It can be quite difficult to locate a dropped pedicle or bleeding vessel via the limited exposure of a flank incision; therefore this approach may not be a good option for the inexperienced surgeon, or for the more difficult spays such as those in obese animals. In addition, the flank approach is not recommended for kittens less than 3 months of age because the uterine body is relatively short in young kittens, making it difficult to expose the uterine bifurcation via a flank incision. Increased postoperative pain also has been reported in queens spayed via a flank approach as compared with those spayed using a ventral midline approach.[75,76] The possibilities of visible scarring or abnormal hair regrowth after surgery may make this approach less desirable when a perfect cosmetic outcome is a primary concern. Finally, when the flank approach is utilized, a spay scar or tattoo that would otherwise be identified by shaving the ventral midline may go undetected.

The flank approach can be performed with the patient in either right or left lateral recumbency based on surgeon preference. One consideration is that the left lateral approach requires caution to avoid damage to the spleen, because of its proximity to the incision. The right lateral approach also affords greater ease of exposure of the contralateral side of the reproductive tract because the left ovary is positioned more caudally and has a longer suspensory ligament than the right side. For these reasons many surgeons prefer the right flank approach over the left flank approach. A small rolled-up towel placed under the patient's lateral lumbar area will remove the concavity of the flank and help to improve visualization. The prepped surgical area should begin at the last rib and extend caudally to the greater trochanter; its dorsoventral limits should be the vertebral transverse processes and the ventral midline. The incision should be located midway between the dorsal and the ventral midline and approximately three centimeters cranial to the greater trochanter. In other words the incision can be placed three to four centimeters caudal to the last rib and two centimeters ventral to the transverse processes (Figure 75-1). The incision can be vertical, horizontal, or oblique and should be about two centimeters long. After making the skin incision, the body wall is grasped with thumb forceps and the fibers of the external abdominal oblique, internal abdominal oblique, and transversus abdominis muscles are separated bluntly to enter the abdomen. The

uterine horn now should be visible and can be withdrawn gently from the abdomen with a spay hook. The remainder of the procedure is performed as in the ventral midline approach. The body wall is closed easily with one or two cruciate mattress sutures passed through all three muscle layers; the subcutis and skin can be closed according to surgeon preference.[66,71-74]

OVARIAN PEDICLE TIE

The ovarian pedicle tie is another useful technique to enhance efficiency for high volume ovariohysterectomy. This technique is analogous to self-ligature of the spermatic cord (cord tie) as performed in castration.[23,70] The feline suspensory ligament contains few blood vessels and a negligible amount of fat, making this procedure safe in cats. In contrast, the pedicle tie is not appropriate for use in other species such as dogs and rabbits. In these species the large amount of fat in the suspensory ligament makes isolation of the vessels and secure knotting problematic. Advantages of the pedicle tie include decreased surgical and anesthetic time, and a reduction in the amount of suture material implanted. Decreased postoperative pain also may be a benefit, because the procedure avoids manual disruption of the suspensory ligament. There are no general limitations on the use of this technique; however, the surgeon should develop skill in its application prior to performing the pedicle tie on cats with larger ovarian vessels such as queens who are in estrus or pregnant.

The technique is performed as follows. After the ovary is grasped and retracted into the incision, the suspensory ligament is sharply divided as close to the ovarian pedicle as possible (Figure 75-2, *A* to *C*). Sharp dissection is recommended in order to aid in isolation of the ovarian pedicle, because any tissue that remains with the pedicle will be integrated into the ligature and could compromise its security. In addition, sharp dissection is thought by some surgeons to be less painful than digital traction and rupture of the ligament. (Many surgeons report anecdotally no reaction from the patient on sharp division of the suspensory ligament, versus an increased heart and respiratory rate and noticeable movement when the ligament is ruptured manually.) Next, using either sharp or blunt dissection, an aperture approximately 2 centimeters long is created in the broad ligament, adjacent to the ovary (Figure 75-2, *D*). Again, this is performed as close to the ovarian pedicle as possible so as to isolate the vascular pedicle completely in preparation for ligation. The surgeon then holds the ovary in the nondominant hand and directs it gently to the far side of the table, while a hemostat held in the dominant hand is passed through the aperture in the broad ligament and behind the pedicle. The hemostat should be held in the closed position with the jaws pointing toward the surgeon (Figure 75-2, *E*). The tip of the hemostat then is directed over the near side of the pedicle, and the entire instrument is turned 180 degrees (Figure 75-2, *F*) so that the jaws are now facing away from the surgeon. The jaws then are opened and the pedicle is clamped loosely (to the first

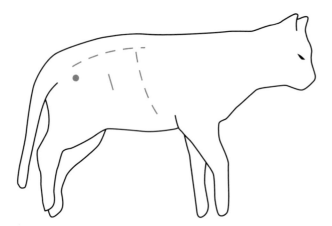

Figure 75-1 When performing a flank spay, the incision is made midway between the dorsal and the ventral midline, approximately three centimeters cranial to the greater trochanter.

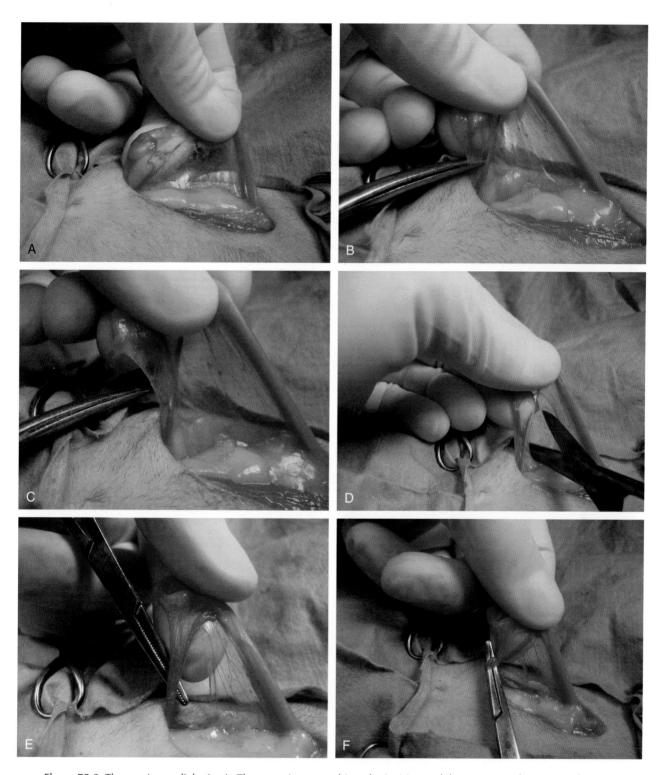

Figure 75-2 The ovarian pedicle tie. **A,** The ovary is retracted into the incision and the suspensory ligament and ovarian artery are identified. **B** and **C,** The suspensory ligament is divided sharply as close to the ovarian pedicle as possible. **D,** An aperture is created in the broad ligament adjacent to the ovary. **E,** The pedicle is now isolated and ready for ligation. The hemostat is held in the closed position with the jaws pointing toward the surgeon; it is passed through the aperture in the broad ligament and behind the pedicle. **F,** The tip of the hemostat is directed over the near side of the pedicle and the entire instrument is turned 180 degrees.

Continued

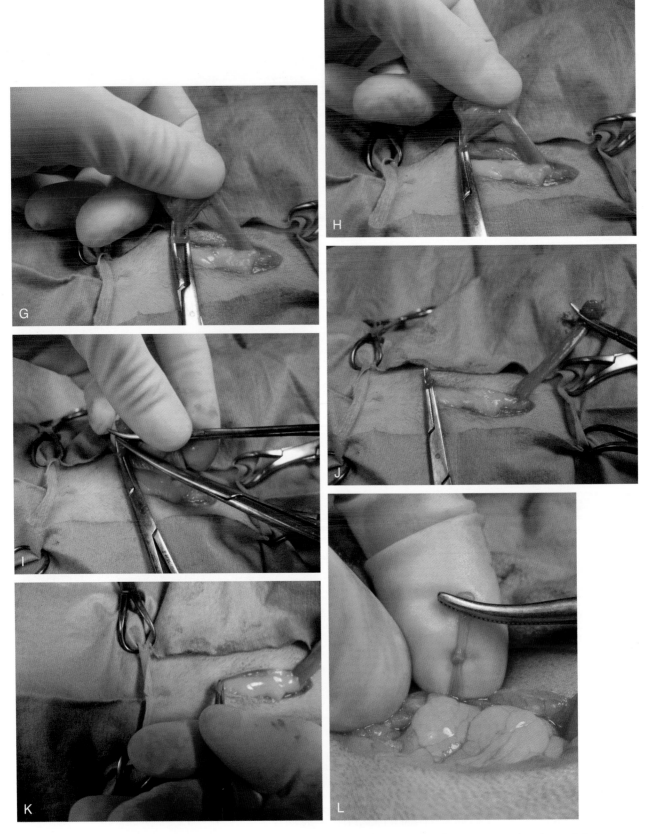

Figure 75-2, cont'd G and **H,** The pedicle is clamped loosely with the tips of the hemostats. **I** and **J,** The pedicle is divided between the ovary and the hemostat, and the ovary and uterus are laid down to one side of the surgery field. Note the placement of the additional hemostat just proximal to the ovary to prevent bleeding after division from the pedicle. **K,** The hemostat is clamped completely shut and the surgeon pushes the knot off the tip of the hemostat. **L,** The knot is tightened manually and the pedicle inspected for hemorrhage.

ratchet; Figure 75-2, *G* and *H*). The pedicle is divided between the ovary and the hemostat, and the ovary and uterus are laid down to one side of the surgical field (Figure 75-2, *I* and *J*). The hemostat then is clamped completely shut and the surgeon pushes the knot off the tip of the hemostat (Figure 75-2, *K*). Pointing the hemostat straight down toward the operating table may make it easier to slide the knot off the end of the instrument. Care should be taken not to place excessive traction on the pedicle. Prior to releasing the hemostat, the knot should be tightened and the pedicle inspected for hemorrhage (Figure 75-2, *L*). The process is repeated on the contralateral pedicle.

In addition to the technique just described, the pedicle tie can be performed in other variations based on the surgeon's comfort with instrument and tissue handling. For example, some surgeons may find it easier to direct the ovary initially to the near side of the table. In this instance the hemostat initially will be directed away from the surgeon with the 180-degree turn resulting in the jaws of the hemostat directed toward the surgeon.

OVARIOHYSTERECTOMY VERSUS OVARIECTOMY

Some surgeons prefer ovariectomy to ovariohysterectomy. The former is less invasive and requires less surgical and anesthetic time. Ovariectomy is the procedure of choice for spaying healthy cats in Europe. Because pyometra is a sex hormone–dependent disease, patients undergoing ovariectomy are not at increased risk for developing this condition compared with patients undergoing ovariohysterectomy.[77]

SPECIAL KNOTS FOR SPAY AND NEUTER SURGERY

The Miller's knot is a binding knot of the friction knot category and, as such, is a very secure tie for ligatures. The Miller's knot (or one of several modifications including the strangle knot) is easily learned and rapid to perform as an instrument tie, and enables the surgeon to apply a secure ligature quickly to thick tissues such as the uterine body, eliminating the need for double ligation.[23,78,79] The Miller's knot can be used to ligate the cat uterus securely and efficiently, and may be particularly helpful when tissues are friable. This is because it distributes pressure over a greater surface area than a single encircling ligature, thereby reducing the tendency to cut or crush friable tissue.

The figure-8 knot is a modification of the more common overhand knot. The additional pass through the knot increases friction within the knot; this leads to increased security against untying when the knot is used for the cord tie for feline castration.[23] The technique for tying the figure-8 knot using the hemostat requires only one simple modification to the cord tie. The surgeon holds the testis in the nondominant hand and wraps the spermatic cord around the hemostat once, then proceeds to perform the cord tie as usual.

IDENTIFICATION OF NEUTERED CATS

According to published guidelines, spay-neuter programs should choose a consistent means of identifying animals who have been neutered.[15] This is especially important for cats, because those with unknown histories are commonly presented to veterinarians and animal shelters for determination of gender and reproductive status.[80] Evidence of an abdominal incision from previous ovariohysterectomy may be lacking, particularly if the animal was spayed at a very young age or if a flank approach was used. In many instances cats undergo unnecessary anesthesia and exploratory surgery, only to reveal that previous ovariohysterectomy was performed. This translates into unnecessary trauma for pets, expense for owners, and frustration for veterinarians. In addition to females, males occasionally may undergo unnecessary exploratory surgery. For instance, this may occur if a neutered tomcat is mistaken for a female cat. In addition, bilateral cryptorchid cats may be mistaken for neutered animals. For all of these reasons, the use of a permanent tattoo is strongly recommended to mark pet cats at the time of spay-neuter surgery.

In contrast, removal of the tip of one of the ears (or pinna) is the accepted global standard for marking or identifying a neutered free-roaming or feral cat (Figure 75-3).[18] Alley Cat Allies, a national humane organization that serves as a resource on feral cats, recommends removal of the left ear tip and this standard is used widely. Yet, some organizations identify cats by removing the right ear tip. Whichever ear is selected for tipping, it is best to be consistent with the standard in that community. For example, the California Veterinary Medical Association recommends removal of the right ear tip.

It often is impossible to get close enough to a feral cat to see a subtle mark or tattoo and collars may be lost;

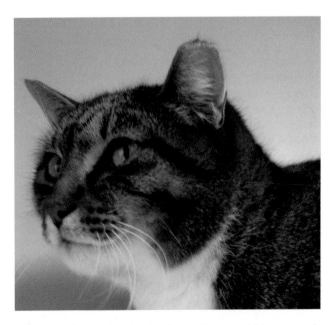

Figure 75-3 Removal of the tip of the left ear is widely accepted as the standard for identifying a neutered free-roaming or feral cat.

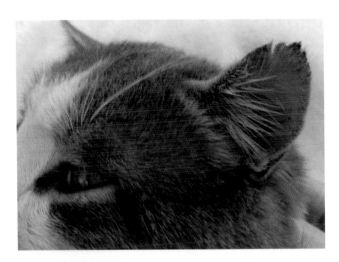

Figure 75-4 The ear flaps may be torn during fighting, leaving the appearance of a notched ear as seen in this photograph of an anesthetized unneutered tomcat. For this reason ear-tipping is used to identify feral cats rather than ear notching.

therefore such methods of identification are not useful. When cats are ear-tipped, animal control officers, shelter workers, and caregivers can identify them easily and reliably as neutered cats. This is important to ensure that all cats in a colony are neutered and it prevents shelter euthanasia of feral cats who are part of managed colonies. It is very important that ears be tipped, rather than notched, because notching may occur as the result of fighting, especially in tomcats, and may be mistaken as a sign of previous neutering (Figure 75-4). In cold climates mild frostbite of the ear tips is common and may be unilateral or bilateral. Frostbitten ear tips may appear to be cropped but often have a thickened, irregular border. However, it often is difficult to distinguish a frostbitten pinna from a tipped pinna especially from a distance. In such climates, some programs apply green tattoo paste to the skin margins at the ear tip site to aid in identification of neutered cats.

Ear-Tipping for Identification of Neutered Free-Roaming and Feral Cats

Ear-tipping should be considered an antiseptic surgical procedure rather than an aseptic one. Hair removal or shaving of the pinna is unnecessary and is not recommended, to avoid abrasion of the tender skin of the earflap. Antiseptic solution (such as chlorhexidine or Betadine) is used to swab both sides of the pinna gently. Care should be taken to avoid introducing moisture into the ear canal, which could predispose the cat to otitis externa. The most practical method for removal of the distal tip of the pinna is simple sharp excision. In most instances, the ear-tipping procedure will be performed using a pair of hemostatic forceps and scissors. Scissors are preferred over a scalpel blade because their crushing action aids hemostasis. Straight scissors and straight hemostats should be used to make it easier to crop the ear in a straight line. This is very important to ensure the desired visual effect: the ear should have a distinct straight edge that is easy to recognize from a distance. If available, an electrosurgical unit or surgical laser also may be used

for ear tipping; both have the potential advantages of improved hemostasis and reduced opportunity for disease transmission via surgical instruments. If either of these methods is employed, care must be taken to prevent collateral thermal damage to the pinna, or severe pinnal necrosis may result. The most important requirement is proper matching of energy setting to excision speed to prevent heat build-up at the excisional margin. A simple plastic spring clamp may be placed across the excised portion of the ear tip as a straightedge. This will facilitate a straight crop and makes it easier to maintain adequate excision speed to minimize collateral thermal damage.

Ear-tipping should be performed after the cat has been anesthetized and has reached a surgical plane of general anesthesia, but before surgical sterilization, to allow adequate time for hemostasis to occur. Most commonly the procedure is performed by placing a straight hemostat across the designated pinna exposing approximately ½ inch of the ear tip. The amount of the ear tip removed may be more or less depending on the size of the cat. Proportionately, approximately one third of the distal pinna is removed (Figure 75-5). Straight scissors are used to excise the ear tip, leaving the hemostat in place until the cat is in recovery. Some bleeding may occur during recovery especially if the cat rubs or bumps the fresh clot. Gluing, suturing, cauterizing, or the use of antibiotics are neither necessary nor recommended. Instruments used in ear-tipping must be cleaned thoroughly, and disinfected or sterilized between patients to prevent the spread of pathogens.

Proper placement of the hemostat on the ear tip is critical for proper healing and appearance of the ear. If the clamp is placed too high, the ear tip will be difficult to visualize and recognize from a distance. If the clamp is placed too low, skin retraction will expose the pinnal cartilage, resulting in prolonged healing and predisposition to surgical-site infection. If the clamp is not placed perpendicular to the long axis of the pinna, the ensuing cut will cause it to appear pointed from a distance, making it difficult to recognize as a tipped ear.

Tattooing to Identify Neutered Pet Cats

Tattoo guns may be used to apply special identifying marks; however, equipment should be cleaned and disinfected carefully between patients to prevent transmission of blood-borne viruses or other infections. In order to make the process more time and cost efficient, several simpler tattoo techniques have been developed that do not require special equipment. These techniques have been used extensively for more than a decade by some spay-neuter programs.[81-83] In these techniques, animal tattoo ink in the form of paste (Ketchum Manufacturing, Inc., Brockville, ON, Canada) is used to create a simple line on the ventral abdomen to mark the animal. Green paste generally is preferred because it is easily recognizable and unlikely to be mistaken for natural pigmentation as with black ink. Examination for a ventral midline scar (spay scar) is a standard practice to determine sterilization status of females; therefore the presence of a green line in this area would be discovered easily and could verify that surgical sterilization had been performed (Figure 75-6). The tattoo should be shown to the owner

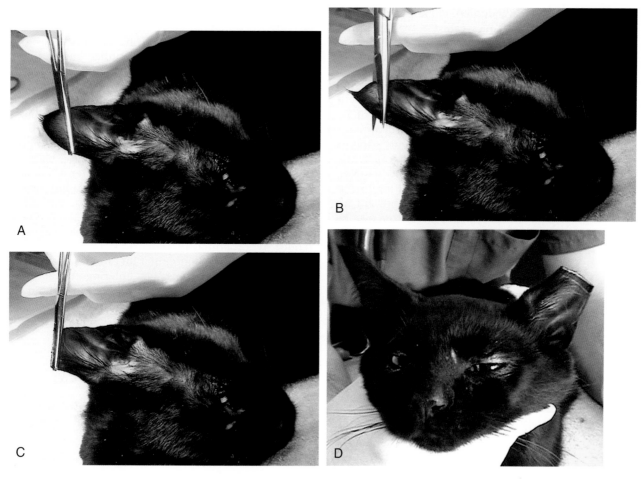

Figure 75-5 Ear-tipping. **A,** A straight hemostat is placed perpendicular to the long axis of the pinna, exposing proportionately approximately ⅓ of the ear tip. **B,** The ear tip is removed using straight scissors to cut over the edge of the hemostats. **C,** The hemostats are left in place until hemostasis occurs. **D,** Proper appearance of an ear after being cropped. Note the distinctive straight edge that is easily recognizable from a distance.

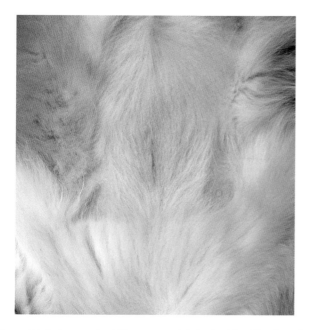

Figure 75-6 A ventral midline tattoo aids in the identification of a "spay scar."

and described in the written discharge instructions to prevent unnecessary concern if the owner notices the green ink.

The specific tattoo technique used is according to the surgeon's preference. Techniques include application of tattoo paste to the incision at the time of surgery, intradermal injection of tattoo paste adjacent to the incision, or creation of a "scoring tattoo" adjacent to the incision. For female cats, a sterile cotton-tipped applicator, or a needle and syringe may be used to apply tattoo paste along the cut edge of the incision after subcuticular or intradermal closure. To apply the ink to the surgical incision using a sterile cotton-tipped applicator, the applicator is simply rolled in ink and then gently drawn between the apposed skin edges. Alternatively, paste may be applied via a 3-mL syringe with a 22-gauge needle by depressing the plunger of the syringe just enough to form a tiny bubble at the end of the needle, and drawing a line with it between the apposed edges of the skin incision. Alternatively, paste may be injected intradermally lateral to the incision. This may be done on one or both sides of the incision to create a single permanent mark or parallel marks. Many surgeons prefer to make a separate superficial skin incision on the abdomen and apply paste into this incision. This is sometimes called a scoring tattoo because the skin is scored with a scalpel blade and paste then is applied. A paper sterility indicator strip from the surgery pack may be used conveniently to apply the paste to the incision. Afterwards, the skin edges are inverted slightly and a drop of tissue adhesive is applied on top of the skin for closure. Regardless of the tattoo technique employed, many surgeons elect to apply a small amount of tissue adhesive over the tattoo. This prevents patients from licking the tattoo and developing a temporary case of "green tongue" in recovery. In addition to females, toms also should be tattooed on their ventral midline at the time of neutering, as this will serve to prevent an unnecessary laparotomy should the neutered tom ever be mistaken for a queen.

SPECIAL CONSIDERATIONS FOR PEDIATRIC SURGERY

Although the safety of administering anesthesia and performing surgery on patients 6 weeks and older has been well established,[38-40,84-86] the surgeon should be aware of the unique physiology and perianesthetic requirements of the pediatric patient (Table 75-2). Given that metabolic development is largely complete by 6 weeks of age, the same anesthetic protocols that are used in adult cats can be administered safely (see Table 75-1 and Box 75-2).

Historically, anticholinergic drugs such as atropine or glycopyrrolate have been recommended for routine use in pediatric patients because heart rate was believed previously to be related directly to cardiac output in these patients. However, clinical studies and experience have not supported this recommendation. In addition, an improved understanding of the potential adverse effects of these drugs makes their routine use undesirable and no longer recommended.[15]

Surgical techniques used to sterilize adult cats also can be used on pediatric patients. As the tissue is elastic and devoid of excessive fat, the procedure often is easier and takes less time to complete than in adult animals, although a few unique features should be emphasized. The surgeon should be cautious to make the incision of a length appropriate for the size of the patient so as to reduce hypothermia. In pediatric kittens most surgeons prefer to center the abdominal incision midway between the umbilicus and pubis. On entering the abdominal cavity, a moderate amount of clear peritoneal fluid often is encountered; this is normal. Tissues are fragile and should be handled gently to minimize trauma and reduce hemorrhage.[37-39,85-87]

NONSURGICAL STERILIZATION OF CATS

Perhaps the most promising advancements in methods employed to increase numbers of sterilized cats will be in

Table 75-2 Unique Physiological and Perianesthetic Requirements for Pediatric Patients

Pediatric Physiology	Potential Complication	Preventive Measures
Poor ability to compensate for blood loss	Anemia	Meticulous tissue-handling Ensure and verify hemostasis
Low glycogen stores	Hypoglycemia	Do not fast for more than 2 to 4 hours preoperatively Administer 50% dextrose or Karo syrup PO postoperatively if slow to recover Feed when standing or within 1 to 2 hours postoperatively
Large surface area to volume ratio Immature thermoregulatory system Lesser fat stores	Hypothermia	Provide bedding and sources of conductive heat and/or convective air warming Use warm prep solutions and avoid the use of isopropyl alcohol in surgical preparation Avoid excessive clipping of the hair coat and large surgical incisions Minimize surgical and anesthetic time
Small body weight	Drug overdose	Obtain accurate body weight for calculation of drug dosages Dilute stock concentrations of drugs as necessary to improve accuracy of dosing
Gradual loss of maternal antibodies	Infectious disease	Vaccinate prior to surgery whenever possible or perioperatively if necessary Use standard protocols to minimize transmission of infectious disease Practice meticulous cleaning and disinfection procedures Minimize stress
Fear imprinting	Phobia development	House littermates together before surgery and as soon as they are able to stand in recovery Minimize stress Consider use of premedication

the area of nonsurgical sterilization. Potential benefits of these agents include the possibility of use with minimal expertise, time, and cost, and lack of need for specialized anesthetic and surgical equipment and facilities compared with surgical techniques. The ideal contraceptive product would induce permanent sterilization rapidly, eliminate breeding behavior as well as fertility, and provide at least as many health benefits as surgical sterilization, while requiring only a single dose. Furthermore, the ideal product would be effective in cats of both genders and all ages, and be safe and easy to administer. To date no single product is able to fulfill all of these criteria; however, several promising products are under development. Even if the ideal formulation can not be produced, safe products that induce sterility in cats, male or female, will be valuable tools for increasing sterilization of this species. Current strategies for nonsurgical agents for cats focus on the use of contraceptive drugs and vaccines that exert their effects through the manipulation of reproductive hormones, the use of immunocontraception, and the use of intratesticular injections. Currently no products are available commercially for use in cats in the United States.[87]

MODEL SPAY-NEUTER PROGRAMS

A variety of programs have been designed and implemented to serve as efficient surgical initiatives providing accessible, targeted sterilization to large numbers of cats. These programs include stationary and mobile spay-neuter clinics, mobile army surgical hospital (MASH)-style operations, shelter services, feral cat programs, and services provided through private practitioners.[15] In order for a community to support a stationary clinic, the National Spay Neuter Response Team (http://www.humanealliance.org) recommends a minimum human population of 250,000 within a 90-mile radius of a proposed clinic site. In order to be self-sufficient, these clinics typically must be capable of performing a minimum of 25 surgeries per day, 5 days per week, 48 weeks per year. Transport systems can be used to bring in cats from surrounding areas for surgery.

Stationary clinics offer many advantages over mobile clinics, including the ability to establish a relationship with local private veterinary practices and community members, the possibility to hospitalize animals if necessary, and the ability to intensify spay-neuter efforts in a particular area of need. Stationary clinics often are able to perform higher numbers of surgeries per day than most mobile services. Disadvantages include time and costs associated with establishing and maintaining a commercial facility, and the potential for geographical limitation of the population in need of services. An alternative model of a stationary clinic that may counteract some of these disadvantages is the use of an existing veterinary hospital for regularly scheduled spay-neuter clinics. These so-called *in clinic clinics* are especially valuable for serving the needs of targeted populations in rural communities.

Mobile spay-neuter clinics often take one of two forms: MASH-style clinics and vehicles outfitted with surgical facilities. These models have the advantages of being able to target any geographical area in which services are needed and lower overhead costs. Disadvantages include limited animal housing and time constraints on spay-neuter efforts at a given location. Client communication and emergency care protocols must be especially well planned, because mobile clinics often leave an area after completing surgeries for the day, potentially leaving animals without the benefit of veterinary care shortly after recovery and release to their owners. In some states, practice acts prohibit or limit mobile neutering services.

OPTIMIZING SUCCESS OF SPAY-NEUTER PROGRAMS

In order to optimize the impact of spay-neuter programs, the individual needs of a specific community must be identified. Factors to consider include both geographical and regional needs, as well as socioeconomic and cultural barriers. A sterilization program should target the subpopulation of cats most responsible for influencing the population dynamics at a given locality (see Chapter 77). In other words efforts should be focused on those cats who contribute the most to shelter impoundment and euthanasia and those who otherwise would not receive veterinary care. For example, in a given community, the number of feral and free-roaming cats entering shelters might exceed the number of relinquished pet cats. In this case efforts should focus most heavily on spay-neuter programs for feral cats. Successful programs also must take into account ethical and political considerations, and should reflect public sentiment, which favors neutering cats over euthanasia.[88,89]

Networking with a variety of humane agencies and veterinarians is critical to ensure the availability of services across regions. SPAY/USA, a program of North Shore Animal League of America, is a nationwide network and referral service for affordable spay-neuter services (http://www.spayusa.org). With the assistance of SPAY/USA, many states have formed their own individual networks in order to provide affordable services collaboratively through a variety of programs throughout their state. These networks frequently utilize state-wide toll-free telephone numbers to facilitate referral to local spay-neuter services.

Support from the local veterinary community also helps to ensure the success of spay-neuter programs. Historically, many veterinarians have been opposed to low-cost spay-neuter services, believing that they represent unfair competition for business.[90] However, pet owner surveys demonstrate that these programs serve those people who do not have a veterinarian or could not otherwise afford surgery.[91] For this reason individuals involved in spay-neuter programs should communicate with local veterinarians about their goals in order to prevent or relieve misconceptions and facilitate collaboration and patient referral.

Developing a plan for sustainable funding of spay-neuter programs also is critical to their success. Models for both private and public funding have been implemented successfully. In some communities, public animal control funds are directed toward neutering pets rather than sheltering and euthanasia. In this way, taxpayer money contributes to proactive measures to decrease shelter euthanasia. Private humane organizations and private veterinarians both have developed sustainable business models to serve targeted populations in need of low-cost or subsidized spay-neuter services. Recruitment and training of veterinarians to staff these clinics is another crucial consideration. With this in mind, the Veterinary Task Force to Advance Spay-Neuter was established in 2006 in order to improve the availability of resources and support for veterinarians in this practice area. Finally, collecting data to track the impact of spay-neuter programs on community cat population dynamics represents another important goal. The ability to demonstrate a measurable effect of spay-neuter efforts on shelter statistics serves to further legitimize programs and could be used to justify additional funding for them.[92]

SUMMARY

Neutering serves to enhance the welfare of the feline species through a reduction in birth rates. In addition, the medical and behavioral benefits to individual cats are numerous. Sterilization efforts should target specific populations that are often underserved or overlooked, and a variety of anesthetic and surgical techniques are available to enable the performance of a high volume of surgeries without compromising patient care. Ensuring the availability of accessible, affordable spay-neuter services provides opportunities to care for more cats, which not only helps individual cats and people, but also promotes veterinary medicine while providing humane alternatives to sheltering and euthanasia. It is important to recognize that within all of these efforts lies a critical message: cats deserve and require responsible care including neutering, vaccination, and regular care-giving.

REFERENCES

1. Humane Society of the United States. HSUS Pet Overpopulation Estimates. Accessed July 22, 2008 at http://www.hsus.org/pets/issues_affecting_our_pets/pet_overpopulation_and_ownership_statistics/hsus_pet_overpopulation_estimates.html.
2. National Council on Pet Population Study and Policy. The Shelter Statistics Survey 1994-97. Accessed July 22, 2008 at http://www.petpopulation.org/statsurvey.html.
3. Lord LK, Wittum TE, Ferketich AK, et al: Search and identification methods that owners use to find a lost cat, *J Am Vet Med Assoc* 230:217, 2007.
4. Lord LK, Wittum TE, Ferketich AK, et al: Search and identification methods that owners use to find a lost dog, *J Am Vet Med Assoc* 230:211, 2006.
5. Salman MD, New Jr. JG, Scarlett JM, et al: Human and animal factors related to the relinquishment of dogs and cats in 12 selected animal shelters in the United States, *J Appl Anim Welf Sci* 1:207, 1998.
6. Slater MR: *Community approaches to feral cats: problems, alternatives, and recommendations*, Washington, DC, 2002, Humane Society Press.
7. Levy JK, Crawford PC: Humane strategies for controlling feral cat populations, *J Am Vet Med Assoc* 225:1354, 2004.
8. Griffin B: Shelter medicine: no more homeless pets. In Proceedings of the 23rd ACVIM Forum, Baltimore, MD, 2005.
9. New JC, Salman MD, King M, et al: Characteristics of shelter-relinquished animals and their owners compared with animals and their owners in U.S. pet owning households, *J Appl Anim Welf Sci* 3:179, 2000.
10. Patronek GJ, Glickman LT, Beck AM, et al: Risk factors for relinquishment of cats to an animal shelter, *J Am Vet Med Assoc* 209:582, 1996.
11. Scarlett JM, Salman MD, New Jr. JG, et al: Reasons for relinquishment of companion animals in U.S. animal shelters: selected health and personal issues, *J Appl Anim Welf Sci* 2:41, 1999.
12. American Pet Products Manufacturers Association (APPMA) 2007-2008 National Pet Owners Survey.
13. Moulton C: Early spay/neuter: risks and benefits for shelters, *American Humane Shoptalk* 7:1, 1990.
14. American Veterinary Medical Association: Policy Statement on Dog and Cat Population Control. Accessed November 1, 2008 at http://www.avma.org/issues/policy/animal_welfare/population_control.asp.
15. Looney AL, Bohling MW, Bushby PA, et al: The Association of Shelter Veterinarians veterinary medical care guidelines for spay-neuter programs, *J Am Vet Med Assoc* 233:74, 2008.
16. American Veterinary Medical Association: Policy Statement on Early-Age (Prepubertal) Spay/Neuter of Dogs and Cats. Accessed July 22, 2008 at http://www.avma.org/issues/policy/animal_welfare/spay_neuter.asp.
17. Griffin B: Prolific cats: the estrous cycle, *Compend Contin Educ Pract Vet* 23:1049, 2001.
18. Griffin B: Prolific cats: the impact of their fertility on the welfare of the species, *Compend Contin Educ Pract Vet* 23:1058, 2001.
19. Luke C: Animal shelter issues, *J Am Vet Med Assoc* 208:524, 1996.
20. Manning AM, Rowan AN: Companion animal demographics and sterilization status: results from a survey in four Massachusetts towns, *Anthrozoos* 5:192, 1992.
21. Root Kustritz MV: Determining the optimal age for gonadectomy of dogs and cats, *J Am Vet Med Assoc* 231:1665, 2007.
22. Howe LM: Short-term results and complications of prepubertal gonadectomy in cats and dogs, *J Am Vet Med Assoc* 211:57, 1997.
23. Fossum TW, editor: *Small animal surgery*, ed 3, St. Louis, 2007, Mosby.
24. Overley B, Shofer FS, Goldschmidt MH, et al: Association between ovarihysterectomy and feline mammary carcinoma, *J Vet Intern Med* 19:560, 2005.
25. Hayes HM, Milne KL, Mandell CP: Epidemiological features of feline mammary carcinoma, *Vet Rec* 108:476, 1981.
26. Kass PH, New Jr. JC, Scarlett JM, et al: Understanding animal companion surplus in the United States: relinquishment of nonadoptables to animal shelters for euthanasia, *J Appl Anim Welf Sci* 4:237, 2001.
27. Lepper M, Kass PH, Hart LA: Prediction of adoption versus euthanasia among dogs and cats in a California animal shelter, *J Appl Anim Welf Sci* 5:29, 2002.
28. Salman MD, Hutchison J, Ruch-Gallie R, et al: Behavioral reasons for relinquishment of dogs and cats to 12 shelters, *J Appl Anim Welf Sci* 3:93, 2000.
29. Hart BL, Barrett RE: Effects of castration on fighting, roaming, and urine spraying in adult male cats, *J Am Vet Med Assoc* 163:290, 1973.
30. Stubbs WP, Bloomberg MS, Scruggs SL, et al: Effects of prepubertal gonadectomy on physical and behavioral development in cats, *J Am Vet Med Assoc* 209:1864, 1996.

31. Hart BL, Eckstein RA: The role of gonadal hormones in the occurrence of objectionable behaviours in dogs and cats, *Appl Anim Behav Sci* 52:331, 1997.

32. Howe LM, Slater MR, Boothe HW: Long-term outcome of gonadectomy performed at an early age or traditional age in cats, *J Am Vet Med Assoc* 217:1661, 2000.

33. Spain CV, Scarlett JM, Houpt KA: Long-term risks and benefits of early-age gonadectomy in cats, *J Am Vet Med Assoc* 224:372, 2004.

34. Root MV, Johnston SD, Olson PN: The effect of prepuberal and postpuberal gonadectomy on radial physeal closure in male and female domestic cats, *Vet Radiol Ultrasound* 38:42, 1997.

35. Root MV, Johnston SD, Johnston GR, et al: The effect of prepuberal and postpuberal gonadectomy on penile extrusion and urethral diameter in the domestic cat, *Vet Radiol Ultrasound* 37:363, 1996.

36. Stubbs WP, Bloomberg MS: Implications of early neutering in the dog and cat, *Semin Vet Med Surg* 10:8, 1995.

37. Herron MA: The effect of prepubertal castration on the penile urethra of the cat, *J Am Vet Med Assoc* 160:208, 1972.

38. Faggella AM, Aronsohn MG: Anesthetic techniques for neutering 6- to 14-week-old kittens, *J Am Vet Med Assoc* 202:56, 1993.

39. Aronsohn MG, Faggella AM: Surgical techniques for neutering 6- to 14-week-old kittens, *J Am Vet Med Assoc* 202:53, 1993.

40. Theran P: Early-age neutering of dogs and cats, *J Am Vet Med Assoc* 202:914, 1993.

41. McNicholas WT, Wilkens BE, Blevins WE, et al: Spontaneous femoral capital physeal fractures in adult cats: 26 cases (1996-2001), *J Am Vet Med Assoc* 221:1731, 2002.

42. Craig LE: Physeal dysplasia with slipped capital femoral epiphysis in 13 cats, *Vet Pathol* 38:92, 2001.

43. Root MV, Johnston SD, Olson PN: The effect of prepuberal and postpuberal gonadectomy on radial physeal closure in male and female cats, *Vet Radiol Ultrasound* 38:42, 1997.

44. Brooke WC: Feline Spay FAQ. Accessed August 1, 2008 at http://www.veterinarypartner.com/Content.plx?P=A&S=0&C=0&A=602.

45. Adey R: Spay/neuter record attempt raises concerns. *DVM Newsmagazine*. March 2008, p 36.

46. Griffin B: Standards of care for high quality, high volume spay-neuter. Proceedings of the North American Veterinary Conference, Orlando, FL, 2008.

47. Pollari FL, Bonnett BN, Bamsey SC, et al: Postoperative complications of elective surgeries in dogs and cats determined by examining electronic and paper medical records, *J Am Vet Med Assoc* 208:1882, 1996.

48. Pollari FL, Bonnett BN: Evaluation of postoperative complications following elective surgeries of dogs and cats in private practice using computerized records, *Can Vet J* 37:672, 1996.

49. American Animal Hospital Association. AAHA Standards of Accreditation. 2008.

50. American Veterinary Medical Association. Model Veterinary Practice Act. Accessed August 1, 2008 at http://www.avma.org/issues/policy/mvpa.asp.

51. American Association of Feline Practitioners. Guidelines Publications. Accessed August 5, 2008 at http://www.catvets.com/professionals/guidelines/publications/.

52. Reese MJ, Patterson EV, Tucker SJ, et al: Effects of anesthesia and surgery on serological responses to vaccination in kittens, *J Am Vet Med Assoc* 233:116, 2008.

53. Fischer SM, Quest CM, Dubovi EJ, et al: Response of feral cats to vaccination at the time of neutering, *J Am Vet Med Assoc* 230:52, 2007.

54. Paddleford RR, editor: *Manual of small animal anesthesia*, Philadelphia, 1999, Saunders.

55. McCobb EC, Patronek GJ, Marder A, et al: Assessment of stress levels among cats in four animal shelters, *J Am Vet Med Assoc* 226:548, 2005.

56. Carlstead K, Brown JL, Strawn W: Behavioral and physiological correlates of stress in laboratory cats, *Appl Anim Behav Sci* 38:143, 1993.

57. McMillan FD: Development of a mental wellness program for animals, *J Am Vet Med Assoc* 220:965, 2002.

58. Griffith CA, Steigerwald ES, Buffington T: Effects of a synthetic facial pheromone on behavior of cats, *J Am Vet Med Assoc* 217:1154, 2000.

59. American College of Veterinary Anesthesiologists: American College of Veterinary Anesthesiologists' position paper on the treatment of pain in animals, *J Am Vet Med Assoc* 213:628, 1998.

60. American Animal Hospital Association and American Association of Feline Practitioners: AAHA/AAFP pain management guidelines for dogs and cats, *J Am Anim Hosp Assoc* 43:235, 2007.

61. Corletto F: Multimodal and balanced analgesia, *Vet Res Commun* 31(suppl 1):59, 2007.

62. Cistola AM, Golder FJ, Levy JK, et al: Comparison of two injectable anesthetic regimes in feral cats at a large-volume spay clinic, *Vet Anaesth Analg* 30:101, 2003.

63. Wiese AJ, Muir WW: Anaesthetic and cardiopulmonary effects of intramuscular morphine, medetomidine and ketamine administered to telemetered cats, *J Feline Med Surg* 9:150, 2007.

64. Williams LS, Levy JK, Robertson SA, et al: Use of the anesthetic combination of tiletamine, zolazepam, ketamine and xylazine for neutering feral cats, *J Am Vet Med Assoc* 220:1491, 2002.

65. Ko JC, Abbo LA, Weil AB, et al: A comparison of anesthetic and cardiorespiratory effects of tiletamine-zolazepam-butorphanol and tiletamine-zolazepam-butorphanol-medetomidine with or without atipamezole in cats. Proceedings of the ACVA Annual Meeting, 2007.

66. Appel LD, Hart RC: Spay and neuter surgical techniques for the animal shelter. In Miller L, Zawistowksi S, editors: *Shelter medicine for veterinarians and staff*, Ames, 2004, Blackwell, p 355.

67. Lascelles BDX, Robertson SA, Taylor PMT, et al: Comparison of the pharmacokinetics and thermal antinociceptive pharmacodynamics of 20 mcg/kg buprenorphine administered sublingually or intravenously in cats, *Vet Anaesth Analg* 30:108, 2003.

68. Humane Alliance: Feline drug protocol. p 81. In Training and Operations Manual. Accessed August 6, 2008 at http://www.humanealliance.org/.

69. Greene CE, editor: *Infectious diseases of the dog and cat*, ed 3, St. Louis, 2006, Saunders.

70. Slatter D, editor: *Textbook of small animal surgery*, ed 3, St. Louis, 2003, Saunders.

71. McGrath H, Hardie RJ, Davis E: Lateral flank approach for ovariohysterectomy in small animals, *Compend Contin Educ Pract Vet* 26:922, 2004.

72. Dorn AS: Ovariohysterectomy by the flank approach, *Vet Med Small Anim Clin* 70:569, 1975.

73. Krzaczynski J: The flank approach to feline ovariohysterectomy (an alternate technique), *Vet Med Small Anim Clin* 69:572, 1974.

74. Wilson FD, Balasubramanian NN: The lateral approach for the spaying of canines and felines, *Ind Vet Jour* 44:1052, 1967.

75. Burrow R, Wawra E, Pinchbeck G, et al: Prospective evaluation of postoperative pain in cats undergoing ovariohyster-

ectomy by a midline or flank approach, *Vet Rec* 158:657, 2006.

76. Grint NJ, Murison PJ, Coe RJ, et al: Assessment of the influence of surgical technique on postoperative pain and wound tenderness in cats following ovariohysterectomy, *J Feline Med Surg* 8:15, 2006.

77. Okkens AC, Kooistra HS, Nickel RF: Comparison of long-term effects of ovariectomy versus ovariohysterectomy in bitches, *J Reprod Fertil Suppl* 51:227, 1997.

78. Hardie RJ: Don't forget the Miller's knot. *DVM Newsmagazine,* July 2008, p 48.

79. Humane Alliance: Feline ovariohysterectomy. In Training and Operations Manual. p 67. Accessed August 6, 2008. http://www.humanealliance.org.

80. August JR, editor: *Consultations in feline internal medicine,* vol 5, St. Louis, 2006, Elsevier Saunders.

81. Personal communication. Marvin Mackie, Animal Birth Control, Los Angeles, CA, October 17, 2008.

82. Personal communication. Tracy Land, Project Spay-Neuter, Cumming, GA, November 11, 2005.

83. Personal communication. Karla Brestle, Humane Alliance, Asheville, NC, October 14, 2007.

84. Howe LM: Prepubertal gonadectomy in dogs and cats—Part 1. *Compend Contin Educ Pract Vet* 21:103, 1999.

85. Howe LM: Prepubertal gonadectomy in dogs and cats—Part 2. *Compend Contin Educ Pract Vet* 21:197, 1999.

86. Grandy JL, Dunlop CI: Anesthesia of pups and kittens, *J Am Vet Med Assoc* 198:1244, 1991.

87. Griffin B, Levy JK: The future is not far away: non-surgical sterilization. In Proceedings of the North American Veterinary Conference, Orlando, FL, 2008.

88. Passanisi WC, Macdonald DW: *The fate of controlled feral cat colonies.* Potters Bar, England, 1990, The Universities Federation for Animal Welfare.

89. Ash SJ: *Ecological and sociological considerations of using TTVAR (Trap, Test, Vaccinate, Alter, Return) method to control free-ranging domestic cat,* Felis catus, *populations.* College Station, Texas, 2001, Texas A&M University.

90. Robinson GW: How to keep a humane society hospital out of your community, *Vet Econ June* 32-41, 1990.

91. Humane Alliance: Statistics. Accessed Dec 5, 2008 at http://www.humanealliance.org.

92. Scarlett JM: Interface of epidemiology, pet population issues and policy, *Prev Vet Med* 86:188, 2008.

76 Genetic Testing in Domestic Cats

Leslie A. Lyons

Genetic techniques and resources for the domestic cat are becoming more sophisticated as cat genomics leap forward. These improvements are allowing genetic diagnostic tools for veterinary practitioners to become more commonplace in the clinical setting. The genomic sequence of the domestic cat is facilitating the analysis of feline genes by scientists interested in feline health and comparative medicine in other species, as well as the overall understanding of biological mechanisms and physiological pathways common to a variety of vertebrate species.

A direct product of diverse interests in cat genetics is the identification of genetic mutations that cause desired traits, such as specific colorations, and undesired traits, such as diseases. These mutations can be used to identify carriers of the traits, predict the incidence of traits from breeding programs, and influence medical prognoses and treatments. An overall goal of identifying these genetic mutations is the correction of the defect using gene therapies and designer drug therapies. Thus genetic testing is an effective preventative medicine and a potential ultimate cure. Genetics also is moving cats towards the veterinary version of designer medicine termed "4P Medicine," which implies using genetics to *p*redict disease in the individual, *p*revent the occurrence of disease by controlled breeding, *p*ersonalize drug selection based on genotype, and to encourage active *p*articipation in pet and population health by the owner/breeders. This chapter will review the available genetic tests for the domestic cat, potential sources of error for genetic testing, and the pros and cons of their use in veterinary medicine.

GENETIC STRUCTURE OF THE CAT

Understanding genetic testing in the feline species begins with understanding the domestic cat itself. The cat is a species that is domesticating itself, actively, right before our very eyes, with a little additional help of course from human beings. Cats represent one of the most recently domesticated animals, the domestication process likely starting within the past 5000 to 10,000 years, initiating around the time of agricultural development. Because the "wild" progenitor of the cat is relatively recent and because "domesticated" cats have been relatively "free-ranging" and uncontrolled, the genetic foundation of cat breeds is relatively diverse, perhaps more diverse than dogs but less diverse than human beings. Genetic diversity studies have shown that not all random-bred cats have the same genetics[1,2] and that the origins of the cat may be important to the validity of a genetic test. Cats in Southeast Asia may have a completely different mutation for a disease than cats in the United States because their populations are quite genetically distinct.

A majority of the cats in the world are still represented by fairly free-ranging, random-bred individuals.[3] Not only is cat domestication a recent event, but so too is the development of cat breeds.[4-6] The cat breeds that were recognized at the initiation of the cat fancy in the late 1800s represented different geographical locales, and hence, different genetic populations of cats such as Siamese from Southeast Asia, Abyssinian from India, and Persians from Western Europe. These breeds remain genetically distinct today and represent the foundation of the cat fancy.[1] However, most cat breeds have developed in the past 50 years, either as derivatives from these foundation breeds or from diverse random-bred populations. The different geographical origins of cat breeds imply highly distinctive genetics; thus, like the random-bred populations, genetic mutations found in cat breeds from Southeast Asia are not likely to be genetically in common (*identical by descent*) with genetic mutations of cats originating from the Mediterranean or Western Europe. Therefore the mutations that cause disease in one breed may not be the same mutation in all breeds, depending on when the mutation occurred in the cat domestication history or if cross-breedings have occurred.

Two studies have analyzed the genetic makeup of cat breeds (Table 76-1).[1,2] Menotti-Raymond et al evaluated 37 breeds, 21 of which were clearly distinct and 15 forming breed groups. Breeds such as Persian and Exotic could not be resolved as distinctly at the basic genetic level common as the other cat breeds. Analyses of these "breed families" managed to show sub-structuring, indicating that subbreeds can be defined in the cat. Lipinski et al found similar genetic demarcations of cat breeds, analyzing 22 breeds, identifying 19 distinct breed populations and three breed groups. In addition, the association of cat breeds with their geographical origins was identified. Thus knowing the association and relationship of cat breeds can help predict the likelihood that the same genetic mutation is causing a trait in one cat population versus another.

DOMESTIC CAT MUTATIONS

Some genetic mutations are quite old and inherent in the domestication process of the cat itself, such as many coat color mutations. The color mutations for solid coloration,[7] brown variants,[8] and dilution[9] have shown to be the exact same mutation in all cat populations, east and west: likely an ancient single mutation event. However, the mutations for albinism probably occurred later in the domestication process because they have a higher prevalence in one geographical location, Southeast Asia.[10] The albinism color variant that causes the Siamese and Burmese pointing pattern on the cat's head, ears, paws, and tail likely originated in Southeast Asia and then spread around the world, once other cat breeds developed that desired the coloration.

Mutations that have occurred in one geographical group of cats can be spread to others by virtue of cross-breeding. Many newly developing breeds often incorporate older, well-established breeds to "short-cut" the time required to obtained desired colorations and morphological traits. One of the oldest breeds, the Persian, has been used in the production of American Shorthairs, Scottish Folds, and Selkirk Rex, quickly "borrowing" the genes responsible for brachycephalia, a desired head-type in each of these breeds. Along with the brachycephalia, these new breeds also suffer from polycystic kidney disease (PKD),[11] a highly prevalent genetic disease in Persian cats.[12-16] The use of Persians in several of these breeds is so intense and/or so recent that they can not be distinguished clearly as separate breeds on the overall genetic level. Even the Exotic Shorthair, a longstanding

short-haired version of the Persian, can not be differentiated from a Persian based on genetic evaluations.[1,2] Therefore the Exotic is just a single gene variety of a Persian. However, if cross-breeding is performed sparingly with established breeds, then newer developing breeds can become genetically distinct. The coloration of the foundation cat breed Siamese is found in many Western European and Mediterranean breeds, such as Ragdolls and Persians. However, the overall genetic structure of these newer breeds is distinctive from Siamese.

The genetics of long fur in the domestic cat is an interesting variation on a theme. At least four genetic mutations in the same gene, fibroblast growth factor 5 (*FGF5*), are causative for long fur in cats.[17,18] Specific long fur mutations are more prevalent than others in particular breeds of cats, meaning some breeds have more than one mutation causing long fur. This implies that independent mutation events for long fur have occurred in the original population sources for a given breed. Therefore not all long-haired cats within a breed have the same mutation and some cats may be *compound heterozygotes*. A compound heterozygote is an individual who has two different mutations, but together those two mutations cause the individual to have the phenotype of interest. Long fur is a recessive trait, thus a cat with only one of any given mutation for long fur will still have short fur, but when two mutations are present, even though they are different mutations, the cat's fur will be long. Therefore for a genetic test to identify carriers of long fur, all *FGF5* mutations must be genotyped in the cats of interest. The same circumstance will occur when different mutations cause the same clinical disease, which is termed *disease heterogeneity*. Thus genetic testing laboratories must account for multiple mutations and this information must be conveyed to the veterinarian and owner appropriately.

Understanding cat breed relationships and disease heterogeneity helps to not only predict the causative factors of a disease, but also to clarify when genetic tests should be recommended and how they should be interpreted. As mentioned previously, the mutation causing PKD is found in most breeds that have used Persians as outcrosses. These breeds also show high similarity in their overall genetic composition. An alternative example is hypertrophic cardiomyopathy (HCM). A mutation for HCM has been identified in the Maine Coon breed[19]; however, Ragdolls have a different mutation in the same gene associated with the same type of cardiac disease[20] (see Chapter 39). The two genetic forms of HCM are a perfect example of *disease heterogeneity*, a similar clinical presentation caused by different genetic factors. Although a few Ragdolls and Maine Coons may interbreed, overall, the crossing of the two breeds is not a common or acceptable practice. Therefore two breeds, both developed from random-bred cats of the United States and not as derivatives of one another, have two unrelated mutations for HCM, even though these mutations are in the same gene. A variety of other breeds and cat populations, such as Siberians and Bengals, are noted to have a prevalence of HCM.[21-25] Only time will tell if their causative mutations are shared with Ragdolls and Maine Coons because of interbreeding, or if each breed has had the "fickle finger

Table 76-1 Genetic Analyses of Cat Breeds

	Breed	Number*	Breed (Family) Grouping	Heterozygosity*
1	Abyssinian	29, 40	Somali	0.62, 0.52
2	American Curl	9, 0	Random bred cats	0.82, —
3	American Shorthair	26, 13	American Wirehair	0.77, 0.63
4	American Wire	9, 0	American Shorthair	0.75, —
5	Balinese	11, 0	Javanese, Colorpoint, Oriental, Siamese	0.58, —
6	Bengal	13, 0		0.80, —
7	Birman	43, 28		0.60, 0.48
8	Bombay	21, 0	Burmese, Singapura, Tonkinese	0.72, —
9	British Shorthair	13, 28	Scottish Fold	0.66, 0.63
10	Burmese	50, 25	Bombay, Singapura, Tonkinese	0.69, 0.51
11	Chartreux	21, 30		0.74, 0.61
12	Colorpoint Shorthair	14, 0	Balinese, Javanese, Oriental, Siamese	0.70, —
13	Cornish Rex	41, 0		0.71, —
14	Devon Rex	57, 0	Sphynx	0.66, —
15	Egyptian Mau	21, 19		0.70, 0.63
16	Exotic	18, 40	Persian	0.75, 0.63
17	Havana Brown	49, 11		0.55, 0.46
18	Japanese Bobtail	16, 32		0.76, 0.67
19	Javanese	13, 0	Balinese, Colorpoint, Oriental, Siamese	0.68, —
20	Korat	11, 39		0.55, 0.57
21	Maine Coon	43, 31		0.79, 0.66
22	Manx	29, 0		0.84, —
23	Norwegian Forest	67, 10		0.84, 0.70
24	Ocicat	19, 0		0.65, —
25	Oriental Shorthair	33, 0	Balinese, Javanese, Colorpoint, Siamese	0.74, —
26	Persian[†]	70, 33	Exotic	0.77, 0.62
27	Ragdoll	43, 0		0.76, —
28	Russian Blue	23, 25		0.71, 0.50
29	Scottish Fold	41, 0	British Shorthair	0.81, —
30	Selkirk Rex	28, 0		0.77, —
31	Siamese	34, 32	Balinese, Javanese, Colorpoint, Oriental	0.64, 0.52
32	Siberian	0, 19		—, 0.73
33	Singapura	14, 24	Bombay, Burmese, Tonkinese	0.57, 0.38
34	Sokoke	0, 14		—, 0.44
35	Somali	24, 0	Abyssinian	0.66, —
36	Sphynx	26, 27	Devon Rex	0.78, 0.64
37	Tonkinese	19, 0	Bombay, Burmese, Singapura	0.71, —
38	Turkish Angora	17, 14	Turkish Van	0.81, 0.66
39	Turkish Van	28, 21	Turkish Angora	0.76, 0.59
	Total Cats	**1040, 555**	**Average Heterozygosity All Breeds**	**0.87, 0.58**

*Data represent Menotti-Raymond, et al. (2008) in left column, which is based on 29 tetranucleotide repeats, and Lipinski et al. (2008) in right column, which is based on 39 dinucleotide repeats.

[†]Includes 19 Himalayan as this is not a recognized breed by CFA or TICA but a color variety.

of fate" alter their genetic material in a unique manner. Overall, a genetic mutation must be proven to be causative in each breed by considering population histories and by confirming that the disease is completely correlated with the known genetic mutations.

TYPES OF GENETIC MUTATIONS

A variety of methods are used to implicate specific gene candidates for a particular trait of interest. However, proving the causative action of a mutation can be even more complicated. *Comparative genetics*, using the knowledge of causative genes and mutations from other species with similar traits and applying this knowledge to the species of interest, is a long-standing technique and often is supportive evidence for declaring a genetic mutation as causative for a trait. Deoxyribonucleic acid (DNA) mutations causing several inborn errors of metabolism, such as gangliosidosis[26-30] or the various types of mucopolysaccharidosis,[31-34] were readily identified by comparative genetic approaches. However, the normal or "wild-type" presentation for any trait or condition can be altered at the genetic level in a variety of manners.

One of the simplest alterations of a gene is termed a *single nucleotide polymorphism* (SNP). Some SNPs are innocuous and never affect the gene and its protein and are general polymorphisms or DNA variants. In the case of a disease-causing SNP, the changed nucleotide needs to alter the genetic code in a manner that will affect the protein produced by that gene. An SNP can cause an amino acid to change to a code that causes the termination of protein construction, a stop codon. The mutation of PKD changes the nucleotide sequence of the gene, which causes nearly a third of the normal protein not to be made during protein synthesis.[11] The genomic sequence of a gene is divided into regions that code for the protein sequence, called exons, which are separated by noncoding sequences, called introns. The exons must be all spliced together to allow a normal protein to be synthesized. Some SNPs can alter the nucleotide signals that are at the beginning and ends of exons and introns, leading to exon skipping and exon splicing errors. A mutation affecting the exon-intron junction in *tyrosine-related protein (TYRP)* causes alterations in the coat coloration of the cat.[8] Mutations that cause stop codons and splicing errors can be clearly implicated as causative mutations for a trait or disease. Insertions and deletions *(indels)* of nucleotides of a gene, both large and small, can alter the reading frame of a protein. They are found in genes such as agouti signaling protein *(ASIP)*, which change a cat coloration from nonsolid to solid.[7,8] A large sequence inversion clearly causes spinal muscular atrophy in the Maine Coon Cat.[35] This sequence inversion is so large that it affects the end of one gene and the beginning of another, complicating the interpretation of which gene actually causes the disease.

Because of the different ways genetic mutations can potentially disrupt a protein, the validation of genetic tests can be a long and arduous process. SNPs that cause an amino acid in the protein to change, but not as drastically as causing a stop codon or splicing error (like both

HCM mutations in cats), may affect some binding site or function of the protein. These mutations often are the most difficult to validate, because one must show cause and effect between the mutation and the disease. Computer modeling can support that the amino acid changes caused by the mutations would significantly alter the protein's secondary and tertiary structures. Often a relative risk will be calculated between having the mutation and the disease in cases in which a cause and effect can not be defined clearly. For example, several DNA variants (SNPs) have been found in the cat HCM gene, myosin-binding protein C (*MYBPC*), but the relative risks associated with these additional mutations and having disease are lower than the mutations identified initially as causing Maine Coon and Ragdoll HCM.[19,20]

In addition, some confusion has arisen over "nomenclature" in regard to HCM. HCM in Maine Coons and Ragdolls is an autosomal dominant trait, implying only one copy of the mutation can cause the disease. Disease onset is unpredictable and some cats are severely affected and die young, while others have minimal cardiac involvement and live long lives. However, for most other dominant traits, when two copies are present and the mutation is homozygous, these individuals are severely compromised and die in utero (see Chapter 39). Taillessness in the Manx cat is a typical example. Breeding experiments suggested that the smaller litters associated with breeding two tailless cats are caused by homozygous lethality.[36] The tailless mutation is still not known, but the mutations for different polydactyly in cats have been identified. Polydactyly is another autosomal dominant condition, but homozygous cats have been identified.[37] In the case of PKD no homozygotes are found, even in severe and early-onset cases.[11] But for HCM, cats homozygous for the Maine Coon mutation have been identified and usually have more severe disease with an earlier onset. Some investigators have erroneously considered the HCM mutation recessive because of the earlier age of onset in homozygotes. Because cats with one copy of the mutation can get disease, albeit generally at an older age, the disease still is an autosomal dominant trait, with variable age of onset and variable expression. These nomenclature disagreements can be very misleading, and can cause confusion and unfounded distrust in genetic testing.

Another reason for confusion and mistrust in genetic testing stems from situations in which more than one mutation in a gene can have equally plausible explanations for producing a trait. The recent identification of mutations associated with blood group B in the cat is a good example of the complications associated with defining causative mutations.[38] Cytidine monophospho-N-acetylneuraminic acid hydroxylase (CMAH) is an enzyme that converts N-acetylneuraminic acid (NeuAc), the blood cell antigen associated with cat blood group A, to N-glycolylneuraminic acid (NeuGc), the antigen associated with cat blood group B. Several mutations have been identified in the *CMAH* gene, all completely associated with cat blood group B. Only one mutation should cause the B blood group; therefore why is there an association with several mutations in one gene? Sometimes extensive validation studies are required to elucidate the truly causative mutations for a trait. (See Chapter 61 for a discussion of feline blood groups.)

GENETIC TESTING VALIDATION

Any mutation study of a candidate gene faces the same problems as those found for *CMAH* and cat blood type. Genetic mutations can always be found in genes, but deciphering the causative mutation for the trait is complicated. As mentioned, some mutations are fairly obvious because of the genetic changes they cause. However, sometimes several mutations appear to be completely associated with a disease. The simplest answer is that only one causes the disease and the rest are just hitchhiking along for the ride. These "hitchhiking" DNA variants may be polymorphisms that are frequent in the population. One way to decipher the various genetic alterations is the analysis of large population sets. However, acquisition of large data sets can be prohibitive, and may only materialize once genetic testing is commercialized and large sample sets are acquired by the testing laboratories. The published study for *CMAH* and cat blood group analyzed over 200 cats, including 14 breeds. Some of the limitations of this study are presented in Chapter 61. The analysis of the 200 cats revealed that several mutations in the *CMAH* gene were not correlated completely with disease, but the mutations could not be narrowed to just one. Since that publication the genetic test has been commercialized. Continued interaction with cat breeders has helped to narrow the truly causative gene, but additional work still needs to be performed. Problems then arise for genetic testing when the mutations that have correlation with the blood type are discordant. Thus one mutation may suggest perhaps Type A and the other mutation suggests Type B. Only with continued correlation with other methods, such as serology, are these issues resolved.

Besides large sample sets, diagnostic tests are used in tandem with genetic analyses to define causative mutations. However, deciphering causative mutations also can be complicated by errors in these same associated diagnostic tests. Serological tests have been used for decades to determine the cat blood types. Detailed studies have shown that even the different methods used to detect cat blood types can be discordant with the current "gold standard" method,[39] which requires modification of standard GEL and TUBE type assays. The mechanisms and pathways that produce and detect antigenic responses are complex and redundant. A cat potentially could have a Type B blood type via serology caused by a different pathway producing the B-type antigen than the pathway involving *CMAH*. Discordant results are expected between diagnostic tests and genetic tests, but should be at a very low prevalence if the mutation is correct and the diagnostic test has high accuracy. Overall, the genetic test for blood type should help cat breeders determine appropriate matings to prevent neonatal isoerythrolysis. However, serology and cross-matching should remain the gold standard testing method prior to transfusions and transplantations.

Prior to the development of the genetic test for PKD, ultrasonic imaging reigned as the best diagnostic procedure to identify cats with PKD.[14,40] However, ultrasound itself was estimated to be only 95 per cent accurate at 11 months of age in predicting PKD. The 5 per cent error was a result of slow progression of the disease and the limits of imaging resolution. However, poor quality imaging and technician error also has caused misdiagnosis and confusion as to which is correct, the genetic test or the imaging. Disease heterogeneity can always be a factor in discordance between a clinical diagnostic test and a genetic test, especially when considering a disease that has not been well-defined in other breeds and random-bred populations. Cystic kidneys have been noted on pathology in cats who were negative by PKD genetic testing.[41] By definition, the discordant cases are animals with polycystic kidneys, but likely a different disease process and/or mutation. Overall, the PKD mutation in Persians is concordant, clearly causing disease. The genetic test is more accurate, cheaper, and provides earlier detection than ultrasound. However, the test can not predict severity; therefore ultrasonographic evaluations are still critical for prognosis in positive cats. In addition, genetic tests still take time and can not be performed in a clinical setting; thus genetic tests should never become a surrogate for veterinary care.

GENETIC TESTING ACCURACY

Genetic tests inherently are considered the definitive and the most accurate tests for a disease or trait because they are supposed to test for the actual causative factor. In addition to alternative biological pathways, nomenclature confusions, disease heterogeneity, variable disease expression, and variable onset of disease, confusion with genetic tests can stem from the error rate in the genetic testing techniques and from the assays themselves. Almost all genetic tests involve some type of amplification of the genetic region of interest. The amplification process, generally known as the polymerase chain reaction (PCR), requires two short DNA pieces for initiation. These two short DNA pieces are known as *primers* because they are produced synthetically and "prime" the DNA amplification. Generally there is one primer on either side of a genetic site of interest; therefore double-stranded DNA can be produced that includes the sequence of the primers, the DNA sequence leading up to the mutation site, and the mutation site itself. By PCR thousands of short copies of DNA are produced that include the site where the genetic mutation of interest should occur. For this process to be accurate, the genetic sequence of the test animal must match the genetic sequence of the primers. If primer site mutation exists, then the primers may not amplify that segment of DNA. Thus once a mutation is found, more research must follow to identify primers that do not have any random genetic variants that could cause nonpriming of one segment of DNA, which is known commonly as a *null allele* or *allele-dropout*. If a primer mismatch happens to occur on a DNA segment that has the mutation, the segment of DNA with the mutation may not amplify and the test would appear as if the cat was clear of the mutation of interest, a false negative. Conversely, if the normal segment of DNA does not amplify, then the animal may appear to have two copies of the mutation because the normal allele is not amplifying, a false positive. If a recessive trait, this result would falsely imply that the animal is going to develop the disease instead of revealing that the cat is only a carrier.

Primer mismatches are rare if conserved genetic regions for a gene can be identified. Primers placed in gene regions that have higher mutation rates, such as introns and untranslated regions, are more likely to have issues with primer mismatches than primers that are placed in exons. Any testing laboratory knows this inherent danger and should try to design primers in the best, most conserved regions; however, a testing laboratory may not have the resources to perform this task or may not want to make the required investment. A researcher may publish a set of primers that will amplify a genetic mutation, which is sufficient for the initial research, but testing laboratories will obtain cats from all over the world; thus they must be leery that the primers are efficient in diverse populations. Because different labs will design their own primers in different areas of a gene for a given mutation test, the primer mismatch rate may be different for different laboratories performing the same genetic test. These errors can only be detected by reported discordances with the disease or trait or by identifying improper Mendelian segregation of the alleles in families. Therefore laboratories with good response to their customer service will have an advantage in identifying their problems.

Most genetic testing involves initial PCR amplification; however, PCR does not actually "detect" the mutation. Another step, the mutation assay step, is required and this step is highly variable between laboratories. Once the genetic segment of interest is amplified by PCR, the most robust method to determine the presence of a mutation is to sequence the segment directly. The same primers for the PCR are used in direct sequencing; therefore no additional concerns with primer mismatches occur. The exact nucleotides of the DNA sequence are determined, indicating the presence of the mutation or the presence of the normal sequence. Direct sequencing generally is considered the most accurate approach and usually is pursued during the research phase of detecting a mutation. However, direct sequencing is a costly endeavor and is not the most conducive for low DNA sources and high throughput assays in commercial services. Thus commercial testing laboratories often find different ways to assay for a mutation, which can be as accurate and robust as direct sequencing but also may have some additional flaws, which are potential additional contributions to the testing error rate. Real-time PCR methods, often known as TaqMan assays, require additional primers, hence another chance for primer mismatch errors. Mutation sites can be "cut" with restriction enzymes producing restriction fragment length polymorphisms (RFLP) in the segment under study. RFLPs are an older but tried and true method, but the enzymes can be costly. Not all genetic sequences are conducive to a RFLP test and high throughput is difficult. Mismatches in the restriction enzyme recognition site that are not at the exact site for the genetic mutation can lead to RFLP test errors. An example of this kind of error has been identified for the test for Siamese points. The restriction enzyme

that can detect the Siamese mutation recognizes 6 DNA bases in the order GGCCAC. If this sequence is present, the DNA is cut into two short fragments, GGC and CAC. If the Siamese mutation is not present, the wild-type sequence reads GGCGAC. Thus the enzyme does not recognize the sequence and does not cut the DNA, leaving a larger DNA fragment. However, some cats have the sequence GG**G**CAC. This sequence is different and does have the mutation site for Siamese, but the restriction enzyme still does not recognize the sequence because of the other SNP in the area. This results in the enzyme not cutting the sequence, suggesting the cat does not have Siamese points. This error was detected in a Siberian cat from Italy because this cat appeared to be pointed by the genetic test but did not have blue eyes. The test was requested because the cat was dominant white and was suspected to be a carrier of the Siamese mutation. The test suggested it should be homozygous, which was wrong because the cat did not have blue eyes, which all pointed cats must have. If a dominant white cat with blue eyes had been submitted, the error would have never been detected. Subsequent direct sequencing of this case revealed the problem and the RFLP test was discontinued.

These types of errors in flanking genetic sequence, sequence that surrounds the causative mutation, that affect genetic tests are predictable and should be anticipated; however, the likelihood of their occurrences is sequence- and population-dependent, and an error rate can not be predicted confidently. Thus genetic testing accuracy improves via a feedback loop. The more testing a laboratory performs, the more likely errors can be detected, and the more likely a testing laboratory can make a better test. Overall, these errors are very minor, perhaps less than 1 per cent. The secondary diagnostic tests that help to confirm the genetic test are thereby very important during the establishment of the test. Laboratories that do not have a research group to help identify the cause of discordances may have higher error rates because, owing to competition, testing laboratories may not share that errors have been identified and testing methods rectified.

Finally, just as is found for any diagnostic laboratory, quality control is always a concern in genetic testing. Mistakes can occur during sample handling, labeling, result interpretation, and reporting. Laboratories with strong reputations and in-depth experience generally have handling and report mistakes well under control. Newer and less invasive sampling techniques, such as the use of buccal swabs and fur can lead to testing problems. When converting to new sampling techniques, tests must be performed in tandem, using both the old and new methods. Some laboratories may convert without this quality control step, potentially not identifying problems with new techniques. An example is the use of fur for DNA testing. Fur is an extremely noninvasive method for DNA sampling, but requires low copy number DNA techniques, which are very sensitive to contamination. Fur can disperse easily in a laboratory, as it does in a household; hence fur generally is not considered the best means for genetic testing in a large scale operation. However, unlike cats, horse mane and tail hair is very thick and coarse, and therefore is an excellent DNA source for genetic testing in horses. Errors also can be made by the submitter of a genetic test. Internal controls, such as gender tests, can be considered along with a test of interest in order to confirm the identity of a submitted animal.

Once a genetic test is performed, how does one prove that the result belongs to a specific cat? Some countries and registries require that a veterinarian collects the DNA sample for genetic test submission, and that a microchip identification number must accompany the genetic tests, thereby linking the result with the cat. An additional means to acquire the same link is to run genetic identification markers with each genetic test, thereby producing a genetic fingerprint for the cat.[42] If a test is then disputed, the test can be rerun and has to match the identification markers as well. A microchip can provide the same check, but the DNA fingerprint does not require the collection by a third party and a microchip, which are two potential extra costs, plus the inconvenience of taking the cat to the third party. Likewise a genetic test may be more expensive if additional markers are analyzed. Both methods are effective. The former promotes interactions with the veterinarian, which also should be encouraged; the latter promotes compliance because costs likely are lower and the procedure is more convenient.

GENETIC TESTING IN HYBRID BREEDS

An additional caveat to genetic testing in cats exists because of the development of breeds that are hybrids with various wildcat species. Bengals are the most common hybrid breed, developed by crossing domestic cats with Asian leopard cats.[43] Savannahs are hybrids between domestic cats and Servals, and Chaussies are hybrids with Jungle cats. Some breeds even intermix

these hybrid breeds. The common ancestor between these various wildcat species and a domestic cat occurred several million years ago[44]; thus the genetic sequence of any given gene of a leopard cat or Serval and a domestic cat will be different. The evolutionary time between cat species is millions of years, not hundreds to thousands between cat breeds and populations. An Asian leopard cat had a common ancestor with the domestic cat about 6 million years ago, the bobcat about 8 million years ago, the Serval about 9.5 million years ago. The Jungle cat is the most closely related wildcat to domestic cats, Jungle cats being a member of the *Felis* lineage. Additionally, for some of these wild cats, different subspecies have been incorporated into the breed. Genetic tests are established with domestic cat populations and few individuals of the wildcat species are available. Therefore the mismatches of genetic sequence between the domestic cat and the wildcat, mismatches caused by the evolutionary distinctness, can cause higher error rates for genetic tests. The genetic sequence of any wildcat species will be more different from a domestic cat than the largest differences that can be found within domestic cats, even if the cats are from the most remote and distinct populations. Thus a very special effort needs to be performed to validate genetic tests in hybrid breeds. Testing laboratories may not recognize this significant source of error if they do not recognize the nature of the cat breed. Because the hybrid breeds may not be highly prevalent and the wildcat progenitors for the breed are not available, some laboratories may not allow testing of hybrid breeds, or at least qualify the accuracy of the test for these breeds.

SUMMARY

A variety of genetic tests has become available for the domestic cat in the past few years (Table 76-2). Because

Table 76-2 Cat Traits and Diseases with Known Gene Mutations

Disease/Coat Color	Gene	Mutation	Breeds	Ref.
Agouti	ASIP	del122-123	All breeds	7
Amber	MC1R	G250A	Norwegian Forest	57
Brown	TYRP1	b = C8G, b^l = C298T	All breeds	8
Dilution	MLPH	T83del	All breeds	9
Color	TYR	c^b = G715T, c^s = G940A c = C975del	All breeds	50, 10
AB blood type (type B)	CMAH	18indel-53	All breeds	38
Gangliosidosis 1	GBL1	G1457C	Korat, Siamese	26
Gangliosidosis 2	HEXB	15bp del (intron)	Burmese	UP
Gangliosidosis 2	HEXB	inv1467-1491	DSH	29
Gangliosidosis 2	HEXB	C667T	DSH (Japan)	27
Gangliosidosis 2	HEXB	C39del	Korat	30
Gangliosidosis 2	GM2A	del390-393	DSH	28

Continued

Table 76-2 Cat Traits and Diseases with Known Gene Mutations—cont'd

Disease/Coat Color	Gene	Mutation	Breeds	Ref.
Glycogen storage disease IV	GBE1	230bp ins 5′-6kb del	Norwegian Forest	53
Hemophilia B	F9	G247A, C1014T	DSH	48
Hyperoxaluria	GRHPR		DSH	55
Hypertrophic cardiomyopathy	MYBPC	G93C, C2460T	Maine Coon, Ragdoll	19, 20
Lipoprotein lipase deficiency	LPL	G1234A	DSH	47
Long fur	FGF5	c.356insT, C406T, c.474delT, A475C	Most breeds	17
Mannosidosis, alpha	LAMAN	del1748-1751	Persian	45
Mucolipidosis II	GNPTA	C2655T	DSH	46
Mucopolysaccharidosis I	IDUA	del1047-1049	DSH	32, 49
Mucopolysaccharidosis VI	ARSB	T1427C	Siamese	34
Mucopolysaccharidosis VI	ARSB	G1558A	Siamese	33
Mucopolysaccharidosis VII	GUSB	A1052G	DSH	31
Muscular dystrophy	DMD	900bpdel M promoter-exon 1	DSH	52
Niemann-Pick C	NPC	G2864C	Persian	51
Progressive retinal atrophy	PRA	IVS50 + 9T>G	Abyssinian	54
Polycystic kidney disease	PKD1	C10063A	Persian	11
Polydactyly	SHH	A479G	Maine Coon, PixieBob	37
		G257C, A481T	DSH	37
Porphyria	HMBS	c.842_844delGAG	Siamese	56
		c.189dupT	Siamese	56
Pyruvate kinase deficiency	PKLR	13bp del in exon 6	Abyssinian	UP
Spinal muscular atrophy	LIX1-LNPEP	140kb del, exons 4-6	Maine Coon	35

UP, Mutations that are unpublished to date; *DSH,* Domestic Shorthair.

many genetic tools have been developed, such as genetic markers and DNA sequence from the cat sequencing project, additional new discoveries will continue at a rapid pace. Finding the genes that cause interesting characteristics and diseases is becoming a rapid and more efficient process. Once a mutation is identified for a gene, which causes a particular coat color or disease, a service laboratory, either associated with the investigator who found the mutation or an independent commercial laboratory, will establish a genetic test for that mutation to offer to the public. Nearly a dozen laboratories around the world now offer genetic testing in cats. All of the laboratories may be technically very good and accurate; however, not all of them "know their cats." The veterinarian now can add genetics to help with diagnostic and prognostic evaluation, but the inherent understanding of the cat's evolution can help to interpret tests, as well as knowing the accuracies and limitations. The veterinarian should be comfortable with contacting laboratories and discussing the methods used for testing and the associated error rates. No test is 100 per cent accurate, but a mutation test in the hands of a strong laboratory can come close to purrfection!

REFERENCES

1. Lipinski MJ, Froenicke L, Baysac KC, et al: The ascent of cat breeds: genetic evaluations of breeds and worldwide random-bred populations, *Genomics* 91:12, 2008.
2. Menotti-Raymond M, David VA, Pflueger SM, et al: Patterns of molecular genetic variation among cat breeds, *Genomics* 91:1, 2008.
3. Louwerens M, London CA, Pedersen NC, et al: Feline lymphoma in the post-feline leukemia virus era, *J Vet Intern Med* 19:329, 2005.
4. Driscoll CA, Menotti-Raymond M, Roca AL, et al: The Near Eastern origin of cat domestication, *Science* 317:519, 2007.
5. Morris D: *Cat breeds of the world,* New York, 1999, Penguin Books.
6. Morris D: *Cat breeds of the world: a complete illustrated encyclopedia,* New York, 1999, Viking Penguin.
7. Eizirik E, Yuhki N, Johnson WE, et al: Molecular genetics and evolution of melanism in the cat family, *Curr Biol* 13:448, 2003.
8. Lyons LA, Foe IT, Rah HC, et al: Chocolate coated cats: TYRP1 mutations for brown color in domestic cats, *Mamm Genome* 16:356, 2005.
9. Ishida Y, David VA, Eizirik E, et al: A homozygous single-base deletion in MLPH causes the dilute coat color pheno-

type in the domestic cat, *Genomics* 88:698, 2006. Epub Jul 24, 2006.

10. Lyons LA, Imes DL, Rah HC, et al: Tyrosinase mutations associated with Siamese and Burmese patterns in the domestic cat *(Felis catus)*, *Animal Genetics* 36:119, 2005.

11. Lyons LA, Biller DS, Erdman CA, et al: Feline polycystic kidney disease mutation identified in PKD1, *J Am Soc Nephrol* 15:2548, 2004.

12. Barthez PY, Rivier P, Begon D: Prevalence of polycystic kidney disease in Persian and Persian related cats in France, *J Feline Med Surg* 5:345, 2003.

13. Beck C, Lavelle RB: Feline polycystic kidney disease in Persian and other cats: a prospective study using ultrasonography, *Aust Vet J* 79:181, 2001.

14. Bonazzi M, Volta A, Gnudi G, et al: Prevalence of the polycystic kidney disease and renal and urinary bladder ultrasonographic abnormalities in Persian and Exotic Shorthair cats in Italy, *J Feline Med Surg* 9:387, 2007.

15. Domanjko-Petric A, Cernec D, Cotman M: Polycystic kidney disease: a review and occurrence in Slovenia with comparison between ultrasound and genetic testing, *J Feline Med Surg* 10:115, 2008.

16. Gubbels EJ, Prins P: Polycystic kidney disease (PKD) in cats, *Tijdschr Diergeneeskd* 130:184, 2005.

17. Drogemuller C, Rufenacht S, Wichert B, et al: Mutations within the FGF5 gene are associated with hair length in cats, *Anim Genet* 38:218, 2007.

18. Kehler JS, David VA, Schaffer AA, et al: Four independent mutations in the feline fibroblast growth factor 5 gene determine the long-haired phenotype in domestic cats, *J Hered* 98:555, 2007.

19. Meurs KM, Sanchez X, David RM, et al: A cardiac myosin binding protein C mutation in the Maine Coon cat with familial hypertrophic cardiomyopathy, *Hum Mol Genet* 14:3587, 2005.

20. Meurs KM, Norgard MM, Ederer MM, et al: A substitution mutation in the myosin binding protein C gene in ragdoll hypertrophic cardiomyopathy, *Genomics* 90:261, 2007.

21. Baty CJ: Feline hypertrophic cardiomyopathy: an update, *Vet Clin North Am Small Anim Pract* 34:1227, 2004.

22. Kraus MS, Calvert CA, Jacobs GJ: Hypertrophic cardiomyopathy in a litter of five mixed-breed cats, *J Am Anim Hosp Assoc* 35:293, 1999.

23. Nakagawa K, Takemura N, Machida N, et al: Hypertrophic cardiomyopathy in a mixed breed cat family, *J Vet Med Sci* 64:619, 2002.

24. Riesen SC, Kovacevic A, Lombard CW, et al: Prevalence of heart disease in symptomatic cats: an overview from 1998 to 2005, *Schweiz Arch Tierheilkd* 149:65, 2007.

25. Rush JE, Freeman LM, Fenollosa NK, et al: Population and survival characteristics of cats with hypertrophic cardiomyopathy: 260 cases (1990-1999), *J Am Vet Med Assoc* 220:202, 2002.

26. De Maria R, Divari S, Bo S, et al: Beta-galactosidase deficiency in a Korat cat: a new form of feline GM1-gangliosidosis, *Acta Neuropathol (Berl)* 96:307, 1998.

27. Kanae Y, Endoh D, Yamato O, et al: Nonsense mutation of feline beta-hexosaminidase beta-subunit (HEXB) gene causing Sandhoff disease in a family of Japanese domestic cats, *Res Vet Sci* 82:54, 2007.

28. Martin DR, Cox NR, Morrison NE, et al: Mutation of the GM2 activator protein in a feline model of GM2 gangliosidosis, *Acta Neuropathol* 110:443, 2005.

29. Martin DR, Krum BK, Varadarajan GS, et al: An inversion of 25 base pairs causes feline GM2 gangliosidosis variant, *Exp Neurol* 187:30, 2004.

30. Muldoon LL, Neuwelt EA, Pagel MA, et al: Characterization of the molecular defect in a feline model for type II GM2-gangliosidosis (Sandhoff disease), *Am J Pathol* 144:1109, 1994.

31. Fyfe JC, Kurzhals RL, Lassaline ME, et al: Molecular basis of feline beta-glucuronidase deficiency: an animal model of mucopolysaccharidosis VII, *Genomics* 58:121, 1999.

32. He X, Li CM, Simonaro CM, et al: Identification and characterization of the molecular lesion causing mucopolysaccharidosis type I in cats, *Mol Genet Metab* 67:106, 1999.

33. Yogalingam G, Hopwood JJ, Crawley A, et al: Mild feline mucopolysaccharidosis type VI. Identification of an N-acetyl-galactosamine-4-sulfatase mutation causing instability and increased specific activity, *J Biol Chem* 273:13421, 1998.

34. Yogalingam G, Litjens T, Bielicki J, et al: Feline mucopolysaccharidosis type VI. Characterization of recombinant N-acetylgalactosamine 4-sulfatase and identification of a mutation causing the disease, *J Biol Chem* 271:27259, 1996.

35. Fyfe JC, Menotti-Raymond M, David VA, et al: An approximately 140-kb deletion associated with feline spinal muscular atrophy implies an essential LIX1 function for motor neuron survival, *Genome Res* 16:1084, 2006.

36. Robinson R: Expressivity of the Manx gene in cats, *J Hered* 84:170, 1993.

37. Lettice LA, Hill AE, Devenney PS, et al: Point mutations in a distant sonic hedgehog cis-regulator generate a variable regulatory output responsible for preaxial polydactyly, *Hum Mol Genet* 17:978, 2008.

38. Bighignoli B, Niini T, Grahn RA, et al: Cytidine monophospho-N-acetylneuraminic acid hydroxylase (CMAH) mutations associated with the domestic cat AB blood group, *BMC Genet* 8:27, 2007.

39. Stieger K, Palos H, Giger U: Comparison of various blood-typing methods for the feline AB blood group system, *Am J Vet Res* 66:1393, 2005.

40. Reichle JK, DiBartola SP, Leveille R: Renal ultrasonographic and computed tomographic appearance, volume, and function of cats with autosomal dominant polycystic kidney disease, *Vet Radiol Ultrasound* 43:368, 2002.

41. Helps C, Tasker S, Harley R: Correlation of the feline PKD1 genetic mutation with cases of PKD diagnosed by pathological examination, *Exp Mol Pathol* 83:264, 2007.

42. Lipinski MJ, Amigues Y, Blasi M, et al: An international parentage and identification panel for the domestic cat *(Felis catus)*, *Anim Genet* 38:371, 2007

43. Johnson G: *Getting to know the Bengal cat*, Greenwell Springs, LA, 1990, Gogees Cattery.

44. Johnson WE, Eizirik E, Pecon-Slattery J, et al: The late Miocene radiation of modern Felidae: a genetic assessment, *Science* 311:73, 2006.

45. Berg T, Tollersrud OK, Walkley SU, et al: Purification of feline lysosomal alpha-mannosidase, determination of its cDNA sequence and identification of a mutation causing alpha-mannosidosis in Persian cats, *Biochem J* 328:863, 1997.

46. Giger U, Tcherneva E, Caverly J, et al: A missense point mutation in N-acetylglucosamine-1-phosphotransferase causes mucolipidosis II in domestic shorthair cats, *J Vet Intern Med* 20:781, 2006.

47. Ginzinger DG, Lewis ME, Ma Y, et al: A mutation in the lipoprotein lipase gene is the molecular basis of chylomicronemia in a colony of domestic cats, *J Clin Invest* 97:1257, 1996.

48. Goree M, Catalfamo JL, Aber S, et al: Characterization of the mutations causing hemophilia B in 2 domestic cats, *J Vet Intern Med* 19:200, 2005.

49. Haskins M, Jezyk P, Giger U: Diagnostic tests for mucopolysaccharidosis, *J Am Vet Med Assoc* 226:1047, 2005.

50. Imes DL, Geary LA, Grahn RA, et al: Albinism in the domestic cat *(Felis catus)* is associated with a tyrosinase (TYR) mutation, *Anim Genet* 37:175, 2006.

51. Somers KL, Royals MA, Carstea ED, et al: Mutation analysis of feline Niemann-Pick C1 disease, *Mol Genet Metab* 79:99, 2003.

52. Winand NJ, Edwards M, Pradhan D: Deletion of the dystrophin muscle promoter in feline muscular dystrophy, *Neuromuscul Disord* 4:433, 1994.

53. Fyfe JC, Kurzhals RL, Hawkins MG, et al: A complex rearrangement in GBE1 causes both perinatal hypoglycemic collapse and late-juvenile-onset neuromuscular degeneration in glycogen storage disease type IV of Norwegian forest cats, *Mol Genet Metab* 90:383, 2007.

54. Menotti-Raymond M, David VA, Schäffer AA, et al: Mutation in CEP290 discovered for cat model of human retinal degeneration, *J Hered* 98:211, 2007. Epub May 16, 2007.

55. Goldstein RE, Narala S, Sabet N, et al: Primary hyperoxaluria in cats caused by a mutation in the feline GRHPR gene, *J Hered* June 16, 2009 [Epub ahead of print].

56. Clavero S, Haskins M, Giger U, et al: Molecular basis of acute intermittent porphyria in the cat. Paper presented at Advances in Canine and Feline Genomics and Inherited Diseases. St. Malo, France, 2008.

57. Peterschmitt M, Grain F, Arnaud B, et al: Mutation in the melanocortin 1 receptor (MC1-R) is associated with amber colour in the Norwegian Forest Cat, *Anim Genet* April 24, 2009 [Epub ahead of print].

CHAPTER

77 Understanding Population Dynamics Models: Implications for Veterinarians

Margaret R. Slater and Christine M. Budke

Population dynamics models are a way to simplify and explain the complex biological systems in which cats, owned or unowned, free-roaming or confined, exist. As veterinarians, we deal primarily with free-roaming cats when they are injured or killed. We are involved with population control through the spay or neuter of our clients' cats as well as cats in shelters and, increasingly, cats living in free-roaming colonies. How do these different populations of cats interact? How do different approaches for sterilization (e.g., surgical versus nonsurgical, early versus traditional age) or depopulation influence cat population size and growth? How does the size of the interbreeding population affect the outcome of population control measures? These are questions that population dynamics models can help illuminate to inform our decisions in regard to caring for populations of cats.

This chapter will provide some background information, definitions, and examples to help the reader understand, evaluate, and interpret published work on cat population dynamics models. The chapter will present (1) definitions of commonly used terminology; (2) types of population dynamics models that have been used for cats (and occasionally dogs); (3) the data needed, including possible sources and limitations; and (4) the components of the model that should be included in an article to help assure quality and validity. Examples and illustrations will be included from recent publications.

BACKGROUND OF POPULATION DYNAMICS MODELS

Population dynamics models have long been used in ecology and agriculture to examine and predict animal population growth or decline.[1,2] This could be in the context of maximizing animal production yields or examining possible extinction or management for different wildlife species. More recently these models have been generalized to dog and cat populations in order to evaluate the percentage of animals that must be sterilized or removed to halt population growth. For example, models can be used to explore the widely cited assertion that 70 per cent of a population must be sterilized to stabilize cat or dog population growth (owned or free-roaming). This 70 per cent goal has been popularized extensively by Merritt Clifton and later by Marvin Mackie.[3-5] Both Clifton and Mackie have pointed out that spay/neuter programs of owned animals in North America seemed to stabilize the population size when the percentage of animals sterilized neared 70 per cent.[6-8] In addition, a few overseas programs seem to have been successful at about 65 per cent sterilization.[9,10]

The impact of free-roaming populations of dogs and cats on the number of animals in the owned population, as well as in shelters, also has been recognized.[11] In recent years the need to target a specific population of dogs or cats so that a high enough percentage can be sterilized

803

quickly has been stated explicitly. However, few studies have been performed specifically on dogs and cats. In addition, the percentage of the population that must be sterilized to halt population growth appears to depend on animal density, social structures, diseases, reproduction, and survival. Therefore a blanket statement for the percentage of the population that must be sterilized probably is unreasonable. Studies in the early 1980s on owned cat populations illustrated the complex interrelationship of different population subgroups (e.g., owned, sheltered, free-roaming).[11] More recent work has used the diagrams generated from these studies to help visualize the subpopulations and demonstrate where additional data are needed.[12-14]

Changes in populations are based on births, deaths, immigration, and emigration.[1] Programs that focus on sterilization of cats try to decrease birth rates. Programs that focus on euthanasia increase death rates. This distinction will be important when comparing different types of population control methods in cats.

DEFINITIONS

Models, in their most basic forms, are simplified representations of a complex ecological system.[1] The population of animals is *dynamic* (or constantly changing): animals find and defend their territory, choose mates, reproduce and raise their young, find food and shelter, and avoid predators, all during certain time periods (e.g., seasonally) and in certain areas. For cats, "ecology" may involve local ordinances and policies, cultural beliefs, local cat breeders, or hunting.[11] Our conceptual models of cat populations, based on verbal, written, or diagrammatic descriptions, become mathematical models when represented with mathematical equations.[2]

Biologically, a *population* of animals is a group of the same species that live together and reproduce. However, a population from a modeling or veterinary perspective is defined much more narrowly. We might talk about owned cats, unowned, free-roaming cats, abandoned cats, kittens in shelters, or a single colony of feral cats. Each population will grow or decrease in different ways for different reasons. Each may or may not interact with one of the other populations.

Changes in populations are based on four "vital statistics." *Birth* (fertility, fecundity) and *death* (mortality, survival) depend on the size and success of the current population. *Immigration* and *emigration* depend on the movement of animals in or out of the population (because of the animals' own movements or the intervention of human beings). For example, the owned cat population of Brazos County, Texas, is increased by the birth of kittens from owned cats, cats or kittens adopted as strays, and owned cats moving in from other counties or states. In this example, owned cats brought in from other counties or states are immigrants, and cats whose owners move out of Brazos County with their cats are emigrants (Figure 77-1). Births and immigration increase the population, and deaths and emigration decrease the population. If there are more births or immigrants than deaths and emigrants, then the population will increase, and vice versa. In a *closed population*, immigration and emigration are zero and only birth and death rates influence population size. In Figure 77-1 the closed population model would not allow for cats to enter or leave the county through shelter transfers of cats, owner movements, cats roaming into or out of neighboring counties, and so forth. For most cat populations, except in rare cases on islands or extremely isolated geographical locations, the populations in which we are interested are not closed, but instead are considered *open populations*.

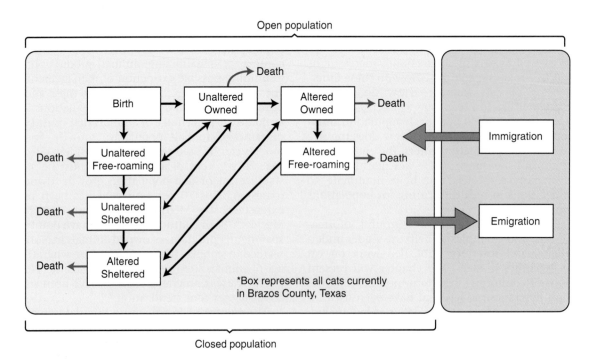

Figure 77-1 A hypothetical flow diagram for the cat population of Brazos County, Texas.

As one can imagine, the constant influx and outflow of animals in an open population complicates the modeling process.

In general in population dynamics modeling, the focus is on female reproduction. This is because there are usually enough males in the population of interest to inseminate all of the females. If this is not true, then male reproductive rates also must be calculated. It also is assumed that the other vital rates for males are the same as for females.[15] *Reproductive rate* (R_0) is an overall measure of female reproduction: the average number of female kittens produced by each queen over her lifetime. There are many external factors that influence reproduction: (1) limited food and resources may drain the queen; (2) there may be less time for finding food during kitten rearing; and (3) there may be poorer growth of the adults or kittens if resources are limited. If R_0 is greater than 1, then there is a net increase in kittens in each generation. Conversely, if R_0 is lower than 1, the population is tending toward extinction. If R_0 is 1, the population is in equilibrium and the kittens produced balance the deaths in each generation.

APPROACHES TO POPULATION DYNAMICS MODELING

Box 77-1 outlines the questions that will help a reader become oriented to a publication on population dynamics. The population of animals evaluated should be defined clearly so it is readily apparent which subgroups are included. The objective should be stated clearly and may include (1) simple descriptions of a biological process or situation; (2) synthesis of current knowledge and understanding to see where the gaps are; (3) guidance for future experimental work; (4) evaluation of different interventions and their effects; (5) risk analysis or decision support; and (6) predictions of future changes in the population.[2] In veterinary medicine we are interested most often in (2) and (4). For example, the effect of an intervention on rabies and population control in dogs can be illustrated by a project that vaccinated and sterilized neighborhood dogs in India.[9] In 8 years 65 per cent of females were sterilized and vaccinated, and the total population of dogs decreased by 28 per cent. Local human cases of rabies subsequently dropped to zero. Most commonly the authors measure numbers of animals or growth rate; sometimes both estimates are included.

The simplest types of mathematical models are *descriptive models*. These models use basic mathematical expressions to represent population growth. *Exponential growth* occurs when a value increases by a multiplicative factor per unit time (e.g., bacterial growth), with an exponential formula used as the model. These models provide a growth rate for the population, which also is called the *intrinsic rate of increase (r)* or the Malthusian parameter. If r is positive, then the population is growing; if r is negative, the population is declining; if zero, then the population size remains constant. The major assumptions made about a population undergoing exponential growth are (1) it is a closed population; (2) birth and death rates are constant throughout the organism's life; and (3) there is no variability in genetics, age, or size that affects birth or death. If these assumptions are not appropriate for the population being studied, then the conclusions will be erroneous. This most basic model and its assumptions are unlikely to be correct for most cat populations. Therefore other, more complex models should be used.

A somewhat more complicated model uses a formula for *logistic growth,* which accounts for the influence of the density of the animals living in the area on births and deaths.[2] Typically, increasing population densities will increase competition for food, mates, and territory, resulting in slower or level population growth. The *carrying capacity* (K) is the maximum number of animals that can be supported in that population at that time and location. The calculation of carrying capacity is sometimes an objective of a model. Basic logistic models otherwise have similar assumptions to the exponential models, except for taking density into account. Variations on the logistic growth models are possible and can account for the influence that time lags may have on reproduction or death as well as different types of density dependence (linear or variable). *Density dependence* is the regulation of the size of the population by mechanisms that themselves are controlled by the size of the population (e.g., the availability of resources like shelter). The effectiveness of these mechanisms increases as population size increases. For example, a variation on the logistic model is the *Ricker* or *exponential logistic model*. This model focuses on growth rate and carrying capacity. However, unlike the basic logistic model, increasing population density results in a linear, density-dependent decrease in the growth rate and prevents the population size from ever being calculated as a negative number.

Age- or stage-structured population growth can be modeled using *demographic models* (also known as structured population models). This approach takes into account the effects that demographic variables like age or life stage might have on birth rate or survival and, hence, population growth. Demographic models allow for inclusion of many different types of population data and therefore provide a flexible approach to modeling.

Box 77-1 Information to Orient the Reader to a Population Dynamics Project

1. What is the population that is being studied?
2. What is the objective of the study? Is it clearly defined?
3. What are the source(s) of data?
4. What type of model is used? What are the model assumptions and do they make sense given the situation and limitations?
5. What is the outcome measurement and how is it interpreted?
6. Have the authors demonstrated which vital rate is most important (sensitivity or elasticity analysis)?
7. How are the authors dealing with variability?
8. Are the results believable given existing knowledge on the subject?
9. What are the take home messages from the study?

However, the simpler versions are not density-dependent and assume there is no ceiling on population growth. The intrinsic growth rate for a population is λ *(lambda)*. If λ is 1 then there is no net change in the population size. If λ is higher than 1, the population is increasing. If λ is lower than 1, the population size is decreasing.

A major assumption thus far is that the population is closed. This may be the case on uninhabited islands and there are studies of cat population dynamics that assume an island population.[16] However, few real-life cat populations are closed and this can be a major limitation for models. For example, abandonment of cats is a common way of increasing cat immigration to the unowned, free-roaming cat population, whereas adoption of strays would be a form of emigration. It is possible to include various rates of immigration and emigration in the models. However, estimating the immigration and emigration rates is very difficult and may introduce more error than assuming a closed population. Movement of animals in and out of populations is often density-dependent. In addition, it is influenced by the biology of the species, local resources, and, of course, people. This issue should be addressed by the authors of the publication and their choices explained and defended.

If age is important, it can be accounted for, most commonly by dividing the ages of the population into classes or groups. Sometimes stage of life is more important than actual age: for example, kitten, reproductive adult, or sterilized adult. Each of these stages would correlate with age, but in terms of birth and death, they may be the most useful way to divide the population.

Demographic models use matrices to perform the calculations. Different approaches are named after the biologists who proposed them and these names often are used to describe the model. *Leslie matrix analyses* include age-related changes in birth and death rates. *Usher matrices* lump all the adults with similar survival rates into one class. *Lefkovitch matrices* collapse age entirely into stages of life where animals within each life stage have similar fecundity and mortality.

There are many other types of population dynamics models. However, those described above have been used most commonly for companion animals.[15,17,18]

The models discussed to this point are all *deterministic*: we use our one best estimate for the included vital statistics and the model gives us a single answer in terms of population change. However, there is variability in everything. *Stochastic models* incorporate variability into the data that are used in the model.[2] For example, we can include data that incorporate a range of litter size in queens. Stochastic models also allow us to include the role of chance and environment in influencing populations. There are four types of stochasticity to consider: (1) environmental; (2) demographic; (3) genetic; and (4) catastrophic. *Environmental stochasticity* is the variability in good and bad years for population growth because of factors like climate and food sources. Human intervention and garbage sources also could be considered in this type. *Demographic stochasticity* is the variation in births and deaths from the normal variability in seasonal and individual patterns. A run of extra litters could influence birth rates for a couple of years and might not be bal-

anced out by extra deaths. Variation in the sex ratios of litters also could have an effect because models often are based solely on female members of the population. *Genetic stochasticity* is the amount of genetic variation in the population and how that affects the vital statistics. For example, inbreeding may decrease genetic diversity and change survival rates. On the other hand, some genetic homogeneity likely will make estimates of vital statistics more stable in the short term. *Catastrophic stochasticity* is variability caused by unpredictable and often substantial influences on populations. Catastrophes may be considered a subtype of environmental influences because natural disasters like floods, droughts, and hurricanes all would fall into this category. However, localized catastrophes such as dog attacks on cat populations, poisonings, or changes to the habitat, like construction, also could influence cat populations strongly.

Metapopulation is a term used in wildlife biology and conservation to refer to groups of interlinked populations where there is immigration and/or emigration between the populations.[1] Usually the context for these analyses is to determine extinction or specific types of population interactions like predation. Other types of models are used to study competition between species for food, shelter, and so forth and are particularly important with limited resources. *Lotka-Volterra models* allow for the kinds of competition between populations that occur in these situations.[1,2] Although no work has been published on cats using this approach, predator-prey models seeking to understand or control predation have been published.[19,20]

The *Allee effect* occurs when the per capita birth rate declines at low population densities.[2] This effect can be important in small or decreasing populations. This may be caused by the inability to hunt as effectively compared with a larger group, difficulties in finding mates, or increased vulnerability to predation. In contrast, some small populations actually may experience improved survival. One project evaluating feline immunodeficiency virus spread in cats included the Allee effect in the modeling.[21] The Allee effect (or its absence) might become worth studying in areas where the numbers of cats have been reduced successfully.

Simulation models are designed specifically to compare the computer model results to the behavior of the population in the real world. They allow us to see how complete our understanding of the population is by looking at parts of the model that do not fit the real world very well. These should be simple models to start with; added complexity can be included if needed. Simulation models often combine density-dependence and population structure (e.g., age) with environmental stochasticity. Few studies utilizing this type of modeling have been conducted for cat and dog populations thus far.

WHAT DATA ARE NEEDED?

The most difficult aspect of population dynamics modeling for cat populations is acquiring accurate data. First, the particular populations of interest can vary substantially from place to place. For example, cat ownership appears to vary regionally in the United States. Second, we often do not have funding or the ability to collect detailed data in the populations of interest, with numbers of free-roaming cats very difficult to obtain. Generally numbers of cats will have to be extrapolated from previous studies if new research using existing wildlife counting techniques is not possible.[22] Finally, sometimes it is just very difficult to actually obtain the data. For example, how do we estimate the number of cats abandoned? Animal shelters in the city of interest may not keep detailed records on the numbers of kittens who enter the shelter and, because of the sensitive nature of the topic, telephone surveys also may not provide accurate information on abandonment rates. It is crucial that the investigators making the model clearly document where they obtained their data and exactly what data they used. This will provide enough information to decide if the data seem realistic and similar to a population in which the reader is interested.

To calculate birth rates, fertility or *fecundity tables* are needed. These tables provide the average number of female kittens for queens in each age class or stage in a particular time period (often 1 year). For death rates, *survivorship tables* (i.e., life tables) provide *age- or stage-specific mortality* for each class or stage (Table 77-1). Age interval, for example 0-1, includes newly born cats through cats about to become 1 year old. To continue this example, the second column, l_x, indicates how many cats survived until they were about to become 1 year old. The third column, d_x, indicates how many cats died in

the first year of life. The fourth column, q_x, is the proportion of cats who died in the first year of life (e.g., the number dying in the first year of life divided by the number of cats born). The fifth column, L_x, is the number of cat-years lived in that time interval (e.g., number of cats born minus half of the number of cats dying in the first year of life). The sixth column, T_x, is the total number of years lived beyond the beginning of the age interval (e.g., the sum of column L_x from this age interval on). The last column, e_x, indicates the mean expected lifespan of cats in that age group.

Survivorship tables are calculated in three ways: (1) follow a group (cohort) of individuals across time and determine their life span; (2) collect data across a shorter time span on all animals who died during that period and their age at death (also requires growth rate of the population); and (3) use cross-sectional data (often from a questionnaire) to estimate survival for each age class or stage.[2] These methods are listed from most to least reliable.

EVALUATING THE MODEL

Each model has its strengths and limitations. Just because a model has not represented reality completely, does not mean we can not learn from it. One way to evaluate the model is to perform a sensitivity or elasticity analysis.[2] This means that if the estimates are not very accurate, we can see how the model changes if the various parameters (e.g., vital statistics) are changed. Even if the estimates

Table 77-1 Example Life Table for Owned Cats

Age Interval (in years) (x, x + n)	Number Living at Age x (l_x)	Number Dying in (x, x + n) (d_x)	Probability of Dying in (x, x + n) (q_x)	Years Lived in (x, x + n) (L_x)	Years Lived Beyond x (T_x)	Expectation of Life at Age x (e_x)
0-1	3936	1323	0.34	3274.5	16353.0	4.2
1-2	2613	590	0.23	2318.0	13078.5	5.0
2-3	2023	346	0.17	1850.0	10760.5	5.3
3-4	1677	319	0.19	1517.5	8910.5	5.3
4-5	1358	195	0.14	1260.5	7393.0	5.4
5-6	1163	185	0.16	1070.5	6132.5	5.3
6-7	978	101	0.10	927.5	5062.0	5.2
7-8	877	112	0.13	821.0	4134.5	4.7
8-9	765	115	0.15	707.5	3313.5	4.3
9-10	650	80	0.12	610.0	2606.0	4.0
10-11	570	155	0.27	492.5	1996.0	3.5
11-12	415	55	0.13	387.5	1503.5	3.6
12-13	360	82	0.23	319.0	1116.0	3.1
13-14	278	77	0.28	239.5	797.0	2.9
14-15	201	32	0.16	185.0	557.5	2.8
15-16	169	65	0.38	136.5	372.5	2.2
≥16	104	—	—	—	—	—

Data from Japanese animal cemetery records, 1981-1982.[23]

are accurate, we can evaluate the relative importance of each of the vital statistics on the results of the model. To do this, the values of the vital statistics are varied up and down to see how big an influence there is on the model and the overall conclusions. One then can determine which of the vital statistics has the greatest effect on the model. This might be useful to know if fecundity is found to be most important and we are talking about a sterilization program. In most mammalian systems, survival has a greater effect than fecundity, because the animal has to survive to reproduce. However, this may not always be true in populations with extreme values for these vital statistics.

Sensitivity analysis changes the vital statistics by a fixed amount that makes sense for the population. *Elasticity analysis* changes each of the vital statistics by the same proportion. The choice depends on the population and what seems logical, but one of these analyses should be done for any model.

Determining if the model is accurate is called *validation*.[2] The simplest way to validate a model is to compare the model results to existing data or a subset of existing data. The more difficult way is to compare the model results and projections to a new independent data set. The latter generally is considered to be more rigorous, but new data sets may be hard to find. Depending on the objective of the model, we may not need to be able to generalize the model's results to other data sets. In the event that different data sets result in different models and results, we should analyze the differences between the methods and data sources carefully. These comparisons may provide valuable insight into the areas where more information is needed, or to times or locations where unusual events occurred. Comparisons also should generate new hypotheses to be tested, which may help explain the difference between models. No model is perfect; it is intended as a simplified representation of reality.

RECENT EXAMPLES

A Ricker model was used to study free-roaming cats in counties in Florida and California with high volume spay/neuter programs.[17] This type of model focuses on the growth rate of the populations, the effect of population density on growth, and the idea that carrying capacity limits growth rate. The model used birth and death rates and assumed a closed population. This type of model can show changes in population size either by slowing growth or by modifying the environment to decrease the carrying capacity. The authors' primary interest was the impact of sterilization on population growth. There were limitations in the data used (e.g., data from county programs and published data) and in the assumptions (e.g., closed population). However, several of their conclusions are worth further consideration. First, they calculated that 94 per cent and 71 per cent of cats in the Florida and California counties, respectively, would need to be sterilized to decrease population growth. At the county level, thousands or tens of thousands of cats would need to be sterilized. Second, targeting smaller

populations should make it possible to reach high levels of sterilization for those particular populations. And third, data on cats re-trapped as part of the sterilization efforts could help with population size and sterilization percentage estimates to evaluate success.

A study in a small area (60 square kilometers) of Western Australia evaluated control measures for feral cats.[18] A logistic model was used based on data from a 58-month study period. Carrying capacity and rate of increase were utilized to examine maximum sustained yield (MSY), which represented the minimum number of cats to be removed each year in order to eliminate the cat population within a designated time frame. The intrinsic rate of increase (r_m) from the model was 0.98 (indicating an approximate doubling of the population every 8.5 months), with a carrying capacity (K) of 1.5 cats/km^2. This resulted in a MSY of 0.6 cats/km^2/year to drive the population to extinction. In other words, it would take 10 years of removing 36 cats/year from the study area to drive the population to extinction, assuming the absence of immigration. Higher removal rates would shorten the time to extinction. However, the authors calculated that in one area of their study region, it took five times the effort to trap the last cat as the first in a 2-year eradication effort. This increase in effort as removal proceeds is typical, and must be taken into account in eradication efforts.[18]

Another model utilized a simple matrix model approach using a hypothetical closed free-roaming cat population and published vital rates for juvenile and adult survival and fecundity.[15] The objective was to compare trap-neuter-return (a change in fecundity) and remove and euthanize (a change in survival) as control methods for free-roaming cats. High and low estimates for each vital rate were used in eight combinations for juveniles and adults. These models resulted in λ from 1.34 to 2.49 with a geometric mean of 1.84. Therefore even the lowest survival and fecundity estimates still resulted in continued growth of the population. Models for different levels (10 per cent to 75 per cent) of sterilization (fecundity) and removal (survival) were run, utilizing the geometric mean λ from the initial models for the baseline population. Even at a sterilization percentage of 75 per cent, λ equaled 1.08, which indicated a slightly increasing population. Removal of more than 50 per cent of both juvenile and adult cats was required to reach λ less than 1. In almost all models, elasticity analysis indicated that juvenile survival was the most important vital rate followed by adult survival. This makes sense because kittens must survive to reproductive age if they are to contribute to population growth. In addition, the authors point out that any program that removes cats from the free-roaming population, such as adoption, would alter the survival rate.

Figure 77-2 provides a simple example, using the data from this article, of what population growth with a 50 per cent decrease in adult and juvenile reproduction (λ = 1.35), a 75 per cent decrease in adult and juvenile reproduction (λ = 1.08), and a 90 per cent decrease in adult and juvenile reproduction (λ = 0.89) would look like starting with 100 adult female intact cats and a baseline population growth rate of λ equaling 1.84.

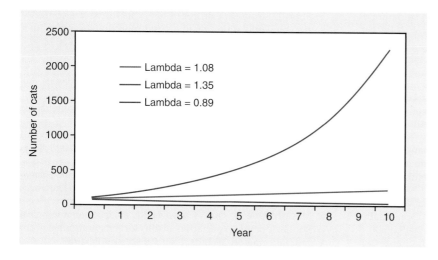

Figure 77-2 The hypothetical 10-year growth of a cat population at three levels of intrinsic growth rate (λ, lambda), which results in a slowly decreasing, slowing increasing, and rapidly increasing population of cats. The lambdas are altered by changing the birth rate of the cats.

Another application of cat population dynamics models is their use for evaluating infectious diseases as control methods. One example was the use of feline panleukopenia virus (FPV) on Marion Island to control (and eventually eradicate) the cats.[16] This approach required both vital rates for the cat population as well as data on disease transmission. Cat densities and contact behavior are crucial for infectious disease models. Data on the cats were obtained from Marion Island and other well-studied subantarctic islands. Birth rate was 1.1/cat/year and mortality rate was 0.89/cat/year before disease introduction. For FPV, both direct contact and environmental contamination were included in the simulation modeling. Results of the modeling were consistent with the 6 years of available data, and provided insight into disease modeling in island populations of cats. The experiment and the modeling both indicated that FPV infection was unable to eradicate the cat population. Although numbers of cats did decline substantially across the 6 years of observation, other methods across many more years were needed to finally eradicate the cats.

SUMMARY

Population dynamics models can be very useful in studying cat and dog populations. Often, ecologists or wildlife biologists will have the most experience in building the models. Models that have been utilized recently for companion animal populations have been based on the same principles as wildlife models. Data for the models can be difficult to find, with the scientific literature one common source. Organizations or individuals who keep detailed records on the population of interest also can provide detailed data for some modeling efforts. Some of the assumptions made for the modeled population and the data used can result in serious limitations. Nonetheless, understanding these limitations may allow for useful conclusions about the population being studied.

Models designed to test interventions should target a manageable population of interest. Often we have based the target population on human locations (e.g., zip codes with the largest number of kittens brought to the shelter) or socioeconomic status (e.g., low income families for subsidized sterilization). However, we also should consider focused cat-related geographically based targets such as a colony of cats or cats living in a park. This may change the percentage and numbers of animals dramatically that need to be sterilized.

Population dynamics modeling is a tool that can help plan or evaluate a potential intervention and help determine if a 70 per cent sterilization rate (and of what population!) really should be our goal.

REFERENCES

1. Gotelli NJ: *A primer of ecology*, ed 3, Sunderland, MA, 2001, Sinauer Associates, Inc.
2. Owen-Smith N: *Introduction to modeling in wildlife and resource management*, Malden, MA, 2007, Blackwell.
3. Clifton M: What RU-487 means for animals, *Animal People* November, 2000. Retrieved July 1, 2008 from http://www.animalpeoplenews.org/ru4861100.html.
4. Clifton M: Sterilization and vaccination: 70% or flunk, *Animal People* October, 2002. Retrieved July 25, 2008 from http://www.bestfriends.org/nomorehomelesspets/pdf/threshold.pdf.
5. Mackie M: Pet overpopulation and the 70% rule, *The Pet Press*, Los Angeles 4(6), March/April, 2003. Retrieved July 25, 2008 from http://www.animalrescue-sf.org/english_area/e_dr_mackie/e_dr_mackie%20_a_2.html.
6. Alberta Spay Neuter Task Force: 70% Solution. Retrieved July 25, 2008 from http://www.abtaskforce.org/70%20per%20cent.html.
7. The Animal Mission, Columbia, SC: The 70% Solution. Retrieved July 25, 2008 from http://www.animalmission.org/public/files/docs/70_percent.pdf.
8. Spay Neuter Kansas City, Kansas City, MO: What you should know about pet overpopulation. Retrieved July 25, 2008 from http://www.snkc.net/petoverpopulation.html.
9. Reece JF, Chawla SK: Control of rabies in Jaipur, India by sterilisation and vaccination of neighbourhood dogs, *Vet Rec* 159:379, 2006.
10. Gioberchio G: A special relationship. *Perspectives in Health—The magazine of the Pan American Health Organization* 10 (November), 2005. Retrieved July 25, 2008 from http://www.paho.org/english/dd/pin/Number21_article05.htm.
11. Slater MR: *Community approaches to feral cats: problems, alternatives and recommendations*, Washington, DC, 2002, The Humane Society Press.

12. Nassar R, Fluke J: Pet population dynamics and community planning for animal welfare and animal control, *J Am Vet Med Assoc* 198:1160, 1991.

13. Patroneck G, Glickman L: Development of a model for estimating the size and dynamics of the pet dog population, *Anthrozöös* 7:25, 1994.

14. Frank J: An interactive model of human and companion animal dynamics: the ecology and economics of dog overpopulation and the human costs of addressing the problem, *Human Ecol* 32:107, 2004.

15. Andersen MC, Martin BJ, Roemer GW: Use of matrix population models to estimate the efficacy of euthanasia versus trap-neuter-return for management of free-roaming cats, *J Am Vet Med Assoc* 225:1871, 2004.

16. Berthier K, Langlais M, Auger P, et al: Dynamics of a feline virus with two transmission modes within exponentially growing host populations, *Proc R Soc Long* 267:2049, 2000.

17. Foley P, Foley JE, Levy JK, et al: Analysis of the impact of trap-neuter-return programs on populations of feral cats, *J Am Vet Med Assoc* 227:1775, 2005.

18. Short J, Turner B: Control of feral cats for nature conservation IV. Population dynamics and morphological attributes of feral cats at Shark Bay Western Australia, *Wildl Res* 32:489, 2005.

19. Baxter PWJ, Sabo JL, Wilcox C, et al: Cost-effective suppression and eradication of invasive predators, *Conserv Biol* 22:89, 2007.

20. Cai GQ, Lin YK: Stochastic analysis of predator-prey type ecosystems, *Ecol Complex* 4:242, 2007.

21. Hilker FM, Langlais M, Petrovskii SV, et al: A diffusive SI model with Allee effect and application to FIV, *Math Biosci* 206:61, 2007.

22. Krebs CJ: Population parameters. In *Ecology: the experimental analysis of distribution and abundance*, ed 5, San Francisco, 2001, Benjamin-Cummings, p 116.

23. Hayashidoni H, Omi Y, Ogawa M, et al: Epidemiological studies on the expectation of life for cats computed from animal cemetery records, *Jpn J Vet Sci* 51:905, 1989.

78 Hospice "Pawspice"

Alice Villalobos

Hospice for ailing cats has been a natural home-oriented behavior in the society of loving pet owners since the Pharaohs ruled the Egyptians. It was customary in ancient Egypt for family members to shave their eyebrows to signify their loss after the death of a beloved family cat. Veterinary medicine always has been involved somewhat unofficially in helping families deal with feline end-of-life issues. The twenty-first century has witnessed an unprecedented open appreciation for the human-animal bond including the feline population that has surpassed the dog population in the United States. Society's love for their cats has driven the demand for modern feline medicine and excellent resources for the profession such as this book. Members of our profession must refine the skills, knowledge, attitude, and aptitude that will properly address the dramatic evolution of relationships that people share with their cats. Because disease and senescence prevail in the end, the demand for feline hospice services is increasing. The profession needs a more formal approach that describes and formats pet hospice "Pawspice" care specifically for the feline patient. The first pet hospice symposium was held at the University of California, Davis, in March 2008. An umbrella organization, the International Association for Animal Hospice and Palliative Care (www.iaahpc.org), was formed in 2009. Pawspice services, to be complete, also would include training the veterinary staff to provide emotional support for the dying patient's families.[1-6]

It is important for the practitioner to recognize and communicate respect and appreciation for the human-animal bond and for special attachments that link a particular cat to family members. We can develop further skills in this "high-touch" aspect of veterinary medicine by understanding the full meaning and the application of "Emotional Intelligence" as described by Dr. Richard Timmins in courses for certification of veterinarians at the University of California, Davis, for the Association of Veterinary Family Practitioners [http://www.avfp.org/].

In addition, we can use the Emotional SOAP (Subjective, Objective, Assessment, Plan) technique to assess the feelings of our clients when they present their sick cats for our help. The E-SOAP technique parallels the typical SOAP patient-assessment format used in medicine worldwide. Carolyn Butler and Laurel Lagoni proposed the

E-SOAP method, when they were counselors at the Argus Center at Colorado State University.*

The Emotional SOAP begins when the veterinary team walks into the examination room and interacts with the client and their cat. The Pawspice team expects to encounter a raft of emotional issues that come along with attachment, such as anxiety, anticipatory grief, worry, and fear of being unable to handle the costs and demands of pet care. The E-SOAP parallels the physical examination system using the Subjective-Objective-Assessment-Plan method.

It is equally important for the pet hospice practitioner to assess and address quality of life issues for the patient to help the pet owner face the realities of their cat's situation. All of these communications must be blended with compassion, concern, and sensitivity for the unique relationship between the owner and their cat. The proposed HHHHHMM Quality of Life Scale for Feline Pawspice may be used by doctors, nursing staff, and pet owners and may serve as the pivotal tool that defines your practice's Pawspice program (Table 78-1).[†]

RATIONALE FOR FELINE PAWSPICE CARE

Tenacious cat lovers have generated an increasing demand to spend the last days with their ailing terminal cats at home, preferring to await the inevitable loss patiently and peacefully. The hospice movement was started by the nursing profession to help people die peacefully and painlessly at home with their families and friends. Hospice is about care when cure is not feasible and it serves as a model for veterinary medicine. Veterinarians can lead the hospice movement conscientiously for pets across America by adopting the hospice philosophy into their practices. When a family can not accept early euthanasia or treatment that has little hope for success, Pawspice becomes a very helpful option. Providing palliative and comfort care for cats, when needed or requested, honors the human-animal bond during the difficult days approaching death. The Pawspice philosophy allows all involved to have quality time to cherish their relationship during an extended farewell.

When a beloved cat has an incurable or terminal condition, many families will, if given the option, choose to provide Pawspice care at home. Surveys have shown that veterinarians underestimate their clientele's needs and wants frequently. How much care are pet owners willing to provide for their beloved ailing cats? For some pet owners, the willingness to care for their cat may have no limits. It is not unusual for clients to change their approach. They might be interested initially in participating in a treatment protocol, but after their cat encounters adverse events, they might decline further treatment and opt for Pawspice care or vice versa.

Entering terminally ill cats into Pawspice programs offers pet owners a buoy. It provides supportive, palliative options for complete care and attention to their cat's special needs as cachexia, dehydration, anorexia, pain, and lethargy pull the patient downstream toward death.

DISMISSED CLIENTS GO ELSEWHERE

The economic downturn, foreclosures, increased prices for gasoline, oil, and commodities have put a financial squeeze on the middle class. Many Americans will be forced to streamline expenses, including pet care. If a cat's illness can not be treated because of financial constraints or a logistical problem, that case should not be dismissed.

It is, and will always be, good medicine to provide medical advice compassionately with meticulous home-care instructions to maintain quality of life for that patient. If a cat's kidneys or heart are in failure; if a previously treated cancer has recurred, metastasized, or has become resistant to treatment; or if a cat was diagnosed in the terminal stages of cancer or diabetes mellitus, in-home hospice care is a wonderful next step that keeps family and cat comfortably in their nest. Offering pet owners a well thought-out, creative, palliative Pawspice plan may be the very best medicine that veterinarians can offer a dying cat to honor the human-feline bond.

Each pet family has their own belief system, personal life style, and tolerance level. They will weigh issues such as their personal finances, the logistics of getting to and from the treatment center, and scheduling for visits and home care requirements. Typically, family members deal with feelings of guilt, sense of duty, and remorse as their cat encounters problems along the bumpy path toward death.

Declining treatment is an emotionally difficult decision for highly bonded caretakers to make. Many old cats have concurrent medical conditions that appeared in their senior years and these conditions can be expected to worsen with time. They also can be expected to complicate treatment of a terminal illness. For example, one third of the pet cat population is overweight and/or obese. When obese cats become burdened with terminal illness and related treatment issues, they are at risk for development of hepatic lipidosis. Studies have shown that having more than one preexisting disorder such as heart disease, chronic kidney disease, or hyperthyroidism, in addition to cancer, is associated with shortened patient survival times.[7] It is important to keep these factors in mind when recommending aggressive definitive therapy for cats with concurrent disease.

Decision-making for cats can be frustrating. Some procedures such as surgical removal of a large vaccine-associated sarcoma or ear ablation or mandibulectomy for squamous cell carcinoma may seem straightforward. However, the prognosis for surgery alone may be poor without follow-up radiation therapy.[8-11] If the cat's prognosis does not yield enough survival time to satisfy the

---

*This handy emotional assessment guide can be accessed on line at the American Association of Human Animal Bond Veterinarians web site [http://www.aah-abv.org]. Click newsletters, choose the Autumn 2002 issue, and review the penultimate page.
[†]Anyone may access and download the original Quality of Life Scale using the URL [http://www.veterinarypracticenews.com/images/pdfs/Quality_of_Life.pdf].

Table 78-1 The HHHHHMM Quality of Life Scale

Score	Criterion
H: 0-10	**HURT** Adequate pain control, including breathing ability, is the first and foremost consideration. Is the cat's pain managed successfully? Is oxygen necessary?
H: 0-10	**HUNGER** Is the cat eating enough? Does hand-feeding help? Does the patient require a feeding tube?
H:0-10	**HYDRATION** For cats not drinking or eating foods containing enough water, use SQ fluids q12-24h to supplement fluid intake. Is the patient dehydrated?
H: 0-10	**HYGIENE** The patient should be kept brushed and cleaned. This is paramount for cats with oral cancer. Check the body for soiling after elimination. Avoid pressure sores and keep all wounds clean.
H: 0-10	**HAPPINESS** Does the cat express joy and interest? Is the cat responsive to things around him (e.g., family, toys)? Does the cat purr when scratched or petted? Is the cat depressed, lonely, anxious, bored, afraid? Can the cat's bed be near the kitchen and moved near family activities so as not to be isolated?
M: 0-10	**MOBILITY** Is the cat having seizures or stumbling? Some caregivers feel euthanasia is preferable to a definitive surgery, yet cats are resilient. Cats with limited mobility may still be alert and responsive and can have a good quality of life if the family is committed to providing quality care.
M: 0-10	**MORE GOOD DAYS THAN BAD** When bad days outnumber good days, quality of life for the dying cat might be too compromised. When a healthy human-animal bond is no longer possible, caregivers must be made aware that their duty is to protect their cat from pain by making the final call for euthanasia. The decision needs to be made if the cat has unresponsive suffering. If death comes peacefully and painlessly at home, that is acceptable.
*TOTAL	*A total score >35 is acceptable quality of life for maintaining a good feline Pawspice.

Feline caregivers can use this scale to evaluate the success of their Pawspice program. Grading each criterion using a scale of 0 to 10 will help caregivers determine quality of life for sick cats.

Adapted from Villalobos A, Kaplan L: *Canine and feline geriatric oncology: honoring the human-animal bond,* Hoboken, NJ, 2007, Wiley-Blackwell; and Villalobos A: Quality of life scale helps make final call, *Oncology Outlook, VPN,* September 2004.

owners, they can not justify the emotional or financial costs. Occasionally clients are regretful but willing to sacrifice their cat's quality of life rather than elect amputation of a limb. Some pet owners have the honest yet teleological feeling that amputation is mutilation and not fair to the cat. Instead, they allow their cat to bear a painful limb for months before euthanasia. It is the attending veterinarian's ethical duty to oversee pain control for patients like these.

When a family declines the ideal treatment plan, the battle should not be over. When a pet owner asks if there is another, less risky and/or less costly option, the veterinarian must offer the option of Pawspice wholeheartedly. When this is not presented as an option, some clients will sneak away from the hospital and pursue alternative treatments without the doctor's knowledge or guidance. They may not want to hurt their family veterinarian's

feelings. They may be embarrassed or think that their veterinarian will be angry with them or disapprove.

If the attending veterinarian refrains from being judgmental and continues to offer options that may be more palatable for the family to accept, the client will remain faithful to the practice. Adjusting options toward maintaining quality of life and providing comfort care is better than no care at all. By creating a protocol for supportive care, Pawspice becomes a very acceptable option for clients who otherwise would seek help for their cats elsewhere.

BARRIERS TO PROVIDING PAWSPICE CARE

Change is not easy, yet change we must. A number of barriers may prevent a practice from moving into providing Pawspice services for their clients' dying pets. Personnel and staffing problems would be at the top of most veterinarians' lists of challenges. Finding a way to associate the special Pawspice services rendered with a fee structure is second.

Dedicated people are essential to help the practice offer an effective Pawspice service. Extra training in client communications, attachment theory, and grief management would be a minimum requirement for staff participants. Other barriers to establishing a Pawspice would be low staff morale, a rushed atmosphere, and a lack of willingness and patience. The Pawspice staff needs to be willing and able to visit client homes to minister to the ailing pet and comfort sad people effectively. If the general practice does not provide for Pawspice house calls, then referral to a house call doctor would be appropriate and much appreciated by many families.

It is somewhat difficult to charge for "high touch" services including the phone consultations and home visits. However, there is a steady demand for end-of-life services. One must realize that cat clients expect and are willing to pay for specialty Pawspice services. Create a special Pawspice fee schedule that includes fees for continuous and repetitive care and for extended consultations or home visits by a nursing staff or the doctor. Charging clients professional fees for end-of-life care services should parallel the practice's normal, established fees, which generally are based on time and services rendered. Some practices are making the noble attempt to have a nonprofit organization to fund pet hospice services. This endeavor may place an unnecessary workload on the staff and constitute a barrier toward offering end-of-life services.

The paperwork and consent forms for Pawspice patients also may become a barrier. If a cat has a poor prognosis and the family desires therapy that is not expected to help, it is appropriate to document the situation in the medical chart. Read the phrases out loud for clarification and then ask the client to initial or sign the statement with the date and time. This process of informed consent will prevent most of the common misunderstandings and keeps everyone on the same page during therapy.

HOW DOES ONE START?

First of all, step away from suggesting utilitarian, premature euthanasia as an option when a feline friend is diagnosed with a potentially terminal disease. Cat lovers present their sick cats to veterinarians seeking help. Many pet owners are offended by the "knee jerk" suggestion of euthanasia for their sick or elderly cat. Society wants something between cure versus kill. They are really seeking and deserve compassionate care and expertise in end-of-life issues.

A good working definition of euthanasia is, "The act or method of causing a painless and peaceful death, so as to end suffering: to deal with those dying of incurable, painful diseases." It is crucial to refrain from suggesting or insisting on euthanasia if the client declines definitive or ideal therapy for their cat. *Clients come to veterinarians for advice. Clients do not expect nor do they want veterinari-*

ans to euthanize their terminally ill cat prematurely without exhausting reasonable options. Offer the client more resourceful options. Inform clients that pain relief and a good quality of life are paramount. Start with pain relief and comfort care. This gives the family more choice and time to do their own research so they can make an informed decision regarding therapy that will satisfy their particular situation. Clients may feel that the recommended ideal procedures must be pursued as an "all-or-none" option. Other clients may be confused because their cat's overall prognosis was poor regardless of which therapy was elected. Veterinarians may say that the cat is in pain, yet the cat may be discharged without adequate pain control or supportive home care recommendations. It is important for veterinarians to know that many cat owners feel dismissed, abandoned, unsupported, and disappointed at this juncture because of lack of care when they need care most. Offering Pawspice care will certainly help to keep our profession more heartfelt, cherished, and celebrated in the eyes of the public. Caring for the feline species' unique needs requires a special form of medical finesse that is greatly needed and appreciated by those who love their cats.[12]

Once the practice is comfortable with the philosophy behind Pawspice, start booking appointments to explain and teach Pawspice care. Through examination room consultations, veterinarians and nursing staff can gracefully and kindly provide the education and support needed for the efficient home-care of ailing cats on a fee-for-service basis. Pet owners will gladly pay for the education that facilitates the control of pain and the art of providing good nutritional and hydration support for their pet. These consultation and demonstration sessions give clients the ability to care for their terminal feline friends with expertise. Daily, weekly, or monthly rechecks and home-care are essential for monitoring and fine-tuning care of the Pawspice patient.

Finally, delete the use of insensitive terms such as "disposal" on all hospital release forms, euthanasia forms, and invoices. Revise the terms for this service with more sensitivity. Clients feel insulted with the literal translation that their deceased cat's body will be disposed of. If the forms in your hospital contain this offensive terminology, be sure to cross it out. Use words such as "making arrangements" for private cremation, group cremation, or burial.

INGREDIENTS FOR PAWSPICE PROGRAMS

Willingness is the essential ingredient to look for in oneself, in the hospital staff, and in the pet owner. Organize a special Pawspice staff meeting. Ask these questions "Do we want to be a compassionate veterinary care facility that offers a Pawspice program? Does the nursing and reception staff agree with the Pawspice philosophy? Is there value in making efforts to preserve the bond between our clients and their terminal pets?"

Find the most interested and willing technician or staff member in your clinic's Pawspice team and invite them to lead the group. You might explain that the position will rotate periodically to prevent compassion fatigue.

Regardless of who is appointed as the leader, if a staff member has a friendly or neighborly relationship with a particular client, then that person should be the Pawspice liaison between the owner and the hospital.

Instruct clients to direct phone calls to a designated staff member or the Pawspice support team. Nursing staff can be trained to handle most of the phone calls regarding home-care problems and maintenance for the best quality of life under the circumstances.

The next ingredient to look for is satisfaction. Ask the client if they are satisfied with their cat's Pawspice care. Ask the staff if they are satisfied with the level of care and supervision that they are providing. Does the client need more help with home-care visits? To assess satisfaction, schedule regular Pawspice rechecks every 5 to 14 days so that the patient can be evaluated properly. At each recheck, the nursing staff can start by reviewing the Quality of Life Scale and using the scoring system to assess the cat's Pawspice. The attending veterinarian should monitor the Pawspice cat's weight, hydration, and health status. The veterinarian should answer major questions to the client's satisfaction. Ask this question at the end of the visit: "Is there anything else we can help you with?" Based on findings during the examination, the doctor can make the necessary changes in care recommendations and prescription medications. If the cat's status has improved or has been stable, be sure to rejoice with the client. Many Pawspice visits can be very upbeat and full of encouragement if the patient is stable and enjoying life. If the cat has lost weight, or has worsened, counsel the family so they realize the decline and help them understand the end may be near.

Veterinarians now work within the paradigm of the pediatrician model and have the social responsibility to provide emotional support to their distressed clients. There may be conflict in the family about how attached the main caregiver is to their Pawspice cat. Some family members feel inconvenienced with the soiling and odors, and the sacrifice, sadness, or diverted attention of the exhausted caregiver. This issue of disapproval creates a double-edged sword with which the patient's main caregiver must deal on a daily basis. It is best to address this issue directly with the family so that they can come to a supportive consensus. If the issue goes beyond the veterinarian's personal counseling ability, it is best to refer them to a family counselor for help. Willingness and satisfaction are the most positive ingredients to make Pawspice a good experience for everyone involved.

VALIDATE "THE BOND"

Each member of the veterinary team must be helpful, kind, and respectful during Pawspice. It is essential for staff members to acquire good communication skills to properly counsel and comfort the emotions of the clients to help them face the final days with their feline best friend. Front desk staff, room attendants, and nurses should be informed to be especially considerate and accommodating to Pawspice clients. Their behavior should be focused to help support the emotional needs of sensitive clients who must say goodbye to their highly bonded pet. Staff members can play an important role to uplift the emotions of sad cat owners by validating their special bond with a few words of empathy such as, "We know that you share a special bond with Fluffy and that you love Fluffy very much."

RECOGNIZE ANTICIPATORY GRIEF

It is important to recognize that some pet owners will be suffering from the torment and anguish of anticipatory grief. Many pet owners do not realize that they are cheating themselves out of enjoyment with their cat because they are so upset. They may respond with a wide range of emotions from panic all the way to shut-down (see Chapter 72).

A trained staff can help these clients by suggesting that they focus on communication with their cat and value the good parts of each day. Point out that the Pawspice cat is still very much alive and actually with them now. Guide clients to feel "an attitude of gratitude" for knowing that these are precious days. Don't let clients be cheated by the angst of anticipatory grief. Say something like this, "We don't want you to cheat yourself from enjoying these precious days with Fluffy. Anticipatory grief takes the joy of the moment away from you. Try your best to focus on Fluffy right now because he is still here."

FEARFUL OWNERS

Some pet owners cringe at the sight of needles and can not handle the thought of giving injections to their cat. Many feline Pawspice patients need subcutaneous fluids to maintain hydration, especially with concurrent renal disease, hypercalcemia, or other electrolyte imbalances. For many, the thought of using a feeding tube to maintain a Pawspice cat is "over the top." Feeding tubes may sound like heroic measures to one person and make perfect sense to another. Let clients know that feeding tubes are used routinely for cats to provide them with proper nutrition during recovery from hepatic lipidosis, oral surgery, or radiation therapy to the oral cavity (see Chapter 12).

Staff can approach the fear of needles with cheerful teaching. It is truly important to always speak to the Pawspice caregiver in a tender, unhurried fashion, because that person most likely is under a tremendous amount of personal, financial, and emotional stress. Ask the owner to consider the usefulness of a pen. Its function is to transfer information to the chart. Explain that the syringe with its needle is like a pen, which transfers medications to the cat without having to struggle with the cat's objections to the oral medications. Consider the syringe to be a tool like a pen and nothing to be afraid of. It is best to give demonstrations using saline and ask the pet owner to actually give mock injections to their cat in the office. If the client is clumsy or reluctant, have them practice at home using syringes to inject teriyaki sauce into chicken or Grand Marnier into strawberries. Practicing will bring confidence.

House call visits are essential for caregivers who are unable to deal with administering injections and subcutaneous fluids to their Pawspice cat. Keep a list for the reception staff that identifies which cats are on Pawspice programs, so they can be sensitive when family members call in for information, updates, appointments, or general concerns. Be sure that Pawspice clients get priority access to appointments with the veterinarian on duty.

EDUCATING CLIENTS FOR HOME CARE

Many pet owners want to nurse their terminally ill cat at home. The veterinary team can train clients to provide their cat with excellent home care. It is obvious that cats are better off psychosocially at home than in the hospital. The most important factors to educate home caregivers to monitor confidently are quality of life (see Table 78-1), minimal pain, adequate nutrition, hydration and respiration, and detection of sepsis. Ask the question, "If this pet owner were trained to take their cat's temperature, administer subcutaneous fluids and necessary injections, and to provide the proper pain control, oral medications, sufficient food, and hygiene, would this cat have some well being and live longer at home?"

Each client has unique inhibitions and concerns that can challenge the veterinary team to tailor client training sessions accordingly. Clients need to know how to maintain their cat's finer points of hygiene and physical maintenance. Most highly bonded cat owners, especially those on a budget, are very motivated and show great fortitude and interest in learning how to administer injections, subcutaneous fluids, oral medications, and nursing care to their pets. They need and want this knowledge for their cat's convenience.

Home care for a cat with incontinence or paresis is a task certain pet owners are willing to provide. They need advice regarding special ramps, soft bedding, and extra towels and diapers. Some cats might need frequent bandage changes. Some will need to have their bladders expressed. Incontinent cats, or those with uncontrollable diarrhea, need frequent bathing to avoid urine scald or fecal contamination. Cats with oral tumors need extra washing of the face, the front legs, and the paws to control odor and matting from thick, fetid salivation and drooling. Cats with head and neck tumors must have effective pain management.

Some Pawspice cats have compromised respiration induced by asthma, heart disease, pulmonary metastases, lymphoma, chylothorax, and other cardiopulmonary diseases. Many owners are willing to acquire portable oxygen units to help their cats breathe more comfortably at home. Instruct the client to use a stethoscope at home. Show them how to monitor respiration rates and to listen for troubled breathing and fluid sounds. Pet owners must realize that dyspnea is painful.

Some clients get distressed when they see a tumor growing. They actually think that if the tumor ruptures, their cat will die. Comfort fearful clients with a kind, soothing tone, and assure them that it would be unusual for this to happen and that, at worst, the tumor might develop an ulcer or drain some necrotic tissue and that there may be a limited discharge like a sliced tomato.

The sight and smell of blood and discharges from epistaxis, oozing wounds, or body orifices may cause some people to overreact with a paralyzing fear or nervousness and disgust. Pawspice cats might be plagued with these problems from radiation therapy–induced mucositis and desquamation, vascular slough sites, ulcerated tumors, and decubital ulcers. Others cringe if they have to watch the nurses give injections or provide medical procedures. These problems might be solved with frequent technician house calls, daily rechecks for bandage changes, or hospitalization. Arrange technician house calls to assist the owner for a reasonable desensitization period until they can get a home-care routine established. Suggest air fresheners, incense, placing the pet's bed near an open window, or placing a low-level fan that will blow the odors out of the house when possible.

This author recalls one Pawspice cat with bladder cancer belonging to a woman whose boyfriend was a house-call veterinarian. Her cat had chronic loose stools and no fecal or bladder control, causing a strong odor in the home. She could not euthanize her perky feline friend and he could not validate her tenacity for the cat or tolerate visiting because of the stench. We suggested using newborn baby diapers, probiotics, and a novel diet, which made a significant difference in quality of life and the environment. This respite allowed the couple to reconcile during the cat's Pawspice.

QUALITY OF LIFE SCALE HELPS DECISION-MAKING

It is important to have good tools to assess various aspects of quality of life for aging, ailing, and terminally ill cats. Veterinarians frequently are asked, "When is the right time to euthanize my beloved pet? How will I know?" Advise the family that their cat will give a sign such as unresponsive vomiting, diarrhea, trouble breathing, crying, a drop in mentation, a moribund state, or more bad days than good days. Put clients at ease by saying something like this, "We will help you make the decision, but you will probably know the right time because Fluffy will tell you with a look or a gesture, a sign, or a series of bad days" (see Chapter 72). The proposed Quality of Life Scale presented in Table 78-1 may help everyone, especially those in denial, to look at issues that are difficult to face. Clients can use this itemized scale to ask themselves if they are able to provide enough help to maintain their cat in the proper manner and cleanliness.

Cats have certain needs and desires that should be recognized and respected. If we can meet these basic needs and desires at a satisfactory level, then we are justified in preserving the cat's life during its steady decline toward death. The Quality of Life Scale provides an easy guideline for assessment of the cat so that pet owners can maintain a rewarding relationship that nurtures the human animal bond. Continuous review of the Quality of Life Scale will relieve guilt feelings and engender the support of the veterinary team to actively help in the care and decision making for end-of-life "Pawspice" patients.

It is up to the veterinary profession and to the pet's individual caretaker to design a Pawspice program that addresses each factor and deals with it openly and honestly. There may be other basic desires that need the attention of both healer and caretaker, but use these criteria as a start.

USING THE HHHHHMM QUALITY OF LIFE SCALE

Think of this scale as the 5-H scale, "HHHHHMM," so it is easy to remember the pet's needs and desires: *Hurt, Hunger, Hydration, Hygiene, Happiness, Mobility,* and *More* good days than bad days. Score patients from 0 to 10 for each criterion. A score of 5 or above for each of these criteria would be acceptable for maintaining a good Pawspice. Each cat's situation needs to be customized. Each pet owner needs to be recognized as an individual who needs a kind, supportive coaching approach to come to terms with the decision to end a best friend's life.

HURT: 0-10

No hurt: Pain control is first and foremost on the scale. This includes the cat's ability to breathe properly. Most people do not realize that not being able to breathe is ranked at the top of the pain scale in human medicine. Cats with pulmonary effusion need thoracentesis on an as-needed basis. Pet owners need to be trained to monitor their pet's respirations and comfort level and to identify dyspnea so that they do not wait too long to provide relief. Some families are willing to provide oxygen therapy at home for their ailing pets. The veterinarian can prescribe oxygen through a medical supply house. Pain control may include oral, transdermal, and injectable medications. Pain control must be given preemptively, because cats do not communicate their pain very clearly and may be suffering silently without their family's awareness.[2]

HUNGER: 0-10

No hunger: If the cat is not getting adequate nutrition with hand-feeding, coaxing, or force-feeding, then placement of a feeding tube must be considered (see Chapter 12). Cats do very well with esophageal feeding tubes. Malnutrition develops quickly in sick cats when the caretaker is not adequately educated to know how much their cat must eat to maintain body weight. Instruct owners to use a blender or liquid diets to help their cat maintain proper nutritional and caloric intake. Many cats will live much longer if offered a variety of wholesome, flavorful foods. It takes patience and gentle concentrated coaxing to get some Pawspice cats to eat. It is hard not to be disappointed when such specially prepared food is rejected.

Just come back with another offering with a different flavor a little later and that meal may be more appealing to the patient. Appetite stimulators such as mirtazapine given PO q72h and monthly Depo-Provera injections can be very helpful in selected patients.

HYDRATION: 0-10

No hydration problems: Educate pet owners about adequate fluid intake per kilogram body weight (22 mL/kg/24h) and to assess for hydration by the pinch method. Subcutaneous fluids are a wonderful way to supplement the fluid intake of ailing pets. It may take a few demonstration sessions for a pet owner to learn how to administer SQ fluids. This helpful procedure saves the client a lot of money and keeps the pet much healthier. Giving SQ fluids can make a very significant difference in quality of life during Pawspice.

HYGIENE: 0-10

Is the sick cat brushed and clean? Is the coat matted? Is the cat able to use the litter box independently or with help? Can the cat be situated properly to avoid soiling after eliminations? Cats with oral cancer, especially squamous cell carcinoma of the tongue, are unable to keep themselves clean. Cats become demoralized when they are dirty. The odor associated with necrotic, oral tumors can be offensive and cause social rejection by family members. Use long-acting injectable antibiotics such as cefovecin (Convenia) to help reduce foul-smelling infections. Dampen a sponge with a very dilute solution of lemon juice and hydrogen peroxide and gently stroke the cat's face, paws and legs. This action is similar to a "mother tongue" and helps to clean the fur while soothing the unkempt cat.

HAPPINESS: 0-10

Is the cat able to experience any joy or mental stimulation? It is obvious to see that cats communicate with their eyes, their body language, and by vocalizing. Is the ailing cat willing to interact with the family and be responsive? Is the cat able to purr and enjoy being on the bed or in a family member's lap? Is there a response to a little catnip or to stroking with a feather? Can the cat bat at toys or look at and follow a laser light? Does the cat enjoy the upbeat greetings and petting of loving family members? Can the cat's bed be moved close to the family's activities and not left in an isolated or neglected area? Is the cat depressed, lonely, anxious, bored, or afraid? Is there a routine fun time that the cat looks forward to? Every good Pawspice program also should provide entertainment. Instruct cat owners to create routines for fun (doing the cat's favorite things). The cat actually may cheer up and began to look forward to these joyful events. This can be as simple as taking the cat outside to sit on the grass and soak up some sunshine. Try catnip and various cat toys to enchant the patient.

MOBILITY: 0-10

Is the cat able to move on its own or with help in order to satisfy basic desires? Does the cat want to hide under the bed or withdraw? Is the pet showing central nervous system signs, seizures, or stumbling? Can the cat be taken outdoors or helped into the litter box to eliminate with assistance? Will a harness be helpful? Is medication helping? If the cat is not able to walk without assistance, advise owners to provide regular assistance to help the cat into the litter box.

For cats, the mobility score is acceptable anywhere in the range from 0 to 10. The need for mobility seems dependent on the species and breed. Cats and small lap dogs can and do enjoy life with much less need for mobility than large and giant breed dogs. If the cat is only able to lie in bed, is there a schedule to change the position and rotate the body at least every 2 to 3 hours? Atelectasis and decubital ulcers must be avoided by frequent rotation and soft bedding. Can the cat's bed be moved around the house to be nearby at meal time and bedtime, so that the cat can be kept entertained in the family's company? Some cats with limited mobility may enjoy a good Pawspice if they are still alert and responsive.

MORE GOOD DAYS THAN BAD DAYS: 0-10

Ask if there are more good days than bad days. If there are more than a few bad days in a row, or if the cat seems to be "turned off" to life, the cat is too compromised to go on. Bad days are those filled with undesirable experiences such as vomiting, nausea, diarrhea, frustration, falling down, seizures, and other distressing events. Bad days could result from a condition that worsens such as cancer cachexia, the profound weakness from anemia, the discomfort caused by gradual tumor pressure or obstruction, or a large, inoperable tumor in the abdomen. If the two-way exchange needed to communicate and maintain a healthy human-animal bond is just not there, the pet owner must decide or be told gently that the end may be near.

It is very difficult for families to make the final decision to end a beloved pet's life by euthanasia. Coming to a decision about euthanasia is especially avoided when euthanasia is against the pet owner's religious beliefs. Sometimes they are not sure about the quality-of-life issues at the very end. It can be made clearer to them if the standard scale for Quality of Life is set ahead of time and reevaluated every week or two, or every few days or hours as the situation requires. If the pet is passing on slowly with a peaceful tranquility, then that may be a satisfactory situation. People often really want their pet to pass on naturally at home in their arms or in their own bed. That is appropriate, as long as the pet is just weakening steadily and not suffering terminally. As veterinarians we need to accept the fact that it is a very personal and natural wish when our clients request us to help their pet

to die naturally at home. We are the ones they turn to for help and we have an oath "to use our scientific knowledge and skills for the benefit of society through the protection of animal health and the relief of animal suffering." We can help our client's pet-loss needs and, at the same time, guarantee that the pet has a pain-free passage by using preemptive pain medications. Here is where a referral for home euthanasia with a kindly house-call veterinarian should be recommended. Hopefully, using this conceptualized user-friendly "HHHHHMM" scale for quality of life will facilitate the heart-wrenching decision that euthanasia truly is. Hopefully our professional guidance can help relieve the angst and regret about a beloved pet's death that often haunts pet owners for the rest of their lives. (See Chapter 72 for a discussion on the use of the Rule of Three in helping owners make decisions concerning euthanasia.)

SPECIFIC DISEASE CONDITIONS

RENAL FAILURE

Cats with end-stage chronic kidney disease (CKD) may be fed special modified diets such as Hill's Feline k/d or home-cooked diets (see Chapter 13) to prolong survival. Affected cats may enjoy a better quality of life if they are supported with educated home Pawspice care, which may include subcutaneous fluids, supplemental potassium (Tumil-K), H_2-blockers (famotidine), phosphate binders (Amphojel), vitamins—especially water-soluble vitamins, and fatty acids (safflower oil or fish oils).[13] Schedule rechecks with laboratory profiles and complete blood counts to monitor renal function, acidosis, and anemia. Erythropoietin, 1000 IU SQ q24h for 3 consecutive days and then weekly, may be used to normalize hematocrit (see Chapter 66).[14,15] One cat with CKD in this author's practice survived 6 happy years at home on daily subcutaneous fluids, passing away at age 22.

INFLAMMATORY INTESTINAL, HEPATIC, AND PANCREATIC DISEASE

Older cats may be afflicted with concurrent inflammatory liver disease, lymphocytic pancreatitis, and inflammatory bowel disease. Pawspice cats with these concurrent problems may be treated palliatively with subcutaneous fluids, oral potassium gluconate, vitamin E, prednisolone, metronidazole, Actigall, pancreatic enzymes, L-carnitine, lactulose, S-adenosylmethionine, SQ vitamin K_1, and prophylactic antimicrobial agents, and feeding tube placement for anorexic cats if vomiting can be controlled[2,16] (see Chapters 12 and 19).

DIABETES MELLITUS

Needle-shy owners of diabetic cats may prefer to use oral hypoglycemic therapy. Be sure to offer this option, because one third of nonketoacidotic cats with early diabetes mellitus may respond to oral therapy and a change to a high-protein diet such as Hill's m/d or a home-prepared meat-based diet (see Chapter 13). The cat is better served when the attending veterinarian listens to the client's concerns and remains sufficiently flexible to help the cat while prioritizing the client's concerns. If hyperglycemia is not controlled with oral medication and diet change, the owner may be more inclined to try an effective injectable insulin therapy as a second choice[12] (see Chapter 27).

ANOREXIA

Anorexic cats may respond to the administration of mirtazapine at 3.75 mg PO q72h. Pawspice cats may need to be hand-fed, coaxed, or force-fed. Staff must teach clients carefully and enthusiastically the proper technique to best hand-feed their ill cat. Cats like their food warmed to body temperature. Expanding oral neoplasia disrupts structures causing infection, loose teeth, ulceration, and pain. Squamous cell carcinoma of the tongue in cats renders the tongue stiff and nonfunctional and causes early starvation despite efforts to eat. If a cat can not or will not eat, it is best to recommend a percutaneous esophageal feeding tube if the upper gastrointestinal tract is functional. This procedure was described originally in 1993.[17] The esophagostomy tube placement procedure may be performed under a short anesthetic with minimal risk[9] (see Chapter 12). After the esophagostomy feeding tube is in place, the cat must be fed successfully with a liquefied diet several times in the hospital. It is essential that a discharge appointment be scheduled for a demonstration on how and what to feed the cat. Select the most informative and helpful nurse/technician for this important discharge teaching appointment. Allow the owner to call their teaching nurse at the hospital for clarification and further instructions. If the nurse who gives this demonstration is accessible to the client by phone, they will be more at ease during the first few days as they adjust to feeding their Pawspice cat with the feeding tube. The diet and supplements for feeding must be detailed in writing on a calendar. The client must know how to avoid clogging the tube. Follow-up calls over the next few days must ensure that the cat is getting enough calories and liquid to maintain body weight. For clogged feeding tubes, instruct the owner to use Sprite or seltzer water to dissolve the clog. Create a treatment schedule for every day of the week, which shows the morning and evening requirements for medications, chemotherapy, amounts of fluid, feeding volumes, and supplements. A written schedule is invaluable for caregivers to keep track of the many medications and supplements that many Pawspice cats require.[7]

NASAL CANCER

Cats with facial deformity and nighttime stridor may be palliated with multimodality pain management using nonsteroidal antiinflammatory drugs such as piroxicam, carprofen, or meloxicam, and gabapentin and an opioid.

Many cats will sleep more comfortably and with less stridor if they receive late night sedation with diazepam, buprenorphine, nalbuphine, or butorphanol.[2]

PARALYSIS

Paralyzed cats may benefit from a wide range of resourceful rehabilitation techniques and home-care items such as ramps to bypass the stairs or to get up on the bed or window sill. Some cats will benefit from rehabilitation slings for assistance while walking, chest and rump lifts to help them stand up, and canvas suspension hammocks. Soft cloth foot covers help to prevent abnormal wearing and ulcers of the metacarpal and metatarsal areas and pads.

DECUBITAL ULCERS

Recumbent cats may be able to avoid decubital ulcers if thoughtful advanced planning includes soft padding, waterbeds, and egg crate mattresses, all with washable covers. Frequent and complete cleaning of the pet's coat and skin is important if the cat is being soiled by urine or feces. If the cat enjoys time outdoors, extreme caution must be taken to prevent fly strike and maggots. Be especially vigilant to look for wounds or maggots in longhair breeds.

BLADDER CANCER

Affected cats may live many months on palliative chemotherapy.[9] It helps to apply diapers or Pampers when the cat is in the house and keep the bed close to the litter pan. This helps the family to endure their pet's problems of stranguria and pollakiuria. If the hematuria is sufficiently severe to cause extreme blood loss, measures to control the hemorrhage are justified. Mix a 1 per cent solution of formalin with a vial of the topical ear solution Synotic, which contains dimethylsulfoxide, and instill the solution into the bladder with a urinary catheter. Keep the mixture in the bladder for 10 to 15 minutes and then void and flush out the clots.[7] This palliative procedure may reduce the hematuria for 7 to 10 days and it may be repeated as indicated. Selected patients with a tumor obstructing urine outflow at the trigone may benefit from a prepubic cystostomy. The cat will leak urine, so it is important to place modified (cut a hole for the tail) newborn baby diapers regularly on the cat. Owners are instructed to void the patient's bladder three to four times a day into the used diaper before changing it. The stoma bypasses the obstruction and maintains a quality of life for selected cats. Piroxicam, 1 mg PO q24h, also has been shown to increase survival times. This author uses mitoxantrone, 4.5 mg/m^2 IV every 21 to 30 days on a 0.5 mg dose escalation schedule not to exceed 6 mg/m^2. It is important to monitor the cat hematologically during the nadir at 7 to 10 days. It also is important to take a complete blood count and platelet count, and to check kidney function, before each treatment. (See

Chapter 51 for a discussion on cancer of the urinary tract.)

BRAIN TUMORS

Cats with brain tumors, who experience periodic seizures, may be able to stay at home with confidence and with fewer emergency visits if the pet owner is given instructions to use injectable diazepam. Instruct the client to introduce diazepam at 0.2 to 0.4 mg/kg into the nasal passages as nose drops or into the rectum as a suppository to control seizures. Prednisone, 5 mg PO q12h, and lomustine, 2.5 mg PO q48h for three to four doses and repeated every 4 to 6 weeks, may be administered. The patient must be monitored for leukopenia before each cycle of lomustine therapy. Oil of Evening Primrose (4 capsules daily), OM-3 fatty acids, and fish oils are reasonable palliative supplements, which complement this author's Pawspice protocol for feline brain tumors[3,7] (see Chapter 55 for a discussion of brain tumors).

If seizure control is not achieved with medication, the cat's quality of life is compromised, forcing the family to yield to hospitalization for intravenous anesthesia. If the patient can not be stabilized, the kindest option would be to provide the gift of euthanasia to release the cat from further suffering. Be sure to counsel families about placing special and clear DNR (Do Not Resuscitate) orders for their Pawspice cat in the event of cardiac or respiratory arrest (see Chapter 54 for a discussion of seizure control).

"PP" was an 18-year-old female Siamese cat who had had two previous brain surgeries. A large meningioma was removed at the first surgery. A recurrent mass was removed in a second surgery 2 years later when PP was 16 years old. PP again developed clinical signs of recurrence of blindness, tremors, and disorientation and was presented to this author for a second opinion. Pawspice and palliative therapy were chosen using the brain tumor protocol and Pawspice care protocol discussed above. The family was pleased with PP's response and she remained at home for 6 more months.

Temozolomide, the oral form of the alkylating agent, dacarbazine, is used in the treatment of human patients with anaplastic astrocytomas. At this writing, there are no published data about the use of temozolomide in cats with brain tumors or lymphoma; however, it may be useful. It is this author's intention to use valproic acid and temozolomide in a metronomic (continuous low-dose) therapy protocol as palliation for brain tumors in cats. Valproic acid (VPA) is used in children to prevent seizures. Valproic acid has anticancer function as a histone deacetylase (HDAC) inhibitor and it enhances chemosensitivity. The relatively low toxicity profiles and ease of oral administration make both of these drugs qualify as good candidate drugs that may be useful to further palliate Pawspice cats diagnosed with brain tumors.

REFRACTORY VOMITING

Cat owners experience anxiety and frustration when their cat has refractory vomiting. If the normal first-line anti-emetic drugs such as metoclopramide fail to control vomiting, then use drugs that influence the chemoreceptor trigger zone. Maropitant (Cerenia), administered by injection or orally q24h, may be very effective in the control of vomiting for Pawspice cats, especially if chemotherapy-induced. (Clients must be notified that maropitant is labeled for use in dogs only.) Cats with refractory vomiting may need hospitalization for intravenous therapy with maropitant, ondansetron, or dolasetron. The injectable solution of ondansetron or dolasetron also may be given orally or mixed with a palatable substrate such as yogurt, baby food, or Hill's Feline a/d (see Chapter 21 for discussion of antiemetic drugs).

PAIN

Chronic and moderate pain may be controlled with transmucosal administration of 90 μg of injectable buprenorphine q6-7h. Opioid-like drugs such as butorphanol and diluted nalbuphine injectable solution may control visceral and somatic pain in cats. Nalbuphine is an inexpensive generic opioid-like drug similar to butorphanol. It provides pain control without the typical sedation effects that accompany most of the powerful opioid analgesic drugs. Nalbuphine doses for cats range from 0.2 to 0.5 mg/kg. For dispensing, dilute 1 mL of the injectable solution with 9 mL of sterile water in a sterile 10-mL vial. Instruct the owner to give 0.1 mL SQ or PO q1-6 h as needed. Nalbuphine is not registered under the controlled substance regulations and may be of great value in pain management for Pawspice cats. Fentanyl transdermal patches are now available in a 12.5 μg size. This smaller size provides a more reliable delivery rate for cats and is effective for two to four days. Using multimodality pain management for severe pain is essential for a good feline Pawspice. Add gabapentin at 25 to 100 mg PO q12h and a nonsteroidal antiinflammatory drug such as meloxicam (Metacam, 1.5 mg/mL) at one drop (0.05 mg) per 1.8 kg body weight PO q24h for multimodal therapy.[2,5,18]

Cats with oral tumors have severe pain on manipulation of the mouth. Therefore they should not be given oral medications or be force-fed. Instead, recommend to the client that a feeding tube be placed so that pain medications and food delivery will not stress the patient. Show the client how to give injections through the rubber port of the Venoset tubing during subcutaneous fluid administration. Use a long-acting injectable antibiotic such as cefovecin with a duration of efficacy of up to 14 days. Use compounding pharmacies to prepare selective medications for transdermal administration. (See Chapter 18 in the fifth volume of this series for a discussion on transdermal therapeutics.) Be resourceful and observant for breakthrough pain, and medicate appropriately.

DIARRHEA

Cats in Pawspice often are afflicted with soft, loose stools. Abnormal stools may result from the illness itself, the treatment, or from eating a highly variable diet from day to day. The concurrent use of multiple medications and erratic food intake may cause bacterial overgrowth, soft or loose stools, and irregular elimination times. It is difficult for some pet owners to manage their cat's loose feces if their cat fails to use the litter box. Practical suggestions include feeding baby food rice cereal mix with an easily digestible recovery diet (Hill's Prescription Diet a/d) and adding more fiber (psyllium, oatmeal, millet) to the diet. Symptomatic treatment using probiotics (see Chapter 11) in combination with metronidazole or tylosin may alleviate the problem. Encourage the caregiver to keep the cat clean with frequent wiping or bathing. (The reader is referred to Chapters 8 and 22 for further discussion on the nutritional and therapeutic management of chronic diarrhea, respectively).

IMMUNONUTRITION AND CHEMOPREVENTION

Palliative care for feline Pawspice candidates often includes nutritional supplements and nutraceuticals. Immunonutrition is an emerging field that supports the concept that diet can actively influence the immune system, which is altered or depressed with age, stress, and nutritional deficiencies.[13] Chemoprevention involves the use of natural or synthetic compounds that may reverse or suppress the process of carcinogenesis, metastasis, and recurrence. Most cats who undergo surgery, chemotherapy, or radiation therapy are still considered to be at moderate to high risk for recurrence of their cancer. A majority of these cats are expected to have recurrence of their disease or die from metastases within 4 to 12 months, with cats who have mammary cancer, vaccine-associated sarcoma, or lymphoma falling into this group. Cats who have inflammatory bowel disease, or are infected with feline leukemia virus and/or feline immunodeficiency virus are at greater risk of developing illness or cancer. These cats, including frail elderly cats, are candidates for palliative Pawspice and may derive benefit from immunonutrition and chemoprevention. Some of the most commonly used immunonutrition agents are derived from mushrooms, such as *Agaricus blasei*, which enhance the immune system. This author also uses lymphocyte T-cell modulator (T-Cyte, Imulan Biotherapeutics), which acts as a T-cell growth factor in cats to enhance T-cell function. OM-3 fatty acids from fish oil have antineoplastic and antiinflammatory effects. Some of the most commonly used chemoprevention agents used in cats are nonsteroidal antiinflammatory drugs such as piroxicam, 1 mg PO q24h, and meloxicam, one drop (0.05 mg)/1.8 kg body weight PO q24h. Because these nonsteroidal antiinflammatory drugs also control pain, they provide dual benefits in Pawspice as long as the cat is not on concurrent corticosteroid therapy.

INTERNET AND NETWORKING

Ask clients if they would like to exchange phone numbers or share their e-mail addresses with another person providing Pawspice care for their cat. This gives owners the opportunity to share their experiences. Clients often use the Internet for information that brings them comfort and support. Dr. Kathleen Carson and volunteer, Christine Grey, both originally from this author's facility, started a chat room on America on Line (AOL) for owners of cats with chronic kidney disease. This informative chat room opens every Sunday at 5:00 PM (PST) and is listed in private chat room, "CRF." This type of on-line networking is very helpful for detailed information and for mutual support and it is a wonderful time saver for the clinic staff.

DAY CARE

Daily help for Pawspice cats can be provided conveniently by the clinic of the primary care veterinarian or a boarding facility while the owners are at work. This service may include taking the pet's temperature and weight, bathing and brushing the soiled pet, administering subcutaneous fluids and injectable medications, and hand feedings. This service can be the key to sustaining a quality Pawspice for the working pet owner. Convenient monthly billing and drop-off and pick-up times that revolve around the owner's schedule may be prearranged with attending staff members before and after regular receiving hours.

EUTHANASIA FOR THE PAWSPICE CAT

More families are expressing the wish for their beloved cat to pass away naturally at home. Explain to the family that natural death may not go smoothly and that it may be unfair to some cats. The slow decline of a sick cat may be too difficult for all family members to accompany all the way to the end of the cat's life. It is best to establish plans A, B, C, and D. Plan A would be that their cat passes peacefully and painlessly at home. Plan B would be house-call euthanasia. Plan C would be euthanasia at the attending doctor's hospital during the day, and Plan D would be euthanasia at an emergency clinic nearby.

When the time approaches for the cat to be euthanized humanely, the emotional pain for the family may be softened if they know that the procedure can be performed at any time of the day or night. Arrangements must be made in advance to cover the patient's needs 24 hours a day. Referrals for house calls, night calls, and after-hour emergency room facilities need to be established so that the decision time for euthanasia is made on behalf of the pet, not the doctor's office hours.

When the time comes for the emotional pain of euthanasia, caregivers who are in a Pawspice program are enabled to make the best decision for the pet. If they are going to bring the dying cat to a facility for euthanasia, ask them to bring their cat's favorite blanket and a candle, and family or friends and other pets, to share in the final goodbye. If the clinic does not have a comfort room, a gentler atmosphere can be created if overhead lights can be softened or turned off and a smaller room lamp turned on. Another option is to turn off the overhead lights in the examination room and turn on the radiograph viewbox to give the room softer lighting. Light a candle and present it to the family during this last visit to show reverence and respect at this time. This author brings flowers and green leaves into the room and places a few near or on the cat's body. Be sure to make arrangements for payment or billing prior to the procedure to avoid undue stress.

The next step in the euthanasia process is to sedate the cat in the presence of the owner. Administering a sedative to the cat allows people to relax while their pet falls gently into sedation. To avoid emesis associated with medetomidine hydrochloride, this author gives a subcutaneous injection of butorphanol as a pretreatment 5 to 10 minutes before administering medetomidine intramuscularly. This allows that big first step of physical separation to be easy for the family to see as they watch their beloved cat fall slowly into a relaxed sleep. Pet owners often comment that they sensed that their cat seemed very peaceful with the sedative. At this time it is kind to ask if each person in the room wants to stay for the final injection. Many families are content to leave their cat in the sedated state with complete trust that euthanasia will be painless and fast. If family members want to be present for the final injection, place a towel over the cat's body to cover the chest area up to the neck. Explain to them that the next injection will not hurt because of the heavy sedation. Also, tell the owners that the injection will be administered directly into the heart and will cause the heart to stop beating; however, there may be reflexive breathing and even a sigh after their cat has passed.

At this time, it is this author's preference to gently lift the towel near the ribs, palpate for heart beats and then give the final euthanasia solution directly into the heart while the family strokes the pet's head lovingly. Some feline practitioners and house-call veterinarians prefer to give the final injection intraperitoneally. The patient takes longer to pass by this method, but the passing is peaceful. Most importantly, there is no struggle to place a catheter or to identify a vein.

Many house-call veterinarians have found this method of sedation and euthanasia to be of great relief to them. House-call doctors often are the providers of Pawspice care services and they have the sad job of many home euthanasia visits.[11] The task of placing an intravenous catheter in the home environment can be extremely challenging. The house-call veterinarian now can bypass the ritual of using an intravenous catheter and use the simpler, more humane presedation and delivery of euthanasia by intracardiac or intraperitoneal injection, as described. The veterinarian then can leave the house while the family conducts their own wake. Clients can be referred to a cremation service that will pick up the pet's remains from their home in a timely fashion.[19]

Many academic institutions teach students that euthanasia must be given as an intravenous injection through an indwelling catheter (see Chapter 72). The catheter often must be placed into the cat only moments before the euthanasia procedure. This exercise runs against the sensitivity and philosophy of Pawspice. Catheter placement may be traumatic for the dying cat behind the scenes. It is best not to take near-death cats away from their grief-stricken owners even for 1 minute. Most near death cats are often anemic, hypovolemic, or hypotensive, and the catheter placement may not go smoothly.

If catheter placement causes any struggle or discomfort for the cat in the last few minutes of life, everyone involved in the process feels distressed. That struggle would be too difficult for caring staff nurses to witness repeatedly, even though the pet owner is not present. Placing that last catheter is a betrayal to the pet. The catheter is placed to make the job of the veterinarian easier at the expense of the pet and family.

All veterinarians should rethink and redesign their procedure for euthanasia. Think only about making every last moment of life easiest for the patient and family. Use subcutaneous or intramuscular sedation as step one. Allow the cat to fall asleep comfortably in the arms of the grieving family as step two. Then, when the cat is completely sedated and pain free, use intravenous, intracardiac, or intraperitoneal delivery of the euthanasia solution as the final step.

ALLOW TIME TO HONOR THE CAT'S LIFE

After the family members are gently assured that their cat's heart has stopped beating, it is appropriate and thoughtful to encourage them to stay and view their deceased cat. This provides special time for a "wake." There is not enough reverence, service, ceremony, or emotional support that can be offered to the family on the occasion of the death of the family cat by the veterinary profession. Providing excellent care for patients is not enough. It is the recognition of the bond between them that holds clients to veterinarians.

As Pawspice becomes commonplace across the country, more hospitals will set aside softly lit rooms for thoughtful euthanasia and afterlife services such as pet wakes on the occasion of a pet's passing. The "wake" time is the special time to read poems and talk compassionately about how important and sweet this dear beloved pet was to its family. One book that is fitting for this situation is *Angel Whiskers*, a wonderful anthology of cat memorial poetry and stories edited by Laurel E. Hunt.

Encourage the family to read a few more poems. Invite them to spend as much time as they need in private to grieve alone with their deceased cat. Every 5 or 10 minutes, check in on the family and see if they need any assistance. Offer to clip a bit of the cat's fur and place it in a windowed envelope as a memento. Place the cat's name and date of birth and death on the envelope. This may be the best time to make a memorial plaster imprint of the deceased cat's paw. Pet owners often treasure these thoughtful gestures.

After the wake, escort the family outside the clinic. Ask them to sit down for a few minutes to regain their composure, especially the person who is the driver. Suggest that they take a personal day off work or take a walk by the seashore, or a lake or river where earth and water and sky meet. Suggest that they create a shrine at home, with pictures of their beloved cat and candles. Suggest that they write an e-mail tribute or a story about their cat that describes what made their relationship so meaningful, and send it to friends and family. Writing about the deceased cat is a big help for the closure process of grief.

THE VETERINARIAN-CLIENT BOND

Realize that your clients also are bonded to you and your staff. They have been coming into your facility and interacting with you for some time. Unfortunately, these interactions that are full of noble purpose will have an abrupt end after their beloved cat dies. When Pawspice comes to an end, there is a parting of meaningful connections and supportive relationships between the veterinary team and the patient's family. Suddenly, the enormity of the caregiving routine and the way things were are gone.

RESPOND TO CRISIS

At times, a client might say that they want to die when their cat dies. The first thing to do in a situation like this, whether on the phone or in the examination room, is to validate the importance of the cat in their life and then say something like this, "Cats were not designed to live as long as we do. They come to us with an internal time clock, like an hourglass, that runs out of life way before ours does. If you love a cat and if you have one to three pets at a time, you will have up to 27 heartbreaks in your lifetime." Let the client know how many pets you have and that you also have sad farewells.

It is appropriate for the Pawspice team to provide on-the-spot emotional and spiritual comfort with comments such as, "Some of the heartbreaks, like with Fluffy, will be harder than others. Take Fluffy's loss and each future loss in the perspective of your life as a person who will probably live to be 90 to 100 years old! Some say that pets like Fluffy come to us with a special mission on earth. Only you know what Fluffy's mission is, because it is very personal. Fluffy's illness and passing will teach you something about life and death that you did not want to know. But you will be a much deeper and richer person for learning this lesson. The love and joy that Fluffy gives you are the reasons for your deep sadness. The cycle of life is round and the highs are always balanced by the lows. Your sadness is a rich emotion, just as beautiful and rich as the love bond that you share with Fluffy."

Explain that euthanasia is a gift that allows animals to pass away with ease and dignity so they do not have to waste away and suffer to death. Recommend pet-loss counseling either in group bereavement sessions or with a qualified counselor. Cat owners in spiritual distress might benefit from the help of a spiritual counselor or pet chaplain. If the client displaying maladaptive grief was referred by another practice, it is the attending doctor's responsibility to inform the referring veterinarian. All involved should encourage the grief stricken owner to seek bereavement counseling. (See Chapter 72 for further discussion on facilitating client grief.)

POSTEUTHANASIA FOLLOW-UP

When a Pawspice patient dies, a little part of the practice goes with them. The staff will miss seeing the family with their cat because they were closely bonded to the practice. Send one or two sympathy cards with staff notes and signatures. Ask the pet owner to stop by the clinic soon and bring some pictures of their deceased cat. Put the client's e-mail address in the hospital's special cat lovers list to stay in contact.

It is appropriate for the veterinarian or the Pawspice nurse to call the client anywhere from a day or two to several weeks after their cat has passed to ask how things are going. This may be a difficult call for some veterinarians to make because it is not about medicine or a protocol. Ask the question, "How is your heart?" and say something like this, "I know you must be missing Fluffy very much. These days of pet loss are difficult and we just wanted you to know that we are thinking of you." Talking about the cat helps the bereaved person. If they are feeling troubled, offer emotional support or a referral to a pet loss counselor or a pet loss hot line. One very helpful tip to pass on to pet owners is to encourage tears and grief feelings, but limit the sad feelings to 30 minutes a day, preferably in the morning or the evening. This helps the pet owner face their work day with more clarity. Tell the pet owner that you and your staff miss them. Encourage clients to get back into the love cycle again by adopting a lovable homeless cat as soon as they are ready.

Staff also may say something like, "It would be hard to imagine you without little paw prints at your side." Invite the pet owner to come back and visit the hospital around their old appointment times or during staff lunch breaks with cookies and pictures. Unconditional kindness and compassion are essential ingredients for the bond-centered philosophy of Pawspice care.[3,20]

SIR WALTER SCOTT'S POEM

When a client enters their beloved cat into a Pawspice program or when euthanasia is being discussed, it is helpful to quote Sir Walter Scott's beautiful poem about the human-animal bond. The poem is featured in *Angel Whiskers* by Laurel Hunt.[21] With one changed word (dog to cat), this poem assuages the emotional pain of pet loss.

"I have sometimes thought of the final cause of cats having such short lives and I am quite satisfied it is in compassion to the human race; for if we suffer so much in loving a cat after an acquaintance of ten or twelve years, what would it be if they were to live double that time?"

REFERENCES

1. Choen SP, Fudin CE, editors: *Problems in veterinary medicine: animal illness and human emotion*, vol 3, Philadelphia, 1991, JB Lippincott.
2. Gaynor JS, Muir WW, editors: *Handbook of veterinary pain management*, St. Louis, 2009, Mosby.
3. Villalobos A: Conceptualized hospice for pet's last days: "Pawspice." Proceedings of the 137th AVMA Convention: 322, 2000.
4. Withrow S, Vail D, editors: *Small animal clinical oncology*, ed 4, Philadelphia, 2007, Saunders.

5. Ogilvie GK: Hospice and bond-centered practice: the future of veterinary care. Proceedings of the 17th ACVIM Forum, Chicago, 1999.

6. Hoskins JD, editor: *Geriatrics and gerontology of the dog and cat*, ed 2, Philadelphia, 2004, Saunders.

7. Villalobos A, Kaplan L: *Canine and feline geriatric oncology: honoring the human-animal bond*, Hoboken, NJ, 2007, Wiley-Blackwell.

8. Kent MS, Gordon IK: Veterinary radiation oncology: technology, imaging, intervention and future applications, Theilen Tribute Symposium, at http://cancer-therapy.org/CT6A/HTML/17._Gordon_and_Kent,_167-176.html.

9. Ogilvie GK, Moore AS: *Feline oncology*, Yardley, PA, 2001, Veterinary Learning Systems.

10. Morrison WB: *Cancer in dogs and cats: medical and surgical management*, ed 2, Jackson, WY, 2002, Teton New Media.

11. Fugimoto NS: *Kindred spirit, kindred care*, Novato, CA, 2005, New World Library.

12. Hodgkins EM: *Your cat: simple new secrets to a longer, stronger life*, New York, 2007, St. Martin's Press.

13. Satyaraj E: Immunonutrition. Nestle Purina Nutrition Forum, 2008.

14. Plotnick A: Anemia: treatment with erythropoietin, Manhattan Cat Specialists, 2006. Available at http://www.manhattancats.com/Articles/erythropoietin.html

15. Feline CRF, anemia, erythropoietin used to stimulate red blood cell production. Feline CRF Information Center, 2006. Available at http://www.felinecrf.com/meds0.htm

16. Hoskins J: *Feline "Triad disease" poses triple threat*. DVM Newsmagazine. February 2000, p 4S.

17. Rawlings C: Percutaneous placement of a midcervical esophagostomy tube: new technique and representative cases, *J Am Anim Hosp Assoc* 29:562, 1993.

18. De Lorimier LP, Fan TM: Understanding and recognizing cancer pain in dogs and cats: treating cancer pain in dogs and cats, *Vet Med* 352, May 2005.

19. Downing R: *Pets living with cancer: a pet owner's resource*, Denver, 2000, American Animal Hospital Association Press.

20. Lagoni L, Morehead D, Butler C: The bond-centered practice: the future of veterinary care. Proceedings of the 17th ACVIM Forum, Chicago, 1999.

21. Hunt LE: *Angel whiskers: reflections on loving and losing a feline companion*, New York, 2001, Hyperion Press.

79 Alternative Modalities in Feline Practice

Michele C. Gaspar

In an era when increasingly sophisticated medical diagnostic tests, advanced surgical procedures, and conventional therapeutics are widely available to feline patients, it may seem ironic that clients' interest in alternative modalities for their cats is increasingly keen. However, it is the rare feline practitioner who has not been asked by at least one client about the feasibility of nonallopathic treatments and alternatives for feline diseases.

What constitutes complementary and alternative veterinary medicine (CAVM)? Broadly speaking, any unconventional treatment that generally is not provided within the context of allopathic veterinary medicine can be included in CAVM. Acupuncture, herbal therapies, chiropractic/spinal manipulation, homeopathy, homotoxicology, Reiki, light/sound/color therapy, massage, and nutraceuticals—as well as other modalities—all can be included under this umbrella. However, as traditional veterinary practices incorporate some of these modalities increasingly into patient care, the line between CAVM and non-CAVM blurs.

Interest in the use of alternative therapies in veterinary medicine in general, and in feline practice in particular, most likely mirrors that seen in human medicine, although few statistics exist on the dollar expenditure for alternative veterinary care and treatments or the number of patient visits. In 2002 it was estimated that 36 per cent of the adult human population in the United States had visited an alternative practitioner.[1] In 1990 (the last year for which such statistics exist), there were 425 million visits to alternative practitioners in the United States, compared with 388 million visits to primary physicians.[1] In that year, an estimated $13.7 billion was spent with alternative practitioners; and of that, 75 per cent was paid out-of-pocket. This compared with $12.8 billion spent

in that same year out-of-pocket for all U.S. human hospitalizations.

Surveys of users of alternative modalities in human medicine showed that these individuals tended to have higher educations, poorer health status, claimed to have had a "transformational experience" that changed their world view, and were more committed to spirituality, feminism, and environmental concerns than the general population.[1] Dissatisfaction with conventional medicine, as well as gender, income, or age did not influence an individual's desire to pursue complementary and alternative medicine (CAM) therapies. In many instances, patients utilized conventional and alternative therapies simultaneously, and it was estimated that 70 per cent of individuals who utilized CAM therapies did not share that information with their primary care physician.[1]

A survey of 254 clients presenting with companion animals to the Animal Cancer Center of Colorado State University was done regarding their use of alternative therapies.[2] Of that sample, 76 per cent reported using some alternative medicine in their pets. Nutritional supplements were used most commonly, with 40 per cent of respondents stating that the supplements were part of the patient's regimen. Only 46 per cent of those responding said that their veterinarian was the source of information on the use of these products. Of those persons surveyed, 57 per cent said they had discussed the use of the products with their pet's veterinarian.

In veterinary medicine there has been a slow, yet steady shift toward acceptance of at least some CAVM modalities as part of patient care. In 2000, 120 personnel at the 27 U.S. veterinary medical schools were surveyed regarding their educational and research programs in alternative modalities.[3] At that time, seven of the schools surveyed had educational programs in alternative modalities, and six had conducted CAVM research. Of the 41 completed surveys (from 23 of the 27 schools), 87 per cent of respondents believed that acupuncture, nutraceuticals, nutritional supplements, and physical therapy should be included in the curriculum; 61 per cent of respondents stated that botanical (herbal) medicine and chiropractic should be included in the curriculum, and 44 per cent believed that homeopathy had a place in veterinary medical education. The majority of the respondents thought CAVM should be offered as elective courses only.

The American Veterinary Medical Association's policy statement on CAVM, written initially in 2001 and revised in 2007, recognized the interest in alternative modalities for nonhuman species and stated that the organization was "open to their consideration."[4] No determination of value was given to individual modalities, and practitioners were advised to exercise caution when extrapolating data from human usage of alternative modalities and to advise clients of "proven treatment methods" when presenting all treatment options. Cautions also were given regarding lack of Food and Drug Administration (FDA) premarketing evaluation of many animal nutritional supplements and botanicals, and that manufacturers of alternative veterinary devices need not be required to obtain premarketing approval by the FDA regarding efficacy and safety issues.

With few exceptions, veterinary medical boards generally limit the practice of alternative modalities in veterinary medicine to licensed veterinarians, or to nonveterinarians who work under the referral of a veterinarian. However, the boards vary on the requirements for veterinarians who utilize and practice alternative medicine, and practitioners who utilize alternative methodologies need to familiarize themselves with their state's requirements. For example, in Texas, before veterinary "holistic medicine," defined as the blending of alternative and conventional therapies, can be performed, the practitioner is required to have a written statement signed by the client that they are aware that holistic therapy is alternative practice.[5] Additionally, the practitioner must inform the client of conventional treatments that are available and their "probable ability to cure the problem."[5] The signed statement becomes part of the patient's permanent medical record.

Why do clients seek alternative therapies for their cats? The reasons are varied and range from seeking treatment for illnesses for which no conventional therapy exists to the desire to treat the cat (a species often viewed as a companion animal that, although domesticated, still possesses many characteristics of wild animals) as naturally as possible. Often clients wish to avoid possible side effects of conventional medications and therapies. Still others desire to combine conventional and alternative therapies in the hope of maximizing a positive outcome. However, despite these intentions, the same limitations often affect CAVM treatment of cats: (1) the reluctance of clients to travel with their cats for repeated treatments; (2) difficulty administering many oral medications; and (3) the cat's perceived inherent dislike of many medical interventions. These either limit the types of alternative modalities that can be utilized, or demand creative use and administration of them in feline patients. Despite these concerns, however, many alternative therapies can be administered to cats and most of these patients are amenable to treatments and therapies. The author utilizes conventional and alternative therapies routinely for a wide range of feline diseases in practice.

It is beyond the scope of this chapter to discuss all possible alternative modalities that can be used in feline practice, and it is not the intent to present arguments regarding the validity of offering alternative therapies to feline patients. Instead, the alternative therapies used most commonly in feline practice will be discussed: acupuncture, chiropractic/spinal manipulation, and herbal medicine (Chinese and Western). These three modalities often are used synergistically in conjunction with conventional veterinary practice.

ACUPUNCTURE

HISTORY AND THEORY

Horses were the first nonhuman beings treated with acupuncture and the first veterinary acupuncture textbook was produced in China in 650 BC. However, it was not until 1975, when the International Veterinary Acupuncture Society (IVAS) was formed and began to offer classes to veterinarians, that dogs and cats, as well as other small mammals and birds, began to receive acupuncture treatments.

Acupuncture can be viewed through its traditionally understood Chinese theory of normalizing the flow of energy (Qi) through the body by using various meridians (invisible channels that course through the body, beginning or ending at the distal points of the upper or lower extremities, as well as the chest or head). Alternatively, acupuncture can be explained using a Western medical approach by which it provides therapy by accessing points that coincide with vascular nerve bundles that contain more mast cells, as well as points that have been identified histologically as being located at motor points, at midline points where bilateral nerves meet, over superficial nerves or plexuses, or at Golgi tendon organs. Segmental anesthesia through stimulation of inhibitor interneurons; release of endorphins, serotonin, reproductive hormones, and cortisol through spinothalamic tracts; autonomic effects through the use of the somatovisceral reflex; and induction of microtrauma with attendant inflammation and healing also have been ascribed to acupuncture.[6]

Acupuncture points are named most commonly by the meridian (Lung, Large Intestine, Kidney, Bladder, Liver, Gallbladder, Heart, Pericardium, Small Intestines, Triple Heater, Stomach, and Spleen), and by a number that corresponds to a specific point along the meridian (Stomach 36; ST 36). The meridian names, which are familiar to practitioners (except for the Triple Heater, which is not associated with any specific anatomical organ or region and functions as a transporter of fluids in the pelvis, abdomen, and chest), do not correspond necessarily with the organ as it is known to Western medicine. Acupunc-

---

Box 79-1   Veterinary Acupuncture References

Nancy Zidonis, Amy Snow: *Acu-Cat: A Guide To Feline Acupressure.* Tallgrass Publishers, LLC, 2000.

Cheryl Schwartz: *Four Paws Five Directions: A Guide for Chinese Medicine for Cats and Dogs.* Celestial Arts, 1996.

Traditional Chinese Veterinary Medicine Fundamental Principles. Reddick, FL, 2007, Chi Institute.

Allen Schoen: *Veterinary Acupuncture: Ancient Art to Modern Medicine.* St. Louis, 2000, Mosby.

Huisheng Xie, Vanessa Preast: *Xie's Veterinary Acupuncture.* Ames, IA, 2007, Blackwell.

---

ture points selected for treatment of certain conditions do not have to be chosen from the meridian named for the organ that is diseased. Hence points on the Bladder, Kidney, and Lung meridians can be used to treat some forms of heart failure. It is recommended that the interested practitioner obtain meridian charts from the books listed in Box 79-1.

Additionally, there are "classical points" that commonly have only a Chinese name and that are specific for certain conditions (for example, Ding-chuan or "Stop Cough/Asthma," located on the dorsolateral cervicothoracic junction, midline between C7-T1).

Cats generally receive acupuncture on a tabletop that is covered by a soft blanket. Acupuncture needles are of very small gauges, with 0.5 inch by 0.2 mm diameter needles used for points along the back and 0.5 inch by 0.16 to 0.22 mm needles used for other points. Very sensitive points, located typically at the tips of the extremities, as well as around the eyes and nose, can be treated with extremely small Korean hand needles. Cats who are intolerant of the needles remaining in place for any period of time can be treated using "aquapuncture," which involves the subcutaneous injection of small quantities (0.1 to 0.3 mL) of vitamin B_{12} into the points. Electrostimulation, which involves the creation of a small electrical circuit linking points, is surprisingly well-tolerated by cats, in the author's experience. Moxibustion, which involves the burning of a small amount of mugwort on the tip of an acupuncture needle or by holding a specialized stick over the area to be treated, can be used on back points in another small subset of cats. Because the smell of burning mugwort is similar to that of some illicit drugs, "smokeless" moxa sticks can be purchased. The author has had selected clients use moxibustion on their cats at home. Low-intensity laser light therapy, involving the use of hand-held small lasers also can be used in feline patients.

Many clients and practitioners question the safety of acupuncture, particularly that done with needles. Pneumothorax, cardiac tamponade, broken needles, syncope, puncture of body cavities and vital organs, and abortion all have been cited by various authors as serious complications of acupuncture therapy.[7]

Using appropriately short needles, placing those needles with proper technique, care in needling areas of the thorax and shoulder muscles, and familiarizing oneself with certain points that can cause strong uterine contractions are all used to provide safe acupuncture treatments, regardless of patient species. Occasionally exaggeration of clinical signs can occur in human beings and animals who receive acupuncture. In human beings this can last up to 1 day posttreatment; in dogs, this may occur for up to 5 days posttreatment. The author has had patients on very rare occasion whose clinical signs were exaggerated after acupuncture treatment.

CLINICAL UTILITY IN FELINE PRACTICE

The traditional Chinese medicine (TCM) perspective holds that patient signs and symptoms are considered as being consistent with a variety of patterns. As such, patients can be described in the broadest sense as having an excessive or deficient condition. Additionally, they may have signs consistent with heat (blood in the stool or urine, or a purulent discharge from the eyes, nose, or urogenital tract) or cold (copious, clear urination, or mucoid diarrhea). Because of this classification system, patients with one Western diagnosis (chronic kidney disease) may not be treated similarly. A cat with chronic kidney disease who is polydipsic and polyuric and heat-seeking, for example, would be treated differently than a similarly azotemic cat who drinks only small amounts of water, urinates small amounts of urine, and prefers to lie on cool tile or avoids warm areas. A kitten who presents with a clear nasal discharge and sneezing, consistent with a presumptive Western diagnosis of viral rhinitis would be diagnosed as having a Wind-Cold pattern, and would be treated with slightly different acupuncture points than a littermate who presents with fever, nasal congestion, and a thick and yellow oculonasal discharge (signs of Wind-Heat by the TCM pattern).

An examination of the tongue and peripheral pulses (best assessed by palpation of the femoral arteries) generally is used prior to initiating acupuncture therapy, and allows for the patterns to be described more specifically. In TCM, the tongue is divided into several regions, each representing a different body organ. The kidney area is located at the most caudal part of the tongue; the spleen in the middle of the tongue, the liver on the lateral aspects, the heart at the most proximal portion, and the lung located just distal to the heart area.[8]

Tongue color, the presence or absence of fluid or phlegm on the dorsal lingual surface, as well as the presence or absence of a coating are all used to make a basic assessment of the patient's underlying physical condition and diagnosis. A cat who presents with a history of watery diarrhea or vomiting may have a pale tongue, noting deficiency. The tongue also may be thick and flabby and often has some fluid located at the area dedicated to the spleen, which in TCM is the organ that "transforms" food and is involved in digestive issues.

Pulse diagnosis is used to characterize deficiency or excess patterns of various organs.[8] In cats the pulses of the femoral arteries are assessed with the cat standing and the practitioner placing her or his fingers on the right and left femoral pulses with the index fingers placed proximally, the middle fingers placed medially on the arteries, and the fourth fingers placed more distally. On the left side, the proximal position is that of the heart; the middle, the liver; and the lowest, the kidney yin (cooling). On the right side, the upper position is dedicated to the lung, the middle to the spleen, and the lowest to the kidney yang (warming). The pulse quality (depth, speed, shape, strength, and rhythm) is assessed by pressing firmly on the pulses until they are obliterated. Very superficial and slow pulses may be consistent with a cold pattern; rapid and surging pulses would be more consistent with a heat pattern.

Another portion of the Traditional Chinese Veterinary Medicine (TCVM) examination is the palpation of various acupoints along the meridians that may allow a practitioner to diagnose certain disorders. These points are divided into Association (back-Shu) points, located along the dorsum and Alarm (Mu) points. The Association and Alarm points each reference certain organs, and pain elicited at the points can be useful in assessing possible internal medicine problems.

For example, the Association (back-Shu) point for the liver is Bladder 18, located about one inch lateral to the lateral aspect of the dorsal spinous process of T10; the Alarm (Mu) point for the liver is Liver 14, located on the lateral thorax in the sixth intercostal space at the level of the mammary glands. The Association (back-Shu) point for the Large Intestine is Bladder 25, located on the dorsolateral aspect of the spine, approximately one inch lateral to the caudal border of the dorsal spinous process of L5; the Alarm (Mu) point of the large intestine is Stomach 25, located on the ventrolateral abdomen, approximately 1.5 inches lateral to the umbilicus, in the center of the rectus abdominis muscle. Cats presenting with liver disease may be sensitive at Liver 14 and Bladder 18; cats with underlying colitis or constipation/megacolon, may have increased sensitivity at Bladder 25 and Stomach 25.[9]

While proper training in acupuncture is recommended before initiating therapy on a feline patient, four acupuncture points may be of benefit to feline patients that can be placed by veterinarians with only familiarity of their anatomical locations. These points are: Shen-Gan, at the junction between the haired and nonhaired area of the dorsal nasal planum, which is useful for stimulating appetite; Governing Vessel (GV) 26 (Jen Chung), a point that may be useful for resuscitation of patients with cardiac arrest or anesthetic complications; GV 20, a calming point that may be useful in cats with inappropriate urination or defecation, as well as stressed cats coming to the hospital; and Pericardium (PC) 6, a point that may be useful in antiemesis. The author uses these points in combination with conventional treatments and not as substitutes for allopathic therapies.

GV 26 is located on the nasal philtrum at the level of the ventral aspect of the nares. This point can be needled with a "pecking" technique, using a 25-gauge (or smaller) hypodermic needle in cats. Another technique is to twirl the needle vigorously at the point while advancing and retracting it. In dogs appropriate stimulation of GV has been shown to increase heart rate, stroke volume, and cardiac output, and produce increases in pulse pressures that are similar to that achieved with injections of epinephrine.[10] Stimulation also causes a significant increase

in mean arterial pressure with a decrease in total peripheral resistance. These changes have been shown to be mediated through alterations in sympathetic tone and are blocked by concurrent use of propranolol. Simultaneous stimulation of Kidney 1 (located between the third and fourth metatarsals under the central pad of the hind limbs) is useful as adjunctive therapy for cardiopulmonary resuscitation and anesthetic overdosage.[10]

GV 20, located on the dorsal midline on a line drawn from the tips of the ears level with the ear canal, has been shown to be a sedating point in many species. The author typically begins acupuncture sessions with a needle placed in this location (Figure 79-1). This point also may be useful in calming stressed cats in the clinical setting, and has been advocated as a point for weekly aquapuncture therapy in cats with inappropriate urination and defecation.[11]

PC 6, located on the medial aspect of the thoracic limb, approximately two inches proximal to the carpal crease in the groove between the flexor carpi radialis and the superficial digital flexor muscles, has been well studied in human beings and dogs for its antiemetic effects. This point is stimulated in the popular antiseasickness bands used by people.[12,13] In 26 human trials involving 3000 patients, stimulation of PC 6 was found superior to sham stimulation for both nausea and vomiting, including postoperative sickness, chemotherapy-associated nausea and vomiting, and pregnancy-related nausea and vomiting.[14] Pooled data of trials including different antiemetics in both adults and children, showed that P6 stimulation was superior to antiemetic medication for nausea and equivalent for vomiting. For chemotherapy-associated vomiting, electroacupuncture, but not manual acupuncture, was shown to be beneficial for first-day vomiting.[14]

In addition to PC 6, other acupuncture points, Conception Vessel (CV) 12 and Stomach (ST) 36 (Figure 79-2) have been shown to benefit functional gastrointestinal

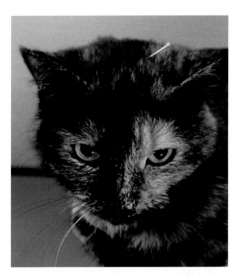

Figure 79-1 Cat receiving acupuncture with needle placed at GV 20. This point is for calming and may help with inappropriate urination.

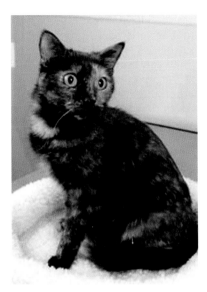

Figure 79-2 Cat receiving acupuncture with needle placed at ST 36 (shown near the lateral aspect of the left stifle joint). This point is helpful for intestinal and stomach problems.

Box 79-2 Acupuncture Training Programs

International Veterinary Acupuncture Society (IVAS)
2625 Redwing Road, Suite 160
Fort Collins, CO 80526
United States
Phone: 970-266-0666. Fax: 970-266-0777
E-mail: office@ivas.org

Chi Institute
9700 West Highway 318
Reddick, FL 32686
United States
Phone: 800-891-1986. Fax: 866-700-8772
E-mail: barbara@tcvm.org

Medical Acupuncture for Veterinarians
Colorado State Veterinary Medical Association
Fort Collins, CO
United States
Phone: 303-318-0447
E-mail: info@colostate.org

symptoms, affect/alter acid secretion, and limit visceral pain in human beings with gastroesophageal reflux (GERD) and irritable bowel syndrome (IBS). As such, these points may be of benefit to feline patients with a wide range of gastrointestinal motility issues (vomiting, diarrhea, and constipation), as well as those cats with pancreatitis. CV-12 is located on the ventrum, halfway between the umbilicus and the xiphoid, and has been shown to cause muscle relaxation via the somatosympathetic pathway. This point also has inhibitory effects on the intestinal tract and may benefit patients with diarrhea and enhanced colonic motility. Acupuncture at CV-12 may inhibit gastric acid secretion via the somatosympathetic pathway and benefit cats with hypergastrinemia, secondary to chronic kidney disease. ST-36, located on the craniolateral aspect of the pelvic limb, approximately one-half inch lateral to the cranial aspect of the tibial crest in the belly of the cranial tibialis muscle, causes muscle contractions via the somatoparasympathetic pathway. The stimulatory effects of ST-36 may benefit cats with constipation who show a delayed colonic transit time.[15] Stimulation of ST-36 and PC-6 has antinociceptive effects and may be beneficial to cats with visceral hypersensitivity,[15] including pancreatitis.

Several textbooks are available for the interested feline practitioner on the subject of acupuncture as adjunctive therapy for feline internal medicine disorders, including hyperthyroidism, diabetes mellitus, hypertension, and asthmatic bronchitis (see Box 79-1). Although a few points can be used by veterinarians without formal training in veterinary acupuncture, it is best that patients be treated by practitioners who have studied at one of the three current veterinary acupuncture programs (Box 79-2). These rigorous programs generally meet for 4 days once-monthly over the course of 4 to 5 months, with final written examinations and point finding examinations prior to certification.

CHIROPRACTIC/SPINAL MANIPULATION

HISTORY AND THEORY

Veterinary chiropractic was founded in the late 1980s by Sharon Willoughby, DVM, who received a chiropractic degree from the Palmer College of Chiropractic in 1986. She founded the American Veterinary Chiropractic Association in 1989. Although most veterinary chiropractic treatments are given to equine and canine patients, the author has referred many cats to veterinary chiropractors for a variety of issues, including musculoskeletal problems, recurrent skin lesions that result from self-trauma and perceived referred pain, radial nerve paralysis secondary to traumatic injuries, and occasional patients with constipation and/or dysuria that appear to have a neurological basis. However, limited formal research exists on the clinical efficacy of small animal chiropractic techniques. In most cases chiropractic or spinal manipulation performed on cats (and dogs, as well as horses) has been borrowed from human chiropractic theories, techniques, and research.

The safety of chiropractic is often questioned, particularly as it relates to the possibility of stroke following manipulation of the cervical spine. In 2001 Canadian researchers writing in Stroke considered 582 cases of vertebrobasilar accidents (VBAs)/vertebral artery dissection, a rare form of stroke, in Ontario, Canada during 1993 to 1998.[16] Results of the study showed that for patients 45 years of age and younger, VBA cases were five times more likely than controls to have visited a chiropractor within 1 week of the VBA. This group also was five times as likely to have had three or more visits to a chiropractor with a cervical diagnosis in the month before the date of the VBA. No significant association was found in those patients over 45 years of age. However, further age/gender-standardized analyses showed that for every

100,000 persons less than 45 years of age receiving chiropractic, there were 1.3 cases of VBA attributable to chiropractic.[16]

No statistics exist for adverse effects related to veterinary chiropractic; however, they are thought to be very uncommon and this author's experience with chiropractic in her patient population has found it to be a safe, gentle, and effective technique. A transient stiffness or worsening of a condition posttreatment may occur within the ensuing 6 to 12 hours, and may last 24 to 48 hours. Potential harmful effects from improperly applied manipulation from poorly trained individuals can include articular damage or loss of function (torn ligaments, injured muscles, luxated joints, fractures, or paralysis). This is particularly true if severe, underlying pathology is present and not diagnosed.[17]

Contraindications for chiropractic include fractures, infectious diseases, neoplasia, metabolic disorders, or non–mechanically related joint disorders. Chiropractic care can not reverse severe degenerative processes or overt pathology, although it can contribute to the rehabilitation of postsurgical patients and some severe medical conditions by helping in the restoration of the normal musculoskeletal function.

Chiropractic treatment involves joint manipulation. The vertebral motion segment is the functional unit of the spine and includes two adjacent vertebrae and the associated soft tissues that bind them together. Joint motion can be categorized into three zones of movement: physiological, paraphysiological, and pathological. The physiological zone includes active and passive ranges of motion and is the site to which mobilization is applied. The paraphysiological zone of movement occurs outside the joint's normal barrier and is the site of joint cavitation. The pathological zone of movement lies outside the limits of normal anatomical joint integrity and is characterized by joint injury (sprain, subluxation, or luxation). Vertebral motion segment injury can cause altered proprioception, protective muscle guarding, altered intervertebral disc and joint biomechanics, and increased tension in the joint capsule.[17]

A thorough patient history must be taken and musculoskeletal examination performed by the veterinarian on cats prior to referral for chiropractic. Generally the author begins by assessing the cat's cervical range of motion (ventroflexion and dorsiflexion, as well as right and left lateral flexion). The spine then is evaluated with gentle palpation to locate areas of apparent soreness, asymmetry, resistance to pressure, and changes in tissue texture (including "trigger points," or "tissue knots"). Care is taken to watch the cat's often subtle movements and reactions to varying degrees of depth of palpation. Tenderness and hypersensitivity are noted particularly. The limbs are placed in extension and flexion, to gauge restricted mobility, soreness, or hypermobility.

With their athletic lifestyles of leaping and jumping, even when confined to small urban homes, cats can incur even minor trauma that can lead to an initial subluxation of a vertebra. In younger animals, the tissues have a resiliency that allows them to recover into a neutral position. Older animals, however, often have poor tissue reliance and this can lead to eventual fixation of the joint. With advanced cases of vertebral fixation, cats can have large blocks of immobile vertebrae. As the spine becomes rigid, the movement of the spine becomes concentrated in a few joints, which can become hypermobile and prone to injury.[18]

Spinal fixation also can occur by the impingement of efferent nerves as they emerge from a compressed intervertebral foramen. This results in increased tendencies for the nerves to depolarize. Depolarization initiates muscle contraction and spasm. Spasms in some muscles can further immobilize the subluxations, progressing to spinal instability.[18]

CLINICAL APPLICATIONS

Cats with degenerative joint disease, limited cervical range of motion, and pain at the lumbosacral area (which can manifest as hyperesthesia syndrome), potentially can be helped by chiropractic care. Unfortunately, anecdotal evidence for the technique predominates, and there is a paucity of controlled studies in canine or feline chiropractic. For these reasons, wider acceptance of this modality has been impeded in veterinary medicine.

The author has successfully referred cats suffering from "hot spots" or focal, self-traumatized areas to veterinary chiropractors. If conventional dermatological tests and other ancillary diagnostic examinations fail to find an underlying cause, it often is helpful to consider these lesions as representative of referred pain from spinal dermatomes.

Spinal dermatomes have been identified in the cat for the cervical and upper thoracic areas, as well as the lower lumbar areas of the spine.[19] Dermatomes are areas of the skin associated with paired dorsal roots of the spinal cord. The most distal area of the forelimbs is innervated by the C8-T1 segment, with more proximal regions of the forelimb innervated by more proximal regions of the cervical spine. A patient with a persistently self-traumatized lesion just distal to the elbow, for example, for which no other underlying cause can be identified, might be helped by an adjustment of the cervical spine at the level of C7.[20]

Cats with lower urinary tract disease who are refractory to treatment and for whom other underlying diseases have been excluded, may receive some benefit from chiropractic adjustment. A 1996 review of the human literature found potential relationships between the biomechanics of the pelvic soft tissues and the pathogenesis of lower urinary tract dysfunction.[21] Urgency and frequency of voiding may have a neurogenic cause, and it is postulated that soft-tissue injury, including scarring and inflammatory states, can lead to altered afferent sensory information to the spinal cord. Movement restrictions in the pelvic articulations may restrict related structures, including the urethra, which can send altered afferent information to the spinal cord.[21]

FURTHER STUDY AND TRAINING

There is a paucity of textbooks on veterinary chiropractic and most of the certification programs utilize human chiropractic texts with additional handouts on particular veterinary applications.

As with acupuncture, cats should be referred to a veterinarian or human chiropractor who has completed one of the three veterinary chiropractic programs (Box 79-3) and has passed the certification examination of the American Veterinary Chiropractic Association (AVCA). Colorado State University also has offered a spinal manipulation program in the past. Some human chiropractors without veterinary-specific training perform manipulations on animal patients; however, without specific knowledge of quadrupedal anatomy and relationships, such treatments can not be recommended. Practitioners should check with their state's appropriate licensing board to see if written referral is required prior to having a cat seen by a human chiropractor.

Several weekend "veterinary adjustment" courses are offered by a variety of human chiropractors and veterinarians who are not affiliated with any AVCA-recognized program and advertise the ability to perform spinal

---

Box 79-3 Veterinary Chiropractic Training Programs

American Veterinary Chiropractic Association
442154 E.140 Rd
Bluejacket, OK 74333
United States
Phone: 918-784-2231. Fax: 918-784-2675

Healing Oasis Wellness Center
2555 Wisconsin Street
Sturtevant, WI 53177
United States
Phone: 262-878-9549. Fax: 262-886-6460
Web site: http://thehealingoasis.com

Options for Animals
Wellsville, KS
United States
Phone: 309-658-2920. Fax: 309-658-2622
Web site: http://www.animalchiro.com

Parker College of Chiropractic
2500 Walnut Hill Lane
Dallas, TX 75229
United States
Phone 800-266-4723
Web site: http://www.parkercc.edu/Index.
    aspx?id=1135&displayid=1137

Healing Oasis Wellness Centre of Canada
124 Charing Cross Street
Brantford, Ontario
Canada
Phone: 519-448-1306. Fax 519-756-1597
Website: http://www.veterinarychiropractic.ca/

BackBone Academy for Veterinary Chiropractic and
    Healing Arts
4, D-27419
Kalbe, Germany
Phone: 49-4282-590688. Fax: 49-721-15136646
Website: http://www.backbone-academy.com

---

manipulations on patients after only a few hours of instruction. Practitioners should be aware of the differences between these programs and the rigorous, AVCA-affiliated programs and make referrals appropriately.

CHINESE AND WESTERN HERBS

HISTORY AND THEORY

For millennia, human beings have used a variety of plant roots, leaves, and seeds selectively as treatments for various external and internal maladies. Most cat clients and veterinarians are familiar with the often amusing side effects of cats sniffing or eating catnip (Nepeta cataria), caused by the affect of nepetalactone (a component of Nepeta cataria and other species of Nepeta) on opioid receptors.[22] The use of herbal treatments in veterinary medicine has been incorporated increasingly into mainstream allopathic practice. Milk thistle (Silybum marianum), for example, is now used routinely for its hepatoprotective effects, including antioxidant properties, inhibition of lipid peroxidation, and increased hepatocyte protein synthesis.

The Materia Medicas of Chinese and Western herbologies are vast and many of the teas, tinctures, and pills available have poor palatability for feline patients. Furthermore, several herbs, including tea tree oil, are toxic to cats. Herbs may be considered "natural remedies" by many clients, but they can exert potent effects on body systems, as well as interact with other drugs. St. John's Wort, which sometimes is used as an anxiolytic, can inhibit a variety of drugs (amitriptyline, digoxin, and cyclosporine) through the cytochrome p450 system.[23]

Essential oils are the volatile, organic constituents of plant matter that contribute to plant fragrance and can be especially toxic to companion animals, including cats. These oils are popular among human beings for a variety of purposes, including relaxation and stress release. Many of these essential oils are not recommended for use in veterinary patients, because of unknown or oral LD50s of less than 1 g/kg. Wintergreen, pennyroyal, menthol, tea tree, and sweet birch are some essential oils that are used commonly by unsuspecting clients. Practitioners should consult Boxes 79-4 and 79-5 for the potentially toxic essential oils and the most toxic essential oils, and counsel clients against their use.

Within the past few years, there has been increasing scrutiny of the safety of herbal medications that come from China. Practitioners are advised to use herbs that are available through large companies that have excellent quality control and to query the herbalists on the sources of their herbal medications. Most reputable companies will conduct their own analysis of imported herbs, and will be able to satisfy safety concerns regarding heavy metals and other toxic compounds.

In general most herbal remedies from these companies are safe for use in cats, and practitioners are encouraged to speak with the herbalists employed by these companies regarding any concerns with the contents of formulas, particularly those that are proprietary. Because cats are sensitive to salicylates, there has been some concern

Box 79-4 Potentially Toxic Essential Oils[24]

Wintergreen	Myrrh
Cornmint	Birch (sweet)
Savory (summer)	Bay leaf (West Indian)
Clove leaf	Oregano
Basil	Sassafras (*S. albidum*)
Hyssop	Tarragon
Sassafras (Brazilian)	Tea tree
Savin	

Box 79-5 Most Toxic Essential Oils[24]

Boldo leaf	Wormwood
Wormseed	Bitter almond
Mustard	Tree wormwood
Arnoise	Large wormwood
Pennyroyal (European)	Buchu
Tansy	Horseradish
Thuja	Lanyana
Calamus	Pennyroyal (North American)
Western red cedar	Southernwood

that salicylate-containing herbals (including dandelion root, which often is used as a diuretic; licorice, which often is prescribed for intestinal upset; and meadowsweet, which is used for diarrhea) may present problems for cats. However, when a standard dose of aspirin in cats is considered to be 10 mg/kg (50 mg of acetylsalicylate acid), even meadowsweet, which has one of the highest salicylate concentrations of herbs (388 µg/mL in a 1:2 extract) would provide a dose of 0.388 mg in 1 mL.[24]

CLINICAL APPLICATIONS

Several herbs are relatively easy to administer and are useful in feline medicine. These herbs are Yunnan Pai Yao, Rehmannia, Shiitake mushrooms, slippery elm, marshmallow, bugleweed, and other antithyroid herbal formulations.

Yunnan Pai Yao is a proprietary Chinese formula (often highly guarded), that is reported to contain a variety of herbs, including *Panax notoginseng* and Chinese yam (in some formulae). This hemostatic herbal remedy can be used topically to stop bleeding and also can be dosed orally, in the case of gastric ulcerations. This herbal formula has been shown to decrease bleeding times in animals and to initiate platelet release.[25]

Rehmannia glutinosa is used traditionally in Chinese medicine in heat disorders (discussed previously under Acupuncture). It can be used in a variety of conditions, including low-grade fever, xerostomia, and constipation, and in cats with chronic kidney disease who are not overtly polydipsic and polyuric. In a rat acute renal failure model, *Rehmannia* improved creatinine clearance, urine sodium excretion, and urine osmolality.[26] The preferred dosage is 17 to 133 mg/kg PO q8h. The herb can be placed

in gel caps for easier administration to cats. Alternatively, a decoction can be made with 5 to 30 grams of herb in eight ounces of water administered at one to two ounces for each 5 kg body weight daily. Tea pills, small coated pills that are easy to administer to most cats, also are available.[24]

Shiitake (*Lentinula edodes*) mushrooms have purported anticancer activity. Lentinan is used in Japan and China for adjuvant cancer treatment, although no double-blind or placebo-controlled trials have been performed. In a study of human patients with advanced colorectal cancer, median survival was 200 days in the group receiving lentinan and 98 days in the control group.[27] Mice given a carcinogen, N-butyl-N-butanolnitrosamine, received either a control diet or a 5 per cent dried, powdered Shiitake diet.[28] All 10 mice in the control group developed bladder cancer; only nine of 17 (52.9 percent) in the lentinan group developed cancer. The dried herb can be placed in gel caps and dosed at 5 to 30 grams PO q8h. Alternatively, an infusion can be made of 5 to 30 grams of herb in eight ounces of water with this administered at 1 to 2 ounces daily.[24]

Slippery elm (*Ulmus rubra*) has anecdotal usefulness for inflammatory bowel disease, as well as fiber-responsive gastrointestinal problems. It has demulcent, emollient, antitussive, astringent, nutritive, and laxative properties, and also may be helpful in some cases of feline lower urinary tract disease. It contains mucilage that forms a hydrocolloid in the gut.[24] This author has used a tincture, with a preferred dosage of 0.33 to 0.66 mL PO q8h for cats with inflammatory bowel disease. This can be added to moist food.

Marshmallow (*Althaea officinalis*) root and leaf are mucilages and have been used in upper respiratory tract infections with irritation of the oral and pharyngeal mucosae, as well as in mild inflammation of the gastrointestinal tract. Decocting destroys mucilage, so this herb is best given as a cold infusion (5 to 30 g in 8 ounces of cold water, and dosed at 1 to 2 ounces for each 5 kg of body weight daily, preferably divided into three equal doses).[24]

Bugleweed (*Lycopus europaeus* or *virginicus*), used as an alcohol extract only, reduces peripheral deiodination of thyroxine, and decreases levels of triiodothyronine and thyroid stimulating hormone.[29] Anecdotally, the combination of *Lycopus* and *Melissa* (lemon balm) has been used to control hyperthyroidism in cats. It should not be combined with other antithyroid medications. The dosage is 5 to 30 grams of herb in eight ounces of water, dosed at 1 to 2 ounces for each 5 kg of body weight daily and divided into three doses, or 8 to 25 mg/kg of the dried herb q8h. The dried herb can be placed in gel caps for ease of administration.[24]

Sargassum Jade Pot, a proprietary herbal formulation from Jing Tang Herbal Company and available in similar preparations from other suppliers, can be used in some cats who are unable to take methimazole and are not candidates for radioactive iodine therapy or surgical thyroidectomy. Although not as efficacious as methimazole, there are anecdotal reports that this formulation does control clinical signs. Another proprietary formulation, Hyper Jia Bing Formula, could be used in hyperthyroid cats with irritability, weight loss, emaciation, diarrhea, and vomiting.[30]

Because Chinese herbal medications in particular are prescribed based on tongue and pulse diagnostics, as well as clinical signs, the practitioner without training in this modality is encouraged to refer the patient to a colleague who has completed herbal training and/or consult with an herbalist employed by one of the larger herbal suppliers.

FURTHER STUDY AND TRAINING

The textbook, Veterinary Herbal Medicine by Susan G. Wynn and Barbara J. Fougere contains a comprehensive review and study of Western, Ayurvedic, and Chinese herbal remedies, as well as suppliers.[24] Training in herbal medicine is offered at a variety of schools worldwide and specific information can be obtained in the appendix of that book, as well as by contacting the Veterinary Botanical Medicine Association at http://www.vbma.org.

REFERENCES

1. Eisenberg DM, Kessler RC, Foster C, et al: Unconventional medicine in the United States: prevalence, costs and patterns of use, *N Engl J Med* 328:246, 1993.
2. Lana SE, Kogan LR, Crisp KA, et al: The use of complementary and alternative therapies in dogs and cats with cancer, *J Am Anim Hosp Assoc* 42:361, 2006.
3. Schoen AM: Results of a survey on educational and research programs in complementary and alternative veterinary medicine at veterinary medical schools in the United States, *J Am Vet Med Assoc* 216:502, 2000.
4. American Veterinary Medical Association: AVMA guidelines for complementary and alternative veterinary medicine. Retrieved January 4, 2009 at http://www.avma.org/issues/policy/comp_alt_medicine.asp
5. Texas State Board of Veterinary Medical Examiners, Rule 573.15, adopted to be effective November 4, 1994. Retrieved January 4, 2009 at http://info.sos.state.tx.us/pls/pub/readtac$ext.TacPage?sl=R&app=9&p_dir=&p_rloc=&p_tloc=&p_ploc=&pg=1&p_tac=&ti=22&pt=24&ch=573&rl=15
6. Clemmons RM: Functional neuroanatomical physiology of acupuncture. In Xie H, Preast V, editors: *Xie's veterinary acupuncture*, Ames, 2007, Blackwell, p 341.
7. Xie H, Preast V: General rules of acupuncture therapy. In Xie H, Preast V, editors: *Xie's veterinary acupuncture*, Ames, 2007, Blackwell, p 235.
8. Xie H, Preast V: *Traditional Chinese veterinary medicine: fundamental principles*, Reddick, FL, 2007, Chi Institute.
9. Xie H, Preast V: Acupuncture for treatment of musculoskeletal and neurological disorders. In Xie H, Preast V, editors: *Xie's veterinary acupuncture*, Ames, 2007, Blackwell, p 247.
10. Lee DC, Lee MO, Clifford DH, et al: The autonomic effects of acupuncture and analgesic drugs on the cardiovascular system of dogs, *Am J Acupunct* 10:5, 1982.
11. Swanson J: Personal communication, October, 1996.
12. Nunley C, Wakim J, Guinn C: The effects of stimulation of acupressure point p6 on postoperative nausea and vomiting: a review of literature, *J Perianesth Nurs* 23:247, 2008.
13. Tatewaki M, Strickland C, Fukoda H, et al: Effects of acupuncture on vasopressin-induced emesis in conscious dogs, *Am J Physiol Regul Integr Comp Physiol* 288:R401, 2005.
14. Ezzo J, Streitberger K, Schneider A: Cochrane systemic reviews examine P6 acupuncture-point stimulation for nausea and vomiting, *J Altern Complement Med* 12:489, 2006.
15. Takahashi T: Acupuncture for functional gastrointestinal disorders, *J Gastroenterol* 41:408, 2006.
16. Rothwell DM, Bondy SJ, Williams TI, et al: Chiropractic manipulation and stroke: a population-based case-control study, *Stroke* 32:2207, 2001.
17. Haussler KK: Small animal chiropractic techniques. Proceedings of the Western Veterinary Conference, Las Vegas, NV, 2006.
18. Marsden SP: Understanding chiropractic. Proceedings of Western Veterinary Conference, Las Vegas, NV, 2003.
19. Hekmatpanah J: Organization of tactile dermatomes, C1 through L4 in the cat, *J Neurophysiol* 24:129, 1961.
20. DeStefano C: Personal communication, September, 2007.
21. Stone C: Links between pelvic biomechanics and urinary tract dysfunction, *Physiotherapy* 82:616, 1996.
22. Aydin S, Beis R, Ozturk Y, et al: Nepetalactone: a new opioid analgesic from Nepeta caesarea Boiss, *J Pharm Pharmacol* 50:813, 1998.
23. Markowitz JS, Donovan JL, DeVane CL, et al: Effects of St. John's wort on drug metabolism by induction of cytochrome p450 3A4 enzyme, *JAMA* 290:1500, 2003.
24. Wynn SG, Fougere BJ: *Veterinary herbal medicine*, St. Louis, 2007, Mosby.
25. Ogle CW, Dai S, Ma JC: The haemostatic effects of the Chinese herbal drug Yunnan Bai Yao: a pilot study, *Am J Chin Med* 4:147, 1976.
26. Kang DG, Sohn EJ, Moon MK, et al: Rehmannia glutinose ameloriates renal function in the ischemia/reperfusion-induced acute renal failure rates, *Biol Pharm Bull* 28:1662, 2005.
27. Taguchi T, Furue H, Kimura T, et al: Life-span prolongation effect of lentinan in patients with advanced or recurrent colorectal cancer, *Int J Immunopharmacol* 4:271, 1982.
28. Kurashie S, Akuzawa Y, Endo F: Effects of *Lentinus edodes*, *Grifola frondosa* and *Pleurotus ostreatus* administration on cancer outbreak and activities of macrophages and lymphocytes in mice treated with carcinogen, N-butyl-N-butanolnitrosamine, *Immunopharmacol Immunotoxicol* 19:175, 1997.
29. Winteroff H, Gumbinger HG, Vahlensieck U, et al: Endocrine effects of Lycopus europaeus L. following oral application, *Arzneimittelforschung* 44:41, 1994.
30. Xie H: Traditional Chinese veterinary medicine clinical approach/herbology: liver/endocrinology, Reddick, FL, 2008, Chi Institute, Course Proceedings, p 149, February 21-24.

80 Catteries: Reproductive Performance and Problems

Eva Axnér

A thorough knowledge about reproductive physiology increases the chances for successful breeding of cats. There are, however, large individual variations in seasonality, length of the estrous cycle, and age of puberty that make it more difficult to set normal ranges than it is for other domestic species. In addition, there are differences between breeds—for example, in age of puberty, seasonality, pregnancy length, litter size, birth weight, and kitten mortality. Many of the problems that can arise can be prevented by proper management. Records of individuals, including observation of estrus, mating, vaccination, health tests, weights of kittens, and medical treatment, facilitate the identification and correction of the underlying causes. Overcrowding increases the risk of behavioral problems associated with stress and facilitates the spread and manifestation of infectious diseases that may cause reproductive problems.

REPRODUCTIVE PHYSIOLOGY

SEASONALITY

The female domestic cat is seasonally polyestrous and a long-day breeder. Increased day length induces estrus. The mean duration of the reproductive season varies with geographical latitude. Near the equator, no seasonality is seen, while the seasonal anestrus typically lasts from September to January in the northern hemisphere.[1,2] However, large individual variations in the length of the reproductive season cause wide normal ranges within the same geographical latitude.[2] Seasonality often is more pronounced in cats allowed outdoors than in cats confined indoors, because artificial light can interfere with the natural photoperiods. Feral cats have a pronounced

834

seasonal pattern, with most pregnancies found in the spring.[3] Although seasonality can be observed in the distribution of litters in pedigree catteries, it is less pronounced than in feral cats, probably because of the influence of artificial light on cats confined indoors and perhaps also because of genetic background.[4,5] A genetic influence on the sensitivity for alterations in daylight is indicated by breed differences in seasonality. The Persian breed, for example, generally has a more pronounced seasonality than the Burmese breed.[4-6]

Light programs can be used to control the estrus cycle. A day length less than 8 hours will suppress estrous activity. To induce cyclicity throughout the year, owners should ensure a constant day length of 12 hours or more.[1] In a room with windows, the changes in natural photoperiods may interfere with a light program; therefore an environment that allows for full control over the amount of light may be necessary for successful control of the estrous cycle.

Although it is known that male cats can produce offspring throughout the year, the effect of season on reproductive function in the male domestic cat has not been explored sufficiently. Recent studies indicate, however, that sperm quality may decrease during the nonreproductive season.[7,8]

PUBERTY

Female

The queen will have her first estrus between 4 and 21 months of age, with a median around 9 to 12 months.[6,9] Because cyclicity is controlled by the day length, age of puberty will be affected by season. Depending on month of birth, the queen may enter her first estrus during the next breeding season or during the season the second year after birth.[2] There seem to be some breed differences in the age of puberty. The Siamese and Burmese breeds reach puberty at an earlier age, on average, than the Persian breed, although individual variations often overlap breed differences.[6,9]

Male

Spermatogenesis is generally established at 6 to 8 months of age, at which time an increase in testicular weight and testosterone production can be observed, but the spermatogenic function usually is not mature until after 8 to 12 months of age.[10] The age when the male starts to mate may, however, vary more than the age of established spermatogenesis. Some individual males in long-haired breeds do not breed until they are 3 years of age.

THE ESTROUS CYCLE

The queen typically is an induced ovulator, which means that a mating stimulus usually is required for ovulation to occur. Spontaneous ovulations, however, also can occur. The phases in the estrous cycle in the nonmated queen can be characterized as the follicular phase (proestrus and estrus) and the nonfollicular phase (interestrus). Estrus is followed by the luteal phase if a sterile mating

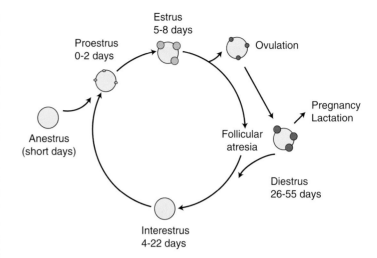

Figure 80-1 The reproductive cycle of the female domestic cat.

induces ovulation or if the queen ovulates spontaneously (Figure 80-1).

Follicular Phase

The follicular phase, determined as the period when estradiol levels are above basal level, has a duration of 3 to 16 days and is not affected by mating or ovulation. The onset of the follicular phase is abrupt, with a twofold increase in estradiol-17β, within 24 hours. When estradiol is increased above basal levels, some queens will show estrous behavior the first day; however, the majority do not exhibit behavioral estrus until day 3 or 4 in the follicular phase.[11]

A short period of proestrus often can be observed. During proestrus, the queen starts to shows estrous behavior but she does not allow mating. Estrus is defined as the period when the queen allows mating. The follicles increase in size and reach a diameter of 2 to 3 mm. The average duration of estrous behavior is 5 to 8 days, with a range of 2 to 19 days.[11,12] The duration is not affected by mating or ovulation.[12,13] Estrous behavior may continue for 1 to 4 days after the end of the follicular phase.[11]

Estrous behavior is induced by an increase in estradiol during the follicular phase. Typical behaviors observed during estrus are increased affection, vocalization, restlessness, loss of appetite, increased frequency of urination, rolling, rubbing of the head, and lordosis.[14] Lordosis may be shown spontaneously or can be provoked by grasping the female by the scruff of the neck and scratching around the tail. The queen then will lower her chest, elevate her pelvis, tread with her legs, and deviate her tail. When the queen is lifted, the back often will be stiff as she tries to stretch and arch it. A clear vaginal discharge often can be observed.[14] Behaviors displayed during estrus also can be seen to some extent when the queen is not in estrus or in neutered females, but their intensity and frequency are more pronounced in estrus. There are, however, individual variations in the intensity of estrous behavior. Intensity also may depend on environment and stress. If the queen is put in an unfamiliar environment, she will often show a less pronounced behavior because of insecurity.

Interestrus

In the absence of a mating stimulus, ovarian follicles regress after estrus.[13] During interestrus the queen shows no estrous behavior. The duration of interestrus varies but is usually 4 to 22 days during the reproductive season.[11]

Diestrus or Pseudopregnancy

Although the queen typically is an induced ovulator, spontaneous ovulations do occur.[15] A nonpregnant luteal phase occurs after a sterile mating or a spontaneous ovulation. The diestrus phase also is called *pseudopregnancy*. Basal level of progesterone is less than 3 nmol/L.[13] The first significant increase in progesterone is seen from days 3 to 4 after mating.[16,17] Peak levels are reached between days 13 and 21, after which concentrations decrease steadily.[13,17] Progesterone concentrations do not differ significantly from those of pregnant animals until around day 30, after which levels are significantly lower in pseudopregnant queens. The duration of diestrus is 26 to 55 days, with a mean of 38 days, giving a cycle length of 6 to 10 weeks in nonpregnant ovulating queens.[13] There is no increase in prolactin concentration in the pseudopregnant cat, in contrast to the pregnant queen.[18]

Anestrus

During anestrus the queen is reproductively inactive, and there are no active structures in the ovaries.

ENDOCRINOLOGY IN THE MALE CAT AND THE EFFECTS OF TESTOSTERONE

In intact males testosterone is released in a pulsatile fashion without any apparent rhythm and varies between nondetectable and 81.5 nmol/L. Testosterone reaches basal levels (0 to 1.7 nmol/L) within 24 hours after castration.[19] The glans penis of the male cat is covered with spines. The development of the penile spines is related directly to testosterone production. The spines start to develop around 2 months of age and are fully developed around 6 to 7 months. The penile spines regress after castration. The presence of penile spines indicates that a male cat produces testosterone.[20,21] In young domestic kittens, the prepuce is attached to the penis by loose connective tissue. The penis and the prepuce are separated under the influence of androgens. This attachment may remain if a male cat is castrated at a young age.[20,22]

MATING AND OVULATION

Mating Behavior

The male grasps the queen firmly in the neck. He often will tread with his legs over the female's pelvis. This will stimulate a more pronounced lordosis. Intromission is rapid, during which the queen emits a characteristic shriek. An experienced male will withdraw quickly; otherwise, the queen will free herself and strike out at him. The queen then will display the typical postcoital reac-

tion, which includes rolling vigorously on the floor and licking the genitals. Mating will be repeated when the queen allows.

Management of Mating

Mating causes a reflex that releases gonadotrophin-releasing hormone (GnRH) from the hypothalamus. In response to the GnRH surge, luteinizing hormone (LH) is released from the pituitary gland, which induces ovulation. When a threshold of LH has been reached, mature oocytes ovulate. Often more than one mating is required to reach the threshold of LH. In one study, only 50 per cent of all queens who were mated only once had an LH release that reached the threshold required for ovulation to occur.[23]

It is necessary to consider the temperament of cats, their mating behavior, and the mechanism of ovulation. Because cats are territorial, it usually is better to bring the female to the male for mating, because the likelihood of a successful mating is increased if the male is in familiar surroundings. If the female is very frightened and nervous, it may be better to move the male to the female. There must be enough space for the male to withdraw from the female's postcoital reaction. The cats should not be separated before day 3 or 4 of estrus, because some queens will not ovulate after a mating in early estrus.[16] Because the release of LH depends on the number of matings, at least four matings should be allowed during the same day. Some cats will not mate when observed, and each mounting may not be followed by a mating. The postcoital reaction is, however, an indication that there has been an intromission.

Breeders sometimes believe that allowing cats to mate for several days during estrus will result in kittens of different ages in the litter; therefore they restrict the number of days for mating. There is, however, no evidence that there will be ovulations on more than one occasion during estrus. Once the threshold of LH has been reached, all mature follicles will ovulate.[24] Fertilization can only take place up to approximately 49 hours after ovulation induction (17 to 24 hours after ovulation); therefore all embryos will be of similar age.[25]

DIAGNOSTIC METHODS TO MONITOR THE ESTROUS CYCLE

Estrous behavior usually is distinct and easy to recognize. Some queens will, however, have a more diffuse behavior. Grasping the queen in the neck skin and scratching around the tail usually results in lordosis and treading of the hind legs in a queen in estrus. Vaginal cytology is a useful method to diagnose elevated estradiol concentrations indirectly, indicating estrus. Estradiol causes cornification of the vaginal cells. The queen is firmly held by the neck skin in order to collect a vaginal cytological sample. A cotton swab is moistened with saline, inserted in the vestibulum, and rolled to catch the vaginal cells. The cotton swab is rolled over a microscopic slide that is then stained with Diff Quick. During estrus more than 80 per cent of the vaginal cells are cornified (Figure 80-2). It is important to remember that vaginal cytology sampling

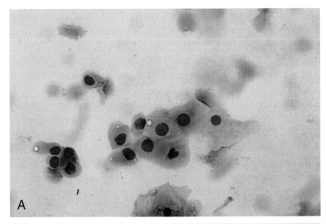

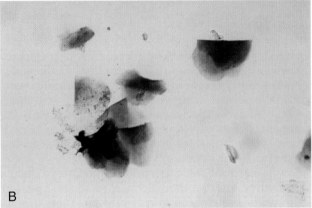

Figure 80-2 A, Vaginal cytology in a queen that is not in estrus. (Stained with Hemacolor.) **B,** Vaginal cytology from a queen in estrus. (Stained with Hemacolor.) (Courtesy Merck, Darmstadt, Germany.)

can cause ovulation as a result of the vaginal stimulation; therefore the queen should be bred within 49 hours after sampling if breeding is intended during the same estrus. Analysis of serum or plasma estradiol also can be used to monitor ovarian function. An estradiol concentration greater than 70 pmol/L is indicative of estrus.[11] Although there are individual variations, the first rise in estradiol often precedes estrous behavior by 1 to 4 days and the cornified vaginal smear by approximately 2 to 3 days. Estrous behavior often continues a few days after estradiol has returned to basal levels.[11]

FERTILIZATION AND IMPLANTATION

Ovulation usually is completed 25 to 32 hours after mating, and fertilization occurs shortly thereafter.[26,27] The embryos have reached the uterus on day 6 after mating.[27] The preimplantation phase lasts from fertilization until approximately day 12.5 after mating, when the embryos are hatched from the zona pellucida and come in contact with the endometrium, leading to initiation of the implantation process.[28] The trophoblast cells start to invade the endometrium on day 14, and on day 16 the embryos are attached and can not be flushed from the uterus.[28,29] The placenta is endotheliochorial and zonary. At either end of the placental girdle are the marginal hematomas forming brown borders.[28]

SUPERFETATION

Superfetation occurs when a mating during pregnancy results in a new pregnancy, leading to fetuses of different ages in the uterus. Ovarian follicular activity also can be observed during the luteal phase, and these follicles therefore may be associated with elevations of estradiol.[13] Females sometimes show estrous behavior and allow mating during pregnancy. There are, however, no confirmed cases of superfetation in cats.

SUPERFECUNDATION

Superfecundation occurs when there are multiple fathers to a litter. Matings up to 49 hours after induction of ovulation can result in pregnancy, and the length of life of spermatozoa must be at least 32 hours (the interval between mating and ovulation) because a single mating may result in pregnancy.[25] Therefore the oocytes can be fertilized by matings up to 49 hours after the mating that caused ovulation, while it is not known how long spermatozoa from matings before this time can survive in the female genital tract. Superfecundation is common in cats allowed to roam freely and is more common in dense populations. In one study, 76 per cent of all litters of free-roaming queens in a dense population had more than one father, and five different fathers for six kittens was observed for one litter.[30]

GESTATION LENGTH

The gestation period ranges between 57 and 71 days, with an average of 63 to 66 days. Although unusual, birth of live kittens has been reported after a gestation length of only 50 days.[31] More than 95 per cent of all pregnancies have been reported to be within the interval of 61 to 69 days, and more than 90 per cent within 63 to 67 days.[31] Large litter sizes may be associated with a shorter gestation length than for small litters.[31] There seems to be some genetic influence in the duration of pregnancy as demonstrated by breed and line differences, with the Korat breed having the shortest mean gestation length (63 days) and the Siamese and Oriental breeds the longest (66 days).[31,32] Increased mortality has been observed in kittens born before day 63, indicating that they may be premature.[4] The more the length of the pregnancy deviates from the normal range, the higher is the risk that the kittens will not be viable.[31]

PREVALENCE AND CAUSES OF DYSTOCIA

Dystocia is not uncommon in the pure-bred queen, although the frequency seems to vary between breeds. In a colony with research cats of mixed origin, the frequency was only 0.4 per cent, while the mean for pure-bred cats is around 8 to 14 per cent, with 6 to 8 per cent of litters delivered by cesarean section.[31,33] The Siamese breed seems to have a higher incidence than other breeds.[31,33,34] In one study, there was no connection between small litter size and dystocia, while another study found that a small litter size increased the risk of dystocia.[31,34] Most dystocias (67 per cent) are of maternal origin, with the majority caused by uterine inertia (61 per cent). A small birth canal is the second most common maternal cause of dystocia (5 per cent) and can be caused by previous fractures, a vaginal tumor, or by the fact that the queen is young and immature. Fetal malpresentations (16 per cent) and fetal malformations (8 per cent) are the most common fetal causes of dystocia.[34]

CONCEPTION RATES, LITTER SIZES, AND BIRTH WEIGHTS

The normal conception rate is 70 to 80 per cent.[9,12,27,35] The number of kittens varies between one and 13, with a mean of four to five.[4,6,12,31,36] Most litters are of one to six kittens, while more than nine kittens is uncommon. Often, the mean number of kittens is lower in the first litter than in subsequent litters.[5,36,37] The mean litter size varies between breeds and is larger for the Burmese, Siamese, and Oriental breeds than for the Abyssinian, Somali, Persian, and Sacred Birman breeds.[5,31] The number of days on which the queen is mated and the number of matings during estrus does not affect litter size.[4] The mean weight of the newborn kittens has been reported to be 100 g ±10 g in the domestic shorthair cat, but often is lower in pedigree breeds and varies with breed from 73 g in the Korat to 116 g for the Maine Coon. Birth weight ranges from 30 to 170 g in all live-born kittens.[31,32,38] Festing and Bleby[37] found no effect of litter size on birth weight, while Sparkes et al[31] found that the birth weight decreased with larger litter sizes.

When cats are bred for optimal production, as in colonies of research cats, two to three litters can be born per year to each queen.[36] A decline in reproduction in older queens has been reported in one study, but was not found in another.[5,31] An association between age and litter size may, however, be difficult to detect because relatively few old queens are kept for breeding.[31] Another reason for a failure to detect a general relationship between old age and low litter size could be that queens who are kept in breeding programs have been shown to be good breeders in their previous litters.

KITTEN MORTALITY FROM BIRTH TO WEANING

The frequency of stillborn kittens varies between catteries and breeds. The mean proportion for all breeds varies from 4.3 to 7.2 per cent.[31,36] The percentage of stillborn kittens has been reported to be higher for the Persian breed (11 to 22 per cent) than for other breeds.[4,31] The risk of stillborn kittens increases with litter size.[31]

The proportion of kittens surviving until weaning is around 84 to 87 per cent; however, the survival rate is lower in general for the Persian breed than for other breeds, with approximately 75 per cent weaned successfully.[6,31,36] The majority of the kittens who die between birth and weaning are either stillborn or die during their first week of life.[31,38] Litters from overweight queens have

increased mortality. A small birth weight also increases the risk of neonatal mortality.[38] Congenital abnormalities account for a proportion of kitten mortality, while trauma and infections are the most common acquired causes of kitten mortality.[38] However, the cause of death often can not be established. The chance of finding an underlying etiological cause increases if whole carcasses are submitted for necropsy examination instead of only tissue samples.[38-40] Kittens reared in a specific pathogen-free (SPF) colony had lower mortality, with only 3.3 per cent stillborn and 8.9 per cent total losses until weaning, indicating that control of infections increases kitten survival.[37] A summary of reproductive performance in the domestic cat can be found in Table 80-1.

NUTRITION

A pregnant queen needs extra energy early in pregnancy. The weight gain is linear until parturition. At the end of gestation, the queen needs 25 to 50 per cent more energy than her normal maintenance needs.[41,42] Free-choice feeding will allow the queen to provide herself with adequate nutrition. Only 40 per cent of the total increase in weight is lost at parturition, while the rest is needed as extra reserves for lactation.[41]

A well-balanced diet is essential for good reproductive performance. The diet should contain at least 32 per cent high-quality protein and 18 per cent fat. Diets that are more calorie-dense (23 per cent vs. 10 to 14 per cent fat) result in slightly larger litter sizes, while depletion of

Table 80-1 Reproductive Performance in the Domestic Cat

Puberty female	4-21 months, median 9-12 months
Puberty male	6-12 months
Duration of estrus	2-19 days, on average 5 to 8 days
Duration of interestrus	Usually 4-22 days
Duration of diestrus	26-55 days, mean 38
Implantation	Days 14-16 after breeding
Duration of pregnancy	95% within 61-69 days
Pregnancy rate	70-80%
Birth weight	Mean 73-116 g depending on breed
Stillbirths	4-7%
Kitten mortality until weaning	13-16% (on average higher for the Persian)
Litter size	Usually 1-6, range 1-13 (more extreme variations are sometimes reported anecdotally)
Dystocia	8-14% for pure bred cats
Weaning	Not before 7-8 weeks. Breeders and cat organizations often prefer that kittens are not re-homed before 12-13 weeks of age.

essential fatty acids will result in a reduced number of viable kittens.[43,44] Long-term taurine insufficiency will result in increased frequency of pseudopregnancies after mating, fetal resorptions, smaller litter sizes, and stillborn kittens.[45] When queens were fed a diet with insufficient copper, the time interval to conception was increased but litter size was not affected.[46]

LACTATION, PASSIVE IMMUNITY, AND NEONATAL ISOERYTHROLYSIS

Lactation and Weaning

Lactation is the most energy-demanding phase in the reproductive cycle of the queen. She will consume two to three times her normal maintenance energy, but will still lose weight because body reserves are needed to provide enough energy.[41,47] Milk production can be observed from 1 to 7 days before parturition. The milk yield varies from 1 to 8 per cent of the queen's body weight depending on the number of kittens and lactation stage, with a mean of 5 to 6 per cent.[47,48] Dentition usually starts around 3 weeks of age, and supplemental kitten food can be given from 3 to 4 weeks of age. Milk alone can support growth until 4 weeks of age.[41,49] The age when the kittens start to eat solid food varies between 3 to 5 weeks, with differences between litters.[49] Homemade diets for weaning should be avoided because these may have an incorrect balance of nutrients (see Chapter 13). Kittens should not be weaned completely before 7 to 8 weeks of age.[41] Some cat organizations recommend that kittens not be separated from their mother before they are 12 to 13 weeks old to promote the proper development of social behavior and immunity before the kitten is sold.[50,51]

Passive Immunity

The endotheliochorial placenta allows transfer of only minimal amounts of antibodies, which is why kittens are born with very low antibody levels. Feline colostrum, however, is rich in antibodies. The total antibody concentrations in milk decrease rapidly during the first week of lactation.[52] Colostral antibodies can only be transferred through the intestinal tract of the kittens for the first 12 to 16 hours after birth.[53] Ingestion of colostrum results in a rapid increase in antibody levels in the kitten's blood during the first day of life. The concentration of maternal antibodies decreases steadily from the first day of the kitten's life due to catabolism and is lowest around 3 to 5 weeks of age, after which the concentration increases due to the kitten's own antibody synthesis.[52,54] If kittens are deprived of colostrum and fostered by a queen in the milk phase of lactation, or fed a milk replacer instead of colostrum, there will be failure of passive immunity.[52] Therefore extra attention is needed to protect such kittens from infections.

Feline Neonatal Isoerythrolysis

Some cat breeds are affected by neonatal isoerythrolysis. There are three blood groups in cats: A, B, and AB. Blood group B is uncommon in most populations of household cats but is more prevalent in some pedigree breeds. Breeds with a high percentage of blood group B include British Shorthair, Devon Rex, and Cornish Rex, while blood group B is absent or very uncommon in the Siamese and Burmese breeds. Blood group AB is the most uncommon blood group.[55] (See Chapter 61 for further discussion on feline blood types.)

Cats with blood group A or B produce alloantibodies against the foreign blood group. These antibodies are transferred to the colostrum. Queens with blood group B have high levels of antibodies with strong affinity for the A antigen on the erythrocytes, while queens with blood group A have low levels of anti-B antibodies with a lower affinity against blood group B. Cats with blood group AB do not produce antibodies against either blood group A or B. Kittens with blood group A (or AB) who nurse from a queen with blood group B during the first hours of life (when antibodies can be absorbed) therefore will be affected by neonatal isoerythrolysis because anti-A antibodies ingested with the colostrum will attack their erythrocytes. After the first day of life, antibodies are no longer absorbed and the kittens can nurse safely from their mother. Typical signs of neonatal isoerythrolysis are kittens who are born healthy but who develop signs such as icterus, pigmenturia, or sudden death after ingestion of colostrum. In less severe cases, there is necrosis of the tail tip.[55]

Neonatal isoerythrolysis can be prevented by blood typing cats from breeds with a high prevalence of B or AB blood types before breeding. Blood group B is recessive to blood group A, while the AB allele is recessive to the A allele but dominant over the B allele, which is why kittens at risk have a mother with blood group B and a father with blood group A or AB.[55,56] In these litters, kittens at risk must be removed from their mother for 24 hours and allowed to nurse from a queen with blood group A or fed a milk replacer. After that time, they can be allowed to nurse safely from their mother.

GROWTH OF KITTENS

Kittens should gain approximately 7 to 10 g/day or 50 to 100 g/week until they are 6 months old. Failure to increase in weight indicates that the kitten is not getting enough milk and immediate intervention is needed.[57] Birth weight does not differ between male and female kittens, but males are heavier at 6 weeks of age.[37]

INFERTILITY

Infertility in the queen may be caused by abnormal estrous cycles, failure to ovulate, failure to conceive, or pregnancy loss after fertilization. The history should include fertility of the male, previous breeding records of the female, estrous length and intervals, estrous interval after breeding, observation of mating and/or postcoital reaction, previous health tests, and vaccination history. Information about general health and reproductive performance in the cattery also is valuable to identify possible herd health problems.

The clinical evaluation depends somewhat on the information in the history and the specific reason for consultation. If it is obvious that the queen has not ovulated after a mating, it may be enough to correct management factors. Depending on the history, it also may be wise to start with evaluation of the male cat. Otherwise, the clinical evaluation generally should include a thorough general health check and a special gynecological examination, with particular attention paid to the presence of vaginal discharge, evaluation of vaginal cytology, abdominal palpation of the uterus, and an ultrasound evaluation of the uterus and ovaries. Unless already included in the routine evaluation of the cattery, tests for feline leukemia virus (FeLV) antigen and, if indicated, feline immunodeficiency virus (FIV) antibody should be performed. Aborted fetuses with their fetal membranes should be sent for autopsy. A postmortem examination also is valuable in kittens who die without an obvious cause.

ABNORMAL ESTROUS CYCLES

Anestrus

A diagnosis of anestrus should not be made before the queen is about 2 years of age. The anestrus may be primary or secondary. In primary anestrus, the queen has never displayed estrous behavior, while in secondary anestrus the interval is prolonged. Because the estrus interval varies considerably between individuals, it is not possible to determine an exact limit for a normal interval. Absence of estrus for a year or more, however, is not normal. It is important to consider the seasonal nature and effect of light on female reproduction. If there is inadequate light, the female will not come into estrus. In primary anestrus, developmental disorders can not be excluded.

Although unusual, chromosomal abnormalities may be a cause of primary anestrus. X-chromosome monosomy (37,XO) will result in ovarian dysgenesis, resulting in primary anestrus. Queens with X-chromosome mosaicism (37,XO/39,XXY or 37,XO/38XX) may be fertile, however.[58,59] Male cats with defective androgen receptors

have female external genitalia, although their karyotype is normal male (38,XY), and they have testosterone-producing testes in their abdomen. The testosterone, however, may not affect the target organs because of defective androgen receptors.[60]

The most common reason for secondary anestrus is likely to be season and/or an insufficient amount of light. This is physiological and can be corrected by increasing the amount of light to more than 12 to 14 hours per day. A light program, however, is not always practical if the cats are kept in a home environment, because full control of the amount of light and changes in the day length may be necessary.

A previous ovariectomy may be the reason for permanent anestrus in a queen with unknown history. In order to diagnose the presence or absence of ovaries, a plasma sample for analysis of estradiol-17β is collected 120 minutes after injection of a GnRH analogue (Busereline, Receptal Vet., Intervet, 0.4 μg/kg IM). At 120 minutes after Busereline stimulation, estradiol-17β ranged between 5 and 9 pmol/L in spayed queens, and between 12 and 41 pmol/L in inactive (not in estrus) intact queens (Figure 80-3). Measurement of resting estradiol levels without previous stimulation with GnRH is not very useful to diagnose the presence of ovaries, because resting concentrations in intact queens overlap the basal concentrations in spayed females.[61] (The reader is referred to Chapter 24 in the fifth volume of this series for further discussion of this subject.)

A thorough history is important to exclude medications as a cause of anestrus. A thorough clinical examination should be performed to rule out intercurrent diseases.

Estrus can be induced artificially by the IM injection of 100 to 150 IU equine chorionic gonadotropin (eCG); however, eCG is not licensed for use in cats.[62] Prepubertal cats should not be treated, and the queen should not be in silent estrus (to avoid hyperstimulation) or in the luteal phase (because the treatment is unlikely to be effective) when treated. Overdosing will lead to ovarian hyperstimulation.

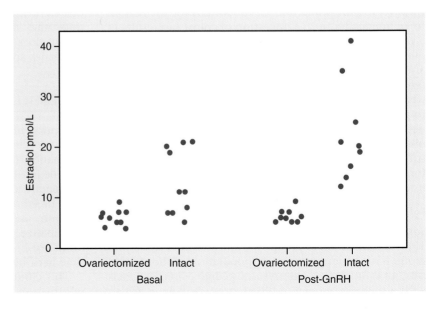

Figure 80-3 Estradiol concentrations in ovariectomized (n=11) and intact (n=11) queens before and 2 hours after injection with a GnRH-analogue. (From Axnér E, Gustavsson T, Ström Holst B: Estradiol measurement after GnRH-stimulation as a method to diagnose the presence of ovaries in the female domestic cat, *Theriogenology* 70:186, 2008.)

Silent Estrus

The queen with silent estrus has normal follicular waves but does not display overt signs of estrus. This condition probably is more common in subordinate queens in multiple-cat households. Vaginal cytology collected twice weekly can be used to identify queens with silent estrus. Affected queens can be bred successfully when the smear is indicative of estrus.[12]

Persistent Estrus

Estrus behavior for more than 19 days may indicate an ovarian abnormality. Generally, follicular waves do not overlap in cats. Occasionally, overlapping waves may cause a prolonged duration of estrus. Another reason for a prolonged estrous behavior is that some queens will continue to show estrous behavior during periods of interestrus. Vaginal cytology can be used to determine if a queen with prolonged estrous behavior has active ovarian follicles.[11]

Follicular cysts may produce estradiol, causing signs of continuous estrus, a cornified vaginal smear, and elevated plasma estradiol. Although the treatment of choice is ovariohysterectomy, successful treatment resulting in restored fertility has been described. Induction of ovulation may be attempted for valuable breeding queens. Administration of 250 IU human chorionic gonadotropin (hCG) IM q24h for 2 days may result in luteinization of the cyst.[63] Surgical resection of the cysts sparing the ovaries, or ovariectomy if the cyst is unilateral, also may be attempted in valuable breeding queens.[63] After excluding other reasons for prolonged estrus, treatment with progestagens might induce cyst atrophy; however, the risk of side effects has to be considered.

Cysts around the ovary that are discovered during ultrasound examination or found at surgery are not always clinically important. Rete ovarii cysts are nonfunctional and usually can be considered as incidental findings unless their size causes compression of the ovarian cortex. Paraovarian cysts are remnants of the mesonephric tubule and also can be considered as incidental findings.[64-66]

Steroid-producing tumors also may cause persistent estrus. The most common feline ovarian tumor is the granulosa-theca cell tumor. Dysgerminomas have been reported to induce estrous behavior in cats but also may cause masculine behavior due to androgen production. Queens with hormone-producing ovarian tumors will not respond to treatment with progestagens or to attempts to induce ovulation. The treatment of choice is ovariohysterectomy unless the tumor has already metastasized at the time of diagnosis.[67,68] A summary of causes of abnormal cyclicity can be found in Box 80-1.

INFERTILITY IN THE QUEEN WITH NORMAL ESTROUS CYCLES

Failure to produce kittens after a mating may be caused by failure to mate and ovulate, failure to conceive after a normal mating, failure of implantation, and resorption or abortion. If the queen comes into estrus within 40 days

---

Box 80-1 Potential Causes of Abnormal Estrus Cycles

ANESTRUS
Primary
Chromosomal disorders (X-chromosome monosomy)
Prepubertal ovario(hyster)ectomy
Pseudohermaphroditism
Late puberty
Secondary
Insufficient light
Seasonal anestrus
Ovario(hyster)ectomy after puberty
Medication with progestagens
Other debilitating disease

PROLONGED ESTRUS
Overlapping ovarian follicles
Behavioral estrus during periods of interestrus
Functional ovarian follicular cysts
Hormone-producing ovarian neoplasia

OTHER
Silent estrus

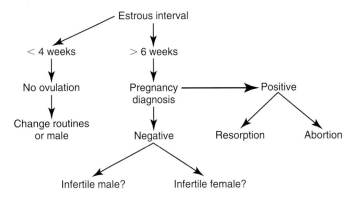

Figure 80-4 Flow chart for evaluation of infertility in the female domestic cat.

---

after a mating, most likely she has not ovulated. The reason for a failure to ovulate usually is that there has been no mating, or a mating occurred too early or late during estrus. Therefore changing the male and/or adjusting the routines for mating may solve the problem (Figure 80-4).

Developmental disorders may be a reason for failure of conception. Congenital malformations of the uterus and vagina are rare and difficult to diagnose because there may be no signs other than infertility. Aplasia of the cranial vagina, parts of the uterine body, or uterine horns may interfere with transport of spermatozoa to the oviducts and are caused by failure in the development of the müllerian duct. Depending on the type and localization of the defect, however, there may be accumulation of secretions in the uterus resulting in mucometra or hydrometra.[69,70]

The possible role of stress in pregnancy failure has not been evaluated in queens. It is known, however, that stress or injection with adrenocorticotrophic hormone (ACTH) induces release of cortisol and progesterone from the adrenal glands.[71] Administration of ACTH and resulting altered progesterone profiles is a potential cause of embryo loss in the sow, so it seems wise to avoid stressful situations for a queen who has been mated.[72]

Cystic Endometrial Hyperplasia

Cystic endometrial hyperplasia (CEH) is a condition in which repeated, hormonally influenced growth of the endometrium results in a hyperplastic growth of the epithelium and cystic dilatation of uterine glands (Figure 80-5). Unless the CEH has been complicated with an infection, affected queens usually show no clinical signs except for infertility.[73] In the normal cycling queen, both estradiol and progesterone contribute to cyclic growth of the endometrium.[74] Normally, this growth regresses in interestrus and anestrus. Frequent estrus cycles, spontaneous ovulation, and treatment with exogenous progestins are believed to predispose to the development of the abnormal endometrial growth. The condition is not unusual, and the frequency increases with age of the queen, with more than 85 per cent of queens more than 5 years of age affected.[73,75,76] In one study, CEH was found to be much more common in colony cats kept indoors than in feral cats, indicating that housing conditions influence the development of the condition.[75] Ultrasonography and hysterography can be used to diagnose CEH; however, it may be difficult to differentiate between normal cyclic changes of the endometrium and CEH if the changes are mild.[77] At this time there is no effective treatment for CEH except ovariohysterectomy.

Endometritis/Metritis

Low-grade uterine infection is a known cause of infertility in other species such as the mare and sow. Because of the difficulties associated with diagnosing this condition in cats, the incidence is unknown in this species. Uterine infections are caused by opportunistic bacteria from the normal vaginal flora; therefore a bacterial culture can not be used to diagnose uterine infection because the same species of bacteria are found in healthy queens and in queens with uterine infections.[78,79] Bacteria are not found normally in the uterus; however, they may enter the uterus from the vagina occasionally during estrus when the cervix is open. Most likely, these bacteria are eliminated normally by the defense mechanisms of the healthy uterus.[78,80]

Vaginal discharge always is an indication of a genital pathology, except for the small amount of clear fluid that can be seen during estrus. To avoid selecting resistant bacterial strains, treatment with antibiotics should be reserved for queens in whom there is a clear indication that there may be a uterine infection, once other causes of infertility have been excluded such as viral infections (e.g., FeLV and FIV), CEH, and poor breeding management resulting in failure of mating and/or ovulation. Treatment with antibiotics may, however, restore fertility in queens in whom there is reason to suspect a mild uterine infection and in whom other causes have been excluded.[77]

Although breeders sometimes report problems with uterine infections in several queens after mating with the same tom, the possible role of the tom in spreading infections has not been evaluated. Uterine infections, however, generally are caused by the same type of bacteria that are present in the normal vaginal flora, so the spread of infectious agents between cats is not likely to be a common cause of metritis.

Pyometra

In the queen with pyometra, the uterine infection has resulted in accumulation of pus in the uterine lumen. In contrast to mild, low-grade infections, pyometra usually is easy to diagnose from clinical findings and ultrasound evaluation. The most common clinical sign is mucopurulent to hemorrhagic vaginal discharge. Other signs include anorexia, lethargy, vomiting, weight loss, abdominal distension, palpable uterus, dehydration, and fever. Polydipsia/polyuria also may be seen but is not observed as frequently as in bitches.[81,82]

In contrast to CEH, which is not associated with any particular phase of the cycle, pyometra occurs most often during the luteal phase. Most cases are diagnosed within

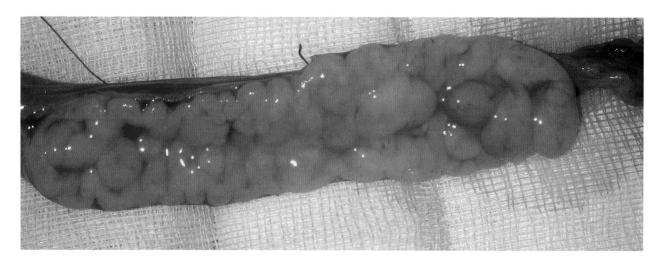

Figure 80-5 A feline uterus with endometrial hyperplasia.

a month after estrus.[81] CEH predisposes queens to pyometra; therefore the disease often, but not always, is seen together with CEH.[73,81] Because of the association between the luteal phase and pyometra, spontaneous ovulation or treatment with endogenous progestins also are likely to be predisposing factors.

Although the treatment of choice for pyometra is ovariohysterectomy, it is often possible to save the breeding value of an affected queen. Good candidates for medical treatment are young breeding queens in good condition and with an open pyometra. Antibiotics should not be used as a sole therapy when there is fluid in the uterine lumen but should be combined with prostaglandins to achieve evacuation of the uterine lumen. Prostaglandins stimulate uterine contractions and also may cause luteolysis during late luteal phase.[82] The treatment is associated with side effects such as vocalization, panting, restlessness, grooming, tenesmus, salivation, diarrhea, kneading, mydriasis, emesis, urination, and lordosis.[82] Side effects usually resolve 2 to 20 minutes after treatment. The side effects after prostaglandin treatment in queens are milder than those observed after the same treatment in bitches.[63,82] Treatment with natural prostaglandins (0.1 mg/kg SQ or IM q12h or q24h), in combination with antibiotics, has been successful, with 80 to 90 per cent of treated queens subsequently producing live kittens. Recurrence of disease occurred in 10 to 14 per cent of treated queens, but could be resolved with repeated treatment.[63,82] Verstegen[83] suggested a treatment regimen with lower doses of 20 to 50 μg/kg natural PGF$_{2\alpha}$ administered three to five times each day for 5 to 7 days to reduce side effects and to achieve more frequent uterine contractions.[83] The queen should be monitored with ultrasound during treatment, and ovariohysterectomy should be performed if uterine diameter is not reduced. Hospitalization is recommended during treatment to monitor side effects and to evaluate response to treatment.

Queens with live fetuses or with the presence of fetal remnants and queens with cardiac or pulmonary disease should not be treated with PGF$_{2\alpha}$.[63,82]

The progesterone blocker aglepristone can be beneficial in queens with pyometra in the luteal phase. Aglepristone is administered at a dose of 15 mg on days 1, 2, and 8 of treatment and may facilitate opening of the cervix in queens with closed pyometra. After the cervix is open, the treatment is combined with PGF$_{2\alpha}$.[84] Before breeding from a queen previously affected with pyometra, the possibility that the predisposition might be hereditary should be considered.

INFECTIOUS DISEASES

Viral Infections

Abortion, resorption, and preimplantation loss have been described in viremic FeLV-infected queens. Queens with reproductive failure due to FeLV usually show no other signs of disease.[85,86] Vaccines are available to protect cats against FeLV infection; however, the best method to prevent infection in a cattery is to introduce only FeLV-negative cats to the facility.

Feline immunodeficiency virus is excreted in the saliva and is spread mainly by bite wounds, making infections most common in free-roaming male cats.[87] FIV can cause transplacental infection of feline fetuses resulting in abortion, arrested fetal development, low birth weight, thymus atrophy, and birth of weak, infected kittens.[88] As with FeLV, cats should be tested before they are introduced to the cattery.

Feline panleukopenia virus (FPV) has an affinity for rapidly dividing cells, making the developing fetus a target for the virus. Transplacental infection can occur in seriously ill queens as well as in queens with subclinical disease. FPV infection in pregnant queens can lead to resorption, abortion, or birth of kittens with cerebellar hypoplasia resulting in ataxia and hydrocephalus depending on at which stage of gestation the fetuses were infected. The virus may infect only part of a litter.[89] Vaccination against FPV is recommended as a core vaccine for all cats and is efficient in protecting against the disease. FPV seems to be an important cause of mortality in pedigree kittens.[40] If there is environmental exposure to large doses of virus, there may be kitten mortality even if the cats in the household are vaccinated.[90] Live FPV vaccine should not be used during pregnancy because this can cause the same lesions in fetuses as natural infection.[91]

Transplacental transfer has been induced by experimental infections with feline herpesvirus (FHV); however, pregnancy failure after natural infections is more likely to be caused by severe debilitating upper respiratory disease of the queen.[92] An association between prevalence of FHV and reproductive disease has been observed. FHV infection also is a cause of kitten mortality.[40,92-94] Serological examination to identify healthy carriers is problematic because most cats are vaccinated routinely against FHV. Vaccination has a protective effect against the disease but does not prevent infection.[87]

In utero infection of feline calicivirus (FCV) resulting in fetal death has been described.[95,96] FCV infection probably is an uncommon cause for abortion in cats considering the paucity of reports; it is more likely to cause kitten mortality.[40] Testing and eliminating infected cats is difficult because of the high prevalence of the disease, routine vaccination, and the occurrence of clinically healthy carriers. Therefore vaccination is the recommended method to control clinical problems associated with FCV. Vaccination protects against the disease but does not prevent infection.[87]

Protozoal Infections

Cats are definitive hosts for the protozoan *Toxoplasma gondii* and are infected commonly although clinical signs usually are not seen. The major concern is that *T. gondii* is a zoonotic pathogen that can infect human fetuses. In utero infection, however, does appear to occur in cats.[97,98] Experimental infection of cats has caused transplacental transmission with abortion of mummified fetuses, premature birth, and birth of weak kittens.[97] Generalized toxoplasmosis has been identified as a cause of preweaning kitten mortality.[39] The risk of infection with *T. gondii* can be reduced by not feeding cats raw meat, keeping them indoors, and not allowing them to hunt.

Bacterial Infections

The most common reason for pregnancy failure after a bacterial infection is likely to be infection with opportunistic pathogens from the normal vaginal flora (see Endometritis, above). *Escherichia coli* is the most common bacterial species isolated from queens with pyometra, and *E. coli* placentitis has been reported as a cause of late abortion.[39,81]

The major clinical sign after infection with *Chlamydophila felis* is conjunctivitis. The organism can be isolated from the vagina and has been believed to be associated with reproductive failure. A clear association between infection and reproductive problems has not been demonstrated.[93]

Salmonella typhimurium infection from ingestion of raw chicken resulted in fetal death after transplacental infection.[99] The risk of *Salmonella* infection can be reduced by not feeding cats raw meat and not allowing them to hunt. A summary of the causes for pregnancy failure can be found in Box 80-2.

INFERTILITY IN THE MALE CAT

Poor Libido and Inability to Mate

Poor libido probably is caused most often by management factors. Stress caused by new surroundings, for example, can depress libido. Inexperienced males often require a longer time to achieve a mating than experienced toms. Partner preference is another cause for mating failure. Some males in long-haired breeds may not mate until they are 2 to 3 years old. A congenital poor libido may be hereditary.

A tom with suspected poor libido should be evaluated for a possible underlying disease and normality of the genital organs. Long-haired males sometimes develop a hair-ring around the penis that prevents mating and has to be removed.[100] Persistent penile frenulum, resulting from an incomplete separation of the prepuce and penis, causes a deviation of the penis and inhibits full extrusion and mating.[101]

Poor Semen Quality

An adequate total number of functionally normal spermatozoa are required to achieve fertilization. However, the limits of different semen parameters for normal fertility have not been established for male cats. Testicular hypoplasia is a congenital condition associated with incomplete development of the seminiferous tubules, while testicular degeneration is caused by some external negative factor. Numerous causes of testicular degeneration have been identified in other species, including heat stress, malnutrition, infections, endocrine disorders, and toxins; however, similar information about cats is scarce. The prognosis for improvement of testicular hypoplasia is hopeless, but testicular degeneration may have a favorable prognosis unless the damage has been too severe. It is not always possible to distinguish testicular hypoplasia from degeneration; however, previous fertility indicates that the condition is acquired. Small testes and complete azoospermia (absence of spermatozoa) are unfavorable signs for improvement.

Chromosomal Disorders

It is well known that tortoiseshell male cats usually are infertile. The reason is that both red and nonred coat colors are linked to the X-chromosome, so two X-chromosomes are needed for a tortoiseshell coat pattern. Extra X-chromosomes can occur in cats who are chimeras (composed of two or more cell populations from different individuals resulting from fusion of embryos) or mosaics (two or more cell populations from the same individual). Sometimes, tortoiseshell male cats are fertile; for example, chimeras who have formed from the fusion of two brother embryos resulting in a normal 38, XY-karyotype.[102] The coat pattern is an indication that there might be a chromosomal abnormality, but these types of abnormalities are not restricted to tortoiseshell males. A brown Burmese cat with a 39,XXY karyotype has been described.[101] Infertile males with abnormal chromosomes often have small testes with complete hypoplasia.

Developmental Disorders

Hypospadia is a congenital condition associated with abnormal localization of the urethral opening and often is accompanied by abnormalities of the scrotum. Although probably rare, this condition has been described in toms.[103]

Box 80-2   Potential Causes of Pregnancy Failure

PREIMPLANTATION
Failure to mate due to inadequate mating regimen, partner preference, pain or presence of hair rings, or anatomical deviations of the male
Failure to ovulate due to inadequate mating regimen
Failure of fertilization due to infertile male
Failure of fertilization due to anatomical deviations of the tubular female genital organs (segmental aplasia)
Stress?
In addition, the same causes as for postimplantation losses

POSTIMPLANTATION
Embryonic or fetal death due to chromosomal abnormalities or congenital defects
Endometrium that can not support pregnancy due to CEH
Embryonic or fetal death due to nonspecific local uterine infection
Feline immunodeficiency virus
Feline leukemia virus
Feline panleukopenia virus
Feline calicivirus
Toxoplasmosis
General debilitating disease of the mother from infectious or other causes
Toxins
Medication of the mother with drugs that are not safe during pregnancy
Nutritional disorders

CEH, Cystic endometrial hyperplasia.

Intersexes

Both hermaphrodites and pseudohermaphrodites have been described in cats.[104-106] True hermaphrodites have both female and male gonads and are rare.[104] Pseudohermaphrodites are more common. Male pseudohermaphrodites have male gonads and chromosomes, but they have various degrees of feminization of the internal and external reproductive organs.[105,106]

Evaluation of Infertility in Male Cats

A general clinical examination can reveal signs of underlying disease that may affect fertility. An andrological examination includes palpation of the testes for location, size, consistency, and symmetry. The penis is inspected for anatomical abnormalities and the presence of spines. Because of the pulsatile manner of testosterone release, the analysis of a single blood sample may or may not reveal basal values in intact males and therefore is not a reliable method to monitor testicular function. Stimulation of testosterone release from the Leydig cells with an hCG or GnRH injection before the blood sample is collected is the preferred method of monitoring testosterone production. Inspection of the penile spines, however, usually will give enough information about the male's testosterone production.[21]

A semen sample is necessary to diagnose poor semen quality. Although semen collection by an artificial vagina is possible in cats, this method is not likely to be successful in a clinical situation. Therefore the method used most commonly for semen collection in cats is electroejaculation. This method requires that the male be anesthetized. Collection of spermatozoa by inserting a catheter into the urethra of cats sedated with medetomidine (130 to 140 μg/kg) has been described recently and could be a useful alternative method for sperm collection in clinical practice.[107]

As an alternative to collection of an ejaculate, a urine sample can be collected after mating and evaluated for the presence of spermatozoa. Fertile males usually have spermatozoa in the urine because there is always some backflow to the bladder. Although the quality of spermatozoa can not be evaluated from a urine sample, absence of spermatozoa in the sediment of a centrifuged urine sample collected after mating, together with small testes, is a strong indication that the male is likely to be azoospermic with a poor prognosis.[107]

COMPONENTS IN A CATTERY HERD HEALTH PROGRAM

As mentioned in the introduction, to manage a cattery, it is essential to keep detailed records and to avoid overcrowding. Any cat who is introduced to the cattery or mated with cats in the cattery should be tested negative for FeLV and FIV (see Chapter 6). In order to control infections with FPV, FHV, and FCV, vaccination is likely to be more efficient than routine testing because these agents are widespread in the cat population and the diseases can be kept under control with proper vaccination programs.[87]

Cats used for breeding should not be fed raw meat or allowed to hunt because raw meat is a potential source of infectious agents that can cause infertility and other diseases.[39,97,99] In cat breeds in which blood group B is prevalent, it is wise to test for blood groups before breeding to avoid kitten losses due to neonatal isoerythrolysis[55] (see Chapter 61). Frequent repeated estrous cycles are a risk factor for the development of cystic endometrial hyperplasia and should be avoided, if possible. Use of progestins to stop queens from cycling are, however, also likely to predispose for CEH.[73-75]

SUMMARY

As information about feline reproduction has improved, more treatment options have become available for different clinical conditions. With more knowledge, it also has become more clear how different management factors can affect the reproductive health of cats. Improved methods for contraception of cats would help control populations of feral cats, and reversible methods would allow a queen to take a rest from breeding without experiencing the harmful effects of repeated cycles or the side effects caused by the contraceptive.

REFERENCES

1. Hurni H: Daylength and breeding in the domestic cat, *Lab Anim* 15:229, 1981.
2. Tsutsui T, Nakagawa K, Hirano T, et al: Breeding season in female cats acclimated under a natural photoperiod and interval until puberty, *J Vet Med Sci* 66:1129, 2004.
3. Wallace JL, Levy JK: Population characteristics of feral cats admitted to seven trap-neuter programs in the United States, *J Feline Med Surg* 8:279, 2006.
4. Prescott CW: Reproduction patterns in the domestic cat, *Aust Vet J* 49:126, 1973.
5. Johnstone I: Reproductive patterns of pedigree cats, *Aust Vet J* 64:197, 1987.
6. Jemmett JE, Evans JM: A survey of sexual behaviour and reproduction of female cats, *J Small Anim Pract* 18:31, 1977.
7. Axnér E, Linde Forsberg C: Sperm morphology in the domestic cat, and its relation with fertility: a retrospective study, *Reprod Domest Anim* 42:282, 2007.
8. Blottner S, Jewgenow K: Moderate seasonality in testis function of domestic cat, *Reprod Dom Anim* 42:536, 2007.
9. Povey RC: Reproduction in the pedigree female cat. A survey of breeders, *Can Vet J* 19:207, 1973.
10. Siemieniuch MJ, Woclawek-Potocka I: Morphological features of the seminiferous epithelium in cat (*Felis catus*, L. 1758) testes, *J Reprod Dev* 53:1125, 2007.
11. Shille VM, Lundström KE, Stabenfeldt GH: Follicular function in the domestic cat as determined by estradiol-17b concentrations in plasma: relation to estrous behaviour and cornification of exfoliated vaginal epithelium, *Biol Reprod* 21:953, 1979.
12. Root MV, Johnston SD, Olson PN: Estrous length, pregnancy rate, gestation and parturition lengths, litter size and juvenile mortality in the domestic cat, *J Am Anim Hosp Assoc* 31:429, 1995.
13. Wildt DE, Chan SYW, Seager SWJ, et al: Ovarian activity, circulating hormones, and sexual behavior in the cat. I. Relationships during the coitus-induced luteal phase

and the estrous period without mating, *Biol Reprod* 25:15, 1981.

14. Stover DG, Sokolowski JH: Estrous behavior of the domestic cat, *Feline Pract* 8:54, 1978.

15. Lawler DF, Johnston SD, Hegstad RL, et al: Ovulation without cervical stimulation in domestic cats, *J Reprod Fertil Suppl* 47:57, 1993.

16. Banks DH, Stabenfeldt G: Luteinizing hormone release in the cat in response to coitus on consecutive days of estrus, *Biol Reprod* 26:603, 1982.

17. Verstegen JP, Onclin K, Silva LD, et al: Regulation of progesterone during pregnancy in the cat: studies on the roles of corpora lutea, placenta and prolactin secretion, *J Reprod Fertil Suppl* 47:165, 1993.

18. Banks DH, Paape SR, Stabenfeldt GH: Prolactin in the cat: I. Pseudopregnancy, pregnancy and lactation, *Biol Reprod* 28:923, 1983.

19. Johnstone IP, Bancroft BJ, McFarlane JR: Testosterone and androstenedione profiles in the blood of domestic tom cats, *Anim Reprod Sci* 7:363, 1984.

20. Aronson LR, Cooper ML: Penile spines of the domestic cat: their endocrine-behaviour relations, *Anat Rec* 157:71, 1967.

21. Johnston SD, Root MV, Olson PN: Ovarian and testicular function in the domestic cat: clinical management of spontaneous reproductive disease, *Anim Reprod Sci* 42:261, 1996.

22. Root MV, Johnston SD, Johnston GR, et al: The effect of prepuberal and postpuberal gonadectomy on penile extrusion and urethral diameter in the domestic cat, *Vet Radiol Ultrasound* 37:363, 1996.

23. Concannon P, Hodgson B, Lein D: Reflex LH release in estrous cats following single and multiple copulations, *Biol Reprod* 23:111, 1980.

24. Wildt DE, Seager SWJ: Laparoscopic determination of ovarian and uterine morphology during the reproductive cycle. In Morrow DA, editor: *Current therapy in theriogenology*, Philadelphia, 1980, WB Saunders, p 828.

25. Sojka NJ, Jennings LL, Hamner CE: Artificial insemination in the cat (Felis catus L), *Lab Anim Care* 20:198, 1970.

26. Shille VM, Munro C, Walker Farmer S, et al: Ovarian and endocrine responses in the cat after coitus, *J Reprod Fertil* 68:29, 1983.

27. Swanson WF, Roth TL, Wildt DE: In vivo embryogenesis, embryo migration, and embryonic mortality in the domestic cat, *Biol Reprod* 51:452, 1994.

28. Leiser R, Koob B: Development and characteristics of placentation in a carnivore, the domestic cat, *J Exp Zool* 266:642, 1993.

29. Thatcher MJD, Shille VM, Fliss MF, et al: Characterisation of feline conceptus proteins during pregnancy, *Biol Reprod* 44:108, 1991.

30. Say L, Pontier D, Natoli E: High variation in multiple paternity of domestic cats (*Felis catus* L.) in relation to environmental conditions, *Proc R Soc Lond B* 266:2071, 1999.

31. Sparkes AH, Rogers K, Henley WE, et al: A questionnaire-based study of gestation, parturition and neonatal mortality in pedigree breeding cats in the UK, *J Feline Med Surg* 8:145, 2006.

32. Munday HS, Davidson HPB: Normal gestation lengths in the domestic shorthair cat (*Felis domesticus*), *J Reprod Fertil* 47(suppl):199, 1993.

33. Gunn-Moore DA, Thrusfield MV: Feline dystocia: prevalence, and association with cranial conformation and breed, *Vet Rec* 136:350, 1995.

34. Ekstrand C, Linde Forsberg C: Dystocia in the cat: a retrospective study of 155 cases, *J Small Anim Pract* 35:459, 1994.

35. Mowrer RT, Conti PA, Rossow CF: Vaginal cytology an approach of improvement of cat breeding, *Vet Med Small Anim Clin* 70:691, 1975.

36. Robinson R, Cox HW: Reproductive performance in a cat colony over a 10-year period, *Lab Anim* 4:99, 1970.

37. Festing MFW, Bleby J: Breeding performance and growth of SPF cats (*Felis catus*), *J Small Anim Pract* 11:533, 1970.

38. Lawler DF, Monti KL: Morbidity and mortality in neonatal kittens, *Am J Vet Res* 45:1455, 1984.

39. Ström Holst B, Karlstam E: Causes of mortality in kittens 0-20 weeks old: A retrospective study. In Verstegen J, Onclin K, Linde Forsberg C, editors: *Proceedings of the 3rd EVSSAR Congress*, Belgium, 2002, Liège, p 176.

40. Cave TA, Thompson H, Reid SWJ, et al: Kitten mortality in the United Kingdom: a retrospective analysis of 274 histopathological examinations (1986 to 2000), *Vet Rec* 151:497, 2002.

41. Case LP, Carey DP, Hirakawa DA, et al: *Canine and feline nutrition*, ed 2, St Louis, 2000, Mosby.

42. Kealy RD: Feline nutrition. In Morrow DA, editor: *Current therapy in theriogenology*, Philadelphia, 1980, WB Saunders, p 853.

43. Kelley RL: The effect of nutrition on feline reproduction. In *Proceedings, Society for Theriogenology*, 2003, Columbus, OH, p 354.

44. Morris JG: Do cats need arachidonic acid in the diet for reproduction, *J Anim Physiol Anim Nutr* 88:131, 2004.

45. Dieter JA, Stewart DR, Haggarty MA, et al: Pregnancy failure in cats associated with long-term dietary taurine insufficiency, *J Reprod Fertil Suppl* 47:457, 1993.

46. Fascetti AJ, Quinton RR, Morris JG: Dietary copper influences reproduction in cats, *J Nutr* 130:1287, 2000.

47. Hendriks WH, Wamberg S: Milk intake of suckling kittens remains relatively constant from one to four weeks of age, *J Nutr* 130:77, 2000.

48. Dobenecker B, Zottman B, Kienzle E, et al: Investigations on milk composition and milk yield in queens, *J Nutr* 128:2618, 1998.

49. Munday H, Earle KE: Energy requirements of the queen during lactation and kittens from birth to 12 weeks, *J Nutr* 121:43, 1991.

50. Fédération Internationale Féline Breeding and Registration Rules date of issue: 01.01. 2008, http://www.fifeweb.org/wp/lib/lib_current.html. Accessed 6/23/2009.

51. The Governing Council of the Cat Fancy: General Code of Ethics for Breeders & Owners. Accessed June 23, 2008, at http://www.gccfcats.org/ethics.html.

52. Claus MA, Levy JK, MacDonald K, et al: Immunoglobulin concentrations in feline colostrum and milk, and the requirement of colostrum for passive transfer of immunity to neonatal kittens, *J Feline Med Surg* 8:184, 2006.

53. Casal ML, Jezyk PF, Giger U: Transfer of colostral antibodies from queens to their kittens, *Am J Vet Res* 57:1653, 1996.

54. Yamada T, Nagai Y, Matsuda M: Changes in serum immunoglobulin values in kittens after ingestion of colostrum, *Am J Vet Res* 52:393, 1991.

55. Giger U, Casal ML: Feline colostrum—friend or foe: maternal antibodies in queens and kittens, *J Reprod Fertil Suppl* 51:313, 1997.

56. Griot-Wenk ME, Callan MB, Casal ML, et al: Blood type AB in the feline AB blood group system, *Am J Vet Res* 57:1438, 1996.

57. Berman E: Growth patterns, fetal and neonatal. In Morrow DA, editor: *Current therapy in theriogenology*, Philadelphia, 1980, WB Saunders, p 850.

58. Johnston SD, Buoen LC, Madl JE, et al: X-Chromosome monosomy (37,XO) in a Burmese cat with gonadal dysgenesis, *J Am Vet Med Assoc* 182:986, 1983.

59. Thomsen PD, Byskov AG, Basse A: Fertility in two cats with X-chromosome mosaicism and unilateral ovarian dysgenesis, *J Reprod Fertil* 80:43, 1987.

60. Meyers-Wallen VN, Wilson JD, Fisher S, et al: Testicular feminization in a cat, *J Am Vet Med Assoc* 195:631, 1989.

61. Axnér E, Gustavsson T, Ström Holst B: Estradiol measurement after GnRH-stimulation as a method to diagnose the presence of ovaries in the female domestic cat, *Theriogenology* 70:186, 2008.

62. Pelican KM, Wildt DE, Pukazhenthi B, et al: Ovarian control for assisted reproduction in the domestic cat and wild felids, *Theriogenology* 66:37, 2006.

63. Feldman EC, Nelson RW: Feline reproduction. In Feldman EC, Nelson RW, editors: *Canine and feline endocrinology and reproduction*, ed 3, St Louis, 2004, WB Saunders, p 1016.

64. Gelberg HB, McEntee K, Heath EH: Feline cystic rete ovarii, *Vet Pathol* 21:304, 1984.

65. McEntee K: *Reproductive pathology of domestic mammals*, San Diego, 1990, Academic Press.

66. Buergelt CD: *Color atlas of reproductive pathology of domestic animals*, St Louis, 1997, Mosby-Year Book.

67. Stein BS: Tumours of the feline genital tract, *J Am Anim Hosp Assoc* 17:1022, 1981.

68. Gelberg HB, McEntee K: Feline ovarian neoplasms, *Vet Pathol* 22:572, 1985.

69. Nash AS, McCandlish AP, Renton JP: Hydrometra in two cats, *J Small Anim Pract* 27:265, 1986.

70. Nomura K, Koreeda T, Kawata M, et al: Vaginal atresia with transverse septum in a cat, *J Vet Med Sci* 59:1045, 1999.

71. Chatdarong K, Ponglowhapan S, Karlsson A, et al: Exogenous ACTH induced progesterone levels in female domestic cats, *Theriogenology* 66:1482, 2006.

72. Brandt Y, Madej A, Rodríguez-Martínez H, et al: Effects of exogenous ACTH during oestrus on early embryo development and oviductal transport in the sow, *Reprod Dom Anim* 42:118, 2007.

73. Dow C: The cystic hyperplasia-pyometra complex in the cat, *Vet Rec* 74:141, 1962.

74. Chatdarong K, Rungsipipat A, Axnér E, et al: Hysterographic appearance and uterine histology at different stages of the reproductive cycle and after progestagen treatment in the domestic cat, *Theriogenology* 64:12, 2005.

75. Perez JF, Conley AJ, Dieter JA, et al: Studies on the origin of ovarian interstitial tissue and the incidence of endometrial hyperplasia in domestic and feral cats, *Gen Comp Endocrinol* 116:10, 1999.

76. Ström Holst B, Karlstam E, Bergström A, et al: Uterine pathology in routinely ovariohysterectomised cats. In Verstegen J, Onclin K, Linde Forsberg C, editors: *Proceedings of the 3rd EVSSAR Congress*, Belgium, 2002, Liège, p 178.

77. Axnér E, Ågren E, Båverud V, et al: Infertility in the cycling queen: seven cases, *J Feline Med Surg*, 10:566, 2008.

78. Clemetson LL, Ward ACS: Bacterial flora of the vagina and uterus of healthy cats, *J Am Vet Med Assoc* 196:902, 1990.

79. Ström Holst B, Bergström A, Lagerstedt AS, et al: Characterization of the bacterial population of the genital tract of adult cats, *Am J Vet Res* 64:963, 2003.

80. Chatdarong K, Rungsipipat A, Axnér E, et al: Investigation of cervical patency and uterine appearance in domestic cats by fluoroscopy and scintigraphy, *Reprod Dom Anim* 37:275, 2002.

81. Kenney KJ, Evans RH, Reimers TJ, et al: Pyometra in cats: 183 cases (1979-1984), *J Am Vet Med Assoc* 191:1130, 1987.

82. Davidson AP, Feldman EC, Nelson RW: Treatment of pyometra in cats, using prostaglandin F$_{2\alpha}$: 21 cases (1982-1990), *J Am Vet Med Assoc* 200:825, 1992.

83. Verstegen J: Contraception and pregnancy termination. In Ettinger SJ, Feldman EC, editors: *Textbook of veterinary internal medicine*, ed 5, Philadelphia, 2000, WB Saunders, p 1542.

84. Lennoz-Roland M: Practical uses of Aglepristone: review of a recent expert meeting—Nice, June 17-18, 2005. In Luvoni GC, Thuróczy J, editors: *Proceedings of the 5th Biannual EVSSAR Congress*, 2006, Budapest, p 152.

85. Goldsmith FG: Habitual abortion and FeLV, *Fel Pract* 5:4, 1975.

86. Cotter SM, Hardy WD, Essex M: Association of feline leukemia virus with lymphosarcoma and other disorders in the cat, *J Am Vet Assoc* 166:449, 1975.

87. Ström Holst B: Disease transmission by mating or artificial insemination in the cat: concerns and prophylaxis. In Concannon PW, England G, Verstegen J, et al, editors: *Recent advances in small animal reproduction*, Ithaca, New York, 2002, International Veterinary Information Service (www.ivis.org).

88. Weaver CC, Burgess SC, Nelson PD, et al: Placental immunopathology and pregnancy failure in the FIV-infected cat, *Placenta* 26:138, 2005.

89. Csiza CK, Scott FW, De Lahunta A, et al: Feline viruses. XIV. Transplacental infections in spontaneous panleukopenia of cats, *Cornell Vet* 61:423, 1971.

90. Addie DD, Toth S, Thompson H, et al: Detection of feline parvovirus in dying pedigree kittens, *Vet Rec* 142:353, 1998.

91. Sharp NHJ, Davis BJ, Guy JS, et al: Hydrancephaly and cerebellar hypoplasia in two kittens attributed to intrauterine parvovirus infection, *J Comp Pathol* 121:39, 1999.

92. Hoover EA, Griesemer RA: Experimental feline herpesvirus infection in the pregnant cat, *Am J Pathol* 65:173, 1971.

93. Gaskell RM, Povey RC: Transmission of feline viral rhinotracheitis, *Vet Rec* 111:359, 1982.

94. Sykes JE, Anderson GA, Studdert VP, et al: Prevalence of feline *Chlamydia psittaci* and feline herpesvirus 1 in cats with upper respiratory tract disease, *J Vet Intern Med* 13:153, 1999.

95. Ellis TM: Jaundice in a Siamese cat with in utero feline calicivirus infection, *Aust Vet J* 57:383, 1981.

96. Van Vuuren M, Gerber D, Nöthling JO, et al: Characterisation of a potentially abortigenic strain of feline calicivirus isolated from a domestic cat, *Vet Rec* 144:636, 1999.

97. Sato K, Iwamoto I, Yoshiki K: Experimental toxoplasmosis in pregnant cats, *J Vet Med Sci* 55:1005, 1993.

98. Dubey JP, Carpenter JL: Neonatal toxoplasmosis in littermate cats, *J Am Vet Med Assoc* 203:1546, 1993.

99. Reilly GA, Bailie NC, Morrow WT, et al: Feline stillbirths associated with mixed salmonella typhimurium and leptospira infection, *Vet Rec* 135:608, 1994.

100. Colby ED, Stein BS: The reproductive system. In Pratt PW, editor: *Feline medicine*, ed 1, Santa Barbara, CA, 1983, American Veterinary Publications, p 511.

101. Axnér E, Ström B, Linde-Forsberg C, et al: Reproductive disorders in 10 domestic male cats, *J Small Anim Pract* 37:394, 1996.

102. Centerwall WR, Benirschke K: An animal model for the XXY Klinefelter's syndrome in man: tortoiseshell and calico male cats, *Am J Vet Res* 36:1275, 1975.

103. Foley RH, Collins KS: Hypospadias in two male cats, *Feline Pract* 27:18, 1999.

104. Felts JF, Randell MG, Greene RW, et al: Hermaphroditism in a cat, *J Am Vet Med Assoc* 181:925, 1982.

105. Bredal WP, Thoresen SI, Kvellestad A, et al: Male pseudo-hermaphroditism in a cat, *J Small Anim Pract* 38:21, 1997.

106. Hakala JE: Reproductive tract anomalies in two male cats, *Modern Vet Pract* 65:629, 1984.

107. Zambelli D, Prati F, Cunto M, et al: Quality and in vitro fertilization ability of cryopreserved cat spermatozoa obtained by urethral catheterization after medetomidine administration, *Theriogenology* 69:485, 2008.

Index

Index entries followed by "f" indicate
figures; "t" tables; "b" boxes.